Great care begins with great
CARE PLANNING!

Doenges, Moorhouse & Murr
NURSING DIAGNOSIS MANUAL
Planning, Individualizing, and Documenting Client Care

Rely on this complete reference to identify interventions commonly associated with specific nursing diagnoses across the lifespan, and to help plan, individualize, and document care for more than 800 diseases and disorders.

Doenges & Moorhouse
APPLICATION OF NURSING PROCESS AND NURSING DIAGNOSIS
An Interactive Text for Diagnostic Reasoning

Master the nursing process with this interactive, step-by-step approach to the whys and hows.

Doenges, Moorhouse & Murr
NURSING CARE PLANS
Guidelines for Individualizing Client Care Across the Life Span

Three care plan resources in one—medical-surgical, maternity, and psychiatric/mental health—170 customizable plans in all! Take a multimedia approach to care planning with guidelines that make it easier to apply the nursing process and to individualize care.

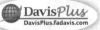

Nurse's Pocket Guide

Diagnoses, Prioritized Interventions, and Rationales

Marilynn E. Doenges, APRN, BC—Retired

Clinical Specialist—Adult Psychiatric/Mental Health Nursing
Retired Adjunct Faculty
Beth-El College of Nursing and Health Sciences, UCCS
Colorado Springs, Colorado

Mary Frances Moorhouse, RN, MSN, CRRN, LNC

Nurse Consultant
TNT-RN Enterprises
Adjunct Faculty
Pikes Peak Community College
Colorado Springs, Colorado

Alice C. Murr, BSN, RN—Retired

Independence, Missouri

EDITION 13

 F. A. DAVIS COMPANY • Philadelphia

F. A. Davis Company
1915 Arch Street
Philadelphia, PA 19103
www.fadavis.com

Printed in the United States of America

Last digit indicates print number: 10 9 8 7 6 5 4 3 2 1

Publisher, Nursing: Joanne Patzek DaCunha, RN, MSN
Project Editor: Elizabeth Hart
Design and Illustration Manager: Carolyn O'Brien

As new scientific information becomes available through basic and clinical research, recommended treatments and drug therapies undergo changes. The author(s) and publisher have done everything possible to make this book accurate, up to date, and in accordance with accepted standards at the time of publication. The author(s), editors, and publisher are not responsible for errors or omissions or for consequences from application of the book and make no warranty, expressed or implied, in regard to the contents of the book. Any practice described in this book should be applied by the reader in accordance with professional standards of care used in regard to the unique circumstances that may apply in each situation. The reader is advised always to check product information (package inserts) for changes and new information regarding dose and contraindications before administering any drug. Caution is especially urged when using new or infrequently ordered drugs.

Library of Congress Cataloging-in-Publication Data

Doenges, Marilynn E., 1922–
Nurse's pocket guide : diagnoses, prioritized interventions, and rationales / Doenges Marilynn E., Moorhouse Mary Frances, Murr Alice C.—Ed. 13
  p. ; cm.
  Includes bibliographical references and index.
  ISBN-13: 978-0-8036-2782-6
  ISBN-10: 0-8036-2782-6
I. Moorhouse, Mary Frances, 1947– II. Murr, Alice C., 1946– III. Title.
  [DNLM: 1. Nursing Diagnosis—Handbooks. 2. Nursing Care—classification—Handbooks. 3. Patient Care Planning—Handbooks. WY 49]
  616.07'5—dc23   2012036506

DEDICATION

This book is dedicated to:

Our families, who helped with the mundane activities of daily living that allowed us to write this book and who provide us with love and encouragement in all our endeavors.

Our friends, who support us in our writing, put up with our memory lapses, and love us still.

Bob Martone, Publisher, Nursing, who germinated the idea for this project so long ago. Joanne DaCunha and Elizabeth Hart, who provided direct support and kept us focused. Robert Allen, who has guided us through the XML maze since the book went high tech. The F. A. Davis production staff, who coordinated and expedited the project through the editing and printing processes, meeting unreal deadlines, and sending pages to us with bated breath.

Robert H. Craven, Jr., and the F. A. Davis family.

And last and most important:

The nurses we are writing for, to those who have found the previous editions of the *Pocket Guide* helpful, and to other nurses who are looking for help to provide quality nursing care in a period of transition and change, we say, "Nursing Diagnosis is the way."

CONTRIBUTORS

Sheila Marquez
Formerly Executive Director
Vice President/Chief Operating Officer
The Colorado SIDS Program, Inc.
Denver, Colorado

Cayrn F. Demaree, RN, BSN, IBCLC
Lactation Specialist
Denver Health Medical Center
Denver, Colorado

Research Assistant
Mary Katherine Blackwell
Mississippi State University

ACKNOWLEDGMENTS

A special acknowledgment to Marilynn's friend, the late Diane Camillone, who provoked an awareness of the role of the patient and continues to influence our thoughts about the importance of quality nursing care, and to our late colleague, Mary Jeffries, who started us on this journey and introduced us to nursing diagnoses.

To our colleagues in NANDA International, who continue to formulate and refine nursing diagnoses to provide nursing with the tools to enhance and promote the growth of the profession.

Marilynn E. Doenges
Mary Frances Moorhouse
Alice C. Murr

CONTENTS

Health Conditions and Client Concerns with Associated Nursing Diagnoses appear on pages 1041–1183.

  Taxonomy II, Domain, Class, Code, Year Submitted/Revised
  Diagnostic Division
  Definition
  Related/Risk Factors, Defining Characteristics: Subjective/Objective
  Desired Outcomes/Evaluation Criteria
  Actions/Interventions
  Nursing Priorities
  Documentation Focus

HOW TO USE THE NURSE'S POCKET GUIDE

The American Nurses Association (ANA) *Social Policy Statement* of 1980 was the first to define nursing as the diagnosis and treatment of human responses to actual and potential health problems. This definition, when combined with the ANA *Standards of Practice*, provided impetus and support for the use of nursing diagnosis. Defining *nursing* and its effect on client care supports the growing awareness that nursing care is a key factor in client survival and in the maintenance, rehabilitative, and preventive aspects of healthcare. Changes and new developments in healthcare delivery in the past 20 years have given rise to the need for a common framework of communication to ensure continuity of care for the client moving between multiple healthcare settings and providers. Evaluation and documentation of care are important parts of this process.

This book is designed to aid the practitioner and student nurse in identifying interventions commonly associated with specific nursing diagnoses as proposed by NANDA International (NANDA-I). These interventions are the activities needed to implement and document care provided to the individual client and can be used in varied settings from acute to community/home care.

Chapters 1 and 2 present brief discussions of the nursing process, data collection, and care plan construction. Chapter 3 contains the Diagnostic Divisions, Assessment Tool, a sample plan of care, concept/mind map, and corresponding documentation and charting examples. For more in-depth information and inclusive plans of care related to specific medical or psychiatric conditions (with rationale and the application of the diagnoses), the nurse is referred to the larger works, all published by the F. A. Davis Company: *Nursing Care Plans: Guidelines for Individualizing Client Care Across the Life Span*, ed. 8 (Doenges, Moorhouse, & Murr, 2010); *Psychiatric Care Plans: Guidelines for Individualizing Care*, ed. 3 (Doenges, Townsend, & Moorhouse, 1998); and *Maternal/Newborn Plans of Care: Guidelines for Individualizing Care*, ed. 3 (Doenges & Moorhouse, 1999), with updated versions included on the CD-ROM provided with *Nursing Care Plans*.

Nursing diagnoses are listed alphabetically in Chapter 4 for ease of reference and include the diagnoses accepted for use by NANDA-I through 2012–2014. Each diagnosis approved for testing includes its definition and information divided into the

NANDA-I categories of Related or Risk Factors and Defining Characteristics. Related/Risk Factors information reflects causative or contributing factors that can be useful for determining whether the diagnosis is applicable to a particular client. Defining Characteristics (signs and symptoms or cues) are listed as subjective and/or objective and are used to confirm actual diagnoses, aid in formulating outcomes, and provide additional data for choosing appropriate interventions. The authors have not deleted or altered NANDA-I's listings; however, on occasion, they have added to their definitions or suggested additional criteria to provide clarification and direction. These additions are denoted with brackets [ ].

With the development and acceptance of Taxonomy II following the biennial conference in 2000, significant changes were made to better reflect the content of the diagnoses within the taxonomy. Taxonomy II was designed to reduce miscalculations, errors, and redundancies. The framework is organized in Domains and Classes, with 13 domains, 47 classes, and 217 diagnoses. (Eight diagnoses have been retired from the NANDA-I taxonomy; one diagnosis [disturbed Sensory Perception] was retired in 2012 but remains in this edition to allow for possible revision and resubmission.) Although clinicians will use the actual diagnoses, understanding the taxonomic structure will help the nurse to find the desired information quickly. Taxonomy II is designed to be multiaxial, with seven axes (see Appendix 2). An *axis* is defined as a dimension of the human response that is considered in the diagnostic process. Sometimes an axis may be included in the diagnostic concept, such as ineffective community Coping, in which the unit of care (e.g., community) is named. Some are implicit, such as Activity Intolerance, in which the individual is the unit of care. On occasion, an axis may not be pertinent to a particular diagnosis and will not be a part of the nursing diagnosis label or code. For example, the time axis may not be relevant to each diagnostic situation. The Taxonomic Domain and Class are noted under each nursing diagnosis heading.

The ANA, in conjunction with NANDA-I, proposed that specific nursing diagnoses currently approved and structured according to Taxonomy I Revised be included in the International Classification of Diseases (ICD) within the section "Family of Health-Related Classifications." Although the World Health Organization did not accept this initial proposal because of lack of documentation of the usefulness of nursing diagnoses at the international level, the NANDA-I list has been accepted by SNOMED (Systemized Nomenclature of Medicine) for inclusion in its international coding system and is included in the Unified Medical Language System of the National Library of Medicine. Today, nurse researchers from around the world have submitted new nursing diagnoses and are validating current diagnoses in support for resubmission and acceptance of the NANDA-I list in future editions of the ICD.

The authors have chosen to categorize the list of nursing diagnoses approved for clinical use and testing into Diagnostic Divisions, which is the framework for an assessment tool (Chapter 3) designed to assist the nurse to readily identify an appropriate nursing diagnosis from data collected during the assessment process. The Diagnostic Division label follows the Taxonomic label under each nursing diagnosis heading.

Desired Outcomes/Evaluation Criteria are identified to assist the nurse in formulating individual client outcomes and to support the evaluation process.

Interventions in this pocket guide are primarily directed to adult care settings (although general age-span considerations are included) and are listed according to nursing priorities. Some interventions require collaborative or interdependent orders (e.g., medical, psychiatric), and the nurse will need to determine when this is necessary and take the appropriate action. In general, interventions that address specialty areas outside the scope of this book are not routinely presented (e.g., obstetrics). For example, when addressing acute Pain, the nurse is directed to administer analgesics as indicated; however, specific direction regarding epidural block is not listed.

The inclusion of Documentation Focus suggestions is to remind the nurse of the importance and necessity of recording the steps of the nursing process.

Finally, in recognition of the ongoing work of numerous researchers over the past 20 years, the authors have referenced the Nursing Interventions and Outcomes labels developed by the Iowa Intervention Projects (Bulechek, Butcher, & Dochterman, Moorhead, Johnson, Mass, & Swanson). These groups have been classifying nursing interventions and outcomes to predict resource requirements and measure outcomes, thereby meeting the needs of a standardized language that can be coded for computer and reimbursement purposes. As an introduction to this work in progress, sample NIC and NOC labels have been included under the heading Sample Nursing Interventions & Outcomes Classifications at the conclusion of each nursing diagnosis section. The reader is referred to the various publications by Joanne C. Dochterman and Marion Johnson for more in-depth information.

Chapter 5 presents 460 disorders/health conditions reflecting all specialty areas, with associated nursing diagnoses written as client diagnostic statements that include the "related to" and "evidenced by" components. This section will facilitate and help validate the assessment and problem or need identification steps of the nursing process.

As noted, with few exceptions, we have presented NANDA-I's recommendations as formulated. We support the belief that practicing nurses and researchers need to study, use, and evaluate the diagnoses as presented. Nurses can be creative as they use the standardized language, redefining and sharing information as the diagnoses are used with individual clients. As new nursing diagnoses are developed, it is important that the data they encompass are added to assessment tools and current database. As part of the process by clinicians, educators, and researchers across practice specialties and academic settings to define, test, and refine nursing diagnosis, nurses are encouraged to share insights and ideas with NANDA-I online at http://www.nanda.org or at the following address: NANDA International, PO Box 157, Kaukauna, WI 54130–0157.

CHAPTER 1

The Nursing Process

Nursing is both a science and an art concerned with the physical, psychological, sociological, cultural, and spiritual concerns of the individual. The science of nursing is based on a broad theoretical framework; its art depends on the caring skills and abilities of the individual nurse. In its early developmental years, nursing did not seek or have the means to control its own practice. In more recent times, the nursing profession has struggled to define what makes nursing unique and has identified a body of professional knowledge unique to nursing practice. In 1980, the American Nurses Association (ANA) developed the first *Social Policy Statement* defining nursing as "the diagnosis and treatment of human responses to actual or potential health problems." Along with the definition of nursing came the need to explain the methods used to provide nursing care.

Years before, nursing leaders had developed a problem-solving process consisting of three steps—assessment, planning, and evaluation—patterned after the scientific method of observing, measuring, gathering data, and analyzing findings. This method, introduced in the 1950s, was called the *nursing process*. Shore (1988) described the nursing process as "combining the most desirable elements of the art of nursing with the most relevant elements of systems theory, using the scientific method." This process incorporates an interactive/interpersonal approach with a problem-solving and decision-making process (Peplau, 1952; King, 1971; Yura & Walsh, 1988).

Over time, the nursing process expanded to five steps and has gained widespread acceptance as the basis for providing effective nursing care. The nursing process is now included in the conceptual framework of all nursing curricula, is accepted in the legal definition of nursing in the *Nurse Practice Acts* of most states, and is included in the ANA *Nursing: Scope and Standards of Practice*.

The five steps of the nursing process consist of the following:

1. *Assessment* is an organized dynamic process involving three basic activities: (a) systematically gathering data, (b) sorting and organizing the collected data, and (c) documenting the data in a retrievable fashion. Subjective and objective data are collected from various sources, such as a client interview

and physical assessment. Subjective data are what the client or significant others (SOs) report, believe, or feel; objective data are what can be observed or obtained from other sources, such as laboratory and diagnostic studies, old medical records, or other healthcare providers. Using a number of techniques, the nurse focuses on eliciting a profile of the client that supplies a sense of the client's overall health status, providing a picture of the client's physical, psychological, sociocultural, spiritual, cognitive, and developmental levels as well as their economic status, functional abilities, and lifestyle. The profile is known as the *client database*.

2. *Diagnosis/need identification* involves the analysis of collected data to identify the client's needs or problems; this process is also known as the nursing diagnosis (ND). The purpose of this step is to draw conclusions regarding the client's specific needs or human responses of concern so that effective care can be planned and delivered. This process of data analysis uses diagnostic reasoning (a form of clinical judgment) in which conclusions are reached about the meaning of the collected data to determine whether nursing intervention is indicated. The end product is the *client diagnostic statement* that combines the specific client need with the related factors or risk factors (etiology), as well as defining characteristics (or cues) as appropriate. The status of the client's needs are categorized as *actual* or currently existing diagnoses, potential or *risk* diagnoses that could develop due to specific vulnerabilities of the client, and *health promotion*-diagnoses reflecting a client's desire to improve his or her well-being. Ongoing changes in healthcare delivery and computerization of client records require a commonality of communication to ensure continuity of care for the client moving from one setting or level of healthcare to another. The use of standardized terminology or NANDA International (NANDA-I) ND labels provides nurses with a common language for identifying client needs. Furthermore, the use of standardized ND labels also promotes identification of appropriate goals, provides acuity information, is useful in creating standards for nursing practice, provides a base for quality improvement, and facilitates research supporting evidence-based nursing practices.

3. *Planning* includes setting priorities, establishing goals, identifying desired client outcomes, and determining specific nursing interventions. These actions are documented as the *plan of care*. This process requires input from the client/SOs to reach agreement regarding the plan to facilitate the taking of responsibility by the client for his or her own care and the achievement of the desired outcomes and goals. Setting priorities for client care is a complex and dynamic challenge

that helps ensure that the nurse's attention and subsequent actions are properly focused. What is perceived today as the top client care need or appropriate nursing intervention could change tomorrow, or, for that matter, within minutes, based on changes in the client's condition or situation. Once client needs are prioritized, goals for treatment and discharge are established that indicate the general direction in which the client is expected to progress in response to treatment. The goals may be short term (those that usually must be met before the client is discharged or moved to a lesser level of care), such as having a *plan in place to meet client needs postdischarge*—and/or long term, such as *controlled weight loss to 145 pounds*, which may continue even after discharge. From these goals, desired outcomes are determined to measure the client's progress toward achieving the goals of treatment or the discharge criteria. To be more specific, outcomes are client responses that are achievable and desired by the client that can be attained within a defined period, given the situation and resources. Outcomes are mindful of the client's age, situation, and individual strengths, when possible. Next, nursing interventions are chosen that are based on the client's ND, the established goals and desired outcomes, the ability of the nurse to successfully implement the intervention, and the ability and the willingness of the client to undergo or participate in the intervention. Nursing interventions are direct-care activities or prescriptions for behaviors, treatments, activities, or actions that assist the client in achieving the measurable outcomes. Nursing interventions, like NDs, are key elements of the knowledge of nursing and continue to grow as research supports the connection between actions and outcomes (McCloskey & Bulechek, 2000). Recording the planning step in a written or computerized plan of care provides for continuity of care, enhances communication, assists with determining agency or unit staffing needs, documents the nursing process, serves as a teaching tool, and coordinates provision of care among disciplines. A valid plan of care demonstrates individualized client care by reflecting the concerns of the client and SOs, as well as the client's physical, psychosocial, and cultural needs and capabilities.

4. *Implementation* occurs when the plan of care is put into action and the nurse performs the planned interventions. Regardless of how well a plan of care has been constructed, it cannot predict everything that will occur with a particular client on a daily basis. Individual knowledge and expertise and agency routines allow the flexibility that is necessary to adapt to the changing needs of the client. Legal and ethical concerns related to interventions must also be considered. For example, the wishes of the client and family/SOs

regarding interventions and treatments must be discussed and respected. Before implementing the interventions in the plan of care, the nurse needs to understand the reason for doing each intervention, its expected effect, and any potential hazards that can occur. The nurse must also be sure that the interventions are (a) consistent with the established plan of care, (b) implemented in a safe and appropriate manner, (c) evaluated for effectiveness, and (d) documented in a timely manner.

5. *Evaluation* is accomplished by determining the client's progress toward attaining the identified outcomes and by monitoring the client's response to and effectiveness of the selected nursing interventions for the purpose of altering the plan as indicated. This is done by direct observation of the client, interviewing the client/SO, and/or reviewing the client's healthcare record. Although the process of evaluation seems similar to the activity of assessment, there are important differences. Evaluation is an ongoing process, a constant measuring and monitoring of the client status to determine (a) the appropriateness of nursing actions, (b) the need to revise interventions, (c) the development of new client needs, (d) the need for referral to other resources, and (e) the need to rearrange priorities to meet changing demands of care. Comparing overall outcomes and noting the effectiveness of specific interventions are the clinical components of evaluation that can become the basis for research for validating the nursing process and supporting evidenced-based practice. The external evaluation process is the key for refining standards of care and determining the protocols, policies, and procedures necessary for the provision of quality nursing care for a specific situation or setting.

When a client enters the healthcare system, whether as an acute-care, clinic, or home-care client, the steps of the process noted above are set in motion. Although these steps are presented as separate or individual activities, the nursing process is an interactive method of practicing nursing, with the components fitting together in a continuous cycle of thought and action.

To effectively use the nursing process, the nurse must possess, and be able to apply, certain skills. Particularly important is a thorough knowledge of science and theory, as applied not only in nursing, but also in other related disciplines, such as medicine and psychology. A sense of caring, intelligence, and competent technical skills are also essential. Creativity is needed in the application of nursing knowledge as well as adaptability for handling constant change in healthcare delivery and the many unexpected happenings that characterize the everyday practice of nursing.

Because decision making is crucial to each step of the process, the following assumptions are important for the nurse to consider:

- The client is a human being of worth and dignity. This entitles the client to participate in his or her own healthcare decisions and delivery. It requires a sense of the personal in each individual and the delivery of competent healthcare.
- There are basic human needs that must be met, and when they are not, problems arise that may require interventions by others until and if the individual can resume responsibility for self. This challenges healthcare providers to anticipate and initiate actions necessary to save another's life or to secure the client's return to health and independence.
- The client has the right to quality health and nursing care delivered with interest, compassion, competence, and with a focus on wellness and prevention of illness. The philosophy of caring encompasses all of these qualities.
- The therapeutic nurse-client relationship is important in this process, providing a milieu in which the client can feel safe to disclose and talk about his or her deepest concerns.

In 1995, the ANA acknowledged that since the release of their original statement, nursing had been influenced by many social and professional changes as well as by the science of caring. Nursing has integrated these changes with the 1980s definition to include treatment of human responses to health and illness (*Nursing's Social Policy Statement,* ANA, 1995). The revised statement provided four essential features of today's contemporary nursing practice:

- Attention to the full range of human experiences and responses to health and illness without restriction to a problem-focused orientation (in short, clients may have needs for wellness or personal growth that are not "problems" to be corrected)
- Integration of objective data with knowledge gained from an understanding of the client's or group's subjective experience
- Application of scientific knowledge to the process of diagnosis and treatment
- Provision of a caring relationship that facilitates health and healing

In 2003, the definition of nursing was further expanded to reflect nursing's role in wellness promotion and responsibility to clients, wherever they may be found. Therefore, "nursing is the protection, promotion, and optimization of health and abilities, prevention of illness and injury, alleviation of suffering through the diagnosis and treatment of human responses, and advocacy in the care of individuals, families, communities, and populations" (*Nursing's Social Policy Statement*, ANA, 2003, p. 6).

Our understanding of what nursing is and what nurses do continues to evolve. Whereas nursing actions were once based on variables such as diagnostic tests and medical diagnoses, use of the nursing process and NDs provides a uniform method of identifying and dealing with specific client needs or responses in which the nurse can intervene. The ND is thus helping to set standards for nursing practice and should lead to improved care delivery.

Nursing and medicine are interrelated and have implications for each other. This interrelationship includes the exchange of data, the sharing of ideas, and the development of plans of care that include all data pertinent to the individual client as well as the family/SOs. Although nurses work within medical and psychosocial domains, nursing's phenomena of concern are the patterns of human response, not disease processes. Thus, the written plan of care should contain more than just nursing actions in response to medical orders and may reflect plans of care encompassing all involved disciplines to provide holistic care for the individual/family.

Summary

Because the nursing process is the basis of all nursing action, it is the essence of nursing. It can be applied in any healthcare or educational setting, in any theoretical or conceptual framework, and within the context of any nursing philosophy. In using ND labels as an integral part of the nursing process, the nursing profession has identified a body of knowledge that contributes to the prevention of illness as well as the maintenance or restoration of health (or the relief of pain and discomfort when a return to health is not possible). Subsequent chapters in this book help the nurse applying the nursing process to review the current NANDA-I list of NDs, their definitions, related/risk factors (etiology), and defining characteristics. Once aware of the desired outcomes and commonly used interventions, the nurse can develop, implement, and document an individualized plan of care.

CHAPTER 2

Application of the Nursing Process

Because of their hectic schedules, many nurses believe that time spent writing a plan of care is time taken away from client care. Plans of care have been viewed as "busy work" to satisfy accreditation requirements or the whims of supervisors. In reality, quality client care must be planned and coordinated. Properly written and applied plans of care can save time by providing direction and continuity of care and by facilitating communication among nurses and other caregivers. They also provide guidelines for documentation and tools for evaluating the care provided.

The components of a plan of care are based on the nursing process presented in the first chapter. Creating a plan of care begins with the collection of data (assessment). The client database consists of subjective and objective information encompassing the various concerns reflected in the current NANDA International (NANDA-I) list of nursing diagnoses (NDs) (Table 2.1). Subjective data are those that are reported by the client (and significant others [SOs]) in the individual's own words. This information includes the individual's perceptions and what he or she wants to share. It is important to accept what is reported because the client is the "expert" in this area. Objective data are those that are observed or described (quantitatively or qualitatively) and include findings from diagnostic testing and physical examination and information from old medical records and other healthcare providers.

Analysis of the collected data leads to the identification or diagnosis of problems or areas of concern or need (including health promotion) specific to the client. These problems or needs are expressed as nursing diagnoses. The diagnosis of client needs has been determined by nurses on an informal basis since the beginning of the profession. The term *nursing diagnosis* came into formal use in the nursing literature during the 1950s (Fry, 1953), although its meaning continued to be viewed in the context of medical diagnosis. In 1973, a national conference was held to identify client needs that fall within the scope of nursing, to label them, and to develop a classification system that could be used by nurses throughout the world. They called the labels *nursing*

Text continued on page 14

TABLE 2.1—Nursing Diagnoses Accepted for Use and Research (2012–2014)

Activity Intolerance [specify level]
Activity Intolerance, risk for
Activity Planning, ineffective
+Activity Planning, risk for ineffective
+Adverse Reaction to Iodinated Contrast Media, risk for
Airway Clearance, ineffective
+Allergy Response, risk for
Anxiety [specify level: mild, moderate, severe, panic]
Aspiration, risk for
Attachment, risk for impaired
Autonomic Dysreflexia
Autonomic Dysreflexia, risk for

Behavior, disorganized infant
Behavior, readiness for enhanced organized infant
Behavior, risk for disorganized infant
Bleeding, risk for
Blood Glucose Level, risk for unstable
Body Image, disturbed
Body Temperature, risk for imbalanced
+Breast Milk, insufficient
Breastfeeding, ineffective
Breastfeeding, interrupted
*Breastfeeding, readiness for enhanced
*Breathing Pattern, ineffective

Cardiac Output, decreased
Caregiver Role Strain
Caregiver Role Strain, risk for
+Childbearing Process, ineffective
Childbearing Process, readiness for enhanced
+Childbearing Process, risk for ineffective
*Comfort, impaired
Comfort, readiness for enhanced
Communication, impaired verbal
Communication, readiness for enhanced
Confusion, acute
Confusion, chronic
Confusion, risk for acute
Constipation
Constipation, perceived
Constipation, risk for

+New ND
*Revised ND

TABLE 2.1—*(continued)*

Contamination
Contamination, risk for
Coping, compromised family
Coping, defensive
Coping, disabled family
Coping, ineffective
Coping, ineffective community
Coping, readiness for enhanced
Coping, readiness for enhanced community
Coping, readiness for enhanced family

Death Anxiety
Decision-Making, readiness for enhanced
Decisional Conflict [specify]
Denial, ineffective
Dentition, impaired
Development, risk for delayed
Diarrhea
Disuse Syndrome, risk for
Diversional Activity, deficient
+Dry Eye, risk for

Electrolyte Imbalance, risk for
Energy Field, disturbed
Environmental Interpretation Syndrome, impaired

Failure to Thrive, adult
Falls, risk for
Family Processes, dysfunctional
Family Processes, interrupted
Family Processes, readiness for enhanced
Fatigue
Fear [specify focus]
Feeding Pattern, ineffective infant
Fluid Balance, readiness for enhanced
[Fluid Volume, deficient hyper/hypotonic]
Fluid Volume, deficient [isotonic]
Fluid Volume, excess
Fluid Volume, risk for deficient
Fluid Volume, risk for imbalanced

Gas Exchange, impaired
Gastrointestinal Motility, dysfunctional

(table continues on page 10)

+New ND
*Revised ND

TABLE 2.1—Nursing Diagnoses Accepted for Use and Research (2012–2014) *(continued)*

Gastrointestinal Motility, risk for dysfunctional
Gastrointestinal Perfusion, risk for ineffective
Grieving
Grieving, complicated
Grieving, risk for complicated
Growth, risk for disproportionate
Growth and Development, delayed

+Health, deficient community
Health Behavior, risk-prone
Health Maintenance, ineffective
Home Maintenance, impaired
Hope, readiness for enhanced
Hopelessness
Human Dignity, risk for compromised
Hyperthermia
Hypothermia

Immunization Status, readiness for enhanced
+Impulse Control, ineffective
Incontinence, bowel
Incontinence, functional urinary
Incontinence, overflow urinary
Incontinence, reflex urinary
Incontinence, stress urinary
Incontinence, urge urinary
Incontinence, risk for urge urinary
*Infection, risk for
Injury, risk for
Insomnia
Intracranial Adaptive Capacity, decreased

*Jaundice, neonatal
+Jaundice, risk for neonatal

Knowledge, deficient [Learning Need (specify)]
Knowledge [specify], readiness for enhanced

Latex Allergy Response
Latex Allergy Response, risk for
Lifestyle, sedentary

+New ND
*Revised ND

TABLE 2.1—*(continued)*

Liver Function, risk for impaired
Loneliness, risk for

Maternal-Fetal Dyad, risk for disturbed
Memory, impaired
Mobility, impaired bed
Mobility, impaired physical
Mobility, impaired wheelchair
Moral Distress

*Nausea
Noncompliance [ineffective Adherence] [specify]
Nutrition: less than body requirements, imbalanced
Nutrition: more than body requirements, imbalanced
Nutrition: more than body requirements, risk for imbalanced
Nutrition, readiness for enhanced

Oral Mucous Membrane, impaired

Pain, acute
Pain, chronic
Parenting, impaired
Parenting, readiness for enhanced
Parenting, risk for impaired
Perioperative Positioning Injury, risk for
Peripheral Neurovascular Dysfunction, risk for
Personal Identity, disturbed
+Personal Identity, risk for disturbed
Poisoning, risk for
Post-Trauma Syndrome [specify stage]
Post-Trauma Syndrome, risk for
Power, readiness for enhanced
*Powerlessness [specify level]
*Powerlessness, risk for
Protection, ineffective

Rape-Trauma Syndrome
+Relationship, ineffective
Relationship, readiness for enhanced
+Relationship, risk for ineffective
Religiosity, impaired

(table continues on page 12)

+New ND
*Revised ND

TABLE 2.1—Nursing Diagnoses Accepted for Use and Research (2012–2014) *(continued)*

Religiosity, readiness for enhanced
Religiosity, risk for impaired
Relocation Stress Syndrome
Relocation Stress Syndrome, risk for
Renal Perfusion, risk for ineffective
Resilience, impaired individual
Resilience, readiness for enhanced
Resilience, risk for compromised
Role Conflict, parental
Role Performance, ineffective

Self-Care, readiness for enhanced
Self-Care Deficit, bathing
Self-Care Deficit, dressing
Self-Care Deficit, feeding
Self-Care Deficit, toileting
Self-Concept, readiness for enhanced
Self-Esteem, chronic low
Self-Esteem, situational low
*Self-Esteem, risk for chronic low
Self-Esteem, risk for situational low
Self-Health Management, ineffective
*Self-Health Management, readiness for enhanced
Self-Mutilation
Self-Mutilation, risk for
Self-Neglect
[Sensory Perception, disturbed (specify: visual, auditory, kinesthetic, gustatory, tactile, olfactory)] (retired 2012)
Sexual Dysfunction
Sexuality Pattern, ineffective
Shock, risk for
Skin Integrity, impaired
*Skin Integrity, risk for impaired
Sleep, readiness for enhanced
Sleep Deprivation
Sleep Pattern, disturbed
Social Interaction, impaired
Social Isolation
Sorrow, chronic
Spiritual Distress
Spiritual Distress, risk for

+New ND
*Revised ND

TABLE 2.1—*(continued)*

Spiritual Well-Being, readiness for enhanced
Stress Overload
Sudden Infant Death Syndrome, risk for
Suffocation, risk for
Suicide, risk for
Surgical Recovery, delayed
Swallowing, impaired

Therapeutic Regimen Management, ineffective family
+Thermal Injury, risk for
Thermoregulation, ineffective
Tissue Integrity, impaired
*Tissue Perfusion, ineffective peripheral
Tissue Perfusion, risk for decreased cardiac
Tissue Perfusion, risk for ineffective cerebral
+Tissue Perfusion, risk for ineffective peripheral
Transfer Ability, impaired
Trauma, risk for

Unilateral Neglect
Urinary Elimination, impaired
Urinary Elimination, readiness for enhanced
Urinary Retention [acute/chronic]

Vascular Trauma, risk for
Ventilation, impaired spontaneous
Ventilatory Weaning Response, dysfunctional
Violence, risk for other-directed
Violence, risk for self-directed

Walking, impaired
Wandering [specify sporadic or continuous]

+New ND
*Revised ND

Used with permission from Herdman, T.H. (2012). NANDA International: Definitions and Classification, 2012–2014. Oxford: Wiley-Blackwell.

Information in brackets added by authors to clarify and enhance the use of the NDs.

Please also see the NANDA diagnoses grouped according to Gordon's Functional Health Patterns on the inside front cover.

diagnoses, which represent clinical judgments about an individual's, family's, or community's responses to actual or potential health problems and life processes. Therefore, an ND is a decision about a need or problem that requires nursing intervention and management. The need may be anything that interferes with the quality of life the client is used to and/or desires. It includes concerns of the client, SOs, and/or nurse. The ND focuses attention on a physical or behavioral response that is either a current need or a problem at risk for developing.

The identification of client needs and selection of an ND label require experience, expertise, and intuition. A six-step diagnostic reasoning or critical thinking process facilitates an accurate analysis of the client assessment data to determine specific client needs. First, data are reviewed to identify cues (signs and symptoms) reflecting client needs that can be described by ND labels. This is called *problem-sensing.* Next, alternative explanations are considered for the identified cues to determine which ND label may be the most appropriate. As relationships among data are compared, etiological factors are identified based on the nurse's understanding of biological, physical, and behavioral sciences, and possible ND choices are *ruled out* until the most appropriate label remains. Next, a comprehensive picture of the client's past, present, and potential health status is *synthesized*, and the suggested nursing diagnosis label is combined with the identified related (or risk) factors and cues to create a hypothesis. *Confirming the hypothesis* is achieved by reviewing the NANDA-I definition, defining characteristics (cues), and determining related factors (etiology) for the chosen ND to ensure the accuracy and objectivity in this diagnostic process. Now, based on the synthesis of the data (step 3) and evaluation of the hypothesis (step 4), the *client's needs are listed* and the correct ND label is combined with the assessed etiology and signs/symptoms to finalize the client diagnostic statement. Once all the NDs are identified, the problem list is *reevaluated,* assessment data are reviewed again, and the client is consulted to ensure that all areas of concern have been addressed.

When the ND label is combined with the individual's specific related or risk factors and defining characteristics (as appropriate), the resulting client diagnostic statement provides direction for nursing care. It is important to remember that the affective tone of the ND can shape expectations of the client's response and/or influence the nurse's behavior toward the client.

The development and classification of NDs have continued through the years spurred on by the need to describe what nursing does in conjunction with changes in healthcare delivery and reimbursement, the expansion of nursing's role, and the evolution of technology. The advent of alternative healthcare settings (e.g., outpatient surgery centers, home health, rehabilitation or subacute units, extended or long-term care facilities, and hospice services) increases the need for a commonality of communication to ensure continuity of care for the client who moves from one setting or level of care to another. The efficient documentation of the client encounter, whether that is a single office visit or a lengthy hospitalization, and the movement toward paperless (computerized or electronic) client records have strengthened the need for standardizing nursing language to better demonstrate what nursing is and what nursing does.

The NANDA-I NDs is one of the standardized nursing languages recognized by the American Nurses Association (ANA) as providing clinically useful terminology that supports nursing practice. NANDA-I has also established a liaison with the International Council of Nursing to support and contribute to the global effort to standardize the language of healthcare with the goal that NANDA-I NDs will be included in the International Classification of Diseases. In the meantime, they are included in the U.S. version of International Classification of Diseases—Clinical Modifications (ICD-10CM). The NANDA-I nursing diagnosis labels have also been combined with Nursing Interventions Classification (NIC) and Nursing Outcomes Classification (NOC) to create a complete nursing language that has been coded into the Systematized Nomenclature of Medicine (SNOMED). Inclusion in an international coded terminology such as SNOMED is essential if nursing's contribution to healthcare is to be recognized in computer databases. Indexing of the entire medical record supports disease management activities, research, and analysis of outcomes for quality improvement for all healthcare disciplines. Coding also supports telehealth (the use of telecommunications technology to remotely provide healthcare information and services) and facilitates access to healthcare data across care settings and various computer systems.

The key to accurate diagnosis is the collection and analysis of data. In Chapter 3, the NDs have been categorized into divisions (Diagnostic Divisions: Nursing Diagnoses Organized According to a Nursing Focus, Section 2), and a sample assessment tool designed to assist the nurse to identify appropriate NDs as the data are collected is provided. Nurses may feel hesitant to commit themselves to documenting a ND for fear they might be wrong. However, unlike medical diagnoses, NDs can change as the client progresses through various stages of illness or maladaptation to resolution of the condition or situation.

Desired outcomes are then formulated to give direction to, as well as to evaluate, the care provided. These outcomes emerge from the diagnostic statement and are what the client hopes to achieve. They serve as the guidelines to evaluate progress toward resolution of needs or problems, providing impetus for revising the plan as appropriate. In this book, outcomes are stated in general terms to permit the practitioner to individualize them by adding timelines and other data according to specific client circumstances. Outcome terminology needs to be concise, realistic, measurable, and stated in words the client can understand, because the terms that are used indicate what the client is expected to do or accomplish. Beginning the outcome statement with an action verb provides measurable direction (e.g., "Verbalizes relationship between diabetes mellitus and circulatory changes in feet within 2 days" or "Performs procedure for home glucose monitoring correctly within 48 hours").

Interventions are the activities taken to achieve the desired outcomes, and because they are communicated to others, they must be clearly stated. A solid nursing knowledge base is vital to this process because the rationale for interventions needs to be sound and feasible with the intention of providing effective, individualized care. The actions may be independent or collaborative and may encompass specific orders from nursing, medicine, and other disciplines. Written interventions that guide ongoing client care need to be dated and signed. To facilitate the planning process, specific nursing priorities have been identified in this text to provide a general ranking of interventions. This ranking would be altered according to individual client situations. The seasoned practitioner may choose to use these as broad-based interventions. The student or beginning practitioner may need to develop a more detailed plan of care by including the appropriate interventions listed under each nursing priority. It is important to remember that because each client usually has a perception of individual needs or problems that he or she faces and an expectation of what could be done about the situation, the plan of care must be congruent with the client's reality or it will fail. In short, the nurse needs to plan care with the client because both are accountable for that care and for achieving the desired outcomes.

The plan of care is the end product of the nursing process and documents client care in areas of accountability, quality assurance, and liability. Therefore, the plan of care is a permanent part of the client's healthcare record. The format for recording the plan of care is determined by agency policy and may be handwritten, standardized forms or clinical pathways, or computer-generated documentation. Before implementing the plan of care, it should be reviewed to ensure the following:

• It is based on accepted nursing practice, reflecting knowledge of scientific principles, nursing standards of care, and agency policies.
• It provides for the safety of the client by ensuring that the care provided will do no harm.
• The client diagnostic statements are supported by the client data.
• The goals and outcomes are measurable, observable, and can be achieved.

- The interventions can benefit the client, family, or SOs in a predictable way in achieving the identified outcomes, and they are arranged in a logical sequence.
- It demonstrates individualized client care by reflecting the concerns of the client and SOs, as well as their physical, psychosocial, and cultural needs and capabilities.

Once the plan of care is put into action, changes in the client's needs must be continually monitored because care is provided in a dynamic environment and flexibility is required to allow changing circumstances. Periodic review of the client's response to nursing interventions and progress toward attaining the desired outcomes helps determine the effectiveness of the plan of care. Based on the findings, the plan may need to be modified or revised, referrals to other resources may be required, or the client may be ready for discharge from the care setting.

Summary

Healthcare providers have a responsibility for planning with the client and family for continuation of care to the eventual outcome of an optimal state of wellness or a dignified death. Today, the act of diagnosing client problems or needs is well established, and the use of standardized nursing language to describe what nursing does is rapidly becoming an integral part of an effective system of nursing practice. Although not yet comprehensive, the current NANDA-I list of diagnostic labels defines and refines professional nursing activity. With repeated use of NANDA-I NDs, strengths and weaknesses of the NDs can be identified, promoting research and further development.

Planning, setting goals, and choosing appropriate interventions are essential to the construction of a plan of care and delivery of quality nursing care. These nursing activities constitute the planning phase of the nursing process and are documented in the plan of care for a particular client. As a part of the client's permanent record, the plan of care not only provides a means for the nurse who is actively caring for the client to be aware of the client's needs (NDs), goals, and actions to be taken, but also substantiates the care provided for review by third-party payers and accreditation agencies while meeting legal requirements.

CHAPTER 3

Putting Theory Into Practice: Sample Assessment Tools, Plans of Care, Mind Mapping, and Documentation

The client assessment is the foundation on which identification of individual needs, responses, and problems are based. To facilitate the steps of assessment and diagnosis in the nursing process, an assessment tool (Assessment Tools for Choosing Nursing Diagnoses, Section 1) has been constructed using a nursing focus instead of the medical approach of "review of systems." This has the advantage of identifying and validating nursing diagnoses (NDs) as opposed to medical diagnoses.

To achieve this nursing focus, we have grouped the NANDA International (NANDA-I) NDs into related categories titled Diagnostic Divisions (Section 2) that reflect a blending of theories, primarily Maslow's Hierarchy of Needs and a self-care philosophy. These divisions serve as the framework or outline for data collection and clustering that focuses attention on the nurse's phenomena of concern—the human responses to health and illness—and directs the nurse to the most likely corresponding NDs.

Because the divisions are based on human responses and needs and not specific "systems," information may be recorded in more than one area. For this reason, the nurse is encouraged to keep an open mind, to pursue all leads, and to collect as much data as possible before choosing the ND label that best reflects the client's situation. For example, when the nurse identifies the cue of restlessness in a client, the nurse may infer that the client is anxious, assuming that the restlessness is psychologically based and thus overlooking the possibility that it is physiologically based.

From the specific data recorded in the database, an individualized client diagnostic statement can be formulated using the problem, etiology, and signs and symptoms (PES) format to accurately represent the client's situation. Whereas a medical diagnosis of diabetes mellitus is the same label used for all individuals with this condition, the diagnostic statement developed by the nurse is individualized to reflect a specific client need. For example, the diagnostic statement may read, "deficient Knowledge regarding diabetic care, related to misinterpretation of information and/or lack of recall, evidenced by inaccurate follow-through of instructions and failure to recognize signs and symptoms of hyperglycemia."

Desired client outcomes are identified to facilitate choosing appropriate interventions and to serve as evaluators of both nursing care and client response. These outcomes also form the framework for documentation.

Interventions are designed to specify the action of the nurse, the client, and/or significant others (SOs). Interventions need to promote the client's movement toward health and independence in addition to achievement of physiological stability. This requires involvement of the client in his or her own care, including participation in decisions about care activities and projected outcomes.

Section 3, Client Situation and Prototype Plan of Care, contains a sample plan of care formulated on data collected with the nursing model assessment tool. Individualized client diagnostic statements and desired client outcomes (with timelines added to reflect anticipated length of stay and individual client and nurse expectations) were identified, and interventions were chosen based on concerns or needs identified by the client and nurse during data collection, as well as by physician orders.

Although not normally included in a written plan of care, rationales are included in this sample for the purpose of explaining or clarifying the choice of interventions to enhance the nurse's learning.

Another way to conceptualize the client's care needs is to create a *Mind Map*. This technique was developed to help visualize the linkages between various client symptoms, interventions, or problems as they impact each other. The parts that are great about traditional care plans (problem-solving and categorizing) are retained, but the linear or columnar nature of the plan is changed to a design that uses the whole brain—a design that brings left-brain, linear problem-solving thinking together with the free-wheeling, interconnected, creative right brain. Joining mind mapping and care planning enables the nurse to create a holistic view of a client, strengthening critical thinking skills and facilitating the creative process of planning client care.

Finally, to complete the learning experience, samples of documentation based on the client situation are presented in Section 4, Documentation Techniques. The plan of care provides documentation of the planning process and serves as a framework or outline for the charting of administered care. The primary nurse needs to periodically review the client's documentation of progress evaluating effectiveness of the treatment plan. Other care providers can also read the notes and obtain a clear picture of what occurred with the client and make appropriate judgments regarding client management. The best way to ensure clarity of the progress notes is through the use of descriptive (or observational) statements. Observations of client behavior and response to therapy provide invaluable information. Through this communication, it can be determined if any of the client's current interventions can be eliminated or altered to achieve desired outcomes. Progress notes are an integral component of the overall medical record and should include all significant events that occur in the daily life of the client. They reflect implementation of the treatment plan and document that appropriate actions have been carried out, precautions taken, and so forth. It is important that both the implementation of interventions and progress toward the desired outcomes be documented. The notes need to be written in a clear and objective fashion, specific as to date and time, and signed by the person making the entry.

Use of clear documentation helps the nurse individualize client care. Providing a picture of what has happened and is happening promotes continuity of care and facilitates evaluation. This reinforces each person's accountability and responsibility for using the nursing process to provide individually appropriate and cost-effective client care.

SECTION 1

Assessment Tools for Choosing Nursing Diagnoses

The following are suggested guidelines or tools for creating assessment databases reflecting Doenges & Moorhouse's Diagnostic Divisions of Nursing Diagnoses. They are intended to provide a nursing focus and should help the nurse think about planning care with the client at the center (following the mind-mapping theory; see page 62). Although the divisions are alphabetized here for ease of presentation, they can be prioritized or rearranged to meet individual needs. In addition, the assessment tool can be adapted to meet the needs of specific client populations. Excerpts of assessment tools adapted for psychiatric and obstetric settings are included at the end of this section.

ADULT MEDICAL/SURGICAL ASSESSMENT TOOL

General Information

Name: _____ ❏ Age: _____ ❏ DOB: _____
Gender: _____ Race: _____
Admission: Date: _____ ❏ Time: _____ ❏ From: _____
Reason for this visit (primary concern): _____
Cultural concerns (relating to healthcare decisions, religious concerns, pain, childbirth, family involvement, communication, etc.): _____
Source of information: _____ ❏ Reliability (1 to 4 with 4 = very reliable): _____

Activity/Rest

Subjective (Reports)
Occupation: _____ ❏ Able to participate in usual activities/ hobbies: _____
Leisure time/diversional activities: _____
Ambulatory: _____ ❏ Gait (describe): _____
Activity level (sedentary to very active): _____ ❏ Regular exercise/type: _____
Muscle mass/tone/strength (e.g., normal, increased, decreased): _____
History of problems/limitations imposed by condition (e.g., immobility, can't transfer, weakness, breathlessness): _____
Feelings (e.g., exhaustion, restlessness, can't concentrate, dissatisfaction): _____
Developmental factors (e.g., delayed/age): _____
Sleep: Hours: _____ ❏ Naps: _____
Insomnia: _____ ❏ related to: _____ ❏ Difficulty falling asleep: _____
Difficulty staying asleep: _____ ❏ Rested on awakening: _____
    ❏ Excessive grogginess: _____
Bedtime rituals: _____
Relaxation techniques: _____
Sleeps on more than one pillow: _____
Oxygen use (type): _____ When used: _____
Medications or herbals for/affecting sleep: _____

Objective (Exhibits)
Observed response to activity: Heart rate: _____
    Rhythm (reg/irreg): _____ ❏ Blood pressure: _____ ❏ Respiration rate: _____ ❏ Pulse oximetry: _____
Mental status (i.e., cognitive impairment, withdrawn/lethargic): _____

Muscle mass/tone: _____ ❑ Posture (e.g., normal, stooped, curved
    spine): _____
    Tremors: _____ ❑ Location: _____
    ROM: _____
    Strength: _____ ❑ Deformity: _____
Uses mobility aid (list): _____

Circulation

Subjective (Reports)

History of/treatment for (date): High blood pressure: _____
    Brain injury: _____ ❑ Stroke: _____
    Heart problems/surgery: _____
    Palpitations: _____ ❑ Syncope: _____
    Cough/hemoptysis: _____ ❑ Blood clots: _____
    Bleeding tendencies/episodes: _____ ❑ Pain in legs
    w/activity: _____
    Extremities: Numbness: _____
      ❑ (location): _____
    Tingling: _____ ❑ (location): _____
Slow healing/describe: _____
Change in frequency/amount of urine: _____
History of spinal cord injury/dysreflexia episodes: _____
Medications/herbals: _____

Objective (Exhibits)

Color (e.g., pale, cyanotic, jaundiced, mottled, ruddy): _____
    Skin: _____
    Mucous membranes: _____ ❑ Lips: _____
    Nailbeds: _____ ❑ Conjunctiva: _____
    Sclera: _____
Skin moisture: (e.g., dry, diaphoretic): _____
BP: Lying: **R** _____ **L** _____ ❑ Sitting: **R** _____ **L** _____
    Standing: **R** _____ **L** _____ ❑ Pulse pressure: _____
    Auscultatory gap: _____
Pulses (palpated 1–4 strength): Carotid: _____ ❑ Temporal: _____
    Jugular: _____ ❑ Radial: _____ ❑ Femoral: _____
    Popliteal: _____ ❑ Post-tibial: _____ ❑ Dorsalis pedis: _____
Cardiac (palpation): Thrill: _____ ❑ Heaves: _____
Heart sounds (auscultation): Rate: _____ ❑ Rhythm: _____
    Quality: _____ ❑ Friction rub: _____
    Murmur (describe location/sounds): _____
Vascular bruit (location): _____
Jugular vein distention: _____
Breath sounds (location/describe): _____
Extremities: Temperature: _____ ❑ Color: _____
    Capillary refill (1–3 sec): _____
    Homans' sign: _____ ❑ Varicosities (location): _____
    Nail abnormalities: _____

Edema (location/severity +1 – +4): _____
Distribution/quality of hair: _____
Trophic skin changes: _____

Ego Integrity

Subjective (Reports)
Relationship status: _____
Expression of concerns (e.g., financial, lifestyle, role changes):
_____
Stress factors: _____
Usual ways of handling stress: _____
Expression of feelings: Anger: _____ ❑ Anxiety: _____
Fear: _____ ❑ Grief: _____
Helplessness: _____ ❑ Hopelessness: _____
Powerlessness: _____
Cultural factors/ethnic ties: _____
Religious affiliation: _____ ❑ Active/practicing: _____
Practices prayer/meditation: _____
Religious/spiritual concerns: _____ ❑ Desires clergy visit: _____
Expression of sense of connectedness/harmony with self and others: _____
Medications/herbals: _____

Objective (Exhibits)
Emotional status (check those that apply): ❑ Calm: _____
❑ Anxious: _____ ❑ Angry: _____ ❑ Withdrawn: _____
❑ Fearful: _____ ❑ Irritable: _____ ❑ Restive: _____
❑ Euphoric: _____
Observed body language: _____
Observed physiological responses (e.g., palpitations, crying, change in voice quality/volume): _____
Changes in energy field: Temperature: _____
Color: _____ Distribution: _____
Movement: _____
Sounds: _____

Elimination

Subjective (Reports)
Usual bowel elimination pattern: _____ ❑ Character of stool (e.g., hard, soft, liquid): _____ ❑ Stool color (e.g., brown, black, yellow, clay colored, tarry): _____
Date of last BM and character of stool: _____
History of bleeding: _____ ❑ Hemorrhoids/fistula: _____
Constipation acute: _____ ❑ or chronic: _____
Diarrhea: acute: _____ ❑ or chronic: _____
Bowel incontinence: _____
Laxative: _____ ❑ how often: _____
Enema/suppository: _____ ❑ how often: _____

Usual voiding pattern and character of urine: _____
   Difficulty voiding: Urgency: _____
   Frequency: _____
   Retention: _____ ❑ Bladder spasms: _____ ❑ Burning: _____
Urinary incontinence (type/time of day usually occurs): _____
History of kidney/bladder disease: _____
Diuretic use: _____ ❑ Herbals: _____

Objective (Exhibits)
Abdomen (palpation): Soft/firm: _____
   Tenderness/pain (quadrant location): _____
   Distention: _____ ❑ Palpable mass/location: _____
   Size/girth: _____
   Abdomen (auscultation): Bowel sounds (location/type): _____
   Costovertebral angle tenderness: _____
Bladder palpable: _____ ❑ Overflow voiding: _____
Rectal sphincter tone (describe): _____
Hemorrhoids/fistulas: Stool in rectum: Impaction: ___ ❑ Occult
   blood (+ or −): _____
Presence/use of catheter or continence devices: _____
Ostomy appliances (describe appliance and location): _____

Food/Fluid

Subjective (Reports)
Usual diet (type): _____
Calorie/carbohydrate/protein/fat intake (g/day): _____ ❑ # of
   meals daily: _____ ❑ Snacks (number/time consumed): _____
Dietary pattern/content:
   B: _____ L: _____ D: _____
   Snacks: _____
Last meal consumed/content: _____
Food preferences: _____
Food allergies/intolerances: _____
Cultural or religious food preparation concerns/prohibitions: ___
   _____Usual appetite: _____ ❑ Change in appetite: _____
Usual weight: _____
Unexpected/undesired weight loss or gain: _____
Nausea/vomiting: ___ ❑ related to: ___ ❑ Heartburn/indiges-
   tion: _____ ❑ related to: _____ ❑ relieved by: _____
Chewing/swallowing problems: _____
   Gag/swallow reflex present: _____
   Facial injury or surgery: _____
   Stroke/other neurological deficit: _____
Teeth: Normal: _____ ❑ Dentures (full/partial): _____
   Loose/absent teeth/poor dental care: _____
Sore mouth/gums: _____
Diabetes: _____ ❑ Controlled with diet/pills/insulin: _____
Vitamin/food supplements: _____

Medications/herbals: _____

Current weight: ____ ❑ Height: ____ ❑ Body build: ____ ❑ Body
    fat %: ____
Skin turgor (e.g., firm, supple, dehydrated): _____ ❑ Mucous
    membranes (moist/dry): _____
Edema: Generalized: ____ ❑ Dependent: ____ ❑ Feet/ankles: ____
    ❑ Periorbital: _____ ❑ Abdominal/ascites: _____
Jugular vein distention: _____
Breath sounds (auscultate)/location: Faint/distant: _____
    Crackles: _____
    Wheezes: _____
Condition of teeth/gums: _____
Appearance of tongue: _____
    Mucous membranes: _____
Abdomen: Bowel sounds (quadrant location/type): _____
    Hernia/masses: _____
Urine S/A or Chemstix: _____
Serum glucose (Glucometer): _____

Hygiene

Subjective (Reports)
Ability to carry out activities of daily living: Independent/depen-
    dent (level 1 = no assistance needed to 4 = completely depen-
    dent):
Mobility: _____ ❑ Assistance needed (describe): _____
    Assistance provided by: _____
    Equipment/prosthetic devices required: _____
Feeding: _____ ❑ Can prepare food: _____
    Can feed self/use eating utensils: _____
    Equipment/prosthetic devices required: _____
Hygiene: _____ ❑ Get supplies: _____
    Wash body or body parts: _____
    Can regulate bath water temperature: _____
    Get in and out alone: _____
    Preferred time of personal care/bath: _____
Dressing: _____ ❑ Can select clothing and dress self: _____
    Needs assistance with (describe): _____
    Equipment/prosthetic devices required: _____
Toileting: _____ ❑ Can get to toilet or commode alone: _____
    Needs assistance with (describe): _____

Objective (Exhibits)
General appearance: Manner of dress: _____
    Grooming/personal habits: _____ ❑ Condition of hair/
    scalp: _____ ❑ Body odor: _____
    Presence of vermin (e.g., lice, scabies): _____

Neurosensory

Subjective (Reports)

History of brain injury, trauma, stroke (residual effects): _____
_____

Fainting spells/dizziness: _____
Headaches (location/type/frequency): _____
Tingling/numbness/weakness (location): _____
Seizures: _____ ❑ History or new onset seizures: _____
    Type (e.g., grand mal, partial): _____
    Frequency: _____ ❑ Aura: _____ ❑ Postictal state: _____
    How controlled: _____
Vision: Loss or changes in vision: _____
    Date last exam: _____ ❑ Glaucoma: _____
    Cataract: _____ ❑ Eye surgery (type/date): _____
Hearing: Loss or change: _____ ❑ Sudden or gradual: _____
    Date last exam: _____
Sense of smell (changes): _____
Sense of taste (changes): _____ ❑ Epistaxis: _____
Other: _____

Objective (Exhibits)

Mental status: (note duration of change): _____
    Oriented: Person: _____ ❑ Place: _____ ❑ Time: _____
    Situation: _____
Check all that apply: ❑ Alert: _____ ❑ Drowsy: _____ ❑ Lethar-
    gic: _____ ❑ Stuporous: _____ ❑ Comatose: _____
    ❑ Cooperative: _____ ❑ Agitated/Restless: _____
    ❑ Combative: _____
    ❑ Follows commands: _____
Delusions (describe): _____ ❑ Hallucinations (describe): _____
Affect (describe): _____ ❑ Speech: _____
Memory: Recent: _____ ❑ Remote: _____
Pupil shape: _____ ❑ Size/reaction: R/L: _____
Facial droop: _____ ❑ Swallowing: _____
Handgrasp/release: R: _____ L: _____
Coordination: _____ ❑ Balance: _____
    Walking: _____
Deep tendon reflexes (present/absent/location): _____
    Tremors: _____ ❑ Paralysis (R/L): _____
    Posturing: _____
Wears glasses: _____ ❑ Contacts: _____ ❑ Hearing aids: _____

Pain/Discomfort

Subjective (Reports)

Primary focus: Location: _____
    Intensity (use pain scale or pictures): _____
    Quality (e.g., stabbing, aching, burning): _____
    Radiation: _____ ❑ Duration: _____

Frequency: _____
Precipitating factors: _____
Relieving factors (including nonpharmaceuticals/therapies): ___
_____
Associated symptoms (e.g., nausea, sleep problems, crying): ___
_____
Effect on daily activities: _____
   Relationships: _____ ❑ Job: _____ ❑ Enjoyment of life: _____
Additional pain focus/describe: _____
Medications: _____ ❑ Herbals: _____

Objective (Exhibits)
Facial grimacing: _____ ❑ Guarding affected area: _____
   Emotional response (e.g., crying, withdrawal, anger): _____
   Narrowed focus: _____
Vital sign changes (acute pain): BP: _____ ❑ Pulse: _____
   Respirations: _____

Respiration

Subjective (Reports)
Dyspnea/related to: _____
   Precipitating factors: _____
   Relieving factors: _____
Airway clearance (e.g., spontaneous/device): _____
Cough/describe (e.g., hard, persistent, croupy): _____
   Produces sputum (describe color/character): _____
   Requires suctioning: _____
History of (year): Bronchitis: _____ ❑ Asthma: _____
   Emphysema: _____ ❑ Tuberculosis: _____
   Recurrent pneumonia: _____
Exposure to noxious fumes/allergens, infectious agents/diseases,
   poisons/pesticides: _____
Smoker: _____ ❑ Packs/day: _____ ❑ # of years: _____
Use of respiratory aids: _____
   Oxygen (type/frequency): _____
Medications/herbals: _____

Objective (Exhibits)
Respirations (spontaneous/assisted): _____ ❑ Rate: _____
   Depth: _____
   Chest excursion (e.g., equal/unequal): _____
   Use of accessory muscles: _____
   Nasal flaring: _____ ❑ Fremitus: _____
Breath sounds (presence/absence; crackle, wheezes): _____
   Egophony: _____
Skin/mucous membrane color (e.g., pale, cyanotic): _____
Clubbing of fingers: _____
Sputum characteristics: _____

Mentation (e.g., calm, anxious, restless): _____

Pulse oximetry: _____

Safety

Subjective (Reports)

Allergies/sensitivity (medications, foods, environment, latex, iodine): _____

  Type of reaction: _____

Exposure to infectious diseases (e.g., measles, influenza, pink
  eye): _____

Exposure to pollution, toxins, poisons/pesticides, radiation (describe reactions): _____

Geographic areas lived in/visited: _____

Immunization history: Tetanus: _____ ❏ Pneumonia: _____

  Influenza: ___ ❏ MMR: ___ ❏ Polio: ___ ❏ Hepatitis: ___

  HPV: _____

Altered/suppressed immune system (list cause): _____

History of sexually transmitted disease (date/type): _____

  Testing: _____

High-risk behaviors: _____

Blood transfusion/number: _____ ❏ Date: _____

  Reaction (describe): _____

Uses seat belt regularly: _____ ❏ Bike helmets: _____

  Other safety devices: _____

Workplace safety/health issues (describe): _____

  Currently working: _____

  Rate working conditions (e.g., safety, noise, heating, water,
  ventilation): _____

History of accidental injuries: _____

Fractures/dislocations: _____

Arthritis/unstable joints. _____

  Back problems: _____

Skin problems (e.g., rashes, lesions, moles, breast lumps, enlarged nodes)/describe: _____

Delayed healing (describe): _____

Cognitive limitations (e.g., disorientation, confusion): _____

Sensory limitations (e.g., impaired vision/hearing, detecting
  heat/cold, taste, smell, touch): _____

Prostheses: _____ ❏ Ambulatory devices: _____

Violence (episodes or tendencies): _____

Objective (Exhibits)

Body temperature/method (e.g., oral, rectal, tympanic): _____

Skin integrity (e.g., scars, rashes, lacerations, ulcerations,
  bruises, blisters, burns [degree/%], drainage)/mark location on
  diagram below:

Musculoskeletal: General strength: _____
    Muscle tone: _____ ❑ Gait: _____
    ROM: _____ ❑ Paresthesia/paralysis: _____
Results of testing (e.g., cultures, immune function, TB, hepatitis): _____
    tis): _____

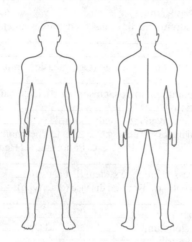

Sexuality [Component of Social Interaction]

Subjective (Reports)

Sexually active: _____ ❑ Birth control method: _____
    Use of condoms: _____
Sexual concerns/difficulties (e.g., pain, relationship, role problems): _____
    lems): _____

    Recent change in frequency/interest: _____

Female: Subjective (Reports)

Menstruation: Age at menarche: _____
    Length of cycle: _____ ❑ Duration: _____
    Number of pads/tampons used/day: _____
    Last menstrual period: ___ ❑ Bleeding between periods: ___
Reproductive: Infertility concerns: _____
    Type of therapy: _____
    Pregnant now: _____ ❑ Para: _____ ❑ Gravida: _____
    Due date: _____
Menopause: Last period: _____
    Hysterectomy (type/date): _____
    Problem with: Hot flashes: _____ ❑ Other: _____
    Vaginal lubrication: _____ ❑ Vaginal discharge: _____
Hormonal therapies: _____

Osteoporosis medications: _____

Breasts: Practices breast self-exam: _____

    Last mammogram, biopsy, or surgery date: _____

Last Pap smear: _____ ❏ Results: _____

Objective (Exhibits)

Breast examination: _____

Genitalia: Warts/lesions: _____

Vaginal bleeding/discharge: _____

STD test results: _____

Male: Subjective (Reports)

Circumcised: _____ ❏ Vasectomy (date): _____

Prostate disorder: _____

Practice self-exam: Breast: _____ ❏ Testicles: _____

Last proctoscopic/prostate exam: _____

    Last PSA/date: _____

Medications/herbals: _____

Objective (Exhibits)

Genitalia: Penis: Circumcised: _____ ❏ Warts/lesions: _____

    Bleeding/discharge: _____

    Testicles (e.g., lumps): _____ ❏ Vasectomy: _____

Breast examination: _____

STD test results: _____

Social Interactions

Subjective (Reports)

Relationship status (check): ❏ Single: _____ ❏ Married: _____

    ❏ Living with partner: _____ ❏ Divorced: _____

    ❏ Widowed: _____ Years in relationship: _____ ❏ Perception

    of relationship: _____ Concerns/stresses: _____

Role within family structure: _____

Number/age of children: _____

Perception of relationship with family members: _____

Extended family: _____ ❏ Other support person(s): _____

Ethnic/cultural affiliations: _____

    Strength of ethnic identity: _____

    Lives in ethnic community: _____

Feelings of (describe): Mistrust: _____

    Rejection: _____ ❏ Unhappiness: _____

    Loneliness/isolation: _____

Problems related to illness/condition: _____

Problems with communication (e.g., speech, another language, brain injury): _____

    Use of speech/communication aids (list): _____

    Is interpreter needed: _____

    Primary language: _____

Genogram: Diagram on separate page

Objective (Exhibits)

Communication/speech: Clear: _____ ❏ Slurred: _____
    Incomprehensible: _____ ❏ Aphasic: _____
    Unusual speech pattern/impairment: _____
    Laryngectomy present: _____
Verbal/nonverbal communication with family/SO(s): _____
    Family interaction (behavioral) pattern: _____

Teaching/Learning

Subjective (Reports)

Communication: Dominant language (specify): _____
    Second language: _____ ❏ Literate (reading/writing): _____
    Education level: _____
    Learning disabilities (specify): _____
    Cognitive limitations: _____
Culture/ethnicity: Where born: _____
    If immigrant, how long in this country: _____
Health and illness beliefs/practices/customs: _____
Which family member makes healthcare decisions/is spokesperson for client: _____
Presence of Advance Directives: _____ ❏ Code status: Durable
    Medical Power of Attorney: _____ ❏ Designee: _____
Health goals: _____
Current health problem: Client understanding of problem: _____
Special healthcare concerns (e.g., impact of religious/cultural
    practices): _____
Familial risk factors (indicate relationship): _____
    Diabetes: _____ ❏ Thyroid (specify): _____
    Tuberculosis: _____ ❏ Heart disease: _____
    Stroke: _____ ❏ Hypertension: _____
    Epilepsy/seizures: _____ ❏ Kidney disease: _____
    Cancer: _____ ❏ Mental illness: _____
    Depression: _____ ❏ Other: _____
Prescribed medications: _____
    Drug: _____ ❏ Dose: _____
    Times (circle last dose): _____
    Take regularly: _____ ❏ Purpose: _____
    Side effects/problems: _____
Nonprescription drugs/frequency: OTC drugs: _____
    Vitamins: _____ ❏ Herbals: _____
    Street drugs: _____
    Alcohol (amount/frequency): _____
    Tobacco: _____ ❏ Smokeless tobacco: _____
Admitting diagnosis per provider: _____
Reason for hospitalization per client: _____
History of current problem: _____

Expectations of this hospitalization: _____
Will admission cause any lifestyle changes (describe): _____
Previous illnesses and/or hospitalizations/surgeries: _____
Evidence of failure to improve: _____
Last complete physical exam: _____

Discharge Plan Considerations
Projected length of stay (days or hours): _____
Anticipated date of discharge: _____
Date information obtained: _____
Resources available: Persons: _____
    Financial: _____ ❑ Community supports: _____
    Groups: _____
Areas that may require alteration/assistance:
    Food preparation: _____ ❑ Shopping: _____
    Transportation: _____ ❑ Ambulation: _____
    Medication/IV therapy: _____
    Treatments: _____
    Wound care: _____
    Supplies/DME: _____
    Self-care (specify): _____
    Homemaker/maintenance (specify): _____
    Socialization: _____
    Physical layout of home (specify): _____
Anticipated changes in living situation after discharge: _____
    Living facility other than home (specify): _____
Referrals (date/source/services): Social services: _____
    Rehab services: _____ ❑ Dietary: _____
    Home care/hospice: _____ ❑ Resp/O_2: _____
    Equipment: _____
    Supplies: _____
Other: _____

EXCERPT FROM PSYCHIATRIC NURSING ASSESSMENT TOOL

Ego Integrity

Subjective (Reports)

What kind of person are you (positive/negative, etc.)? _____

What do you think of your body? _____

How would you rate your self-esteem (1 to 10, with 10 the highest)? _____

What are your problematic moods? Depressed: _____

    Guilty: _____ ❏ Unreal: _____

    Ups/downs: _____ ❏ Apathetic: _____

    Separated from the world: _____

    Detached: _____

Are you a nervous person? ____ ❏ Are your feelings easily hurt?

    _____ Report of stress factors: _____

    Previous patterns of handling stress: _____

Financial concerns: _____

Relationship status: _____

Work history/military service: _____

Cultural/ethnic factors: _____

Religion: _____ ❏ Practicing: _____

Lifestyle: _____ ❏ Recent changes: _____

    Significant losses/changes (dates): _____

Stages of grief/manifestations of loss: _____

Feelings of (check those that apply): ❏ Helplessness: _____

❏ Hopelessness: _____ ❏ Powerlessness: _____

❏ Restive: _____ ❏ Passive: _____ ❏ Dependent: _____

❏ Euphoric: ____ ❏ Angry/hostile: ____ ❏ Other (specify): ____

Objective (Exhibits)

Emotional status (check those that apply): ❏ Calm: _____

❏ Friendly: _____ ❏ Cooperative: _____ ❏ Evasive: _____

❏ Fearful: _____ ❏ Anxious: _____ ❏ Irritable: _____

❏ Withdrawn: _____

Defense mechanisms: _____

    Projection: _____ ❏ Denial: _____ ❏ Undoing: _____

    Rationalization: _____ ❏ Repression: _____

    Regression: _____

    Passive/aggressive: _____ ❏ Sublimation: _____

    Intellectualization: _____ ❏ Somatization: _____

    Identification: _____ ❏ Introjection: _____

    Reaction formation: _____

    Isolation: _____ ❏ Displacement: _____

    Substitution: _____

Consistency of behavior: Verbal: _____ ❏ Nonverbal: _____

Characteristics of speech: _____

    Slow/rapid: _____ ❏ Pressured: _____

    Volume: _____ ❏ Impairments: _____

    Aphasia: _____

Motor behaviors: _____ ❏ Posturing: _____
  Restless: _____
  Underactive/overactive: _____
  Stereotypical: _____ ❏ Tics/tremors: _____
  Gait patterns: _____
Observed physiological response(s): _____

Neurosensory

Subjective (Reports)
Dreamlike states: _____ ❏ Walking in sleep: _____
  Automatic writing: _____
Believe/feel you are another person: _____
Perception different than others: _____
Ability to follow directions: _____
  Perform calculations: _____
  Accomplish ADLs: _____
Fainting spells/dizziness: _____ ❏ Blackouts: _____
  Seizures: _____

Objective (Exhibits)
Mental status (note duration of change): _____
Oriented: Person: _____ ❏ Place: _____ ❏ Time: _____
Check all that apply: ❏ Alert: _____ ❏ Drowsy: _____
  ❏ Lethargic: _____
  ❏ Stuporous: _____ ❏ Comatose: _____ ❏ Cooperative: _____
  ❏ Combative: _____ ❏ Delusions: _____ ❏ Hallucinations: _____
Memory: Immediate: _____ ❏ Recent: _____ ❏ Remote: _____
  Comprehension: _____
Thought processes (assessed through speech): Patterns of speech
  (e.g., spontaneous/sudden silences): _____
  Content: _____ ❏ Change in topic: _____
  Delusions: _____ ❏ Hallucinations: _____
  Illusions: _____
  Rate or flow: _____ ❏ Clear, logical progression: _____
  Expression: _____ ❏ Flight of ideas: _____
  Ability to concentrate: _____ ❏ Attention span: _____
Mood: Affect: _____ ❏ Appropriateness: _____
  Intensity: _____
  Range: _____
Insight: _____ ❏ Misperceptions: _____
Attention/calculation skills: _____
  Judgment: _____
  Ability to follow directions: _____
  Problem-solving: _____
Impulse control: Aggression: _____ ❏ Hostility: _____
  Affection: _____
Sexual feelings: _____

EXCERPT FROM PRENATAL ASSESSMENT TOOL

Safety

Subjective (Reports)

Allergies/sensitivity: _____

  Reaction: _____

Previous alteration of immune system: _____

  Cause: _____

History of sexually transmitted diseases/gynecological infections (date/type): _____

  Testing/date: _____

High-risk behaviors: _____

Blood transfusion/number: _____ ❑ When: _____

  Reaction: _____

  Describe: _____

Childhood diseases: _____

  Immunization history/date: Tetanus: _____

  Pneumonia: _____

  Influenza: _____ ❑ Hepatitis: _____ ❑ MMR: _____

  Polio: _____ ❑ HPV: _____

Recent exposure to German measles: _____

  Other viral infections: _____

  X-ray/radiation: _____ ❑ House pets: _____

Previous obstetric problems: PIH: _____ ❑ Kidney: _____

  Hemorrhage: _____ ❑ Cardiac: _____

  Diabetes: _____ ❑ Infection/UTI: _____ ❑ ABO/Rh sensitivity: _____ ❑ Uterine surgery: _____

  Anemia: _____ ❑ Explain "yes" responses: _____

Length of time since last pregnancy: _____

  Type of previous delivery: _____

History of accidental injuries: Fractures/dislocations: _____

  Physical abuse: _____

  Arthritis/unstable joints: _____

  Back problems: _____

Changes in moles: _____ ❑ Enlarged nodes: _____

Impaired vision: _____ ❑ Hearing: _____

Prostheses: _____ ❑ Ambulatory devices: _____

Objective (Exhibits)

Temperature: _____ ❑ Diaphoresis: _____

Skin integrity: _____ ❑ Scars: _____ ❑ Rashes: _____

  Ecchymosis: _____ ❑ Genital warts/lesions: _____

General strength: _____ ❑ Muscle tone: _____

  Gait: _____

  ROM: _____ ❑ Paresthesia/paralysis: _____

Fetal: Heart rate: _____ ❑ Location: _____

  Method of auscultation: _____ ❑ Fundal height: _____

  Estimated gestation (weeks): _____ ❑ Movement: _____

Ballottement: _____

Fetal testing: Date: _____ ❑ Test: _____ ❑ Result: _____

   AFT: _____ ❑ Ultrasound: _____

Screenings: Serology: _____ ❑ Syphilis: _____

   Sickle cell: _____ ❑ Rubella: _____

   Hepatitis: _____ ❑ HIV: _____ ❑ AFP: _____

Results of cultures (cervical/rectal): _____

   Immune system testing: _____

Blood type: Maternal: _____ ❑ Paternal: _____

Sexuality (Component of Social Interactions)

Subjective (Reports)

Sexual concerns: _____

Menarche: _____ ❑ Length of cycle (days): _____

   Duration (days): _____

First day of last menstrual period (LMP): _____ ❑ Amount: _____

   Bleeding/cramping since LMP: _____

   Vaginal discharge: _____

Client's belief of when conception occurred: _____

Estimated date of delivery: _____

Last Pap smear: _____ ❑ Practices breast self-examination: _____

Recent contraceptive method: _____

OB history (GPTPAL): Gravida: _____ ❑ Para: _____ ❑ Term: _____

   Preterm: _____ ❑ Abortions: _____ ❑ Living: _____ ❑ Multiple

   births: _____

Delivery history: Year: _____ ❑ Place of delivery: _____

   Length of gestation (weeks): _____

   Length of labor (hours): _____ ❑ Type of delivery: _____

   Born (alive): _____ ❑ Weight: _____ ❑ Apgar scores: _____

Complications (maternal/fetal): _____

Objective (Exhibits)

Pelvic: Vulva: _____ ❑ Perineum: _____ ❑ Vagina: _____

   Cervix: _____ ❑ Uterus: _____ ❑ Adnexal: _____

   Diagonal conjugate: _____

   Transverse: _____ ❑ Diameter: _____ ❑ Outlet (cm): _____

   Shape of sacrum: _____ ❑ Arch: _____ ❑ Coccyx: _____

   SS notch: _____

   Ischial spines: _____

   Adequacy of inlet: _____ ❑ Mid: _____ ❑ Outlet: _____

Prognosis for delivery: _____

Breast exam: _____ ❑ Nipples: _____

Pregnancy test: _____ ❑ Serology test (date): _____

Pap smear results: _____

EXCERPT FROM INTRAPARTAL ASSESSMENT TOOL

Pain/Discomfort

Subjective (Reports)

Uterine contractions began: _____ ❑ Became regular: _____
    Character: ____ ❑ Frequency (minutes): ____ ❑ Duration: ____
Location of contractile pain (check): ❑ Front: _____
    ❑ Sacral area: _____
Degree of discomfort (check): ❑ Mild: _____ ❑ Moderate: _____
    ❑ Severe: _____
How relieved: Breathing/relaxation techniques: _____
    Positioning: _____ ❑ Sacral rubs: _____ ❑ Effleurage: _____
    Other: _____

Objective (Exhibits)

Facial expression: _____ ❑ Narrowed focus: _____
Body movement: _____ ❑ Change in BP: _____ ❑ Pulse: _____

Safety

Subjective (Reports)

Allergies/sensitivity: _____
    Reaction (specify): _____
History of STD (date/type): _____
Month of first prenatal visit: _____
Previous/current obstetric problems/treatment:
    PIH: ____ ❑ Kidney: ____ ❑ Hemorrhage: ____ ❑ Cardiac: ____
    Diabetes: _____ ❑ Infection/UTI: _____
    ABO/Rh sensitivity: _____ ❑ Anemia: _____
    Uterine surgery: _____
Length of time since last pregnancy: _____
Type of previous delivery: _____
Health status of living children: _____
Blood transfusion: _____ ❑ When: _____
    Reaction (describe): _____
Maternal stature/build: _____
    Pelvis: _____
Fractures/dislocations: _____ ❑ Arthritis/unstable joints: _____
Spinal problems/deformity: Kyphosis: _____ ❑ Scoliosis: _____
    Trauma: _____
    Surgery: _____
Prosthesis: _____ ❑ Ambulatory devices: _____

Objective (Exhibits)

Temperature: _____
Skin integrity: _____ ❑ Rashes: _____ ❑ Sores: _____
    Bruises: _____ ❑ Scars: _____
Paresthesia/paralysis: _____

Fetal status: Heart rate: _____ ❏ Location: _____
   Method of auscultation: _____
   Fundal height: _____ ❏ Estimated gestation (weeks): _____
   Activity/movement: _____
   Fetal assessment/testing: Test: _____
   Date: _____ ❏ Results: _____
Labor status: Cervical dilation: _____ ❏ Effacement: _____
   Fetal descent: _____ ❏ Engagement: _____
   Presentation: _____ ❏ Lie: _____ ❏ Position: _____
Membranes: Intact: _____ ❏ Ruptured/time: _____
   Nitrazine test (+/−): _____
   Amount of drainage: _____ ❏ Character: _____
Blood type/Rh: Maternal: _____ ❏ Paternal: _____
Screens (check): ❏ Sickle cell: _____ ❏ Rubella: _____
   ❏ Hepatitis: _____ ❏ HIV: _____ ❏ TB: _____ ❏ HPV: _____
Serology: Syphilis (+/−): _____ ❏ Cervical/rectal culture
   (+/−): _____
Vaginal warts/lesions: _____ ❏ Perineal varicosities: _____

SECTION 2

Diagnostic Divisions: Nursing Diagnoses Organized According to a Nursing Focus

After data are collected and areas of concern or need are identified, the nurse is directed to the Diagnostic Divisions to review the list of NDs that fall within the individual categories. This will assist the nurse in choosing the specific diagnostic label to accurately describe the data. Then, with the addition of etiology or related/risk factors and signs and symptoms or cues (defining characteristics) when present, the client diagnostic statement emerges.

ACTIVITY/REST—Ability to engage in necessary or desired activities of life (work and leisure) and to obtain adequate sleep or rest

Activity Intolerance [specify level]
Activity Intolerance, risk for
Activity Planning, ineffective
Activity Planning, risk for ineffective
Disuse Syndrome, risk for
Diversional Activity, deficient
Fatigue
Insomnia
Lifestyle, sedentary
Mobility, impaired bed
Mobility, impaired wheelchair
Sleep, readiness for enhanced
Sleep Deprivation
Sleep Pattern, disturbed
Transfer Ability, impaired
Walking, impaired

CIRCULATION—Ability to transport oxygen and nutrients necessary to meet cellular needs

Autonomic Dysreflexia
Autonomic Dysreflexia, risk for
Bleeding, risk for
Cardiac Output, decreased
Gastrointestinal Perfusion, risk for ineffective

Intracranial Adaptive Capacity, decreased
Renal Perfusion, risk for ineffective
Shock, risk for
Tissue Perfusion, ineffective peripheral
Tissue Perfusion, risk for decreased cardiac
Tissue Perfusion, risk for ineffective cerebral
Tissue Perfusion, risk for ineffective peripheral

EGO INTEGRITY—Ability to develop and use skills and behaviors to integrate and manage life experiences*

Anxiety [specify level]
Body Image, disturbed
Coping, defensive
Coping, ineffective
Coping, readiness for enhanced
Death Anxiety
Decision-Making, readiness for enhanced
Decisional Conflict
Denial, ineffective
Energy Field, disturbed
Fear
Grieving
Grieving, complicated
Grieving, risk for complicated
Health Behavior, risk-prone
Hope, readiness for enhanced
Hopelessness
Human Dignity, risk for compromised
Impulse Control, ineffective
Moral Distress
Personal Identity, disturbed
Personal Identity, risk for disturbed
Post-Trauma Syndrome [specify stage]
Post-Trauma Syndrome, risk for
Power, readiness for enhanced
Powerlessness
Powerlessness, risk for
Rape-Trauma Syndrome
Relationship, ineffective
Relationship, readiness for enhanced
Relationship, risk for ineffective
Religiosity, impaired
Religiosity, readiness for enhanced
Religiosity, risk for impaired
Relocation Stress Syndrome
Relocation Stress Syndrome, risk for
Resilience, impaired individual
Resilience, readiness for enhanced
Resilience, risk for compromised

Self-Concept, readiness for enhanced
Self-Esteem, chronic low
Self-Esteem, risk for chronic low
Self-Esteem, situational low
Self-Esteem, risk for situational low
Sorrow, chronic
Spiritual Distress
Spiritual Distress, risk for
Spiritual Well-Being, readiness for enhanced

ELIMINATION—Ability to excrete waste products*

Constipation
Constipation, perceived
Constipation, risk for
Diarrhea
Gastrointestinal Motility, dysfunctional
Gastrointestinal Motility, risk for dysfunctional
Incontinence, bowel
Incontinence, functional urinary
Incontinence, overflow urinary
Incontinence, reflex urinary
Incontinence, risk for urge urinary
Incontinence, stress urinary
Incontinence, urge urinary
Urinary Elimination, impaired
Urinary Elimination, readiness for enhanced
Urinary Retention [acute/chronic]

FOOD/FLUID—Ability to maintain intake of and utilize nutrients and liquids to meet physiological needs*

Blood Glucose Level, risk for unstable
Breast Milk, insufficient
Breastfeeding, ineffective
Breastfeeding, interrupted
Breastfeeding, readiness for enhanced
Dentition, impaired
Electrolyte Imbalance, risk for
Failure to Thrive, adult
Feeding Pattern, ineffective infant
Fluid Balance, readiness for enhanced
[Fluid Volume, deficient hyper/hypotonic]
Fluid Volume, deficient [isotonic]
Fluid Volume, excess
Fluid Volume, risk for deficient
Fluid Volume, risk for imbalanced
Liver Function, risk for impaired
Nausea
Nutrition: less than body requirements, imbalanced
Nutrition: more than body requirements, imbalanced
Nutrition: more than body requirements, risk for imbalanced

Nutrition, readiness for enhanced
Oral Mucous Membrane, impaired
Swallowing, impaired

HYGIENE—Ability to perform activities of daily living

Self-Care, readiness for enhanced
Self-Care Deficit, bathing
Self-Care Deficit, dressing
Self-Care Deficit, feeding
Self-Care Deficit, toileting
Self-Neglect

NEUROSENSORY—Ability to perceive, integrate, and respond to internal and external cues

Behavior, disorganized infant
Behavior, readiness for enhanced organized infant
Behavior, risk for disorganized infant
Confusion, acute
Confusion, risk for acute
Confusion, chronic
Memory, impaired
Peripheral Neurovascular Dysfunction, risk for
[Sensory Perception, disturbed (specify: visual, auditory, kinesthetic, gustatory, tactile, olfactory)]
Stress Overload
Unilateral Neglect

PAIN/DISCOMFORT—Ability to control internal and external environment to maintain comfort

Comfort, impaired
Comfort, readiness for enhanced
Pain, acute
Pain, chronic

RESPIRATION—Ability to provide and use oxygen to meet physiological needs

Airway Clearance, ineffective
Aspiration, risk for
Breathing Pattern, ineffective
Gas Exchange, impaired
Ventilation, impaired spontaneous
Ventilatory Weaning Response, dysfunctional

SAFETY—Ability to provide safe, growth-promoting environment

Adverse Reaction to Iodinated Contrast Media, risk for
Allergy Response, risk for
Body Temperature, risk for imbalanced
Contamination
Contamination, risk for
Dry Eye, risk for

Environmental Interpretation Syndrome, impaired
Falls, risk for
Health Maintenance, ineffective
Home Maintenance, impaired
Hyperthermia
Hypothermia
Immunization Status, readiness for enhanced
Infection, risk for
Injury, risk for
Jaundice, neonatal
Jaundice, risk for neonatal
Latex Allergy Response
Latex Allergy Response, risk for
Maternal-Fetal Dyad, risk for disturbed
Mobility, impaired physical
Perioperative Positioning Injury, risk for
Poisoning, risk for
Protection, ineffective
Self-Mutilation
Self-Mutilation, risk for
Skin Integrity, impaired
Skin Integrity, risk for impaired
Sudden Infant Death Syndrome, risk for
Suffocation, risk for
Suicide, risk for
Surgical Recovery, delayed
Thermal Injury, risk for
Thermoregulation, ineffective
Tissue Integrity, impaired
Trauma, risk for
Vascular Trauma, risk for
Violence, risk for other-directed
Violence, risk for self-directed
Wandering [specify sporadic or continual]

SEXUALITY—[Component of Ego Integrity and Social Interaction] Ability to meet requirements/characteristics of male/female roles*

Childbearing Process, ineffective
Childbearing Process, readiness for enhanced
Childbearing Process, risk for ineffective
Sexual Dysfunction
Sexuality Pattern, ineffective

SOCIAL INTERACTION—Ability to establish and maintain relationships*

Attachment, risk for impaired
Caregiver Role Strain
Caregiver Role Strain, risk for
Communication, impaired verbal

Communication, readiness for enhanced
Coping, compromised family
Coping, disabled family
Coping, ineffective community
Coping, readiness for enhanced community
Coping, readiness for enhanced family
Family Processes, dysfunctional
Family Processes, interrupted
Family Processes, readiness for enhanced
Loneliness, risk for
Parenting, impaired
Parenting, readiness for enhanced
Parenting, risk for impaired
Role Conflict, parental
Role Performance, ineffective
Social Interaction, impaired
Social Isolation

TEACHING/LEARNING—Ability to incorporate and use information to achieve healthy lifestyle/optimal wellness*

Development, risk for delayed
Growth, risk for disproportionate
Growth and Development, delayed
Health, deficient community
Knowledge, deficient [Learning Need (specify)]
Knowledge, readiness for enhanced
Noncompliance [ineffective Adherence] [specify]
Self-Health Management, ineffective
Self-Health Management, readiness for enhanced
Therapeutic Regimen Management, ineffective family

Please also see the NANDA-I diagnoses grouped according to Gordon's Functional Health Patterns on the inside front cover.

*Information that appears in brackets has been added by authors to clarify and enhance the use of NDs.

Client Situation and Prototype Plan of Care

Client Situation

Mr. R. S., a client with type 2 diabetes (noninsulin dependent) for 10 years, presented to his physician's office with a nonhealing ulcer of 3 weeks' duration on his left foot. Screening studies done in the doctor's office revealed blood glucose of 356/fingerstick and urine Chemstix of 2%. Because of distance from medical provider and lack of local community services, he is admitted to the hospital.

Admitting Physician's Orders

Culture/sensitivity and Gram's stain of foot ulcer
Random blood glucose on admission and fingerstick BG qid
CBC, electrolytes, serum lipid profile, glycosylated Hb in AM
Chest x-ray and ECG in AM
DiaBeta 10 mg, PO bid
Glucophage 500 mg, PO daily to start—will increase gradually
Humulin N 10 units SC q AM. Begin insulin instruction for post-discharge self-care if necessary
Dicloxacillin 500 mg PO q6h, start after culture obtained
Darvocet-N 100 mg PO q4h prn pain
Diet—2,400 calories, 3 meals with 2 snacks
Consult with dietitian
Up in chair ad lib with feet elevated
Foot cradle for bed
Irrigate lesion L foot with NS tid, cover with sterile dressing
Vital signs qid

Client Assessment Database

Name: R. S.   Informant: client
Reliability (Scale 1 to 4): 3
Age: 73   DOB: 5/3/39   Race: Caucasian   Gender: M
Adm. date: 6/28/2012   Time: 7 PM   From: home

Activity/Rest

Subjective (Reports)

Occupation: farmer
Usual activities/hobbies: reading, playing cards. "Don't have time to do much. Anyway, I'm too tired most of the time to do anything after the chores."

Limitations imposed by illness: "Have to watch what I order if I eat out."

Sleep: Hours: 6 to 8 hr/night   Naps: no   Aids: no

Insomnia: "Not unless I drink coffee after supper."

Usually feels rested when awakens at 4:30 AM

Objective (Exhibits)

Observed response to activity: limps, favors L foot when walking

Mental status: alert/active

Neuromuscular assessment: Muscle mass/tone: bilaterally equal/
firm Posture: erect

ROM: full Strength: equal 4 extremities/(favors L foot currently)

Circulation

Subjective (Reports)

History of slow healing: lesion L foot, 3 weeks' duration

Extremities: Numbness/tingling: "My feet feel cold and tingly like sharp pins poking the bottom of my feet when I walk the quarter mile to the mailbox."

Cough/character of sputum: occ./white

Change in frequency/amount of urine: yes/voiding more lately

Objective (Exhibits)

Peripheral pulses: radials 3+; popliteal, dorsalis, post-tibial/
pedal, all 1+

BP: R: Lying: 146/90   Sitting: 140/86   Standing: 138/90
    L: Lying: 142/88   Sitting: 138/88   Standing: 138/84

Pulse: Apical: 86   Radial: 86   Quality: strong
    Rhythm: regular

Chest auscultation: few wheezes clear with cough, no murmurs/
rubs

Jugular vein distention: 0

Extremities:

Temperature: feet cool bilaterally/legs warm

Color: Skin: legs pale

Capillary refill: slow both feet (approx. 4 sec)

Homans' sign: 0

Varicosities: few enlarged superficial veins on both calves

Nails: toenails thickened, yellow, brittle

Distribution and quality of hair: coarse hair to midcalf; none on
ankles/toes

Color:

General: ruddy face/arms

Mucous membranes/lips: pink

Nailbeds: pink

Conjunctiva and sclera: white

Ego Integrity

Subjective (Reports)

Report of stress factors: "Normal farmer's problems: weather, pests, bankers, etc."

Ways of handling stress: "I get busy with the chores and talk things over with my livestock. They listen pretty good."

Financial concerns: Medicare only and needs to hire someone to do chores while here

Relationship status: married

Cultural factors: rural/agrarian, eastern European descent, "American," no ethnic ties

Religion: Protestant/practicing

Lifestyle: middle class/self-sufficient farmer

Recent changes: no

Feelings: "I'm in control of most things, except the weather and this diabetes now."

Concerned re possible therapy change "from pills to shots."

Objective (Exhibits)

Emotional status: generally calm, appears frustrated at times

Observed physiological response(s): occasionally sighs deeply/ frowns, fidgeting with coin, shoulders tense/shrugs shoulders, throws up hands

Elimination

Subjective (Reports)

Usual bowel pattern: almost every PM

Last BM: last night Character of stool: firm/brown
 Bleeding: 0   Hemorrhoids: 0   Constipation: occ.

Laxative used: hot prune juice on occ.

Urinary: no problems Character of urine: pale yellow

Objective (Exhibits)

Abdomen tender: no Soft/firm: soft Palpable mass: 0

Bowel sounds: active all 4 quads

Food/Fluid

Subjective (Reports)

Usual diet (type): 2,400 calorie (occ. "cheats" with dessert; "My wife watches it pretty closely.")

No. of meals daily: 3/1 snack

Dietary pattern:

  B: fruit juice/toast/ham/decaf coffee

  L: meat/potatoes/veg/fruit/milk

  D: $\frac{1}{2}$ meat sandwich/soup/fruit/decaf coffee

  Snack: milk/crackers at HS. Usual beverage: skim milk, 2 to 3 cups decaf coffee, drinks "lots of water"—several quarts

Last meal/intake: Dinner: $\frac{1}{2}$ roast beef sandwich, vegetable soup, pear with cheese, decaf coffee

Loss of appetite: "Never, but lately I don't feel as hungry as usual."

Nausea/vomiting: 0   Food allergies: none

Heartburn/food intolerance: cabbage causes gas, coffee after supper causes heartburn

Mastication/swallowing problems: 0
  Dentures: partial upper plate—fits well

Usual weight: 175 lb Recent changes: has lost about 6 lb this month

Diuretic therapy: no

Objective (Exhibits)

Wt: 169 lb   Ht: 5 ft 10 in.   Build: stocky

Skin turgor: good/leathery Mucous membranes: moist

Condition of teeth/gums: good, no irritation/bleeding noted

Appearance of tongue: midline, pink

Mucous membranes: pink, intact

Breath sounds: few wheezes cleared with cough

Bowel sounds: active all 4 quads

Urine Chemstix: 2%   Fingerstick: 356 (Dr. office) 450 random BG on adm

Hygiene

Subjective (Reports)

Activities of daily living: independent in all areas

Preferred time of bath: PM

Objective (Exhibits)

General appearance: clean-shaven, short-cut hair; hands rough and dry; skin on feet dry, cracked, and scaly

Scalp and eyebrows: scaly white patches

No body odor

Neurosensory

Subjective (Reports)

Headache: "Occasionally behind my eyes when I worry too much."

Tingling/numbness: feet, 4 or 5 times/week (as noted)

Eyes: Vision loss, farsighted, "Seems a little blurry now." Examination: 2 yrs ago

Ears: Hearing loss R: "Some." L: no (has not been tested)

Nose: Epistaxis: 0   Sense of smell: "No problem."

Objective (Exhibits)

Mental status: alert, oriented to person, place, time, situation
Affect: concerned   Memory: Remote/recent: clear and intact
Speech: clear/coherent, appropriate
Pupil reaction: PERRLA/small
Glasses: reading   Hearing aid: no
Handgrip/release: strong/equal

Pain/Discomfort

Subjective (Reports)

Primary focus: Location: medial aspect, L heel
Intensity (0 to 10): 4 to 5   Quality: dull ache with occ. sharp
  stabbing sensation
Frequency/duration: "Seems like all the time."
  Radiation: no
Precipitating factors: shoes, walking
  How relieved: ASA, not helping
Other complaints: sometimes has back pain following chores/
  heavy lifting, relieved by ASA/liniment rubdown

Objective (Exhibits)

Facial grimacing: when lesion border palpated
Guarding affected area: pulls foot away
Narrowed focus: no
Emotional response: tense, irritated

Respiration

Subjective (Reports)

Dyspnea: 0   Cough: occ. morning cough, white sputum
Emphysema: 0   Bronchitis: 0   Asthma: 0   Tuberculosis: 0
Smoker: filters Pk/day: $\frac{1}{2}$ No. yrs: 50+
Use of respiratory aids: 0

Objective (Exhibits)

Respiratory rate: 22   Depth: good   Symmetry: equal, bilateral
Auscultation: few wheezes, clear with cough
Cyanosis: 0   Clubbing of fingers: 0
Sputum characteristics: none to observe
Mentation/restlessness: alert/oriented/relaxed

Safety

Subjective (Reports)

Allergies: 0   Blood transfusions: 0
Sexually transmitted disease: 0
Wears seat belt
Fractures/dislocations: L clavicle, 1960s, fell getting off tractor

Arthritis/unstable joints: "Some in my knees."

Back problems: occ. lower back pain

Vision impaired: requires glasses for reading

Hearing impaired: slightly (R), compensates by turning "good ear" toward speaker

Immunizations: current flu/pneumonia 3 yrs ago/tetanus maybe 8 yrs ago

Objective (Exhibits)

Temperature: 99.4°F (37.4°C) Tympanic

Skin integrity: impaired L foot   Scars: R inguinal, surgical

Rashes: 0   Bruises: 0   Lacerations: 0   Blisters: 0

Ulcerations: medial aspect L heel, 2.5 cm diameter, approx. 3 mm deep, wound edges inflamed, draining small amount cream-color/pink-tinged matter, slight musty odor noted

Strength (general): equal all extremities   Muscle tone: firm

ROM: good   Gait: favors L foot   Paresthesia/paralysis: tingling, prickly sensation in feet after walking $\frac{1}{4}$ mile

Sexuality: Male

Subjective (Reports)

Sexually active: yes   Use of condoms: no (monogamous)

Recent changes in frequency/interest: "I've been too tired lately."

Penile discharge: 0   Prostate disorder: 0   Vasectomy: 0

Last proctoscopic examination: 2 yrs ago   Prostate examination: 1 yr ago

Practice self-examination: Breasts/testicles: no

Problems/complaints: "I don't have any problems, but you'd have to ask my wife if there are any complaints."

Objective (Exhibits)

Examination: Breasts: no masses   Testicles: deferred
Prostate: deferred

Social Interactions

Subjective (Reports)

Marital status: married 45 yrs   Living with: wife

Report of problems: none

Extended family: 1 daughter lives in town (30 miles away); 1 daughter married with a son, living out of state

Other: several couples, he and wife play cards/socialize with 2 to 3 times/mo, church fellowship weekly

Role: works farm alone; husband/father/grandfather

Report of problems related to illness/condition: none until now

Coping behaviors: "My wife and I have always talked things out. You know the 11th commandment is 'Thou shalt not go to bed angry.'"

Speech: clear, intelligible

Verbal/nonverbal communication with family/SO(s): speaks quietly with wife, looking her in the eye; relaxed posture

Family interaction patterns: wife sitting at bedside, relaxed, both reading paper, making occasional comments to each other

Teaching/Learning

Subjective (Reports)

Dominant language: English   Second language: 0   Literate: yes

Education level: 2 yr college

Health and illness/beliefs/practices/customs: "I take care of the minor problems and see the doctor only when something's broken."

Presence of Advance Directives: yes—wife to bring in

Durable Medical Power of Attorney: wife

Familial risk factors/relationship:

  Diabetes: maternal uncle

  Tuberculosis: brother died, age 27

  Heart disease: father died, age 78, heart attack

  Strokes: mother died, age 81

  High BP: mother

Prescribed medications:

  Drug: DiaBeta Dose: 10 mg bid

  Schedule: 8 AM/6 PM, last dose 6 PM today

  Purpose: control diabetes

  Takes medications regularly? yes

  Home urine/glucose monitoring: Only using test strips, stopped some months ago when he ran out. "It was always negative, anyway, and I don't like sticking my finger."

Nonprescription (OTC) drugs: occ. ASA

Use of alcohol (amount/frequency): socially, occ. beer

Tobacco: $\frac{1}{2}$ pk/day

Admitting diagnosis (physician): hyperglycemia with nonhealing lesion L foot

Reason for hospitalization (client): "Sore on foot and the doctor is concerned about my blood sugar, and says I'm supposed to learn this finger stick test now."

History of current complaint: "Three weeks ago I got a blister on my foot from breaking in my new boots. It got sore so I lanced it, but it isn't getting any better."

Client's expectations of this hospitalization: "Clear up this infection and control my diabetes."

Other relevant illness and/or previous hospitalizations/surgeries: 1960s, R inguinal hernia repair, tonsils age 5 or 6

Evidence of failure to improve: lesion L foot, 3 wks
Last physical examination: complete 1 yr ago, office follow-up 5 mo ago

Discharge Considerations (as of 6/28)

Anticipated discharge: 7/1/12 (3 days)

Resources: self, wife

Financial: "If this doesn't take too long to heal, we got some savings to cover things."

Community supports: diabetic support group (has not participated)

Anticipated lifestyle changes: become more involved in management of condition

Assistance needed: may require farm help for several days

Teaching: learn new medication regimen and wound care; review diet; encourage smoking cessation

Referral: Supplies: the Downtown Pharmacy or AARP

Equipment: Glucometer—AARP

Follow-up: primary care provider 1 wk after discharge to evaluate wound healing and potential need for additional changes in diabetic regimen

PLAN OF CARE FOR CLIENT WITH DIABETES MELLITUS

Client Diagnostic Statement:

impaired Skin Integrity related to pressure, altered metabolic state, circulatory impairment, and decreased sensation, as evidenced by draining wound L foot.

Outcome: Wound Healing: Secondary Intention (NOC) Indicators: Client Will:

Be free of purulent drainage within 48 hrs (6/30 1900).

Display signs of healing with wound edges clean/pink within 60 hrs (7/1 0700).

ACTIONS/ INTERVENTIONS	RATIONALE
Wound Care (NIC)	
Irrigate wound with room temperature sterile NS tid.	Cleans wound without harming delicate tissues.
Assess wound with each dressing change. Obtain wound tracing on adm and at discharge.	Provides information about effectiveness of therapy, and identifies additional needs.
Apply sterile dressing.	Keeps wound clean/minimizes cross contamination.
Use paper tape.	Adhesive tape may be abrasive to fragile tissues.
Infection Control (NIC)	
Follow wound precautions.	Use of gloves and proper handling of contaminated dressings reduces likelihood of spread of infection.
Obtain sterile specimen of wound drainage on admission.	Culture/sensitivity identifies pathogens and therapy of choice.
Administer dicloxacillin 500 mg PO q6h, starting 10 PM.	Treatment of infection and prevention of complications.
	Food interferes with drug absorption, requiring scheduling around meals.
Observe for signs of hypersensitivity: pruritus, urticaria, rash.	Although no history of penicillin reaction, it may occur at any time.

Client Diagnostic Statement:

risk for unstable Blood Glucose Level related to lack of adherence to diabetes management and inadequate blood glucose monitoring with fingerstick 450/adm.

Outcome: Blood Glucose Level (NOC)
Indicators: Client Will:

Demonstrate correction of metabolic state as evidenced by FBS less than 120 mg/dL within 36 hrs (6/30 0700).

ACTIONS/ INTERVENTIONS	RATIONALE
Hyperglycemia Management (NIC)	
Perform fingerstick BG qid.	Bedside analysis of blood glucose levels is a more timely method for monitoring effectiveness of therapy and provides direction for alteration of medications.
Administer antidiabetic medications:	Treats underlying metabolic dysfunction, reducing hyperglycemia and promoting healing.
10 U Humulin N insulin SC q AM after fingerstick BG;	Intermediate-acting preparation with onset of 2 to 4 hrs, peaks at 6 to 12 hrs, with a duration of 18 to 24 hrs. Increases transport of glucose into cells and promotes the conversion of glucose to glycogen.
DiaBeta 10 mg PO bid;	Lowers blood glucose by stimulating the release of insulin from the pancreas and increasing the sensitivity to insulin at the receptor sites.
Glucophage 500 mg PO daily; note onset of side effects.	Glucophage lowers serum glucose levels by decreasing hepatic glucose production and intestinal glucose absorption and increasing sensitivity to insulin. By using in conjunction with DiaBeta, client may be able to discontinue insulin once target dosage is achieved (e.g., 2,000 mg/day). An increase of 1 tablet per week is necessary to limit side effects of diarrhea, abdominal cramping, vomiting, possibly leading to dehydration and prerenal azotemia.

ACTIONS/ INTERVENTIONS	RATIONALE
Provide diet of 2,400 cals—3 meals/2 snacks.	Proper diet decreases glucose levels/insulin needs, prevents hyperglycemic episodes, can reduce serum cholesterol levels and promote satiation.
Schedule consultation with dietitian to restructure meal plan and evaluate food choices.	Calories are unchanged on new orders but have been redistributed to 3 meals and 2 snacks. Dietary choices (e.g., increased vitamin C) may enhance healing.

Client Diagnostic Statement:
acute Pain related to physical agent (open wound L foot), as evidenced by verbal report of pain and guarding behavior.

Outcome: Pain Control (NOC) Indicators: Client Will:
Report pain is minimized/relieved within 1 hr of analgesic administration (ongoing).
Report absence or control of pain by discharge (7/1).

Outcome: Pain Disruptive Effects (NOC) Indicators: Client Will:
Ambulate normally, full weight bearing by discharge (7/1).

ACTIONS/ INTERVENTIONS	RATIONALE
Pain Management (NIC)	
Determine pain characteristics through client's description.	Establishes baseline for assessing improvement/changes.
Place foot cradle on bed; encourage use of loose- fitting slipper when up.	Avoids direct pressure to area of injury, which could result in vasoconstriction/increased pain.
Administer Darvocet-N 100 mg PO q4h as needed. Document effectiveness.	Provides relief of discomfort when unrelieved by other measures.

Client Diagnostic Statement:
ineffective peripheral Tissue Perfusion related to deficient knowledge of disease process/aggravating factors and diabetes mellitus as evidenced by diminished pulses, pale/cool feet; capillary refill of 4 seconds; parathesia of feet "when walks $\frac{1}{4}$ mile."

Verbalize understanding of relationship between chronic disease (diabetes mellitus) and circulatory changes within 48 hrs (6/30 1900).

Demonstrate awareness of safety factors and proper foot care within 48 hrs (6/30 1900).

Maintain adequate level of hydration to maximize perfusion, as evidenced by balanced intake/output, moist skin/mucous membranes, and capillary refill less than 3 sec (ongoing).

ACTIONS/ INTERVENTIONS	RATIONALE
Circulatory Care: Arterial Insufficiency (NIC)	
Elevate feet when up in chair. Avoid long periods with feet in a dependent position.	Minimizes interruption of blood flow, reduces venous pooling.
Assess for signs of dehydration.	Glycosuria may result in dehydration with consequent reduction of circulating volume and further impairment of peripheral circulation.
Monitor intake/output. Encourage oral fluids.	
Instruct client to avoid constricting clothing/socks and ill-fitting shoes.	Compromised circulation and decreased pain sensation may precipitate or aggravate tissue breakdown.
Reinforce safety precautions regarding use of heating pads, hot water bottles, or soaks.	Heat increases metabolic demands on compromised tissues. Vascular insufficiency alters pain sensation, increasing risk of injury.
Recommend cessation of smoking.	Vascular constriction associated with smoking and diabetes impairs peripheral circulation.
Discuss complications of disease that result from vascular changes: ulceration, gangrene, muscle or bony structure changes.	Although proper control of diabetes mellitus may not prevent complications, severity of effect may be minimized. Diabetic foot complications are the leading cause of nontraumatic lower extremity amputations.

	Note: Skin dry, cracked, scaly; feet cool; and pain when walking a distance suggest mild to moderate vascular disease (autonomic neuropathy) that can limit response to infection, impair wound healing, and increase risk of bony deformities.
Review proper foot care as outlined in teaching plan.	Altered perfusion of lower extremities may lead to serious or persistent complications at the cellular level.

Client Diagnostic Statement:

deficient Knowledge/Learning Need regarding diabetic condition related to misinterpretation of information and/or lack of recall as evidenced by inaccurate follow-through of instructions regarding home glucose monitoring and foot care and failure to recognize signs/symptoms of hyperglycemia.

Outcome: Knowledge: Diabetes Management (NOC) Indicators: Client Will:

Perform procedure for home glucose monitoring correctly within 36 hrs (6/30 0700).

Verbalize basic understanding of disease process and treatment within 38 hrs (6/30 0900).

Explain reasons for actions within 38 hrs (6/30 0900).

Perform insulin administration correctly within 60 hrs (7/1 0700).

Teaching: Disease Process (NIC)	
Determine client's level of knowledge, priorities of learning needs, desire/need for including wife in instruction.	Establishes baseline and direction for teaching/planning. Involvement of wife, if desired, will provide additional resource for recall/understanding and may enhance client's follow through.

ACTIONS/ INTERVENTIONS	RATIONALE
Provide teaching guide, "Understanding Your Diabetes," 6/29 AM. Show film "Living with Diabetes" 6/29 4 PM, when wife is visiting. Include in group teaching session 6/30 AM. Review information and obtain feedback from client/wife.	Provides different methods for accessing/reinforcing information and enhances opportunity for learning/ understanding.
Discuss factors related to altering diabetic control such as stress, illness, exercise.	Drug therapy/diet may need to be altered in response to both short-term and long-term stressors and changes in activity level.
Review signs/symptoms of hyperglycemia (e.g., fatigue, nausea, vomiting, polyuria, polydipsia). Discuss how to prevent and evaluate this situation and when to seek medical care. Have client identify appropriate interventions.	Recognition and understanding of these signs/symptoms and timely intervention will aid client in avoiding recurrences and preventing complications.
Review and provide information about necessity for routine examination of feet and proper foot care (e.g., daily inspection for injuries, pressure areas, corns, calluses; proper nail cutting; daily washing and application of good moisturizing lotion such as Eucerin, Keri, Nivea bid). Recommend wearing loose-fitting socks and properly fitting shoes (break new shoes in gradually) and avoiding going barefoot. If foot injury/skin break occurs, wash with soap/dermal cleanser and water, cover with sterile dressing, and inspect wound and change dressing daily; report redness, swelling, or presence of drainage.	Reduces risk of tissue injury; promotes understanding and prevention of stasis ulcer formation and wound-healing difficulties.

ACTIONS/ INTERVENTIONS	RATIONALE
Teaching: Prescribed Medication (NIC)	
Instruct regarding prescribed insulin therapy:	May be a temporary treatment of hyperglycemia with infection or may be permanent replacement of oral hypoglycemic agent.
Humulin N Insulin, SC.	Intermediate-acting insulin generally lasts 18 to 24 hrs, with peak effect between 6 to 12 hrs.
Keep vial in current use at room temperature (if used within 30 days).	Cold insulin is poorly absorbed.
Store extra vials in refrigerator.	Refrigeration prevents wide fluctuations in temperature, prolonging the drug shelf life.
Roll bottle and invert to mix, or shake gently, avoiding bubbles.	Vigorous shaking may create foam, which can interfere with accurate dose withdrawal and may damage the insulin molecule.
	Note: New research suggests that shaking the vial may be more effective in mixing suspension. Refer to Procedure Manual.
Choice of injection sites (e.g., across lower abdomen in a Z pattern).	Provides for steady absorption of medication. Site is easily visualized and accessible by client, and a Z pattern minimizes tissue damage.
Demonstrate, then observe client drawing insulin into syringe, reading syringe markings, and administering dose. Assess for accuracy.	May require several instruction sessions and practice before client/wife feel comfortable drawing up and injecting medication.
Instruct in signs/symptoms of insulin reaction or hypoglycemia: fatigue, nausea, headache, hunger, sweating, irritability, shakiness, anxiety, or difficulty concentrating.	Knowing what to watch for and appropriate treatment such as $\frac{1}{2}$ cup of grape juice for immediate response and a snack within $\frac{1}{2}$ hr (e.g., one slice of bread with peanut butter or cheese or fruit and slice of cheese for sustained effect) may prevent or minimize complications.

ACTIONS/INTERVENTIONS	RATIONALE
Review "Sick Day Rules" (e.g., call the doctor if too sick to eat normally or stay active) and take insulin as ordered. Keep record as noted in Sick Day Guide.	Understanding of necessary actions in the event of mild-to-severe illness promotes competent self-care and reduces risk of hyper/hypoglycemia.
Instruct client/wife in finger-stick glucose monitoring to be done qid until stable, then bid, rotating times such as FBS and before dinner or before lunch and HS. Observe return demonstrations of the procedure.	Fingerstick monitoring provides accurate and timely information regarding diabetic status. Return demonstration verifies correct learning.
Recommend client maintain record/log of finger stick testing, antidiabetic medication, insulin dosage/site, unusual physiological response, and dietary intake. Outline desired goals of FBS 80–110, premeal 80–130.	Provides accurate record for review by caregivers for assessment of therapy effectiveness/needs.
Discuss other healthcare issues, such as smoking habits, self-monitoring for cancer (breasts/testicles), and reporting changes in general well-being.	Encourages client involvement, awareness, and responsibility for own health; promotes wellness. **Note:** Smoking tends to increase client's resistance to insulin.

ANOTHER APPROACH TO PLANNING CLIENT CARE— MIND OR CONCEPT MAPPING

Mind mapping starts in the center of the page with a representation of the main concept—the client. (This helps keep in mind that the client is the focus of the plan, not the medical diagnosis or condition.) From that central thought, other main ideas that relate to the client are added. Different concepts can be grouped together by geometric shapes, color coding, or by placement on the page. Connections and interconnections between groups of ideas are represented by the use of arrows or lines with defining phrases added that explain how the interconnected thoughts relate to one another. In this manner, many different pieces of information *about* the client can be connected directly *to* the client.

Whichever piece is chosen becomes the first layer of connections—clustered assessment data, NDs, or outcomes. For example, a map could start with NDs featured as the first "branches," each one being listed separately in some way on the map. Next, the signs and symptoms or data supporting the diagnoses could be added, or the plan could begin with the client outcomes to be achieved with connections then to NDs. When the plan is completed, there should be an ND (supported by subjective and objective assessment data), nursing interventions, desired client outcomes, and any evaluation data, all connected in a manner that shows there is a relationship between them. It is critical to understand that there is no preset order for the pieces because one cluster is not more or less important than another (or one is not "subsumed" under another). It is important, however, that those pieces within a branch be in the same order in each branch.

Figure 3.1 shows a Mind Map for Mr. R. S., the client with type 2 diabetes in our Client Situation at the beginning of this section of the chapter.

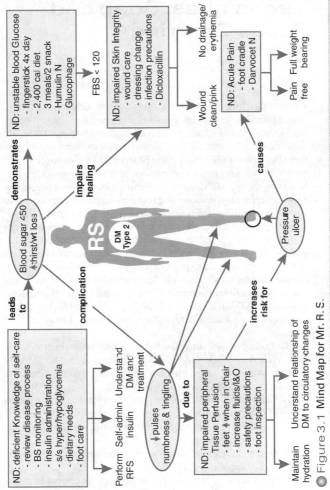

ND: unstable Blood Glucose
- fingerstick 4x day
- 2,400 cal diet
- 3 meals/2 snack
- Humulin N
- Glucophage

FBS < 120

ND: impaired Skin Integrity
- wound care
- dressing change
- infection precautions
- Dicloxacillin

No drainage/erythemia

Wound clean/pink

ND: Acute Pain
- foot cradle
- Darvocet N

Full weight bearing

Pain free

demonstrates

impairs healing

causes

Blood sugar <50
↑thirst/wt loss

RS

DM Type 2

Pressure ulcer

leads to

complication

increases risk for

ND: deficient Knowledge of self-care
- review disease process
- BS monitoring
- insulin administration
- s/s hyper/hypoglycemia
- dietary needs
- foot care

Perform RFS

Self-admin insulin

Understand DM and treatment

↓pulses numbness & tingling

due to

ND: impaired peripheral Tissue Perfusion
- feet ↑ when in chair
- increase fluids/I&O
- safety precautions
- foot inspection

Maintain hydration

Understand relationship of DM to circulatory changes

Figure 3.1 Mind Map for Mr. R. S.

SECTION 4

Documentation Techniques: Soap and Focus Charting®

Several charting formats are currently used for documentation. These include block notes, with a single entry covering an entire shift (e.g., 7 AM to 3 PM), narrative timed notes (e.g., "0830, ate breakfast well"), and the problem-oriented medical record system (POMR or PORS) using the SOAP/SOAPIER approach, to name a few. The latter can provide thorough documentation; however, the SOAP/SOAPIER charting system was designed by physicians for episodic care and requires that the entries be tied to a problem identified from a problem list. (See Example 1.)

The Focus Charting® system (see Example 2) has been designed by nurses for documentation of frequent or repetitive care and to encourage viewing the client from a positive rather than a negative (problem-only) perspective. Charting is focused on client and nursing concerns, with the focal point of client status and the associated nursing care. A Focus is usually a client problem, concern, or ND but is not a medical diagnosis or a nursing task or treatment (e.g., wound care, indwelling catheter insertion, tube feeding).

Recording of assessment, interventions, and evaluation using Data, Action, and Response (DAR) categories facilitates tracking what is happening to the client at any given moment. Thus, the four components of this charting system are:

1. *Focus:* ND, client problem or concern, signs or symptoms of potential importance (e.g., fever, dysrhythmia, edema), a significant event or change in status, or specific standards of care or agency policy.
2. *Data:* Subjective and objective information describing and/or supporting the Focus.
3. *Action:* Immediate and future nursing actions based on assessment and consistent with, or complementary to, the goals and nursing action recorded in the client plan of care.
4. *Response:* Describes the effects of interventions and whether the goal was met.

The following charting examples are based on the data within the client situation of Mr. R. S. in Chapter 3, Section 3, pages 46–53.

EXAMPLE 1 **SAMPLE SOAP/IER CHARTING FOR PROTOTYPE PLAN OF CARE**

S = Subjective   O = Objective   A = Analysis   P = Plan
I = Implementation   E = Evaluation   R = Revision

Date	Time	Number/ Problem*	Note
6/29/12	1900	No. 1 (impaired Skin Integrity)*	S: "That hurts" (when tissue surrounding wound is palpated).
			O: Scant amount of serous drainage on dressing. Wound borders pink. No odor present.
			A: Wound shows early signs of healing, free of infection.
			P: Continue skin care per plan of care.

To document more of the nursing process, some institutions have added the following: Implementation, Evaluation, and Revision (if plan was ineffective).

			I: NS irrig. as ordered. Applied sterile dressing with paper tape.
			E: Wound clean, no drainage present.
			R: None required. Signed: E. Moore, RN
6/29/12	2100	No. 3 (acute Pain)*	3. "Dull, throbbing pain in left foot." 4/10 States there is no radiation to other areas.
			O: Muscles tense. Moving about bed, appears uncomfortable.
			A: Persistent pain.
			P: Per plan of care.
			I: Foot cradle on bed. Darvocet-N given PO. Signed: M. Siskin, RN
	2200		E: Reports pain relieved 0/10. Appears relaxed. Signed: M. Siskin, RN

(table continues on page 66)

S = Subjective   O = Objective   A = Analysis   P = Plan
I = Implementation   E = Evaluation   R = Revision

Date	Time	Number/ Problem*	Note
6/30/12	1100	No. 5 (Learning Need, Diabetic Care)*	S: "My wife and I have some questions and concerns we wish to discuss."
			O: Copy of list of questions attached to teaching plan.
			A: R. S. and wife need review of information and practice for insulin administration.
			P: Attended group teaching session with wife and read "Understanding Your Diabetes." To meet with dietitian.
			I: R. S. demonstrated insulin administration techniques for wife to observe. Procedure handout sheet for future reference provided to couple. Scheduled meeting for them with dietitian at 1300 today to discuss remaining questions
			E: R. S. more confident in demonstration, performed activity correctly without hesitation or hand tremors. R. S. explained steps of procedure and reasons for actions to wife. Couple identified resources to contact if questions/ problems arise. Signed: B. Briner, RN

*As noted on Plan of Care.

EXAMPLE 2 **SAMPLE OF FOCUS CHARTING® FOR PROTOTYPE PLAN OF CARE**

D = Data   A = Action   R = Response

Date	Time	Focus*	
6/29/12	1900	Skin integrity	D: Scant amount of serous drainage on dressing, wound borders pink, no odor present, denies discomfort except with direct palpation of surrounding tissue. A: NS irrig. as ordered. Sterile dressing applied with paper tape. R: Wound clean—no drainage present. Signed: E. Moore, RN
6/29/12	2100	Pain L foot	D: Reports dull/throbbing ache L foot 4/10—no radiation. Muscles tense, restless in bed. A: Foot cradle on bed. Darvocet-N 100 mg given PO. Signed: M. Siskin, RN
	2200	Pain L foot	R: Reports pain relieved 0/10. Appears relaxed. Signed: M. Siskin, RN
6/30/12	1100	Learning Need, Diabetic Teaching	D: Attended group teaching session with wife. Both have read "Understanding Your Diabetes." A: Reviewed list of questions/concerns from R. S. and wife. (Copy attached to teaching plan.) R. S. demonstrated insulin administration technique for wife to observe.

(table continues on page 68)

D = Data	A = Action	R = Response

Date	Time	Focus[a]

Procedure handout sheet for future reference provided to couple.
Meeting scheduled with dietitian for 1300 today to discuss remaining questions.

R: R. S. more confident in demonstration, performed activity correctly without hesitation or hand tremors. He explained steps of procedure and reasons for actions to wife. Couple identified resources to contact if questions/problems arise.

The following is an example of documentation of a client need/concern that currently does not require identification as a client problem (ND) or inclusion in the plan of care and therefore is not easily documented in the SOAP format:

6/28/12   2120   Gastric distress

D: Awakened from light sleep by "indigestion/burning sensation." Places hand over epigastric area. Skin warm/dry, color pink, vital signs unchanged.

A: Given Mylanta 30 mL PO. Head of bed elevated approximately 15 degrees.

R: Reports pain relieved. Appears relaxed, resting quietly.
Signed: E. Moore, RN

[a]FOCUS Charting®, Susan Lampe, RN, MS: Creative Nursing Management, Inc., 614 East Grant Street, Minneapolis, MN 55404.

CHAPTER 4

Nursing Diagnoses in Alphabetical Order

Activity Intolerance [specify level]

Taxonomy II: Activity/Rest—Class 4 Cardiovascular/
Pulmonary Responses (00092)
[Diagnostic Division: Activity/Rest]
Submitted 1982

Definition: Insufficient physiological or psychological energy to endure or complete required or desired daily activities

Related Factors

Generalized weakness
Sedentary lifestyle
Bedrest/immobility
Imbalance between oxygen supply and demand; [anemia]

Defining Characteristics

Subjective
Reports fatigue, feeling weak
Exertional discomfort/dyspnea

Objective
Abnormal heart rate or blood pressure response to activity
Electrocardiographic changes reflecting arrhythmias or ischemia

Functional Level Classification (Gordon, 2010):

Level I: Walk, regular pace, on level indefinitely; climb one flight or more but more short of breath than normal

---

Information that appears in brackets has been added by the authors to clarify and enhance the use of nursing diagnoses.

Level II: Walk one city block [or] 500 ft on level; climb one flight slowly without stopping
Level III: Walk no more than 50 ft on level without stopping; unable to climb one flight of stairs without stopping
Level IV: Dyspnea and fatigue at rest

Desired Outcomes/Evaluation Criteria— Client Will:

• Identify negative factors affecting activity tolerance and eliminate or reduce their effects when possible.
• Use identified techniques to enhance activity tolerance.
• Participate willingly in necessary/desired activities.
• Report measurable increase in activity tolerance.
• Demonstrate a decrease in physiological signs of intolerance (e.g., pulse, respirations, and blood pressure remain within client's normal range).

Actions/Interventions

Nursing Priority No. 1.

To identify causative/precipitating factors:

• Note presence of acute or chronic illness, such as heart failure, pulmonary disorders, hypothyroidism, diabetes mellitus, AIDS, anemias, cancers, pregnancy-induced hypertension (PID), acute and chronic pain. **Many factors cause or contribute to fatigue, but the term "activity intolerance" implies that the client cannot endure or adapt to increased energy or oxygen demands caused by an activity.** (Refer to ND Fatigue.)
• Evaluate client's actual and perceived limitations and severity of deficit in light of usual status. **Provides comparative baseline and information about needed education or interventions regarding quality of life.**
• Note client reports of weakness, fatigue, pain, difficulty accomplishing tasks, and/or insomnia. **Symptoms may be result of or contribute to intolerance of activity.**
• Assess cardiopulmonary response to physical activity, including vital signs, before, during, and after activity. Note accelerating fatigue. **Dramatic changes in heart rate and rhythm, changes in usual blood pressure, and progressively worsening fatigue result from an imbalance of oxygen supply and demand.**
• Ascertain ability to stand and move about and degree of assistance necessary or use of equipment **to determine current**

Information that appears in brackets has been added by the authors to clarify and enhance the use of nursing diagnoses.

status and needs associated with participation in needed/ desired activities.

- Identify activity needs versus desires **to evaluate appropriateness (e.g., is barely able to walk upstairs but would like to play tennis).**
- Assess emotional and psychological factors affecting the current situation (**e.g., stress and/or depression may be increasing the effects of an illness or depression might be the result of forced inactivity**).
- Note treatment-related factors, such as side effects and interactions of medications, **which can affect nature and degree of activity intolerance.**

Nursing Priority No. 2.

To assist client to deal with contributing factors and manage activities within individual limits:

- Monitor vital and cognitive signs, watching for changes in blood pressure, heart, and respiratory rates; note skin pallor and/or cyanosis and presence of confusion.
- Reduce intensity level or discontinue activities that cause undesired physiological changes **to prevent overexertion.**
- Provide and monitor response to supplemental oxygen, medications, and changes in treatment regimen.
- Increase exercise/activity levels gradually; teach methods **to conserve energy,** such as stopping to rest for 3 minutes during a 10-minute walk or sitting down to brush hair instead of standing.
- Plan care to carefully balance rest periods with activities **to reduce fatigue.**
- Provide positive atmosphere, while acknowledging the difficulty of the situation for the client. **Helps to minimize frustration and rechannel energy.**
- Encourage expression of feelings contributing to or resulting from the condition.
- Involve client/SO(s) in planning of activities as much as possible.
- Assist with activities and provide/monitor client's use of assistive devices (e.g., crutches, walker, wheelchair, or oxygen tank) **to protect client from injury.**
- Promote comfort measures and provide for relief of pain **to enhance ability to participate in activities.** (Refer to NDs acute Pain; chronic Pain.)
- Provide referral to other disciplines, such as exercise physiologist, psychological counseling/therapy, occupational/

Information that appears in brackets has been added by the authors to clarify and enhance the use of nursing diagnoses.

physical therapists, and recreation/leisure specialists, as indicated, **to develop individually appropriate therapeutic regimens.**

Nursing Priority No. 3.

To promote wellness (Teaching/Discharge Considerations):

- Plan for maximal activity within the client's ability. **Promotes the idea of normalcy of progressive abilities in this area.**
- Review expectations of client/SO(s)/providers **to establish individual goals.** Explore conflicts and differences **to reach agreement for the most effective plan.**
- 🏠• Instruct client/SO(s) in monitoring response to activity and in recognizing signs/symptoms that **indicate need to alter activity level.**
- 🏠• Plan for progressive increase of activity level/participation in exercise training, as tolerated by client. **Both activity tolerance and health status may improve with progressive training.**
- 🏠• Give client information that provides evidence of daily/ weekly progress **to sustain motivation.**
- 🏠• Assist client in learning and demonstrating appropriate safety measures **to prevent injuries.**
- 🏠• Provide information about the effect of lifestyle and overall health factors on activity tolerance (e.g., nutrition, adequate fluid intake, getting sufficient rest and sleep, exercise, smoking cessation, and mental health status).
- 🏠• Encourage client to maintain positive attitude; suggest use of relaxation techniques, such as visualization or guided imagery, as appropriate, **to enhance sense of well-being.**
- 🏠• Encourage participation in recreation, social activities, and hobbies appropriate for situation. (Refer to ND deficient Diversional Activity.)

Documentation Focus

Assessment/Reassessment
- Level of activity as noted in Functional Level Classification.
- Causative or precipitating factors.
- Client reports of difficulty or change.
- Vital signs before, during, and following activity.

Planning
- Plan of care and who is involved in planning.

Information that appears in brackets has been added by the authors to clarify and enhance the use of nursing diagnoses.

Implementation/Evaluation
- Response to interventions, teaching, and actions performed.
- Implemented changes to plan of care based on assessment/reassessment findings.
- Teaching plan and understanding of material presented.
- Attainment or progress toward desired outcome(s).

Discharge Planning
- Referrals to other resources.
- Long-term needs and who is responsible for actions.

Sample Nursing Outcomes & Interventions Classifications (NOC/NIC)

NOC—Activity Tolerance
NIC—Energy Management

risk for Activity Intolerance

Taxonomy II: Activity/Rest—Class 4 Cardiovascular/Pulmonary Response (00094)
[Diagnostic Division: Activity/Rest]
Submitted 1982

Definition: At risk of experiencing insufficient physiological or psychological energy to endure or complete required or desired daily activities

Risk Factors

History of previous activity intolerance
Circulatory/respiratory problems; [dysrhythmias]
Deconditioned status; [aging]
Inexperience with an activity

NOTE: A risk diagnosis is not evidenced by signs and symptoms, as the problem has not yet occurred; rather, nursing interventions are directed at prevention.

Desired Outcomes/Evaluation Criteria—Client Will:

- Verbalize understanding of potential loss of ability in relation to existing condition.

Information that appears in brackets has been added by the authors to clarify and enhance the use of nursing diagnoses.

- Participate in conditioning/rehabilitation program to enhance ability to perform.
- Identify alternative ways to maintain desired activity level (e.g., walking in a shopping mall if weather is bad).
- Identify conditions or symptoms that require medical reevaluation.

Actions/Interventions

Nursing Priority No. 1.
To assess factors affecting current situation:

- Note presence of medical diagnosis and/or therapeutic regimens (e.g., AIDS, chronic obstructive pulmonary disease [COPD], cancer, heart failure/other cardiac problems, anemia, multiple medications or treatment modalities, extensive surgical interventions, musculoskeletal trauma, neurological disorders, or renal failure) **that have potential for interfering with client's ability to perform at a desired level of activity.**
- Ask client/SO(s) about usual level of energy **to identify potential problems and/or client's/SO's perception of client's energy and ability to perform needed or desired activities.**
- Identify factors, such as age, functional decline, client resistive to efforts, painful conditions, breathing problems, vision or hearing impairments, climate or weather, unsafe areas to exercise, and need for mobility assistance, **that could block/affect desired level of activity.**
- Determine current activity level and physical condition with observation, exercise-capacity testing, or use of functional level classification system (e.g., Gordon's), as appropriate. **Provides baseline for comparison and an opportunity to track changes.**

Nursing Priority No. 2.
To develop alternative ways to remain active within the limits of the disabling condition/situation:

- Implement physical therapy/exercise program in conjunction with the client and other team members (e.g., physical and/or occupational therapist, exercise/rehabilitation physiologist). **A collaborative program with short-term achievable goals enhances likelihood of success and may motivate the client to adopt a lifestyle of physical exercise for the enhancement of health.**
- Promote and implement conditioning program. Support inclusion in exercise and activity groups **to prevent/limit deterioration.**

Information that appears in brackets has been added by the authors to clarify and enhance the use of nursing diagnoses.

⊕ Cultural 🌐 Collaborative 🏠 Community/Home Care

- Instruct client in proper performance of unfamiliar activities and in alternate ways of doing familiar activities **to conserve energy and promote safety.**

Nursing Priority No. 3.

To promote wellness (Teaching/Discharge Considerations):

- Discuss with client/SO(s) the relationship of the illness or debilitating condition and ability to perform desired activities. **Understanding this relationship can help with acceptance of limitations or reveal opportunity for changes of practical value.**
- Provide information regarding potential interfering factors with activity, such as smoking when one has respiratory problems or lack of motivation/interest in exercise, **which may be amenable to modification.**
- Assist client/SO(s) with planning for changes that may become necessary, such as use of supplemental oxygen **to improve client's ability to participate in desired activities.**
- Identify and discuss symptoms for which client needs to seek medical assistance/evaluation, **providing for timely intervention.**
- Refer to appropriate resources for assistance and/or equipment, as needed, **to sustain activity level.**

Documentation Focus

Assessment/Reassessment
- Identified or potential risk factors for individual.
- Current level of activity tolerance and blocks to activity.

Planning
- Treatment options, including physical therapy or exercise program, other assistive therapies and devices.
- Lifestyle changes that are planned, who is to be responsible for each action, and monitoring methods.

Implementation/Evaluation
- Responses to interventions, teaching, and actions performed.
- Attainment or progress toward desired outcome(s).
- Modification of plan of care.

Discharge Planning
- Referrals for medical assistance/evaluation.

Information that appears in brackets has been added by the authors to clarify and enhance the use of nursing diagnoses.

Sample Nursing Outcomes & Interventions Classifications (NOC/NIC)

NOC—Endurance
NIC—Energy Management

ineffective Activity Planning

Taxonomy II: Coping/Stress Tolerance—Class 2 Coping Response (00199)
[Diagnostic Division: Activity/Rest]
Submitted 2008

Definition: Inability to prepare for a set of actions fixed in time and under certain conditions

Related Factors

Unrealistic perception of events or personal competence
Lack of family/friend support
Compromised ability to process information
Defensive flight behavior when faced with the proposed solution
Hedonism [motivated by pleasure and/or pain]

Defining Characteristics

Subjective
Reports fear toward a task to be undertaken
Reports worries/excessive anxieties about a task to be undertaken

Objective
Failure pattern of behavior
Lack of plan, resources, and/or sequential organization
History of procrastination
Unmet goals for chosen activity

Desired Outcomes/Evaluation Criteria— Client Will: (Include Specific Time Frame)

- Acknowledge difficulty with follow-through of activity plan.
- Identify negative factors affecting ability to plan activities.
- Develop own plan for activity.
- Report lessened anxiety and fear toward planning.
- Be aware of and make plan to deal with procrastination.

Information that appears in brackets has been added by the authors to clarify and enhance the use of nursing diagnoses.

Actions/Interventions

Nursing Priority No. 1.

To identify causative/precipitating factors:

- Determine individual problems with planning and follow-through with activity plan. **Identifies individual difficulties (e.g., anxiety regarding what kind of activity to choose, lack of resources, lack of confidence in own ability).**
- Perform complete physical examination. **May have underlying problems such as allergies, hypertension, or asthma that are contributing to fatigue and difficulty with undertaking a task.**
- Review medication regimen **for possible side effects affecting client's desire to become involved in any activity.**
- Assess mental status; use Beck's Depression Inventory as indicated.
- Identify client's personal values and perception of self including strengths and weaknesses.
- Determine client's need to be in control, fear of dependency on others (although may need assistance from others), or belief he or she cannot do the task. **Indicative of external locus of control, where client sees others as having the control and ability.**
- Identify culture/religious issues **that may affect how individuals deal with issues of life or how they see their ability to make choices or manage their own life.**
- Discuss awareness of procrastination, need for perfection, fear of failure. **Although client may not acknowledge it as a problem, this may be a factor in their difficulty in planning for, choosing, and following through with activities that might be enjoyed.**
- Assess client's ability to process information. **This may interfere with perception of the world and self.**
- Discuss possibility that client is motivated by pleasure to avoid pain (hedonism). **Individual may seek activities that bring pleasure to avoid painful experiences.**
- Note availability and use of resources.

Nursing Priority No. 2.

To assist client to recognize and deal with individual factors and begin to plan appropriate activities:

- Encourage expression of feelings contributing/resulting from a situation. Maintain a positive atmosphere without seeming overly cheerful.

Information that appears in brackets has been added by the authors to clarify and enhance the use of nursing diagnoses.

- Discuss client's perception of self as worthless and not deserving of success and happiness. **This belief is common among individuals who struggle with feelings of low self-esteem and self-confidence. Sometimes the underlying feelings are those of wanting to be perfect, and it is difficult to finish the task because of the fear that it will not be perfect (perfectionism). They believe that anything they do is bound to fail, and feelings of anxiety and worry contribute to failure.**
- Gently confront client's ambivalent, angry, or depressed feelings.
- Help client learn how to reframe negative thoughts about self into a positive view of what is happening.
- Involve client/SOs in planning an activity. **Having the support of family and nurse will help promote success.**
- Direct client to break down desired activity into specific steps. **Makes activity more manageable, and as each step is accomplished, the client feels more confident about their ability to finish the task.**
- Encourage client to recognize procrastinating behaviors and make a decision to change. **Procrastination is a learned behavior and serves many purposes for the individual.**
- Accompany client to activity of own choosing, encouraging participation together if appropriate. **Support from caregiver may enable client to begin participating and gain confidence.**
- Assist client in developing skills of relaxation, imagery/visualization, and mindfulness. **Using these techniques can help the client learn to overcome stress and be able to manage life's difficulties more effectively.**
- Assist client to investigate the idea that seeking pleasure (hedonism) is interfering with motivation to accomplish goals. **Some philosophers believe that pleasure is the only good for a person and that the individual does not see other aspects of life, which interferes with accomplishments.**

Nursing Priority No. 3.
To promote wellness (Teaching/Discharge Criteria):

🏠• Assist client in identifying life goals and priorities.
🏠• Review treatment goals and expectations of client/SOs. **Helps clarify what has been discussed and decisions that have been made; provides an opportunity to change goals as needed.**
🏠• Discuss progress in learning to relax and deal productively with anxieties and fears. **As client sees that progress is being made, feelings of worthwhileness will be enhanced and individual will be encouraged to continue working toward goals.**

Information that appears in brackets has been added by the authors to clarify and enhance the use of nursing diagnoses.

- Identify community resources such as social services, senior centers, or classes **to provide support and options for activities and change.**
- Refer for cognitive therapy as indicated. **This structured therapy can help the individual identify, evaluate, and modify any underlying assumptions and dysfunctional beliefs and begin the process of change. Learning to set one's own schedule with reminders can also help a client to get tasks done in a timely manner.**

Documentation Focus

Assessment/Reassessment
- Specific problems exhibited by client.
- Causative or precipitating factors.
- Client reports of difficulty making and following through with plans.

Planning
- Plan of care and who is involved in planning.
- Teaching plan.

Implementation/Evaluation
- Response to interventions, teaching, and actions performed.
- Attainment or progress toward desired outcome(s).

Discharge Planning
- Referrals to other resources.
- Long-term needs and who is responsible for actions.

Sample Nursing Outcomes & Interventions Classifications (NOC/NIC)

NOC—Motivation
NIC—Self-Awareness Enhancement

---

risk for ineffective Activity Planning

Taxonomy II: Coping/Stress Tolerance—Class 2 Coping Responses
[Diagnostic Division: Activity/Rest]
Submitted 2010

Definition: At risk for an inability to prepare for a set of actions fixed in time and under certain conditions

---

Information that appears in brackets has been added by the authors to clarify and enhance the use of nursing diagnoses.

Risk Factors

Unrealistic perception of events or personal competence
Insufficient/ineffective support systems
Compromised ability to process information
Defensive flight behavior when faced with proposed solution
History of procrastination
Hedonism

Desired Outcomes/Evaluation Criteria–Client Will: (Include Specific Time Frame)

- Express awareness of negative factors or actions that can interfere with planning.
- Establish mindfulness and relaxation activities to lessen anxiety.
- Develop a plan, including the time frame, for a task to be completed.

Actions/Interventions

Nursing Priority No. 1.

To identify causative/precipitating factors related to risk:

- Determine circumstances of client's situation that may impact participating in selective activities.
- Note client's ability to process information. **Compromised mental ability, low self-esteem, and anxiety can interfere with dealing with planning activities.**
- Review health history and medications. **Underlying physical problems such as fatigue or medication side effects can affect ability to engage in tasks.**
- Evaluate mental status, using Beck's Depression scale or other inventories as indicated.
- Discuss religious/cultural and personal values and perception of self, including view of strengths and weaknesses that may **affect client's willingness to undertake planning.**
- Ascertain need for control, fear of dependency on others, or belief they will not be able to do the task. **Although client may need assistance, he/she may have external control and see others as having control and ability to do things they are not able to do.**
- Investigate client's awareness of procrastination, need for perfection, or fear of failure.
- Discuss issue of avoiding pain by seeking pleasure (hedonism). **People sometimes avoid pain by choosing activities**

Information that appears in brackets has been added by the authors to clarify and enhance the use of nursing diagnoses.

  Cultural 🌐 Collaborative 🏠 Community/Home Care

that provide pleasure but then they do not get needed tasks accomplished.
- Note availability and use of resources and support.

Nursing Priority No. 2.

To assist client to recognize and deal with risk factors that interfere with appropriate activities:

- Encourage recognition of feelings associated with issues that may prevent client from planning desired activities. **Awareness of frustration and/or anxiety will help client redirect energy into productive activities.**
- Help client to reframe negative thoughts about self into a positive view of what they are able to achieve.
- Encourage client to recognize procrastinating behaviors and make a decision to change.
- Develop a plan with the client to deal with activities in small steps. **Learning to do this will help client to feel more organized and successful in completing the desired task.**
- Encourage client to engage in an activity of choice with a friend, family member, or therapist.
- Investigate with the client the possibility that seeking pleasure (hedonism) may interfere with achieving life goals. **Individual may believe that pleasure is the only good and avoid tasks or activities viewed as not fun or pleasurable.**

Nursing Priority No. 3.

To promote wellness (Teaching/Discharge Criteria):

- Identify life goals and priorities. **If the individual has never thought about setting goals, they may begin to think about the possibility of being successful.**
- Discuss use of relaxation techniques and mindfulness to deal with anxieties and life stressors.
- Identify community resources, such as social services, senior centers, or classes. **Provides an opportunity to be involved in different activities and be successful in trying new activities.**
- Refer for cognitive therapy as indicated. **May help client deal with basic assumptions or dysfunctional beliefs.**

Documentation Focus

Assessment/Reassessment

- Individual risk factors identified.
- Client concerns or difficulty making and following through with plans.

Information that appears in brackets has been added by the authors to clarify and enhance the use of nursing diagnoses.

Planning
- Plan of care and who is involved in planning.
- Teaching plan.

Implementation/Evaluation
- Response to interventions, teaching, and actions performed.
- Attainment or progress toward outcomes.
- Client's plan for the future.

Discharge Planning
- Referrals to other resources.
- Long-term need and who is responsible for actions.

Sample Nursing Outcomes & Interventions Classification (NOC/NIC)

NOC—Motivation
NIC—Self-Modification Assistance

risk for Adverse Reaction to Iodinated Contrast Media

Taxonomy II: Defensive Processes—Class 5 Environmental Hazards
[Diagnostic Division: Safety]
Submitted 2010

Definition: At risk for any noxious or unintended reaction associated with the use of iodinated contrast media that can occur within 7 days after contrast agent injection

Risk Factors

History of allergies, previous adverse effect from iodinated contrast media [ICM]

Physical and chemical properties of the contrast media (e.g., iodine concentration, viscosity, high osmolality, ion toxicity)

Underlying disease (e.g., heart or pulmonary disease, blood dyscrasias, endocrine or renal disease, pheochromocytoma, autoimmune disease), concurrent use of medications (e.g., interleukin-2, metformin or nephrotoxic medications)

Fragile veins (e.g., prior or actual chemotherapy treatment or radiation in the limb to be injected, multiple attempts to ob-

---

Information that appears in brackets has been added by the authors to clarify and enhance the use of nursing diagnoses.

🌐 Cultural   ⊗ Collaborative   🏠 Community/Home Care

tain intravenous access, indwelling intravenous lines in place for more than 24 hours, previous axillary lymph node dissection in the limb to be injected, distal intravenous access sites—hand, wrist, foot, or ankle)

Extremes of age, generalized debilitation

Dehydration

Unconsciousness

Anxiety

> **NOTE:** A risk diagnosis is not evidenced by signs and symptoms, as the problem has not occurred; the nursing interventions are directed at prevention.

Desired Outcomes/Evaluation Criteria– Client Will:

- Experience no adverse reaction from ICM.
- Verbalize understanding of individual risks and responsibilities to avoid exposure.
- Recognize need for/seek assistance to limit allergic response/complications

Actions/Interventions

Nursing Priority No. 1.

To identify causative/precipitating factors related to risk:

- Identify the client at risk for adverse reaction prior to procedures (e.g., history of allergies, asthma, diabetes, renal insufficiency, including solitary kidney with elevated creatinine, thyroid dysfunction, hypertension, heart failure, current or recent use of nephrotoxic medications, or reaction to previous ICM administration).
- Ascertain type of reaction client experienced when there is a history of past reaction. **There are two types of reactions, idiosyncratic and nonidiosyncratic, both of which could change decisions about using ICM for diagnostic purposes.**

Nursing Priority No. 2.

To assist client/caregiver to reduce or correct individual risk factors:

- Administer infusions using "6 rights" system (right client, right medication, right route, right dose, right time, and right

---

Information that appears in brackets has been added by the authors to clarify and enhance the use of nursing diagnoses.

documentation) **to prevent client from receiving improper contrast agent or dosage.**

⊕• Administer intravenous fluids as appropriate **to reduce incidence of contrast medium-induced nephropathy.**

⊕• Perform imaging tests that do not require contrast media where possible **when client is at high risk for reaction.**

🗴• Administer medications (e.g., prednisone [Deltasone] or Benadryl) before, during, and after injection or procedures **to reduce risk or severity of reaction.**

• Observe intravenous injection site frequently **to ascertain that no extravasation of contrast solution is occurring.**

• Halt infusion immediately if client reports site discomfort or redness or swelling is noted **to prevent tissue damage from contrast agent**.

• Monitor results of lab studies (e.g., creatinine clearance) **to ascertain status of kidney function**.

Nursing Priority No. 3.
To promote wellness (Teaching/Discharge Criteria):

• Instruct client regarding signs and symptoms that should be reported to physician after a procedure. **Any delayed signs of reaction should be reported to physician immediately for timely intervention**.

• Instruct client/care provider about puncture sites and to report redness, soreness, or pain **to reduce risk of complications associated with extravasation.**

• Encourage client to use Medic Alert bracelet **to alert healthcare providers of history of prior reaction to contrast media**.

Documentation Focus

Assessment/Reassessment
• Individual risk factors identified.
• Client concerns or difficulty making and following through with plans.

Planning
• Plan of care and who is involved in planning.
• Teaching plan.

Implementation/Evaluation
• Response to interventions, teaching, and actions performed.
• Attainment or progress toward outcomes.

Information that appears in brackets has been added by the authors to clarify and enhance the use of nursing diagnoses.

🌐 Cultural   ⊛ Collaborative   🏠 Community/Home Care

Discharge Planning
- Referrals to other resources.
- Long-term need and who is responsible for actions.

Sample Nursing Outcomes & Interventions Classifications (NOC/NIC)

NOC—Allergic Response: Systemic
NIC—Allergy Management

ineffective Airway Clearance
Taxonomy II: Safety/Protection—Class 2 Physical Injury (00031)
[Diagnostic Division: Respiration]
Submitted 1980; Revised 1996, and Nursing Diagnosis Extension and Classification (NDEC) 1998

Definition: Inability to clear secretions or obstructions from the respiratory tract to maintain a clear airway

Related Factors

Environmental
Smoking; secondhand smoke; smoke inhalation

Obstructed Airway
Retained secretions; secretions in the bronchi; exudate in the alveoli; excessive mucus; airway spasm; foreign body in airway; presence of artificial airway

Physiological
Chronic obstructive pulmonary disease [COPD]; asthma; allergic airways; hyperplasia of the bronchial walls
Neuromuscular dysfunction
Infection

Defining Characteristics

Subjective
Dyspnea

Objective
Diminished/adventitious breath sounds (rales, crackles, rhonchi, or wheezes)

Information that appears in brackets has been added by the authors to clarify and enhance the use of nursing diagnoses.

Cough ineffective/absent, excessive sputum
Changes in respiratory rate/rhythm
Difficulty vocalizing
Wide-eyed, restlessness
Orthopnea
Cyanosis

Desired Outcomes/Evaluation Criteria— Client Will:

- Maintain airway patency.
- Expectorate/clear secretions readily.
- Demonstrate absence/reduction of congestion with breath sounding clear, noiseless respirations, and improved oxygen exchange (e.g., absence of cyanosis and arterial blood gas [ABG]/pulse oximetry results within client norms).
- Verbalize understanding of cause(s) and therapeutic management regimen.
- Demonstrate behaviors to improve or maintain clear airway.
- Identify potential complications and how to initiate appropriate preventive or corrective actions.

Actions/Interventions

Nursing Priority No. 1.
To maintain adequate, patent airway:

- Identify client populations at risk. **Persons with impaired ciliary function (e.g., cystic fibrosis, lung transplant recipients); those with excessive or abnormal mucus production (e.g., asthma, emphysema, pneumonia, dehydration, bronchiectasis, mechanical ventilation); those with impaired cough function (e.g., neuromuscular diseases, such as muscular dystrophy; multiple sclerosis neuromotor conditions, such as cerebral palsy; spinal cord injury); those with swallowing abnormalities (e.g., poststroke, seizures, head/neck cancer, coma/sedation, tracheostomy, facial burns/trauma/surgery); those who are immobile (e.g., sedated individual, frail elderly, developmentally delayed, institutionalized client with multiple high-risk conditions; infant/child (e.g., feeding intolerance, abdominal distention, and emotional stressors that may compromise airway) are all at risk for problems with the maintenance of open airways.**

Information that appears in brackets has been added by the authors to clarify and enhance the use of nursing diagnoses.

- Assess level of consciousness/cognition and ability to protect own airway. **Information is essential for identifying potential for airway problems, providing baseline level of care needed, and influencing choice of interventions**
- Monitor respirations and breath sounds, noting rate and sounds (e.g., tachypnea, stridor, crackles, or wheezes) **indicative of respiratory distress and/or accumulation of secretions.**
- Evaluate client's cough/gag reflex, amount and type of secretions, and swallowing ability **to determine ability to protect own airway.**
- Position head appropriate for age and condition **to open or maintain open airway in an at-rest or compromised individual.**
- Suction nose, mouth, and trachea prn **to clear airway when excessive or viscous secretions are blocking airway or client is unable to swallow or cough effectively.**
- Elevate head of bed, encourage early ambulation, or change client's position every 2 hours **to take advantage of gravity decreasing pressure on the diaphragm and enhancing drainage of/ventilation to different lung segments.**
- ∞ Monitor infant/child for feeding intolerance, abdominal distention, and emotional stressors **that may compromise airway.**
- Insert oral airway (using correct size for adult or child) when needed **to maintain anatomical position of tongue and natural airway, especially when tongue/laryngeal edema or thick secretions may block airway.**
- Assist with appropriate testing (e.g., pulmonary function or sleep studies) **to identify causative/precipitating factors.**
- Instruct in/review postoperative breathing exercises, effective coughing, and use of adjunct devices (e.g., IPPB or incentive spirometer) in preoperative teaching.
- Assist with procedures (e.g., bronchoscopy or tracheostomy) **to clear/maintain open airway.**
- Keep environment allergen free (e.g., dust, feather pillows, or smoke) according to individual situation.

Nursing Priority No. 2.
To mobilize secretions:

- Mobilize client as soon as possible. **Reduces risk or effects of atelectasis, enhancing lung expansion and drainage of different lung segments**

Information that appears in brackets has been added by the authors to clarify and enhance the use of nursing diagnoses.

- Encourage deep-breathing and coughing exercises or splint chest/incision **to maximize effort.**
- Administer analgesics **to improve cough when pain is inhibiting effort. (Caution: Overmedication can depress respirations and cough effort.**)
- Administer medications (e.g., expectorants, anti-inflammatory agents, bronchodilators, and mucolytic agents), as indicated, **to relax smooth respiratory musculature, reduce airway edema, and mobilize secretions.**
- Increase fluid intake to at least 2,000 mL/day within cardiac tolerance (may require IV in acutely ill, hospitalized client). Encourage/provide warm versus cold liquids as appropriate. Provide supplemental humidification, if needed (ultrasonic nebulizer, room humidifier). **Hydration can help prevent accumulation of viscous secretions and improve secretion clearance.** Monitor for signs/symptoms of congestive heart failure (crackles, edema, weight gain) when client is at risk.
- Perform or assist client in learning airway clearance techniques, such as postural drainage and percussion (CPT), flutter devices, high-frequency chest compression with an inflatable vest, intrapulmonary percussive ventilation administered by a percussinator, and active cycle breathing (ACB). **Various therapies/modalities may be required to acquire and maintain adequate airways and improve respiratory function and gas exchange.** (Refer to NDs ineffective Breathing Pattern; impaired Gas Exchange; impaired spontaneous Ventilation.)
- Support reduction/cessation of smoking **to improve lung function.**
- Position appropriately (e.g., head of bed elevated, side lying) and discourage use of oil-based products around nose **to prevent vomiting with aspiration into lungs.** (Refer to NDs risk for Aspiration; impaired Swallowing.)

Nursing Priority No. 3.

To assess changes, note complications:

- Auscultate breath sounds and assess air movement **to ascertain current status and note effects of treatment in clearing airways.**
- Monitor vital signs, noting changes in blood pressure and heart rate.

Information that appears in brackets has been added by the authors to clarify and enhance the use of nursing diagnoses.

- Observe for signs of respiratory distress (increased rate, restlessness/anxiety, use of accessory muscles for breathing).
- Evaluate changes in sleep pattern, noting insomnia or daytime somnolence, **which may be evidence of nighttime airway incompetence or sleep apnea.** (Refer to NDs Insomnia, Sleep Deprivation.)
- Document response to drug therapy and/or development of adverse side effects or interactions with antimicrobials, steroids, expectorants, and bronchodilators.
- Observe for signs/symptoms of infection (e.g., increased dyspnea with onset of fever or change in sputum color, amount, or character) **to identify the infectious process and promote timely intervention.**
- Obtain sputum specimen, preferably before antimicrobial therapy is initiated, **to verify appropriateness of therapy.**
- Monitor/document serial chest x-rays, ABGs, pulse oximetry readings.

Nursing Priority No. 4.

To promote wellness (Teaching/Discharge Considerations):

- Assess client's/SO's knowledge of contributing causes, treatment plan, specific medications, and therapeutic procedures **to determine educational and support needs.**
- Provide information about the necessity of raising and expectorating secretions versus swallowing them **to report changes in color and amount in the event that medical intervention may be needed to prevent or treat infection.**
- Demonstrate/assist client/SO in performing specific airway clearance techniques (e.g., forced expiratory breathing [also called huffing] or respiratory muscle strength training, chest percussion, or use of a vest), as indicated.
- Encourage/provide opportunities for rest; limit activities to level of respiratory tolerance. **Prevents/reduces fatigue.**
- Refer to appropriate support groups (e.g., stop smoking clinic, COPD exercise group, weight reduction, the American Lung Association, the Cystic Fibrosis Foundation, or the Muscular Dystrophy Association).
- Determine that client has equipment and is informed in use of nocturnal continuous positive airway pressure (CPAP) **for treatment of obstructive sleep apnea, when indicated.** (Refer to NDs Insomnia, Sleep Deprivation.)

Information that appears in brackets has been added by the authors to clarify and enhance the use of nursing diagnoses.

Documentation Focus

Assessment/Reassessment
* Related factors for individual clients.
* Breath sounds, presence and character of secretions, use of accessory muscles for breathing.
* Character of cough and sputum.
* Respiratory rate, pulse oximetry/O_2 saturation, vital signs.

Planning
* Plan of care and who is involved in planning.
* Teaching plan.

Implementation/Evaluation
* Client's response to interventions, teaching, and actions performed.
* Use of respiratory devices/airway adjuncts.
* Response to medications administered.
* Attainment or progress toward desired outcome(s).
* Modifications to plan of care.

Discharge Planning
* Long-term needs and who is responsible for actions to be taken.
* Specific referrals made.

Sample Nursing Outcomes & Interventions Classifications (NOC/NIC)

NOC—Respiratory Status: Airway Patency
NIC—Airway Management

risk for Allergy Response

Taxonomy II: Safety/Protection—Class 5 Defensive Processes
[Diagnostic Division: Safety]
Submitted 2010

Definition: Risk of an exaggerated immune response or reaction to substances

Information that appears in brackets has been added by the authors to clarify and enhance the use of nursing diagnoses.

🌐 Cultural   🔵 Collaborative   🏠 Community/Home Care

Risk Factors

Chemical products (e.g., bleach, cosmetics)
Environmental substances (e.g., mold, dust, pollen); dander; repeated exposure to environmental substances
Foods (e.g., peanuts, shellfish, mushrooms)
Insect stings
Pharmaceutical agents (e.g., penicillins)

> **NOTE:** A risk diagnosis is not evidenced by signs and symptoms, as the problem has not occurred; rather, nursing interventions are directed at prevention.

Desired Outcomes/Evaluation Criteria– Client Will:

* Be free of signs of hypersensitive response
* Verbalize understanding of individual risks and responsibilities in avoiding exposure
* Identify signs/symptoms requiring prompt response

Actions/Interventions

Nursing Priority No. 1.

To identify causative/precipitating factors related to risk:

* Question client regarding known allergies upon admission to healthcare facility. **Basic safety information will help healthcare providers prepare a safe environment for client while providing care.**
* Ascertain type of allergy and usual symptoms if client reports history of allergies (e.g., seasonal rhinitis ["hay fever"], allergic dermatitis, conjuctavitis, environmental asthma, environmental substances [e.g., mold, dust, pet dander], insect stings reactions, food intolerance, immunodeficiency such as Addison's Disease, drug or transfusion reaction). **Allergies can manifest as local reactions (as may occur in skin rashes) or be systemic. Client/caregiver may be aware of some, but not all, allergies.**
* Obtain a written list of drug allergies upon first contact with client. **Helps prevent adverse drug events while client is in facility care.**
* Discuss possibility of latex allergy when entering facility care, especially when procedures are anticipated (e.g., laboratory,

---

Information that appears in brackets has been added by the authors to clarify and enhance the use of nursing diagnoses.

emergency department, operating room, wound care management, one-day surgery, dental) **so that proper precautions can be taken by healthcare providers.** (Refer to ND Latex Allergy Response for related interventions.)

∞• Note client's age. **Although allergies can occur at any time in client's life span, there are some that can start early in life. These include food allergies (e.g., peanuts) and respiratory ailments (e.g., asthma).**

• Perform challenge or patch test, if appropriate, **to identify specific allergens in a client with known type IV hypersensitivity.**

Nursing Priority No. 2.

To take measures to avoid exposure and reduce/limit allergic response:

• Discuss client's current symptoms, noting reports of rash, hives, itching; teary eyes; localized swelling (e.g., of lips) or diarrhea; nausea; a feeling of faintness. Ascertain if client/care provider associates these symptoms with certain food, substances, or environmental factors. **May help isolate cause for a reaction.**

• Provide allergen-free environment (e.g., clean dust-free room or use air filters to reduce mold and pollens in air) **to reduce client exposure to allergens.**

• Collaborate with all healthcare providers to administer medications and perform procedures with client's allergies in mind.

• Encourage client to wear medical ID bracelet/necklace **to alert providers to condition if client is unresponsive or unable to relay information for any reason.**

• Refer to physician/allergy specialists as indicated **for interventions related to specific allergy conditions.**

Nursing Priority No. 3.

To promote wellness (Teaching/Discharge Criteria):

• Instruct/review with client and care provider(s) ways to prevent or limit client exposures.

• Instruct in signs of reaction and emergency treatment needs. **Allergic reactions range from skin irritation to anaphylaxis. Reaction may be gradual but progressive, affecting multiple body systems, or may be sudden, requiring life-saving treatment.**

Information that appears in brackets has been added by the authors to clarify and enhance the use of nursing diagnoses.

🌐 Cultural 🤝 Collaborative 🏠 Community/Home Care

- Emphasize the critical importance of taking immediate action for moderate to severe hypersensitivity reactions **to limit life-threatening symptoms**.
- Demonstrate equipment and injection procedure and recommend client carry auto-injectable epinephrine **to provide timely emergency treatment, as needed**.
- Emphasize necessity of informing all new care providers of allergies.
- Provide educational resources and assistance numbers for emergencies. **When allergy is suspected or the potential for allergy exists, protection must begin with identification and removal of possible sources.**

Documentation Focus

Assessment/Reassessment
- Individual risk factors identified.
- Client concerns or difficulty making and following through with plans.

Planning
- Plan of care and who is involved in planning.
- Teaching plan.

Implementation/Evaluation
- Response to interventions, teaching, and actions performed.
- Attainment or progress toward outcomes.

Discharge Planning
- Referrals to other resources.
- Long-term need and who is responsible for actions.

Sample Nursing Outcomes & Interventions Classifications (NOC/NIC)

NOC—Allergy Response: Systemic
NIC—Allergy Management

Information that appears in brackets has been added by the authors to clarify and enhance the use of nursing diagnoses.

Anxiety [specify level]

Taxonomy II: Coping/Stress Tolerance—Class 2 Coping
    Responses (00146)
[Diagnostic Division: Ego Integrity]
Submitted 1973; Revised 1982, 1998 (by small group
    work 1996)

Definition: Vague uneasy feeling of discomfort or dread
accompanied by an autonomic response (the source often nonspecific or unknown to the individual); a feeling
of apprehension caused by anticipation of danger. It is
an alerting signal that warns of impending danger and
enables the individual to take measures to deal with
threat.

Related Factors

Unconscious conflict about essential beliefs, goals, values of
    life
Situational/maturational crises
Stress
Familial association; heredity
Interpersonal transmission/contagion
Threat to self-concept
Threat of death [perceived or actual]
Threat to/change in health status, interaction patterns, role
    function/status, environment, and economic status
Unmet needs
Exposure to toxins; substance abuse

Defining Characteristics

Subjective

Behavioral
Reports concerns due to change in life events; insomnia

Affective
Regretful; rattled; distressed; apprehensive; fear; feelings of in-
    adequacy; uncertainty; jittery; worried; painful/persistent in-
    creased helplessness

Cognitive
Fear of unspecified consequences; awareness of physiological
    symptoms

Information that appears in brackets has been added by the authors to clarify
and enhance the use of nursing diagnoses.

Physiological
Shakiness

Sympathetic
Dry mouth; heart pounding; weakness; respiratory difficulties; anorexia, diarrhea

Parasympathetic
Tingling in extremities; nausea; abdominal pain; diarrhea; urinary frequency/hesitancy; faintness; fatigue; sleep disturbance

Objective

Behavioral
Poor eye contact; glancing about; scanning; vigilance; extraneous movement; fidgeting; restlessness; diminished productivity

Affective
Increased wariness; focus on self; irritability; overexcited; anguish

Cognitive
Preoccupation; impaired attention; difficulty concentrating; forgetfulness; diminished ability to learn or problem-solve; rumination; tendency to blame others; blocking of thought; confusion; decreased perceptual field

Physiological
Voice quivering, trembling/hand tremors; increased tension; facial tension; increased perspiration

Sympathetic
Cardiovascular excitation; facial flushing; superficial vasoconstriction; increased pulse, respiration, blood pressure; pupil dilation; twitching; increased reflexes

Parasympathetic
Urinary urgency; decreased blood pressure/pulse

Desired Outcomes/Evaluation Criteria— Client Will:

* Verbalize awareness of feelings of anxiety.
* Appear relaxed and report that anxiety is reduced to a manageable level.
* Identify healthy ways to deal with and express anxiety.

Information that appears in brackets has been added by the authors to clarify and enhance the use of nursing diagnoses.

- Demonstrate problem-solving skills.
- Use resources/support systems effectively.

Actions/Interventions

Nursing Priority No. 1.

To assess level of anxiety:

- Review familial and physiological factors (e.g., genetic depressive factors), psychiatric illness, active medical conditions (e.g., thyroid problems, metabolic imbalances, cardiopulmonary disease, anemia, or dysrhythmias), and recent/ongoing stressors (e.g., family member illness or death, spousal conflict/abuse, or loss of job). **These factors can cause/exacerbate anxiety and anxiety disorders.**
- Determine current prescribed medications and recent drug history of prescribed or over-the-counter (OTC) medications (e.g., steroids, thyroid preparations, weight loss pills, or caffeine). **These medications can heighten feelings and sense of anxiety.**
- Identify client's perception of the threat represented by the situation.
- Note cultural factors that may influence anxiety. **Individual responses are influenced by cultural values and beliefs and culturally learned patterns of their family of origin.**
- Monitor vital signs (e.g., rapid or irregular pulse, rapid breathing/hyperventilation, changes in blood pressure, diaphoresis, tremors, or restlessness) **to identify physical responses associated with both medical and emotional conditions.**
- Observe behaviors **that can point to the client's level of anxiety:**

Mild

Alert; more aware of environment; attention focused on environment and immediate events

Restless; irritable; wakeful; reports of insomnia

Motivated to deal with existing problems in this state

Moderate

Perception narrower; concentration increased; able to ignore distractions in dealing with problem(s)

Voice quivers or changes pitch

Trembling; increased pulse/respirations

Information that appears in brackets has been added by the authors to clarify and enhance the use of nursing diagnoses.

   🌐 Cultural   🔄 Collaborative   🏠 Community/Home Care

Severe

Range of perception is reduced; anxiety interferes with effective functioning

Preoccupied with feelings of discomfort; sense of impending doom

Increased pulse/respirations with reports of dizziness, tingling sensations, headaches, and so forth

Panic

Ability to concentrate is disrupted; behavior is disintegrated; client distorts the situation and does not have realistic perceptions of what is happening. Client may be experiencing terror or confusion or be unable to speak or move (paralyzed with fear).

- Note reports of insomnia or excessive sleeping, limited/ avoidance of interactions with others, and use of alcohol or other drugs that can be abused, **which may be behavioral indicators of use of withdrawal to deal with problems.**
- Review results of diagnostic tests (e.g., drug screens, cardiac testing, complete blood count, and chemistry panel), **which may point to physiological sources of anxiety.**
- Be aware of defense mechanisms being used (e.g., denial or regression) **that interfere with ability to deal with problem.**
- Identify coping skills the individual is currently using, such as anger, daydreaming, forgetfulness, overeating, smoking, or lack of problem-solving.
- Review coping skills used in past **to determine those that might be helpful in current circumstances.**

Nursing Priority No. 2.

To assist client with identifying feelings and beginning to deal with problems:

- Establish a therapeutic relationship, conveying empathy and unconditional positive regard. **Note:** Nurse needs to be aware of own feelings of anxiety or uneasiness, exercising care **to avoid the contagious effect or transmission of anxiety.**
- Be available to client for listening and talking.
- Encourage client to acknowledge and to express feelings, such as crying (sadness), laughing (fear or denial), or swearing (fear or anger).
- Assist client in developing self-awareness of verbal and nonverbal behaviors.
- Clarify meaning of feelings and actions by providing feedback and checking meaning with the client.

Information that appears in brackets has been added by the authors to clarify and enhance the use of nursing diagnoses.

- Acknowledge anxiety/fear. Do not deny or reassure client that everything will be all right.
- Provide accurate information about the situation. **Helps client identify what is reality based.**
- Be truthful, avoid bribing, and provide physical comfort (e.g., hugging or rocking) when dealing with a child **to soothe fears and provide assurance.**
- Provide comfort measures (e.g., calm/quiet environment, soft music, a warm bath, or a back rub).
- Modify procedures as much as possible (e.g., substitute oral for intramuscular medications or combine blood draws/use finger stick method) **to limit degree of stress and avoid overwhelming a child or anxious adult.**
- Manage environmental factors, such as harsh lighting and high traffic flow, which may be confusing and stressful to older individuals.
- Accept client as is. **The client may need to be where he or she is at this point in time, such as in denial after receiving the diagnosis of a terminal illness.**
- Allow the behavior to belong to the client; do not respond personally. **The nurse may respond inappropriately, escalating the situation to a nontherapeutic interaction.**
- Assist client to use anxiety for coping with the situation, if helpful. **Moderate anxiety heightens awareness and permits the client to focus on dealing with problems.**

Panic

- Stay with client, maintaining a calm, confident manner.
- Speak in brief statements using simple words.
- Provide for nonthreatening, consistent environment/atmosphere. Minimize stimuli. Monitor visitors and interactions **to lessen the effect of transmission of feelings.**
- Set limits on inappropriate behavior and help client to develop acceptable ways of dealing with anxiety.

> **NOTE:** Staff may need to provide safe controls and environment until client regains control.

- Gradually increase activities/involvement with others as anxiety is decreased.
- Use cognitive therapy **to focus on or correct faulty catastrophic interpretations of physical symptoms.**
- Administer medications (anti-anxiety agents/sedatives), as ordered.

Information that appears in brackets has been added by the authors to clarify and enhance the use of nursing diagnoses.

🌐 Cultural   🤝 Collaborative   🏠 Community/Home Care

Nursing Priority No. 3.

To promote wellness (Teaching/Discharge Considerations):

- Assist client in identifying precipitating factors and new methods of coping with disabling anxiety.
- Review happenings, thoughts, and feelings preceding the anxiety attack.
- Identify actions and activities the client has previously used to cope successfully when feeling nervous/anxious.
- List helpful resources and people, including available "hotline" or crisis managers **to provide ongoing/timely support.**
- Encourage client to develop an exercise/activity program, **which may serve to reduce level of anxiety by relieving tension.**
- Assist in developing skills (e.g., awareness of negative thoughts, saying "Stop," and substituting a positive thought) **to eliminate negative self-talk. Mild phobias tend to respond well to behavioral therapy.**
- Review strategies, such as role-playing, use of visualizations to practice anticipated events, and prayer/meditation. **Useful for being prepared for/dealing with anxiety-provoking situations.**
- Review medication regimen and possible interactions, especially with OTC drugs, other prescription drugs, and alcohol. Discuss appropriate drug substitutions, changes in dosage, or time of dose **to minimize side effects.**
- Refer to physician for drug management alteration of prescription regimen. **Drugs that often cause symptoms of anxiety include aminophylline/theophylline, anticholinergics, dopamine, levodopa, salicylates, and steroids.**
- Refer to individual and/or group therapy, as appropriate, **to deal with chronic anxiety states.**

Documentation Focus

Assessment/Reassessment
- Level of anxiety and precipitating/aggravating factors.
- Description of feelings (expressed and displayed).
- Awareness and ability to recognize and express feelings.
- Related substance use, if present.

Planning
- Treatment plan and individual responsibility for specific activities.
- Teaching plan.

Information that appears in brackets has been added by the authors to clarify and enhance the use of nursing diagnoses.

Implementation/Evaluation
- Client involvement and response to interventions, teaching, and actions performed.
- Attainment or progress toward desired outcome(s).
- Modifications to plan of care.

Discharge Planning
- Referrals and follow-up plan.
- Specific referrals made.

Sample Nursing Outcomes & Interventions Classifications (NOC/NIC)

NOC—Anxiety Level
NIC—Anxiety Reduction

risk for **Aspiration**

Taxonomy II: Safety/Protection—Class 2 Physical Injury (00039)
[Diagnostic Division: Respiration]
Submitted 1988

Definition: At risk for entry of gastrointestinal secretions, oropharyngeal secretions, or (exogenous food) solids or fluids into the tracheobronchial passages

Risk Factors

Reduced level of consciousness [sedation/anesthesia]

Depressed cough/gag reflexes

Impaired swallowing [inability of the epiglottis and true vocal cords to move to close off trachea]

Facial/oral/neck surgery or trauma; wired jaws; [congenital malformations]

Situation hindering elevation of upper body

Incompetent lower esophageal sphincter; delayed gastric emptying; decreased gastrointestinal motility; increased intragastric pressure; increased gastric residual

Presence of tracheostomy or endotracheal [ET] tube

Presence of gastrointestinal tubes; tube feedings

Treatment-related side effects (e.g., pharmaceutical agents)

Information that appears in brackets has been added by the authors to clarify and enhance the use of nursing diagnoses.

> **NOTE:** A risk diagnosis is not evidenced by signs and symptoms, as the problem has not occurred; rather, nursing interventions are directed at prevention.

Desired Outcomes/Evaluation Criteria— Client Will:

- Experience no aspiration as evidenced by noiseless respirations; clear breath sounds; clear, odorless secretions.
- Identify causative/risk factors.
- Demonstrate techniques to prevent and/or correct aspiration.

Actions/Interventions

Nursing Priority No. 1.

To assess causative/contributing factors:

- Identify at-risk clients according to condition or disease process, as listed in Risk Factors, **to determine when observation and/or interventions may be required.**
- ∞ Assess for age-related risk factors potentiating risk of aspiration (e.g., premature infant, elderly infirm). **Aspiration pneumonia is more common in extremely young or old patients and commonly occurs in individuals with chronically impaired airway defense mechanisms.**
- Note client's level of consciousness, awareness of surroundings, and cognitive function, **as impairments in these areas increase client's risk of aspiration owing to the inability to cough or swallow well and/or the presence of an artificial airway, mechanical ventilation, and/or tube feedings.**
- Determine the presence of neuromuscular disorders, noting muscle groups involved, degree of impairment, and whether they are of an acute or progressive nature (e.g., stroke, Parkinson's disease, progressive supranuclear palsy and similar disabling brain diseases; Guillain-Barré syndrome, or amyotrophic lateral sclerosis).
- Assess client's ability to swallow and presence and strength of gag/cough reflex. Evaluate amount/consistency of secretions. **Helps to determine effectiveness of protective mechanisms.**
- Observe for neck and facial edema. **Client with a head/neck surgery or a tracheal/bronchial injury (e.g., upper torso burns or inhalation/chemical injury) is at particular risk**

Information that appears in brackets has been added by the authors to clarify and enhance the use of nursing diagnoses.

for airway obstruction and an inability to handle secretions.

- Note administration of enteral feedings **because of potential for regurgitation and/or displacement of tube with aspiration of gastric contents.**
- Ascertain lifestyle habits; for example, use of alcohol, tobacco, and other central nervous system suppressant drugs, **which can affect awareness and impair gag/swallow mechanisms.**
- Assist with/review diagnostic studies (e.g., videofluoroscopy or fiberoptic endoscopy), **which may be done to assess for presence/degree of impairment.**

Nursing Priority No. 2.

To assist in correcting factors that can lead to aspiration:

- Monitor use of oxygen masks in clients at risk for vomiting. Refrain from using oxygen masks for comatose individuals.
- Keep wire cutters/scissors with client at all times when jaws are wired/banded **to facilitate clearing the airway in emergency situations.**
- Maintain operational suction equipment at bedside/chairside.
- Suction (oral cavity, nose, and ET/tracheostomy tube), as needed, and avoid triggering gag mechanism when performing suction or mouth care **to clear secretions while reducing potential for aspiration of secretions.**
- Avoid keeping client supine/flat when on mechanical ventilation (especially when also receiving enteral feedings). **Supine positioning and enteral feedings have been shown to be independent risk factors for the development of aspiration pneumonia.**
- Perform scrupulous oral care **to prevent accumulation of thickened secretions in the oral pharynx and to remove secretions that may interfere with the movement of air.**
- Auscultate lung sounds frequently, especially in a client who is coughing frequently or not coughing at all, or in a client on a ventilator being tube-fed, **to determine decreased breath sounds, rales, or dullness to percussion that could indicate presence of aspirated food or secretions, as well as "silent aspiration."**
- Elevate client to highest or best possible position (e.g., sitting upright in chair) for eating and drinking and during tube feedings. **Adults and children should be upright for meals or placed on their right side to decrease the likelihood of**

Information that appears in brackets has been added by the authors to clarify and enhance the use of nursing diagnoses.

drainage into trachea and to reduce reflux and improve gastric emptying.

🏠• Provide a rest period prior to feeding time. **The rested client may have less difficulty with swallowing.**

• Feed slowly, using small bites, instructing client to chew slowly and thoroughly.

🏠• Vary placement of food in client's mouth according to type of deficit (e.g., place food in right side of mouth if facial weakness is present on left side).

🏠• Provide soft foods that stick together/form a bolus (e.g., casseroles, puddings, or stews) **to aid swallowing effort.**

🏠• Determine liquid viscosity best tolerated by client. Add thickening agent to liquids, as appropriate. **Some individuals may swallow thickened liquids better than thin liquids.**

🏠• Offer very warm or very cold liquids. **Activates temperature receptors in the mouth that help to stimulate swallowing.**

🏠• Avoid washing solids down with liquids.

🔏• Ascertain that the feeding tube (when used) is in the correct position. **Placement may be done under fluoroscopy and/or measurement of aspirate pH following placement of feeding tube may be indicated.** Ask client about feeling of fullness and/or measure residuals (just prior to feeding and several hours after feeding), when appropriate, **to reduce risk of aspiration.**

∞• Determine best resting position for infant/child (e.g., with the head of bed elevated 30 degrees and infant propped on right side after feeding). **Upper airway patency is facilitated by an upright position and turning to right side decreases likelihood of drainage into trachea.**

💊• Provide oral medications in elixir form or crush, if appropriate.

💊• Minimize use of sedatives/hypnotics whenever possible. **These agents can impair coughing and swallowing.**

🔏• Refer to physician and/or speech/language therapist for medical or surgical interventions and/or exercises **to strengthen muscles and learn specific techniques to enhance swallowing/reduce potential aspiration.**

Nursing Priority No. 3.
To promote wellness (Teaching/Discharge Considerations):

🏠• Review with client/SO individual risk or potentiating factors.

🏠• Provide information about the signs and effects of aspiration on the lungs. **Note: Severe coughing and cyanosis**

Information that appears in brackets has been added by the authors to clarify and enhance the use of nursing diagnoses.

associated with eating or drinking or changes in vocal quality after swallowing indicate onset of respiratory symptoms associated with aspiration and require immediate intervention.

🏠 • Instruct in safety concerns regarding oral or tube feeding. (Refer to ND impaired Swallowing.)

🏠 • Train client how to self-suction or train family members in suction techniques (especially if client has constant or copious oral secretions) **to enhance safety/self-sufficiency.**

🏠 • Instruct individual/family member to avoid or limit activities after eating that increase intra-abdominal pressure (straining, strenuous exercise, or tight/constrictive clothing), **which may slow digestion/increase risk of regurgitation.**

Documentation Focus

Assessment/Reassessment
- Assessment findings, conditions that could lead to problems of aspiration.
- Verification of tube placement, observations of physical findings.

Planning
- Interventions to prevent aspiration or reduce risk factors and who is involved in the planning.
- Teaching plan.

Implementation/Evaluation
- Client's responses to interventions, teaching, and actions performed.
- Foods/fluids client handles with ease or difficulty.
- Amount and frequency of intake.
- Attainment or progress toward desired outcome(s).
- Modifications to plan of care.

Discharge Planning
- Long-term needs and who is responsible for actions to be taken.

Sample Nursing Outcomes & Interventions Classifications (NOC/NIC)

NOC—Aspiration Prevention
NIC—Aspiration Precautions

Information that appears in brackets has been added by the authors to clarify and enhance the use of nursing diagnoses.

risk for impaired Attachment

Taxonomy II: Role Relationships—Class 2 Family Relationships (00058)
[Diagnostic Division: Social Interaction]
Submitted as Risk for Impaired Parent/Infant/Child Attachment 1994

Definition: At risk for disruption of the interactive process between parent/significant other and child that fosters the development of a protective and nurturing reciprocal relationship

Risk Factors

Inability of parents to meet personal needs
Anxiety associated with the parent role [parents who themselves experienced altered attachment]
Premature infant or ill child who is unable to effectively initiate parental contact; disorganized infant behavior
Parental conflict resulting from altered behavioral organization
Parent-child separation; physical barriers; lack of privacy
Substance abuse
Difficult pregnancy and/or birth
Uncertainty of paternity; conception as a result of rape/sexual abuse

> **NOTE:** A risk diagnosis is not evidenced by signs and symptoms, as the problem has not occurred; rather, nursing interventions are directed at prevention.

Desired Outcomes/Evaluation Criteria— Parent Will:

* Identify and prioritize family strengths and needs.
* Exhibit nurturing and protective behaviors toward child.
* Identify and use resources to meet needs of family members.
* Demonstrate techniques to enhance behavioral organization of the infant/child.
* Engage in mutually satisfying interactions with child.

Information that appears in brackets has been added by the authors to clarify and enhance the use of nursing diagnoses.

Actions/Interventions

Nursing Priority No. 1.
To identify causative/contributing factors:

- Interview parents, noting their perception of situation and individual concerns.
- Assess parent/child interactions.
- Ascertain availability and use of resources to include extended family, support groups, and financial resources.
- Evaluate parents' ability to provide protective environment and participate in a reciprocal relationship.

Nursing Priority No. 2.
To enhance behavioral organization of child:

- ∞ Identify infant's strengths and vulnerabilities. **Each child is born with his or her own temperament that affects interactions with caregivers.**
- ∞ Educate parents regarding child growth and development, addressing parental perceptions. **Helps clarify realistic or unrealistic expectations.**
- ∞ Assist parents in modifying the environment **to provide appropriate stimulation.**
- Model care-giving techniques that best support behavioral organization.
- ∞ Respond consistently with nurturing to infant/child.

Nursing Priority No. 3.
To enhance best functioning of parents:

- Develop therapeutic nurse-client relationship. Provide a consistently warm, nurturing, and nonjudgmental environment.
- Assist parents in identifying and prioritizing family strengths and needs. **Promotes positive attitude by looking at what they already do well and using those skills to address needs.**
- Support and guide parents in the process of assessing resources.
- ∞ Involve parents in activities with the child that they can accomplish successfully. **Promotes sense of confidence, thus enhancing self-concept.**
- Recognize and provide positive feedback for nurturing and protective parenting behaviors. **Reinforces continuation of desired behaviors.**

Information that appears in brackets has been added by the authors to clarify and enhance the use of nursing diagnoses.

- Minimize number of professionals on team with whom parents must have contact **to foster trust in relationships.**

Nursing Priority No. 4.

To support parent/child attachment during separation:
- Provide parents with telephone contact, as appropriate.
- Establish a routine time for daily phone calls/initiate calls, as indicated. **Provides sense of consistency and control and allows for planning of other activities.**
- Invite parents to use Ronald McDonald House or provide them with a listing of a variety of local accommodations and restaurants when child is hospitalized out of town.
- Arrange for parents to receive photos and progress reports from the child.
- Suggest parents provide a photo and/or audiotape of themselves for the child.
- Consider use of contract with parents **to clearly communicate expectations of both family and staff.**
- Suggest parents keep a journal of infant/child progress.
- Provide "homelike" environment for situations requiring supervision of visits.

Nursing Priority No. 5.

To promote wellness (Teaching/Discharge Considerations):
- Refer to individual counseling, family therapies, or addiction counseling/treatment, as indicated.
- Identify services for transportation, financial resources, housing, and so forth.
- Develop support systems appropriate to situation (e.g., extended family, friends, or social worker).
- Explore community resources (e.g., church affiliations, volunteer groups, or day/respite care).

Documentation Focus

Assessment/Reassessment
- Identified behaviors of both parents and child.
- Specific risk factors, individual perceptions and concerns.
- Interactions between parent and child.

Planning
- Plan of care and who is involved in planning.
- Teaching plan.

Information that appears in brackets has been added by the authors to clarify and enhance the use of nursing diagnoses.

Implementation/Evaluation
- Parents'/child's responses to interventions, teaching, and actions performed.
- Attainment or progress toward desired outcomes.
- Modifications to plan of care.

Discharge Planning
- Long-term needs and who is responsible.
- Plan for home visits to support parents and to ensure infant/child safety and well-being.
- Specific referrals made.

Sample Nursing Outcomes & Interventions Classifications (NOC/NIC)

NOC—Parent-Infant Attachment
NIC—Attachment Promotion

Autonomic Dysreflexia

Taxonomy II: Coping/Stress Tolerance—Class 3 Neuro-behavioral Stress (00009)
[Diagnostic Division: Circulation]
Submitted 1988

Definition: Life-threatening, uninhibited sympathetic response of the nervous system to a noxious stimulus after a spinal cord injury at T7 or above

Related Factors

Bladder/bowel distention; [catheter insertion/obstruction; irrigation; constipation]
Skin irritation
Deficient patient/caregiver knowledge
[Sexual excitation; menstruation; pregnancy; labor and delivery]
[Environmental temperature extremes]

Defining Characteristics

Subjective
Headache (a diffuse pain in different portions of the head and not confined to any nerve distribution area)

Information that appears in brackets has been added by the authors to clarify and enhance the use of nursing diagnoses.

Paresthesia; chilling; blurred vision; chest pain; metallic taste in mouth; nasal congestion

Objective

Paroxysmal hypertension (sudden periodic elevated blood pressure in which systolic pressure is greater than 140 mm Hg and diastolic pressure is greater than 90 mm Hg)

Bradycardia or tachycardia

Diaphoresis (above the injury), red splotches on skin (above the injury), or pallor (below the injury)

Horner's syndrome (contraction of the pupil, partial ptosis of the eyelid, enophthalmos, and sometimes loss of sweating over the affected side of the face); conjunctival congestion

Pilomotor reflex (goosebump formation when skin is cooled)

Desired Outcomes/Evaluation Criteria— Client/Caregiver Will:

- Identify precipitating factors.
- Recognize signs/symptoms of syndrome.
- Demonstrate corrective techniques.
- Experience no episodes of dysreflexia or will seek medical intervention in a timely manner.

Actions/Interventions

Nursing Priority No. 1.

To assess for precipitating factors:

- Note timing and specifics of injury. **Autonomic dysreflexia (AD) does not occur in the acute phase of spinal cord injury. However, some studies have identified factors that may point toward a client's likelihood of developing AD, perhaps early in recovery. These include higher levels of injury (e.g., cervical versus thoracic involvement) and more complete lesions.**
- Monitor for bladder distention, presence of bladder spasms, stones, or infection. **The most common stimulus for AD is bladder irritation or overstretch associated with urinary retention or infection, blocked catheter, overfilled collection bag, or noncompliance with intermittent catheterization.**
- Assess for bowel distention, fecal impaction, or problems with bowel management program. **Bowel irritation or overstretch is associated with constipation or impaction;**

Information that appears in brackets has been added by the authors to clarify and enhance the use of nursing diagnoses.

digital stimulation, suppository, or enema use during bowel program; hemorrhoids or fissures; and/or infection of gastrointestinal tract, such as might occur with ulcers or appendicitis.

• Observe skin and tissue pressure areas, especially following prolonged sitting. **Skin and tissue irritants include direct pressure (e.g., object in chair or shoe, leg straps, abdominal support, orthotics), wounds (e.g., bruise, abrasion, laceration, pressure ulcer), ingrown toenails, tight clothing, sunburn, or other burn.**

• Inquire about sexual activity and/or determine if reproductive issues are involved. **Overstimulation, vibration, sexual intercourse, ejaculation, scrotal compression, menstrual cramps, and/or pregnancy (especially labor and delivery) are known precipitants.**

∞• Note onset of crying, irritability, or somnolence in an infant or child **who may present with nonspecific symptoms; they may not be able to verbalize discomforts**.

• Inform client/care providers of additional precipitators during course of care. **Client is prone to numerous physical conditions or treatments (e.g., intolerance to temperature extremes; deep vein thrombosis; kidney stones; fractures/other trauma; or surgical, dental, and diagnostic procedures), any of which can precipitate AD.**

Nursing Priority No. 2.

To provide for early detection and immediate intervention:

• Investigate associated complaints/symptoms (e.g., sudden severe headache, chest pains, blurred vision, facial flushing, nausea, or a metallic taste). **AD is a potentially life-threatening condition that requires immediate intervention.**

• Eliminate causative stimulus immediately when possible, moving in a step-wise fashion (e.g., perform immediate catheterization or restore urine flow if blocked, remove bowel impaction or stop digital stimulation, reduce skin pressure by changing position or removing restrictive clothing, and protect from temperature extremes).

• Elevate head of bed as high as tolerated or place client in sitting position with legs dangling **to lower blood pressure.**

• Monitor vital signs frequently during an acute episode, **as blood pressure can fluctuate quickly due to impaired**

Information that appears in brackets has been added by the authors to clarify and enhance the use of nursing diagnoses.

🌐 Cultural   🅒 Collaborative   🏠 Community/Home Care

autonomic regulation. Continue to monitor blood pressure at intervals after symptoms subside **to evaluate effectiveness of interventions.**

- Administer medications as required **to block excessive autonomic nerve transmission, normalize heart rate, and reduce hypertension.**

- Know contraindications and cautions associated with antihypertensive medications; adjust dosage of antihypertensive medications carefully for children, the elderly, individuals with known heart disease, male client using sildenafil for sexual activity, or pregnant women. **Prevents complications such as untoward side effects, while maintaining blood pressure within desired range.**

Nursing Priority No. 3.

To promote wellness (Teaching/Discharge Considerations):

- Discuss warning signs and how to avoid onset of syndrome with client/SO(s). **Knowledge can support adherence to preventive measures and promote prompt intervention when required.**

- Instruct client/caregivers in preventive care (e.g., safe and timely bowel and bladder care; prevention of skin breakdown; care of existing skin breaks; prevention of infection).

- Instruct family member/caregiver in blood pressure monitoring, and client's usual blood pressure range; discuss plan for monitoring, reporting, and treatment of high blood pressure during acute episodes.

- Review proper use/administration of medication if indicated. **Client may have medication(s) both for emergent situations and/or prevention of AD.**

- Assist client/family in identifying emergency referrals (e.g., physician, rehabilitation nurse, home care supervisor). Place phone number(s) in a prominent place or program into client's/caregiver's cell phone.

- Recommend wearing medical alert bracelet/necklace and carrying information card reviewing client's typical signs/symptoms and usual methods of treatment. **Provides vital information to care providers in emergent situation.**

- Refer for advice or treatment of sexual and reproductive concerns as indicated.

- Refer to ND risk for Autonomic Dysreflexia.

Information that appears in brackets has been added by the authors to clarify and enhance the use of nursing diagnoses.

Documentation Focus

Assessment/Reassessment
- Individual findings, noting previous episodes, precipitating factors, and individual signs/symptoms.

Planning
- Plan of care and who is involved in planning.
- Teaching plan.

Implementation/Evaluation
- Client's responses to interventions and actions performed, understanding of teaching.
- Attainment or progress toward desired outcome(s).
- Modifications to plan of care.

Discharge Planning
- Long-term needs and who is responsible for actions to be taken.

Sample Nursing Outcomes & Interventions Classifications (NOC/NIC)

NOC—Neurological Status: Autonomic
NIC—Dysreflexia Management

risk for Autonomic Dysreflexia

Taxonomy II: Coping/Stress Tolerance—Class 3 Neuro-behavioral Stress (00010)
[Diagnostic Division: Circulation]
Nursing Diagnosis Extension and Classification Submission 1998; Revised 2000

Definition: At risk for life-threatening, uninhibited response of the sympathetic nervous system postspinal shock, in an individual with a spinal cord injury [SCI] or lesion at T6 or above (it has been demonstrated in patients with injuries at T7 and T8)

Risk Factors

An injury at T6 or above or a lesion at T6 or above and at least one of the following noxious stimuli:

Information that appears in brackets has been added by the authors to clarify and enhance the use of nursing diagnoses.

Musculoskeletal—Integumentary Stimuli

Cutaneous stimulations (e.g., pressure ulcer, ingrown toenail, dressing, burns, or rash); sunburn; wounds

Pressure over bony prominences/genitalia; range-of-motion exercises; spasms

Fractures; heterotrophic bone

Gastrointestinal Stimuli

Constipation; difficult passage of feces; fecal impaction; bowel distention; hemorrhoids

Digital stimulation; suppositories; enemas

Gastrointestinal system pathology; esophageal reflux; gastric ulcers; gallstones

Urological Stimuli

Bladder distention, spasm

Detrusor sphincter dyssynergia

Catheterization; instrumentation; surgery; calculi

Urinary tract infection; cystitis; urethritis; epididymitis

Regulatory Stimuli

Temperature fluctuations; extreme environmental temperatures

Situational Stimuli

Positioning; surgical procedure; [diagnostic procedures]

Constrictive clothing (e.g., straps, stockings, or shoes)

Reactions to pharmaceutical agents (e.g., decongestants, sympathomimetics, vasoconstrictors); narcotic/opiate withdrawal

Surgical or diagnostic procedures

Neurological Stimuli

Painful or irritating stimuli below the level of injury

Cardiac/Pulmonary Stimuli

Pulmonary emboli; deep vein thrombosis

Reproductive [and Sexuality] Stimuli

Sexual intercourse; ejaculation; [vibrator overstimulation]

Menstruation; pregnancy; labor and delivery; ovarian cyst

> **NOTE:** A risk diagnosis is not evidenced by signs and symptoms as the problem has not occurred; rather, nursing interventions are directed at prevention.

Information that appears in brackets has been added by the authors to clarify and enhance the use of nursing diagnoses.

Desired Outcomes/Evaluation Criteria—Client Will:

- Identify risk factors present.
- Demonstrate preventive or corrective techniques.
- Free of episodes of dysreflexia.

Actions/Interventions

Nursing Priority No. 1.

To assess risk factors present:

- Monitor for potential precipitating factors, including urological (e.g., bladder distention, acute urinary tract infection, or kidney stones), gastrointestinal (e.g., bowel overdistention, hemorrhoids, or digital stimulation), cutaneous (e.g., pressure ulcers, extreme external temperatures, or dressing changes), reproductive (e.g., sexual activity, menstruation, or pregnancy/delivery), and miscellaneous (e.g., pulmonary emboli, drug reaction, or deep vein thrombosis). (Refer to ND Autonomic Dysreflexia for a more complete listing of precipitating factors if indicated.)

Nursing Priority No. 2.

To prevent occurrence:

- Monitor vital signs routinely, noting elevation in blood pressure, heart rate, and temperature, especially during times of physical stress, **to identify trends and intervene in a timely manner. Note:** The baseline blood pressure in clients with spinal cord injuries (adults and children) is lower than the general population; therefore, an elevation of 20 to 40 mm Hg above baseline may be indicative of autonomic dysreflexia (AD).
- Instruct in appropriate interventions (e.g., regularly timed catheter and bowel care, appropriate padding for skin and tissues, proper positioning with frequent pressure-relief actions, checking frequently for tight clothes/leg straps, routine foot/toenail care, temperature control, sunburn/other burn prevention, compliance with preventive medications when used) **to prevent occurrence/limit severity.**
- Instruct all caregivers in safe bowel and bladder care and immediate and long-term care for the prevention of skin stress/breakdown. **These problems are associated most frequently with AD.**

Information that appears in brackets has been added by the authors to clarify and enhance the use of nursing diagnoses.

🔧• Administer antihypertensive medications when at-risk client is placed on a routine "maintenance dose," **as might occur when noxious stimuli cannot be removed (presence of chronic sacral pressure sore, fracture, or acute postoperative pain).**

• Refer to ND Autonomic Dysreflexia.

Nursing Priority No. 3.
To promote wellness (Teaching/Discharge Considerations):

🏠• Discuss warning signs of AD with client/caregiver (i.e., sudden, severe pounding headache; flushed red face; increased blood pressure/acute hypertension; nasal congestion; anxiety; blurred vision; metallic taste in mouth; sweating and/or flushing above the level of SCI; goosebumps; bradycardia; cardiac irregularities). **AD can develop rapidly (in minutes), requiring quick intervention.**

∞• Be aware of client's communication abilities. **AD can occur at any age, from infants to the elderly, and the individual may not be able to verbalize a pounding headache, which is often the first symptom during onset of AD.**

🏠• Ascertain that client/caregiver understands ways to avoid onset of syndrome. Provide an information card and instruct and periodically reinforce teaching, as needed, regarding the following:

Keeping indwelling catheter free of kinks, keeping bag empty and situated below bladder level, and checking daily for deposits (bladder grit) inside catheter
Catheterizing as often as necessary **to prevent overfilling**
Monitoring voiding patterns for adequate frequency and amount
Performing a regular bowel evacuation program
Performing routine skin assessments
Monitoring all systems for signs/symptoms of infection and reporting promptly.

🔧• Review proper use and administration of medication if preventive medications are anticipated.

• Emphasize importance of regularly scheduled medical evaluations **to monitor status and to identify developing problems.**

🏠• Recommend wearing a medical alert bracelet or necklace with information card about signs/symptoms of AD and usual

---

Information that appears in brackets has been added by the authors to clarify and enhance the use of nursing diagnoses.

methods of treatment. **Provides vital information in emergencies.**

@• Assist client/family in identifying emergency referrals (e.g., healthcare provider's contact number in a prominent place or program it into client's/caregiver's cell phone).

Documentation Focus

Assessment/Reassessment
• Individual risk factors.
• Previous episodes, precipitating factors, and individual signs/symptoms.

Planning
• Plan of care and who is involved in planning.
• Teaching plan.

Implementation/Evaluation
• Client's responses to interventions and actions performed; understanding of teaching.
• Attainment or progress toward desired outcome(s).
• Modifications to plan of care.

Discharge Planning
• Long-term needs and who is responsible for actions to be taken.

Sample Nursing Outcomes & Interventions Classifications (NOC/NIC)

NOC—Risk Control
NIC—Dysreflexia Management

---

disorganized infant Behavior

Taxonomy II: Coping/Stress Tolerance—Class 3 Neurobehavioral Stress (00116)
[Diagnostic Division: Neurosensory]
Submitted 1994; Nursing Diagnosis Extension and Classification Revision 1998

Definition: Disintegrated physiological and neurobehavioral responses of an infant to the environment

---

Information that appears in brackets has been added by the authors to clarify and enhance the use of nursing diagnoses.

🌐 Cultural @ Collaborative 🏠 Community/Home Care

Related Factors

Prenatal
Congenital or genetic disorders; teratogenic exposure

Postnatal
Oral or motor problems; feeding intolerance; malnutrition
Invasive procedures; pain

Individual
Low postconceptual age; prematurity; immature neurological system
Illness; [hypoxia, birth asphyxia]

Environmental
Physical environment inappropriateness
Sensory inappropriateness; overstimulation; deprivation
Lack of containment within environment

Caregiver
Cue misreading; deficient knowledge regarding behavioral cues
Environmental stimulation contribution

Defining Characteristics

Objective

Regulatory Problems
Inability to inhibit startle irritability

State-Organization System
Active-awake (fussy, worried gaze); quiet awake (staring, gaze aversion)
Diffuse sleep; state-oscillation
Irritable crying

Attention-Interaction System
Abnormal response to sensory stimuli (e.g., difficult to soothe, unable to sustain alert status)

Motor System
Finger splaying, fisting; hands to face; hyperextension of extremities
Tremors, startles, twitches; jittery; uncoordinated movement
Changes to motor tone; altered primitive reflexes

Information that appears in brackets has been added by the authors to clarify and enhance the use of nursing diagnoses.

Physiological
Bradycardia; tachycardia; arrhythmias
Skin color changes; desaturation
"Time-out signals" (e.g., gaze, grasp, hiccough, cough, sneeze, sigh, slack jaw, open mouth, tongue thrust)
Feeding intolerances

Desired Outcomes/Evaluation Criteria— Infant Will:

• Exhibit organized behaviors that allow the achievement of optimal potential for growth and development as evidenced by modulation of physiological, motor, state, and attentional-interactive functioning.

Parent/Caregiver Will:

• Recognize individual infant cues.
• Identify appropriate responses (including environmental modifications) to infant's cues.
• Verbalize readiness to assume caregiving independently.

Actions/Interventions

Nursing Priority No. 1.
To assess causative/contributing factors:
• Determine infant's chronological and developmental age; note length of gestation.
• Observe for cues suggesting presence of situations that may result in pain/discomfort.
• Determine adequacy of physiological support.
• Evaluate level and appropriateness of environmental stimuli.
• Ascertain parents' understanding of infant's needs and abilities.
• Listen to parents' concerns about their capabilities to meet infant's needs.

Nursing Priority No. 2.
To assist parents in providing coregulation to the infant:
• Provide a calm, nurturing physical and emotional environment.
• Encourage parents to hold infant, including skin-to-skin contact, using kangaroo care (KC) as appropriate. **Research suggests KC may have a positive effect on infant development**

Information that appears in brackets has been added by the authors to clarify and enhance the use of nursing diagnoses.

🌐 Cultural 🤝 Collaborative 🏠 Community/Home Care

by enhancing neurophysiological organization as well as an indirect effect by improving parental mood, perceptions, and interactive behavior.

- Model gentle handling of baby and appropriate responses to infant behavior. **Provides cues to parent.**
- Support and encourage parents to be with infant and participate actively in all aspects of care. **Situation may be overwhelming, and support may enhance coping and strengthen attachment.**
- Encourage parents refrain from social interaction during feedings as appropriate. **Infant may have difficulty/lack necessary energy to manage feeding and social stimulation simultaneously.**
- Provide positive feedback for progressive parental involvement in caregiving process. **Transfer of care from staff to parents progresses along a continuum as parents' confidence level increases and they are able to take on more complex care activities.**
- Discuss infant growth and development, pointing out current status and progressive expectations, as appropriate. **Augments parents' knowledge of coregulation.**
- Incorporate the parents' observations and suggestions into plan of care. **Demonstrates valuing of parents' input and encourages continued involvement.**

Nursing Priority No. 3.

To deliver care within the infant's stress threshold:

- Provide a consistent caregiver. **Facilitates recognition of infant cues or changes in behavior.**
- Identify infant's individual self-regulatory behaviors (e.g., sucking, mouthing, grasp, hand-to-mouth, face behaviors, foot clasp, brace, limb flexion, trunk tuck, boundary seeking).
- Support hands to mouth and face; offer pacifier or nonnutritive sucking at the breast with gavage feedings. **Provides opportunities for infant to suck.**
- Avoid aversive oral stimulation, such as routine oral suctioning; suction ET tube only when clinically indicated.
- Use Oxyhood large enough to cover the infant's chest so arms will be inside the hood. **Allows for hand-to-mouth activities during this therapy.**
- Provide opportunities for infant to grasp.
- Provide boundaries and/or containment during all activities. Use swaddling, nesting, bunting, and caregiver's hands as indicated.

Information that appears in brackets has been added by the authors to clarify and enhance the use of nursing diagnoses.

- Allow adequate time and opportunities to hold infant. Handle infant very gently, move infant smoothly, slowly, and contained, avoiding sudden or abrupt movements.
- Maintain normal alignment, position infant with limbs softly flexed and with shoulders and hips adducted slightly. Use appropriate-sized diapers.
- Evaluate chest for adequate expansion, placing rolls under trunk if prone position is indicated.
- Avoid restraints, including at IV sites. If IV board is necessary, secure to limb positioned in normal alignment.
- Provide a sheepskin, egg-crate mattress, water bed, and/or gel pillow or mattress for infant who does not tolerate frequent position changes. **Minimizes tissue pressure, lessens risk of tissue injury.**
- Visually assess color, respirations, activity, and invasive lines without disturbing infant. Assess with "hands on" every 4 hours as indicated and prn. **Allows for undisturbed rest and quiet periods.**
- Schedule care activities to allow time for rest and organization of sleep and wake states to maximize tolerance of infant. Defer routine care when infant is in quiet sleep.
- Provide care with baby in side-lying position. Begin by talking softly to the baby, then place hands in a containing hold on the baby, **which allows baby to prepare.** Proceed with least-invasive manipulations first.
- Respond promptly to infant's agitation or restlessness. Provide a "time out" when infant shows early cues of overstimulation. Comfort and support the infant after stressful interventions.
- Remain at infant's bedside for several minutes after procedures and caregiving **to monitor infant's response and provide necessary support.**
- Administer analgesics as individually appropriate.

Nursing Priority No. 4.

To modify the environment to provide appropriate stimulation:

- Introduce stimulation as a single mode and assess individual tolerance.

Light/Vision

- Reduce lighting perceived by infant; introduce diurnal lighting (and activity) when infant achieves physiological stability.

Information that appears in brackets has been added by the authors to clarify and enhance the use of nursing diagnoses.

🌐 Cultural   🅒 Collaborative   🏠 Community/Home Care

(Daylight levels of 20 to 30 candles and night light levels of less than 10 candles are suggested.) Change light levels gradually **to allow infant time to adjust.**

- Protect the infant's eyes from bright illumination during examinations and procedures, as well as from indirect sources, such as neighboring phototherapy treatments, **to prevent retinal damage.**
- Deliver phototherapy (when required) with biliblanket devices if available **(alleviates need for eye patches).**
- Provide caregiver face (preferably parent's) as visual stimulus when infant shows readiness (awake, attentive).
- Evaluate/readjust placement of pictures, stuffed animals, etc., within the infant's immediate environment. **Promotes state maintenance and smooth transition by allowing infant to look away easily when visual stimuli become stressful.**

Sound
- Identify sources of noise in environment and eliminate/reduce them (e.g., speak in a low voice; reduce volume on alarms and telephones to safe but not excessive volumes; pad metal trash can lids; open paper packages, such as IV tubing and suction catheters slowly and at a distance from bedside; conduct rounds or report away from bedside; place soft, thick fabric, such as blanket rolls and toys, near infant's head to absorb sound).
- Keep all incubator portholes closed, closing with two hands **to avoid a loud snap and associated startle response.**
- Refrain from playing musical toys or tape players inside incubator.
- Avoid placing items on top of incubator; if necessary to do so, pad surface well.
- Conduct regular decibel (dB) checks of interior noise level in incubator (recommended not to exceed 60 dB).
- Provide auditory stimulation **to console and support infant before and through handling or to reinforce restfulness.**

Olfactory
- Be cautious in exposing infant to strong odors (e.g., alcohol, Betadine, perfumes), **as olfactory capability of the infant is very sensitive.**
- Place a cloth or gauze pad scented with milk near the infant's face during gavage feeding. **Enhances association of milk with act of feeding and gastric fullness.**

Information that appears in brackets has been added by the authors to clarify and enhance the use of nursing diagnoses.

- Invite parents to leave a handkerchief that they have scented by wearing close to their body near infant. **Strengthens infant recognition of parents.**

Vestibular
- Move and handle the infant slowly and gently. Do not restrict spontaneous movement.
- Provide vestibular stimulation **to console, stabilize breathing and heart rate, or enhance growth.** Use a water bed (with or without oscillation), a motorized or moving bed or cradle, or rocking in the arms of a caregiver.

Gustatory
- Dip pacifier in milk and offer to infant during gavage feeding **for sucking and to stimulate tasting.**

Tactile
- Maintain skin integrity and monitor closely. Limit frequency of invasive procedures.
- Minimize use of chemicals on skin (e.g., alcohol, Betadine, solvents) and remove afterward with warm water **because skin is very sensitive/fragile.**
- Limit use of tape and adhesives directly on skin. Use DuoDerm under tape **to prevent dermal injury.**
- Touch infant with a firm containing touch; avoid light stroking. Provide a sheepskin pad or soft linen. **Note: Tactile experience is the primary sensory mode of the infant.**
- Encourage frequent parental holding of infant (including skin-to-skin). Supplement activity with extended family, staff, and volunteers.

Nursing Priority No. 5.
🏠 To promote wellness (Teaching/Discharge Considerations):
- Evaluate home environment **to identify appropriate modifications.**
- Identify community resources (e.g., early stimulation programs, qualified childcare facilities, respite care, visiting nurse, home-care support, specialty organizations).
- Determine sources for equipment and therapy needs.
- Refer to support or therapy groups, as indicated, **to provide role models, facilitate adjustment to new roles/responsibilities, and enhance coping.**
- Provide contact number, as appropriate (e.g., primary nurse), **to support adjustment to home setting.**
- Refer to additional NDs, such as risk for impaired Attachment; compromised/disabled or readiness for enhanced family

---

Information that appears in brackets has been added by the authors to clarify and enhance the use of nursing diagnoses.

Coping; delayed Growth and Development; risk for Caregiver Role Strain.

Documentation Focus

Assessment/Reassessment
- Findings, including infant's cues of stress, self-regulation, and readiness for stimulation, and chronological and developmental age.
- Parents' concerns/level of knowledge.

Planning
- Plan of care and who is involved in the planning.
- Teaching plan.

Implementation/Evaluation
- Infant's responses to interventions and actions performed.
- Parents' participation and response to interactions and teaching.
- Attainment or progress toward desired outcome(s).
- Modifications of plan of care.

Discharge Planning
- Long-term needs and who is responsible for actions to be taken.
- Specific referrals made.

Sample Nursing Outcomes & Interventions Classifications (NOC/NIC)

NOC—Preterm Infant Organization
NIC—Environmental Management

---

risk for disorganized infant Behavior

Taxonomy II: Coping/Stress Tolerance—Class 3 Neuro-behavioral Stress (00115)
[Diagnostic Division: Neurosensory]
Submitted 1994

Definition: At risk for alteration in integration and modulation of the physiological and behavioral systems of functioning (i.e., autonomic, motor, state-organization, self-regulatory, and attentional-interactional systems)

Information that appears in brackets has been added by the authors to clarify and enhance the use of nursing diagnoses.

Risk Factors

Pain; invasive or painful procedures
Oral or motor problems
Environmental overstimulation
Lack of containment within environment
Prematurity (hypoxia or birth asphyxia)

> **NOTE:** A risk diagnosis is not evidenced by signs and symptoms, as the problem has not occurred; rather, nursing interventions are directed at prevention.

Desired Outcomes/Evaluation Criteria—Infant Will:

• Exhibit organized behaviors that allow the achievement of optimal potential for growth and development as evidenced by modulation of physiological, motor, state, and attentional-interactive functioning.

Parent/Caregiver Will:

• Identify cues reflecting infant's stress threshold and current status.
• Develop or modify responses (including environment) to promote infant adaptation and development.
• Verbalize readiness to assume caregiving independently.

Refer to ND disorganized infant Behavior for Actions/Interventions and Documentation Focus.

Sample Nursing Outcomes & Interventions Classifications (NOC/NIC)

NOC—Neurological Status
NIC—Environmental Management

Information that appears in brackets has been added by the authors to clarify and enhance the use of nursing diagnoses.

readiness for enhanced organized infant Behavior

Taxonomy II: Coping/Stress Tolerance—Class 3 Neuro-
behavioral Stress (00117)
[Diagnostic Division: Neurosensory]
Submitted 1994

Definition: A pattern of modulation of the physiological
and behavioral systems of functioning (i.e., autonomic,
motor, state-organization, self-regulatory, and attentional-
interactional systems) in an infant that is sufficient for
well-being and can be improved

Defining Characteristics

Objective
Stable physiological measures
Definite sleep-wake states
Use of some self-regulatory behaviors
Response to stimuli (e.g., visual and auditory)

Desired Outcomes/Evaluation Criteria—
Infant Will:

• Continue to modulate physiological and behavioral systems
  of functioning.
• Achieve higher levels of integration in response to environmental stimuli.

Parent/Caregiver Will:

• Identify cues reflecting infant's stress threshold and current
  status.
• Develop or modify responses (including environment) to promote infant adaptation and development.

Actions/Interventions

Nursing Priority No. 1.
To assess infant status and parental skill level:
• Determine infant's chronological and developmental age;
  note length of gestation.
• Identify infant's individual self-regulatory behaviors, such as
  suck, mouth, grasp, hand-to-mouth, face behaviors, foot clasp,
  brace, limb flexion, trunk tuck, and boundary seeking.

Information that appears in brackets has been added by the authors to clarify
and enhance the use of nursing diagnoses.

- Observe for cues suggesting presence of situations that may result in pain/discomfort.
- Evaluate level and appropriateness of environmental stimuli.
- Ascertain parents' understanding of infant's needs and abilities.
- Listen to parents' perceptions of their capabilities to promote infant's development.

Nursing Priority No. 2.
To assist parents to enhance infant's integration:

- Review infant growth and development, pointing out current status and progressive expectations.
- Identify cues reflecting infant stress.
- Discuss possible modifications of environmental stimuli, handling, activity schedule, sleep, and pain control needs based on infant's behavioral cues. **Stimulation that is properly timed and appropriate in complexity and intensity allows the infant to maintain a stable balance of his/her subsystems and enhances development.**
- Provide positive feedback for parental involvement in caregiving process. **Transfer of care from staff to parents progresses along a continuum as parents' confidence level increases and they are able to take on more responsibility.**
- Discuss use of skin-to-skin contact (kangaroo care [KC]), as appropriate. **Research suggests KC may have a positive effect on infant development by enhancing neurophysiological organization as well as an indirect effect by improving parental mood, perceptions, and interactive behavior.**
- Incorporate parents' observations and suggestions into plan of care. **Demonstrates value of and regard for parents' input and enhances sense of ability to deal with situation.**

Nursing Priority No. 3.
To promote wellness (Teaching/Learning Considerations):

- Identify community resources (e.g., visiting nurse, home-care support, childcare).
- Refer to support group or individual role model **to facilitate adjustment to new roles/responsibilities.**
- Refer to additional NDs, such as readiness for enhanced family Coping.

Information that appears in brackets has been added by the authors to clarify and enhance the use of nursing diagnoses.

🌐 Cultural 😊 Collaborative 🏠 Community/Home Care

Documentation Focus

Assessment/Reassessment
- Findings, including infant's self-regulation and readiness for stimulation; chronological and developmental age.
- Parents' concerns/level of knowledge.

Planning
- Plan of care and who is involved in the planning.
- Teaching plan.

Implementation/Evaluation
- Infant's responses to interventions and actions performed.
- Parents' participation and response to interactions and teaching.
- Attainment or progress toward desired outcome(s).
- Modifications of plan of care.

Discharge Planning
- Long-term needs and who is responsible for actions to be taken.
- Specific referrals made.

Sample Nursing Outcomes & Interventions Classifications (NOC/NIC)

NOC—Neurological Status
NIC—Developmental Care

risk for Bleeding

Taxonomy II: Safety/Protection—Class 2: Physical Injury (00206)
[Diagnostic Division: Circulation]
Submitted 2008

Definition: At risk for a decrease in blood volume that may compromise health

Risk Factors

Aneurysm; trauma; history of falls
Gastrointestinal disorders (e.g., gastric ulcer disease, polyps, varices)

Information that appears in brackets has been added by the authors to clarify and enhance the use of nursing diagnoses.

Impaired liver function (e.g., cirrhosis, hepatitis)

Pregnancy-related complications (e.g., placenta previa, molar pregnancy, abruption placenta); postpartum complications (e.g., uterine atony, retained placenta)

Inherent coagulopathies (e.g., thrombocytopenia, hereditary hemorrhagic telangiectasia [HHT])

Treatment-related side effects (e.g., surgery, medications, administration of platelet-deficient blood products, chemotherapy); circumcision

Disseminated intravascular coagulopathy

Deficient knowledge

> **NOTE:** A risk diagnosis is not evidenced by signs and symptoms, as the problem has not occurred; rather, nursing interventions are directed at prevention.

Desired Outcomes/Evaluation Criteria— Client Will:

- Be free of signs of active bleeding, such as hemoptysis, hematuria, hematemesis, or excessive blood loss, as evidenced by stable vital signs, skin and mucous membranes free of pallor, and usual mentation and urinary output.
- Display laboratory results for clotting times and factors within normal range for individual.
- Identify individual risks and engage in appropriate behaviors or lifestyle changes to prevent or reduce frequency of bleeding episodes.

Actions/Interventions

Nursing Priority No. 1.

- Assess client risk, noting possible medical diagnoses or disease processes that may lead to bleeding as listed in risk factors.
- Note type of injury/injuries when client presents with trauma. **The pattern and extent of injury and bleeding may or may not be readily determined. For example, unbroken skin can hide a significant injury where large amount of blood is lost within soft tissues; or a crush injury resulting in interruption of the integrity of the pelvic ring can cause life-threatening bleeding from three sources: arterial, venous, and bone edge bleeding.**

Information that appears in brackets has been added by the authors to clarify and enhance the use of nursing diagnoses.

🌐 Cultural   😊 Collaborative   🏠 Community/Home Care

- Determine presence of hereditary factors, obtain detailed history if a familial bleeding disorder is suspected, such as HHT, hemophilia, other factor deficiencies, or thrombocytopenia. **Hereditary bleeding or clotting disorders predispose client to bleeding complications, necessitating specialized testing and/or referral to hematologist.**
- Note client's gender. **While bleeding disorders are common in both men and women, women are affected more owing to the increased risk of blood loss related to menstrual cycle and child delivery procedures.**
- Identify pregnancy-related factors such as overdistention of the uterus, lacerations of birth canal, or retained placenta.
- Evaluate client's medication regimen. **Use of medications, such as nonsteroidal anti-inflammatory drugs, anticoagulants, corticosteroids, and certain herbals (e.g., gingko biloba), predispose client to bleeding.**

Nursing Priority No. 2.

- Monitor perineum and fundal height in postpartum client and wounds, dressings, or tubes in client with trauma, surgery, or other invasive procedures **to identify active blood loss. Note: Hemorrhage may occur because of inability to achieve hemostasis in the setting of injury or may result from the development of a coagulopathy**.
- Evaluate and mark boundaries of soft tissues in enclosed structures, such as a leg or abdomen, **to document expanding bruises or hematomas.**
- Assess vital signs, including blood pressure, pulse, and respirations. Measure blood pressure lying/sitting/standing as indicated to evaluate for orthostatic hypotension; monitor invasive hemodynamic parameters when present **to determine if intravascular fluid deficit exists.**
- Hematest all secretions and excretions for occult blood **to determine possible sources of bleeding.**
- Note client report of pain in specific areas, whether pain is increasing, diffuse, or localized. **Can help identify bleeding into tissues, organs, or body cavities.**
- Assess skin color and moisture, urinary output, level of consciousness, or mentation. **Changes in these signs may be indicative of blood loss affecting systemic circulation or local organ function such as kidneys or brain.**
- Review laboratory data (e.g., complete blood count [CBC], platelet numbers and function, and other coagulation factors such as Factor I, Factor II, prothrombin time [PT], partial

---

Information that appears in brackets has been added by the authors to clarify and enhance the use of nursing diagnoses.

thromboplastin time [PTT], and fibrinogen) **to evaluate bleeding risk. An abrupt drop in Hb of 2 g/dLl can indicate active bleeding**.

• Prepare client for or assist with diagnostic studies such as x-rays, computed tomography (CT) or magnetic resonance imaging (MRI) scans, ultrasound, or colonoscopy **to determine presence of injuries or disorders that could cause internal bleeding.**

Nursing Priority No. 3.

To prevent bleeding/correct potential causes of excessive blood loss:

• Apply direct pressure and cold pack to bleeding site, insert nasal packing, or perform fundal massage as appropriate.

• Restrict activity, encourage bedrest or chair rest until bleeding abates.

• Maintain patency of vascular access **for fluid administration or blood replacement as indicated.**

• Assist with treatment of underlying conditions causing or contributing to blood loss such as medical treatment of systemic infections or balloon tamponade of esophageal varices prior to sclerotherapy; use of proton pump inhibitor medications or antibiotics for gastric ulcer; surgery for internal abdominal trauma or retained placenta.

• Provide special intervention for at-risk client, such as an individual with bone marrow suppression, chemotherapy, or uremia, **to prevent bleeding associated with tissue injury:**

Monitor closely for overt bleeding.

Observe for diffuse oozing from tubes, wounds, or orifices with no observable clotting.

Maintain direct pressure or pressure dressings as indicated for longer period of time over arterial puncture sites **to prevent oozing or active bleeding.**

Hematest secretions and excretions for occult blood **for early identification of internal bleeding**.

Protect client from trauma such as falls, accidental or intentional blows, or lacerations.

Use soft toothbrush or toothettes for oral care **to reduce risk of injury to oral mucosa.**

• Collaborate in evaluating need for replacing blood loss or specific components and be prepared for emergency interventions.

Information that appears in brackets has been added by the authors to clarify and enhance the use of nursing diagnoses.

- Administer hemostatic agents **to promote clotting and diminish bleeding by increasing coagulation factors,** or medications to prevent bleeding such as proton pump inhibitors to reduce risk of gastrointestinal bleeding.
- Provide information to client/family about hereditary or familial problems that predispose to bleeding complications.
- Instruct at-risk client and family regarding:

Specific signs of bleeding requiring healthcare provider notification, such as active bright bleeding anywhere, prolonged epistaxis or trauma in client with known factor bleeding tendencies, black tarry stools, weakness, vertigo, and syncope.

Need to inform healthcare providers when taking aspirin and other anticoagulant-type agents (e.g., Coumadin or Plavix), especially when elective surgery or other invasive procedure is planned. **These agents will most likely be held for a period of time prior to elective procedures to reduce potential for excessive blood loss.**

Importance of periodic review of client's medication regimen **to identify medications that might cause or exacerbate bleeding problems.**

Necessity of regular medical and laboratory follow-up when on anticoagulants, such as Coumadin, **to determine needed dosage changes or client management issues requiring monitoring and/or modification.**

Dietary measures **to promote blood clotting, when indicated, such as foods rich in vitamin K.**

Need to avoid alcohol in diagnosed liver disorders or seek treatment for alcoholism in presence of alcoholic varices.

Techniques for postpartum client to check her own fundus and perform fundal massage as indicated and the need to contact physician for postdischarge bleeding that is bright red or dark red with large clots. **May prevent blood loss complications, especially if client is discharged early from hospital.**

Documentation Focus

Assessment/Reassessment
- Individual factors that may potentiate blood loss—type of injuries, obstetrical complications, and so on.
- Baseline vital signs, mentation, urinary output, and subsequent assessments.
- Results of laboratory tests or diagnostic procedures.

Information that appears in brackets has been added by the authors to clarify and enhance the use of nursing diagnoses.

Planning
- Plan of care and who is involved in the planning.
- Teaching plan.

Implementation/Evaluation
- Responses to interventions, teaching, and actions performed.
- Attainment or progress toward desired outcome(s).
- Modifications to plan of care.

Discharge Planning
- Long-term needs, identifying who is responsible for actions to be taken.
- Community resources or support for chronic problems.
- Specific referrals made.

Sample Nursing Outcomes & Interventions Classifications (NOC/NIC)

NOC—Blood Loss Severity
NIC—Bleeding Precautions

---

risk for unstable Blood Glucose Level

Taxonomy II: Nutrition—Class 4 Metabolism (00179)
[Diagnostic Division: Food/Fluid]
Submitted 2006

Definition: At risk for variation of blood glucose/sugar levels from the normal range that may compromise health

---

Risk Factors

Lack of acceptance of diagnosis; deficient knowledge of diabetes management (e.g., action plan)

Lack of diabetes management or adherence to diabetes management plan (e.g., adhering to the action plan); inadequate blood glucose monitoring; medication management

Dietary intake; weight gain or loss; rapid growth periods; pregnancy

Physical health status or activity level

Stress; mental health status

Developmental level

Information that appears in brackets has been added by the authors to clarify and enhance the use of nursing diagnoses.

🌐 Cultural   🌀 Collaborative   🏠 Community/Home Care

> **NOTE:** A risk diagnosis is not evidenced by signs and symptoms, as the problem has not occurred; rather, nursing interventions are directed at prevention.

Desired Outcomes/Evaluation Criteria— Client/Caregivers Will:

- Acknowledge factors that may lead to unstable glucose.
- Verbalize understanding of body and energy needs.
- Verbalize plan for modifying factors to prevent or minimize shifts in glucose level.
- Maintain glucose within satisfactory range.

Actions/Interventions

Nursing Priority No. 1.

To assess risk/contributing factors:

- Determine individual factors that may contribute to unstable glucose as listed in risk factors. **Client or family history of diabetes, known diabetic with poor glucose control, eating disorders (e.g., morbid obesity), poor exercise habits, or a failure to recognize changes in glucose needs or control due to adolescent growth spurts or pregnancy can result in problems with glucose stability.**
- Ascertain client's/SO's knowledge and understanding of condition and treatment needs.
- Identify individual perceptions and expectations of treatment regimen.
- Note influence of cultural, ethnic origin, socioeconomic, or religious factors impacting diabetes recognition and care, including how person with diabetes is viewed by family and community; the seeking and receiving of healthcare; management of factors such as dietary practices, weight, blood pressure, and lipids; and expectations of outcomes. **These factors influence a client's ability to manage their condition and must be considered when planning care.**
- Determine client's awareness and ability to be responsible for dealing with situation. **Age, maturity, current health status, and developmental stage all affect a client's ability to provide for their own safety.**
- Assess family/SO(s) support of client. **Client may need assistance with lifestyle changes (e.g., food preparation or**

Information that appears in brackets has been added by the authors to clarify and enhance the use of nursing diagnoses.

consumption, timing of intake and/or exercise, or administration of medications).

🏠• Note availability and use of resources.

Nursing Priority No. 2.

To assist client to develop preventive strategies to avoid glucose instability:

• Ascertain whether client/SOs are certain they are obtaining accurate readings on their glucose-monitoring device and are adept at using the device. **In addition to checking blood glucose more frequently when it is unstable, it is wise to ascertain that equipment is functioning properly and being used correctly. All available devices will provide accurate readings if properly used, maintained, and routinely calibrated. However, there are many other factors that may affect the accuracy of numbers, such as the size of blood drop with finger-sticking, forgetting a bolus from insulin pump, and injecting insulin into a lumpy subcutaneous site.**

🏠• Provide information on balancing food intake, antidiabetic agents, and energy expenditure.

✎• Review medical necessity for regularly scheduled lab screening and monitoring tests for diabetes. **Screening tests may include fasting plasma glucose or oral glucose tolerance tests. In the known or sick diabetic, tests can include fasting and daily (or numerous times in a day) finger-stick glucose levels. Also, in diabetics, regular testing of hemoglobin (Hgb) A_1C and the estimated average glucose (eAG) helps determine glucose control over several months.**

🏠• Discuss home glucose monitoring according to individual parameters (e.g., six times a day for a normal day and more frequently during times of stress) **to identify and manage glucose variations.**

🏠• Review client's common situations that contribute to glucose instability on daily, occasional, or crisis basis. **Multiple factors can play a role at any time, such as missing meals, adolescent growth spurt, or infection or other illness.**

🏠• Review client's diet, especially carbohydrate intake. **Glucose balance is determined by the amount of carbohydrates consumed, which should be determined in needed grams per day.**

🏠• Encourage client to read labels and choose carbohydrates described as having a low glycemic index (GI), and foods with adequate protein, higher fiber, and low-fat content. **These**

Information that appears in brackets has been added by the authors to clarify and enhance the use of nursing diagnoses.

foods produce a slower rise in blood glucose and more stable release of insulin.

- Discuss how client's antidiabetic medication(s) work. **Drugs and combinations of drugs work in varying ways with different blood glucose control and side effects. Understanding drug actions can help client avoid or reduce risk of potential for hypoglycemic reactions.**

For Client Receiving Insulin

- Emphasize importance of checking expiration dates of medications, inspecting insulin for cloudiness if it is normally clear, and monitoring proper storage and preparation (when mixing required). **Affects insulin absorbability.**
- Review type(s) of insulin used (e.g., rapid, short, intermediate, long-acting, premixed) and delivery method (e.g., subcutaneous, intramuscular injection, prefilled pen, pump). Note time when short- and long-acting insulins are administered. Remind client that only short-acting insulin is used in pump. **Affects timing of effects and provides clues to potential timing of glucose instability.**
- Check injection sites periodically. **Insulin absorption can vary from day to day in healthy sites and is less absorbable in lipohypertrophic (lumpy) tissues.**
- Ascertain that all injections are being given. **Children, adolescents, and elderly clients may forget injections or be unable to self-inject and may need reminders and supervision.**

Nursing Priority No. 3.

To promote wellness (Teaching/Discharge Considerations):

- Review individual risk factors and provide information to assist client in efforts to avoid complications, such as those caused by chronic hyperglycemia and acute hypoglycemia. **Note: Hyperglycemia is most commonly caused by alterations in nutrition needs, inactivity, and/or inadequate use of antidiabetic medications. Hypoglycemia is the most common complication of antidiabetic therapy, stress, and exercise.**
- Emphasize consequences of actions and choices—both immediate and long term.
- Engage client/family/caregiver in formulating a plan to manage blood glucose level incorporating lifestyle, age and developmental level, and physical and psychological ability to manage condition.

Information that appears in brackets has been added by the authors to clarify and enhance the use of nursing diagnoses.

- Consult with dietitian about specific dietary needs based on individual situation (e.g., growth spurt, pregnancy, change in activity level following injury).
- Encourage client to develop a system for self-monitoring to provide a sense of control and enable client to follow own progress and assist with making choices.
- Refer to appropriate community resources, diabetic educator, and/or support groups, as needed, **for lifestyle modification, medical management, referral for insulin pump or glucose monitor, financial assistance for supplies, and so forth.**

Documentation Focus

Assessment/Reassessment
- Findings related to individual situation, risk factors, current caloric intake, and dietary pattern; prescription medication use; monitoring of condition.
- Client's/caregiver's understanding of individual risks and potential complications.
- Results of laboratory tests and finger-stick testing.

Planning
- Plan of care and who is involved in planning.
- Teaching plan.

Implementation/Evaluation
- Individual responses to interventions, teaching, and actions performed.
- Specific actions and changes that are made.
- Attainment or progress toward desired outcomes.
- Modifications to plan of care.

Discharge Planning
- Long-term plans for ongoing needs, monitoring and management of condition, and who is responsible for actions to be taken.
- Sources for equipment/supplies.
- Specific referrals made.

Sample Nursing Outcomes & Interventions Classifications (NOC/NIC)

NOC—Blood Glucose Level
NIC—Hyperglycemia Management

Information that appears in brackets has been added by the authors to clarify and enhance the use of nursing diagnoses.

disturbed Body Image

Taxonomy II: Perception/Cognition—Class 3 Body Image (00118)
[Diagnostic Division: Ego Integrity]
Submitted 1973; Revised 1998 (by small group work 1996)

Definition: Confusion [and/or dissatisfaction] in mental picture of one's physical self

Related Factors

Biophysical; illness; trauma; injury; surgery; [mutilation, pregnancy]
Treatment regimen
Psychosocial
Cultural; spiritual
Cognitive; perceptual
Developmental changes [maturational changes]
[Significance of body part or functioning with regard to age, gender, developmental level, or basic human needs]

Defining Characteristics

Subjective

Reports feelings that reflect an altered view of one's body (e.g., appearance, structure, function)
Reports perceptions that reflect an altered view of one's body in appearance
Reports change in lifestyle
Reports fear of reaction by others
Focus on past strength, function, appearance
Reports negative feelings about body (e.g., feelings of helplessness, hopelessness, or powerlessness)
Preoccupation with change/loss
Refusal to verify actual change
Emphasis on remaining strengths
Heightened achievement
Personalization of body part/loss by name
Depersonalization of part/loss by use of impersonal pronouns

Objective

Behaviors of: acknowledgment of one's body; avoidance of one's body; monitoring one's body

---

Information that appears in brackets has been added by the authors to clarify and enhance the use of nursing diagnoses.

Nonverbal response to actual or perceived change in body (e.g., appearance, structure, function)

Missing body part

Actual change in structure or function

Not looking at/not touching body part

Trauma to nonfunctioning part

Change in ability to estimate spatial relationship of body to environment

Extension of body boundary to incorporate environmental objects

Intentional/unintentional hiding or overexposing of body part

Change in social involvement

Aggression; low frustration tolerance level

Desired Outcomes/Evaluation Criteria— Client Will:

• Verbalize understanding of body changes.
• Recognize and incorporate body image change into self-concept in accurate manner without negating self-esteem.
• Verbalize acceptance of self in situation (e.g., chronic progressive disease, amputee, decreased independence, weight as is, effects of therapeutic regimen).
• Verbalize relief of anxiety and adaptation to actual/altered body image.
• Seek information and actively pursue growth.
• Acknowledge self as an individual who has responsibility for self.
• Use adaptive devices/prosthesis appropriately.

Actions/Interventions

Nursing Priority No. 1.

To assess causative/contributing factors:

• Discuss pathophysiology present and/or situation affecting the individual and refer to additional NDs as appropriate. For example, when alteration in body image is related to neurological deficit (e.g., cerebrovascular accident—CVA), refer to ND Unilateral Neglect; in the presence of severe, ongoing pain, refer to ND chronic Pain; or in loss of sexual desire/ability, refer to ND Sexual Dysfunction.
• Determine whether condition is permanent with no expectation for resolution (May be associated with other NDs, such as Self-Esteem [specify] or risk for impaired Attachment, when child is affected.) **There is always something that can**

Information that appears in brackets has been added by the authors to clarify and enhance the use of nursing diagnoses.

be done to enhance acceptance, and it is important to hold out the possibility of living a good life with the disability.

• Assess mental and physical influence of illness or condition on the client's emotional state (e.g., diseases of the endocrine system, use of steroid therapy).

• Evaluate level of client's knowledge of and anxiety related to situation. Observe emotional changes, **which may indicate acceptance or nonacceptance of situation.**

• Recognize behavior indicative of overconcern with body and its processes.

• Have client describe self, noting what is positive and what is negative. Be aware of how client believes others see self.

∞• Discuss meaning of loss/change to client. **A small (seemingly trivial) loss may have a big impact (such as the use of a urinary catheter or enema for continence). A change in function (such as immobility in elderly) may be more difficult for some to deal with than a change in appearance. Or the change could be devastating, such as permanent facial scarring of child.**

∞• Use developmentally appropriate communication techniques for determining exact expression of body image in child (e.g., puppet play or constructive dialogue for toddler). **Developmental capacity must guide interaction to gain accurate information.**

⊕• Note signs of grieving or indicators of severe or prolonged depression **to evaluate need for counseling and/or medications.**

⊕• Determine ethnic background and cultural and religious perceptions or considerations. **May influence how individual deals with what has happened.**

• Identify social aspects of illness or condition (e.g., sexually transmitted diseases, sterility, chronic conditions).

• Observe interaction of client with SO(s). **Distortions in body image may be unconsciously reinforced by family members and/or secondary gain issues may interfere with progress.**

Nursing Priority No. 2.

To determine coping abilities and skills:

• Assess client's current level of adaptation and progress.

• Listen to client's comments and responses to the situation. **Different situations are upsetting to different people, depending on individual coping skills and past experiences.**

Information that appears in brackets has been added by the authors to clarify and enhance the use of nursing diagnoses.

- Note withdrawn behavior and the use of denial. **May be normal response to situation or may be indicative of mental illness (e.g., schizophrenia).** (Refer to ND ineffective Denial.)
- Note use of addictive substances, such as alcohol or other drugs, **which may reflect dysfunctional coping.**
- Identify previously used coping strategies and effectiveness.
- Determine individual/family/community resources available to client.

Nursing Priority No. 3.

To assist client and SO(s) to deal with/accept issues of self-concept related to body image:

- Establish therapeutic nurse-client relationship, conveying an attitude of caring and developing a sense of trust.
- Visit client frequently and acknowledge the individual as someone who is worthwhile. **Provides opportunities for listening to concerns and questions.**
- Assist in correcting underlying problems **to promote optimal healing and adaptation.**
- Provide assistance with self-care needs as necessary, while promoting individual abilities and independence.
- Work with client's self-concept, avoiding moral judgments regarding client's efforts or progress (e.g., "You should be progressing faster"; "You're weak or not trying hard enough"). **Positive reinforcement encourages client to continue efforts and strive for improvement.**
- Discuss concerns about fear of mutilation, prognosis, rejection when client is facing surgery or potentially poor outcome of procedure/illness, **to address realities and provide emotional support.**
- Acknowledge and accept feelings of dependency, grief, and hostility.
- Encourage verbalization of and role play anticipated conflicts **to enhance handling of potential situations.**
- Encourage client and SO(s) to communicate feelings to each other.
- Assume all individuals are sensitive to changes in appearance but avoid stereotyping.
- Alert staff to monitor own facial expressions and other nonverbal behaviors **because they need to convey acceptance and not revulsion when the client's appearance is affected.**
- Encourage family members to treat client normally and not as an invalid.

Information that appears in brackets has been added by the authors to clarify and enhance the use of nursing diagnoses.

⊕ Cultural   ⊛ Collaborative   🏠 Community/Home Care

- Encourage client to look at/touch affected body part **to begin to incorporate changes into body image.**
- Allow client to use denial without participating (e.g., client may at first refuse to look at a colostomy; the nurse says "I am going to change your colostomy now" and proceeds with the task). **Provides individual with time to adapt to situation.**
- Set limits on maladaptive behavior and assist client to identify positive behaviors **to aid in recovery.**
- Provide accurate information as desired/requested. Reinforce previously given information.
- Discuss the availability of prosthetics, reconstructive surgery, and physical/occupational therapy or other referrals as dictated by individual situation.
- Help client select and use clothing or makeup **to minimize body changes and enhance appearance.**
- Discuss reasons for infectious isolation and treatment procedures when used and make time to sit down and talk/listen to client while in the room **to decrease sense of isolation/loneliness.**

Nursing Priority No. 4.

To promote wellness (Teaching/Discharge Considerations):

- Begin counseling/other therapies (e.g., biofeedback, relaxation) as soon as possible **to provide early/ongoing sources of support.**
- Provide information at client's level of acceptance and in small segments **to allow easier assimilation.** Clarify misconceptions. Reinforce explanations given by other health team members.
- Include client in decision-making process and problem-solving activities.
- Assist client in incorporating therapeutic regimen into activities of daily living (e.g., including specific exercises and housework activities). **Promotes continuation of program.**
- Identify/plan for alterations to home and work environment/activities **to accommodate individual needs and support independence.**
- Assist client in learning strategies for dealing with feelings and venting emotions.
- Offer positive reinforcement for efforts made (e.g., wearing makeup or using a prosthetic device).
- Refer to appropriate support groups.

Information that appears in brackets has been added by the authors to clarify and enhance the use of nursing diagnoses.

Documentation Focus

Assessment/Reassessment
- Observations, presence of maladaptive behaviors, emotional changes, stage of grieving, level of independence.
- Physical wounds, dressings; use of life support–type machine (e.g., ventilator, dialysis machine).
- Meaning of loss or change to client.
- Support systems available (e.g., SOs, friends, groups).

Planning
- Plan of care and who is involved in planning.
- Teaching plan.

Implementation/Evaluation
- Client's response to interventions, teaching, and actions performed.
- Attainment or progress toward desired outcome(s).
- Modifications of plan of care.

Discharge Planning
- Long-term needs and who is responsible for actions.
- Specific referrals made (e.g., rehabilitation center, community resources).

Sample Nursing Outcomes & Interventions Classifications (NOC/NIC)

NOC—Body Image
NIC—Body Image Enhancement

---

risk for imbalanced **Body Temperature**

Taxonomy II: Safety/Protection—Class 6 Thermoregulation (00005)
[Diagnostic Division: Safety]
Submitted 1986; Revised 2000

Definition: At risk for failure to maintain body temperature within normal range

---

Risk Factors

Extremes of age/weight
Exposure to extremes of environmental temperature; inappropriate clothing for environmental temperature

---

Information that appears in brackets has been added by the authors to clarify and enhance the use of nursing diagnoses.

🌐 Cultural ㊂ Collaborative 🏠 Community/Home Care

Dehydration

Inactivity or vigorous activity

Pharmaceutical agents causing vasoconstriction or vasodilation; sedation

Illness or trauma affecting temperature regulation (e.g., infections; neoplasms or tumors; collagen/vascular disease) or altered metabolic rate

> **NOTE:** A risk diagnosis is not evidenced by signs and symptoms as the problem has not occurred; rather, nursing interventions are directed at prevention.

Desired Outcomes/Evaluation Criteria—Client Will:

- Maintain body temperature within normal range.
- Verbalize understanding of individual risk factors and appropriate interventions.
- Demonstrate behaviors for monitoring and maintaining appropriate body temperature.

Actions/Interventions

Nursing Priority No. 1.

To identify causative/risk factors present:

- Determine if present illness/condition results from exposure to environmental factors, surgery, infection, trauma. **Helps in determining the scope of interventions that may be needed (e.g., simple addition of warm blankets after surgery or hypothermia therapy following brain trauma).**
- Monitor laboratory values (e.g., tests indicative of infection, thyroid or other endocrine tests, drug screens) **to identify potential internal causes of temperature imbalances.**
- Note client's age (e.g., premature neonate, young child, or aging individual), **as it can directly impact ability to maintain/regulate body temperature and respond to changes in environment.**
- Assess nutritional status **to determine metabolism effect on body temperature and to identify foods or nutrient deficits that affect metabolism.**

Nursing Priority No. 2.

To prevent occurrence of temperature alteration:

- Monitor temperature regularly, measuring core body temperature whenever needed to observe this vital sign. Exercise care

---

Information that appears in brackets has been added by the authors to clarify and enhance the use of nursing diagnoses.

in selecting an appropriate thermometer for client's age and clinical condition and observe for inconsistencies in readings obtained with various instruments. Observe temperature reading for trends and do not make therapeutic decisions based solely on thermometer readings. **Tympanic thermometer may be most commonly used, as it is the most accurate noninvasive method, except in critically ill adults, or in infants, where skin or internal electrodes may be preferred.**

- Monitor and maintain comfortable ambient environment (e.g., provide heating/cooling measures such as space heaters/fans) as indicated **to reduce the effect on body temperature alterations**.

- Supervise use of heating pads, electric blankets, ice bags, and hypothermia blankets, especially in clients who cannot self-protect.

🏠• Dress client or discuss with client/caregiver(s) appropriate dressing (e.g., layering clothing, use of hat and gloves in cold weather, light loose clothing in warm weather, water-resistant outer gear for rainy weather).

∞• Cover infant's head with knit cap, place under adequate blankets, and provide for skin-to-skin contact with mother. Place newborn infant under radiant warmer. **Heat loss in newborns/infants, especially very low weight neonates, is greatest through head and by evaporation and convection.**

∞• Limit clothing or remove blanket from premature infant placed in incubator **to prevent overheating in climate-controlled environment.**

⊛• Restore/maintain core temperature within client's normal range. **Client may require interventions to treat hypothermia or hyperthermia.** (Refer to NDs Hypothermia; Hyperthermia.)

- Maintain good nutrition and adequate fluid intake. Offer cool or warm liquids, as appropriate. **Good nutrition and hydration assist in maintaining normal body temperature.**

🌡• Review client's medications (e.g., diuretics, certain sedatives and antipsychotic agents, some heart and blood pressure medications, or anesthesia) **for possible thermoregulatory side effects.**

🏠• Recommend lifestyle changes, such as cessation of smoking or substance use (such as methamphetamines), normalization of body weight, nutritious meals, and regular exercise **to prevent overheating and loss of regulatory body mechanisms, and to maximize metabolism to meet individual needs.**

Information that appears in brackets has been added by the authors to clarify and enhance the use of nursing diagnoses.

🌐 Cultural ⊛ Collaborative 🏠 Community/Home Care

⊕• Refer at-risk persons to appropriate community resources (e.g., home care, social services, foster adult care, and housing agencies) **to provide assistance to meet individual needs.**

Nursing Priority No. 3.
To promote wellness (Teaching/Discharge Considerations):

🏠• Discuss potential problem/individual risk factors with client/SO(s).

∞• Review age and gender issues, as appropriate. **Older or debilitated persons, babies, and young children typically feel more comfortable in higher ambient temperatures. Women notice feeling cooler quicker than men, which may be related to body size, or to differences in metabolism and the rate that blood flows to extremities to regulate body temperature.**

🏠• Instruct in appropriate self-care measures (e.g., adding or removing clothing, adding or removing heat sources, reviewing medication regimen with physician to identify those which can affect thermoregulation, evaluating home/shelter for ability to manage heat and cold, addressing nutritional and hydration status) **to protect from identified risk factors.**

🏠• Review ways to prevent accidental temperature alterations, such as hypothermia resulting from overzealous cooling to reduce fever or maintaining too warm an environment for client who has lost the ability to perspire.

Documentation Focus

Assessment/Reassessment
• Identified individual causative and risk factors.
• Record of core temperature, initially and prn.
• Results of diagnostic studies and laboratory tests.

Planning
• Plan of care and who is involved in planning.
• Teaching plan, including best ambient temperature, and ways to prevent hypothermia or hyperthermia.

Implementation/Evaluation
• Response to interventions, teaching, and actions performed.
• Attainment or progress toward desired outcome(s).
• Modifications to plan of care.

Information that appears in brackets has been added by the authors to clarify and enhance the use of nursing diagnoses.

Discharge Planning
• Long-term needs and who is responsible for actions.
• Specific referrals made.

Sample Nursing Outcomes & Interventions Classifications (NOC/NIC)

NOC—Thermoregulation
NIC—Temperature Regulation

insufficient Breast Milk

Taxonomy II: Nutrition—Class 1 Ingestion (00216)
[Diagnostic Division: Food/Fluid]
Submitted 2010

Definition: Low production of maternal breast milk

Related Factors

Mother:
Fluid volume depletion (e.g., dehydration, hemorrhage)
Tobacco smoking; alcohol intake
Malnutrition
Medication side effects (e.g., contraceptives, diuretics)
Pregnancy
Infant:
Ineffective latching or sucking
Insufficient opportunity to suckle; short sucking time
Rejection of breast

Defining Characteristics

Objective
Mother:
Volume of expressed breast milk is less than prescribed volume
Milk production does not progress
No milk appears when mother's nipple is pressed
Infant:
Long breastfeeding time; wants to suck very frequently
Does not seem satisfied after sucking time; frequent crying
Voids small amounts of concentrated urine (less than four to six times a day); constipation
Weight gain is lower than 500 g in a month (comparing two measures)

Information that appears in brackets has been added by the authors to clarify and enhance the use of nursing diagnoses.

🌐 Cultural 🤝 Collaborative 🏠 Community/Home Care

Desired Outcomes/Evaluation Criteria– Client Will:

- Develop plan to correct/change contributing factors.
- Demonstrate techniques to enhance milk production.
- Achieve mutually satisfactory breastfeeding pattern with infant content after feedings and gaining weight appropriately.

Actions/Interventions

Nursing Priority No. 1.

To identify maternal causative or contributing factors:

- Assess mother's knowledge about breastfeeding and extent of instruction that has been provided.
- Identify cultural expectations and conflicts about breastfeeding and beliefs or practices regarding lactation, let-down techniques, and maternal food preferences.
- Note incorrect myths/misunderstandings especially in teenage mothers, **who are more likely to have limited knowledge and more concerns about body image issues.**
- Perform physical examination, noting appearance of breasts and nipples, marked asymmetry of breasts, obvious inverted or flat nipples, minimal or no breast enlargement during pregnancy. **Inadequate mammary gland tissue, breast surgery that has damaged the nipple, areola enervation result in irremediable primary lactation failure.**
- Assess for other causes of primary lactation failure. **Maternal prolactin deficiency/serum prolactin levels, pituitary or thyroid disorders, and anemia may be corrected with medication.**
- Review lifestyle for common causes of secondary lactation failure. **Smoking, caffeine/alcohol use, birth control pills containing estrogen, medications (e.g., antihistamines, decongestants, diuretics), stress, and fatigue are known to inhibit milk production.**
- Determine desire/motivation to breastfeed. **Increasing milk supply can be intense, requiring commitment to therapeutic regimen and possible lifestyle changes.**

Nursing Priority No. 2.

To identify infant causative or contributing factors:

- Observe infant at breast to evaluate latching-on skill and presence of suck/swallow difficulties. **Poor latching on, and lack of audible swallowing/gulp are associated with inadequate**

Information that appears in brackets has been added by the authors to clarify and enhance the use of nursing diagnoses.

intake. **The infant gets substantial amounts of milk when drinking with an open—pause—close type of suck. Note: Open—pause—close is one suck; the pause is not a pause between sucks.**

- Evaluate signs of inadequate infant intake. **Infant arching and crying at the breast with resistance to latching on, decreased urinary output/frequency of stools, inadequate weight gain indicate need for further evaluation and intervention.**
- Review feeding schedule—frequency, length of feeding, taking one or both breasts at each feeding.

Nursing Priority No. 3.

To increase mother's milk supply:

- Instruct on how to differentiate between perceived and actual insufficient milk supply. **Normal breastfeeding frequencies, suckling times, and amounts vary not only between mothers but are also based on infant's needs/moods. Milk production is likely to be a reflection of the infant's appetite, rather than the mother's ability to produce milk.**
- Provide emotional support to mother. Use one-to-one instruction with each feeding during hospital stay and clinic or home visits. Refer adoptive mothers choosing to breastfeed to a lactation consultant **to assist with induced lactation techniques.**
- Inform mother how to assess and correct a latch if needed. Demonstrate asymmetric latch aiming infant's lower lip as far from base of the nipple as possible, then bringing infant's chin and lower jaw in contact with breast while mouth is wide open and before upper lip touches breast. **Correct latching on is the most effective way to stimulate milk supply.**
- Demonstrate breast massage technique to increase milk supply naturally. **Gently massaging breast while infant feeds from it can improve the release of higher calorie hindmilk from the milk glands.**
- Use breast pump 8 to 12 times a day. **Expressing with a hospital-grade, double (automatic) pump is ideal for stimulation/reestablishing milk supply.**
- Suggest using a breast pump or hand expression after infant finishes breastfeeding. **Continued breast stimulation cues the mother's body that more milk is needed, increasing supply.**
- Monitor increased filling of breasts in response to nursing and/ or pumping **to help evaluate effectiveness of interventions.**

Information that appears in brackets has been added by the authors to clarify and enhance the use of nursing diagnoses.

🌐 Cultural ⊛ Collaborative 🏠 Community/Home Care

- Discuss appropriate/safe use of herbal supplements. **Herbs such as sage, parsley, oregano, peppermint, jasmine, and yarrow may have a negative affect on milk supply if taken in large quantities.** A number of herbs have been used for centuries to stimulate milk production, such as fenugreek (*Trigonella foenum-graecum*), the most commonly recommended herbal galactogogue to facilitate lactation.
- Discuss the possible use of prescribed medications (galactogogues) to increase milk production. **Domperidone (Motilium) is approved by the American Academy of Pediatrics for use in breastfeeding mothers and has fewer side effects. Metoclopramide (Reglan) has been shown to increase milk supply anywhere from 72% to 110%, depending on how many weeks postpartum a mother is.**

Nursing Priority No. 4.

To promote optimal success and satisfaction of breastfeeding process for mother and infant:

- Encourage frequent rest periods, sharing household and childcare tasks. **Having assistance can limit fatigue (known to impact milk production) and facilitate relaxation at feeding time.**
- Discuss with spouse/SO mother's requirement for rest, relaxation, and time together with family members. **This enhances understanding of mother's needs, and family members feel included and are therefore more willing to support breastfeeding activity/treatment plan.**
- Arrange a dietary consult to review nutritional needs and vitamin/mineral supplements, such as vitamin C, as indicated. **During lactation, there is an increased need for energy requiring supplementation of protein, vitamins, and minerals to provide nourishment for the infant.**
- Stress importance of adequate fluid intake. **Alternating types of fluids (e.g., water, juice, decaffeinated tea/coffee, and milk) enhances intake, promoting milk production. Note: Beer and wine are not recommended for increasing lactation.**
- Promote peer counseling for teen mothers. **This provides positive role model that teen can relate to and feel comfortable with discussing concerns and feelings.**
- Recommend monitoring number of infant's wet and soiled diapers. **Stools should be yellow in color, and infant should have at least six wet diapers a day to determine that infant is receiving sufficient intake.**

Information that appears in brackets has been added by the authors to clarify and enhance the use of nursing diagnoses.

- Weigh infant every three days, or as directed by primary provider/lactation consultant, and record. **Monitors weight gain, verifying adequacy of intake or need for additional interventions.**
- Identify products/programs for cessation of smoking. **Smoking can interfere with the release of oxytocin, which stimulates the let-down reflex.**
- Refer to support groups (e.g., La Leche League, parenting support groups, stress reduction, or other community resources), as indicated.

Documentation Focus

Assessment/Reassessment
- Identified maternal assessment factors—hydration level, medication use, lifestyle choices.
- Infant assessment factors—latching-on technique, hydration level/number of wet diapers, weight gain/loss.
- Use of supplemental feedings.

Planning
- Plan of care, specific interventions, and who is involved in planning.
- Individual teaching plan.

Implementation/Evaluation
- Mother's/infant's responses to interventions, teaching, and actions performed.
- Change in infant's weight.
- Attainment or progress toward desired outcomes.
- Modification to plan of care.

Discharge Planning
- Specific referrals made.

Sample Nursing Outcomes & Interventions Classifications (NOC/NIC)

NOC—Breastfeeding Maintenance
NIC—Breastfeeding Assistance

Information that appears in brackets has been added by the authors to clarify and enhance the use of nursing diagnoses.

🌐 Cultural   ⓒ Collaborative   🏠 Community/Home Care

ineffective Breastfeeding

Taxonomy II: Role Relationships—Class 1 Caregiving
Roles (00104)
[Diagnostic Division: Food/Fluid]
Submitted 1988

Definition: Dissatisfaction or difficulty that a mother, infant, or child experiences with the breastfeeding process

Related Factors

Prematurity; [late preterm (35 to 37 weeks]; poor infant sucking reflex
Infant anomaly [cleft palate/lip, Down Syndrome, ankyloglossia (tongue tied)]
Infant receiving supplemental feedings with artificial nipple
Maternal anxiety or ambivalence
Deficient knowledge
Previous history of breastfeeding failure
Interrupted breastfeeding
Nonsupportive partner or family
Maternal breast anomaly; previous breast surgery; [infections]

Defining Characteristics

Subjective
Unsatisfactory breastfeeding process
Persistence of sore nipples beyond the first week of breastfeeding
Insufficient emptying of each breast per feeding
Inadequate/perceived inadequate milk supply

Objective
Insufficient opportunity for suckling at the breast
Infant inability to latch onto maternal breast correctly; unsustained suckling at the breast
Infant arching/crying at the breast; resisting latching on
Infant exhibiting fussiness/crying within the first hour after breastfeeding; unresponsive to other comfort measures
No observable signs of oxytocin release
Lack of infant weight gain; sustained infant weight loss

Information that appears in brackets has been added by the authors to clarify and enhance the use of nursing diagnoses.

Desired Outcomes/Evaluation Criteria— Client Will:

- Verbalize understanding of causative or contributing factors.
- Demonstrate techniques to enhance breastfeeding experience.
- Assume responsibility for effective breastfeeding.
- Achieve mutually satisfactory breastfeeding regimen with infant content after feedings, gaining weight appropriately, and output within normal range.

Actions/Interventions

Nursing Priority No. 1.

To identify maternal causative or contributing factors:

- Assess client knowledge about breastfeeding and extent of instruction that has been given.
- Identify cultural expectations and conflicts about breastfeeding and beliefs or practices regarding lactation, let-down techniques, and maternal food preferences.
- Note incorrect myths/misunderstandings especially in teenage mothers, **who are more likely to have limited knowledge and more concerns about body image issues.**
- Encourage discussion of current and previous breastfeeding experience(s).
- Note previous unsatisfactory experience (including self or others) **because it may lead to negative expectations.**
- Perform physical assessment, noting appearance of breasts and nipples, marked asymmetry of breasts, obvious inverted or flat nipples, or minimal or no breast enlargement during pregnancy.
- Determine whether lactation failure is primary (**i.e., maternal prolactin deficiency/serum prolactin levels, inadequate mammary gland tissue, breast surgery that has damaged the nipple, areola enervation [irremediable], and pituitary disorders**) or secondary (**i.e., sore nipples, severe engorgement, plugged milk ducts, mastitis, inhibition of let-down reflex, and maternal/infant separation with disruption of feedings [treatable]**). *Note:* **Overweight or obese women are 2.5 and 3.6 times less successful, respectively, in initiating breastfeeding than the general population.**
- Note history of pregnancy, labor, and delivery (vaginal or cesarean section), other recent or current surgery, preexisting medical problems (e.g., diabetes, seizure disorder, cardiac diseases, or presence of disabilities), or adoptive mother.

Information that appears in brackets has been added by the authors to clarify and enhance the use of nursing diagnoses.

- Identify maternal support systems or presence and response of SO(s), extended family, friends. **Infant's father and maternal grandmother (in addition to caring healthcare providers) are important factors that contribute to successful breastfeeding.**
- Ascertain mother's age, number of children at home, and need to return to work.
- Determine maternal feelings (e.g., fear/anxiety, ambivalence, depression).

Nursing Priority No. 2.

To assess infant causative/contributing factors:

- Determine suckling problems, as noted in Related Factors/Defining Characteristics.
- Note prematurity and/or infant anomaly (e.g., cleft lip/palate) **to determine special equipment/feeding needs.**
- Review feeding schedule to note increased demand for feeding (at least eight times a day, taking both breasts at each feeding for more than 15 minutes on each side) or use of supplements with artificial nipple.
- Evaluate observable signs of inadequate infant intake (e.g., baby latches onto mother's nipples with sustained suckling but minimal audible swallowing or gulping noted, infant arching and crying at the breasts with resistance to latching on, decreased urinary output and frequency of stools, inadequate weight gain).
- Determine whether baby is content after feeding or exhibits fussiness and crying within the first hour after breastfeeding, **suggesting unsatisfactory breastfeeding process.**
- Note any correlation between maternal ingestion of certain foods and "colicky" response of infant.

Nursing Priority No. 3.

To assist mother to develop skills of successful breastfeeding:

- Provide emotional support to mother. Use one-to-one instruction with each feeding during hospital stay and clinic or home visit. Refer adoptive mothers choosing to breastfeed to a lactation consultant **to assist with induced lactation techniques.**
- Discuss early infant feeding cues (e.g., rooting, lip smacking, and sucking fingers/hand) versus late cue of crying. **Early recognition of infant hunger promotes timely/more rewarding feeding experience for infant and mother.**

Information that appears in brackets has been added by the authors to clarify and enhance the use of nursing diagnoses.

- Inform mother how to assess and correct a latch if needed. Demonstrate asymmetric latch aiming infant's lower lip as far from base of the nipple as possible, then bringing infant's chin and lower jaw in contact with breast while mouth is wide open and before upper lip touches breast.
- Recommend avoidance or overuse of supplemental feedings and pacifiers (unless specifically indicated), **which can lessen infant's desire to breastfeed/increase risk of early weaning. Note: Adoptive mothers may not develop a full breast milk supply, necessitating supplemental feedings.**
- Restrict use of nipple shields (i.e., only temporarily to help draw the nipple out) and then place baby directly on nipple.
- Demonstrate use of hand expression, hand pump, and piston-type electric breast pump with bilateral collection chamber when necessary **to maintain or increase milk supply.**
- Discuss/demonstrate breastfeeding aids (e.g., infant sling, nursing pillows, or footstool).
- Suggest using a variety of nursing positions **to find the most comfortable for mother and infant. Positions particularly helpful for plus-sized women or those with large breasts include the "football" hold with infant's head to mother's breast and body curved around behind mother or lying down to nurse.**
- Encourage frequent rest periods, sharing household/childcare duties **to limit fatigue and facilitate relaxation at feeding times.**
- Recommend abstinence/restriction of tobacco, caffeine, alcohol, drugs, and excess sugar, as appropriate, **because they may affect milk production and let-down reflex or be passed on to the infant.**
- Promote early management of breastfeeding problems. For example:

  Engorgement: Wear a supportive bra, apply heat and/or cool applications to the breasts, and massage from chest wall down to nipple **to enhance let-down reflex;** soothe "fussy baby" before latching on the breast; properly position baby on breast/nipple; alternate the side baby starts nursing on; nurse round the clock and/or pump with piston-type electric breast pump with bilateral collection chambers at least 8 to 12 times a day; and avoid using bottle, pacifier, or supplements.

  Sore nipples: Wear 100% cotton fabrics; do not use soap or alcohol/other drying agents on nipples; avoid use of nipple shields or nursing pads that contain plastic; cleanse and then pat dry with a clean cloth; apply a thin layer of USP

Information that appears in brackets has been added by the authors to clarify and enhance the use of nursing diagnoses.

modified lanolin on the nipple, and administer a mild pain reliever as appropriate. **Note:** Infant should latch on least sore side or begin with hand expression **to establish let-down reflex;** properly position infant on breast/nipple and use a variety of nursing positions. Break suction after breastfeeding is complete.

Clogged ducts: Use larger bra or extender to avoid pressure on site; use moist or dry heat; gently massage from above plug down to nipple; nurse infant, hand express, or pump after massage; nurse more often on affected side.

Inhibited let-down: Use relaxation techniques before nursing (e.g., maintain quiet atmosphere, massage the breast, apply heat to breasts, have beverage available, assume a position of comfort, place infant on mother's chest skin-to-skin). Develop a routine for nursing, and encourage mother to enjoy her baby.

Mastitis: Promote bedrest (with infant) for several days; administer antibiotics; provide warm, moist heat before and during nursing; empty breasts completely, continuing to nurse baby at least 8 to 12 times a day or pump breasts for 24 hours and then resume breastfeeding as appropriate.

Nursing Priority No. 4.

To condition infant to breastfeed:

- Scent breast pad with breast milk and leave in bed with infant along with mother's photograph when separated from mother for medical purposes (e.g., prematurity).
- Increase skin-to-skin contact (kangaroo care).
- Provide practice times at breast for infant to "lick and learn."
- Express small amounts of milk into baby's mouth.
- Have mother pump breast after feeding to enhance milk production.
- Use supplemental nutrition system cautiously when necessary.
- Identify special interventions for feeding in presence of cleft lip/palate. **These measures promote optimal interaction between mother and infant and provide adequate nourishment for the infant, enhancing successful breastfeeding.**

Nursing Priority No. 5.

To promote wellness (Teaching/Discharge Considerations):

- Schedule follow-up visit with healthcare provider 48 hours after hospital discharge and 2 weeks after birth **for evaluation of milk intake/breastfeeding process and to answer mother's questions.**

Information that appears in brackets has been added by the authors to clarify and enhance the use of nursing diagnoses.

- Recommend monitoring number of infant's wet/soiled diapers. **Stools should be yellow in color, and infant should have at least six wet diapers a day to determine that the infant is receiving sufficient intake.**
- Weigh infant at least every third day initially as indicated and record **to verify adequacy of nutritional intake.**
- Educate father/SO about benefits of breastfeeding and how to manage common lactation challenges. **Enlisting support of father/SO is associated with a higher ratio of successful breastfeeding at 6 months.**
- Promote peer and cultural group counseling for teen mothers. **Provides positive role model that teen can relate to and feel comfortable discussing concerns/feelings.**
- Review mother's need for rest, relaxation, and time with other children as appropriate.
- Discuss importance of adequate nutrition and fluid intake, prenatal vitamins, or other vitamin/mineral supplements, such as vitamin C, as indicated.
- Address specific problems (e.g., suckling problems, prematurity facial anomalies).
- Discuss timing of introduction of solid foods and importance of delaying until infant is at least 4 months, preferably 6 months old. If supplementation is necessary, infant can be finger fed, spoon fed, cup fed, or syringe fed.
- Inform mother that return of menses within first 3 months after infant's birth may indicate inadequate prolactin levels.
- Refer to support groups (e.g., La Leche League, parenting support groups, stress reduction, or other community resources, as indicated).
- Provide bibliotherapy/appropriate Web sites for further information.

Documentation Focus

Assessment/Reassessment
- Identified assessment factors, both maternal and infant (e.g., engorgement present, infant demonstrating adequate weight gain without supplementation).

Planning
- Plan of care, specific interventions, and who is involved in planning.
- Teaching plan.

Information that appears in brackets has been added by the authors to clarify and enhance the use of nursing diagnoses.

Implementation/Evaluation
- Mother's/infant's responses to interventions, teaching, and actions performed.
- Changes in infant's weight and output.
- Attainment or progress toward desired outcome(s).
- Modifications to plan of care.

Discharge Planning
- Referrals that have been made and mother's choice of participation.

Sample Nursing Outcomes & Interventions Classifications (NOC/NIC)

NOC—Breastfeeding Establishment: Maternal [or] Infant
NIC—Breastfeeding Assistance

---

interrupted Breastfeeding

Taxonomy II: Role Relationships—Class 1 Caregiving
  Roles (00105)
[Diagnostic Division: Food/Fluid]
Submitted 1992

Definition: Break in the continuity of the breastfeeding process as a result of inability or inadvisability to put baby to breast for feeding

Related Factors

Maternal/infant illness
Infant prematurity
Maternal employment
Contraindications to breastfeeding (e.g., certain pharmaceutical agents, substance abuse, true breast milk jaundice, HIV positive)
Need to abruptly wean infant

Defining Characteristics

Subjective
Infant receives no nourishment at the breast for some or all feedings
Maternal desire to maintain breastfeeding for child's nutritional needs

---

Information that appears in brackets has been added by the authors to clarify and enhance the use of nursing diagnoses.

Maternal desire to provide breast milk for child's nutritional needs

Deficient knowledge about expression/storage of breast milk

Objective
Mother-child separation

Desired Outcomes/Evaluation Criteria— Client Will:

- Identify and demonstrate techniques to sustain lactation until breastfeeding is reinitiated.
- Achieve mutually satisfactory feeding regimen, with infant content after feedings and gaining weight appropriately.
- Achieve weaning and cessation of lactation if desired or necessary.

Actions/Interventions

Nursing Priority No. 1.
To identify causative/contributing factors:

- Assess client knowledge and perceptions about breastfeeding and extent of instruction that has been given.
- ∞• Note myths/misunderstandings, especially in some cultures and in teenage mothers, **who are more likely to have limited knowledge and concerns about body image issues.**
- • Ascertain cultural expectations/conflicts.
- Encourage discussion of current/previous breastfeeding experience(s). **Useful for determining efforts needed to continue breastfeeding, if desired, while circumstances interrupting process are resolved, if possible.**
- Determine maternal responsibilities, routines, and scheduled activities (e.g., caretaking of siblings, employment in/out of home, work/school schedules of family members, ability to visit hospitalized infant).
- Identify factors necessitating interruption, or occasionally cessation, of breastfeeding (e.g., maternal illness, drug use) and desire or need to wean infant. **In general, infants with chronic diseases benefit from breastfeeding. Only a few maternal infections (e.g., HIV, active/untreated tuberculosis for initial 2 weeks of multidrug therapy, active herpes simplex of the breasts, and development of chickenpox within 5 days prior to delivery or 2 days after delivery) are hazardous to breastfeeding infants. Also, the use of**

Information that appears in brackets has been added by the authors to clarify and enhance the use of nursing diagnoses.

⊕ Cultural ⊗ Collaborative 🏠 Community/Home Care

antiretroviral medications/chemotherapy agents or maternal substance abuse usually requires weaning of infant. Exposure to radiation therapy requires interruption of breastfeeding for length of time radioactivity is known to be present in breast milk and is therefore dependent on agent used. Note: Mother can "pump and dump" her breast milk to maintain supply and continue to breastfeed after her condition has resolved (e.g., chicken pox).

🏠• Determine support systems available to mother/family. **Infant's father and maternal grandmother, in addition to caring healthcare providers, are important factors that contribute to successful breastfeeding.**

Nursing Priority No. 2.

To assist mother to maintain breastfeeding if desired:

• Provide information as needed regarding need/decision to interrupt breastfeeding.

• Give emotional support to mother and support her decision regarding cessation or continuation of breastfeeding. **Many women are ambivalent about breastfeeding and providing information about the pros and cons of both breastfeeding and bottle feeding, along with support for the mother's/couple's decision, will promote a positive experience.**

∞• Promote peer counseling for teen mothers. **Provides positive role model that teen can relate to and feel comfortable with discussing concerns/feelings.**

🏠• Educate father/SO about benefits of breastfeeding and how to manage common lactation challenges. **Enlisting support of father/SO is associated with a higher ratio of successful breastfeeding at 6 months.**

• Discuss/demonstrate breastfeeding aids (e.g., infant sling, nursing footstool/pillows, hand expression, manual and/or piston-type electric breast pumps). **Enhances comfort and relaxation for breastfeeding. When circumstances dictate that the mother and infant are separated for a time, whether by illness, prematurity, or returning to work or school, the milk supply can be maintained by use of the pump. Storing the milk for future use enables the infant to continue to receive the value of breast milk. Learning the correct technique is important for successful use of the pump.**

• Suggest abstinence/restriction of tobacco, caffeine, excess sugar, alcohol, certain medications, all illicit drugs, as appropriate, when breastfeeding is reinitiated **because they may**

Information that appears in brackets has been added by the authors to clarify and enhance the use of nursing diagnoses.

affect milk production/let-down reflex or be passed on to the infant.

🏠 • Review techniques for expression and storage of breast milk **to provide optimal nutrition and promote continuation of breastfeeding process.**

• Problem-solve return-to-work (or school) issues or periodic infant care requiring bottle/supplemental feeding.

• Provide privacy/calm surroundings when mother breastfeeds in hospital/work setting. **Note: Federal Law 2010 requires an employer to provide a place and reasonable break time for an employee to express her breast milk for her baby for 1 year after birth.**

• Determine if a routine visiting schedule or advance warning can be provided **so that infant will be hungry/ready to feed.**

• Recommend using expressed breast milk instead of formula or at least partial breastfeeding for as long as mother and child are satisfied. **Prevents permanent interruption in breast-feeding, decreasing the risk of premature weaning.**

• Encourage mother to obtain adequate rest, maintain fluid and nutritional intake, continue her prenatal vitamins, and schedule breast pumping every 3 hours while awake as indicated **to sustain adequate milk production and breastfeeding process.**

Nursing Priority No. 3.
To promote successful infant feeding:

• Recommend/provide for infant sucking on a regular basis, especially if gavage feedings are part of the therapeutic regimen. **Reinforces that feeding time is pleasurable and enhances digestion.**

• Discuss proper use and choice of supplemental nutrition and alternate feeding methods (e.g., bottle/syringe) if desired.

• Review safety precautions (e.g., proper flow of formula from nipple, frequency of burping, holding bottle instead of propping, formula preparation, and sterilization techniques).

Nursing Priority No. 4.
🏠 To promote wellness (Teaching/Discharge Considerations):

• Identify other means (other than breastfeeding) of nurturing and strengthening infant attachment (e.g., comforting, consoling, play activities).

Information that appears in brackets has been added by the authors to clarify and enhance the use of nursing diagnoses.

- Explain anticipated changes in feeding needs/frequency. **Growth spurts require increased intake/more feedings by infant.**
- Refer to support groups (e.g., La Leche League or Lact-Aid), community resources (e.g., a public health nurse; a lactation specialist; Women, Infants, and Children program; and electric pump rental programs).
- Promote use of bibliotherapy/appropriate Web sites for further information.
- Discuss timing of introduction of solid foods and importance of delaying until infant is at least 4 months, preferably 6 months old, if possible. **American Academy of Pediatrics and the World Health Organization (WHO) recommend delaying solids until at least 6 months. If supplementation is necessary, infant can be finger fed, spoon fed, cup fed, or syringe fed.**

Nursing Priority No. 5.

To assist mother in the weaning process when desired:

- Provide emotional support to mother and accept decision regarding cessation of breastfeeding. **Feelings of sadness are common even if weaning is the mother's choice.**
- Discuss reducing frequency of daily feedings and breast pumping by one session every 2 to 3 days. **Preferred method of weaning, if circumstance permits, to reduce problems associated with engorgement.**
- Encourage wearing a snug, well-fitting bra, but refrain from binding breasts **because of increased risk of clogged milk ducts and inflammation.**
- Recommend expressing some milk from breasts regularly each day over a period of 1 to 3 weeks, if necessary, **to reduce discomfort associated with engorgement until milk production decreases.**
- Suggest holding infant differently during bottle feeding/ interactions or having another family member give infant's bottle feeding **to prevent infant rooting for breast and to prevent stimulation of nipples.**
- Discuss use of ibuprofen/acetaminophen **for discomfort during weaning process.**
- Suggest use of ice packs to breast tissue (not nipples) for 15 to 20 minutes at least four times a day **to help reduce swelling during sudden weaning.**

Information that appears in brackets has been added by the authors to clarify and enhance the use of nursing diagnoses.

Documentation Focus

Assessment/Reassessment

* Baseline findings of maternal and infant factors, including mother's milk supply and infant nourishment.
* Reason for interruption or cessation of breastfeeding.
* Number of wet/soiled diapers daily, log of intake and output, as appropriate; periodic measurement of weight.

Planning

* Method of feeding chosen.
* Plan of care and who is involved in planning.
* Teaching plan.

Implementation/Evaluation

* Maternal response to interventions, teaching, and actions performed.
* Infant's response to feeding and method.
* Whether infant appears satisfied or still seems to be hungry.
* Attainment or progress toward desired outcome(s).
* Modifications to plan of care.

Discharge Planning

* Plan for follow-up and who is responsible.
* Specific referrals made.

Sample Nursing Outcomes & Interventions Classifications (NOC/NIC)

NOC—Breastfeeding Maintenance
NIC—Lactation Counseling

---

readiness for enhanced **Breastfeeding**

Taxonomy II: Role Relationships—Class 1 Caregiving Roles (00106)
[Diagnostic Division: Food/Fluid]
Submitted 1990; Revision 2012

Definition: A pattern of proficiency and satisfaction of the mother-infant dyad that is sufficient to support the breastfeeding process and can be strengthened

---

Information that appears in brackets has been added by the authors to clarify and enhance the use of nursing diagnoses.

Defining Characteristics

Subjective
Mother reports satisfaction with the breastfeeding process

Objective
Mother able to position infant at breast to promote a successful latching-on response
Infant content after feedings
Regular/sustained suckling/swallowing at the breast
Appropriate infant weight patterns for age
Effective mother/infant communication patterns (infant feeding cues and maternal interpretation and response)
Signs/symptoms of oxytocin release are present
Adequate infant elimination patterns for age
Eagerness of infant to nurse

Desired Outcomes/Evaluation Criteria— Client Will:

- Verbalize understanding of breastfeeding techniques; good latch and lactogenesis.
- Demonstrate effective techniques for breastfeeding.
- Demonstrate family involvement and support.
- Attend classes, read appropriate materials, and access resources as necessary.
- Verbalizes understanding of the benefits of breast milk.

Actions/Interventions

Nursing Priority No. 1.
To determine individual learning needs:

- Assess mother's desires/plan for feeding infant. **Provides information for developing plan of care.**
- Assess mother's knowledge and previous experience with breastfeeding.
- Identify cultural beliefs/practices regarding lactation, let-down techniques, and maternal food preferences. **In Western cultures, the breast has taken on a sexual connotation, and some mothers may be embarrassed to breastfeed. While breastfeeding may be accepted, in some cultures, certain beliefs may affect specific feeding practices (e.g., in Mexican-American, Navajo, Filipino, and Vietnamese cul-**

Information that appears in brackets has been added by the authors to clarify and enhance the use of nursing diagnoses.

tures, colostrum is not offered to the newborn; breast-feeding begins only after the milk flow is established).

∞• Note myths/misunderstandings, especially in teenage mothers, **who are more likely to have limited knowledge, as well as concerns about body image issues.**

🏠• Monitor effectiveness of current breastfeeding efforts.

🏠• Determine support systems available to mother/family. **In addition to caring healthcare providers, infant's father and maternal grandmother are important factors in whether breastfeeding is successful.**

Nursing Priority No. 2.

To promote effective breastfeeding behaviors:

• Initiate breastfeeding within first hour after birth. **Throughout the first 2 hours after birth, the infant is usually alert and ready to nurse. Early feedings are of great benefit to mother and infant because oxytocin release is stimulated, helping to expel the placenta and prevent excessive maternal blood loss; the infant receives the immunological protection of colostrum, peristalsis is stimulated, lactation is accelerated, and maternal-infant bonding is enhanced.**

• Encourage skin-to-skin contact. Place infant on mother's stomach, skin-to-skin, after delivery.

• Demonstrate asymmetric latch aiming infant's lower lip as far from base of the nipple as possible, then bringing infant's chin and lower jaw in contact with breast while mouth is wide open and before upper lip touches breast. **This position allows the infant to use both tongue and jaw more effectively to obtain milk from the breast.**

• Demonstrate how to support and position infant (e.g., infant sling or nursing footstool or pillows).

• Observe mother's return demonstration. **Provides practice and the opportunity to correct misunderstandings and add additional information to promote optimal experience for breastfeeding.**

• Keep infant with mother **for unrestricted breastfeeding duration and frequency.**

• Encourage mother to follow a well-balanced diet containing an extra 500 calories/day, continue her prenatal vitamins, and to drink at least 2,000 to 3,000 mL of fluid/day. **There is an increased need for maternal energy, protein, minerals, and vitamins, as well as increased fluid intake during lactation.**

Information that appears in brackets has been added by the authors to clarify and enhance the use of nursing diagnoses.

🌐 Cultural   🔄 Collaborative   🏠 Community/Home Care

- Provide information as needed about early infant feeding cues (e.g., rooting, lip smacking, sucking and fingers/hand) versus the late cue of crying. **Early recognition of infant hunger promotes timely/more rewarding feeding experience for infant and mother.**
- Promote peer counseling for teen mothers. **Provides positive role model that teen can relate to and feel comfortable discussing concerns/feelings.**

Nursing Priority No. 3.

To enhance optimum wellness (Teaching/Discharge Considerations):

- Provide for follow-up contact or home visit 48 hours after discharge, as indicated or desired; repeat visits as necessary **to provide support and assist with problem-solving.**
- Recommend monitoring number of infant's wet diapers. **(Some pediatric care providers suggest that six wet diapers in 24 hours indicate adequate hydration.)**
- Encourage mother/other family members to express feelings/concerns, and Active-listen **to determine nature of concerns.**
- Educate father/SO about benefits of breastfeeding and how to manage common lactation challenges. **Enlisting support of father/SO is associated with higher ratio of successful breastfeeding at 6 months.**
- Review techniques for expression (breast pumping) and storage of breast milk **to help sustain breastfeeding activity.**
- Problem-solve return-to-work issues or periodic infant care requiring bottle/supplemental feeding.
- Recommend using expressed breast milk instead of formula or at least partial breastfeeding for as long as mother and child are satisfied.
- Explain changes in feeding needs/frequency. **Growth spurts require increased intake/more feedings by infant.**
- Review normal nursing behaviors of older breastfeeding infants/toddlers.
- Discuss importance of delaying introduction of solid foods until infant is at least 4 months, preferably 6 months old. **(Recommended by the American Academy of Pediatrics and the World Health Organization).**
- Recommend avoidance of specific medications or substances (e.g., estrogen-containing contraceptives, bromocriptine, nicotine, and alcohol) **that are known to decrease milk supply. Note: Small amounts of alcohol have not been shown to be detrimental.**

Information that appears in brackets has been added by the authors to clarify and enhance the use of nursing diagnoses.

- Emphasize the importance of client notifying healthcare providers, dentists, and pharmacists of breastfeeding status.
- Problem-solve return-to-work issues or periodic infant care requiring bottle or supplemental feeding. **Enables mothers who need or desire to return to work (for economic or personal reasons) or who simply want to attend activities without the infant to deal with these issues, thus allowing more freedom while maintaining adequate breastfeeding.**
- Refer to support groups, such as La Leche League, as indicated. Provide mother with phone number of support person or group prior to leaving the hospital.
- Refer to ND ineffective Breastfeeding for more specific information addressing challenges to breastfeeding, as appropriate.

Documentation Focus

Assessment/Reassessment
- Identified assessment factors (maternal and infant).
- Number of wet diapers daily and periodic weight measurement.

Planning
- Plan of care, specific interventions, and who is involved in the planning.
- Teaching plan.

Implementation/Evaluation
- Mother's response to actions, teaching plan, and actions performed.
- Effectiveness of infant's efforts to feed.
- Attainment or progress toward desired outcome(s).
- Modifications to plan of care.

Discharge Planning
- Long-term needs, referrals, and who is responsible for follow-up actions.

Sample Nursing Outcomes & Interventions Classifications (NOC/NIC)

NOC—Breastfeeding Maintenance
NIC—Lactation Counseling

Information that appears in brackets has been added by the authors to clarify and enhance the use of nursing diagnoses.

🌐 Cultural   🔄 Collaborative   🏠 Community/Home Care

ineffective Breathing Pattern

Taxonomy II: Activity/Rest—Class 4 Cardiovascular/
Pulmonary Responses (00032)
[Diagnostic Division: Respiration]
Submitted 1980; Revised 1996; Nursing Diagnosis Extension and Classification 1998, 2010

Definition: Inspiration and/or expiration that does not provide adequate ventilation

Related Factors

Neuromuscular dysfunction; spinal cord injury; neurological immaturity

Musculoskeletal impairment; bony/chest wall deformity

Anxiety; [panic attacks]

Pain

Neurological damage

Fatigue; [deconditioning]; respiratory muscle fatigue

Body position; obesity

Hyperventilation; hypoventilation syndrome [alteration of client's normal $O_2:CO_2$ ratio (e.g., lung diseases, pulmonary hypertension, airway obstruction, or O_2 therapy in chronic obstructive pulmonary disease (COPD)]

Defining Characteristics

Subjective
Feeling breathless

Objective
Dyspnea; orthopnea

Bradypnea; tachypnea

Alterations in depth of breathing

Prolonged expiration phases; pursed-lip breathing

Decreased minute ventilation; vital capacity

Decreased inspiratory/expiratory pressure

Use of accessory muscles to breathe; assumption of the three-point position

Altered chest excursion; [paradoxical breathing patterns]

Nasal flaring; [grunting]

Increased anterior-posterior diameter

Information that appears in brackets has been added by the authors to clarify and enhance the use of nursing diagnoses.

Desired Outcomes/Evaluation Criteria— Client Will:

- Establish a normal, effective respiratory pattern as evidenced by absence of cyanosis and other signs/symptoms of hypoxia, with arterial blood gasses (ABGs) within client's normal or acceptable range.
- Verbalize awareness of causative factors.
- Initiate needed lifestyle changes.
- Demonstrate appropriate coping behaviors.

Actions/Interventions

Nursing Priority No. 1.

To identify etiology/precipitating factors:

- Determine presence of factors/physical conditions as noted in Related Factors **that would cause breathing impairments.**
- ∞ ⊕ Identify age and ethnic group of client that may be at increased risk. **Respiratory ailments in general are increased in infants and children with neuromuscular disorders, the frail elderly, and persons living in highly polluted environments. Smoking (and potential for smoking-related disorders) is prevalent among such groups as Appalachians, African Americans, Chinese men, Latinos, and Arabs. Communities of color are especially vulnerable as they tend to live in areas (such as close to freeways or high traffic areas) with high levels of air toxins. People most at risk for infectious pneumonias include the very young and frail elderly.**
- Auscultate and percuss chest **to evaluate presence/characteristics of breath sounds and secretions.**
- Note rate and depth of respirations, type of breathing pattern (e.g., tachypnea, grunting, Cheyne-Stokes, other irregular patterns).
- Evaluate cough (e.g., tight or moist) and presence of secretions, **indicating possible obstruction.**
- Assist with/review results of necessary testing (e.g., chest x-rays, lung volumes/flow studies, and pulmonary function/sleep studies) **to diagnose presence/severity of lung diseases.**
- Review laboratory data, such as ABGs **(determines degree of oxygenation and carbon dioxide [CO_2] retention),** drug screens, and pulmonary function studies **(determines vital capacity/tidal volume).**

Information that appears in brackets has been added by the authors to clarify and enhance the use of nursing diagnoses.

- Note emotional responses (e.g., gasping, crying, reports of tingling fingers). **Anxiety may be causing or exacerbating acute or chronic hyperventilation.**
- Assess for concomitant pain/discomfort **that may restrict respiratory effort.**

Nursing Priority No. 2.

To provide for relief of causative factors:

- Administer oxygen at lowest concentration indicated and prescribed respiratory medications **for management of underlying pulmonary condition, respiratory distress, or cyanosis.**
- Suction airway, as needed, **to clear secretions.**
- Assist with bronchoscopy or chest tube insertion as indicated.
- Elevate head of bed and/or have client sit up in chair, as appropriate, **to promote physiological and psychological ease of maximal inspiration.**
- Encourage slower/deeper respirations, use of pursed-lip technique, and so on, **to assist client in "taking control" of the situation.**
- Monitor pulse oximetry, as indicated, **to verify maintenance/ improvement in O_2 saturation.**
- Maintain calm attitude while dealing with client and SO(s) **to limit level of anxiety.**
- Assist client in the use of relaxation techniques.
- Deal with fear/anxiety that may be present. (Refer to NDs Fear; Anxiety.)
- Encourage position of comfort. Reposition client frequently if immobility is a factor.
- Splint rib cage during deep-breathing exercises/cough, if indicated.
- Medicate with analgesics, as appropriate, **to promote deeper respiration and cough.** (Refer to NDs acute Pain; chronic Pain.)
- Encourage ambulation/exercise, as individually indicated.
- Avoid overeating/gas-forming foods **that may cause abdominal distention and impair breathing efforts.**
- Provide/encourage use of adjuncts, such as incentive spirometer, **to facilitate deeper respiratory effort.**
- Supervise use of respirator/diaphragmatic stimulator, rocking bed, apnea monitor, and so forth **when neuromuscular impairment is present.**

Information that appears in brackets has been added by the authors to clarify and enhance the use of nursing diagnoses.

🏠• Ascertain that client possesses and properly operates continuous positive airway pressure (CPAP) machine **when obstructive sleep apnea is causing breathing problems.**

∞• Maintain emergency equipment in readily accessible location and include age/size appropriate endotrachial/trach tubes (e.g., infant, child, adolescent, or adult) **when ventilatory support might be needed.**

Nursing Priority No. 3.

To promote wellness (Teaching/Discharge Considerations):

🏠• Review etiology of respiratory distress, treatment options, and possible coping behaviors.

🏠• Emphasize importance of good posture and effective use of accessory muscles **to maximize respiratory effort.**

🏠• Teach conscious control of respiratory rate, as appropriate.

🏠• Assist client in breathing retraining (e.g., diaphragmatic, abdominal breathing, inspiratory resistive, and pursed-lip), as indicated.

🏠• Recommend energy conservation techniques and pacing of activities.

⊕• Refer for general exercise program (e.g., upper and lower extremity endurance and strength training), as indicated, **to maximize client's level of functioning.**

🏠• Encourage adequate rest periods between activities **to limit fatigue.**

🏠• Discuss relationship of smoking to respiratory function. Stress importance of smoking cessation and a smoke-free environment.

⊕• Encourage client/SO(s) to develop a plan **for smoking cessation.** Provide appropriate referrals.

🏠• Review environmental factors (e.g., exposure to dust, high pollen counts, severe weather, perfumes, animal dander, household chemicals, fumes, secondhand smoke; insufficient home support for safe care) **that may require avoidance of triggers or modification of lifestyle or environment to limit impact on client's breathing.**

🏠• Encourage self-assessment and symptom management:

Use of equipment to identify respiratory decompensation, such as a peak flow meter.

Appropriate use of oxygen (dosage, route, and safety factors).

🔧 Medication regimen, including actions, side effects, and potential interactions of medications, over-the-counter (OTC) drugs, vitamins, and herbal supplements.

Adhere to home treatments such as metered-dose inhalers (MDIs), compressors, nebulizers, and chest physiotherapies.

Information that appears in brackets has been added by the authors to clarify and enhance the use of nursing diagnoses.

Dietary patterns and needs; access to foods and nutrients supportive of health and breathing.

Management of personal environment, including stress reduction, rest and sleep, social events, travel, and recreation issues.

Avoidance of known irritants, allergens, and sick persons.

 Immunizations against influenza and pneumonia.

Early intervention when respiratory symptoms occur, knowing what symptoms require reporting to medical providers, and seeking emergency care.

• Make referral to pulmonary rehabilitation programs, supply resources, and support groups/contact with individuals who have encountered similar problems.

Documentation Focus

Assessment/Reassessment
- Relevant history of problem.
- Respiratory pattern, breath sounds, use of accessory muscles.
- Laboratory values.
- Use of respiratory aids or supports, ventilator settings, and so forth.

Planning
- Plan of care, specific interventions, and who is involved in the planning.
- Teaching plan.

Implementation/Evaluation
- Response to interventions, teaching, actions performed, and treatment regimen.
- Mastery of skills; level of independence.
- Attainment or progress toward desired outcome(s).
- Modifications to plan of care.

Discharge Planning
- Long-term needs, including appropriate referrals and action taken, available resources.
- Specific referrals provided.

Sample Nursing Outcomes & Interventions Classifications (NOC/NIC)

NOC—Respiratory Status: Ventilation
NIC—Ventilation Assistance

Information that appears in brackets has been added by the authors to clarify and enhance the use of nursing diagnoses.

decreased Cardiac Output

Taxonomy II: Activity/Rest—Class 4 Cardiovascular/
   Pulmonary Responses (00029)
[Diagnostic Division: Circulation]
Submitted 1975; Revised 1996, 2000

Definition: Inadequate blood pumped by the heart to
meet the metabolic demands of the body. [**Note:** In a hypermetabolic state, although cardiac output may be
within normal range, it may still be inadequate to meet
the needs of the body's tissues. Cardiac output and tissue perfusion are interrelated, although there are differences. When cardiac output is decreased, tissue perfusion problems will develop; however, tissue perfusion
problems can exist without decreased cardiac output.]

Related Factors

Altered heart rate or rhythm
Altered stroke volume
Altered preload [e.g., decreased venous return]
Altered afterload [e.g., systemic vascular resistance]
Altered contractility [e.g., ventricular-septal rupture, ventricular
   aneurysm, papillary muscle rupture, and valvular disease]

Defining Characteristics

Subjective

Altered heart rate/rhythm: palpitations
Altered preload: fatigue
Altered afterload: [feeling breathless]
Altered contractility: orthopnea/paroxysmal nocturnal dyspnea
   [PND]
Behavioral/emotional: anxiety

Objective

Altered heart rate/rhythm: arrhythmias; tachycardia; bradycardia; EKG [electrocardiogram (ECG)] changes
Altered preload: Jugular vein distention (JVD); edema; weight
   gain; increased/decreased central venous pressure (CVP);
   increased/decreased pulmonary artery wedge pressure
   (PAWP); murmurs
Altered afterload: dyspnea; clammy skin; skin [and mucous
   membrane] color changes [cyanosis, pallor]; prolonged cap-

---

Information that appears in brackets has been added by the authors to clarify
and enhance the use of nursing diagnoses.

illary refill; decreased peripheral pulses; variations in blood pressure readings; increased/decreased systemic vascular resistance (SVR); increased/decreased pulmonary vascular resistance (PVR); oliguria

Altered contractility: crackles; cough; decreased cardiac output/cardiac index; decreased ejection fraction; decreased stroke volume index (SVI)/left ventricular stroke work index (LVSWI); S_3 or S_4 sounds [gallop rhythm]

Behavioral/emotional: restlessness

Desired Outcomes/Evaluation Criteria— Client Will:

- Display hemodynamic stability (e.g., blood pressure, cardiac output, renal perfusion/urinary output, peripheral pulses).
- Report/demonstrate decreased episodes of dyspnea, angina, and dysrhythmias.
- Demonstrate an increase in activity tolerance.
- Verbalize knowledge of the disease process, individual risk factors, and treatment plan.
- Participate in activities that reduce the workload of the heart (e.g., stress management or therapeutic medication regimen program, weight reduction, balanced activity/rest plan, proper use of supplemental oxygen, cessation of smoking).
- Identify signs of cardiac decompensation, alter activities, and seek help appropriately.

Actions/Interventions

Nursing Priority No. 1.

To identify causative/contributing factors:

- Review clients at risk as noted in Related Factors and Defining Characteristics, as well as individuals with conditions that stress the heart. **Acute or chronic conditions (e.g., multiple trauma, renal failure, brainstem trauma, spinal cord injures at T8 or above, alcohol or other drug abuse/overdose, and pregnancy with hypertensive state) may compromise circulation and place excessive demands on the heart.**
- ∞ Note age and ethnic-related cardiovascular considerations. **In infants, failure to thrive with poor ability to suck and feed can be indications of heart problems. Children with poor cardiac function are tachypneic, exercise intolerant, and may have episodes of syncope. When in the supine**

Information that appears in brackets has been added by the authors to clarify and enhance the use of nursing diagnoses.

position, pregnant women incur decreased vascular return during the second and third trimesters, potentially compromising cardiac output. Contractile force is naturally decreased in the elderly with reduced ability to increase cardiac output in response to increased demand. Also, arteries are stiffer, veins are more dilated, and heart valves are less competent, often resulting in systemic hypertension and blood pooling. Generally, higher risk populations for decreased cardiac output due to heart failure include African Americans, Hispanics, Native Americans, and recent immigrants from developing nations, directly related to the higher incidence and prevalence of hypertension and diabetes.

- Assess potential for/type of developing shock states: hematogenic, septicemic, cardiogenic, vasogenic, and psychogenic.
- Review diagnostic studies, including/not limited to: chest radiograph, cardiac stress testing, ECG, echocardiogram, cardiac output and ventricular ejection studies, and heart scan or catheterization. **For example, ECG may show previous or evolving MI, left ventricular hypertrophy, and valvular stenosis. Doppler flow echocardiogram showing an ejection fraction (EF) less than 40% is indicative of systolic dysfunction.**
- Review laboratory data (e.g., cardiac biomarkers, CBC, electrolytes, ABGs, blood urea nitrogen/creatinine (BUN/Cr), and cultures, such as blood/wound/secretions).

Nursing Priority No. 2.

To assess degree of debilitation:

- Evaluate client reports and evidence of extreme fatigue, intolerance for activity, sudden or progressive weight gain, swelling of extremities, and progressive shortness of breath **to assess for signs of poor ventricular function and/or impending cardiac failure.**
- Determine vital signs/hemodynamic parameters including cognitive status. Note vital sign response to activity or procedures and time required to return to baseline. **Provides baseline for comparison to follow trends and evaluate response to interventions.**
- Review signs of impending failure/shock, noting decreased cognition and unstable or subnormal blood pressure or hemodynamic parameters; tachypnea; labored respirations; changes in breath sounds (e.g., crackles, wheezing); distant or altered heart sounds (e.g., murmurs, dysrythmias); neck vein

---

Information that appears in brackets has been added by the authors to clarify and enhance the use of nursing diagnoses.

and peripheral edema; and reduced urinary output. **Early detection of changes in these parameters promotes timely intervention to limit degree of cardiac dysfunction.**
- Note presence of pulsus paradoxus, especially in the presence of distant heart sounds, **suggesting cardiac tamponade.**

Nursing Priority No. 3.
To minimize/correct causative factors, maximize cardiac output:

Acute Phase
- Keep client on bed or chair rest in position of comfort. (In a congestive state, semi-Fowler's position is preferred.) May raise legs 20 to 30 degrees in shock situation. **Decreases oxygen consumption and risk of decompensation.**
- Administer high-flow oxygen via mask or ventilator, as indicated, **to increase oxygen available for cardiac function/ tissue perfusion.**
- Monitor vital signs frequently **to note response to activities and interventions.**
- Perform periodic hemodynamic measurements, as indicated (e.g., arterial, CVP, pulmonary, and left atrial pressures and cardiac output).
- Monitor cardiac rhythm continuously **to note effectiveness of medications and/or assistive devices, such as implanted pacemaker or defibrillator.**
- Administer blood or fluid replacement, antibiotics, diuretics, inotropic drugs, antidysrhythmics, steroids, vasopressors, and/or dilators, as indicated. Evaluate response **to determine therapeutic, adverse, or toxic effects of therapy.**
- Restrict or administer fluids (IV/PO), as indicated. Provide adequate fluid/free water, depending on client needs,
- Assess urine ouput hourly or periodically; weigh daily, noting total fluid balance **to allow for timely alterations in therapeutic regimen.**
- Monitor rate of IV drugs closely, using infusion pumps, as appropriate, **to prevent bolus or overdose.**
- Decrease stimuli; provide quiet environment **to promote adequate rest.**
- Schedule activities and assessments **to maximize rest periods.**
- Assist with or perform self-care activities for client.
- Avoid the use of restraints whenever possible if client is confused. **May increase agitation and increase the cardiac workload.**

Information that appears in brackets has been added by the authors to clarify and enhance the use of nursing diagnoses.

- Use sedation and analgesics, as indicated, with caution **to achieve desired effect without compromising hemodynamic readings.**
- Maintain patency of invasive intravascular monitoring and infusion lines. Tape connections **to prevent air embolus and/or exsanguination.**
- Maintain aseptic technique during invasive procedures. Provide site care, as indicated.
- Alter environment/bed linens and administer antipyretics or cooling measures, as indicated, **to maintain body temperature in near-normal range.**
- Instruct client to avoid/limit activities that may stimulate a Valsalva response (e.g., isometric exercises, rectal stimulation, bearing down during bowel movement, spasmodic coughing), **which can cause changes in cardiac pressures and/or impede blood flow.**
- Encourage client to breathe in/out during activities that increase risk for the Valsalva effect; limit suctioning/stimulation of coughing reflex in intubated client; administer stool softeners when indicated.
- Provide psychological support. Maintain calm attitude, but admit concerns if questioned by the client. **Honesty can be reassuring when so much activity and "worry" are apparent to the client.**
- Provide information about testing procedures and client participation.
- Assist with special procedures, as indicated (e.g., invasive line placement, intra-aortic balloon pump insertion, pericardiocentesis, cardioversion, and pacemaker insertion).
- Explain dietary or fluid restrictions, as indicated.
- Refer to NDs risk for decreased cardiac Tissue Perfusion; risk for Autonomic Dysreflexia.

Nursing Priority No. 4.
To promote venous return:

Postacute/Chronic Phase
- Provide for adequate rest, positioning client for maximum comfort.
- Administer analgesics, as appropriate, **to promote comfort/rest.**
- Encourage relaxation techniques **to reduce anxiety and conserve energy.**
- Elevate legs when in a sitting position; apply sequential compression devices (SCDs), if indicated, **to enhance venous re-**

Information that appears in brackets has been added by the authors to clarify and enhance the use of nursing diagnoses.

🌐 Cultural 🅒 Collaborative 🏠 Community/Home Care

turn; use a tilt table or other circulatory support bed, as needed, **to prevent orthostatic hypotension.**

- Give skin care, provide sheepskin or special flotation mattress (e.g., air, water, gel, or foam), and assist with frequent position changes **to avoid the development of pressure sores.**
- Elevate edematous extremities and avoid restrictive clothing. Assure that support hose are individually fitted and appropriately applied.
- Increase activity levels as permitted by individual condition/physiological response.

Nursing Priority No. 5.
To maintain adequate nutrition and fluid balance:

- Provide for diet restrictions (e.g., low-sodium, bland, soft, low-calorie/fat diet, with frequent small feedings), as indicated.
- Note reports of anorexia or nausea and withhold oral intake, as indicated.
- Provide fluids and electrolytes, as indicated, **to minimize dehydration and dysrhythmias.**
- Monitor intake/output and calculate 24-hour fluid balance.

Nursing Priority No. 6.
To promote wellness (Teaching/Discharge Considerations):

- Note individual risk factors present (e.g., smoking, stress, obesity), and specify interventions for reduction of identified factors.
- Review specifics of drug regimen, diet, exercise/activity plan. Emphasize necessity for long-term medical management of cardiac conditions.
- Discuss significant signs/symptoms that require prompt reporting to healthcare provider (e.g., muscle cramps, headaches, dizziness, skin rashes), **which may be signs of drug toxicity and/or electrolyte loss, especially potassium.**
- Emphasize importance of regular medical follow-up care. Review "danger" signs requiring immediate physician notification (e.g., unrelieved or increased chest pain, functional decline, dyspnea, edema), **which may indicate deteriorating cardiac function, heart failure.**
- Encourage changing positions slowly, dangling legs before standing **to reduce risk for orthostatic hypotension.**
- Give information about positive signs of improvement, such as decreased edema, improved vital signs/circulation, **to provide encouragement.**

Information that appears in brackets has been added by the authors to clarify and enhance the use of nursing diagnoses.

🏠 • Teach home monitoring of weight, pulse, and/or blood pressure, as appropriate, **to detect change and allow for timely intervention.**

🌐 • Arrange time with dietitian **to determine/adjust individually appropriate diet plan.**

• Promote visits from family/SO(s) who provide positive social interaction.

🏠 • Encourage relaxing environment, using relaxation techniques, massage therapy, soothing music, and quiet activities.

🏠 • Instruct in stress management techniques, as indicated, including an appropriate rehabilitation and graded exercise program.

🌐 • Direct client and/or caregivers to resources for emergency assistance, financial help, durable medical supplies, and psychosocial support and respite, especially when client has impaired functional capabilities or requires supporting equipment (e.g., pacemaker, LVAD, or 24-hour oxygen).

🌐 • Identify resources for weight reduction, cessation of smoking, and so forth, **to provide support for change.**

• Refer to NDs Activity Intolerance [specify level]; deficient Diversional Activity; ineffective Coping; compromised family Coping; Sexual Dysfunction; acute or chronic Pain; imbalanced Nutrition; deficient or excess Fluid Volume; as indicated.

Documentation Focus

Assessment/Reassessment
• Baseline and subsequent findings and individual hemodynamic parameters, heart and breath sounds, ECG pattern, presence/strength of peripheral pulses, skin/tissue status, renal output, and mentation.

Planning
• Plan of care and who is involved in planning.
• Teaching plan.

Implementation/Evaluation
• Client's responses to interventions, teaching, and actions performed.
• Status and disposition at discharge.
• Attainment or progress toward desired outcome(s).
• Modifications to plan of care.

Information that appears in brackets has been added by the authors to clarify and enhance the use of nursing diagnoses.

Discharge Planning

- Discharge considerations and who will be responsible for carrying out individual actions.
- Long-term needs and available resources.
- Specific referrals made.

Sample Nursing Outcomes & Interventions Classifications (NOC/NIC)

NOC—Cardiac Pump Effectiveness
NIC—Hemodynamic Regulations

Caregiver Role Strain

Taxonomy II: Role Relationships—Class 1 Caregiving Roles (00061)
[Diagnostic Division: Social Interaction]
Submitted 1992; Nursing Diagnosis Extension and Classification Revision 1998, 2000

Definition: Difficulty in performing family/SO caregiver role

Related Factors

Care Receiver Health Status

Illness severity/chronicity
Unpredictability of illness course; instability of care receiver's health
Increasing care needs; dependency
Problem behaviors; psychological or cognitive problems
Addiction; substance abuse; codependency

Caregiving Activities

Discharge of family member to home with significant care needs (e.g., premature birth/congenital defect, frail elder poststroke)
Unpredictability of care situation; 24-hour care responsibilities; amount/complexity of activities; years of caregiving
Ongoing changes in activities

Caregiver Health Status

Physical problems; psychological or cognitive problems
Inability to fulfill one's own or others' expectations; unrealistic expectations of self

---

Information that appears in brackets has been added by the authors to clarify and enhance the use of nursing diagnoses.

Marginal coping patterns
Substance abuse; codependency

Socioeconomic
Competing role commitments
Alienation or isolation from others
Insufficient recreation

Caregiver-Care Receiver Relationship
Unrealistic expectations of caregiver by care receiver
History of poor relationship
Mental status of elder inhibiting conversation
Presence of abuse or violence

Family Processes
History of marginal family coping or family dysfunction

Resources
Inadequate physical environment for providing care (e.g., housing, temperature, safety)
Inadequate equipment for providing care; inadequate transportation
Insufficient finances
Inexperience with caregiving; insufficient time; physical energy; emotional strength; lack of support
Lack of caregiver privacy
Deficient knowledge about or difficulty accessing community resources; difficulty accessing formal assistance/support; inadequate community services (e.g., respite services or recreational resources)
Inadequate informal assistance/support
Caregiver is not developmentally ready for caregiver role

> **NOTE:** The presence of this problem may encompass other numerous problems/high-risk concerns, such as deficient Diversional Activity; Insomnia; Fatigue; Anxiety; ineffective Coping; compromised family Coping; disabled family Coping; Decisional Conflict [specify]; ineffective Denial; Grieving; Hopelessness; Powerlessness; Spiritual Distress; ineffective Health Maintenance; impaired Home Maintenance; ineffective Sexuality Pattern; readiness for enhanced family Coping; interrupted Family Processes; and Social Isolation. Careful attention to data gathering will identify and clarify the client's specific needs, which can then be coordinated under this single diagnostic label.

Information that appears in brackets has been added by the authors to clarify and enhance the use of nursing diagnoses.

🌐 Cultural   ✜ Collaborative   🏠 Community/Home Care

Defining Characteristics

Subjective

Caregiving Activities
Apprehension about possible institutionalization of care receiver, the future regarding care receiver's health or caregiver's ability to provide care, care receiver's care if caregiver is unable to provide care

Caregiver Health Status—Physical
Gastrointestinal upset; weight change
Headaches; fatigue

Caregiver Health Status—Emotional
Reports feeling depressed; anger; stress; frustration; increased nervousness
Disturbed sleep pattern; sleep deprivation
Lack of time to meet personal needs

Caregiver Health Status—Socioeconomic
Changes in leisure activities; refuses career advancement

Caregiver-Care Receiver Relationship
Reports difficulty watching care receiver go through the illness
Reports grief or uncertainty regarding changed relationship with care receiver

Family Processes—Caregiving Activities
Reports concerns about family members

Objective

Caregiving Activities
Difficulty performing/completing required tasks
Preoccupation with care routine
Dysfunctional change in caregiving activities

Caregiver Health Status—Physical
Rash
Hypertension; cardiovascular disease; diabetes

Caregiver Health Status—Emotional
Impatience; increased emotional lability; somatization
Ineffective coping

Information that appears in brackets has been added by the authors to clarify and enhance the use of nursing diagnoses.

Caregiver Health Status—Socioeconomic
Low work productivity; withdraws from social life

Family Processes
Family conflict

Desired Outcomes/Evaluation Criteria— Client Will:

- Identify resources within self to deal with situation.
- Provide opportunity for care receiver to deal with situation in own way.
- Express more realistic understanding and expectations of the care receiver.
- Demonstrate behavior/lifestyle changes to cope with and/or resolve problematic factors.
- Report improved general well-being, ability to deal with situation.

Actions/Interventions

Nursing Priority No. 1.
To assess degree of impaired function:

- Inquire about and observe physical condition of care receiver and surroundings, as appropriate.
- Assess caregiver's current state of functioning (e.g., hours of sleep, nutritional intake, personal appearance, demeanor).
- Determine use of prescription/over-the-counter drugs or alcohol to deal with situation.
- Identify safety issues concerning caregiver and care receiver.
- Assess current actions of caregiver and how they are viewed by the care receiver (e.g., caregiver may be trying to be helpful, but is not perceived as helpful; may be too protective or may have unrealistic expectations of care receiver). **May lead to misunderstanding and conflict.**
- Note choice and frequency of social involvement and recreational activities.
- Determine use and effectiveness of resources and support systems.

Nursing Priority No. 2.
To identify the causative or contributing factors relating to the impairment:

∞• Note presence of high-risk situations (e.g., elderly client with total self-care dependence or family with several small chil-

---

Information that appears in brackets has been added by the authors to clarify and enhance the use of nursing diagnoses.

dren with one child requiring extensive assistance due to physical condition/developmental delays). **May necessitate role reversal, resulting in added stress or place excessive demands on parenting skills.**

- Determine current knowledge of the situation, noting misconceptions and lack of information. **May interfere with caregiver/care receiver response to illness/condition.**
- Identify relationship of caregiver to care receiver (e.g., spouse/lover, parent/child, sibling, friend).
- Ascertain proximity of caregiver to care receiver. **Caregiver could be living in the home of care receiver (e.g., spouse or parent of disabled child) or be an adult child stopping by to check on elderly parent each day, providing support, food preparation/shopping, and assistance in emergencies. Either situation can be taxing.**
- Note care receiver's physical and mental condition, as well as the complexity of required therapeutic regimen. **Caregiving activities can be complex, requiring hands-on care, problem-solving skills, clinical judgment, and organizational and communication skills that can tax the caregiver.**
- Determine caregiver's level of involvement in/preparedness for the responsibilities of caring for the client and anticipated length of care.
- Ascertain caregiver's physical and emotional health and developmental level, as well as additional responsibilities of caregiver (e.g., job, raising family). **Provides clues to potential stressors and possible supportive interventions.**
- Use assessment tool, such as Burden Interview, when appropriate, **to further determine caregiver's coping abilities.**
- Identify individual cultural factors and impact on caregiver. **Helps clarify expectations of caregiver/receiver, family, and community.**
- Note codependency needs and enabling behaviors of caregiver.
- Determine availability/use of support systems and resources.
- Identify presence and degree of conflict between caregiver, care receiver, and family.
- Determine pre-illness and current behaviors that may be interfering with the care or recovery of the care receiver.

Nursing Priority No. 3.
To assist caregiver in identifying feelings and in beginning to deal with problems:

- Establish a therapeutic relationship, conveying empathy and unconditional positive regard. **A compassionate approach,**

Information that appears in brackets has been added by the authors to clarify and enhance the use of nursing diagnoses.

blending the nurse's expertise in healthcare with the caregiver's firsthand knowledge of the care receiver can provide encouragement, especially in a long-term difficult situation.

- Acknowledge difficulty of the situation for the caregiver/family. **Research shows that the two greatest predictors of caregiver strain are poor health and the feeling that there is no choice but to take on additional responsibilities.**

- Discuss caregiver's view of and concerns about situation, including quality of couple's relationship/presence of intimacy issues.

- Encourage caregiver to acknowledge and express feelings. Discuss normalcy of the reactions without using false reassurance.

- Discuss caregiver's and family members' life goals, perceptions, and expectations of self **to clarify unrealistic thinking and identify potential areas of flexibility or compromise.**

- Discuss impact of and ability to handle role changes necessitated by situation.

Nursing Priority No. 4.

To enhance caregiver's ability to deal with current situation:

- Identify strengths of caregiver and care receiver.

- Discuss strategies to coordinate caregiving tasks and other responsibilities (e.g., employment, care of children/dependents, or housekeeping activities).

- Facilitate family conference, as appropriate, **to share information and develop plan for involvement in care activities.**

- Identify classes and/or needed specialists (e.g., first aid/CPR classes, enterostomal/physical therapist).

- Determine need for, and sources of, additional resources (e.g., financial, legal, respite care, social, and spiritual).

- Provide information and/or demonstrate techniques for dealing with acting out, violent, or disoriented behavior. **Enhances safety of caregiver and care receiver.**

- Identify equipment needs or adaptive aids and resources **to enhance the independence and safety of the care receiver.**

- Provide contact person/case manager **to partner with care provider(s) in coordinating care, providing physical/social support, and assisting with problem-solving, as needed/desired.**

Information that appears in brackets has been added by the authors to clarify and enhance the use of nursing diagnoses.

Nursing Priority No. 5.

🏠 To promote wellness (Teaching/Discharge Considerations):

- Advocate for/assist caregiver to plan for and implement changes that may be necessary (e.g., home care providers, adult day care, placement in long-term care facility, hospice care).
- Support caregiver in setting practical goals for self (and care receiver) that are realistic for care receiver's condition/prognosis and caregiver's own abilities.
- Review signs of burnout (e.g., emotional/physical exhaustion; changes in appetite and sleep; and withdrawal from friends, family, life interests).
- Discuss/demonstrate stress management techniques (e.g., accepting own feelings/frustrations and limitations, talking with trusted friend, taking a break from situation) and importance of self-nurturing (e.g., eating and sleeping regularly and pursuing self-development interests, personal needs, hobbies, social activities, spiritual enrichment). **May provide care provider with options to look after self.**
- Encourage involvement in caregiver support group.
- 💊• Refer to classes/other therapies, as indicated.
- 💊• Identify available 12-step program, when indicated, **to provide tools to deal with enabling/codependent behaviors that impair level of function.**
- 💊• Refer to counseling or psychotherapy, as needed.
- Provide bibliotherapy of appropriate references **for self-paced learning** and encourage discussion of information.

Documentation Focus

Assessment/Reassessment

- Assessment findings, functional level or degree of impairment, caregiver's understanding and perception of situation.
- Identified risk factors.

Planning

- Plan of care and individual responsibility for specific activities.
- Needed resources, including type and source of assistive devices and durable equipment.
- Teaching plan.

Implementation/Evaluation

- Caregiver/receiver response to interventions, teaching, and actions performed.

Information that appears in brackets has been added by the authors to clarify and enhance the use of nursing diagnoses.

- Identification of inner resources, behavior, and lifestyle changes to be made.
- Attainment or progress toward desired outcome(s).
- Modifications to plan of care.

Discharge Planning
- Plan for continuation and follow-through of needed changes.
- Referrals for assistance and reevaluation.

Sample Nursing Outcomes & Interventions Classifications (NOC/NIC)

NOC—Caregiver Role Endurance
NIC—Caregiver Support

risk for Caregiver Role Strain

Taxonomy II: Role Relationships—Class 1 Caregiving Roles (00062)
[Diagnostic Division: Social Interaction]
Submitted 1992; Revised 2010

Definition: At risk for caregiver vulnerability for felt difficulty in performing the family caregiver role

Risk Factors

Illness severity of the care receiver; psychological or cognitive problems in care receiver; substance abuse codependency

Discharge of family member with significant home care needs; premature birth; congenital defect

Unpredictable illness course; instability in the care receiver's health

Duration of caregiving required; inexperience with caregiving; complexity/amount of caregiving tasks; caregiver's competing role commitments

Caregiver health impairment; psychological problems in caregiver

Caregiver is female, spouse

Caregiver is not developmentally ready for caregiver role [e.g., a young adult needing to provide care for middle-aged parent]; developmental delay of the care receiver or caregiver

Presence of situational stressors that normally affect families (e.g., significant loss, disaster or crisis, economic vulnerability, major life events)

Information that appears in brackets has been added by the authors to clarify and enhance the use of nursing diagnoses.

🌐 Cultural 😊 Collaborative 🏠 Community/Home Care

Inadequate physical environment for providing care (e.g., housing, transportation, community services, and equipment)

Family or caregiver isolation

Lack of respite or recreation for caregiver

Marginal family adaptation; family dysfunction prior to the caregiving situation

Marginal caregiver's coping patterns

Past history of poor relationship between caregiver and care receiver

Care receiver exhibits bizarre or deviant behavior

Presence of abuse or violence

> **NOTE:** A risk diagnosis is not evidenced by signs and symptoms, as the problem has not occurred; rather, nursing interventions are directed at prevention.

Desired Outcomes/Evaluation Criteria— Client Will:

- Identify individual risk factors and appropriate interventions.
- Demonstrate and initiate behaviors or lifestyle changes to prevent development of impaired function.
- Use available resources appropriately.
- Report satisfaction with current situation.

Actions/Interventions

Nursing Priority No. 1.

To assess factors affecting current situation:

∞• Note presence of high-risk situations (e.g., elderly client with total self-care dependence or several small children with one child requiring extensive assistance due to physical condition/developmental delays). **May necessitate role reversal, resulting in added stress or place excessive demands on parenting skills.**

- Identify relationship and proximity of caregiver to care receiver (e.g., spouse/lover, parent/child, friend).
- Note therapeutic regimen and physical and mental condition of care receiver **to ascertain potential areas of need (e.g., teaching, direct care support, respite).**
- Determine caregiver's level of responsibility, involvement in, and anticipated length of caring role.
- Ascertain physical and emotional health and developmental level, as well as additional responsibilities of caregiver (e.g.,

---

Information that appears in brackets has been added by the authors to clarify and enhance the use of nursing diagnoses.

job, school, raising family). **Provides clues to potential stressors and possible supportive interventions.**

- Use assessment tool, such as Burden Interview, when appropriate, **to further determine caregiver's abilities.**
- Identify strengths and weaknesses of caregiver and care receiver.
- Verify safety of caregiver/receiver.
- Discuss caregiver's and care receiver's views of and concerns about situation.
- Determine available supports and resources currently used.
- Note any codependency needs of caregiver.

Nursing Priority No. 2.
To enhance caregiver's ability to deal with current situation:

- Discuss strategies to coordinate care and other responsibilities (e.g., employment, care of children/dependents, housekeeping activities).
- Facilitate family conference, as appropriate, **to share information and develop plan for involvement in care activities.**
- Refer to classes and/or specialists (e.g., first aid/CPR classes, enterostomal/physical therapist) **for special training,** as indicated.
- Identify additional resources to include financial, legal, and respite care.
- Identify equipment needs/resources, adaptive aids **to enhance the independence and safety of the care receiver.**
- Identify contact person or case manager as needed **to coordinate care, provide support, and assist with problem solving.**
- Provide information and/or demonstrate techniques for dealing with acting out, violent, or disoriented behavior **to protect/prevent injury to caregiver and care receiver.**
- Assist caregiver to recognize codependent behaviors (e.g., doing things for others that others are able to do for themselves) and how these behaviors affect the situation.

Nursing Priority No. 3.
To promote wellness (Teaching/Discharge Considerations):

- Stress importance of self-nurturing (e.g., pursuing self-development interests, personal needs, hobbies, and social activities) **to improve/maintain quality of life for caregiver.**
- Advocate for and assist caregiver to plan and implement changes that may be necessary (e.g., home care providers,

---

Information that appears in brackets has been added by the authors to clarify and enhance the use of nursing diagnoses.

🌐 Cultural 😊 Collaborative 🏠 Community/Home Care

adult day care, eventual placement in long-term care facility, or hospice care).
- Review signs of burnout (e.g., emotional or physical exhaustion; changes in appetite and sleep; withdrawal from friends, family, or life interests).
- Discuss and demonstrate stress management techniques and importance of self-nurturing (e.g., pursuing self-development interests, personal needs, hobbies, social activities, spiritual enrichment). **May provide care provider with options to protect self/promote well-being.**
- Encourage involvement in caregiver/other specific support group(s).
- Provide bibliotherapy of appropriate references and encourage discussion of information.
- Refer to classes/therapists as indicated.
- Identify available 12-step program, when indicated, **to provide tools to deal with codependent behaviors that impair level of function.**
- Refer to counseling or psychotherapy as needed.

Documentation Focus

Assessment/Reassessment
- Identified risk factors and caregiver perceptions of situation.
- Reactions of care receiver and family.
- Involvement of family members and others.

Planning
- Treatment plan and individual responsibility for specific activities.
- Teaching plan.

Implementation/Evaluation
- Caregiver/receiver response to interventions, teaching, and actions performed.
- Attainment or progress toward desired outcome(s).
- Modifications to plan of care.

Discharge Planning
- Long-term needs and who is responsible for actions to be taken.
- Specific referrals provided for assistance/evaluation.

Information that appears in brackets has been added by the authors to clarify and enhance the use of nursing diagnoses.

Sample Nursing Outcomes & Interventions Classifications (NOC/NIC)

NOC—Caregiver Stressors
NIC—Caregiver Support

ineffective Childbearing Process

Taxonomy II: Sexuality—Class 3 Reproduction (00221)
[Diagnostic Division: Safety]
Submitted 2010

Definition: Pregnancy and childbirth process and care of the newborn that does not match the environmental context, norms, and expectations*

Related Factors

Deficient knowledge (e.g., of labor and delivery, newborn care); lack of realistic birth plan
Unplanned/unwanted pregnancy
Inconsistent/lack of prenatal health visits
Suboptimal maternal nutrition
Substance abuse
Lack of sufficient support systems
Lack of maternal confidence
Maternal powerlessness/psychological distress
Unsafe environment/domestic violence
Lack of appropriate role models or cognitive readiness for parenthood

Defining Characteristics

Subjective

During Pregnancy

Does not report appropriate prenatal lifestyle (e.g., nutrition, elimination, sleep, bodily movement, exercise, personal hygiene), managing unpleasant symptoms in pregnancy, appro-

---

*The original Japanese term for "childbearing" (*shussan ikujikoudou*), which encompasses both childbirth and rearing of the neonate. It is one of the main concepts of Japanese midwifery.

Information that appears in brackets has been added by the authors to clarify and enhance the use of nursing diagnoses.

priate physical preparations, realistic birth plan, availability of support systems

During Labor and Delivery

Does not report lifestyle (e.g., diet, elimination, sleep, bodily movement, personal hygiene) that is appropriate for the stage of labor, availability of support systems

After Birth

Does not report appropriate postpartum lifestyle (e.g., diet, elimination, sleep, bodily movement, exercise, or personal hygiene) or availability of support systems

Objective

During Pregnancy

Inconsistent/lack of prenatal health visits

Does not seek necessary knowledge (e.g., of labor and delivery, newborn care)

Does not access support systems appropriately

Failure to prepare necessary newborn care items; lack of respect for unborn baby

During Labor and Delivery

Does not respond appropriately to onset of labor; lacks proactivity during labor and delivery

Does not demonstrate attachment behavior to the newborn baby

Does not access support systems appropriately

After Birth

Does not demonstrate attachment behavior to the baby, appropriate baby feeding techniques, basic baby care techniques; does not provide safe environment for the baby

Does not demonstrate appropriate breast care

Does not access support systems appropriately

Desired Outcomes/Evaluation Criteria— Client Will:

- Demonstrate healthy pregnancy free of preventable complications.
- Engage in activities to prepare for birth process and care of newborn.
- Experience complication-free labor and childbirth.
- Verbalize understanding of care requirements to promote health of self and infant.

Information that appears in brackets has been added by the authors to clarify and enhance the use of nursing diagnoses.

Actions/Interventions

Nursing Priority No. 1.

To determine causative factors and individual needs:

Prenatal Concerns

• Determine maternal health/nutritional status, usual pregravid weight, and dietary pattern. **Research studies have found a positive correlation between pregravid maternal obesity and increased perinatal morbidity rates (e.g., hypertension and gestational diabetes) associated with preterm births and macrosomia.**

🖉• Note use of alcohol/other drugs and nicotine. **Maternal pregnancy complications and negative effects on the developing fetus are increased with the use of tobacco, alcohol, and illicit drugs. Note: Prescription medications may also be dangerous to the fetus, requiring a risk/benefit analysis for therapeutic choices and appropriate dosage.**

• Evaluate current knowledge regarding physiological and psychological changes associated with pregnancy.

• Identify involvement/response of child's father to pregnancy.

• Determine individual family stressors, economic situation/financial needs, and availability/use of resources **to identify necessary referrals**.

• Verify environmental well-being and safety of client/family. **Women experiencing intimate partner violence both prior to and/or during pregnancy are at higher risk for multiple poor maternal and infant health outcomes.**

🌐• Determine cultural expectations/beliefs about child bearing, self-care, and so on. Identify who provides support/instruction within the client's culture (e.g., grandmother/other family member, cuerandero/doula, or other cultural healer). Work with support person(s) as desired by client, using interpreter as needed. **Helps ensure quality and continuity of care because support person(s) can reinforce information provided.**

• Ascertain client's commitments to work, family, and self; roles/responsibilities within family unit; and use of supportive resources. **Helps in setting realistic priorities to assist client in making adjustments, such as changing work hours, shifting of household chores, curtailing some outside commitments.**

🌐• Determine client's/couple's perception of fetus as a separate entity and extent of preparations being made for this infant.

Information that appears in brackets has been added by the authors to clarify and enhance the use of nursing diagnoses.

🌐 Cultural   🐝 Collaborative   🏠 Community/Home Care

Absence of activities such as choosing a name or nicknaming the baby in utero and home preparations indicate lack of completion of psychological tasks of pregnancy. Note: Cultural or familial beliefs may limit visible preparations out of concern that a bad outcome might result.

Labor and Delivery Concerns

• Ascertain client's understanding and expectations of the labor process and who will participate/provide support.
• Determine presence/appropriateness of birth plan developed by client/couple and any associated cultural expectations/preferences. **Identifies areas to address to ensure that choices made are amenable to the specific care setting, reflect reality of client/fetal status, and accommodate individual wishes.**

Postpartum/Newborn Care Concerns

• Determine plan for discharge after delivery and home care support/needs. **Important to facilitate discharge and ensure client/infant needs will be met.**
• Assess mother's strengths and needs, noting age, relationship status, reactions of family members. **Identifies potential risk factors that may influence the client's/couple's ability to assume role of parenthood. For example, an adolescent still formulating goals and identity may have difficulty accepting the infant as a person. The single parent who lacks support systems may have difficulty assuming sole responsibility for parenting.**
• Ascertain nature of emotional and physical parenting that client/couple received during their childhood. **Parenting role is learned, and individuals use their own parents as role models. Those who experienced a negative upbringing or poor parenting may require additional support to meet the challenges of effective parenting.**

Nursing Priority No. 2.
To promote optimal maternal well-being:

Prenatal

• Emphasize importance of maternal well-being including discussion of nutrition, regular moderate exercise, comfort measures, rest, breast care, and sexual activity. **Fetal well-being is directly related to maternal health, especially during first trimester, when developing organ systems are most**

Information that appears in brackets has been added by the authors to clarify and enhance the use of nursing diagnoses.

vulnerable to injury from environmental or hereditary factors:

Review nutrition requirements and optimal prenatal weight gain to support maternal-fetal needs. **Inadequate prenatal weight gain and/or below normal prepregnancy weight increases the risk of intrauterine growth retardation (IUGR) in the fetus and delivery of a low-birth-weight (LBW) infant.**

Encourage moderate exercise such as walking or non-weight-bearing activities (e.g., swimming, bicycling) in accordance with client's physical condition and cultural beliefs. **Exercise tends to shorten labor, increases likelihood of a spontaneous vaginal delivery, and decreases need for oxytocin augmentation.**

Recommend a consistent sleep and rest schedule (e.g., 1- to 2-hour daytime nap and 8 hours of sleep each night) in a dark, comfortable room.

- Provide necessary referrals (e.g., dietitian, social services, supplemental nutrition assistance programs) as indicated. **Federal/state food programs promote optimal maternal, fetal, and infant nutrition.**

- Explain psychological reactions including ambivalence, introspection, stress reactions, and emotional lability as characteristic of pregnancy. **Helps client/couple understand mood swings and may provide opportunity for partner to offer support and affection at these times. Note: However, the stressors associated with pregnancy may lead to abuse/exacerbate existing abusive behavior.**

- Discuss personal situation and options, providing information about resources available to client. **Partner may be upset about an unplanned pregnancy, have financial concerns regarding supporting the child, or may even be jealous that attention is shifting to the unborn child, creating safety issues for client/family.**

- Identify reportable potential danger signals of pregnancy, such as bleeding, cramping, acute abdominal pain, backache, edema, visual disturbances, headaches, and pelvic pressure. **Helps client distinguish normal from abnormal findings, thus assisting her in seeking timely, appropriate healthcare.** (Refer to ND risk for disturbed Maternal-Fetal Dyad for additional interventions.)

Labor and Delivery

- Monitor labor progress, maternal and fetal well-being per protocol. Provide continuous intrapartal professional support/doula. **Fear of abandonment can intensify as labor pro-**

Information that appears in brackets has been added by the authors to clarify and enhance the use of nursing diagnoses.

gresses, and client may experience increased anxiety and or loss of control when left unattended.

- Identify client's support person/coach and ascertain that the individual is providing support the client requires. **The coach may be the client's husband/SO or doula and needs to provide physical and emotional support for the mother and aid in initiation of bonding with the neonate.**

Postpartum

- Promote sleep and rest. **Reduces metabolic rate and allows energy and oxygen to be used for healing process.**
- Ascertain client's perception of labor and delivery, length of labor, and client's fatigue level. **There is a correlation between length of labor and the ability of some clients to assume responsibility for self-care/infant-care tasks and activities.**
- Assess client's readiness for learning. Assist client in identifying needs. **The postpartum period provides an opportunity to foster maternal growth, maturation, and competence.**
- Provide information about self-care, including perineal care and hygiene; physiological changes, including normal progression of lochial flow; needs for sleep and rest; importance of progressive postpartum exercise program; role changes.
- Review nipple and breast care, special dietary needs for lactating mother, factors that facilitate or interfere with successful breastfeeding, use of breast pump and appropriate suppliers, proper storage of expressed milk or preparation/storage of formula, as indicated.
- Discuss normal psychological changes and needs associated with the postpartal period. **Client's emotional state may be somewhat labile at this time and often is influenced by physical well-being.**
- Discuss sexuality needs and plans for contraception. Provide information about available methods, including advantages/disadvantages.
- Reinforce importance of postpartum examination by healthcare provider and interim follow-up as appropriate. **A follow-up visit is necessary to evaluate recovery of reproductive organs, healing of episiotomy/laceration repair, general well-being, and adaptation to life changes.**

Nursing Priority No. 3.

To promote appropriate participation in childbearing process:

Prenatal

- Develop nurse-client relationship and maintain an open attitude toward beliefs of client/couple. **Acceptance is important**

Information that appears in brackets has been added by the authors to clarify and enhance the use of nursing diagnoses.

to developing and maintaining relationship and support-ing independence.

- Explain office visit routine and rationale for ongoing screen-ing and close monitoring (e.g., urine testing, blood pressure monitoring, weight, fetal growth). Emphasize importance of keeping regular appointments. **Reinforces relationship be-tween health assessment and positive outcomes for mother and baby.**

- Suggest father/siblings attend office visits and listen to fetal heart tones (FHT) as appropriate. **Promotes a sense of in-volvement and helps make baby a reality for family mem-bers.**

- Provide anticipatory guidance regarding health habits/lifestyle and employment concerns:

    Review physical changes to be expected during each trimes-ter. **Prepares client/couple for managing common dis-comforts associated with pregnancy.**

    Discuss signs/symptoms requiring evaluation by primary pro-vider during prenatal period (e.g., excessive vomiting, fe-ver, unresolved illness of any kind, and decreased fetal movement). **Allows for timely intervention.**

    Identify anticipatory adaptations for SO/family necessitated by pregnancy. **Family members will need to be flexible in adjusting own roles and responsibilities in order to assist client to meet her needs related to the demands of pregnancy.**

    Provide information about potential teratogens, such as al-cohol, nicotine, illicit drugs, the STORCH group of viruses (syphilis, toxoplasmosis, other, rubella, cytomegalovirus [CMV], herpes simplex), and HIV. **Helps client make in-formed decisions/choices about behaviors/environment that can promote healthy offspring. Note: Research sup-ports the attribution of a wide range of negative effects in the neonate to alcohol, recreational drug use, and smoking.**

- Provide information about need for additional laboratory stud-ies, diagnostic tests, or procedure(s). Review risks and poten-tial side effects **to facilitate decision-making process.**

- Discuss signs of labor onset; how to distinguish between false and true labor, when to notify healthcare provider, and when to leave for birth center/hospital as appropriate; and stages of labor and delivery. **Helps ensure timely arrival and en-hances coping with labor/delivery process.**

Information that appears in brackets has been added by the authors to clarify and enhance the use of nursing diagnoses.

- Determine anticipated infant feeding plan. Discuss physiology and benefits of breastfeeding.
- Encourage attendance at prenatal and childbirth classes. Provide information about father/sibling or grandparent participation in classes and delivery if client desires.

Labor and Delivery

- Support use of positive coping mechanisms. **Enhances feelings of competence and fosters self-esteem.**
- Demonstrate behaviors and techniques (e.g., breathing, focused imagery, music, other distractions; aromatherapy; abdominal effleurage, back or leg rubs, sacral pressure, repositioning, back rest; oral care, linen changes, shower/tub use) that partner can use **to assist with pain control and relaxation.**
- Discuss available analgesics, appropriate timing, usual responses and side effects (client and fetal), and duration of analgesia effect in light of current situation. **Allows client to make informed choices about means of pain control and can allay client's fears and anxieties about medication use**.
- Honor client's decision about the use or nonuse of medication in a nonjudgmental manner. Continue encouragement for efforts and use of relaxation techniques. **Enhances client's sense of control and may prevent or decrease need for medication.**

After Birth

- Monitor and document the client's/couple's interactions with infant. Note presence of bonding acquaintance behaviors (e.g., making eye contact, using a high-pitched voice and en face [face-to-face] position as culturally appropriate, calling infant by name, and holding infant closely).
- Initiate early breastfeeding or oral feeding according to facility protocol and client preference. **Initiating feeding for breastfed infants usually occurs in the delivery room. Otherwise, 5 to 15 mL of sterile water may be offered in the nursery to assess effectiveness of sucking, swallowing, gag reflexes, and patency of esophagus.**
- Provide for unlimited participation of father and siblings. Ascertain whether siblings attended orientation program. **Facilitates family development and ongoing process of acquaintance.**

Information that appears in brackets has been added by the authors to clarify and enhance the use of nursing diagnoses.

ineffective CHILDBEARING PROCESS

To promote optimal well-being of newborn (Teaching/ Discharge Considerations):

• Provide information about newborn interactional capabilities, states of consciousness, and means of stimulating cognitive development. **Helps parents recognize and respond to infant cues during interactional process and fosters optimal interaction, attachment behaviors, and cognitive development in infant.**

• Note father's/partner's response to birth and to parenting role. **Client's ability to adapt positively to parenting may be strongly influenced by partner's reaction.**

• Discuss normal variations and characteristics of infant, such as caput succedaneum, cephalohematoma, pseudomenstruation, breast enlargement, physiological jaundice, and milia. **Helps parents recognize normal variations and may reduce anxiety.**

• Demonstrate/supervise infant care activities related to feeding and holding; bathing, diapering, and clothing; care of umbilical cord stump; and care of circumcised male infant.

• Note frequency, amount, and length of feedings. Encourage demand feedings instead of scheduled feedings. Note frequency, amount, and appearance of regurgitation. **Hunger and length of time between feedings vary from feeding to feeding, and excessive regurgitation increases replacement needs.**

• Evaluate neonate and maternal satisfaction following feedings. **Provides opportunity to answer client questions, offer encouragement for efforts, identify needs, and problem-solve situations.**

• Appraise level of parent's understanding of physiological needs and adaptation to extrauterine life associated with maintenance of body temperature, nutrition, respiratory needs, and bowel and bladder functioning.

• Emphasize newborn's need for follow-up laboratory tests, regular evaluations by healthcare provider, and timely immunizations.

• Identify manifestations of illness and infection and when to contact healthcare provider. Demonstrate proper technique for taking temperature, administering oral medication, or providing other care activities for infant as required. **Early recognition of illness and prompt use of healthcare facilitate timely treatment and positive outcomes.**

Information that appears in brackets has been added by the authors to clarify and enhance the use of nursing diagnoses.

- Provide oral and written/pictorial information and reliable Web sites about infant care and development, feeding, and safety issues. Offer appropriate resources in client's dominant language and reflecting cultural beliefs. **Maximizes learning, providing opportunity to review information as needed.**
- Refer breastfeeding client to lactation consultant/support group (e.g., La Leche League, Lact-Aid) **to promote a successful breastfeeding outcome.**
- Discuss available community support groups/parenting class as indicated. **Increases parents' knowledge of child rearing and child development and provides supportive atmosphere while parents incorporate new roles.**

Documentation Focus

Assessment/Reassessment
- Assessment findings, general health, previous pregnancy experience, any safety concerns.
- Knowledge of pre/postpartum needs and newborn care.
- Cultural beliefs and expectations.
- Specific birth plan and individuals to be involved in delivery.
- Arrangement for postpartum period and preparation for newborn.

Planning
- Plan of care and who is involved in planning.
- Individual teaching plans for pregnancy, labor/delivery, postpartum self-care, and infant care.

Implementation/Evaluation
- Response to interventions, teaching, and actions performed.
- Attainment or progress toward desired outcomes.
- Modifications to plan of care.

Discharge Planning
- Long-term needs and who is responsible for actions to be taken.
- Available resources, specific referrals made.

Sample Nursing Outcomes & Interventions Classifications (NOC/NIC)

NOC—Childbirth Preparation
NIC—Knowledge: Pregnancy

Information that appears in brackets has been added by the authors to clarify and enhance the use of nursing diagnoses.

readiness for enhanced Childbearing Process

Taxonomy II: Sexuality—Class 3 Reproduction (00208)
[Diagnostic Division: Safety]
Submitted 2008

Definition: A pattern of preparing for and maintaining a healthy pregnancy, childbirth process, and care of the newborn that is sufficient for ensuring well-being and can be strengthened

Defining Characteristics

During Pregnancy

Subjective
Reports appropriate prenatal lifestyle (e.g., nutrition, elimination, sleep, bodily movement, exercise, personal hygiene), a realistic birth plan, appropriate physical preparations, availability of support systems
Reports managing unpleasant symptoms in pregnancy

Objective
Attends regular prenatal health visits
Demonstrates respect for unborn baby; prepares necessary newborn care items
Seeks necessary knowledge (e.g., of labor and delivery, newborn care)

During Labor and Delivery

Subjective
Reports lifestyle (e.g., diet, elimination, sleep, bodily movement, personal hygiene) that is appropriate for the stage of labor

Objective
Responds appropriately to onset of labor
Is proactive in labor and delivery; uses relaxation techniques appropriate for stage of labor; utilizes support systems appropriately
Demonstrates attachment behavior to the newborn baby

After Birth

Subjective
Reports appropriate postpartum lifestyle (e.g., diet, elimination, sleep, bodily movement, exercise, personal hygiene)

Information that appears in brackets has been added by the authors to clarify and enhance the use of nursing diagnoses.

🌐 Cultural   ㊂ Collaborative   🏠 Community/Home Care

Objective

Demonstrates attachment behavior to the baby, basic baby care techniques, appropriate baby feeding techniques

Provides safe environment for the baby

Utilizes support systems appropriately

Demonstrates appropriate breast care

Desired Outcomes/Evaluation Criteria— Client Will (Include Specific Time Frame)

* Demonstrate healthy pregnancy free of preventable complications.
* Engage in activities to prepare for birth process and care of newborn.
* Experience complication-free labor and childbirth.
* Verbalize understanding of care requirements to promote health of self and infant.

Actions/Interventions

Nursing Priority No. 1.

To determine individual needs:

Prenatal

* Evaluate current knowledge and cultural beliefs regarding normal physiological and psychological changes of pregnancy, as well as beliefs about activities, self-care, and so on.
* Determine degree of motivation for learning. **Client may have difficulty learning unless the need for it is clear.**
* Identify who provides support/instruction within the client's culture (e.g., grandmother/other family member, cuerandero/doula, other cultural healer). Work with support person(s) when possible, using interpreter as needed. **Helps ensure quality and continuity of care because support person(s) may be more successful than the healthcare provider in communicating information.**
* Determine client's commitments to work, family, community, and self; roles/responsibilities within family unit; and use of supportive resources. **Helps in setting realistic priorities to assist client in making adjustments, such as changing work hours, shifting of household chores, curtailing some outside commitments.**
* Evaluate the client's/couple's response to pregnancy, individual and family stressors, and cultural implications of pregnancy/childbirth. **The ability to adapt positively**

Information that appears in brackets has been added by the authors to clarify and enhance the use of nursing diagnoses.

depends on support systems, cultural beliefs, resources, and effective coping mechanisms developed in dealing with past stressors.

- Determine client's/couple's perception of fetus as a separate entity and extent of preparations being made for this infant. **Activities such as choosing a name or nicknaming the baby in utero and home preparations indicate completion of psychological tasks of pregnancy. Note: Cultural or familial beliefs may limit visible preparations out of concern that a bad outcome might result.**

- Assess economic situation and financial needs to make necessary referrals.

- Determine usual pregravid weight and dietary patterns. **Research studies have found a positive correlation between pregravid maternal obesity and increased perinatal morbidity rates (e.g., hypertension and gestational diabetes) associated with preterm births and macrosomia.**

Labor and Delivery

- Ascertain client's understanding and expectations of the labor process.

- Review birth plan developed by client/partner. Note cultural expectations and preferences. **Verifies that choices made are amenable to the specific care setting, accommodate individual wishes, and reflect client/fetal status.**

Postpartum/Newborn Care

- Determine plan for discharge after delivery and home care support/needs. **Early planning can facilitate discharge and help ensure that client/infant needs will be met.**

- Ascertain client's perception of labor and delivery, length of labor, and client's fatigue level. **There is a correlation between length of labor and the ability of some clients to assume responsibility for self-care/infant care tasks and activities.**

- Assess mother's strengths and needs, noting age, marital status/relationship, presence and reaction of siblings and other family members, available sources of support, and cultural background. **Identifies potential risk factors and sources of support, which influence the client's/couple's ability to assume role of parenthood. For example, an adolescent still formulating goals and an identity may have difficulty accepting the infant as a person. The single parent who lacks support systems may have difficulty assuming sole responsibility for parenting.**

Information that appears in brackets has been added by the authors to clarify and enhance the use of nursing diagnoses.

Cultural   Collaborative   Community/Home Care

- Appraise level of parent's understanding of infant's physiological needs and adaptation to extrauterine life associated with maintenance of body temperature, nutrition, respiratory needs, and bowel and bladder functioning.
- Evaluate nature of emotional and physical parenting that client/couple received during their childhood. **The parenting role is learned, and individuals use their own parents as role models. Those who experienced a negative upbringing or poor parenting may require additional support to meet the challenges of effective parenting.**
- Note father's/partner's response to birth and to parenting role. **Client's ability to adapt positively to parenting may be strongly influenced by the father's/partner's reaction.**
- Assess client's readiness and motivation for learning. Assist client/couple in identifying needs. **The postpartal period provides an opportunity to foster maternal growth, maturation, and competence.**

Nursing Priority No. 2.

To promote maximum participation in childbearing process:

Prenatal

- Maintain open attitude toward beliefs of client/couple. **Acceptance is important to developing and maintaining relationship and supporting independence.**
- Explain office visit routine, rationale for ongoing screening and close monitoring (e.g., urine testing, blood pressure monitoring, weight, and fetal growth). Emphasize importance of keeping regular appointments. **Reinforces relationship between health assessment and positive outcome for mother and baby.**
- Suggest father and siblings attend prenatal office visits and listen to fetal heart tones (FHT) as appropriate. **Promotes a sense of involvement and helps make baby a reality for family members.**
- Provide information about need for additional laboratory studies, diagnostic tests, or procedure(s). Review risks and potential side effects.
- Discuss any medications that may be needed to control or treat medical conditions. **Helpful in choosing treatment options because need must be weighed against possible harmful effects on the fetus.**
- Provide anticipatory guidance, including discussion of nutrition, regular moderate exercise, comfort measures, rest,

---

Information that appears in brackets has been added by the authors to clarify and enhance the use of nursing diagnoses.

employment, breast care, sexual activity, and health habits/lifestyle. **Information encourages acceptance of responsibility and promotes self-care:**

Review nutrition requirements and optimal prenatal weight gain to support maternal-fetal needs. **Inadequate prenatal weight gain and/or below normal prepregnancy weight increases the risk of intrauterine growth restriction (IUGR) in the fetus and delivery of a low-birth-weight (LBW) infant.**

Encourage moderate exercise such as walking, or non-weight-bearing activities (e.g., swimming or bicycling) in accordance with client's physical condition and cultural beliefs. **Tends to shorten labor, increases likelihood of a spontaneous vaginal delivery, and decreases need for oxytocin augmentation.**

Recommend a consistent sleep and rest schedule (e.g., 1- to 2-hour daytime nap and 8 hours of sleep each night) in a dark, comfortable room.

Identify anticipatory adaptations for SO/family necessitated by pregnancy. **Family members will need to be flexible in adjusting own roles and responsibilities in order to assist client to meet her needs related to the demands of pregnancy.**

Provide/reinforce information about potential teratogens, such as alcohol, nicotine, illicit drugs, the STORCH group of viruses (syphilis, toxoplasmosis, other, rubella, cytomegalovirus, herpes simplex), and HIV. **Helps client make informed decisions/choices about behaviors/environment that can promote healthy offspring. Note: Research supports the attribution of a wide range of negative effects in the neonate to alcohol, recreational drug use, and smoking.**

- Use various methods for learning, including pictures, to discuss fetal development. **Visualization enhances reality of child and strengthens learning process.**

- Discuss signs of labor onset, how to distinguish between false and true labor, when to notify healthcare provider and to leave for hospital/birth center, and stages of labor/delivery. **Helps ensure timely arrival and enhances coping with labor/delivery process.**

- Review signs/symptoms requiring evaluation by primary provider during prenatal period (e.g., excessive vomiting, fever, unresolved illness of any kind, decreased fetal movement). **Allows for timely intervention.**

Information that appears in brackets has been added by the authors to clarify and enhance the use of nursing diagnoses.

🌐 Cultural 🅐 Collaborative 🏠 Community/Home Care

Labor and Delivery
- Identify client's support person/coach and ascertain that the individual is providing support that client requires. **Coach may be client's husband/SO or doula, and support can take the form of physical and emotional support for the mother and aid in initiation of bonding with the neonate.**
- Demonstrate or review behaviors and techniques (e.g., breathing, focused imagery, music, other distractions; aromatherapy; abdominal effleurage, back or leg rubs, sacral pressure, repositioning, and back rest; oral and perineal care and linen changes; and shower/hot tub use) that the partner can use **to assist with pain control and relaxation.**
- Discuss available analgesics, usual responses and side effects (client and fetal), and duration of analgesic effect in light of current situation. **Allows client to make informed choice about means of pain control; can allay client's fears and anxieties about medication use.**
- Support client's decision about the use or nonuse of medication in a nonjudgmental manner. Continue encouragement for efforts and use of relaxation techniques. **Enhances client sense of control and may prevent or decrease need for medication.**

Postpartum/Newborn Care
- Initiate early breastfeeding or oral feeding according to hospital protocol. **Initial feeding for breastfed infants usually occurs in the delivery room. Otherwise, 5 to 15 mL of sterile water may be offered in the nursery to assess effectiveness of suckling, swallowing, gag reflexes, and patency of esophagus.**
- Note frequency, amount, and length of feedings. Encourage demand feedings instead of scheduled feedings. Note frequency, amount, and appearance of regurgitation. **Hunger and length of time between feedings vary from feeding to feeding, and excessive regurgitation increases replacement needs.**
- Evaluate neonate and maternal satisfaction following feedings. **Provides opportunity to answer client questions, offer encouragement for efforts, identify needs, and problem-solve situations.**
- Demonstrate and supervise infant care activities related to feeding and holding; bathing, diapering, and clothing; care of circumcised male infant; and care of umbilical cord stump. Provide written/pictorial information for parents to refer to after discharge.

Information that appears in brackets has been added by the authors to clarify and enhance the use of nursing diagnoses.

- Provide information about newborn interactional capabilities, states of consciousness, and means of stimulating cognitive development. **Helps parents recognize and respond to infant cues during interactional process; fosters optimal interaction, attachment behaviors, and cognitive development in infant.**
- Promote sleep and rest. **Reduces metabolic rate and allows nutrition and oxygen to be used for healing process rather than for energy needs.**
- Provide for unlimited participation for father and siblings. Ascertain whether siblings attended an orientation program. **Facilitates family development and ongoing process of acquaintance and attachment.**
- Monitor and document the client's/couple's interactions with infant. Note presence of bonding or acquaintance behaviors (e.g., making eye contact, using high-pitched voice and en face [face-to-face] position as culturally appropriate, calling infant by name, and holding infant closely).

Nursing Priority No. 3.
To enhance optimal well-being:

Prenatal
- Emphasize importance of maternal well-being. **Fetal well-being is directly related to maternal well-being, especially during the first trimester, when developing organ systems are most vulnerable to injury from environmental or hereditary factors.**
- Review physical changes to be expected during each trimester. **Prepares client/couple for managing common discomforts associated with pregnancy.**
- Explain psychological reactions including ambivalence, introspection, stress reactions, and emotional lability as characteristic of pregnancy. **Helps client/couple understand mood swings and may provide opportunities for partner to offer support and affection at these times.**
- Provide necessary referrals (e.g., dietitian, social services, food stamps, or Women, Infants, and Children [WIC] food programs) as indicated. **Supplemental federally funded food program helps promote optimal maternal, fetal, and infant nutrition.**
- Review reportable danger signals of pregnancy, such as bleeding, cramping, acute abdominal pain, backache, edema, visual disturbance, headaches, and pelvic pressure. **Helps client dis-**

Information that appears in brackets has been added by the authors to clarify and enhance the use of nursing diagnoses.

tinguish normal from abnormal findings, thus assisting her in seeking timely, appropriate healthcare.

- Encourage attendance at prenatal and childbirth classes. Provide information about father/sibling or grandparent participation in classes and delivery if client desires.
- Provide list of appropriate reading materials for client, couple, and siblings regarding adjusting to newborn. **Information helps individual realistically analyze changes in family structure, roles, and behaviors.**

Labor and Delivery

- Monitor labor progress and maternal and fetal well-being per protocol. Provide continuous intrapartal professional support/doula. **Fear of abandonment can intensify as labor progresses, and client may experience increased anxiety and/or loss of control when left unattended.**
- Reinforce use of positive coping mechanisms. **Enhances feelings of competence and fosters self-esteem.**

Postpartum/Newborn Care

- Provide information about self-care, including perineal care and hygiene; physiological changes, including normal progression of lochial discharge; needs for sleep and rest; importance of progressive postpartal exercise program; role changes.
- Review normal psychological changes and needs associated with the postpartal period. **Client's emotional state may be somewhat labile at this time and often is influenced by physical well-being.**
- Discuss sexuality needs and plans for contraception. Provide information about available methods, including advantages and disadvantages.
- Reinforce importance of postpartal examination by healthcare provider and interim follow-up as appropriate. **Follow-up visit is necessary to evaluate recovery of reproductive organs, healing of episiotomy/laceration repair, general well-being, and adaptation to life changes.**
- Provide oral and written information about infant care and development, feeding, and safety issues.
- Offer appropriate references reflecting cultural beliefs.
- Discuss physiology and benefits of breastfeeding, nipple and breast care, special dietary needs, factors that facilitate or interfere with successful breastfeeding, use of breast pump, and appropriate suppliers. **Helps ensure adequate milk supply, prevents nipple cracking and soreness, facilitates comfort, and establishes role of breastfeeding mother.**

Information that appears in brackets has been added by the authors to clarify and enhance the use of nursing diagnoses.

- Refer client to support groups (e.g., La Leche League, Lact-Aid) or lactation consultant **to promote a successful breast-feeding outcome.**
- Identify available community resources as indicated (e.g., WIC program). **WIC and other federal programs support well-being through client education and enhanced nutritional intake for infant.**
- Discuss normal variations and characteristics of infant, such as caput succedaneum, cephalohematoma, pseudomenstruation, breast enlargement, physiological jaundice, and milia. **Helps parents recognize normal variations and may reduce anxiety.**
- Emphasize newborn's need for follow-up evaluation by healthcare provider and timely immunizations.
- Identify manifestations of illness and infection and the times at which a healthcare provider should be contacted. Demonstrate proper technique for taking temperature, administering oral medications, or providing other care activities for infant as required. **Early recognition of illness and prompt use of healthcare facilitate treatment and positive outcome.**
- Refer client/couple to community postpartal parent groups. **Increases parent's knowledge of child rearing and child development and provides supportive atmosphere while parents incorporate new roles.**

Documentation Focus

Assessment/Reassessment
- Assessment findings, general health, previous pregnancy experience.
- Cultural beliefs and expectations.
- Specific birth plan and individuals to be involved in delivery.
- Arrangements for postpartal recovery period.

Planning
- Plan of care and who is involved in planning.
- Teaching plan.

Implementation/Evaluation
- Response to interventions, teaching, and actions performed.
- Attainment or progress toward desired outcome(s).
- Modifications to plan of care.

Discharge Planning
- Long-term needs and who is responsible for actions to be taken.
- Available resources, specific referrals made.

Information that appears in brackets has been added by the authors to clarify and enhance the use of nursing diagnoses.

Sample Nursing Outcomes & Interventions Classifications (NOC/NIC)

NOC—Knowledge: Pregnancy
NIC—Childbirth Preparation

risk for ineffective Childbearing Process

Taxonomy II: Sexuality—Class 3 Reproduction (00227)
[Diagnostic Division: Safety]
Submitted 2010

Definition: Risk for a pregnancy and childbirth process and care of the newborn that does not match the environmental context, norms, and expectations*

Risk Factors

Deficient knowledge (e.g., of labor and delivery, newborn care); lack of realistic birth plan
Unplanned/unwanted pregnancy
Inconsistent/lack of prenatal health visits
Suboptimal maternal nutrition
Substance abuse
Lack of sufficient support systems
Lack of maternal confidence
Maternal powerlessness/psychological distress
Domestic violence
Lack of appropriate role models/cognitive readiness for parenthood

Desired Outcomes/Evaluation Criteria— Client Will:

* Acknowledge and address individual risk factors.
* Demonstrate healthy pregnancy free of preventable complications.
* Engage in activities to prepare for birth process and care of newborn.
* Experience complication-free labor and childbirth.

*The original Japanese term for "childbearing" (*shussan ikujikoudou*), which encompasses both childbirth and rearing of the neonate. It is one of the main concepts of Japanese midwifery.

Information that appears in brackets has been added by the authors to clarify and enhance the use of nursing diagnoses.

• Verbalize understanding of care requirements to promote health of self and infant.

Refer to ND ineffective Childbearing Process, for Interventions and Documentation Focus.

impaired Comfort

Taxonomy II: Comfort—Class 1 Physical Comfort/Class 2 Environmental Comfort/Class 3 Social Comfort (00214)
[Diagnostic Division: Pain/Discomfort]
Submitted 2008; Revised 2010

Definition: Perceived lack of ease, relief, and transcendence in physical, psychospiritual, environmental, cultural, and social dimensions

Related Factors

Illness-related symptoms; treatment-related side effects (e.g., medication, radiation)
Lack of environmental/situational control
Lack of privacy
Noxious environmental stimuli
Insufficient resources (e.g., financial, social support)

Defining Characteristics

Subjective
Reports distressing symptoms, lack of contentment/ease in situation, hunger, itching, being uncomfortable, cold or hot
Disturbed sleep pattern; inability to relax
Anxiety; fear

Objective
Restlessness; irritability; sighing, moaning, crying

Desired Outcomes/Evaluation Criteria— Client Will:

• Engage in behaviors or lifestyle changes to increase level of ease.
• Verbalize sense of comfort or contentment.
• Participate in desirable and realistic health-seeking behaviors.

Information that appears in brackets has been added by the authors to clarify and enhance the use of nursing diagnoses.

Actions/Interventions

Nursing Priority No. 1.

To assess etiology/precipitating contributory factors:

- Determine the type of discomfort client is experiencing, such as physical pain, feeling of discontent, lack of ease with self, environment, or sociocultural settings, or inability to rise above one's problems or pain (lack of transcendence). Have client rate total comfort, using a scale of 0 to 10, with 10 being as comfortable as possible, or a "general comfort" questionnaire using a Likert-type scale. **A comfort scale is similar to pain rating scale and can help client identify focus of discomfort (e.g., physical, emotional, social).**
- Note cultural/religious beliefs and values that impact perceptions and expectations of comfort.
- Ascertain locus of control. **Presence of external locus of control may hamper efforts to achieve sense of peace or contentment.**
- Discuss concerns with client and Active-listen to identify underlying issues (e.g., physical and emotional stressors or external factors such as environmental surroundings; social interactions) that could impact client's ability to control own well-being. **Helps to determine client's specific needs and ability to change own situation.**
- Establish context(s) in which lack of comfort is realized: physical (pertaining to bodily sensations); psychospiritual (pertaining to internal awareness of self and meaning in one's life, relationship to a higher order or being), environmental (pertaining to external surroundings, conditions, and influences), or sociocultural (pertaining to interpersonal, family, and societal relationships).

Physical

- Determine how client is managing pain and pain components. **Lack of control may be related to other issues or emotions such as fear, loneliness, anxiety, noxious stimuli, anger.**
- Ascertain what has been tried or is required for comfort or rest (e.g., head of bed up/down, music on/off, white noise, rocking motion, certain person or thing).

Psychospiritual

- Determine how psychological and spiritual indicators overlap (e.g., meaningfulness, faith, identity, self-esteem) for client.
- Ascertain if client/SO desires support regarding spiritual enrichment, including prayer, meditation, or access to spiritual counselor of choice.

Information that appears in brackets has been added by the authors to clarify and enhance the use of nursing diagnoses.

Environmental
- Determine that client's environment both respects privacy and provides natural lighting with readily accessible view to out-doors—**an aspect that can be manipulated to enhance comfort.**

Sociocultural
- Ascertain meaning of comfort in context of interpersonal, family, cultural values, and societal relationships.
- Validate client/SO understanding of client's situation and on-going methods of managing condition, as appropriate and/or desired by client. **Considers client/family needs in this area and/or shows appreciation for their desires.**

Nursing Priority No. 2.
To assist client to alleviate discomfort:
- Review knowledge base and note coping skills that have been used previously to change behavior/promote well-being. **Brings these to client's awareness and promotes use in current situation.**
- Acknowledge client's strengths in present situation and build on these in planning for future.

Physical
- Collaborate in treating or managing medical conditions in-volving oxygenation, elimination, mobility, cognitive abili-ties, electrolyte balance, thermoregulation, and hydration **to promote physical stability.**
- Work with client to prevent pain, nausea, itching, and thirst/other physical discomforts.
- Review medications or treatment regimen **to determine pos-sible changes or options to reduce side effects.**
- Suggest parent be present during procedures **to comfort child.**
- Provide age-appropriate comfort measures (e.g., back rub, change of position, cuddling, and use of heat/cold) **to provide nonpharmacological pain management.**
- Discuss interventions/activities such as Therapeutic Touch (TT), massage, healing touch, biofeedback, self-hypnosis, guided imagery, and breathing exercises; play therapy; and humor **to promote ease and relaxation and to refocus at-tention.**
- Assist client to use and modify medication regimen **to make best use of pharmacological pain or symptom manage-ment.**

Information that appears in brackets has been added by the authors to clarify and enhance the use of nursing diagnoses.

⊕ Cultural   ⊗ Collaborative   🏠 Community/Home Care

- Assist client/SO(s) to develop plan for activity and exercise within individual ability, emphasizing necessity of allowing sufficient time to finish activities.
- Maintain open and flexible visitation with client's desired persons.
- Encourage/plan care to allow individually adequate rest periods **to prevent fatigue.** Schedule activities for periods when client has the most energy **to maximize participation.**
- Discuss routines to promote restful sleep.

Psychospiritual
- Interact with client in therapeutic manner. **The nurse could be the most important comfort intervention for meeting client's needs. For example, assuring client that nausea can be treated successfully with both pharmacological and nonpharmacological methods may be more effective than simply administering antiemetic without reassurance and a comforting presence.**
- Encourage verbalization of feelings and make time for listening/interacting.
- Identify ways (e.g., meditation, sharing oneself with others, being out in nature/garden, other spiritual activities) to achieve connectedness or harmony with self, others, nature, higher power.
- Establish realistic activity goals with client. **Enhances commitment to promoting optimal outcomes.**
- Involve client/SO(s) in schedule planning and decisions about timing and spacing of treatments **to promote relaxation/reduce sense of boredom.**
- Encourage client to do whatever possible (e.g., self-care, sit up in chair, walk). **Enhances self-esteem and independence.**
- ∞• Use age-appropriate distraction with music, reading, chatting or texting with family and friends, watching TV or movies, or playing video or computer games **to limit dwelling on and transcend unpleasant sensations and situations.**
- Encourage client to develop assertiveness skills, prioritizing goals/activities, and to make use of beneficial coping behaviors. **Promotes sense of control and improves self-esteem.**
- Identify opportunities for client to participate in experiences that enhance control and independence.

Environmental
- Provide quiet environment, calm activities.
- Provide for periodic changes in the personal surroundings when client is confined. Use the individual's input in creating the changes (e.g., seasonal bulletin boards, color changes,

Information that appears in brackets has been added by the authors to clarify and enhance the use of nursing diagnoses.

rearranging furniture, pictures). **Promotes client's sense of self-control and environmental comfort.**

• Suggest activities, such as bird feeders or baths for bird-watching, a garden in a window box/terrarium, or a fish bowl/aquarium, **to stimulate observation as well as involvement and participation in activity.**

Sociocultural

∞• Encourage age-appropriate diversional activities (e.g., TV/radio, computer games, play time, socialization/outings with others).

• Avoid overstimulation/understimulation (cognitive and sensory).

⊕• Make appropriate referrals to available support groups, hobby clubs, service organizations.

Nursing Priority No. 3.

🏠 To promote wellness (Teaching/Discharge Considerations):

• Provide information about conditions/health risk factors or concerns in desired format (e.g., pictures, TV programs, articles, handouts, or audio/visual materials; classes, group discussions, Internet Web sites, and other databases) as appropriate. **Use of multiple modalities enhances acquisition/retention of information and gives client choices for accessing and applying information.**

Physical

• Promote overall health measures (e.g., nutrition, adequate fluid intake, elimination, and appropriate vitamin and iron supplementation).

⊕• Discuss potential complications and possible need for medical follow-up or alternative therapies. **Timely recognition and intervention can promote wellness.**

• Assist client/SO(s) to identify and acquire necessary equipment (e.g., lifts, commode chair, safety grab bars, personal hygiene supplies) to meet individual needs. Refer to appropriate suppliers.

Psychospiritual

⊕• Collaborate with others when client expresses interest in lessons, counseling, coaching, and/or mentoring **to meet/enhance emotional and/or spiritual comfort.**

• Promote and encourage client's contributions toward meeting realistic goals.

• Encourage client take time to be introspective in the search for contentment/transcendence.

Information that appears in brackets has been added by the authors to clarify and enhance the use of nursing diagnoses.

Environmental

∞• Create a compassionate, supportive, and therapeutic environ-
🌐 ment incorporating client's cultural and age or developmental
factors.
• Correct environmental hazards that could influence safety or
negatively affect comfort.
• Arrange for home visit or evaluation as needed.
• Discuss long-term plan for taking care of environmental
needs.

Sociocultural
• Advocate for growth-promoting environment in conflict situations and consider issues from client/family and cultural
perspective.
• Identify resources or referrals (e.g., knowledge and skills, financial resources or assistance, personal or psychological support group, social activities).

Documentation Focus

Assessment/Reassessment
• Individual findings including client's description of current
status/situation and factors impacting sense of comfort.
• Pertinent cultural and religious beliefs and values.
• Medication use and nonpharmacological measures.

Planning
• Plan of care, specific interventions, and who is involved in
planning.
• Teaching plan.

Implementation/Evaluation
• Responses to interventions, teaching, and actions performed.
• Attainment or progress toward desired outcome(s).
• Modifications to plan of care.

Discharge Planning
• Long-term needs and who is responsible for actions to be
taken.
• Specific referrals made.

Sample Nursing Outcomes & Interventions Classifications (NOC/NIC)

NOC—Comfort Status
NIC—Environmental Management: Comfort

Information that appears in brackets has been added by the authors to clarify
and enhance the use of nursing diagnoses.

Taxonomy II: Comfort—Class 1 Physical Comfort/Class 2
  Environmental Comfort (00183)
[Diagnostic Division: Pain/Discomfort]
Submitted 2006

Definition: A pattern of ease, relief, and transcendence in
physical, psychospiritual, environmental, and/or social
dimensions that is sufficient for well-being and can be
strengthened

Defining Characteristics

Subjective

- Expresses desire to enhance comfort; feeling of contentment
- Expresses desire to enhance relaxation
- Expresses desire to enhance resolution of complaints

Objective

Appears relaxed, calm
Participating in comfort measures of choice

Desired Outcomes/Evaluation Criteria—
Client Will:

- Verbalize sense of comfort or contentment.
- Demonstrate behaviors of optimal level of ease.
- Participate in desirable and realistic health-seeking behaviors.

Actions/Interventions

Nursing Priority No. 1.

To determine current level of comfort and motivation for
  change:

- Determine the type of comfort client is experiencing: (1) relief
  (as from pain), (2) ease (a state of calm or contentment), or
  (3) transcendence (a state in which one rises above one's problems or pain).
- Ascertain motivation or expectations for improvement.
- Establish context(s) in which comfort is realized: (1) physical
  (pertaining to bodily sensations), (2) psychospiritual (pertaining to internal awareness of self and meaning in one's life,
  relationship to a higher order or being), (3) environmental

---

Information that appears in brackets has been added by the authors to clarify
and enhance the use of nursing diagnoses.

(pertaining to external surroundings, conditions, and influences), and (4) sociocultural (pertaining to interpersonal, family, and societal relationships).

Physical

- Verify that client is managing pain and pain components effectively. **Success in this area usually addresses other issues and emotions (e.g., fear, loneliness, anxiety, noxious stimuli, anger).**
- Ascertain what is used or required for comfort or rest (e.g., head of bed up or down, music on or off, white noise, rocking motion, certain person or thing, or ability to express and/or manage conflicts).

Psychospiritual

- Determine how psychological and spiritual indicators overlap (e.g., meaningfulness, faith, identity, self-esteem) for client in enhancing comfort.
- Determine influence of cultural beliefs and values.
- Ascertain that client/SO has received desired support regarding spiritual enrichment, including prayer, meditation, and access to spiritual counselor of choice.

Environmental

- Determine that client's environment respects privacy and provides natural lighting and readily accessible view to outdoors **(an aspect that can be manipulated to enhance comfort).**

Sociocultural

- Ascertain meaning of comfort in context of interpersonal, family, cultural values, spatial, and societal relationships.
- Validate client/SO understanding of client's diagnosis and prognosis and ongoing methods of managing condition, as appropriate and/or desired by client. **Considers client/family needs in this area and/or shows appreciation for their desires.**

Nursing Priority No. 2.

To assist client in developing plan to improve comfort:

- Review knowledge base and note coping skills that have been used previously to change behavior and promote well-being. **Brings these to client's awareness and promotes use in the current situation.**
- Acknowledge client's strengths in the present situation that can be used to build on in planning for future.

Information that appears in brackets has been added by the authors to clarify and enhance the use of nursing diagnoses.

Physical

- ⓐ• Collaborate in treating and managing medical conditions involving oxygenation, elimination, mobility, cognitive abilities, electrolyte balance, thermoregulation, hydration **to promote physical stability.**
- Work with client to prevent pain, nausea, itching, thirst, or other physical discomforts.
- ∞• Suggest parent be present during procedures **to comfort child.**
- ∞• Suggest age-appropriate comfort measures (e.g., back rub, change of position, cuddling, use of heat/cold) **to provide nonpharmacological pain management.**
- ⓐ• Review interventions and activities such as therapeutic touch, biofeedback, self-hypnosis, guided imagery, breathing exercises, play therapy, and humor **that promote ease and relaxation, and can refocus attention.**
- 🖊• Assist client to use or modify medication regimen **to make best use of pharmacological pain management.**
- Assist client/SO(s) to develop or modify plan for activity and exercise within individual ability, emphasizing necessity of allowing sufficient time to finish activities.
- Maintain open and flexible visitation with client's desired persons.
- Encourage adequate rest periods **to prevent fatigue.**
- Plan care to allow individually adequate rest periods. Schedule activities for periods when client has the most energy **to maximize participation.**
- Discuss routines to promote restful sleep.

Psychospiritual

- Interact with client in therapeutic manner. **The nurse could be the most important comfort intervention for meeting client's needs. For example, assuring client that nausea can be treated successfully with both pharmacological and nonpharmacological methods may be more effective than simply administering antiemetic without reassurance and comforting presence.**
- Encourage verbalization of feelings and make time for listening and interacting.
- Identify ways (e.g., meditation, sharing oneself with others, being out in nature/garden, other spiritual activities) **to achieve connectedness or harmony with self, others, nature, or a higher power**.
- Establish realistic activity goals with client. **Enhances commitment to promoting optimal outcomes.**

Information that appears in brackets has been added by the authors to clarify and enhance the use of nursing diagnoses.

🌐 Cultural ⓒ Collaborative 🏠 Community/Home Care

- Involve client/SO(s) in schedule planning and decisions about timing and spacing of treatments **to promote relaxation and involvement in plan.**
- Encourage client to do whatever possible (e.g., self-care, sit up in chair, walk, etc.). **Enhances self-esteem and independence.**
∞• Use age-appropriate distraction with music, chatting or texting with family and friends, watching TV, or playing video or computer games **to limit dwelling on, or transcend unpleasant sensations and situations.**
- Encourage client to make use of beneficial coping behaviors and assertiveness skills, prioritizing goals and activities. **Promotes sense of control and improves self-esteem.**
- Offer or identify opportunities for client to participate in experiences that enhance control and independence.

Environmental

- Provide quiet environment and calm activities.
🏠• Provide for periodic changes in the personal surroundings when client is confined. Use the individual's input in creating the changes (e.g., seasonal bulletin boards, color changes, rearranging furniture, pictures). **Enhances sense of comfort and control over environment.**
🏠• Suggest activities, such as bird feeders or baths for bird-watching, a garden in a window box/terrarium, or a fish bowl/aquarium **to stimulate observation as well as involvement and participation in activity.**

Sociocultural

∞• Encourage age-appropriate diversional activities (e.g., TV/radio, play time/games, socialization/outings with others).
- Avoid cognitive or sensory overstimulation and understimulation.
🌐• Make appropriate referrals to available support groups, hobby clubs, service organizations.

Nursing Priority No. 3.
🏠To promote optimum wellness (Teaching/Discharge Considerations):

Physical

- Promote overall health measures (e.g., nutrition, adequate fluid intake, elimination, appropriate vitamin/iron supplementation).

Information that appears in brackets has been added by the authors to clarify and enhance the use of nursing diagnoses.

- Discuss potential complications and possible need for medical follow-up care or alternative therapies. **Timely recognition and intervention can promote wellness.**
- Assist client/SO(s) in identifying and acquiring necessary equipment (e.g., lifts, commode chair, safety grab bars, and personal hygiene supplies) **to meet individual needs.**

Psychospiritual
- Collaborate with others when client expresses interest in lessons, counseling, coaching, and/or mentoring **to meet/enhance emotional and/or spiritual comfort.**
- Encourage client's contributions toward meeting realistic goals.
- Encourage client to take time to be introspective in the search for contentment/transcendence.

Environmental
- Promote a compassionate, supportive, and therapeutic environment incorporating client's cultural, age, and developmental factors.
- Correct environmental hazards **that could influence safety or negatively affect comfort.**
- Arrange for home visit/evaluation, as needed.
- Discuss long-term plan for taking care of environmental needs.

Sociocultural
- Advocate for growth-promoting environment in conflict situations and consider issues from client/family and cultural perspective.
- Support client/SO access to resources (e.g., knowledge and skills, financial resources/assistance, personal/psychological support, social systems).

Documentation Focus

Assessment/Reassessment
- Individual findings, including client's description of current status/situation.
- Motivation and expectations for change.
- Medication use/nonpharmacological measures.

Planning
- Plan of care, specific interventions, and who is involved in planning.
- Teaching plan.

Information that appears in brackets has been added by the authors to clarify and enhance the use of nursing diagnoses.

Cultural Collaborative Community/Home Care

Implementation/Evaluation
- Responses to interventions, teaching, and actions performed.
- Attainment or progress toward desired outcome(s).
- Modifications to plan of care.

Discharge Planning
- Long-term needs and who is responsible for actions to be taken.
- Specific referrals made.

Sample Nursing Outcomes & Interventions Classifications (NOC/NIC)

NOC—Comfort Status
NIC—Self-Modification Assistance

---

impaired verbal Communication

Taxonomy II: Perception/Cognition—Class 5 Communication (00051)
[Diagnostic Division: Social Interaction]
Submitted 1983; Revised 1996, 1998

Definition: Decreased, delayed, or absent ability to receive, process, transmit, and/or use a system of symbols

---

Related Factors

Decreased circulation to brain; brain tumor
Anatomical deficit (e.g., cleft palate, alteration of the neuromuscular visual system, auditory system, or phonatory apparatus)
Difference related to developmental age
Physical barrier (e.g., tracheostomy, intubation)
Physiological conditions [e.g., dyspnea]; alteration of central nervous system (CNS); weakened musculoskeletal system
Psychological barriers (e.g., psychosis, lack of stimuli); emotional conditions; stress
Environmental barriers
Cultural difference
Lack of information
Treatment-related side effects (e.g., pharmaceutical agents)
Alteration in self-concept; situational/chronic low self-esteem
Altered perceptions
Absence of SO(s)

Information that appears in brackets has been added by the authors to clarify and enhance the use of nursing diagnoses.

Defining Characteristics

Subjective

[Reports of difficulty expressing self]

Objective

Inability to speak language of caregiver

Speaks/verbalizes with difficulty; stuttering; slurring

Does not/cannot speak; willful refusal to speak

Difficulty forming sentences or words (e.g., aphonia, dyslalia, dysarthria)

Difficulty expressing thoughts verbally (e.g., aphasia, dysphasia, apraxia, dyslexia)

Inappropriate verbalization [incessant, loose association of ideas; flight of ideas]

Difficulty in comprehending or maintaining usual communication pattern

Absence of eye contact; difficulty in selective attending; partial/ total visual deficit

Inability/difficulty in use of facial or body expressions

Dyspnea

Disorientation to person, space, time

[Inability to modulate speech; message inappropriate to content]

[Use of nonverbal cues (e.g., pleading eyes, gestures, turning away)]

Desired Outcomes/Evaluation Criteria— Client Will:

- Verbalize or indicate an understanding of the communication difficulty and plans for ways of handling.
- Establish method of communication in which needs can be expressed.
- Participate in therapeutic communication (e.g., using silence, acceptance, restating, reflecting, Active-listening, and I-messages).
- Demonstrate congruent verbal and nonverbal communication.
- Use resources appropriately.

Actions/Interventions

Nursing Priority No. 1.

To assess causative/contributing factors:

- Identify physiological or neurological conditions impacting speech such as severe shortness of breath, cleft palate, facial

---

Information that appears in brackets has been added by the authors to clarify and enhance the use of nursing diagnoses.

trauma, neuromuscular weakness, stroke, brain tumors or infections, dementia, brain trauma, deafness, or hard of hearing.

- ∞ Determine age and developmental considerations: (1) child too young for language or has developmental delays affecting speech and language skills or comprehension; (2) autism or other mental impairments; (3) older client doesn't or isn't able to speak, verbalizes with difficulty, or has difficulty hearing or comprehending language or concepts.

- Review history for neurological conditions that could affect speech, such as stroke, tumor, MS, hearing or vision impairment.

- Note results of neurological tests (e.g., electroencephalogram [EEG]; or CT/MRI scans; language/speech tests [e.g., Boston Diagnostic Aphasia Examination, the Action Naming Test]) **to assess and delineate underlying conditions affecting verbal communication.**

- Note whether aphasia is motor (**expressive: loss of images for articulated speech**), sensory (**receptive: unable to understand words and does not recognize the defect**), conduction (**slow comprehension: uses words inappropriately but knows the error**), and/or global (**total loss of ability to comprehend and speak**). Evaluate the degree of impairment.

- Evaluate mental status and note presence of psychiatric conditions (e.g., bipolar, schizoid/affective behavior). Assess psychological response to communication impairment and willingness to find alternate means of communication.

- Note presence of endotracheal tube/tracheostomy or other physical blocks to speech (e.g., cleft palate, jaws wired).

- Assess environmental factors that may affect ability to communicate (e.g., room noise level).

- Identify environmental barriers: recent or chronic exposure to hazardous noise in home, job, recreation, and healthcare setting (e.g., rock music, jackhammer, snowmobile, lawn mower, truck traffic or busy highway, heavy equipment, or medical equipment). **Noise not only affects hearing, but it also increases blood pressure and breathing rate, can have negative cardiovascular effects, disturbs digestion, increases fatigue, causes irritability, and reduces attention to tasks**.

- Determine primary language spoken. **Knowing the client's primary language and fluency in other languages is important to communication. For example, while some individuals may seem to be fluent in conversational English, they may still have limited understanding, especially the**

Information that appears in brackets has been added by the authors to clarify and enhance the use of nursing diagnoses.

language of health professionals, and have difficulty answering questions, describing symptoms, or following directions.

⊕• Ascertain whether client is recent immigrant, their country of origin, and what cultural/ethnic group client identifies with (e.g., recent immigrant may identify with home country and its people, beliefs, and healthcare practices).

⊕• Determine cultural factors affecting communication such as beliefs concerning touch and eye contact. Certain cultures may prohibit client from speaking directly to healthcare provider; some Native Americans, Appalachians, or young African Americans may interpret direct eye contact as disrespectful, impolite, an invasion of privacy, or aggressive; Latinos, Arabs, and Asians may shout and gesture when excited.

• Assess style of speech (as outlined in Defining Characteristics).

• Determine presence of psychological or emotional barriers, history or presence of psychiatric conditions (e.g., manic-depressive illness, schizoid or affective behavior); high level of anxiety, frustration, or fear; presence of angry, hostile behavior. Note effect on speech and communication.

∞• Interview parent to determine child's developmental level of speech and language comprehension.

∞• Note parental speech patterns and manner of communicating with child, including gestures.

Nursing Priority No. 2.

To assist client to establish a means of communication to express needs, wants, ideas, and questions:

• Ascertain that you have client's attention before communicating.

• Establish rapport with client, initiate eye contact, shake hands, address by preferred name, and meet family members present; ask simple questions, smile, and engage in brief social conversation if appropriate. Helps establish a trusting relationship with client/family, demonstrating caring about the client as a person.

• Determine ability to read and write. Evaluate musculoskeletal states, including manual dexterity (e.g., ability to hold a pen and write).

• Advise other healthcare providers of client's communication deficits (e.g., deafness, aphasia, presence of mechanical

---

Information that appears in brackets has been added by the authors to clarify and enhance the use of nursing diagnoses.

⊕ Cultural ⊛ Collaborative 🏠 Community/Home Care

ventilation) and needed means of communication (e.g., writing pad, signing, yes/no responses, gestures, picture board) **to minimize client's frustration and promote understanding.**

- Obtain a translator or provide written translation or picture chart **when writing is not possible or client speaks a different language than that spoken by healthcare provider.**
- Facilitate hearing and vision examinations **to obtain necessary aids.**
- Ascertain that hearing aid(s) are in place and batteries are charged and/or glasses are worn when needed **to facilitate and improve communication.** Assist client to learn to use and adjust to aids.
- Reduce environmental noise that can interfere with comprehension. Provide adequate lighting, especially if client is reading lips or attempting to write.
- Establish relationship with the client, listening carefully and attending to client's verbal/nonverbal expressions. **Conveys interest and concern.**
- Maintain eye contact, preferably at client's level. Be aware of cultural factors that may preclude eye contact (e.g., found in some American Indians, Indo-Chinese, Arabs, and natives of Appalachia).
- Keep communication simple, speaking in short sentences, using appropriate words, and using all modes for accessing information: visual, auditory, and kinesthetic.
- Refrain from shouting when directing speech to confused, deaf, or hearing-impaired client. Speak slowly and clearly, pitching voice low **to increase likelihood of being understood.**
- Maintain a calm, unhurried manner. Provide sufficient time for client to respond. Downplay errors and avoid frequent corrections. **Individuals with expressive aphasia may talk more easily when they are rested and relaxed and when they are talking to one person at a time.**
- Determine meaning of words used by the client and congruency of communication and nonverbal messages.
- Validate meaning of nonverbal communication; do not make assumptions **because they may be wrong.** Be honest; if you do not understand, seek assistance from others.
- Individualize techniques using breathing for relaxation of the vocal cords, rote tasks (such as counting), and singing or melodic intonation **to assist aphasic clients in relearning speech.**

Information that appears in brackets has been added by the authors to clarify and enhance the use of nursing diagnoses.

- Anticipate needs and stay with client until effective communication is reestablished, and/or client feels safe/comfortable.
- Plan for and provide alternative methods of communication, incorporating information about type of disability present:

  Provide pad and pencil or slate board **when client is able to write but cannot speak**.

  Use letter or picture board **when client can't write and picture concepts are understandable to both parties**.

  Establish hand or eye signals **when client can understand language but cannot speak or has physical barrier to writing**.

  Remove isolation mask **when client is deaf and reads lips**.

  Obtain or provide access to tablet or computer **if communication impairment is long-standing or client is used to this method.**

- Identify and use previous successful communication solutions used if situation is chronic or recurrent.
- Provide reality orientation by responding with simple, straightforward, honest statements.
- Provide environmental stimuli, as needed, **to maintain contact with reality,** or reduce stimuli **to lessen anxiety that may worsen problem.**
- Use confrontation skills, when appropriate, within an established nurse-client relationship **to clarify discrepancies between verbal and nonverbal cues.**
- Refer for appropriate therapies and support services. **Client and family may have multiple needs (e.g., sources for further examinations and rehabilitation services, local community or national support groups and services for disabled, or financial assistance with obtaining necessary aids for improving communication).**

Nursing Priority No. 3.
To promote wellness (Teaching/Discharge Considerations):

- Review information about condition, prognosis, and treatment with client/SO(s).
- Teach client and family the needed techniques for communication, whether it be speech or language techniques, or alternate modes of communicating. Encourage family to involve client in family activities using enhanced communication techniques **Reduces stress of difficult situation and promotes earlier return to more normal life patterns.**
- Reinforce that loss of speech does not imply loss of intelligence.

Information that appears in brackets has been added by the authors to clarify and enhance the use of nursing diagnoses.

🌐 Cultural 🔵 Collaborative 🏠 Community/Home Care

- Discuss individual methods of dealing with impairment, capitalizing on client's and caregiver's strengths.
- Discuss ways to provide environmental stimuli as appropriate **to maintain contact with reality or reduce environmental stimuli or noise. Unwanted sound affects physical health, increases fatigue, reduces attention to tasks, and makes speech communication more difficult.**
- Recommend placing a tape recorder with a prerecorded emergency message near the telephone. Information to include: client's name, address, telephone number, and critical information (e.g., type of airway, person cannot speak) and a request for immediate emergency assistance.
- Use and assist client/SO(s) to learn therapeutic communication skills of acknowledgment, Active-listening, and I-messages. **Improves general communication skills.**
- Involve family/SO(s) in plan of care as much as possible. **Enhances participation and commitment to communication with loved one.**
- Refer to appropriate resources (e.g., speech/language therapist, support groups such as stroke club, individual/family, and/or psychiatric counseling).
- Refer to NDs ineffective Coping; disabled family Coping; Anxiety; Fear.

Documentation Focus

Assessment/Reassessment
- Assessment findings, pertinent history information (i.e., physical, psychological, cultural concerns).
- Meaning of nonverbal cues, level of anxiety client exhibits.

Planning
- Plan of care and interventions (e.g., type of alternative communication/translator).
- Teaching plan.

Implementation/Evaluation
- Response to interventions, teaching, and actions performed.
- Attainment or progress toward desired outcome(s).
- Modifications to plan of care.

Discharge Planning
- Discharge needs, referrals made; additional resources available.

Information that appears in brackets has been added by the authors to clarify and enhance the use of nursing diagnoses.

Sample Nursing Outcomes & Interventions Classifications (NOC/NIC)

NOC—Communication
NIC—Communication Enhancement: Speech Deficit

readiness for enhanced Communication

Taxonomy II: Perception/Cognition—Class 5 Communication (00161)
[Diagnostic Division: Teaching/Learning]
Submitted 2002

Definition: A pattern of exchanging information and ideas with others that is sufficient for meeting one's needs and life goals and can be strengthened

Defining Characteristics

Subjective
Expresses willingness to enhance communication
Expresses thoughts/feelings
Expresses satisfaction with ability to share information or ideas with others

Objective
Able to speak or write a language
Forms words, phrases, sentences
Uses and interprets nonverbal cues appropriately

Desired Outcomes/Evaluation Criteria— Client/SO/Caregiver Will:

• Verbalize or indicate an understanding of the communication process.
• Identify ways to improve communication.

Actions/Interventions

Nursing Priority No. 1.
To assess how client is managing communication/challenges:

• Ascertain circumstances that result in client's desire to improve communication. **Many factors are involved in communication, and identifying specific needs/expectations**

Information that appears in brackets has been added by the authors to clarify and enhance the use of nursing diagnoses.

 Cultural   Collaborative   🏠 Community/Home Care

helps in developing realistic goals and determining likelihood of success.

- Evaluate mental status. **Disorientation, acute or chronic confusion, or psychotic conditions may be affecting speech and the communication of thoughts, needs, and desires.**
- Determine client's developmental level of speech and language comprehension. **Provides baseline information for developing plan for improvement.**
- Determine ability to read and write preferred language. **Evaluating grasp of language as well as musculoskeletal states, including manual dexterity (e.g., ability to hold a pen and write), provides information about nature of client's situation. Educational plan can address language skills. Neuromuscular deficits will require individual program in order to improve.**
- Determine country of origin, dominant language, whether client is recent immigrant, and what cultural/ethnic group client identifies with. **Recent immigrant may identify with home country and its people, language, beliefs, and healthcare practices, thus affecting language skills and ability to improve interactions in a new country.**
- Ascertain if interpreter is needed/desired. **Law mandates that interpretation services be made available. A trained, professional interpreter who translates precisely and possesses a basic understanding of medical terminology and healthcare ethics is preferred to enhance client and provider satisfaction.**
- Determine comfort level in expression of feelings and concepts in nonproficient language. **Concern about language skills can impact perception of own ability to communicate.**
- Note any physical barriers to effective communication (e.g., talking tracheostomy, wired jaws) or physiological or neurological conditions (e.g., severe shortness of breath, neuromuscular weakness, stroke, brain trauma, hearing impairment, cleft palate, facial trauma). **Client may be dealing with speech/language comprehension difficulties or have voice production problems (pitch, loudness, or quality) that call attention to voice rather than what speaker is saying. These barriers may need to be addressed to enable client to improve communication skills.**
- Clarify meaning of words used by the client to describe important aspects of life and health/well-being (e.g., pain, sorrow, anxiety). **Words can easily be misinterpreted when**

Information that appears in brackets has been added by the authors to clarify and enhance the use of nursing diagnoses.

sender and receiver have different ideas about their meanings. **Restating what one has heard can clarify whether an expressed statement has been correctly understood or misinterpreted.**

- Determine presence of emotional lability (e.g., anger outbursts) and frequency of unstable behaviors. **Emotional and psychiatric issues can affect communication and interfere with understanding.**
- Evaluate congruency of verbal and nonverbal messages. **Communication is enhanced when verbal and nonverbal messages are congruent.**
- Evaluate need or desire for pictures or written communications and instructions as part of treatment plan. **Alternative methods of communication can help client feel understood and promote feelings of satisfaction with interaction.**

Nursing Priority No. 2.

To improve client's ability to communicate thoughts, needs, and ideas:

- Maintain a calm, unhurried manner. Provide sufficient time for client to respond. **An atmosphere in which client is free to speak without fear of criticism provides the opportunity to explore all the issues involved in making decisions to improve communication skills.**
- Pay attention to speaker. Be an active listener. **The use of Active-listening communicates acceptance and respect for the client, establishing trust and promoting openness and honest expression. It communicates a belief that the client is a capable and competent person.**
- Sit down, maintain eye contact as culturally appropriate, preferably at client's level, and spend time with the client. **Conveys message that the nurse has time and interest in communicating.**
- Observe body language, eye movements, and behavioral cues. **May reveal unspoken concerns; for example, when pain is present, client may react with tears, grimacing, stiff posture, turning away, or angry outbursts.**
- Help client identify and learn to avoid use of nontherapeutic communication. **These barriers are recognized as detriments to open communication, and learning to avoid them maximizes the effectiveness of communication between client and others.**
- Obtain interpreter with language or signing abilities, as needed. **May be needed to enhance understanding of words**

Information that appears in brackets has been added by the authors to clarify and enhance the use of nursing diagnoses.

  Cultural   Collaborative   Community/Home Care

and language concepts or to ascertain that interpretation of communication is accurate.

- Suggest use of pad and pencil, slate board, letter/picture board when interacting or attempting to interface in new situations. **When client has physical impairments that challenge verbal communication, alternate means can provide clear concepts that are understandable to both parties.**

🏠• Obtain or provide access to a voice-enabled computer, when indicated. **Use of these devices may be more helpful when communication challenges are long-standing and/or when client is used to working with them.**

🌐• Respect client's cultural communication needs. **Culture can dictate beliefs of what is normal or abnormal (i.e., in some cultures, eye-to-eye contact is considered disrespectful, impolite, or an invasion of privacy; silence and tone of voice have various meanings, and slang words can cause confusion).**

- Encourage use of glasses, hearing aids, dentures, electronic speech devices, as needed. **These devices maximize sensory perception or speech formation and can improve understanding and enhance speech patterns.**

- Reduce distractions and background noises (e.g., close the door, turn down the radio or TV). **A distracting environment can interfere with communication, limiting attention to tasks and making speech and communication more difficult. Reducing noise can help both parties hear clearly, thus improving understanding.**

- Associate words with objects—using repetition and redundancy—and point to objects or demonstrate desired actions if communication requires visual aids. **Speaker's own body language can be used to enhance client's understanding.**

- Use confrontation skills carefully, when appropriate, within an established nurse-client relationship. **Can be used to clarify discrepancies between verbal and nonverbal cues, enabling client to look at areas that may require change.**

Nursing Priority No. 3.

🏠 To promote optimum communication:

- Discuss with family/SO and other caregivers effective ways in which the client communicates. **Identifying positive aspects of current communication skills enables family members and other caregivers to learn and move forward in desire to enhance ways of interacting.**

Information that appears in brackets has been added by the authors to clarify and enhance the use of nursing diagnoses.

- Encourage client/SO(s) to familiarize themselves with and use new communication technologies. **Enhances family relationships and promotes self-esteem for all members as they are able to communicate regardless of the problems (e.g., progressive disorder) that could interfere with ability to interact.**
- Reinforce client/SO(s) learning and using therapeutic communication skills of acknowledgment, Active-listening, and I-messages. **Improves general communication skills, emphasizes acceptance, and conveys respect, enabling family relationships to improve.**
- Refer to appropriate resources (e.g., speech therapist, language classes, individual/family and/or psychiatric counseling). **May be needed to help overcome challenges as family reaches toward desired goal of enhanced communication.**

Documentation Focus

Assessment/Reassessment
- Assessment findings, pertinent history information (i.e., physical, psychological, cultural concerns).
- Meaning of nonverbal cues, level of anxiety client exhibits.

Planning
- Plan of care and interventions (e.g., type of alternative communication, use of translator).
- Teaching plan.

Implementation/Evaluation
- Progress toward desired outcome(s).
- Modifications to plan of care.

Discharge Planning
- Discharge needs, referrals made, additional resources available.

Sample Nursing Outcomes & Interventions Classifications (NOC/NIC)

NOC—Communication
NIC—Communication Enhancement [specify]

Information that appears in brackets has been added by the authors to clarify and enhance the use of nursing diagnoses.

🌐 Cultural 😊 Collaborative 🏠 Community/Home Care

acute Confusion

Taxonomy II: Perception/Cognition—Class 4 Cognition (00128)
[Diagnostic Division: Neurosensory]
Submitted 1994; Revised 2006

Definition: Abrupt onset of reversible disturbances of consciousness, attention, cognition, and perception that develop over a short period of time

Related Factors

Substance abuse; [medication reaction/interaction; anesthesia/surgery]
Fluctuation in sleep-wake cycle
Over 60 years of age
[Endocrine or metabolic crisis; liver or renal failure; shock]
Delirium [including mania/other psychiatric disorder; febrile epilepticum]
Dementia
[Exacerbation of a chronic illness; hypoxemia]
[Severe pain]

Defining Characteristics

Subjective
Hallucinations [visual or auditory]
Exaggerated emotional responses

Objective
Fluctuation in cognition or level of consciousness
Fluctuation in psychomotor activity
Increased agitation or restlessness
Misperceptions; [inappropriate responses]
Lack of motivation to initiate or follow-through with purposeful behavior
Lack of motivation to initiate or follow-through with goal-directed behavior

Desired Outcomes/Evaluation Criteria—Client Will:

• Regain and maintain usual reality orientation and level of consciousness.

Information that appears in brackets has been added by the authors to clarify and enhance the use of nursing diagnoses.

- Verbalize understanding of causative factors when known.
- Initiate lifestyle or behavior changes to prevent or minimize recurrence of problem.

Actions/Interventions

Nursing Priority No. 1.

To assess causative/contributing factors:

- Identify factors present such as recent surgery or trauma; use of large numbers of medications (polypharmacy); intoxication with/withdrawal from a substance (e.g. prescription and over-the-counter [OTC] drugs; alcohol or illicit drugs); history or current seizure activity; episodes of fever or pain, or presence of acute infection (especially occult urinary tract infection [UTI] in elderly clients); traumatic events; person with dementia experiencing sudden change in environment, unfamiliar surroundings, or people. **Acute confusion is a symptom associated with numerous causes (e.g., hypoxia; metabolic/endocrine/neurological conditions, toxins; electrolyte abnormalities; systemic or central nervous system [CNS] infections; nutritional deficiencies; acute psychiatric disorders).**
- Investigate possibility of alcohol or other drug intoxication or withdrawal.
- Evaluate vital signs **for indicators of poor tissue perfusion (i.e., hypotension, tachycardia, tachypnea) or stress response (tachycardia, tachypnea).**
- Determine current medications/drug use—especially anti-anxiety agents, barbiturates, certain antipsychotic agents, methyldopa, disulfiram, cocaine, alcohol, amphetamines, hallucinogens, or opiates **associated with high risk of confusion and delirium**—and schedule of use, such as cimetidine + antacid or digoxin + diuretics **(combinations can increase risk of adverse reactions and interactions).**
- Assess diet and nutritional status **to identify possible deficiencies of essential nutrients and vitamins (e.g., thiamine) that could affect mental status.**
- Note presence of anxiety, agitation, or fear.
- Evaluate for exacerbation of psychiatric conditions (e.g., mood or dissociative disorders, dementia).
- Evaluate sleep and rest status, noting insomnia, sleep deprivation, or oversleeping. (Refer to NDs Insomnia; Sleep Deprivation, as appropriate.)

Information that appears in brackets has been added by the authors to clarify and enhance the use of nursing diagnoses.

- Monitor laboratory values (e.g., CBC, blood cultures; oxygen saturation and, in some cases, ABGs with carbon monoxide; BUN and Cr levels; electrolytes; thyroid function studies; liver function studies, ammonia levels; serum glucose; urinalysis for infection and drug analysis; specific drug toxicologies and drug levels [including peak and trough, as appropriate]).

Nursing Priority No. 2.

To determine degree of impairment:

- Talk with SO(s) to determine historic baseline, observed changes, and onset or recurrence of changes **to understand and clarify current situation.**
- Collaborate with medical and psychiatric providers. Review results of diagnostic studies (e.g., delirium assessment tools, such as the Confusion Assessment Method [CAM], delirium index [DI], Mini Mental State Examination [MMSE]; brain scans or imaging studies; electroencephalogram [EEG]; or lumbar puncture and cerebrospinal fluid [CSF] studies) **to evaluate extent of impairment in orientation, attention span, ability to follow directions, send and receive communication, and appropriateness of response.**
- Note occurrence and timing of agitation, hallucinations, and violent behaviors. **("Sundown syndrome" may occur, with client oriented during daylight hours but confused during nighttime.)**
- Determine threat to safety of client/others. **Delirium can cause client to become verbally and physically aggressive, resulting in behavior threatening to safety of self and others.**

Nursing Priority No. 3.

To maximize level of function, prevent further deterioration:

- Assist with treatment of underlying problem (e.g., drug intoxication/substance abuse, infectious process, hypoxemia, biochemical imbalances, nutritional deficits, or pain management).
- Monitor/adjust medication regimen and note response. Determine medications that can be changed or eliminated **when polypharmacy, side effects, or adverse reactions are determined to be associated with current condition.**

Information that appears in brackets has been added by the authors to clarify and enhance the use of nursing diagnoses.

- Orient client to surroundings, staff, necessary activities, as needed. Present reality concisely and briefly. Avoid challenging illogical thinking—**defensive reactions may result.**
- Encourage family/SO(s) to participate in reorientation as well as providing ongoing input (e.g., current news and family happenings). **Client may respond positively to a well-known person and familiar items.**
- Maintain calm environment and eliminate extraneous noise or other stimuli **to prevent overstimulation.** Provide normal levels of essential sensory and tactile stimulation—include personal items, pictures, and so forth.
- Mobilize elderly client (especially after orthopedic injury) as soon as possible. **An older person with low level of activity prior to crisis is at particular risk for acute confusion and may fare better when out of bed.**
- Encourage client to use vision or hearing aids when needed.
- Give simple directions. Allow sufficient time for client to respond, communicate, and make decisions.
- Provide for safety needs (e.g., supervision, seizure precautions, placing call bell within reach, positioning needed items within reach/clearing traffic paths, and ambulating with devices).
- Establish and maintain elimination patterns. **Disruption of elimination may be a cause for confusion, or changes in elimination may also be a symptom of acute confusion.**
- Note behavior that may be indicative of potential for violence and take appropriate actions. (Refer to ND risk for other-directed/self-directed Violence.)
- Assist with treatment of alcohol or drug intoxication and/or withdrawal, as indicated.
- Administer psychotropics cautiously **to control restlessness, agitation, hallucinations.**
- Avoid or limit use of restraints—**they may worsen the situation and increase the likelihood of untoward complications.**
- Provide undisturbed rest periods.
- Refer to NDs impaired Memory; impaired verbal Communication, for additional interventions.

Nursing Priority No. 4.
To promote wellness (Teaching/Discharge Considerations):
- Explain reason(s) for confusion, if known. **Although acute confusion usually subsides over time as client recovers**

Information that appears in brackets has been added by the authors to clarify and enhance the use of nursing diagnoses.

Cultural   Collaborative   Community/Home Care

from underlying cause and/or adjusts to situation, it can initially be frightening to client/SO. Therefore, information about the cause and appropriate treatment to improve condition may be helpful in managing sense of fear and powerlessness.

- Discuss need for ongoing medical review of client's medications **to limit possibility of misuse and/or potential for dangerous side effects/interactions.**
- Assist in identifying ongoing treatment needs and emphasize necessity of periodic evaluation **to support early intervention.**
- Educate SO/caregivers to monitor client at home for sudden change in cognition and behavior. **An acute change is a classic presentation of delirium and should be considered a medical emergency. Early intervention can often prevent long-term complications.**
- Emphasize importance of keeping vision/hearing aids in good repair **to improve client's interpretation of environmental stimuli and communication.**
- Review ways to maximize sleep environment (e.g., preferred bedtime rituals, comfortable room temperature, bedding and pillows, and elimination or reduction of extraneous noise or stimuli and interruptions.)
- Provide appropriate referrals (e.g., cognitive retraining, substance abuse treatment and support groups, medication monitoring program, Meals on Wheels, home health, or adult day care).

Documentation Focus

Assessment/Reassessment
- Nature, duration, frequency of problem.
- Current and previous level of function and effect on independence and lifestyle (including safety concerns).

Planning
- Plan of care and who is involved in planning.
- Teaching plan.

Implementation/Evaluation
- Response to interventions and actions performed.
- Attainment or progress toward desired outcomes.
- Modifications to plan of care.

Information that appears in brackets has been added by the authors to clarify and enhance the use of nursing diagnoses.

Discharge Planning

* Long-term needs and who is responsible for actions to be taken.
* Available resources and specific referrals.

Sample Nursing Outcomes & Interventions Classifications (NOC/NIC)

NOC—Acute Confusion Level
NIC—Delirium Management

risk for acute Confusion

Taxonomy II: Perception/Cognition—Class 4 Cognition (00173)
[Diagnostic Division: Neurosensory]
Submitted 2006

Definition: At risk for reversible disturbances of consciousness, attention, cognition, and perception that develop over a short period of time

Risk Factors

Substance abuse
Infection; urinary retention
Pain
Fluctuation in sleep-wake cycle
Pharmaceutical agents—anesthesia, anticholinergics, diphenhydramine, opioids, psychoactive drugs, multiple medications
Metabolic abnormalities—decreased hemoglobin, electrolyte imbalances, dehydration, increased blood urea nitrogen (BUN)/creatinine, azotemia, malnutrition
Decreased mobility; decreased restraints
History of stroke; impaired cognition; dementia; sensory deprivation
Over 60 years of age; male gender

NOTE: A risk diagnosis is not evidenced by signs and symptoms, as the problem has not occurred; rather, nursing interventions are directed at prevention.

Information that appears in brackets has been added by the authors to clarify and enhance the use of nursing diagnoses.

🌐 Cultural 🌐 Collaborative 🏠 Community/Home Care

Desired Outcomes/Evaluation Criteria— Client Will:

- Maintain usual level of consciousness and cognition.
- Verbalize understanding of individual cause and risk factor(s).
- Identify interventions to prevent or reduce risk of confusion.

Actions/Interventions

Nursing Priority No. 1.

To assess causative/contributing factors:

- Identify factors present such as recent trauma, fall; use of large numbers of medications (polypharmacy); intoxication with/ withdrawal from a substance (e.g., prescription and over-the-counter drugs; alcohol, illicit drugs); history of seizures or current seizure activity; episodes of fever, pain; presence of acute infection; exposure to toxic substances; traumatic events in client's/SO's life; person with dementia experiencing sudden change in environment, unfamiliar surroundings, or people. **Acute confusion is a symptom associated with numerous causes (e.g., hypoxia, abnormal metabolic conditions, ingestion of toxins or medications, electrolyte abnormalities, sepsis, nutritional deficiencies, endocrine disorders, central nervous system infections or other neurological pathology, and acute psychiatric disorders).**
- Investigate possibility of alcohol or other drug withdrawal, exacerbation of psychiatric conditions (e.g., mood disorder, dissociative disorders, dementia).
- Determine client's functional level, including ability to provide self-care and move about at will. **Conditions and situations that limit client's mobility and independence (e.g., acute or chronic physical or psychiatric illnesses and their therapies, trauma or extensive immobility, confinement in unfamiliar surroundings, sensory deprivation) potentiate prospect of acute confusional state.**
- Ascertain life events (e.g., death of spouse/other family member, absence of known care provider, move from lifelong home, catastrophic natural disaster) **that can affect client's perceptions, attention, and concentration.**
- Assess diet and nutritional status **to identify possible deficiencies of essential nutrients and vitamins that could affect mental status.**
- Evaluate sleep and rest status, noting insomnia, sleep deprivation, or oversleeping. (Refer to NDs Insomnia; Sleep Deprivation, as appropriate.)

Information that appears in brackets has been added by the authors to clarify and enhance the use of nursing diagnoses.

- Monitor laboratory values (e.g., complete blood count, blood cultures; oxygen saturation and, in some cases, ABGs with carbon monoxide; BUN and Cr levels; electrolytes; thyroid function studies; liver function studies, ammonia levels; serum glucose; urinalysis for infection and drug analysis; specific drug toxicologies, and drug levels [including peak and trough, as appropriate]) **to identify imbalances that have potential for causing confusion.**

Nursing Priority No. 2.
To reduce/correct existing risk factors:

- Assist with treatment of underlying problem (e.g., drug intoxication/substance abuse, infectious processes, hypoxemia, biochemical imbalances, nutritional deficits, pain management).
- Monitor/adjust medication regimen and note response. **May identify medications that can be changed or eliminated in client who is prone to adverse or exaggerated responses (including confusion) to medications.**
- Administer medications, as appropriate (e.g., relieving pain in elderly client with hip fracture can improve cognitive responses).
- Orient client to surroundings, staff, necessary activities.
- Encourage family/SO(s) to participate in orientation by providing ongoing input (e.g., current news and family happenings).
- Maintain calm environment and eliminate extraneous noise or other stimuli **to prevent overstimulation.**
- Provide normal levels of essential sensory and tactile stimulation—include personal items, pictures, desired music, activities, contacts, and so on.
- Encourage client to use vision/hearing aids/other adaptive equipment, as needed, **to assist client in interpretation of environment and communication.**
- Promote early ambulation activities **to enhance well-being and reduce effects of prolonged bedrest or inactivity.**
- Provide for safety needs (e.g., supervision; seizure precautions; placing needed items, such as a call bell, within reach; clearing traffic paths; ambulating with assistance; providing clear directions and instructions).

Nursing Priority No. 3.
To promote wellness (Teaching/Discharge Considerations):

- Assist with treatment of underlying medical conditions and/or management of risk factors **to reduce or limit conditions associated with confusion.**

Information that appears in brackets has been added by the authors to clarify and enhance the use of nursing diagnoses.

- Emphasize importance of ongoing monitoring of medication regimen **to limit possibility of misuse for potential adverse actions or reactions.**
- Provide undisturbed rest periods.
- Review ways to maximize sleep environment (e.g., preferred bedtime rituals, room temperature, bedding/pillows, and elimination or reduction of extraneous noise/stimuli and interruptions).
- Provide appropriate referrals (e.g., medical or psychiatric specialists, medication monitoring program, nutritionist, substance abuse treatment, support groups, home health care, and adult day care).

Documentation Focus

Assessment/Reassessment
- Existing conditions, risk factors for individual.
- Current level of function, effect on independence and ability to meet own needs, including food and fluid intake, and medication use.

Planning
- Plan of care and who is involved in planning.
- Teaching plan.

Implementation/Evaluation
- Response to interventions and actions performed.
- Attainment or progress toward desired outcomes.
- Modifications to plan of care.

Discharge Planning
- Long-term needs and who is responsible for actions to be taken.
- Available resources and specific referrals.

Sample Nursing Outcomes & Interventions Classifications (NOC/NIC)

NOC—Cognition
NIC—Reality Orientation

Information that appears in brackets has been added by the authors to clarify and enhance the use of nursing diagnoses.

chronic **Confusion**

Taxonomy II: Perception/Cognition—Class 4 Cognition (00129)
[Diagnostic Division: Neurosensory]
Submitted 1994

Definition: Irreversible, long-standing, and/or progressive deterioration of intellect and personality characterized by a decreased ability to interpret environmental stimuli and decreased capacity for intellectual thought processes manifested by disturbances of memory, orientation, and behavior

Related Factors

Alzheimer's disease
Korsakoff's psychosis
Multi-infarct dementia
Cerebral vascular attack
Head injury

Defining Characteristics

Objective
Clinical evidence of organic impairment
Altered interpretation
Altered response to stimuli
Progressive/long-standing cognitive impairment
No change in level of consciousness
Impaired socialization
Impaired short-term/long-term memory
Altered personality

Desired Outcome/Evaluation Criteria—Client Will:

- Remain safe and free from harm.
- Maintain usual level of orientation.

Family/SO Will:

- Verbalize understanding of disease process, prognosis, and client's needs.
- Identify and participate in interventions to deal effectively with situation.

Information that appears in brackets has been added by the authors to clarify and enhance the use of nursing diagnoses.

- Provide for maximal independence while meeting safety needs of client.

Actions/Interventions

Nursing Priority No. 1.
To assess degree of impairment:

- Evaluate responses on diagnostic examinations (e.g., memory impairments, reality orientation, attention span, calculations, quality of life). **A combination of tests (e.g., Confusion Assessment Method [CAM], the Mini-Mental State Examination [MMSE], the Alzheimer's Disease Assessment Scale [ADAS-cog], the Brief Dementia Severity Rating Scale [BDSRS], or the Neuropsychiatric Inventory [NPI]) is often needed to complete an evaluation of the client's overall condition relating to a chronic/irreversible condition.**
- Test ability to receive and send effective communication. **Client may be nonverbal or require assistance with/interpretation of verbalizations.**
- Talk with SO(s) regarding baseline behaviors, length of time since onset, and progression of problem, their perception of prognosis, and other pertinent information and concerns for client. **If the history reveals an insidious decline over months to years, and if abnormal perceptions, inattention, and memory problems are concurrent with confusion, a diagnosis of dementia is likely.**
- Ascertain interventions previously used or tried.
- Evaluate response to care providers and receptiveness to interventions **to determine areas of concern to be addressed.**
- Determine anxiety level in relation to situation and problem behaviors **that may be indicative of potential for violence.**

Nursing Priority No. 2.
To limit effects of deterioration/maximize level of function:

- Assist in treating conditions (e.g., infections, malnutrition, electrolyte imbalances, and adverse medication reactions) **that may contribute to/exacerbate confusion, discomfort, and agitation.**
- Provide calm environment, minimize relocations, eliminate extraneous noise/stimuli **that may increase client's level of agitation/confusion.**
- Be open and honest in discussing client's disease, abilities, and prognosis.

Information that appears in brackets has been added by the authors to clarify and enhance the use of nursing diagnoses.

- Use touch judiciously. Tell client what is being done before initiating contact **to reduce sense of surprise and negative reaction.**
- Avoid challenging illogical thinking **because defensive reactions may result.**
- Use positive statements; offer guided choices between two options. Simplify client's tasks and routines **to accommodate fluctuating abilities and to reduce agitation associated with multiple options or demands.**
- Be supportive when client is attempting to communicate and be sensitive to increasing frustration, fears, and misperceived threats.
- Encourage family/SO(s) to provide ongoing orientation and input to include current news and family happenings.
- ⌂ Maintain reality-oriented relationship and environment (e.g., clocks, calendars, personal items, and seasonal decorations). Encourage participation in resocialization groups.
- Allow client to reminisce or exist in own reality, if not detrimental to well-being.
- ⌂ Provide safety measures (e.g., close supervision, identification bracelet, alarm on unlocked exits; medication lockup, removal of car or car keys; lower temperature on hot water tank).
- Set limits on unsafe and/or inappropriate behavior, being alert to potential for violence.
- Avoid use of restraints as much as possible. Use vest (instead of wrist) restraints, or investigate use of alternatives (such as bed nets, electronic bed pads, laptop trays) when required. **Although restraints may prevent falls, they can increase client's agitation and distress and are a safety risk.**
- Administer medications, as ordered (e.g., antidepressants, antipsychotics). Monitor for therapeutic action, as well as adverse reactions, side effects, and interactions. **Medications may be used judiciously to manage symptoms of psychosis, depression, or aggressive behavior.**
- Refer to NDs acute Confusion; impaired Memory; impaired verbal Communication, for additional interventions.

Nursing Priority No. 3.
To assist SO(s) to develop coping strategies:

- Determine family resources, availability, and willingness to participate in meeting client's needs.
- Involve family/SO(s) in planning and care activities as needed/desired. Maintain frequent interactions with SO(s) **in**

Information that appears in brackets has been added by the authors to clarify and enhance the use of nursing diagnoses.

order to relay information, change care strategies, obtain SO feedback, and offer support.

- Discuss caregiver burden and signs of burnout, when appropriate. (Refer to NDs Caregiver Role Strain; risk for Caregiver Role Strain.)
- Provide educational materials, bibliographies, list of available local resources, help lines, Web sites, and so on, as desired, **to assist SO(s) in dealing and coping with long-term care issues.**
- Identify appropriate community resources (c.g., Alzheimer's Disease and Related Disorders Association [ARDA], stroke or brain injury support groups, senior support groups, specialist day services, home care, and respite care; adult placement and short-term residential care; clergy, social services, occupational and physical therapists; assistive technology and tele-care; attorney services for advance directives, and durable power of attorney) **to provide client/SO with support and assist with problem-solving.**

Nursing Priority No. 4.
To promote wellness (Teaching/Discharge Considerations):

- Discuss nature of client's condition (e.g., chronic stable, progressive, or degenerative), treatment concerns, and follow-up needed **to promote maintaining client at highest possible level of functioning.**
- Determine age-appropriate ongoing treatment and socialization needs and appropriate resources.
- Review medications with SO/caregiver(s), including dosage, route, action, expected and reportable side effects, and potential drug interactions **to prevent or limit complications associated with multiple psychiatric and central nervous system medications.**
- Develop plan of care with family **to meet client's and SO's individual needs.**
- Provide appropriate referrals (e.g., Meals on Wheels, adult day care, home care agency, respite care).

Documentation Focus

Assessment/Reassessment
- Individual findings, including current level of function and rate of anticipated changes.
- Safety issues.

Information that appears in brackets has been added by the authors to clarify and enhance the use of nursing diagnoses.

Planning
• Plan of care and who is involved in planning.

Implementation/Evaluation
• Response to interventions and actions performed.
• Attainment or progress toward desired outcomes.
• Modifications to plan of care.

Discharge Planning
• Long-term needs, referrals made and who is responsible for actions to be taken.
• Available resources, specific referrals made.

Sample Nursing Outcomes & Interventions Classifications (NOC/NIC)

NOC—Cognitive Orientation
NIC—Dementia Management

Constipation

Taxonomy II: Elimination and Exchange—Class 2 Gastrointestinal Function (00011)
[Diagnostic Division: Elimination]
Submitted 1975; Nursing Diagnosis Extension and Classification Revision 1998

Definition: Decrease in normal frequency of defecation accompanied by difficult or incomplete passage of stool and/or passage of excessively hard, dry stool

Related Factors

Functional
Irregular defecation habits; inadequate toileting (e.g., timeliness, positioning for defecation, privacy)
Insufficient physical activity; abdominal muscle weakness
Recent environmental changes
Habitual ignoring of urge to defecate

Psychological
Emotional stress; depression; mental confusion

Information that appears in brackets has been added by the authors to clarify and enhance the use of nursing diagnoses.

Pharmacological

Antilipemic agents; laxative abuse; calcium carbonate; aluminum-containing antacids; nonsteroidal anti-inflammatory agents (NSAIDs); opiates; anticholinergics; diuretics; iron salts; phenothiazides; sedatives; sympathomimetics; bismuth salts; antidepressants; calcium channel blockers; anticonvulsants

Mechanical

Hemorrhoids; pregnancy; obesity

Rectal abscess, ulcer, or prolapse; rectal anal fissures or strictures; rectocele

Prostate enlargement; postsurgical obstruction

Neurological impairment; Hirschsprung's disease; tumors

Electrolyte imbalance

Physiological

Poor eating habits; change in usual foods or eating patterns; insufficient fiber or fluid intake; dehydration

Inadequate dentition or oral hygiene

Decreased motility of gastrointestinal tract

Defining Characteristics

Subjective

Change in bowel pattern; unable to pass stool; decreased frequency, decreased volume of stool

Increased abdominal pressure; feeling of rectal fullness or pressure

Abdominal pain; pain with defecation; nausea; vomiting; headache; indigestion; generalized fatigue

Objective

Hard, formed stool

Straining with defecation

Hypoactive or hyperactive bowel sounds; borborygmi

Distended abdomen; abdominal tenderness with or without palpable muscle resistance; palpable abdominal or rectal mass

Percussed abdominal dullness

Presence of soft paste-like stool in rectum; oozing liquid stool; bright red blood with stool

Severe flatus; anorexia

Information that appears in brackets has been added by the authors to clarify and enhance the use of nursing diagnoses.

Atypical presentations in older adults (e.g., change in mental status, urinary incontinence, unexplained falls, elevated body temperature)

Desired Outcomes/Evaluation Criteria—Client Will:

- Establish or regain normal pattern of bowel functioning.
- Verbalize understanding of etiology and appropriate interventions or solutions for individual situation.
- Demonstrate behaviors or lifestyle changes to prevent recurrence of problem.
- Participate in bowel program as indicated.

Actions/Interventions

Nursing Priority No. 1.

To identify causative/contributing factors:

- Review medical, surgical, and social history **to identify conditions commonly associated with constipation, including (1) problems with colon or rectum (e.g., obstruction, scar tissue or stricture, diverticulitis, irritable bowel syndrome, tumors, anal fissure); (2) metabolic or endocrine disorders (e.g., diabetes mellitus, hypothyroidism, uremia); (3) limited physical activity (e.g., bedrest, poor mobility, chronic disability); (4) chronic pain problems (especially when client is on pain medications); (5) pregnancy and childbirth, recent abdominal or perianal surgery; and (6) neurological disorders (e.g., stroke, traumatic brain injury, Parkinson's disease, MS, and spinal cord abnormalities).**
- ∞ Note client's age. **Constipation is more likely to occur in individuals older than 65 but can occur in any age from infant to elderly. A bottle-fed infant is more prone to constipation than a breastfed infant, especially when formula contains iron. Toddlers are at risk because of developmental factors (e.g., too young, too interested in other things, rigid schedule during potty training), and children and adolescents are at risk because of unwillingness to take break from play, poor eating and fluid intake habits, and withholding because of perceived lack of privacy. Many older adults experience constipation as a result of duller nerve sensations, immobility, dehydration and electrolyte imbalances; incomplete emptying of the bowel, or failing to attend to signals to defecate.**

Information that appears in brackets has been added by the authors to clarify and enhance the use of nursing diagnoses.

- Review daily dietary regimen, noting if diet is deficient in fiber. **Inadequate dietary fiber (vegetable, fruits, and whole grains) and highly processed foods contribute to poor intestinal function.**
- Note general oral/dental health issues **that can impact dietary intake.**
- Determine fluid intake. **Most individuals do not drink enough fluids, even when healthy, reducing the speed at which stool moves through the colon. Active fluid loss through sweating, vomiting, diarrhea, or bleeding can greatly increase chances for constipation.**
- Evaluate client's medication/drug regimen (e.g., opioids, pain relievers, antidepressants, anticonvulsants, aluminum-containing antacids, chemotherapy, iron supplements, contrast media, steroids) **that could cause/exacerbate constipation.**
- Note energy and activity levels and exercise pattern. **Lack of physical activity or regular exercise is often a factor in constipation.**
- Identify areas of stress (e.g., personal relationships, occupational factors, financial problems). **Individuals may fail to allow time for good bowel habits and/or suffer gastrointestinal effects from stress.**
- Determine access to bathroom, privacy, and ability to perform self-care activities.
- Investigate reports of pain with defecation. Inspect perianal area for hemorrhoids, fissures, skin breakdown, or other abnormal findings.
- Determine laxative/enema use. Note signs and reports of overuse of stimulant laxatives. **This is most common among older adults preoccupied with having daily bowel movements.**
- Palpate abdomen **for presence of distention or masses.**
- Check rectum for presence of fecal impaction, as indicated.
- Assist with medical work-up (e.g., x-rays, abdominal imaging, proctosigmoidoscopy, anorectal function tests, colonic transit studies, and stool sample tests) **for identification of other possible causative factors.**

Nursing Priority No. 2.

To determine usual pattern of elimination:

- Discuss usual elimination habits (e.g., normal urge time) and problems (e.g., client unable to eliminate unless in own home, passing hard stool after prolonged effort, anal pain).

Information that appears in brackets has been added by the authors to clarify and enhance the use of nursing diagnoses.

• Identify elements that usually stimulate bowel activity (e.g., caffeine, walking, laxative use) and any interfering factors (e.g., taking opioid pain medications, unable to ambulate to bathroom, pelvic surgery).

Nursing Priority No. 3.
To assess current pattern of elimination:

• Note color, odor, consistency, amount, and frequency of stool. **Provides a baseline for comparison, promotes recognition of changes.**

• Ascertain duration of current problem and client's degree of concern (e.g., long-standing condition that client has "lived with" may not cause undue concern, whereas an acute post-surgical occurrence of constipation can cause great distress). **Client's response may or may not reflect severity of condition.**

• Auscultate abdomen for presence, location, and characteristics of bowel sounds **reflecting bowel activity.**

• Note treatments client has tried to relieve current situation (e.g., laxatives, suppositories, enemas) and document failure or lack of effectiveness.

• Encourage client to maintain elimination diary, if appropriate, **to facilitate monitoring of long-term problem.**

Nursing Priority No. 4.
To facilitate return to usual/acceptable pattern of elimination:

• Instruct in and encourage a diet of balanced fiber and bulk (e.g., fruits, vegetables, whole grains) and fiber supplements (e.g., wheat bran, psyllium) **to improve consistency of stool and facilitate passage through colon. Note:** Improvement in elimination as a result of dietary changes takes time and is not a treatment for acute constipation.

• Promote adequate fluid intake, including high-fiber fruit juices, fruit/vegetable smoothies, and popsicles; suggest drinking warm, stimulating fluids (e.g., coffee, hot water, tea) **to avoid dehydration and promote passage of soft stool.**

• Encourage activity and regular exercise within limits of individual ability **to stimulate contractions of the intestines.**

• Provide privacy and routinely scheduled time for defecation (bathroom or commode preferable to bedpan) **so client can respond to urge.**

Information that appears in brackets has been added by the authors to clarify and enhance the use of nursing diagnoses.

- Encourage/support treatment of underlying medical causes where appropriate **to improve organ function, including the bowel.**
- Administer stool softeners, mild stimulants, or bulk-forming agents, as ordered or routinely, when appropriate (e.g., for client receiving opiates, decreased level of activity/ immobility).
- Apply lubricant/anesthetic ointment to anus, if needed.
- Administer enemas; digitally remove impacted stool.
- Encourage sitz bath after stools **for soothing effect to rectal area.**
- Establish bowel program to include predictable interval timing for toileting and privacy; use of particular position for defecation; abdominal massage; biofeedback for pelvic floor dysfunction; and stool softeners, glycerin suppositories, and digital stimulation, as appropriate, **when long-term or permanent bowel dysfunction is present.**
- Refer to primary care provider for medical therapies (e.g., added emolient, saline, or hyperosmolar laxatives, enemas, or suppositories) **to best treat acute situation.**
- Discuss client's current medication regimen with physician **to determine if drugs contributing to constipation can be discontinued or changed.**

Nursing Priority No. 5.
To promote wellness (Teaching/Discharge Considerations):

- Discuss client's particular physiology and acceptable variations in elimination.
- Provide information about relationship of diet, exercise, fluid, and appropriate use of laxatives, as indicated.
- Discuss rationale for and encourage continuation of successful interventions.
- Refer client/care provider to physician if problem does not resolve **to reduce risk of complications, and to promote timely intervention, thereby enhancing client's independence.**

Documentation Focus

Assessment/Reassessment
- Usual and current bowel pattern, duration of the problem, and individual contributing factors, including diet and exercise/ activity level.

Information that appears in brackets has been added by the authors to clarify and enhance the use of nursing diagnoses.

- Characteristics of stool.
- Underlying dynamics.

Planning

- Plan of care, specific interventions, and changes in lifestyle that are necessary to correct individual situation, and who is involved in planning.
- Teaching plan.

Implementation/Evaluation

- Responses to interventions, teaching, and actions performed.
- Change in bowel pattern, character of stool.
- Attainment or progress toward desired outcomes.
- Modifications to plan of care.

Discharge Planning

- Individual long-term needs, noting who is responsible for actions to be taken.
- Recommendations for follow-up care.
- Specific referrals made.

Sample Nursing Outcomes & Interventions Classifications (NOC/NIC)

NOC—Bowel Elimination
NIC—Constipation/Impaction Management

perceived Constipation

Taxonomy II: Elimination and Exchange—Class 2 Gastrointestinal Function (00012)
[Diagnostic Division: Elimination]
Submitted 1988

Definition: Self-diagnosis of constipation combined with abuse of laxatives, enemas, and/or suppositories to ensure a daily bowel movement

Related Factors

Cultural or family health beliefs
Faulty appraisal
Impaired thought processes

Information that appears in brackets has been added by the authors to clarify and enhance the use of nursing diagnoses.

🌐 Cultural 😊 Collaborative 🏠 Community/Home Care

Defining Characteristics

Subjective
Expectation of a daily bowel movement
Expectation of passage of stool at same time every day
Overuse of laxatives, enemas, or suppositories

Desired Outcomes/Evaluation Criteria— Client Will:

- Verbalize understanding of physiology of bowel function.
- Identify acceptable interventions to promote adequate bowel function.
- Decrease reliance on laxatives or enemas.
- Establish individually appropriate pattern of elimination.

Actions/Interventions

Nursing Priority No. 1.
To identify factors affecting individual beliefs:

- Determine client's understanding of a "normal" bowel pattern and cultural expectations. **Helps to identify areas for discussion or intervention. For example, what is considered "normal" varies with the individual, cultural, and familial factors with differences in expectations and dietary habits. In addition, individuals can think they are constipated when, in fact, their bowel movements are regular and soft, possibly revealing a problem with thought processes or perception. Some people believe they are constipated, or irregular, if they do not have a bowel movement every day, because of ideas instilled from childhood. The elderly client may believe that laxatives or purgatives are necessary for elimination, when in fact the problem may be long-standing habits (e.g., insufficient fluids, lack of exercise and/or fiber in the diet).**

- Discuss client's use of laxatives. **Perceived constipation typically results in self-medicating with various laxatives. Although laxatives may correct the acute problem, chronic use leads to habituation, requiring ever-increasing doses that result in drug dependency and, ultimately, a hypotonic colon.**

- Identify interventions used by client to correct perceived problem **to identify strengths and areas of concern to be addressed.**

Information that appears in brackets has been added by the authors to clarify and enhance the use of nursing diagnoses.

Nursing Priority No. 2.

🏠To promote wellness (Teaching/Discharge Considerations):

- Discuss physiology and acceptable variations in elimination.
- Identify detrimental effects of habitual laxative and/or enema use and discuss alternatives.
- Review relationship of diet, hydration, and exercise to bowel elimination.
- Provide support by Active-listening and discussing client's concerns/fears.
- Encourage use of stress-reduction activities and refocusing of attention while client works to establish individually appropriate pattern.
- Offer educational materials and resources for client/SO **to peruse at home to assist them in making informed decisions regarding constipation and management options.**
- Refer to medical and psychiatric providers, as indicated. **Client with fixed perception of constipation where none actually exists, may require further assessment and intervention.**
- Refer to ND Constipation for additional interventions, as appropriate.

Documentation Focus

Assessment/Reassessment
- Assessment findings, client's perceptions of the problem.
- Current bowel pattern, stool characteristics.

Planning
- Plan of care, specific interventions, and who is involved in the planning.
- Teaching plan.

Implementation/Evaluation
- Client's responses to interventions, teaching, and actions performed.
- Changes in bowel pattern, character of stool.
- Attainment or progress toward desired outcome(s).
- Modifications to plan of care.

Discharge Planning
- Referral for follow-up care.

Information that appears in brackets has been added by the authors to clarify and enhance the use of nursing diagnoses.

🌐 Cultural   ⊛ Collaborative   🏠 Community/Home Care

Sample Nursing Outcomes & Interventions Classifications (NOC/NIC)

NOC—Health Beliefs
NIC—Bowel Management

risk for Constipation

Taxonomy II: Elimination and Exchange—Class 2 Gastrointestinal Function (00015)
[Diagnostic Division: Elimination]
Nursing Diagnosis Extension and Classification Submission 1998

Definition: At risk for a decrease in normal frequency of defecation accompanied by difficult or incomplete passage of stool and/or passage of excessively hard, dry stool

Risk Factors

Functional

Irregular defecation habits; inadequate toileting (e.g., timeliness, positioning for defecation, privacy)
Insufficient physical activity; abdominal muscle weakness
Recent environmental changes
Habitual ignoring of urge to defecate

Psychological

Emotional stress; depression; mental confusion

Physiological

Change in usual foods or eating patterns; insufficient fiber/fluid intake, dehydration; poor eating habits
Inadequate dentition or oral hygiene
Decreased motility of gastrointestinal tract

Pharmacological

Phenothiazines; nonsteroidal anti-inflammatory agents; sedatives; aluminum-containing antacids; laxative overuse; bismuth salts; iron salts; anticholinergics; antidepressants; anticonvulsants; antilipemic agents; calcium channel blockers; calcium carbonate; diuretics; sympathomimetics; opiates

---

Information that appears in brackets has been added by the authors to clarify and enhance the use of nursing diagnoses.

Mechanical

Hemorrhoids; pregnancy; obesity

Rectal abscess or ulcer; rectal anal stricture or fissures; rectal prolapse; rectocele

Prostate enlargement; postsurgical obstruction

Neurological impairment; Hirschsprung's disease; tumors

Electrolyte imbalance

> **NOTE:** A risk diagnosis is not evidenced by signs and symptoms, as the problem has not occurred; rather, nursing interventions are directed at prevention.

Desired Outcomes/Evaluation Criteria— Client Will:

* Maintain effective pattern of bowel functioning.
* Verbalize understanding of risk factors and appropriate interventions or solutions related to individual situation.
* Demonstrate behaviors or lifestyle changes to prevent developing problem.

Actions/Interventions

Nursing Priority No. 1.

To identify individual risk factors/needs:

* Review medical, surgical, and social history (e.g., altered cognition; metabolic, endocrine, or neurological disorders; certain medications; surgery; bowel disorders such as irritable bowel syndrome, intestinal obstructions or tumors, hemorrhoids/rectal bleeding; pregnancy; advanced age; weakness/debilitation; conditions associated with immobility; recent travel; stressors/changes in lifestyle; depression) **to identify conditions commonly associated with constipation.**
* Note client's age. **Constipation is more likely to occur in individuals older than 65 but can occur in any age from infant to elderly. A bottle-fed infant is more prone to constipation than a breastfed infant, especially when formula contains iron. Toddlers are at risk because of developmental factors (e.g., too young, too interested in other things, rigid schedule during potty training), and children and adolescents are at risk because of unwillingness to take break from play, poor eating and fluid intake habits, and withholding because of perceived lack of privacy. Many older adults experience constipation as a result of**

Information that appears in brackets has been added by the authors to clarify and enhance the use of nursing diagnoses.

🌐 Cultural ⚘ Collaborative 🏠 Community/Home Care

blunted nerve sensations, immobility, dehydration and electrolyte imbalances, incomplete emptying of the bowel, or failing to attend to signals to defecate.

- Auscultate abdomen for presence, location, and characteristics of bowel sounds **reflecting bowel activity.**
- Discuss usual elimination pattern and use of laxatives.
- Ascertain client's beliefs and practices about bowel elimination, such as "must have a bowel movement every day or I need an enema." **Familial or cultural thinking about elimination affects client's lifetime patterns.**
- Evaluate current dietary and fluid intake and implications for effect on bowel function.
- Review medications (new and chronic use) **for impact on/effects of changes in bowel function.**
- Note energy and activity level and exercise pattern. **Lack of physical activity or regular exercise is often a factor in constipation.**

Nursing Priority No. 2.
To facilitate normal bowel function:

- Instruct in/encourage balanced fiber and bulk in diet (e.g., fruits, vegetables, whole grains) and fiber supplements (c.g., wheat bran, psyllium) **to improve consistency of stool and facilitate passage through colon.**
- Promote adequate fluid intake, including water and high-fiber fruit juices; also suggest drinking warm fluids (e.g., coffee, hot water, tea) **to promote soft stool and stimulate bowel activity.**
- Encourage activity and exercise within limits of individual ability **to stimulate contractions of the intestines.**
- Provide privacy and routinely scheduled time for defecation (bathroom or commode preferable to bedpan) **so client can respond to urge.**
- Administer routine stool softeners, mild stimulants, or bulk-forming agents as needed, or routinely, as appropriate (e.g., for client taking pain medications, especially opiates, or who is inactive, immobile, or unconscious).
- Ascertain frequency, color, consistency, amount of stools. **Provides a baseline for comparison; promotes recognition of changes.**

Nursing Priority No. 3.
To promote wellness (Teaching/Discharge Considerations):

- Discuss physiology and acceptable variations in elimination. **May help reduce concerns/anxiety about situation.**

Information that appears in brackets has been added by the authors to clarify and enhance the use of nursing diagnoses.

- Review individual risk factors, potential problems, and specific interventions.
- Educate client/SO about safe and risky practices for managing constipation. **Information can help client to make beneficial choices when need arises.**
- Encourage client to maintain elimination diary, if appropriate, **to help monitor bowel pattern.**
- Educate client/SO about safe and risky practices for managing constipation. **Information can assist client to make beneficial choices when need arises.**
- Review appropriate use of medications. Discuss client's current medication regimen with physician **to determine if drugs contributing to constipation can be discontinued or changed.**
- Refer for/support treatment of underlying medical causes, where appropriate, **to improve organ function, including the bowel.**
- Refer to NDs Constipation; perceived Constipation for additional interventions as appropriate.

Documentation Focus

Assessment/Reassessment
- Current bowel pattern, characteristics of stool, medications and herbals used.
- Dietary intake.
- Exercise and activity level.

Planning
- Plan of care and who is involved in planning.
- Teaching plan.

Implementation/Evaluation
- Responses to interventions, teaching, and actions performed.
- Attainment or progress toward desired outcomes.
- Modifications to plan of care.

Discharge Planning
- Individual long-term needs, noting who is responsible for actions to be taken.
- Specific referrals made.

Information that appears in brackets has been added by the authors to clarify and enhance the use of nursing diagnoses.

⊕ Cultural Collaborative 🏠 Community/Home Care

Sample Nursing Outcomes & Interventions Classifications (NOC/NIC)

NOC—Bowel Elimination
NIC—Constipation/Impaction Management

Contamination

Taxonomy II: Safety/Protection—Class 4 Environmental Hazards (00181)
[Diagnostic Division: Safety]
Submitted 2006

Definition: Exposure to environmental contaminants in doses sufficient to cause adverse health effects

Related Factors

External

Chemical contamination of food or water; presence of atmospheric pollutants

Inadequate municipal services (trash removal, sewage treatment facilities)

Geographical area (living in area where high levels of contaminants exist)

Playing in outdoor areas where environmental contaminants are used

Personal or household hygiene practices

Economically disadvantaged (increases potential for multiple exposure, lack of access to healthcare, and poor diet)

Use of environmental contaminants in the home (e.g., pesticides, chemicals, environmental tobacco smoke)

Lack of breakdown of contaminants once indoors (breakdown is inhibited without sun and rain exposure)

Flooring surface (carpeted surfaces hold contaminant residue more than hard floor surfaces)

Flaking, peeling paint or plaster in presence of young children

Paint/lacquer in poorly ventilated areas or without effective protection

Inappropriate use/lack of protective clothing

Unprotected contact with heavy metals (e.g., arsenic, chromium, lead)

Exposure to radiation (occupation in radiography, employment in or living near nuclear industries and electrical generating

---

Information that appears in brackets has been added by the authors to clarify and enhance the use of nursing diagnoses.

plants); exposure through ingestion of radioactive material (e.g., food/water contamination)

Exposure to a disaster (natural or man made); exposure to bioterrorism

Internal

Age (children less than 5 years, older adults); gestational age during exposure; developmental characteristics of children

Female gender; pregnancy

Nutritional factors (e.g., obesity, vitamin and mineral deficiencies)

Preexisting disease states; smoking

Concomitant exposure; previous exposures

Defining Characteristics

Defining characteristics are dependent on the causative agent. Agents cause a variety of individual organ responses as well as systemic responses.

Subjective/Objective

Pesticides: (Major categories of pesticides: insecticides, herbicides, fungicides, antimicrobials, rodenticides; major pesticides: organophosphates, carbamates, organochlorines, pyrethrum, arsenic, glycophosphates, bipyridyis, chlorophenoxy compounds)

Dermatological, gastrointestinal, neurological, pulmonary, or renal effects of pesticide

Chemicals: (Major chemical agents: petroleum-based agents, anticholinesterases; type I agents act on proximal tracheobronchial portion of the respiratory tract, type II agents act on alveoli, type III agents produce systemic effects)

Dermatological, gastrointestinal, immunological, neurological, pulmonary, or renal effects of chemical exposure

Biologicals: (Toxins from living organisms—bacteria, viruses, fungi)

Dermatological, gastrointestinal, neurological, pulmonary, or renal effects of exposure to biologicals

Pollution: (Major locations: air, water, soil; major agents: asbestos, radon, tobacco [smoke], heavy metal, lead, noise, exhaust fumes)

Neurological or pulmonary effects of pollution exposure

Information that appears in brackets has been added by the authors to clarify and enhance the use of nursing diagnoses.

Waste: (Major categories of waste: trash, raw sewage, industrial waste

Dermatological, gastrointestinal, hepatic, or pulmonary effects of waste exposure

Radiation: (External exposure through direct contact with radioactive material)

Immunological, genetic, neurological or oncological effects of radiation exposure

Desired Outcomes/Evaluation Criteria— Client Will:

- Be free of injury.
- Verbalize understanding of individual factors that contributed to injury and plans for correcting situation(s) where possible.
- Modify environment, as indicated, to enhance safety.

Client/Community Will:

- Identify hazards that lead to exposure or contamination.
- Correct environmental hazards, as identified.
- Demonstrate necessary actions to promote community safety.

Actions/Interventions

In reviewing this ND, it is apparent there is overlap with other diagnoses. We have chosen to present generalized interventions. Although there are commonalities to contamination situations, we suggest that the reader refer to other primary diagnoses as indicated, such as ineffective Airway Clearance; ineffective Breathing Pattern; impaired Gas Exchange; ineffective Home Maintenance; risk for Infection; risk for Injury; risk for Poisoning; impaired/risk for impaired Skin Integrity; risk for Suffocation; ineffective Tissue Perfusion [specify]; risk for Trauma.

Nursing Priority No. 1.

To evaluate degree/source of exposure:

- Ascertain: (1) type of contaminant(s) to which client has been exposed (e.g., chemical, biological, air pollutant), (2) manner of exposure (e.g., inhalation, ingestion, topical), (3) whether exposure was accidental or intentional, and (4) immediate/delayed reactions. **Determines course of action to be taken by all emergency/other care providers. Note:** Intentional exposure to hazardous materials requires notification of law

---

Information that appears in brackets has been added by the authors to clarify and enhance the use of nursing diagnoses.

enforcement for further investigation and possible prosecution.

∞• Note age and gender: **Children less than 5 years are at greater risk for adverse effects from exposure to contaminants because (1) smaller body size causes them to receive a more concentrated "dose" than adults; (2) they spend more time outside than most adults, increasing exposure to air and soil pollutants; (3) they spend more time on the floor, increasing exposure to toxins in carpets and low cupboards; (4) they consume more water and food per pound than adults, increasing their body weight to toxin ratio; and (5) fetus's/infant's and young children's developing organ systems can be disrupted. Older adults have a normal decline in function of immune, integumentary, cardiac, renal, hepatic, and pulmonary systems; an increase in adipose tissue mass; and a decline in lean body mass. Females, in general, have a greater proportion of body fat, increasing the chance of accumulating more lipid-soluble toxins than males.**

• Ascertain geographical location (e.g., home, work) where exposure occurred. **Individual and/or community intervention may be needed to correct problem.**

• Note socioeconomic status and availability and use of resources. **Living in poverty increases potential for multiple exposures, delayed/lack of access to healthcare, and poor general health, potentially increasing the severity of adverse effects of exposure.**

• Determine factors associated with particular contaminant:

Pesticides: Determine if client has ingested contaminated foods (e.g., fruits, vegetables, commercially raised meats), or inhaled agent (e.g., aerosol bug sprays, in vicinity of crop spraying).

Chemicals: Ascertain if client uses environmental contaminants in the home or at work (e.g., pesticides, chemicals, chlorine household cleaners), and fails to use/inappropriately uses protective clothing.

Biologicals: Determine if client may have been exposed to biological agents (bacteria, viruses, fungi) or bacterial toxins (e.g., botulinum, ricin). **Exposure occurring as a result of an act of terrorism would be rare; however, individuals may be exposed to bacterial agents or toxins through contaminated or poorly prepared foods.**

Information that appears in brackets has been added by the authors to clarify and enhance the use of nursing diagnoses.

🌐 Cultural 🌐 Collaborative 🏠 Community/Home Care

Pollution air/water: Determine if client has been exposed/is sensitive to atmospheric pollutants (e.g., radon, benzene [from gasoline], carbon monoxide, automobile emissions [numerous chemicals], chlorofluorocarbons [refrigerants, solvents], ozone or smog particles [acids, organic chemicals; particles in smoke; commercial plants, such as pulp and paper mills]).

Investigate possibility of home-based exposure to air pollution—carbon monoxide (e.g., poor ventilation, especially in the winter months [poor heating systems, use of charcoal grill indoors, car left running in garage]; cigarette or cigar smoke indoors; ozone [spending a lot of time outdoors, such as playing children, adults participating in moderate to strenuous work or recreational activities]).

Waste: Determine if client lives in area where trash or garbage accumulates or is exposed to raw sewage or industrial wastes that **can contaminate soil and water.**

Radiation: Ascertain if client/household member experienced accidental exposure (e.g., occupation in radiography; living near, or working in, nuclear industries or electrical generation plants).

- Observe for signs and symptoms of infective agent and sepsis such as fatigue, malaise, headache, fever, chills, diaphoresis, skin rash, and altered level of consciousness. **Initial symptoms of some diseases that mimic influenza may be misdiagnosed if healthcare providers do not maintain an index of suspicion.**
- Note presence and degree of chemical burns and initial treatment provided.
- Obtain/assist with diagnostic studies, as indicated. **Provides information about type and degree of exposure/organ involvement or damage.**
- Identify psychological response (e.g., anger, shock, acute anxiety, confusion, denial) to accidental or mass exposure incident. **Although these are normal responses, they may recycle repeatedly and result in post-trauma syndrome if not dealt with adequately.**
- Alert proper authorities to presence of or exposure to contamination, as appropriate. **Depending on agent involved, there may be reporting requirements to local, state, or national agencies, such as the local health department, the Environmental Protection Agency (EPA), and Centers for Disease Control and Prevention (CDC).**

Information that appears in brackets has been added by the authors to clarify and enhance the use of nursing diagnoses.

Nursing Priority No. 2.

To assist in treating effects of exposure:

- Implement a coordinated decontamination plan (e.g., removal of clothing, showering with soap and water), when indicated, following consultation with medical toxicologist, hazardous materials team, and industrial hygiene and safety officer **to prevent further harm to client and to protect healthcare providers.**

- Ensure availability and use of personal protective equipment (PPE) (e.g., high-efficiency particulate air [HEPA] filter masks, special garments, and barrier materials including gloves/face shield) **to protect from exposure to biological, chemical, and radioactive hazards.**

- Provide for isolation or group/cohort individuals with same diagnosis or exposure, as resources require. **Limited resources may dictate open ward-like environment; however, the need to control the spread of infection still exists. Only plague, smallpox, and viral hemorrhagic fevers require more than standard infection-control precautions.**

- Provide/assist with therapeutic interventions, as individually appropriate. **Specific needs of the client and the level of care available at a given time/location determine response.**

- Refer pregnant client for individually appropriate diagnostic procedures or screenings. **Helps to determine effects of teratogenic exposure on fetus, allowing for informed choices/preparations.**

- Screen breast milk in lactating client following radiation exposure. **Depending on type and amount of exposure, breastfeeding may need to be briefly interrupted or, occasionally, terminated.**

- Cooperate with and refer to appropriate agencies (e.g., CDC; U.S. Army Medical Research Institute of Infectious Diseases [USAMRIID]; Federal Emergency Management Agency [FEMA]; U.S. Department of Health and Human Services [DHHS]; Office of Emergency Preparedness [OEP]; EPA) **to prepare for/manage mass casualty incidents.**

Nursing Priority No. 3.

To promote wellness (Teaching/Discharge Considerations):

🏠 *Client/Caregiver*

- Identify individual safety needs and injury/illness prevention in home, community, and work setting.
- Install carbon monoxide monitors and other indoor air pollutant detectors in the home, as appropriate.

Information that appears in brackets has been added by the authors to clarify and enhance the use of nursing diagnoses.

- Review individual nutritional needs, appropriate exercise program, and need for rest. **These are essentials for well-being and recovery.**
- Repair, replace, or correct unsafe household items or situations (e.g., storage of solvents in soda bottles, flaking or peeling paint or plaster, filtering unsafe tap water).
- Emphasize importance of supervising infant/child or individuals with cognitive limitations.
- Encourage removal of or cleaning of carpeted floors, especially for small children and persons with respiratory conditions. **Carpets hold up to 100 times as much fine-particle material as a bare floor and can contain metals and pesticides.**
- Identify commercial cleaning resources, if appropriate, **for safe cleaning of contaminated articles/surfaces.**
- Install dehumidifier in damp areas **to retard growth of molds.**
- Encourage timely replacement of air filters on furnace and/or air-conditioning unit. **Good ventilation cuts down on indoor air pollution from carpets, machines, paints, solvents, cleaning materials, and pesticides.**
- Discuss protective actions for specific "bad air" days (e.g., limiting or avoiding outdoor activities) **especially in sensitive groups (e.g., children who are active outdoors, adults involved in moderate or strenuous outdoor activities, persons with respiratory diseases).**
- Review effects of secondhand smoke and importance of refraining from smoking in home/car where others are likely to be exposed.
- Recommend periodic inspection of well water and tap water **to identify possible contaminants.**
- Encourage client/caregiver to develop a personal/family disaster plan, to gather needed supplies to provide for self and family during a community emergency, and to learn how specific public health threats might affect client and actions **to reduce the risk to health and safety.**
- Instruct client to always refer to local authorities and health experts for specific up-to-date information for the community and to follow their advice.
- Refer to counselor/support groups **for ongoing assistance in dealing with traumatic incident/aftereffects of exposure.**
- Provide bibliotherapy including written resources and appropriate Web sites **for review and self-paced learning.**
- Refer to smoking-cessation program, as needed.

Information that appears in brackets has been added by the authors to clarify and enhance the use of nursing diagnoses.

Community

- Promote community education programs in different modalities, languages, cultures, and educational levels geared to increasing awareness of safety measures and resources available to individuals/community.
- Review pertinent job-related health department and Occupational Safety and Health Administration regulations.
- Refer to local resources that provide information about air quality (e.g., pollen index, "bad air days").
- Encourage community members/groups to engage in problem-solving activities.
- Ascertain that there is a comprehensive disaster plan in place in the community **to ensure an effective response for any emergency** (e.g., flood, toxic spill, infectious disease outbreak, radiation release), including a chain of command, equipment, communication, training, decontamination area(s), and safety and security plans.

Documentation Focus

Assessment/Reassessment
- Details of specific exposure including location and circumstances.
- Client's/caregiver's understanding of individual risks and safety concerns.

Planning
- Plan of care and who is involved in planning.
- Teaching plan.

Implementation/Evaluation
- Individual responses to interventions, teaching, and actions performed.
- Specific actions and changes that are made.
- Attainment or progress toward desired outcome(s).
- Modifications to plan of care.

Discharge Planning
- Long-range plans for discharge needs, lifestyle and community changes, and who is responsible for actions to be taken.
- Specific referrals made.

Information that appears in brackets has been added by the authors to clarify and enhance the use of nursing diagnoses.

🌐 Cultural 🄲 Collaborative 🏠 Community/Home Care

Sample Nursing Outcomes & Interventions Classifications (NOC/NIC)

NOC—Symptom Severity
NIC—Environmental Risk Protection

risk for Contamination

Taxonomy II: Safety/Protection—Class 4 Environmental Hazards (00180)
[Diagnostic Division: Safety]
Submitted 2006

Definition: At risk of exposure to environmental contaminants in doses sufficient to cause adverse health effects

Risk Factors

External
Chemical contamination of food/water; presence of atmospheric pollutants

Inadequate municipal services (e.g., trash removal, sewage treatment facilities)

Geographical area (living in area where high levels of contaminants exist)

Playing in outdoor areas where environmental contaminants are used

Personal/household hygiene practices

Economically disadvantaged (increases potential for multiple exposure, lack of access to healthcare, and poor diet)

Use of environmental contaminants in the home (e.g., pesticides, chemicals, environmental tobacco smoke)

Lack of breakdown of contaminants once indoors (breakdown is inhibited without sun and rain exposure)

Flooring surface (carpeted surfaces hold contaminant residue more than hard floor surfaces)

Flaking, peeling paint/plaster in presence of young children

Paint, lacquer, etc., in poorly ventilated areas or without effective protection

Inappropriate use or lack of protective clothing

Unprotected contact with heavy metals or chemicals (e.g., chromium, lead)

Exposure to radiation (occupation in radiography, employment in/living near nuclear industries and electrical generating plants)

Information that appears in brackets has been added by the authors to clarify and enhance the use of nursing diagnoses.

Exposure to disaster (natural or man made); exposure to bio-terrorism

Internal

Age (children less than 5 years, older adults); gestational age during exposure; developmental characteristics of children

Female gender; pregnancy

Nutritional factors (e.g., obesity, vitamin and mineral deficiencies)

Preexisting disease states; smoking

Concomitant exposure; previous exposures

> **NOTE:** A risk diagnosis is not evidenced by signs and symptoms, as the problem has not occurred; rather, nursing interventions are directed at prevention.

Desired Outcomes/Evaluation Criteria— Client Will:

- Verbalize understanding of individual factors that contribute to possibility of injury and take steps to correct situation(s).
- Demonstrate behaviors or lifestyle changes to reduce risk factors and protect self from injury.
- Modify environment, as indicated, to enhance safety.
- Be free of injury.
- Support community activities for disaster preparedness.

Client/Community Will:

- Identify hazards that could lead to exposure or contamination.
- Correct environmental hazards, as identified.
- Demonstrate necessary actions to promote community safety and disaster preparedness.

Actions/Interventions

Nursing Priority No. 1.

To evaluate degree/source of risk inherent in the home, community, and worksite:

- Ascertain type of contaminant(s) and exposure routes posing a potential hazard to client and/or community (e.g., air, soil, or water pollutants; food source, chemical, biological, radia-

---

Information that appears in brackets has been added by the authors to clarify and enhance the use of nursing diagnoses.

🌐 Cultural 🆇 Collaborative 🏠 Community/Home Care

tion) as listed in Risk Factors. **Determines course of action to be taken by client, community, and care providers.**

∞• Note age and gender of client/community base (e.g., community health clinic serving primarily poor children or elderly; school near large industrial plant; family living in smog-prone area). **Young children, frail elderly, and females have been found to be at higher risk for effects of exposure to many toxins.** (Refer to ND Contamination.)

• Ascertain client's geographical location at home or work (e.g., lives where crop spraying is routine; works in nuclear plant; contract worker/soldier in combat area). **Individual and/or community intervention may be needed to reduce risks of accidental/intentional exposures.**

• Note socioeconomic status and availability and use of resources. **Living in poverty increases the potential for multiple exposures, delayed/lack of access to healthcare, and poor general health.**

• Determine client's/SO's understanding of potential risk and appropriate protective measures.

Nursing Priority No. 2.

🔒 To assist client to reduce or correct individual risk factors:

• Assist client to develop plan to address individual safety needs and injury/illness prevention in home, community, and work setting.

• Repair or replace unsafe household items and situations (e.g., flaking/peeling paint or plaster; filter for unsafe tap water).

• Review effects of secondhand smoke and importance of refraining from smoking in home/car **where others are likely to be exposed.**

• Encourage removal or proper cleaning of carpeted floors, especially for small children and persons with respiratory conditions. **Carpets hold up to 100 times as much fine-particle material as a bare floor and can contain metals and pesticides.**

• Encourage timely cleaning and replacement of air filters on furnace and/or air-conditioning unit. **Good ventilation cuts down on indoor air pollution from carpets, machines, paints, solvents, cleaning materials, and pesticides.**

• Recommend periodic inspection of well water or tap water **to identify possible contaminants.**

• Encourage client to install carbon monoxide monitors and other air pollutant detectors in home, as appropriate.

Information that appears in brackets has been added by the authors to clarify and enhance the use of nursing diagnoses.

- Recommend placing dehumidifier in damp areas **to retard growth of molds.**
- Review proper handling of household chemicals:
  - Read chemical labels. Know primary hazards (especially in commonly used household cleaning and gardening products).
  - Follow directions printed on product label (e.g., avoid use of certain chemicals on food preparation surfaces, refrain from spraying garden chemicals on windy days).
  - Use products labeled "nontoxic" wherever possible. Choose least hazardous products for the job, preferably multiuse products **to reduce number of different chemicals used and stored.**
  - Use form of chemical that most reduces risk of exposure (e.g., cream instead of liquid or aerosol).
  - Wear protective clothing, gloves, and safety glasses when using chemicals. Avoid mixing chemicals at all times, and use in well-ventilated areas.
  - Store chemicals in locked cabinets. Keep chemicals in original labeled containers and do not pour into other containers.
  - ∞ Place safety stickers on chemicals **to warn children of harmful contents.**
- Review proper food handling, storage, and cooking techniques.
- ∞ Stress importance of pregnant or lactating women following fish and wildlife consumption guidelines provided by state and U.S. territorial or Native American tribes. **Ingestion of noncommercial fish or wildlife can be a significant source of pollutants.**

Nursing Priority No. 3.
To promote wellness (Teaching/Discharge Considerations):
🏠 *Home*

- Discuss general safety concerns with client/SO **to ensure that people are educated about potential risks and ways to manage risks**.
- ∞ Stress importance of supervising infant, child, or individuals with cognitive limitations **to protect those who are unable to protect themselves**.
- 🪐 Stress importance of posting emergency and poison control numbers in a visible location.
- Encourage learning CPR and first aid.
- Discuss protective actions for specific "bad air days" (e.g., limiting or avoiding outdoor activities).

Information that appears in brackets has been added by the authors to clarify and enhance the use of nursing diagnoses.

🌐 Cultural   🤝 Collaborative   🏠 Community/Home Care

- Review pertinent job-related safety regulations. Emphasize necessity of wearing appropriate protective equipment.
- Encourage client/caregiver to develop a personal/family disaster plan, to gather needed supplies to provide for self and family during a community emergency, to learn how specific public health threats might affect client, and actions **to promote preparedness and reduce the risk to health and safety.**
- Provide information and refer to appropriate resources about potential toxic hazards and protective measures. Provide bibliotherapy including written resources and appropriate Web sites **for client review and self-paced learning.**
- Refer to smoking cessation program as needed.

Community

- Promote education programs **geared to increasing awareness of safety measures and resources available to individuals/community.**
- Review pertinent job-related health department and Occupational Safety and Health Administration regulations **to safeguard the workplace and the community.**
- Ascertain that there is a comprehensive plan in place for the community that includes a chain of command, equipment, communication, training, decontamination area(s), and safety and security protocol **to ensure an effective response to any emergency (e.g., flood, toxic spill, infectious disease outbreak, radiation release).**
- Refer to appropriate agencies (e.g., Centers for Disease Control; U.S. Army Medical Research Institute of Infectious Diseases; Federal Emergency Management Agency; U.S. Department of Health and Human Services; Office of Emergency Preparedness; Environmental Protection Agency) **to prepare for and manage mass casualty incidents.**

Documentation Focus

Assessment/Reassessment
- Client's/caregiver's understanding of individual risks and safety concerns.

Planning
- Plan of care and who is involved in planning.
- Teaching plan.

Information that appears in brackets has been added by the authors to clarify and enhance the use of nursing diagnoses.

Implementation/Evaluation

- Individual responses to interventions, teaching, and actions performed.
- Specific actions and changes that are made.
- Attainment or progress toward desired outcome(s).
- Modifications to plan of care.

Discharge Planning

- Long-range plans, lifestyle and community changes, and who is responsible for actions to be taken.
- Specific referrals made.

Sample Nursing Outcomes & Interventions Classifications (NOC/NIC)

NOC—Risk Control
NIC—Environmental Risk Protection

---

compromised family Coping

Taxonomy II: Coping/Stress Tolerance—Class 2 Coping Responses (00074)
[Diagnostic Division: Social Interaction]
Submitted 1980; Revised 1996

Definition: A usually supportive primary person (family member, SO, or close friend) provides insufficient, ineffective, or compromised support, comfort, assistance, or encouragement that may be needed by the client to manage or master adaptive tasks related to his or her health challenge

---

Related Factors

Coexisting situations affecting the significant person
Developmental/situational crises the significant person may be facing
Prolonged disease (or disability progression) that exhausts the supportive capacity of SO(s)
Exhaustion of supportive capacity of significant people
Inadequate/incorrect understanding of information by a primary person
Inadequate information available to a primary person; incorrect information obtained by a primary person

---

Information that appears in brackets has been added by the authors to clarify and enhance the use of nursing diagnoses.

Lack of reciprocal support; little support provided by client, in turn, for primary person

Temporary preoccupation by a significant person

Temporary family disorganization/role changes

Defining Characteristics

Subjective

Client reports a complaint/concern about SO(s)' response to health problem

SO(s) expresses an inadequate knowledge base/understanding, which interferes with effective supportive behaviors

SO(s) reports preoccupation with personal reaction (e.g., fear, anticipatory grief, guilt, or anxiety) to client's need

Objective

SO(s) attempts assistive/supportive behaviors with unsatisfactory results

SO(s) displays protective behavior disproportionate to the client's abilities/need for autonomy

SO(s) enters into limited personal communication with client

SO(s) withdraws from client

Desired Outcomes/Evaluation Criteria—
Family Will:

* Identify and verbalize resources within themselves to deal with the situation.
* Interact appropriately with the client, providing support and assistance as indicated.
* Provide opportunity for client to deal with situation in own way.
* Verbalize knowledge and understanding of illness, disability, or disease.
* Express feelings honestly.
* Identify need for outside support and seek such.

Actions/Interventions

Nursing Priority No. 1.
To assess causative/contributing factors:

* Identify underlying situation(s) that may contribute to the inability of family to provide needed assistance to the client. **Circumstances may have preceded the illness and now**

Information that appears in brackets has been added by the authors to clarify and enhance the use of nursing diagnoses.

have a significant effect (e.g., client had a heart attack during sexual activity; mate is afraid any activity may cause repeat).

- Note cultural factors related to family relationships that may be involved in problems of caring for member who is ill.
- Note the length of illness, such as cancer, MS, and/or other long-term situations that may exist.
- Assess information available to and understood by the family/SO(s).
- Discuss family perceptions of situation. **Expectations of client and family members may differ and/or be unrealistic.**
- Identify role of the client in family and how illness has changed the family organization.
- Note other factors besides the client's illness that are affecting abilities of family members **to provide needed support.**

Nursing Priority No. 2.

To assist family to reactivate/develop skills to deal with current situation:

- Listen to client's/SO(s)' comments, remarks, and expression of concern(s). Note nonverbal behaviors and/or responses and congruency.
- Encourage family members to verbalize feelings openly and clearly.
- Discuss underlying reasons for behaviors with family **to help them understand and accept and deal with client behaviors.**
- Assist the family and client to understand "who owns the problem" and who is responsible for resolution. Avoid placing blame or guilt.
- Encourage client and family to develop problem-solving skills **to deal with the situation.**

Nursing Priority No. 3.

To promote wellness (Teaching/Discharge Considerations):

- Provide information for family/SO(s) about specific illness or condition.
- Involve client and family in planning care as often as possible. **Enhances commitment to plan.**
- Promote assistance of family in providing client care, as appropriate. **Identifies ways of demonstrating support while maintaining client's independence (e.g., providing favorite foods, engaging in diversional activities).**

Information that appears in brackets has been added by the authors to clarify and enhance the use of nursing diagnoses.

- Refer to appropriate resources for assistance, as indicated (e.g., counseling, psychotherapy, financial, spiritual).
- Refer to NDs Fear; Anxiety; Death Anxiety; ineffective Coping; readiness for enhanced family Coping; disabled family Coping; Grieving, as appropriate.

Documentation Focus

Assessment/Reassessment
- Assessment findings, including current and past coping behaviors, emotional response to situation and stressors, and support systems available.

Planning
- Plan of care, who is involved in planning, and areas of responsibility.
- Teaching plan.

Implementation/Evaluation
- Responses of family members/client to interventions, teaching, and actions performed.
- Attainment or progress toward desired outcome(s).
- Modifications to plan of care.

Discharge Planning
- Long-term plan and who is responsible for actions.
- Specific referrals made.

Sample Nursing Outcomes & Interventions Classifications (NOC/NIC)

NOC—Family Coping
NIC—Family Involvement Promotion

---

defensive Coping

Taxonomy II: Coping/Stress Tolerance—Class 2 Coping Responses (00071)
[Diagnostic Division: Ego Integrity]
Submitted 1988; Revised 2008

Definition: Repeated projection of falsely positive self-evaluation based on a self-protective pattern that defends against underlying perceived threats to positive self-regard

---

Information that appears in brackets has been added by the authors to clarify and enhance the use of nursing diagnoses.

Related Factors

Conflict between self-perception and value system; uncertainty
Fear of failure, humiliation, or repercussions; low level of self-confidence
Unrealistic expectations of self
Lack of resilience
Low level of confidence in others; deficient support system

Defining Characteristics

Subjective
Denial of obvious problems/weaknesses
Projection of blame/responsibility
Hypersensitive to slight/criticism
Grandiosity
Rationalizes failures

Objective
Superior attitude toward others; ridicule of others; hostile laughter
Difficulty establishing/maintaining relationships
Difficulty in perception of reality testing; reality distortion
Lack of participation or follow-through in treatment/therapy

Desired Outcomes/Evaluation Criteria—Client Will:

- Verbalize understanding of own problems and stressors.
- Identify areas of concern or problems.
- Demonstrate acceptance of responsibility for own actions, successes, and failures.
- Participate in treatment program or therapy.
- Maintain involvement in relationships.

Actions/Interventions

- Refer to ND ineffective Coping for additional interventions.

Nursing Priority No. 1.
To determine degree of impairment:

- Assess ability to comprehend current situation and/or developmental level of functioning.
- Determine level of anxiety and effectiveness of current coping mechanisms.

Information that appears in brackets has been added by the authors to clarify and enhance the use of nursing diagnoses.

🌐 Cultural ④ Collaborative 🏠 Community/Home Care

- Perform or review results of testing such as Taylor Manifest Anxiety Scale and Marlowe-Crowne Social Desirability Scale, as indicated, to identify coping styles.
- Determine coping mechanisms used (e.g., projection, avoidance, rationalization) and purpose of coping strategy (e.g., may mask low self-esteem) **to note how these behaviors affect current situation.**
- Observe interactions with others **to note difficulties and ability to establish satisfactory relationships.**
- Note availability of family/friends support for client in current situation. **SO(s) may not be supportive when a person is denying problems or exhibiting unacceptable behaviors.**
- Note expressions of grandiosity in the face of contrary evidence (e.g., "I'm going to buy a new car" when the individual has no job or available finances).
- Assess physical condition. **Defensive coping style has been connected with a decline or alteration in physical well-being and illnesses, especially chronic health concerns (e.g., congestive heart failure, diabetes, chronic fatigue syndrome).**

Nursing Priority No. 2.
To assist client to deal with current situation:

- Develop therapeutic relationship to enable client **to test new behaviors in a safe environment.** Use positive, nonjudgmental approach and "I" language **to promote sense of self-esteem.**
- Assist client to identify and consider need to address problem differently.
- Use therapeutic communication skills such as Active-listening to assist client to describe all aspects of the problem.
- Acknowledge individual strengths and incorporate awareness of personal assets and strengths in plan.
- Provide explanation of the rules of the treatment program, when indicated, and consequences of lack of cooperation.
- Set limits on manipulative behavior; be consistent in enforcing consequences when rules are broken and limits tested.
- Encourage control in all situations possible, include client in decisions and planning **to preserve autonomy.**
- Convey attitude of acceptance and respect (unconditional positive regard) **to avoid threatening client's self-concept and to preserve existing self-esteem.**
- Encourage identification and expression of feelings.

Information that appears in brackets has been added by the authors to clarify and enhance the use of nursing diagnoses.

- Provide healthy outlets for release of hostile feelings (e.g., punching bags, pounding boards). Involve client in outdoor recreation program or activities.
- Provide opportunities for client to interact with others in a positive manner, **promoting self-esteem.**
- Identify and discuss responses to situation, maladaptive coping skills. Suggest alternative responses to situation **to help client select more adaptive strategies for coping.**
- Use confrontation judiciously **to help client begin to identify defense mechanisms (e.g., denial/projection) that are hindering development of satisfying relationships.**
- Assist with treatments for physical illnesses, as appropriate.

Nursing Priority No. 3.
To promote wellness (Teaching/Discharge Considerations):

- Use cognitive-behavioral therapy. **Helps change negative thinking patterns when rigidly held beliefs are used by client to defend against low self-esteem.**
- Encourage client to learn relaxation techniques, use of guided imagery, and positive affirmation of self **in order to incorporate and practice new behaviors.**
- Promote involvement in activities or classes where client can practice new skills and develop new relationships.
- Refer to additional resources (e.g., substance rehabilitation, family/marital therapy), as indicated.

Documentation Focus

Assessment/Reassessment
- Assessment findings, presenting behaviors.
- Client perception of the present situation and usual coping methods, degree of impairment.
- Health concerns.

Planning
- Plan of care and interventions and who is involved in development of the plan.
- Teaching plan.

Implementation/Evaluation
- Response to interventions, teaching, and actions performed.
- Attainment or progress toward desired outcome(s).
- Modifications to plan of care.

Information that appears in brackets has been added by the authors to clarify and enhance the use of nursing diagnoses.

🌐 Cultural   🄰 Collaborative   🏠 Community/Home Care

Discharge Planning
• Referrals and follow-up program.

Sample Nursing Outcomes & Interventions Classifications (NOC/NIC)

NOC—Acceptance: Health Status
NIC—Self-Awareness Enhancement

disabled family Coping

Taxonomy II: Coping/Stress Tolerance—Class 2 Coping Responses (00073)
[Diagnostic Division: Social Interaction]
Submitted 1980; Revised 1996, 2008

Definition: Behavior of significant person (family member, SO, or close friend) that disables his or her capacities and the client's capacities to effectively address tasks essential to either person's adaptation to the health challenge

Related Factors

SO(s) with chronically unexpressed feelings (e.g., guilt, anxiety, hostility, despair)
Dissonant coping styles for dealing with adaptive tasks by the SO(s) and client
Dissonant coping styles among SO(s)
Highly ambivalent family relationships
Arbitrary handling of family's resistance to treatment
High-risk family situations, such as single or adolescent parent, abusive relationship, substance abuse, acute or chronic disabilities, or a member with terminal illness

Defining Characteristics

Subjective
Expresses despair regarding family reactions or lack of involvement

Objective
Psychosomaticism
Intolerance; rejection; abandonment; desertion; agitation; aggression; hostility; depression

---

Information that appears in brackets has been added by the authors to clarify and enhance the use of nursing diagnoses.

Carrying on usual routines without regard for client's needs; disregarding client's needs

Neglectful care of the client in regard to basic human needs or illness treatment

Neglectful relationships with other family members

Family behaviors that are detrimental to well-being

Distortion of reality regarding the client's health problem

Impaired restructuring of a meaningful life for self; impaired individualization; prolonged overconcern for client

Taking on illness signs of client

Client's development of dependence

Desired Outcomes/Evaluation Criteria— Family Will:

- Verbalize more realistic understanding and expectations of the client.
- Visit or contact client regularly.
- Participate positively in care of client, within limits of family's abilities and client's needs.
- Express feelings and expectations openly and honestly, as appropriate.
- Access available resources/services to assist with required care.

Actions/Interventions

Nursing Priority No. 1.

To assess causative/contributing factors:

- Ascertain pre-illness behaviors and interactions of the family. **Provides comparative baseline.**
- Identify current behaviors of the family members (e.g., withdrawal—not visiting, brief visits, and/or ignoring client when visiting; anger and hostility toward client and others; ways of touching between family members, expressions of guilt).
- Discuss family perceptions of situation. **Expectations of client and family members may/may not be realistic.**
- Note cultural factors related to family relationships that may be involved in problems of caring for member who is ill.
- Note other factors that may be stressful for the family (e.g., financial difficulties or lack of community support, as when illness occurs when out of town). **Provides opportunity for appropriate referrals.**
- Determine readiness of family members to be involved with care of the client.

Information that appears in brackets has been added by the authors to clarify and enhance the use of nursing diagnoses.

Nursing Priority No. 2.

To provide assistance to enable family to deal with the current situation:

- Establish rapport with family members who are available. **Promotes therapeutic relationship and support for problem-solving solutions.**
- Acknowledge difficulty of the situation for the family. **Reduces blaming/feelings of guilt.**
- Active-listen concerns; note both overconcern and lack of concern, which may interfere with ability to resolve situation.
- Allow free expression of feelings, including frustration, anger, hostility, and hopelessness. Place limits on acting-out/inappropriate behaviors **to minimize risk of violent behavior.**
- Give accurate information to SO(s) from the beginning.
- Act as liaison between family and healthcare providers **to provide explanations and clarification of treatment plan.**
- Provide brief, simple explanations about use and alarms when equipment (such as a ventilator) is involved. Identify appropriate professional(s) **for continued support/problem solving.**
- Provide time for private interaction between client/family.
- Include SO(s) in the plan of care; provide instruction **to assist them to learn necessary skills to help client.**
- Accompany family when they visit, **to be available for questions, concerns, and support.**
- Assist SO(s) to initiate therapeutic communication with client.
- Refer client to protective services as necessitated by risk of physical harm. **Removing client from home enhances individual safety and may reduce stress on family to allow opportunity for therapeutic intervention.**

Nursing Priority No. 3.

To promote wellness (Teaching/Discharge Considerations):

- Assist family to identify coping skills being used and how these skills are/are not helping them deal with current situation.
- Answer family's questions patiently and honestly. Reinforce information provided by other healthcare providers.
- Reframe negative expressions into positive, whenever possible. **A positive frame contributes to supportive interactions and can lead to better outcomes.**
- Respect family needs for withdrawal and intervene judiciously. **Situation may be overwhelming and time away can be beneficial to continued participation.**

Information that appears in brackets has been added by the authors to clarify and enhance the use of nursing diagnoses.

- Encourage family to deal with the situation in small increments rather than the whole picture at one time.
🏠• Assist the family to identify familiar items that would be helpful to the client (e.g., a family picture on the wall), especially when hospitalized for long period of time, **to reinforce/maintain orientation.**
🤝• Refer family to appropriate resources, as needed (e.g., family therapy, financial counseling, spiritual advisor).
- Refer to ND Grieving, as appropriate.

Documentation Focus

Assessment/Reassessment
- Assessment findings, current and past behaviors, including family members who are directly involved and support systems available.
- Emotional response(s) to situation or stressors.
- Specific health or therapy challenges.

Planning
- Plan of care, specific interventions, and who is involved in planning.
- Teaching plan.

Implementation/Evaluation
- Responses of individuals to interventions, teaching, and actions performed.
- Attainment or progress toward desired outcome(s).
- Modifications to plan of care.

Discharge Planning
- Ongoing needs, resources, other follow-up recommendations, and who is responsible for actions.
- Specific referrals made.

Sample Nursing Outcomes & Interventions Classifications (NOC/NIC)

NOC—Family Normalization
NIC—Family Therapy

Information that appears in brackets has been added by the authors to clarify and enhance the use of nursing diagnoses.

ineffective Coping

Taxonomy II: Coping/Stress Tolerance—Class 2 Coping
Responses (00069)
[Diagnostic Division: Ego Integrity]
Submitted 1978; Nursing Diagnosis Extension and Clas-
sification Revision 1998

Definition: Inability to form a valid appraisal of the stressors, inadequate choices of practiced responses, and/or
inability to use available resources

Related Factors

Situational or maturational crises
High degree of threat
Inadequate opportunity to prepare for stressor; disturbance in
pattern of appraisal of threat
Inadequate level of confidence in ability to cope; inadequate
level of perception of control; uncertainty
Inadequate resources available; inadequate social support cre-
ated by characteristics of relationships
Disturbance in pattern of tension release
Inability to conserve adaptive energies
Gender differences in coping strategies
Work overload; too many deadlines
Impairment of nervous system; cognitive/sensory/perceptual
impairment or memory loss
Severe/chronic pain

Defining Characteristics

Subjective
Reports inability to cope or ask for help
Sleep pattern disturbance; fatigue
Substance abuse

Objective
Lack of goal-directed behavior or resolution of problem; in-
ability to attend to information; difficulty organizing infor-
mation
Use of forms of coping that impede adaptive behavior
Inadequate problem-solving

Information that appears in brackets has been added by the authors to clarify
and enhance the use of nursing diagnoses.

Inability to meet role expectations/basic needs
Decreased use of social support
Poor concentration
Change in usual communication patterns
High illness rate
Risk-taking behavior
Destructive behavior toward self/others

Desired Outcomes/Evaluation Criteria—Client Will:

- Assess the current situation accurately.
- Identify ineffective coping behaviors and consequences.
- Verbalize awareness of own coping abilities.
- Verbalize feelings congruent with behavior.
- Meet psychological needs as evidenced by appropriate expression of feelings, identification of options, and use of resources.

Actions/Interventions

Nursing Priority No. 1.

To determine degree of impairment:

- Determine individual stressors (e.g., family, social, work environment, life changes, or nursing or healthcare management).
- Evaluate ability to understand events; provide a realistic appraisal of situation.
- Identify developmental level of functioning. (**People tend to regress to a lower developmental stage during illness or crisis.**)
- Assess current functional capacity and note how it is affecting the individual's coping ability.
- Determine alcohol intake, drug use, smoking habits, and sleeping and eating patterns. **These mechanisms are often used when individual is not coping effectively with stressors.**
- Ascertain impact of illness on sexual needs and relationship.
- Assess level of anxiety and coping on an ongoing basis.
- Note speech and communication patterns. Be aware of negative/catastrophizing thinking.
- Observe and describe behavior in objective terms. Validate observations.

Information that appears in brackets has been added by the authors to clarify and enhance the use of nursing diagnoses.

🌐 Cultural   🅒 Collaborative   🏠 Community/Home Care

Nursing Priority No. 2.

To assess coping abilities and skills:

- Ascertain client's understanding of current situation and its impact on life and work.
- Active-listen and identify client's perceptions of what is happening.
- Evaluate client's decision-making ability.
- Determine previous methods of dealing with life problems **to identify successful techniques that can be used in the current situation.**

Nursing Priority No. 3.

To assist client to deal with current situation:

- Call client by name. Ascertain how client prefers to be addressed. **Using client's name enhances sense of self and promotes individuality and self-esteem.**
- Encourage communication with staff/SO(s).
- Use reality orientation (e.g., clocks, calendars, bulletin boards) and make frequent references to time and place, as indicated. Place needed and familiar objects within sight for visual cues.
- Provide for continuity of care with same personnel taking care of the client as often as possible.
- Explain disease process, procedures, and events in a simple, concise manner. Devote time for listening. **May help client to express emotions, grasp situation, and feel more in control.**
- Provide for a quiet environment and position equipment out of view as much as possible **when anxiety is increased by noisy surroundings or the sight of medical equipment.**
- Schedule activities so periods of rest alternate with nursing care. Increase activity slowly.
- Assist client in use of diversion, recreation, and relaxation techniques.
- Emphasize positive body responses to medical conditions, but do not negate the seriousness of the situation (e.g., stable blood pressure during gastric bleed or improved body posture in depressed client).
- Encourage client to try new coping behaviors and gradually master situation.
- Confront client when behavior is inappropriate, pointing out difference between words and actions. **Provides external locus of control, enhancing safety.**

Information that appears in brackets has been added by the authors to clarify and enhance the use of nursing diagnoses.

• Assist in dealing with change in concept of body image, as appropriate. (Refer to ND disturbed Body Image.)

Nursing Priority No. 4.

To provide for meeting psychological needs:

• Treat the client with courtesy and respect. Converse at client's level, providing meaningful conversation while performing care. **Enhances therapeutic relationship.**
• Help client learn how to substitute positive thoughts for negative ones (i.e., "I can do this"; "I am in charge of myself"). Take advantage of teachable moments.
• Allow client to react in own way without judgment by staff. Provide support and diversion, as indicated.
• Encourage verbalization of fears and anxieties and expression of feelings of denial, depression, and anger. Let the client know that these are normal reactions.
• Provide opportunity for expression of sexual concerns.
• Help client to set limits on acting-out behaviors and learn ways to express emotions in an acceptable manner. **Promotes internal locus of control.**

Nursing Priority No. 5.

🏠 To promote wellness (Teaching/Discharge Considerations):

• Give updated or additional information needed about events, cause (if known), and potential course of illness as soon as possible. **Knowledge helps reduce anxiety/fear and allows client to deal with reality.**
• Provide and encourage an atmosphere of realistic hope.
• Give information about purposes and side effects of medications/ treatments.
• Stress importance of follow-up care.
• Encourage and support client in evaluating lifestyle, occupation, and leisure activities.
• Discuss ways to deal with identified stressors (e.g., family, social, work environment, or nursing or healthcare management).
• Provide for gradual implementation and continuation of necessary behavior/lifestyle changes. **Enhances commitment to plan.**
• Discuss or review anticipated procedures and client concerns, as well as postoperative expectations when surgery is recommended.
• Refer to outside resources and/or professional therapy, as indicated or ordered.

Information that appears in brackets has been added by the authors to clarify and enhance the use of nursing diagnoses.

🌐 Cultural   🅒 Collaborative   🏠 Community/Home Care

- Determine need/desire for religious representative/spiritual counselor and arrange for visit.
- Provide information and/or refer for consultation, as indicated, for sexual concerns. Provide privacy when client is not in own home.
- Refer to other NDs, as indicated (e.g., chronic Pain; Anxiety; impaired verbal Communication; risk for other-/self-directed Violence).

Documentation Focus

Assessment/Reassessment
- Baseline findings, specific stressors, degree of impairment, and client's perceptions of situation.
- Coping abilities and previous ways of dealing with life problems.

Planning
- Plan of care, specific interventions, and who is involved in planning.
- Teaching plan.

Implementation/Evaluation
- Client's responses to interventions, teaching, and actions performed.
- Medication dose, time, and client's response.
- Attainment or progress toward desired outcome(s).
- Modifications to plan of care.

Discharge Planning
- Long-term needs and actions to be taken.
- Support systems available, specific referrals made, and who is responsible for actions to be taken.

Sample Nursing Outcomes & Interventions Classifications (NOC/NIC)

NOC—Coping
NIC—Coping Enhancement

Information that appears in brackets has been added by the authors to clarify and enhance the use of nursing diagnoses.

ineffective community Coping

Taxonomy II: Coping/Stress Tolerance—Class 2 Coping
   Responses (00077)
[Diagnostic Division: Social Interaction]
Submitted 1994; Nursing Diagnosis Extension and Clas-
   sification Revision 1998

Definition: Pattern of community activities for adaptation
and problem-solving that is unsatisfactory for meeting
the demands or needs of the community

Related Factors

Deficits in community social support services/resources
Inadequate resources for problem-solving
Ineffective or nonexistent community systems (e.g., lack of
   emergency medical system, transportation system, disaster
   planning systems)
Natural/man-made disasters

Defining Characteristics

Subjective
Community does not meet its own expectations
Reports of community vulnerability/powerlessness
Stressors perceived as excessive

Objective
Deficits of community participation
Excessive community conflicts
High illness rates
Increased social problems (e.g., homicides, vandalism, arson,
   terrorism, robbery, infanticide, abuse, divorce, unemploy-
   ment, poverty, militancy, mental illness)

Desired Outcomes/Evaluation Criteria—
Community Will:

* Recognize negative and positive factors affecting community's ability to meet its own demands or needs.
* Identify alternatives to inappropriate activities for adaptation/
  problem-solving.
* Report a measurable increase in necessary/desired activities
  to improve community functioning.

Information that appears in brackets has been added by the authors to clarify
and enhance the use of nursing diagnoses.

Actions/Interventions

Nursing Priority No. 1.

To identify causative or precipitating factors:

- Evaluate community activities **as related to meeting collective needs within the community itself and between the community and the larger society.**
- Note community reports of community functioning (e.g., transportation, financial needs, emergency response), including areas of weakness or conflict.
- Identify effects of Related Factors on community activities.
- Determine availability and use of resources.
- Identify unmet demands or needs of the community.

Nursing Priority No. 2.

To assist the community to reactivate/develop skills to deal with needs:

- Determine community strengths. **Provides a base upon which to build additional effective coping strategies.**
- Identify and prioritize community goals.
- Encourage community members to join groups and engage in problem-solving activities **to strengthen efforts and broaden base of support.**
- Develop a plan jointly with community **to deal with deficits in support to meet identified goals.**

Nursing Priority No. 3.

To promote wellness as related to community health:

- Create plans managing interactions within the community itself and between the community and the larger society **to meet collective needs.**
- Assist the community to form partnerships within the community and between the community and the larger society. **Promotes long-term development of the community to deal with current and future problems.**
- Promote community involvement in developing a comprehensive disaster plan **to ensure an effective response to any emergency (e.g., flood, tornado, toxic spill, infectious disease outbreak).** (Refer to ND Contamination for additional interventions.)
- Provide channels for dissemination of information to the community as a whole (e.g., print media; radio/television reports and community bulletin boards; speakers' bureau; and reports

---

Information that appears in brackets has been added by the authors to clarify and enhance the use of nursing diagnoses.

to committees, councils, and advisory boards), keeping material on file and accessible to the public.

🏠• Make information available in different modalities and geared
🌐 to differing educational levels and cultural and ethnic populations of the community.

🏠• Seek out and evaluate underserved populations, including the homeless.

Documentation Focus

Assessment/Reassessment
• Assessment findings, including perception of community members regarding problems.
• Availability and use of resources.

Planning
• Plan of care and who is involved in planning.
• Teaching plan.

Implementation/Evaluation
• Response of community entities to plan, interventions, and actions performed.
• Attainment or progress toward desired outcome(s).
• Modifications to plan of care.

Discharge Planning
• Long-term plans and who is responsible for actions to be taken.

Sample Nursing Outcomes & Interventions Classifications (NOC/NIC)

NOC—Community Competence
NIC—Community Health Development

---

readiness for enhanced Coping

Taxonomy II: Coping/Stress Tolerance—Class 2 Coping Responses (00158)
[Diagnostic Division: Ego Integrity]
Submitted 2002

Definition: A pattern of cognitive and behavioral efforts to manage demands that is sufficient for well-being and can be strengthened

---

Information that appears in brackets has been added by the authors to clarify and enhance the use of nursing diagnoses.

🌐 Cultural 🤝 Collaborative 🏠 Community/Home Care

Defining Characteristics

Subjective
Defines stressors as manageable
Seeks social support/knowledge of new strategies
Acknowledges power
Aware of possible environmental changes

Objective
Uses a broad range of problem- or emotion-oriented strategies
Uses spiritual resources

Desired Outcomes/Evaluation Criteria—Client Will:

- Assess current situation accurately.
- Identify effective coping behaviors currently being used.
- Verbalize feelings congruent with behavior.
- Meet psychological needs as evidenced by appropriate expression of feelings, identification of options, and use of resources.

Actions/Interventions

Nursing Priority No. 1.
To determine needs and desire for improvement:

- Evaluate ability to understand events and provide realistic appraisal of situation. **Provides information about client's perception and cognitive ability and whether the client is aware of the facts of the situation. This is essential for facilitating growth.**
- Determine stressors that are currently affecting client. **Accurate identification of situation that client is dealing with provides information for planning interventions to enhance coping abilities.**
- Ascertain motivation/expectations for change.
- Identify social supports available to client. **Available support systems, such as family and friends, can provide client with ability to handle current stressful events, and often "talking it out" with an empathetic listener will help client move forward to enhance coping skills.**
- Review coping strategies client is aware of and currently using. **The desire to improve one's coping ability is based on an awareness of the current status of the stressful situation.**

Information that appears in brackets has been added by the authors to clarify and enhance the use of nursing diagnoses.

- Determine alcohol intake, other drug use, smoking habits, and sleeping and eating patterns. **Use of these substances impairs ability to deal with anxiety and affects ability to cope with life's stressors. Identification of impaired sleeping and eating patterns provides clues to need for change.**

- Assess level of anxiety and coping on an ongoing basis. **Provides information for baseline to develop plan of care to improve coping abilities.**

- Note speech and communication patterns. **Assesses ability to understand and provides information necessary to help client make progress in desire to enhance coping abilities.**

- Evaluate client's decision-making ability. **Understanding client's ability provides a starting point for developing plan and determining what information client needs to develop more effective coping skills.**

Nursing Priority No. 2.
To assist client to develop enhanced coping skills:

- Active-listen and clarify client's perceptions of current status. **Reflecting client's statements and thoughts can provide a forum for understanding perceptions in relation to reality for planning care and determining accuracy of interventions needed.**

- Review previous methods of dealing with life problems. **Enables client to identify successful techniques used in the past, promoting feelings of confidence in own ability.**

- Discuss desire to improve ability to manage stressors of life. **Understanding client's desire to seek new information to enhance life will help client determine what is needed to learn new skills of coping.**

- Discuss understanding of concept of knowing what can and cannot be changed. **Acceptance of reality that some things cannot be changed allows client to focus energies on dealing with things that can be changed.**

🏠• Help client develop problem-solving skills. **Learning the process for problem solving will promote successful resolution of potentially stressful situations that arise.**

Nursing Priority No. 3.
🏠To promote optimum wellness:

- Discuss predisposing factors related to any individual's response to stress. **Understanding that genetic influences, past experiences, and existing conditions determine whether a person's response is adaptive or maladaptive**

Information that appears in brackets has been added by the authors to clarify and enhance the use of nursing diagnoses.

will give client a base on which to continue to learn what is needed to improve life.

- Encourage client to create a stress management program. **An individualized program of relaxation, meditation, involvement with caring for others/pets will enhance coping skills and strengthen client's ability to manage challenging situations.**
- Recommend involvement in activities of interest, such as exercise/sports, music, art. **Individuals must decide for themselves what coping strategies are adaptive for them. Most people find enjoyment and relaxation in these kinds of activities.**
- Discuss possibility of doing volunteer work in an area of the client's choosing. **Many people report satisfaction in helping others, and client may find pleasure in such involvement.**
- Refer to classes and/or reading material, as appropriate. **May be helpful to further learning and pursuing goal of enhanced coping ability.**

Documentation Focus

Assessment/Reassessment
- Baseline information, client's perception of need to enhance abilities.
- Coping abilities and previous ways of dealing with life problems.
- Motivation and expectations for change.

Planning
- Plan of care, specific interventions, and who is involved in planning.
- Teaching plan.

Implementation/Evaluation
- Client's responses to interventions, teaching, and actions performed.
- Attainment or progress toward desired outcome(s).
- Modifications to plan of care.

Discharge Planning
- Long-term needs and actions to be taken.
- Support systems available, specific referrals made, and who is responsible for actions to be taken.

Information that appears in brackets has been added by the authors to clarify and enhance the use of nursing diagnoses.

Sample Nursing Outcomes & Interventions Classifications (NOC/NIC)

NOC—Coping
NIC—Coping Enhancement

readiness for enhanced community Coping

Taxonomy II: Coping/Stress Tolerance—Class 2 Coping Responses (00076)
[Diagnostic Division: Social Interaction]
Submitted 1994

Definition: A pattern of community activities for adaptation and problem-solving that is satisfactory for meeting the demands or needs of the community for the management of current and future problems/stressors and can be improved

Defining Characteristics

One or more characteristics that indicate effective coping

Subjective
Agreement that community is responsible for stress management

Objective
Active planning by community for predicted stressors
Active problem-solving by community when faced with issues
Positive communication among community members
Positive communication between community/aggregates and larger community
Programs available for recreation or relaxation
Resources sufficient for managing stressors

Desired Outcomes/Evaluation Criteria— Community Will:

- Identify positive and negative factors affecting management of current and future problems and stressors.
- Have an established plan in place to deal with identified problems and stressors.
- Describe management of challenges in characteristics that indicate effective coping.
- Report a measurable increase in ability to deal with problems and stressors.

Information that appears in brackets has been added by the authors to clarify and enhance the use of nursing diagnoses.

⚫ Cultural 😊 Collaborative 🏠 Community/Home Care

Actions/Interventions

Nursing Priority No. 1.

To determine existence of and deficits or weaknesses in management of current and future problems/stressors:

- Review community plan for dealing with problems and stressors.
- Determine community's strengths and weaknesses.
- Identify limitations in current pattern of community activities (such as transportation, water needs, roads) **that can be improved through adaptation and problem-solving.**
- Evaluate community activities as related to management of problems and stressors within the community itself and between the community and the larger society.

Nursing Priority No. 2.

To assist the community in adaptation and problem-solving for management of current and future needs/stressors:

- Define and discuss current needs and anticipated or projected concerns. **Agreement on scope/parameters of needs is essential for effective planning.**
- Prioritize goals **to facilitate accomplishment.**
- Identify available resources (e.g., persons, groups, financial, and governmental, as well as other communities).
- Make a joint plan with the community to deal with adaptation and problem-solving **for management of problems and stressors.**
- Seek out and involve underserved and at-risk groups within the community. **Supports communication and commitment of community as a whole.**

Nursing Priority No. 3.

To promote well-being of community:

- Assist the community to form partnerships within the community and between the community and the larger society **to promote long-term developmental growth of the community.**
- Support development of plans for maintaining these interactions.
- Establish mechanism for self-monitoring of community needs and evaluation of efforts. **Facilitates proactive rather than reactive responses by the community.**
- Use multiple formats, such as TV, radio, print media, billboards and computer bulletin boards, speakers' bureaus, and

---

Information that appears in brackets has been added by the authors to clarify and enhance the use of nursing diagnoses.

reports to community leaders/groups on file and accessible to the public **to keep community informed regarding plans, needs, and outcomes.**

Documentation Focus

Assessment/Reassessment
- Assessment findings and community's perception of situation.
- Identified areas of concern, community strengths and challenges.

Planning
- Plan of care and who is involved and responsible for each action.
- Teaching plan.

Implementation/Evaluation
- Response of community entities to the actions performed.
- Attainment or progress toward desired outcomes.
- Modifications to plan of care.

Discharge Planning
- Short- and long-term plans to deal with current, anticipated, and potential needs and who is responsible for follow-through.
- Specific referrals made, coalitions formed.

Sample Nursing Outcomes & Interventions Classifications (NOC/NIC)

NOC—Community Competence
NIC—Program Development

---

readiness for enhanced family Coping

Taxonomy II: Coping/Stress Tolerance—Class 2 Coping Responses (00075)
[Diagnostic Division: Social Interaction]
Submitted 1980

Definition: A pattern of management of adaptive tasks by primary person (family member, SO, or close friend) involved with the client's health challenge that is sufficient for health and growth in regard to self and in relation to the client and can be strengthened

---

Information that appears in brackets has been added by the authors to clarify and enhance the use of nursing diagnoses.

🌐 Cultural   😊 Collaborative   🏠 Community/Home Care

Defining Characteristics

Subjective
SO(s) attempts to describe growth impact of crisis
Individual expresses interest in making contact with others who have experienced a similar situation

Objective
SO(s) moves in direction of health-promotion/enriching lifestyle
Chooses experiences that optimize wellness

Desired Outcomes/Evaluation Criteria— Family Member Will:

* Express willingness to look at own role in the family's growth.
* Verbalize desire to undertake tasks leading to change.
* Report feelings of self-confidence and satisfaction with progress being made.

Actions/Interventions

Nursing Priority No. 1.
To assess situation and adaptive skills being used by the family members:

* Determine individual situation and stage of growth family is experiencing or demonstrating. **Changes that are occurring may help family adapt, grow, and thrive when faced with these transitional events.**
* Ascertain motivation and expectations for change.
* Note expressions such as "Life has more meaning for me since this has occurred," **to identify changes in values.**
* Observe communication patterns of family. Listen to family's expressions of hope and planning and their effects on relationships and life.
* Identify cultural/religious health beliefs and expectations. **For example, Navajo parents may define family as nuclear, extended, or a clan, and it is important to identify who are the primary child-rearing persons.**

Nursing Priority No. 2.
To assist family member to develop/strengthen potential for growth:

* Provide time to talk with family **to discuss their view of the situation.**

Information that appears in brackets has been added by the authors to clarify and enhance the use of nursing diagnoses.

- Establish a relationship with family/client **to foster trust and growth.**
- Provide a role model with which the family member may identify.
- Discuss importance of open communication and of not having secrets.
- Demonstrate techniques, such as Active-listening, I-messages, and problem-solving, **to facilitate effective communication.**
- Establish social goals of achieving and maintaining harmony with oneself, family, and community.

Nursing Priority No. 3.
🏠 To promote wellness (Teaching/Discharge Considerations):

- Assist family member to support the client in meeting own needs within ability and/or constraints of the illness or situation.
- Provide experiences for the family **to help them learn ways of assisting or supporting client.**
- Identify other individuals or groups with similar conditions (e.g., Reach for Recovery, CanSurmount, Al-Anon, MS Society) and assist client/family member to make contact. **Provides ongoing support for sharing common experiences, problem-solving, and learning new behaviors.**
- Assist family member to learn new, effective ways of dealing with feelings and reactions.
- Encourage family member to pursue personal interests, hobbies, and leisure activities **to promote individual well-being and strengthen coping abilities.**

Documentation Focus ————————————————

Assessment/Reassessment
- Adaptive skills being used, stage of growth.
- Family communication patterns.
- Motivation and expectations for change.

Planning
- Plan of care, specific interventions, and who is involved in planning.
- Teaching plan.

Implementation/Evaluation
- Client's/family's responses to interventions, teaching, and actions performed.

———————————

Information that appears in brackets has been added by the authors to clarify and enhance the use of nursing diagnoses.

- Attainment or progress toward desired outcome(s).
- Modifications to plan of care.

Discharge Planning

- Identified needs/referrals for follow-up care and/or support systems.
- Specific referrals made.

Sample Nursing Outcomes & Interventions Classifications (NOC/NIC)

NOC—Family Normalization
NIC—Normalization Promotion

Death Anxiety

Taxonomy II: Coping/Stress Tolerance—Class 2 Coping Response (00147)
[Diagnostic Division: Ego Integrity]
Submitted 1998; Revised 2006

Definition: Vague uneasy feeling of discomfort or dread generated by perceptions of a real or imagined threat to one's existence

Related Factors

Anticipating: pain, suffering, adverse consequences of general anesthesia, impact of death on others
Confronting reality of terminal disease; experiencing dying process; perceived proximity of death
Discussions on topic of death; observations related to death; near-death experience
Uncertainty of prognosis; nonacceptance of own mortality
Uncertainty about the existence of a higher power, life after death, an encounter with a higher power

Defining Characteristics

Subjective

Reports fear of developing a terminal illness, the process of dying, pain/suffering related to dying, loss of mental/[physical] abilities when dying, premature death, or prolonged dying

---

Information that appears in brackets has been added by the authors to clarify and enhance the use of nursing diagnoses.

Reports negative thoughts related to death and dying
Reports deep sadness; feeling powerlessness over dying
Reports concerns of overworking the caregiver; worry about the
impact of one's own death on SO(s)

Desired Outcomes/Evaluation Criteria— Client Will:

- Identify and express feelings (e.g., sadness, guilt, fear) freely/effectively.
- Look toward/plan for the future one day at a time.
- Formulate a plan dealing with individual concerns and eventualities of dying as appropriate.

Actions/Interventions

Nursing Priority No. 1.
To assess causative/contributing factors:

- Determine how client sees self in usual lifestyle role functioning and perception and meaning of anticipated loss to him or her and SO(s).
- Ascertain current knowledge of situation **to identify misconceptions, lack of information, and other pertinent issues.**
- Determine client's role in family constellation. Observe patterns of communication in family and response of family/SO to client's situation and concerns. **In addition to identifying areas of need/concern, also reveals strengths useful in addressing the concerns.**
- Assess impact of client reports of subjective experiences and past experience with death (or exposure to death); for example, witnessed violent death, viewed body in casket as a child, and so on.
- Identify cultural factors/expectations and impact on current situation and feelings.
- Note physical and mental condition and complexity of therapeutic regimen.
- Determine ability to manage own self-care, end-of-life and other affairs, and awareness/use of available resources.
- Observe behavior indicative of the level of anxiety present (mild to panic) **as it affects client's/SO(s)' ability to process information and participate in activities.**
- Identify coping skills currently used and how effective they are. Be aware of defense mechanisms being used by the client.

Information that appears in brackets has been added by the authors to clarify and enhance the use of nursing diagnoses.

Cultural   Collaborative   Community/Home Care

- Note use of alcohol or other drugs of abuse, reports of insomnia, excessive sleeping, and avoidance of interactions with others, **which may be behavioral indicators of use of withdrawal to deal with problems.**
- Note client's religious and spiritual orientation and involvement in religious activities; presence of conflicts regarding spiritual beliefs.
- Listen to client/SO reports/expressions of anger and concern, alienation from God, or belief that impending death is a punishment for wrongdoing.
- Determine sense of futility; feelings of hopelessness or helplessness; lack of motivation to help self. **May indicate presence of depression and need for intervention.**
- Active-listen comments regarding sense of isolation.
- Listen for expressions of inability to find meaning in life or suicidal ideation.

Nursing Priority No. 2.

To assist client to deal with situation:

- Provide an open and trusting relationship.
- Use therapeutic communication skills of Active-listening, silence, acknowledgment. Respect client's desire or request not to talk. Provide hope within parameters of the individual situation.
- Encourage expressions of feelings (anger, fear, sadness, etc.). Acknowledge anxiety/fear. Do not deny or reassure client that everything will be all right. Be honest when answering questions/providing information. **Enhances trust and therapeutic relationship.**
- Provide information about normalcy of feelings and individual grief reaction.
- Make time for nonjudgmental discussion of philosophical issues and questions about spiritual impact of illness/situation.
- Review life experiences of loss and previous use of coping skills, noting client's strengths and successes.
- Provide calm, peaceful setting and privacy as appropriate. **Promotes relaxation and ability to deal with situation.**
- Assist client to engage in spiritual growth activities and experience prayer/meditation and forgiveness to heal past hurts. Provide information that anger with God is a normal part of the grieving process. **Reduces feelings of guilt/conflict, allowing client to move forward toward resolution.**

Information that appears in brackets has been added by the authors to clarify and enhance the use of nursing diagnoses.

- Refer to therapists, spiritual advisors, and counselors **to facilitate grief work.**
- Refer to community agencies/resources **to assist client/SO(s) for planning for eventualities (legal issues, funeral plans, etc.).**

Nursing Priority No. 3.
To promote independence:

- Support client's efforts to develop realistic steps to put plans into action.
- Direct client's thoughts beyond present state to enjoyment of each day and the future when appropriate.
- Provide opportunities for the client to make simple decisions. **Enhances sense of control.**
- Develop individual plan using client's locus of control **to assist client/family through the process.**
- Treat expressed decisions and desires with respect and convey to others as appropriate.
- Assist with completion of Advance Directives, CPR instructions, and durable medical power of attorney.

Documentation Focus

Assessment/Reassessment
- Assessment findings, including client's fears and signs/symptoms being exhibited.
- Responses and actions of family/SO(s).
- Availability and use of resources.

Planning
- Plan of care and who is involved in planning.

Implementation/Evaluation
- Client's response to interventions, teaching, and actions performed.
- Attainment or progress toward desired outcome(s).
- Modifications to plan of care.

Discharge Planning
- Identified needs and who is responsible for actions to be taken.
- Specific referrals made.

Information that appears in brackets has been added by the authors to clarify and enhance the use of nursing diagnoses.

⦿ Cultural   ◎ Collaborative   ⌂ Community/Home Care

Sample Nursing Outcomes & Interventions Classifications (NOC/NIC)

NOC—Dignified Life Closure
NIC—Dying Care

---

readiness for enhanced Decision-Making

Taxonomy II: Life Principles—Class 3 Value/Belief/Action Congruence (00184)
[Diagnostic Division: Ego Integrity]
Submitted 2006

Definition: A pattern of choosing courses of action that is sufficient for meeting short- and long-term health-related goals and can be strengthened

Defining Characteristics

Subjective

Expresses desire to enhance decision-making, use of reliable evidence for decisions, risk-benefit analysis of decisions, understanding of choices for decision-making, understanding of the meaning of choices

Expresses desire to enhance congruency of decisions with personal and sociocultural values and goals

Desired Outcomes/Evaluation Criteria— Client Will:

• Explain possible choices for decision-making.
• Identify risks and benefit of decisions.
• Express beliefs about the meaning of choices.
• Make decisions that are congruent with personal and sociocultural values or goals.
• Use reliable evidence in making decisions.

Actions/Interventions

Nursing Priority No. 1.

To assess causative/contributing factors:

• Determine usual ability to manage own affairs. **Provides baseline for understanding client's decision-making process and measures growth.**

Information that appears in brackets has been added by the authors to clarify and enhance the use of nursing diagnoses.

- Note expressions of decision, dependability, and availability of support persons.
- Active-listen and identify reason(s) client would like to improve decision-making abilities and expectations of change. **As client articulates/clarifies reasons for improvement, direction is provided for change.**
- Note presence of physical signs of excitement. **Enhances energy for quest for improvement and personal growth.**
- Discuss meaning of life and reasons for living, belief in God or higher power, and how these relate to current desire for improvement.

Nursing Priority No. 2.
To assist client to improve/effectively use problem-solving skills:

- Promote safe and hopeful environment. **Provides opportunity for client to discuss concerns/thoughts freely.**
- Provide opportunities for client to recognize own inner control in decision-making process. **Individuals with an internal locus of control believe they have some degree of control in outcomes and that their own actions/choices help determine what happens in their lives.**
- Encourage verbalization of ideas, concerns, particular decisions that need to be made.
- Clarify and prioritize individual's goals, noting possible conflicts or challenges that may be encountered.
- Identify positive aspects of this experience, encouraging client to view it as a learning opportunity.
- Assist client in learning how to find factual information (e.g., use of the library or reliable Internet Web sites).
- Review the process of problem solving and how to do a risk-benefit analysis of decisions.
- ∞ Encourage children to make age-appropriate decisions. **Learning problem solving at an early age will enhance sense of self-worth and ability to exercise coping skills.**
- 🌐 Discuss and clarify spiritual beliefs, accepting client's values in a nonjudgmental manner.

Nursing Priority No. 3.
🏠 To promote optimum wellness:

- Identify opportunities for using conflict-resolution skills, emphasizing each step as it is used.

Information that appears in brackets has been added by the authors to clarify and enhance the use of nursing diagnoses.

- Provide positive feedback for efforts. **Enhances use of skills and learning efforts.**
- Encourage involvement of family/SO(s), as desired or appropriate, in decision-making process **to help all family members improve conflict-resolution skills**.
- Suggest participation in stress management or assertiveness classes, as appropriate.
- Refer to other resources, as necessary (e.g., clergy, psychiatric clinical nurse specialist or psychiatrist, or family or marital therapist).

Documentation Focus

Assessment/Reassessment
- Assessment findings, behavioral responses.
- Motivation and expectations for change.
- Individuals involved in improving conflict skills.
- Personal values and beliefs.

Planning
- Plan of care, intervention, and who is involved in the planning.
- Teaching plan.

Implementation/Evaluation
- Clients and involved individual's responses to interventions, teaching, and actions performed.
- Ability to express feelings, identify options, and use resources.
- Attainment or progress toward desired outcome(s).
- Modifications to plan of care.

Discharge Planning
- Long-term needs, noting who is responsible for actions to be taken.
- Specific referrals made.

Sample Nursing Outcomes & Interventions Classifications (NOC/NIC)

NOC—Decision-Making
NIC—Decision-Making Support

Information that appears in brackets has been added by the authors to clarify and enhance the use of nursing diagnoses.

Decisional Conflict

Taxonomy II: Life Principles—Class 3 Value/Belief/Action
 Congruence (00083)
[Diagnostic Division: Ego Integrity]
Submitted 1988; Revised 2006

Definition: Uncertainty about course of action to be
taken when choice among competing actions involves
risk, loss, or challenge to values and beliefs

Related Factors

Unclear personal values/beliefs; perceived threat to value sys-
 tem
Lack of experience or interference with decision-making
Lack of relevant information; multiple or divergent sources of
 information
Moral obligations require performing/not performing actions
Moral principles, rules, values support mutually inconsistent
 courses of action
Support system deficit
Age; developmental state
Family system; sociocultural factors
Cognitive, emotional, behavioral level of functioning

Defining Characteristics

Subjective

Verbalizes uncertainty about choices and undesired consequences of alternative actions being considered
Verbalizes feeling of distress while attempting a decision
Questioning moral principles, rules, values, or personal beliefs/
 values while attempting a decision

Objective

Vacillation between alternative choices; delayed decision-
 making
Self-focusing
Physical signs of tension or distress (e.g., increased heart rate
 or restlessness)

Information that appears in brackets has been added by the authors to clarify
and enhance the use of nursing diagnoses.

Desired Outcomes/Evaluation Criteria— Client Will:

- Verbalize awareness of positive and negative aspects of choices and alternative actions.
- Acknowledge and ventilate feelings of anxiety and distress associated with making a difficult decision.
- Identify personal values and beliefs concerning issues.
- Make decision(s) and express satisfaction with choices.
- Meet psychological needs as evidenced by appropriate expression of feelings, identification of options, and use of resources.
- Display relaxed manner or calm demeanor free of physical signs of distress.

Actions/Interventions

Nursing Priority No. 1.
To assess causative/contributing factors:

- Determine usual ability to manage own affairs. Clarify who has legal right to intervene on behalf of a child, elder, impaired individual (e.g., parent/spouse, other relative, designee for durable medical power of attorney, or court appointed guardian/advocate). **Family disruption and conflicts can complicate decision process.**
- Note expressions of indecision, dependence on others, availability/involvement of support persons (e.g., client may have lack of/conflicting advice). Ascertain dependency of other(s) on client and/or issues of codependency.
- Active-listen/identify reason for indecisiveness. **Helps client to clarify problem and work toward a solution.**
- Determine effectiveness of current problem-solving techniques.
- Note presence/intensity of physical signs of anxiety (e.g., increased heart rate, muscle tension).
- Listen for expressions of client's inability to find meaning in life/reason for living, feelings of futility, or alienation from God and others around them. (Refer to ND Spiritual Distress, as indicated.)
- Review information client has about the healthcare decision. **Accurate and clearly understood information about situation will help the client make the best decision for self.**

Information that appears in brackets has been added by the authors to clarify and enhance the use of nursing diagnoses.

Nursing Priority No. 2.

To assist client to develop/effectively use problem-solving skills:

• Promote safe and hopeful environment, as needed, while client regains inner control.

• Encourage verbalization of conflicts or concerns.

• Accept verbal expressions of anger or guilt, setting limits on maladaptive behavior **to promote client safety.**

• Clarify and prioritize individual goals, noting where the subject of the "conflict" falls on this scale. **Choices may have risky, uncertain outcomes; may reflect a need to make value judgments or may generate regret over having to reject positive choice and accept negative consequences.**

• Identify strengths and presence of positive coping skills (e.g., use of relaxation technique, willingness to express feelings).

• Identify positive aspects of this experience and assist client to view it as a learning opportunity **to develop new and creative solutions.**

• Correct misperceptions client may have and provide factual information. **Provides for better decision-making.**

• Provide opportunities for client to make simple decisions regarding self-care and other daily activities. Accept choice not to do so. Advance complexity of choices, as tolerated.

∞• Encourage child to make developmentally appropriate decisions concerning own care. **Fosters child's sense of self-worth, enhances ability to learn and exercise coping skills.**

• Discuss time considerations, setting time line for small steps and considering consequences related to not making/postponing specific decisions **to facilitate resolution of conflict.**

• Have client list some alternatives to present situation or decisions, using a brainstorming process. Include family in this activity as indicated (e.g., placement of parent in long-term care facility, use of intervention process with addicted member). (Refer to NDs interrupted Family Processes; dysfunctional Family Processes; compromised family Coping; Moral Distress.)

• Practice use of problem-solving process with current situation/decision.

⊕• Discuss or clarify cultural or spiritual concerns, accepting client's values in a nonjudgmental manner.

Nursing Priority No. 3.

To promote wellness (Teaching/Discharge Considerations):

🏠• Promote opportunities for using conflict-resolution skills, identifying steps as client does each one.

Information that appears in brackets has been added by the authors to clarify and enhance the use of nursing diagnoses.

- Provide positive feedback for efforts and progress noted. **Promotes continuation of efforts.**
- Encourage involvement of family/SO(s), as desired/available, **to provide support for the client.**
- Support client for decisions made, especially if consequences are unexpected and/or difficult to cope with.
- Encourage attendance at stress reduction or assertiveness classes.
- Refer to other resources, as necessary (e.g., clergy, psychiatric clinical nurse specialist/psychiatrist, family/marital therapist, addiction support groups).

Documentation Focus

Assessment/Reassessment
- Assessment findings, behavioral responses, degree of impairment in lifestyle functioning.
- Individuals involved in the conflict.
- Personal values and beliefs.

Planning
- Plan of care, specific interventions, and who is involved in the planning process.
- Teaching plan.

Implementation/Evaluation
- Client's and involved individual's responses to interventions, teaching, and actions performed.
- Ability to express feelings, identify options; use of resources.
- Attainment or progress toward desired outcome(s).
- Modifications to plan of care.

Discharge Planning
- Long-term needs, referrals made, actions to be taken, and who is responsible for doing.
- Specific referrals made.

Sample Nursing Outcomes & Interventions Classifications (NOC/NIC)

NOC—Decision-Making
NIC—Decision-Making Support

Information that appears in brackets has been added by the authors to clarify and enhance the use of nursing diagnoses.

ineffective Denial

Taxonomy II: Coping/Stress Tolerance—Class 2 Coping
  Responses (00072)
[Diagnostic Division: Ego Integrity]
Submitted 1988; Revised 2006

Definition: Conscious or unconscious attempt to disavow
the knowledge or meaning of an event to reduce anxiety
and/or fear, leading to the detriment of health

Related Factors

Anxiety; threat of inadequacy in dealing with strong emotions
Lack of control of life situation; fear of loss of autonomy
Overwhelming stress; lack of competency in using effective
  coping mechanisms
Threat of unpleasant reality
Fear of separation/death
Lack of emotional support from others

Defining Characteristics

Subjective

Minimizes symptoms; displaces source of symptoms to other
  organs
Unable to admit impact of disease on life pattern
Displaces fear of impact of the condition
Does not admit fear of death/invalidism

Objective

Delays seeking or refuses healthcare attention
Does not perceive personal relevance of symptoms
Does not perceive personal relevance of danger
Makes dismissive gestures or comments when speaking of dis-
  tressing events
Displays inappropriate affect
Uses self-treatment

Desired Outcomes/Evaluation Criteria—
Client Will:

- Acknowledge reality of situation or illness.
- Express realistic concern or feelings about symptoms/illness.

Information that appears in brackets has been added by the authors to clarify
and enhance the use of nursing diagnoses.

🌐 Cultural   🌐 Collaborative   🏠 Community/Home Care

- Seek appropriate assistance for presenting problem.
- Display appropriate affect.

Actions/Interventions

Nursing Priority No. 1.
To assess causative/contributing factors:

- Identify situational crisis or problem and client's perception of the situation.
- Determine stage and degree of denial.
- Compare client's description of symptoms or conditions to reality of clinical picture.
- Note client's comments about impact of illness or problem on lifestyle.

Nursing Priority No. 2.
To assist client to deal appropriately with situation:

- Use therapeutic communication skills of Active-listening and I-messages **to develop trusting nurse-client relationship.**
- Provide a safe, nonthreatening environment. **Encourages client to talk freely without fear of judgment.**
- Encourage expressions of feelings, accepting client's view of the situation without confrontation. Set limits on maladaptive behavior **to promote safety.**
- Present accurate information, as appropriate, without insisting that the client accept what has been presented. **Avoids confrontation, which may further entrench client in denial.**
- Discuss client's behaviors in relation to illness (e.g., diabetes, hypertension, alcoholism) and point out the results of these behaviors.
- Encourage client to talk with SO(s)/friends. **May clarify concerns and reduce isolation and withdrawal.**
- Involve client in group sessions **so client can hear other views of reality and test own perceptions.**
- Avoid agreeing with inaccurate statements/perceptions **to prevent perpetuating false reality.**
- Provide positive feedback for constructive moves toward independence **to promote repetition of behavior.**

Nursing Priority No. 3.
To promote wellness (Teaching/Discharge Considerations):

- Provide written information about illness or situation **for client and family to refer to as they consider options.**

Information that appears in brackets has been added by the authors to clarify and enhance the use of nursing diagnoses.

- 🏠 Involve family members/SO(s) in long-range planning for meeting individual needs.
- 🤝 Refer to appropriate community resources (e.g., Diabetes Association, MS Society, Alcoholics Anonymous) **to help client with long-term adjustment.**
- Refer to ND ineffective Coping.

Documentation Focus

Assessment/Reassessment
- Assessment findings, degree of personal vulnerability and denial.
- Impact of illness or problem on lifestyle.

Planning
- Plan of care and who is involved in the planning.
- Teaching plan.

Implementation/Evaluation
- Client's response to interventions, teaching, and actions performed.
- Use of resources.
- Attainment or progress toward desired outcome(s).
- Modifications to plan of care.

Discharge Planning
- Long-term needs and who is responsible for actions taken.
- Specific referrals made.

Sample Nursing Outcomes & Interventions Classifications (NOC/NIC)

NOC—Acceptance: Health Status
NIC—Anxiety Reduction

---

impaired **Dentition**

Taxonomy II: Safety/Protection—Class 2 Physical Injury (00048)
[Diagnostic Division: Food/Fluid]
Nursing Diagnosis Extension and Classification Submission 1998

Definition: Disruption in tooth development/eruption patterns or structural integrity of individual teeth

---

Information that appears in brackets has been added by the authors to clarify and enhance the use of nursing diagnoses.

Related Factors

Dietary habits; nutritional deficits

Selected prescription medications; chronic use of tobacco, coffee, tea, or red wine

Ineffective oral hygiene, sensitivity to heat/cold; chronic vomiting

Deficient knowledge regarding dental health; excessive intake of fluorides or use of abrasive cleaning agents

Barriers to self-care; lack of access to professional care

Economically disadvantaged

Genetic predisposition; bruxism

[Traumatic injury to face/jaw; surgical intervention]

Defining Characteristics

Subjective

Toothache

Objective

Halitosis

Tooth enamel discoloration; erosion of enamel; excessive plaque

Worn down or abraded teeth; crown or root caries; tooth fracture(s); loose teeth; missing teeth; absent teeth

Premature loss of primary teeth; incomplete eruption for age (primary or permanent teeth)

Excessive calculus

Malocclusion; tooth misalignment; asymmetrical facial expression

Desired Outcomes/Evaluation Criteria—Client Will:

- Display healthy gums, mucous membranes, and teeth in good repair.
- Report adequate nutritional and fluid intake.
- Verbalize and demonstrate effective dental hygiene skills.
- Follow through on referrals for appropriate dental care.

Action/Interventions

Nursing Priority No. 1.

To assess causative/contributing factors:

- Inspect oral cavity. Note presence or absence of teeth and/or dentures and ascertain significance of finding in terms of nutritional needs and aesthetics.

Information that appears in brackets has been added by the authors to clarify and enhance the use of nursing diagnoses.

• Evaluate current status of dental hygiene and oral health **to determine need for instruction or coaching, assistive devices, and/or referral to dental care providers.**

∞• Document age, developmental and cognitive status, and manual dexterity. Evaluate nutritional and health state, noting presence of conditions such as bulimia or chronic vomiting, musculoskeletal impairments, or problems with mouth (e.g., bleeding disorders, cancer lesions, abscesses, and facial trauma), **which are factors affecting a client's dental health and the ability to provide effective oral care.**

• Document presence of factors affecting dentition (e.g., chronic use of tobacco, coffee, or tea; bulimia/chronic vomiting; abscesses; tumors; braces; bruxism [chronic grinding of teeth]) **to determine possible interventions and/or treatment needs.**

• Note current situation that could impact dental health (e.g., presence of endotrachial [ET] intubation, facial fractures, or chemotherapy) **and that require special mouth care procedures.**

• Document (photograph) facial injuries before treatment **to provide a "pictorial baseline" for future comparison and evaluation.**

Nursing Priority No. 2.

To treat/manage dental care needs:

• Ascertain client's usual method of oral care **to provide continuity of care or to build on client's existing knowledge base and current practices in developing plan of care.**

• Assist with or provide oral care, as indicated:

   Offer tap water or saline rinses and diluted alcohol-free mouthwashes.

   Provide gentle gum massage and tongue brushing with soft toothbrush, using fluoride toothpaste to manage tartar buildup, if appropriate.

   Use foam sticks **to swab gums and oral cavity when brushing is not possible or inadvisable.**

   Assist with brushing and flossing **when client is unable to do self-care.**

   Demonstrate and assist with electric or battery-powered mouth care devices (e.g., toothbrush, plaque remover, waterpik), as indicated.

∞ Remind client to brush teeth as indicated. **Cues, modeling, or pantomime may be helpful if client is young, elderly, or cognitively or emotionally impaired.**

Information that appears in brackets has been added by the authors to clarify and enhance the use of nursing diagnoses.

Assist with or provide denture care, when indicated (e.g., remove and clean after meals and at bedtime).

- Provide appropriate diet for optimal nutrition, considering client's special needs, such as pregnancy, age and developmental concerns, and ability to chew (e.g., liquids or soft foods), and offer low-sugar, low-starch foods and snacks; limit between-meal eating, sugary foods, and bedtime snacks **to minimize tooth decay and to improve overall health.**
- Increase fluids, as needed, **to enhance hydration and general well-being of oral mucous membranes.**
- Reposition ET tubes and airway adjuncts routinely, carefully padding and protecting teeth or prosthetics. Suction with care, when indicated.
- Avoid thermal stimuli when teeth are sensitive. Recommend use of specific toothpastes **designed to reduce sensitivity of teeth.**
- Maintain good jaw and facial alignment when fractures are present.
- Administer antibiotics, as needed, **to treat dental and gum infections.**
- Recommend use of analgesics and topical analgesics, as needed, **when dental pain is present.**
- Administer antibiotic therapy prior to dental procedures in susceptible individuals (e.g., prosthetic heart valve clients) and/or ascertain that bleeding disorders or coagulation deficits are not present **to prevent excess bleeding.**
- Refer to appropriate care providers (e.g., dental hygienists, dentists, periodontists, oral surgeons).

Nursing Priority No. 3.

To promote wellness (Teaching/Discharge Considerations):

- Instruct client/caregiver in home-care interventions **to treat condition and/or prevent further complications.**
- Review resources that are needed for the client to perform adequate dental hygiene care (e.g., toothbrush/paste, clean water, dental floss, and/or personal care assistant).
- Recommend that client (of any age) limit sugary and high-carbohydrate foods in diet and snacks **to reduce buildup of plaque and risk of cavities caused by acids associated with breakdown of sugar and starch.**
- Instruct older client and caregiver(s) concerning special needs and importance of daily mouth care and regular dental follow-up.
- Advise mother regarding age-appropriate concerns (e.g., refrain from letting baby fall asleep with milk or juice in bottle;

Information that appears in brackets has been added by the authors to clarify and enhance the use of nursing diagnoses.

use water and pacifier during night; avoid sharing eating utensils and tooth brushes among family members; teach children to brush teeth while young; provide child with safety devices such as helmet, face mask, or mouth guard to prevent facial injuries.

∞• Discuss with pregnant women special needs and regular dental care **to maintain maternal dental health and promote strong teeth and bones in fetal development.**

• Encourage cessation of tobacco, especially smokeless, and enrollment in smoking-cessation classes **to reduce incidence of gum disorders, oral cancer, and other health problems.**

⊕• Discuss advisability of dental checkup and care prior to initiating chemotherapy or radiation treatments **to minimize oral and dental tissue damage.**

⊕• Refer to resources to maintain dental hygiene (e.g., dental care providers, oral health care supplies, and/or financial assistance programs).

Documentation Focus

Assessment/Reassessment
• Individual findings, including individual factors influencing dentition problems.
• Baseline photos; description of oral cavity and structures.

Planning
• Plan of care and who is involved in planning.
• Teaching plan.

Implementation/Evaluation
• Responses to interventions, teaching, and actions performed.
• Attainment or progress toward desired outcome(s).
• Modifications to plan of care.

Discharge Planning
• Individual long-term needs, noting who is responsible for actions to be taken.
• Specific referrals made.

Sample Nursing Outcomes & Interventions Classifications (NOC/NIC)

NOC—Oral Hygiene
NIC—Oral Health Restoration

Information that appears in brackets has been added by the authors to clarify and enhance the use of nursing diagnoses.

risk for delayed Development

Taxonomy II: Growth/Development—Class 2 Development (00112)
[Diagnostic Division: Teaching/Learning]
Nursing Diagnosis Extension and Classification Submission 1998

Definition: At risk for delay of 25% or more in one or more of the areas of social or self-regulatory behavior or in cognitive, language, or gross or fine motor skills

Risk Factors

Prenatal
Maternal age of less than 15 or more than 35 years
Unplanned or unwanted pregnancy; inadequate, late, or poor prenatal care
Inadequate nutrition; economically disadvantaged
Illiteracy
Genetic or endocrine disorders; infections; substance abuse

Individual
Prematurity; congenital or genetic disorders
Vision or hearing impairment; frequent otitis media
Inadequate nutrition; failure to thrive
Chronic illness; treatment related side-effects (e.g., chemotherapy; radiation therapy, or pharmaceutical agents)
Brain damage (e.g., hemorrhage in postnatal period, shaken baby, abuse, or accident); seizures
Positive drug screening(s); substance abuse; lead poisoning
Foster or adopted child
Behavior disorders
Technology dependent
Natural disaster

Environmental
Economically disadvantaged
Violence

Caregiver
Learning disabilities
Mental retardation; severe learning disability

Information that appears in brackets has been added by the authors to clarify and enhance the use of nursing diagnoses.

Abuse
Mental illness

> **NOTE:** A risk diagnosis is not evidenced by signs and symptoms, as the problem has not occurred; rather, nursing interventions are directed at prevention.

Desired Outcomes/Evaluation Criteria— Client Will:

- Perform self-regulatory behavior and motor, social, cognitive, and language skills appropriate for age within scope of present capabilities.

Caregiver Will:

- Verbalize understanding of age-appropriate development and expectations.
- Identify individual risk factors for developmental delay or deviation.
- Formulate plan(s) for prevention of developmental deviation.
- Initiate interventions and lifestyle changes promoting appropriate development.

Actions/Interventions

Nursing Priority No. 1.
To assess causative/contributing factors:

- Identify condition(s) that could contribute to developmental deviations; e.g., a genetic condition (e.g., Down syndrome, cerebral palsy) or complications of a high-risk pregnancy (e.g., prematurity, extremes of maternal age, maternal substance abuse, brain injury or damage), chronic severe illness, infections, mental illness, poverty, shaken baby syndrome or child abuse, violence, failure to thrive, inadequate nutrition, and/or others as listed in Risk Factors.
- Collaborate in a multidisciplinary screening evaluation to assess client's development in areas of gross motor, fine motor, cognitive, social, emotional, adaptive, and communicative development **to determine area(s) of need/possible intervention.**
- Identify cultural beliefs, norms, and values **as they may impact parent/caregiver view of situation. Note: Culture**

Information that appears in brackets has been added by the authors to clarify and enhance the use of nursing diagnoses.

shapes parenting practices, understanding of health and illness, perceptions related to development, and beliefs about individuals affected by developmental disorders. **These cultural implications underscore the importance of having a broad array of tools for assessment and instruction as well as a good understanding of the child's culture.**

- Ascertain nature of caregiver-required activities and abilities to perform needed activities.
- Note severity and pervasiveness of situation (e.g., potential for long-term stress leading to abuse or neglect, versus situational disruption during period of crisis or transition). **Situations require different interventions in terms of the intensity and length of time that assistance and support may be critical to the parent/caregiver.**
- Evaluate environment in which long-standing care will be provided **to determine ongoing services/other needs of child and care provider(s).**

Nursing Priority No. 2.

To assist in preventing and/or limiting developmental delays:

- Avoid blame when discussing contributing factors. **Blame engenders negative feelings and contributes nothing to solution of the situation.**
- Note chronological age and review expectations for "normal" development at this age **to help determine developmental expectations.**
- Review expected skills and activities using an authoritative text (e.g., Gesell, Mussen-Congor) or assessment tools (e.g., Ages and Stages Questionnaire [ASQ-3], Parents Evaluation of Developmental Status [PEDS], Temperament and Atypical Behavior Scale [TABS], Denver II Developmental Screening Test, or Bender's Visual Motor Gestalt Test). **Provides guide for comparative measurement as child/individual progresses. Note: Often there is no single diagnostic test for a specific developmental delay. There are tools to evaluate child's skills in certain areas, such as motor development, speech, language, math, etc. However, a diagnosis is often determined over months or years. Also, a child who is delayed in an area at a certain age may "catch up" in later years.**
- Consult professional resources (e.g., physical, occupational, rehabilitation, and speech therapists; home healthcare agencies; social services; nutritionists; special education teachers; family therapists; technological and adaptive equipment

---

Information that appears in brackets has been added by the authors to clarify and enhance the use of nursing diagnoses.

sources; and vocational counselors) **to formulate a plan and address specific individual needs and eligibility for intervention home- and/or community-based services.**

• Encourage setting of short-term realistic goals for achieving developmental potential. **Small incremental steps are often easier to deal with.**

• Identify equipment needs (e.g., adaptive/growth-stimulating computer programs, communication devices).

Nursing Priority No. 3.
🏠 To promote wellness (Teaching/Discharge Considerations):

🌐• Engage in and encourage prevention strategies (e.g., abstinence from drugs, alcohol and tobacco for pregnant women/child, referral for treatment programs, referral for violence prevention counseling, anticipatory guidance for potential handicaps [vision, hearing, or failure to thrive]). **Promoting wellness starts with preventing complications and/or limiting severity of anticipated problems. Such strategies can often be initiated by nurses where the potential is first identified, in the community setting.**

• Evaluate client's progress on continual basis. Identify target symptoms requiring intervention **to make referrals in a timely manner and/or to make adjustments in plan of care, as indicated**.

• Provide information regarding development, as appropriate, including pertinent reference materials.

🌐• Emphasize importance of follow-up screening appointments and encourage attendance at appropriate educational programs (e.g., parenting classes, infant stimulation sessions, seminars on life stresses and the aging process) **to promote ongoing evaluation, support, or management of situation**.

• Provide information as appropriate, including pertinent reference materials and reliable Web sites. **Bibliotherapy provides an opportunity to review data at own pace, enhancing likelihood of retention.**

🌐• Identify available community resources, as appropriate (e.g., early intervention programs, seniors' activity/support groups, gifted and talented programs, sheltered workshop, children's services, and medical equipment/supplier). **Provides additional assistance to support family efforts and coping if interventions are required.**

Information that appears in brackets has been added by the authors to clarify and enhance the use of nursing diagnoses.

Documentation Focus

Assessment/Reassessment
- Assessment findings, individual needs including developmental level and potential for improvement.
- Caregiver's understanding of situation and individual role.

Planning
- Plan of care and who is involved in the planning.
- Teaching plan.

Implementation/Evaluation
- Client's response to interventions, teaching, and actions performed.
- Caregiver response to teaching.
- Attainment or progress toward desired outcome(s).
- Modifications to plan of care.

Discharge Planning
- Identified long-range needs and who is responsible for actions to be taken.
- Specific referrals made, sources for assistive devices, educational tools.

Sample Nursing Outcomes & Interventions Classifications (NOC/NIC)

NOC—Child Development [specify age]
NIC—Developmental Enhancement: Child [or] Adolescent

Diarrhea

Taxonomy II: Elimination and Exchange—Class 2 Gastrointestinal Function (0013)
[Diagnostic Division: Elimination]
Submitted 1975; Nursing Diagnosis Extension and Classification Revision 1998

Definition: Passage of loose, unformed stools

Related Factors

Psychological
High stress levels; anxiety

Information that appears in brackets has been added by the authors to clarify and enhance the use of nursing diagnoses.

Situational
Laxative or alcohol abuse; toxins; contaminants
Adverse effects of pharmaceutical agents; radiation
Tube feedings
Travel

Physiological
Inflammation; irritation
Infectious processes; parasites
Malabsorption

Defining Characteristics

Subjective
Abdominal pain
Urgency; cramping

Objective
Hyperactive bowel sounds
At least three loose liquid stools per day

Desired Outcomes/Evaluation Criteria— Client Will:

- Reestablish and maintain normal pattern of bowel functioning.
- Verbalize understanding of causative factors and rationale for treatment regimen.
- Demonstrate appropriate behavior to assist with resolution of causative factors (e.g., proper food preparation or avoidance of irritating foods).

Actions/Interventions

Nursing Priority No. 1.
To assess causative factors/etiology:

- Ascertain onset and pattern of diarrhea, noting whether acute or chronic. **Acute diarrhea (caused by viral, bacterial, or parasitic infections [e.g., *Norwalk, Rotavirus; Salmonella, Shigella, Giardia;* amebiasis, respectively]; bacterial food-borne toxins [e.g., *Staphylococcus aureus, Escherichia coli*]; medications [e.g., antibiotics, chemotherapy agents, cholchicine, laxatives]; and enteral tube feedings) lasts from a few days up to a week. Chronic diarrhea (caused**

Information that appears in brackets has been added by the authors to clarify and enhance the use of nursing diagnoses.

🌐 Cultural   😊 Collaborative   🏠 Community/Home Care

by irritable bowel syndrome, infectious diseases affecting the colon [e.g., inflammatory bowel disease], colon cancer and treatments, severe constipation, malabsorption disorders, laxative abuse, certain endocrine disorders [e.g., hyperthyroidism, Addison's disease]) almost always lasts more than 3 weeks.

- Obtain history and observe stools for volume, frequency (e.g., more than normal number of stools per day), characteristics (e.g., slightly soft to watery stools), and precipitating factors (e.g., travel, recent antibiotic use, day care center attendance) related to occurrence of diarrhea.

∞• Note client's age. **Diarrhea in infant or young child and older or debilitated client can cause complications of dehydration and electrolyte imbalances.**

- Determine if incontinence is present. (Refer to ND bowel Incontinence.)

- Note reports of abdominal or rectal pain associated with episodes. **Pain is often present with inflammatory bowel disease, irritable bowel syndrome, and mesenteric ischemia.**

- Auscultate abdomen **for presence, location, and characteristics of bowel sounds.**

- Observe for presence of associated factors, such as fever or chills, abdominal pain and cramping, bloody stools, emotional upset, physical exertion, and so forth.

- Evaluate diet history, noting food allergies or intolerances and food and water safety issues, and note general nutritional intake and fluid and electrolyte status.

∞• Review medications, noting side effects and possible interactions. **Many drugs (e.g., antibiotics [e.g., cephalosporins, erythromycin, penicillins, quinolones, tetracyclines], digitalis, angiotensin-converting enzyme [ACE] inhibitors, nonsteroidal anti-inflammatory drugs [NSAIDs], hypoglycemia agents, and cholesterol-lowering drugs) can cause or exacerbate diarrhea, particularly in the elderly and in those who have had surgery on the intestinal tract.**

- Determine recent exposure to different or foreign environments, change in drinking water or food intake, and similar illness of others **that may help identify causative environmental factors.**

- Note history of recent gastrointestinal surgery, concurrent or chronic illnesses and treatment, food or drug allergies, and lactose intolerance.

- Review results of laboratory testing (**e.g., parasites, cultures for bacteria, toxins, fat, blood) for acute diarrhea. Chronic**

Information that appears in brackets has been added by the authors to clarify and enhance the use of nursing diagnoses.

diarrhea testing may include upper and lower gastrointestinal studies, stool examination for parasites, colonoscopy with biopsies, and so forth.

Nursing Priority No. 2.

To eliminate causative factors:

- Restrict solid food intake, as indicated, **to allow for bowel rest and reduced intestinal workload.**
- Provide for changes in dietary intake **to avoid foods or substances that precipitate diarrhea.**
- Limit caffeine and high-fiber foods; avoid milk and fruits, as appropriate.
- Adjust strength or rate of enteral tube feedings; change formula, as indicated, **when diarrhea is associated with tube feedings.**
- Assess for and remove fecal impaction, especially in an elderly client **where impaction may be accompanied by diarrhea.** (Refer to NDs Constipation; bowel Incontinence.)
- Recommend change in drug therapy, as appropriate (e.g., choice of antibiotic).
- Assist in treatment of underlying conditions (e.g., infections, malabsorption syndrome, cancer) and complications of diarrhea. **Therapies can include treatment of fever, pain, and infectious or toxic agents; rehydration; oral refeeding; and so forth.**
- Promote use of relaxation techniques (e.g., progressive relaxation exercise, visualization techniques) **to decrease stress and anxiety.**

Nursing Priority No. 3.

To maintain hydration/electrolyte balance:

- Note reports of thirst, less frequent or absent urination, dry mouth and skin, weakness, light-headedness, and headaches. **These are signs/symptoms of dehydration and need for rehydration.**
- Observe for or question parents about young child crying with no tears, fever, decreased urination, or no wet diapers for 6 to 8 hours; listlessness or irritability; sunken eyes; dry mouth and tongue; and suspected or documented weight loss. **Child needs urgent or emergency treatment for dehydration if these signs are present and child is not taking fluids.**
- Assess for presence of postural hypotension, tachycardia, skin hydration/turgor, and condition of mucous membranes **indicating dehydration.**

Information that appears in brackets has been added by the authors to clarify and enhance the use of nursing diagnoses.

∞• Weigh infant's diapers **to determine amount of output and fluid replacement needs.**

✎• Review laboratory studies for abnormalities. **Chronic diarrhea may require more invasive testing, including upper and/or lower gastrointestinal radiographs, ultrasound, endoscopic evaluations, biopsy, etc.**

💊• Administer antidiarrheal medications, as indicated, **to decrease gastrointestinal motility and minimize fluid losses.**

• Encourage oral intake of fluids containing electrolytes, such as juices, bouillon, or commercial preparations, as appropriate.

🖉• Administer enteral and parenteral fluids, as indicated.

Nursing Priority No. 4.
To maintain skin integrity:

• Assist, as needed, with pericare after each bowel movement.
• Provide prompt diaper/incontinence brief change and gentle cleansing, **because skin breakdown can occur quickly when diarrhea is present.**
• Apply lotion or ointment as skin barrier, as needed.
• Provide dry linen, as necessary.
• Expose perineum and buttocks to air; use heat lamp with caution, if needed to keep area dry.
• Refer to ND impaired Skin Integrity.

Nursing Priority No. 5.
To promote return to normal bowel functioning:

• Increase oral fluid intake and return to normal diet, as tolerated.
• Encourage intake of nonirritating liquids.
∞• Discuss possible change in infant formula. **Diarrhea may be result of or be aggravated by intolerance to a specific formula.**
• Recommend products such as natural fiber, plain natural yogurt, and Lactinex **to restore normal bowel flora.**
💊• Administer medications, as ordered, **to treat infectious process, decrease motility, and/or absorb water.**
• Provide privacy during defecation and psychological support, as necessary.

Nursing Priority No. 6.
🏠 To promote wellness (Teaching/Discharge Considerations):

• Review causative factors and appropriate interventions **to prevent recurrence.**

Information that appears in brackets has been added by the authors to clarify and enhance the use of nursing diagnoses.

- Discuss individual stress factors and coping behaviors.
- Review food preparation, emphasizing adequate cooking time and proper refrigeration or storage **to prevent bacterial growth and contamination.**
- Emphasize importance of hand hygiene **to prevent spread of infectious causes of diarrhea such as** *Clostridium difficile* **or** *S. aureus.*
- Discuss possibility of dehydration and the importance of proper fluid replacement.
- Suggest use of incontinence pads **to protect bedding or furniture, depending on the severity of the problem.**

Documentation Focus

Assessment/Reassessment
- Assessment findings, including characteristics and pattern of elimination.
- Causative and aggravating factors.
- Methods used to treat problem.

Planning
- Plan of care and who is involved in planning.
- Teaching plan.

Implementation/Evaluation
- Client's response to treatment, teaching, and actions performed.
- Attainment or progress toward desired outcome(s).
- Modifications to plan of care.

Discharge Planning
- Recommendations for follow-up care.

Sample Nursing Outcomes & Interventions Classifications (NOC/NIC)

NOC—Bowel Elimination
NIC—Diarrhea Management

Information that appears in brackets has been added by the authors to clarify and enhance the use of nursing diagnoses.

🌐 Cultural   😊 Collaborative   🏠 Community/Home Care

risk for Disuse Syndrome

Taxonomy II: Activity/Rest—Class 2 Activity/Exercise (00040)
[Diagnostic Division: Activity/Rest]
Submitted 1988

Definition: At risk for deterioration of body systems as the result of prescribed or unavoidable musculoskeletal inactivity

NOTE: Complications from immobility can include pressure ulcer, constipation, stasis of pulmonary secretions, thrombosis, urinary tract infection and/or retention, decreased strength or endurance, orthostatic hypotension, decreased range of joint motion, disorientation, body image disturbance, and powerlessness.

Risk Factors

Severe pain; [chronic pain]
Paralysis; [other neuromuscular impairment]
Mechanical or prescribed immobilization
Altered level of consciousness

NOTE: A risk diagnosis is not evidenced by signs and symptoms, as the problem has not occurred; rather, nursing interventions are directed at prevention.

Desired Outcomes/Evaluation Criteria— Client Will:

- Display intact skin and tissues or achieve timely wound healing.
- Maintain or reestablish effective elimination patterns.
- Be free of signs/symptoms of infectious processes.
- Demonstrate absence of pulmonary congestion with breath sounds clear.
- Demonstrate adequate peripheral perfusion with stable vital signs, skin warm and dry, palpable peripheral pulses.
- Maintain usual reality orientation.

Information that appears in brackets has been added by the authors to clarify and enhance the use of nursing diagnoses.

- Maintain or regain optimal level of cognitive, neurosensory, and musculoskeletal functioning.
- Express sense of control over the present situation and potential outcome.
- Recognize and incorporate change into self-concept in accurate manner without negative self-esteem.

Actions/Interventions

Nursing Priority No. 1.

To evaluate probability of developing complications:

- Identify underlying conditions/pathology (e.g., cancer, trauma, fractures with casting, immobilization devices, surgery, chronic disease conditions, malnutrition, neurological conditions [e.g., stroke/other brain injury, postpolio syndrome, MS, or spinal cord injury], chronic pain conditions, or use of predisposing medications [e.g., steroids]) **that cause or exacerbate problems associated with inactivity and immobility.**
- Note specific and potential concerns including client's age, cognition, mobility and exercise status, and whether current condition is acute or short term or may be long term or permanent. **Age-related physiological changes along with limitations imposed by illness or confinement predispose older adults to deconditioning and functional decline.**
- Assess and document client's ongoing functional status, including cognition, vision, and hearing; social support; psychological well-being; abilities in performance of activities of daily living **for comparative baseline; evaluate response to treatment and identify preventive interventions or necessary services.**
- Evaluate client's risk for injury. **Risk is greater in client with cognitive difficulties, lack of safe or stimulating environment, inadequate or unsafe use of mobility aids, and/or sensory-perception problems.**
- Ascertain availability and use of support systems.
- Review psychological assessment of client's emotional status. **Potential problems that may arise from presence of condition need to be identified and dealt with to avoid further debilitation. Common associated psychological changes include depression, anxiety, and avoidance behaviors.**
- Evaluate client's/family's understanding and ability to manage care for long period. **Caregivers may be influenced by their own physical or emotional limitations, degree of**

Information that appears in brackets has been added by the authors to clarify and enhance the use of nursing diagnoses.

🌐 Cultural 🔵 Collaborative 🏠 Community/Home Care

commitment to assisting the client toward optimal independence, or available time.

Nursing Priority No. 2.
To identify individually appropriate preventive/corrective interventions:

♠Skin
- Inspect skin on a frequent basis, noting changes. Monitor skin over bony prominences.
- Reposition frequently as individually indicated **to relieve pressure.**
- Provide skin care daily and prn, drying well and using gentle massage and lotion **to stimulate circulation.**
- Use pressure-reducing devices (e.g., egg crate, gel, water, or air mattress or cushions).
- Review nutritional status and promote diet with adequate protein, calorie, and vitamin and mineral intake **to aid in healing and promote general good health of skin and tissues.**
- Provide or reinforce teaching regarding dietary needs, position changes, and cleanliness.
- Refer to NDs impaired Skin Integrity; impaired Tissue Integrity.

♠Elimination
- Observe elimination pattern, noting changes and potential problems.
- Encourage balanced diet, including fruits and vegetables high in fiber and with adequate fluids **for optimal stool consistency and to facilitate passage through colon.**
- Encourage intake of adequate fluids, including water and cranberry juice **to reduce risk of urinary infections.**
- Maximize mobility at earliest opportunity.
- Evaluate need for stool softeners or bulk-forming laxatives.
- Implement consistent bowel management or bladder training programs, as indicated.
- Monitor urinary output and characteristics **to identify changes associated with infection.**
- Refer to NDs Constipation; Diarrhea; bowel Incontinence; impaired Urinary Elimination; Urinary Retention.

♠Respiration
- Monitor breath sounds and characteristics of secretions **for early detection of complications (e.g., atelectasis, pneumonia).**

Information that appears in brackets has been added by the authors to clarify and enhance the use of nursing diagnoses.

Diagnostic Studies ∞ Pediatric/Geriatric/Lifespan Medications **329**

- Encourage ambulation and an upright position. Reposition, cough, and deep breathe on a regular schedule **to facilitate clearing of secretions and to improve lung function.**
- Encourage use of incentive spirometry. Suction, as indicated, **to clear airways.**
- Demonstrate techniques for, and assist with, postural drainage.
- Assist with, and instruct family and caregivers in, quad coughing techniques and diaphragmatic weight training **to maximize ventilation in presence of a spinal cord injury.**
- Discourage smoking. Encourage client to join a smoking-cessation program, as indicated.
- Refer to NDs ineffective Airway Clearance; ineffective Breathing Pattern.

🛡Vascular (Tissue Perfusion)
- Monitor cognition and mental status. **Changes can reflect state of cardiac health or cerebral oxygenation impairment or can be indicative of mental or emotional state that could adversely affect safety and self-care.**
- Determine core and skin temperature. Investigate development of cyanosis or changes in mentation **to identify changes in oxygenation status.**
- Evaluate circulation and nerve function of affected body parts on a routine, ongoing basis. **Changes in temperature, color, sensation, and movement can be the effect of immobility, disease, aging, or injury.**
- Institute peripheral vascular support measures (e.g., elastic hose, Ace wraps, sequential compression devices [SCDs]) **to enhance venous return.**
- Encourage adequate fluid intake **to prevent dehydration and circulatory stasis.**
- Monitor blood pressure before, during, and after activity—sitting, standing, and lying—if possible, **to ascertain response to and tolerance of activity.**
- Assist with position changes as needed. Raise head gradually. Institute use of tilt table where appropriate. **Injury may occur as a result of orthostatic hypotension.**
- Maintain proper body position; avoid use of constricting garments/restraints **to prevent vascular congestion.**
- Provide range-of-motion exercises for bed or chair. Ambulate as quickly and often as possible, using mobility aids and frequent rest stops **to assist client in continuing activity and prevent circulatory problems related to inactivity.**

Information that appears in brackets has been added by the authors to clarify and enhance the use of nursing diagnoses.

* Refer to physical therapy **for strengthening and restoration of optimal range of motion (ROM) and prevention of circulatory problems.**
* Refer to NDs ineffective peripheral Tissue Perfusion; risk for Peripheral Neurovascular Dysfunction.

♠ Musculoskeletal (Mobility/Range of Motion, Strength/Endurance)

* Perform ROM exercises and involve client in active exercises with physical or occupational therapy (e.g., muscle strengthening) **to promote bone health, muscle strengthening, flexibility, optimal conditioning, and functional ability.**
* Maximize involvement in self-care **to restore or maintain strength and functional abilities.**
* Pace activities as possible **to increase strength and endurance.**
* Apply functional positioning splints as appropriate.
* Evaluate role of physiological and psychological pain in mobility problem.
* Implement pain management program as individually indicated.
* Monitor the use of restraints, if required, and immobilize client as little as possible **to reduce possibility of agitation and injury.** Remove restraints periodically and assist with ROM exercises.
* Refer to NDs Activity Intolerance; risk for Falls; impaired physical Mobility; acute or chronic Pain.

♠ Sensory-Perception

* Orient client as necessary to time, place, person, and situation. Provide cues for orientation (e.g., clock, calendar). **Disturbances of sensory interpretation and thought processes are associated with immobility as well as aging, being ill, disease processes/treatments, and medication effects.**
* Provide appropriate level of environmental stimulation (e.g., music, TV/radio, personal possessions, visitors) **to decrease the sensory deprivation associated with immobility and isolation.**
* Encourage participation in recreational and diversional activities and regular exercise program, as tolerated.
* Suggest use of sleep aids or presleep rituals **to promote normal sleep or rest.**
* Refer to NDs chronic Confusion; Insomnia; Social Isolation; deficient Diversional Activity.

Information that appears in brackets has been added by the authors to clarify and enhance the use of nursing diagnoses.

♠ Self-Esteem, Powerlessness, Hopelessness, Social Isolation

- Determine factors that may contribute to impairment of client's self-esteem and social interactions. **Many factors can be involved, including the client's age, relationship status, usual health state; presence of disabilities, including pain; financial, environmental, and physical problems; or current situation causing immobility and client's state of mind concerning the importance of the current situation in regard to the rest of client's life and desired lifestyle.**
- Ascertain if changes in client's situation are likely to be short term and temporary, or long term, or permanent. **Can affect both the client and care provider's coping abilities and willingness to engage in activities that prevent or limit effects of immobility.**
- Explain or review all care procedures. **Involves client in own care, enhances sense of control, and promotes independence.**
- Provide for, and assist with, mutual goal setting involving SO(s). **Promotes sense of control and enhances commitment to goals.**
- Provide consistency in caregivers whenever possible.
- Ascertain that client can communicate needs adequately (e.g., call light, writing tablet, picture/letter board, interpreter).
- Encourage verbalization of feelings and questions.
- ⊛ Refer for mental, psychological, or spiritual services as indicated **to provide counseling, support, and medications.**
- Refer to NDs Powerlessness; impaired verbal Communication; ineffective Role Performance; Self-Esteem [specify]; impaired Social Interaction.

♠ Body Image

- Evaluate for presence or potential for physical, emotional, and behavioral conditions that may contribute to isolation and degeneration. **Disuse syndrome often affects those individuals who are already isolated for one reason or another (e.g., serious illness or injury with disfigurement, frail elderly living alone, individual with severe depression, or a person with unacceptable behavior or without a support system).**
- Orient to body changes through verbal description, written information; encourage looking at and discussing changes **to promote acceptance and understanding of needs.**
- Promote interactions with peers and normalization of activities within individual abilities.

Information that appears in brackets has been added by the authors to clarify and enhance the use of nursing diagnoses.

- Refer to NDs disturbed Body Image; situational low Self-Esteem; Social Isolation; disturbed Personal Identity.

Nursing Priority No. 3.

🏠 To promote wellness (Teaching/Discharge Considerations):

- Promote self-care and SO-supported activities **to gain or maintain independence.**
- Provide or review information about individual needs and areas of concerns (e.g., client's mental status, living environment, nutritional needs) **to enhance safety and prevent or limit effects of disuse.**
- Encourage involvement in regular exercise program, including isometric or isotonic activities and active or assistive ROM, **to limit consequences of disuse and maximize level of function.**
- Review signs/symptoms requiring medical evaluation or follow-up to promote timely interventions.
- Identify community support services (e.g., financial, counseling, home maintenance, respite care, and transportation).
- Refer to appropriate rehabilitation/home-care resources **to provide assistance (e.g., help with care activities, exercise, meal preparation, financial help, transportation, or respite care; nutritionist).**
- Note sources for assistive devices and necessary equipment.

Documentation Focus ────────────

Assessment/Reassessment

- Assessment findings, noting individual areas of concern, functional level, degree of independence, support systems, and available resources.

Planning

- Plan of care and who is involved in planning.
- Teaching plan.

Implementation/Evaluation

- Client's response to interventions, teaching, and actions performed.
- Changes in level of functioning.
- Attainment or progress toward desired outcome(s).
- Modifications to plan of care.

───────────

Information that appears in brackets has been added by the authors to clarify and enhance the use of nursing diagnoses.

Discharge Planning
- Long-term needs and who is responsible for actions to be taken.
- Specific referrals made, resources for specific equipment needs.

Sample Nursing Outcomes & Interventions Classifications (NOC/NIC)

NOC—Immobility Consequences: Physiological
NIC—Exercise Promotion

deficient Diversional Activity

Taxonomy II: Health Promotion—Class 1 Health Awareness (00097)
[Diagnostic Division: Activity/Rest]
Submitted 1980

Definition: Decreased stimulation from (or interest or engagement in) recreational or leisure activities [**Note:** Internal/external factors may be beyond the individual's control.]

Related Factors

Environmental lack of diversional activity (e.g., long-term hospitalization; frequent, lengthy treatments; homebound; lack of resources)
[Physical limitations; bedridden; fatigue; chronic pain]

Defining Characteristics

Subjective
Reports feeling bored (e.g., wishes there were something to do, to read)
[Changes in abilities/physical limitations]

Objective
Usual hobbies cannot be undertaken in the current setting

Desired Outcomes/Evaluation Criteria— Client Will:

- Recognize own psychological response (e.g., hopelessness and helplessness, anger, depression) and initiate appropriate coping actions.
- Engage in satisfying activities within personal limitations.

Information that appears in brackets has been added by the authors to clarify and enhance the use of nursing diagnoses.

Nursing Priority No. 1.

To assess precipitating/etiological factors:

- Assess client's physical, cognitive, emotional, and environmental status. **Validates reality of environmental deprivation when it exists or considers potential for loss of desired diversional activities in order to plan for prevention or early interventions. Note: Studies show that key problems faced by clients who are hospitalized (or immobilized) for extended periods of time include boredom, stress, and depression. These negative states can impede recovery and lead clients to report symptoms more frequently.**
- ∞• Note impact of disability or illness on lifestyle (e.g., young child with leukemia, elderly person with fractured hip, individual with severe depression). **Provides comparative baseline for assessments and interventions.**
- ∞• Note age and developmental level, gender, cultural factors, and the importance of a given activity in client's life. **Cultural issues include gender roles, communication styles, privacy and personal space, expectations and views regarding time and activities, control of the immediate environment family traditions, and social patterns. When illness interferes with individual's ability to engage in usual activities, the person may have difficulty engaging in meaningful substitute activities.**
- Determine client's actual ability to participate and interest in available activities, noting attention span, physical limitations and tolerance, level of interest or desire, and safety needs. **Presence of acute illness, depression, problems of mobility, protective isolation, or sensory deprivation may interfere with desired activity.**

Nursing Priority No. 2.

To motivate and stimulate client involvement in solutions:

- Institute and continue appropriate actions to deal with concomitant conditions such as anxiety, depression, grief, dementia, physical injury, isolation and immobility, malnutrition, or acute or chronic pain. **These interfere with the individual's ability to engage in meaningful diversional activities.**
- Acknowledge reality of situation and feelings of the client **to establish therapeutic relationship and support hopeful emotions.**

Information that appears in brackets has been added by the authors to clarify and enhance the use of nursing diagnoses.

- Review history of lifelong activities and hobbies client has enjoyed. Discuss reasons client is not doing these activities now and determine whether client can and would like to resume these activities.
- Encourage mix of desired activities and stimuli (e.g., music, news, educational presentations—TV/tapes, movies, computer or Internet access, books and other reading materials, visitors, games, arts and crafts, sensory enrichment [e.g., massage, aromatherapy], grooming and beauty care, cooking, social outings, gardening, or discussion groups, as appropriate). **Activities need to be personally meaningful and not physically or emotionally overwhelming for client to derive the most benefit.**
- Participate in decisions about timing and spacing of visitors, leisure and care activities **to promote relaxation and reduce sense of boredom, as well as to prevent overstimulation and exhaustion.**
- Encourage client to assist in scheduling required and optional activity choices (e.g., if client's favorite TV show occurs at bath time, reschedule bath for a later time), **enhancing client's sense of control.**
- Refrain from making changes in schedule without discussing with client. **It is important for staff to be responsible in making and following through on commitments to client.**
- Provide change of scenery (indoors and outdoors where possible) to **provide positive sensory stimulation, reduce sense of boredom, improve sense of normalcy and control.**
- Identify requirements for mobility (wheelchair, walker, van, volunteers, etc.) **to make it possible for individual to participate safely in desired activities.**
- Provide for periodic changes in the personal environment when the client is confined. Use the individual's input in creating the changes (e.g., seasonal bulletin boards, color changes, rearranging furniture, or pictures).
- Suggest activities, such as bird feeders or baths for bird watching, a garden in a window box or terrarium, or a fish bowl or aquarium **to stimulate observation as well as involvement and participation in activity, such as identification of birds, choice of seeds, and so forth.**
- Accept hostile expressions while limiting aggressive acting-out behavior. **Permission to express feelings of anger and hopelessness allows for beginning resolution. However, destructive behavior is counterproductive to self-esteem and problem-solving.**

Information that appears in brackets has been added by the authors to clarify and enhance the use of nursing diagnoses.

⊕• Involve recreational, occupational, play, music, and/or movement therapist as appropriate **to help identify enjoyable activities for client; procure assistive devices and/or modify activities for individual situation.**

Nursing Priority No. 3.

To promote wellness (Teaching/Discharge Considerations):

🏠• Explore options for useful activities using the person's strengths and abilities.

⊕• Make appropriate referrals to available support groups, hobby clubs, or service organizations.

• Refer to NDs ineffective Coping; Hopelessness; Powerlessness; Social Isolation.

Documentation Focus

Assessment/Reassessment

• Specific assessment findings, including blocks to desired activities.

• Individual choices for activities.

Planning

• Plan of care, specific interventions, and who is involved in planning.

Implementation/Evaluation

• Client's responses to interventions, teaching, and actions performed.

• Attainment or progress toward desired outcome(s).

• Modifications to plan of care.

Discharge Planning

• Long-term needs and who is responsible for actions to be taken.

• Referrals and community resources.

Sample Nursing Outcomes & Interventions Classifications (NOC/NIC)

NOC—Leisure Participation
NIC—Recreation Therapy

Information that appears in brackets has been added by the authors to clarify and enhance the use of nursing diagnoses.

risk for Dry Eye

Taxonomy II: Safety/Protection—Class 5 Physical Injury (00219)
[Diagnostic Division: Safety]
Submitted 2010

Definition: At risk for eye discomfort or damage to the cornea and conjunctiva due to reduced quantity or quality of tears to moisten the eye

Risk Factors

Aging; female gender; hormones; vitamin A deficiency

Autoimmune diseases (rheumatoid arthritis, diabetes mellitus, thyroid disease, gout, osteoporosis, etc.); history of allergy

Contact lenses; ocular surface damage

Environmental factors (air conditioning, excessive wind/sunlight exposure, air pollution, low humidity); place of living

Lifestyle (e.g., smoking, caffeine use, prolonged reading/[computer use])

Neurological lesions with sensory or motor reflex loss (lagophthalmos, lack of spontaneous blink reflex due to decreased consciousness and other medical conditions)

Treatment-related side effects (e.g., pharmaceutical agents such as angiotensin-converting enzyme inhibitors, antihistamines, diuretics, steroids, antidepressants, tranquilizers, analgesics, sedatives, neuromuscular blocking agents; surgical operations); mechanical ventilation therapy

NOTE: A risk diagnosis is not evidenced by signs and symptoms, as the problem has not occurred; rather, nursing interventions are directed at prevention.

Desired Outcomes/Evaluation Criteria– Client Will:

• Be free of discomfort or damage to eye related to dryness.
• Verbalize understanding of risk factors and ways to prevent dry eye.

Information that appears in brackets has been added by the authors to clarify and enhance the use of nursing diagnoses.

Nursing Priority No. 1.

To identify causative/precipitating factors related to risk:

- Obtain history of eye conditions when assessing client concerns overall. Note reports of dry sensation, burning, itching, pain, foreign body sensation, light sensitivity (photophobia), and blurred vision. **These symptoms can be associated with dry eye syndrome and, if present, require further evaluation and possible treatment.**
- Note presence of conditions listed in risk factors above **to identify client with possible dry eye syndrome. Dry eye is most commonly caused by insufficient aqueous tear production. This can occur because of damage to eye surface (e.g., chemical burn) or be associated with disease conditions, neurological disorders, or environmental factors.**
- ∞• Note client's gender and age. **Studies show larger number of dry eye syndrome in females than males, especially aged over 50.**
- Determine client's current situation (e.g., admitted to facility for procedures/surgery, recent neurological event, mechanical ventilation, facial or eye trauma; eye infections, lower eyelid malposition) **that places client at high risk for dry eye associated with low or absent blink reflex and/or decreased tear production.**
- Determine client's history/presence of seasonal or environmental allergies, **which may cause or exacerbate conjunctivitis.**
- Review living and work environment to identify factors (e.g., exposure to smoke, wind, or chemicals; poor lighting; long periods of computer use or eye-straining work)
- Assess client's medications, noting use of certain drugs (e.g., antihistamines, beta-blockers, antidepressants, and oral contraceptives) **known to decrease tear production.**
- Refer for diagnostic evaluation and interventions as indicated.

Nursing Priority No. 2.

To promote eye health/comfort:

- Assist in/refer for treatment of underlying cause of dry eyes.
- Administer artificial tears, lubricating eye drops, or ointments as indicated, **when client is unable to blink or otherwise protect eyes while in healthcare facility.**

Information that appears in brackets has been added by the authors to clarify and enhance the use of nursing diagnoses.

Nursing Priority No. 3.

🏠To promote wellness (Teaching/Discharge Criteria):

- Instruct high-risk client in self-management interventions **to prevent or limit symptoms of dry eye**:

  Avoid air blowing in eyes **such as might occur with hair dryers, car heaters, air conditioners, or fans directed toward eyes.**

  Wear eye glasses or safety shield glasses on windy days **to reduce effects of the wind** and goggles while swimming **to protect eyes from chemicals in the water**.

  Take proper care of contact lenses and adhere to prescribed wearing time.

  Add moisture to indoor air, especially in winter.

  Take eye breaks during long reading and computer tasks or when watching TV for long periods of time.

  Blink repeatedly for a few seconds **to help spread your tears evenly over eye.**

  Position computer screen below eye level. **This may help slow the evaporation of tears between eye blinks.**

  Cessation of smoking and avoidance of smoking environments. **Smoke can worsen dry eye symptoms.**

Documentation Focus

Assessment/Reassessment

- Individual risk factors identified.
- Client concerns or difficulty making and following through with plan.

Planning

- Plan of care and who is involved in planning.
- Teaching plan.

Implementation/Evaluation

- Response to interventions, teaching, and actions performed.
- Attainment or progress toward outcomes.

Discharge Planning

- Referrals to other resources.
- Long-term need and who is responsible for actions.

Information that appears in brackets has been added by the authors to clarify and enhance the use of nursing diagnoses.

Sample Nursing Outcomes & Interventions Classifications (NOC/NIC)

NOC—Risk Control
NIC—Eye Care

risk for Electrolyte Imbalance

Taxonomy II: Nutrition—Class 5 Hydration (00195)
[Diagnostic Division: Food/Fluid]]
Submitted 2008

Definition: At risk for change in serum electrolyte levels that may compromise health

Risk Factors

Deficient fluid volume; diarrhea; vomiting
Excess fluid volume
Endocrine or renal dysfunction
Impaired regulatory mechanisms (e.g., diabetes insipidus, syndrome of inappropriate secretion of antidiuretic hormone)
Treatment-related side effects (e.g., medications, drains)

> **NOTE:** A risk diagnosis is not evidenced by signs and symptoms, as the problem has not occurred; rather, nursing interventions are directed at prevention.

Desired Outcomes/Evaluation Criteria— Client Will:

• Display laboratory results within normal range for individual.
• Be free of complications resulting from electrolyte imbalance.
• Identify individual risks and engage in appropriate behaviors or lifestyle changes to prevent or reduce frequency of electrolyte imbalances.

Actions/Interventions

Nursing Priority No. 1.

To assess causative/contributing factors:

• Identify client with current or newly diagnosed condition commonly associated with electrolyte imbalances, such as

---

Information that appears in brackets has been added by the authors to clarify and enhance the use of nursing diagnoses.

inability to eat or drink, febrile illness, active bleeding or other fluid loss, including vomiting, diarrhea, gastrointestinal drainage, or burns.

• Assess specific client risk, noting chronic disease processes that may lead to electrolyte imbalances, including kidney disease, metabolic or endocrine disorders, chronic alcoholism, cancer or cancer treatments, conditions causing hemolysis such as massive trauma, multiple blood transfusions, and sickle cell disease.

∞• Note client's age and developmental level, which may increase risk for electrolyte imbalance. **This risk group can include the very young or premature infant, the elderly, or individuals unable to meet their own needs or monitor their health status, including clients who are unconscious for an unknown cause or period of time, a trauma victim, and so on.**

• Review client's medications **for those associated with electrolyte imbalance, such as diuretics, laxatives, corticosteroids, barbiturates, certain antidepressants (e.g., SSRIs), some hormones/birth control pills, and some antibiotics and antifungal agents.**

Nursing Priority No. 2.

To identify potential electrolyte deficit:

• Assess mental status, noting client/caregiver report of change—altered attention span, recall of recent events, and other cognitive functions. **Can be associated with electrolyte imbalance; for example, it is the most common problem of hypernatremia.**

• Monitor heart rate and rhythm by palpation and auscultation. **Tachycardia, bradycardia, and other dysrhythmias are associated with potassium, calcium, and magnesium imbalances. Note: Weak pulse and thready pulse can be associated with hypokalemia.**

• Auscultate breath sounds, assess rate and depth of respirations and ease of respiratory effort, observe color of nailbeds and mucous membranes, and note pulse oximetry or blood gas measurement, as indicated. **Certain electrolyte imbalances, such as hypokalemia, can cause or exacerbate respiratory insufficiency.**

• Review electrocardiogram (ECG). **Because the ECG reflects electrophysiological, anatomical, metabolic, and hemodynamic alterations, it is routinely used for the diagnosis of electrolyte and metabolic disturbances, as well as myocar-**

Information that appears in brackets has been added by the authors to clarify and enhance the use of nursing diagnoses.

dial ischemia, cardiac dysrhythmias, structural changes of the myocardium, and drug effects.

- Assess gastrointestinal symptoms, noting presence, absence, and character of bowel sounds; presence of acute or chronic diarrhea; persistent vomiting, high nasogastric tube output. **Any disturbance of the gastrointestinal functioning carries with it the potential for electrolyte imbalances.**
- Review client's food intake. Note presence of anorexia, vomiting, or recent fad or unusual diet; look for signs of chronic malnutrition.
- Evaluate motor strength and function, noting steadiness of gait, hand grip strength, and reactivity of reflexes. **These neuromuscular functions can provide clues to electrolyte imbalances, including calcium, magnesium, phosphorus, sodium, and potassium.**
- Assess fluid intake and output. **Many factors, such as inability to drink, large diuresis or chronic kidney failure, trauma, and surgery, affect an individual's fluid balance, disrupting electrolyte transport, function, and excretion.**
- Review laboratory results for abnormal findings. **Electrolytes include sodium, potassium, calcium, chloride, bicarbonate (carbon dioxide), and magnesium. These chemicals are essential in many bodily functions including fluid balance, movement of fluid within and between body compartments, nerve conduction, muscle contraction—including the heart, blood clotting, and pH balance.**
- Assess for specific imbalances:
  - Sodium (Na^+) **Dominant extracellular cation and cannot freely cross the cell membrane.**

    Review laboratory results—normal range in adults is 135 to 145 mEq/L. **Elevated sodium (hypernatremia) can occur if client has an overall deficit of total body water owing to inadequate fluid intake or water loss and can be associated with low potassium, metabolic acidosis, and hypoglycemia.**

    Monitor for physical or mental disorders impacting fluid intake. **Impaired thirst sensation or an inability to express thirst or obtain needed fluids may lead to hypernatremia.**

    Note presence of medical conditions that may impact sodium level. **Hyponatremia may be associated with disorders such as congestive heart failure, liver and kidney failure, pneumonia, metabolic acidosis, and intestinal conditions**

Information that appears in brackets has been added by the authors to clarify and enhance the use of nursing diagnoses.

resulting in prolonged gastrointestinal suction. **Hypernatremia can result from simple conditions such as febrile illness, causing fluid loss and/or restricted fluid intake, or complicated conditions such as kidney and endocrine diseases, affecting sodium intake or excretion.**

Note presence of cognitive dysfunction such as confusion, restlessness, and abnormal speech (**which may be a cause or effect of sodium imbalance**).

Assess for orthostatic blood pressure changes, tachycardia, or low urine output, or other clinical findings, such as generalized weakness, swollen tongue, weight loss, and seizures. **Signs suggest hypernatremia.**

Assess for nausea, abdominal cramping, lethargy, orthostatic blood pressure changes—if fluid volume is also depleted; confusion, decreased level of consciousness, or headache. **Signs and symptoms suggestive of hyponatremia, which can lead to seizures and a coma if untreated.**

Review drug regimen. **Drugs such as anabolic steroids, angiotensin, cisplatin, and mannitol may increase sodium level. Diuretics, laxatives, theophylline, and trimeterine can decrease sodium level.**

• Potassium (K⁺) **Most abundant intracellular cation, obtained through diet, excreted via the kidneys.**

Review laboratory results—normal range in adults is 3.5 to 5.0 mEq/L.

Note current medical conditions that may impact potassium level. **Metabolic acidosis, burn or crush injuries, massive hemolysis, diabetes, kidney disease/renal failure, cancer, and sickle cell trait are associated with hyperkalemia, fasting, diarrhea or nasogastric suctioning, alkalosis, administration of IV potassium boluses, or transfusions of whole blood or packed cells increases the risk of hypokalemia.**

Identify conditions or situations **that potentiate risk for hyperkalemia, including ingestion of an unusual diet with high-potassium, low-sodium foods or use of potassium supplements, including over-the-counter (OTC) herbals or salt substitutes.**

Monitor ECG, as indicated. **Abnormal potassium levels, both low and high, are associated with changes in the ECG.**

Information that appears in brackets has been added by the authors to clarify and enhance the use of nursing diagnoses.

🌐 Cultural 🅒 Collaborative 🏠 Community/Home Care

Evaluate reports of abdominal cramping, fatigue, hyperactive bowel motility, muscle twitching, and cramps, followed by muscle weakness. Note presence of depressed reflexes, ascending flaccid paralysis of legs and arms. **Signs/symptoms suggesting hyperkalemia.**

Note presence of anorexia, abdominal distention, diminished bowel sounds, postural hypotension, muscle weakness, flaccid paralysis. **May be manifestations of hypokalemia.**

Review drug regimen. **Use of potassium-sparing diuretics, other medications, such as nonsteroidal anti-inflammatory agents (NSAIDs), angiotensin-converting enzyme (ACE) inhibitors, and certain antibiotics such as pentamidine may increase potassium level. Medications such as albuterol, terbutaline, or some diuretics may decrease potassium level.**

- Calcium (Ca^{2+}) **Most abundant cation in the body, participates in almost all vital processes, working with sodium to regulate depolarization and the generation of action potentials.**

Review laboratory results—normal range for adults is 8.5 to 10.5 mg/dL.

Note presence of medical conditions impacting calcium level. **Acidosis, Addison's disease, cancers (e.g., bone, lymphoma, leukemias), hyperparathyroidism, lung disease (e.g., TB, histoplasmosis), thyrotoxicosis, and polycythemia may lead to an increased calcium level. Chronic diarrhea, intestinal disorders such as Crohn's disease; pancreatitis, alcoholism, renal failure, or renal tubular disease; recent orthopedic surgery or bone healing, history of thyroid surgery or irradiation of upper middle chest and neck; and psychosis may result in decreased calcium levels.**

Monitor for excessive urination (polyuria), constipation, lethargy, muscle weakness, anorexia, headache, and coma, **which can be associated with hypercalcemia.**

Monitor for cardiac dysrhythmias, hypotension, and heart failure; muscle cramps, facial spasms—positive Chvostek's sign; numbness and tingling sensations, muscle twitching—positive Trousseau's sign; seizures or tetany, **which suggest hypocalcemia.**

Review drug regimen. **Drugs such as anabolic steroids, some antacids, lithium, oral contraceptives, vitamins A and D, and amoxapine, can increase calcium levels. Drugs such**

Information that appears in brackets has been added by the authors to clarify and enhance the use of nursing diagnoses.

as albuterol, anticonvulsants, glucocorticoids, insulin, phosphates, trazadone, laxative overuse, or long-term anticonvulsant therapy can decrease calcium levels.

- Magnesium (Mg^{2+}) Second most abundant intracellular cation after potassium, magnesium controls absorption or function of sodium, potassium, calcium, and phosphorus.

Review laboratory results—normal range in adults is 1.5 to 2.0 mEq/L.

Note presence of medical condition impacting magnesium level. Diabetic acidosis, multiple myeloma, renal insufficiency, eclampsia, asthma, GI hypomotility; adrenal insufficiency, extensive soft tissue injury, severe burns, shock, sepsis, and cardiac arrest are associated with hypermagnesemia. Conditions resulting in decreased intake (starvation, alcoholism, parenteral feeding) excess gastrointestinal losses (diarrhea, vomiting, nasogastric suction, and malabsorption) renal losses (inherited renal tubular defects among others) or miscellaneous causes (including calcium abnormalities, chronic metabolic acidosis, and diabetic ketoacidosis) can lead to hypomagnesemia.

Note GI and renal function. Main controlling factors of magnesium are GI absorption and renal excretion. Low levels of magnesium, potassium, calcium, and phosphorus may be manifest at the same time if absorption is impaired. High levels of magnesium, calcium, phosphate, and potassium often occur together in the setting of kidney disease.

Monitor for nausea, vomiting, weakness, and vasodilation, which suggest a mild to moderate elevation of magnesium level (from 3.5 to 5.0 mEq/L).

Monitor ECG, as indicated. Presence of heart blocks, especially if accompanied by ventilatory failure and stupor, suggests severe hypermagnesemia (more than 10.0 mEq/L). Hypomagnesemia can lead to potentially fatal ventricular dysrhythmias, coronary artery vasospasm, and sudden death.

Review drug regimen. Drugs such as aspirin and progesterone may increase magnesium level; albuterol, digoxin, diuretics, oral contraceptives, aminoglycosides, proton-pump inhibitors, immunosuppressants, cisplatin, and cyclosporines are some of the medications that may decrease magnesium levels.

Information that appears in brackets has been added by the authors to clarify and enhance the use of nursing diagnoses.

🌐 Cultural 🔵 Collaborative 🏠 Community/Home Care

Nursing Priority No. 3.

To prevent imbalances:

- Collaborate in treatment of underlying conditions **to prevent or limit effects of electrolyte imbalances caused by disease or organ dysfunction.**

- Observe and intervene with elderly hospitalized person upon admission and during facility stay. **Elderly are more prone to electrolyte imbalances related to fluid imbalances, use of multiple medications including diuretics, heart and blood pressure medications, lack of appetite or interest in eating or drinking; or lack of appropriate dietary and/or medication supervision.**

- Provide or recommend balanced nutrition, using best route for feeding. Monitor intake, weight and bowel function. **Obtaining and utilizing electrolytes and other minerals depends on client regularly receiving them in a readily available form, including food and supplements via ingestion, enteral, or parenteral routes.**

- Measure and report all fluid losses, including emesis, diarrhea, wound, or fistula drainage. **Loss of fluids rich in electrolytes can lead to imbalances.**

- Maintain fluid balance **to prevent dehydration and shifts of electrolytes.**

- Use pump or controller device when administering intravenous electrolyte solutions **to provide medication at desired rate and prevent untoward effects of excessive or too rapid delivery.**

Nursing Priority No. 4.

To promote wellness (Teaching/Discharge Considerations):

- Discuss ongoing concerns for client with chronic health problems, such as kidney disease, diabetes, cancer; individuals taking multiple medications, and/or client deciding to take medications or drugs differently than prescribed. **Early intervention can help prevent serious complications.**

- Consult with dietitian or nutritionist for specific teaching needs. **Learning how to incorporate foods that increase electrolyte intake or identifying food or condiment alternatives increases client's self-sufficiency and likelihood of success.**

- Review client's medications at each visit **for possible change in dosage or drug choice based on client's response, change in condition, or development of side effects.**

Information that appears in brackets has been added by the authors to clarify and enhance the use of nursing diagnoses.

⊕• Discuss medications with primary care provider **to determine if different pharmaceutical intervention is appropriate. For example, changing to potassium-sparing diuretic or withholding a diuretic may correct imbalance.**

🖋• Teach client/caregiver to take or administer drugs as prescribed—especially diuretics, antihypertensives, and cardiac drugs **to reduce potential of complications associated with medication-induced electrolyte imbalances.**

🏠• Instruct client/caregiver in reportable symptoms. **For example, a sudden change in mentation or behavior two days after starting a new diuretic could indicate hyponatremia, or an elderly person taking digitalis (for atrial fibrillation) and a diuretic may be hypokalemic.**

🏠• Provide information regarding calcium supplements, as indicated. **It is popular wisdom to instruct people, women in particular, to take calcium for prevention of osteoporosis. However, calcium absorption cannot take place without vitamins D and K and magnesium. Client taking calcium may need additional information or resources.**

Documentation Focus

Assessment/Reassessment
- Identified or potential risk factors for individual.
- Assessment findings, including vital signs, mentation, muscle strength and reflexes, presence of fatigue, respiratory distress.
- Results of laboratory tests and diagnostic studies.

Planning
- Plan of care, specific interventions, and who is involved in the planning.
- Teaching plan.

Implementation/Evaluation
- Client's responses to treatment, teaching, and actions performed.
- Attainment or progress toward desired outcome(s).
- Modifications to plan of care.

Discharge Planning
- Long-term needs, identifying who is responsible for actions to be taken.
- Specific referrals made.

Information that appears in brackets has been added by the authors to clarify and enhance the use of nursing diagnoses.

Sample Nursing Outcomes & Interventions Classifications (NOC/NIC)

NOC—Electrolyte and Acid/Base Balance
NIC—Electrolyte Monitoring

disturbed Energy Field

Taxonomy II: Activity/Rest—Class 3 Energy Balance (00050)
[Diagnostic Division: Ego Integrity]
Submitted 1994; Revised 2004

Definition: Disruption of the flow of energy [aura] surrounding a person's being that results in a disharmony of the body, mind, and/or spirit

Related Factors

Slowing or blocking of energy flows secondary to:

Pathophysiological factors—Illness, injury, or pregnancy
Treatment-related factors—Immobility, labor and delivery, perioperative experience, or chemotherapy
Situational factors—Pain, fear, anxiety, or grieving
Maturational factors—Age-related developmental difficulties or crisis

Defining Characteristics

Objective

Perception of changes in patterns of energy flow, such as:

Movement (wave, spike, tingling, dense, flowing)
Sounds (tones, words)
Temperature change (warmth, coolness)
Visual changes (image, color)
Disruption of the field (deficient, hole, spike, bulge, obstruction, congestion, diminished flow in energy field)

Desired Outcomes/Evaluation Criteria— Client Will:

- Acknowledge feelings of anxiety and distress.
- Verbalize sense of relaxation and well-being.
- Display reduction in severity or frequency of symptoms.

Information that appears in brackets has been added by the authors to clarify and enhance the use of nursing diagnoses.

Actions/Interventions

Nursing Priority No. 1.

To determine causative/contributing factors:

- Review current situation and concerns of client. Provide opportunity for client to talk about condition, past history, emotional state, or other relevant information. Note body gestures, tone of voice, and words chosen to express feelings or issues.
- Determine client's motivation or desire for treatment. **Although attitude can affect success of therapy, therapeutic touch (TT) is often successful, even when the client is skeptical. Recent studies reported that TT produced positive outcomes by decreasing levels of anxiety and pain perception and improving sense of well-being/quality of life; TT may also be beneficial in reducing behavioral symptoms of dementia (e.g., manual manipulation/restlessness, vocalization, pacing).**
- Note use of medications, other drug use (e.g., alcohol). **TT may be helpful in reducing anxiety level in individuals undergoing alcohol withdrawal.**
- Perform/review results of testing, as indicated, such as the State-Trait Anxiety Inventory (STAI) or the Affect Balance Scale (ABS), **to provide measures of the client's anxiety.**

Nursing Priority No. 2.

To evaluate energy field:

- Develop therapeutic nurse-client relationship, initially accepting role of healer/guide as client desires.
- Place client in sitting or supine position with legs and arms uncrossed. Place pillows or other supports to enhance comfort and relaxation.
- Center self physically and psychologically **to quiet mind and turn attention to the healing intent.**
- Move hands slowly over the client at level of 2 to 6 inches above skin to assess state of energy field and flow of energy within the system.
- Identify areas of imbalance or obstruction in the field (i.e., areas of asymmetry; feelings of heat or cold, tingling, congestion, or pressure).

Nursing Priority No. 3.

To provide therapeutic intervention:

- Explain the process of TT and answer questions, as indicated, **to prevent unrealistic expectations. Fundamental focus of**

Information that appears in brackets has been added by the authors to clarify and enhance the use of nursing diagnoses.

🌐 Cultural   🤝 Collaborative   🏠 Community/Home Care

TT is on healing and wholeness, not curing signs/ symptoms of disease.

- Discuss findings of evaluation with client.
- Assist client with exercises to promote "centering" and increase potential to self-heal, enhance comfort, and reduce anxiety.
- Perform unruffling process, keeping hands 2 to 6 inches from client's body **to dissipate impediments to free flow of energy within the system and between nurse and client.**
- Focus on areas of disturbance identified, holding hands over or on skin, and/or place one hand in back of body with other hand in front. **Allows client's body to pull or repattern energy as needed.** At the same time, concentrate on the intent to help the client heal.
- Shorten duration of treatment to 2 to 3 minutes, as appropriate. **Children, elderly individuals, those with head injuries, and others who are severely debilitated are generally more sensitive to overloading energy fields.**
- Make coaching suggestions (e.g., pleasant images or other visualizations, deep breathing) in a soft voice **for enhancing feelings of relaxation.**
- Use hands-on massage/apply pressure to acupressure points, as appropriate, during process.
- Note changes in energy sensations as session progresses. Stop when the energy field is symmetric and there is a change to feelings of peaceful calm.
- Hold client's feet for a few minutes at end of session **to assist in "grounding" the body energy.**
- Provide client time following procedure **for a period of peaceful rest.**

Nursing Priority No. 4.
To promote wellness (Teaching/Discharge Considerations):

- Allow period of client dependency, as appropriate, **for client to strengthen own inner resources.**
- Encourage ongoing practice of the therapeutic process.
- Instruct in use of stress-reduction activities (e.g., centering/ meditation, relaxation exercises) **to promote mind-body-spirit harmony.**
- Discuss importance of integrating techniques into daily activity plan **for sustaining/enhancing sense of well-being.**
- Have client practice each step and demonstrate the complete TT process following the session as client displays readiness to assume responsibilities for self-healing.

Information that appears in brackets has been added by the authors to clarify and enhance the use of nursing diagnoses.

- Promote attendance at a support group, **where members can help each other practice and learn the techniques of TT.**
- Reinforce that TT is a complementary intervention and stress importance of seeking timely evaluation and continuing other prescribed treatment modalities, as appropriate.
- Refer to other resources, as identified (e.g., psychotherapy, clergy, medical treatment of disease processes, hospice), **for the individual to address total well-being or facilitate peaceful death.**

Documentation Focus

Assessment/Reassessment
- Assessment findings, including characteristics and differences in the energy field.
- Client's perception of problem or need for treatment.

Planning
- Plan of care and who is involved in planning.
- Teaching plan.

Implementation/Evaluation
- Changes in energy field.
- Client's response to interventions, teaching, and actions performed.
- Attainment or progress toward desired outcomes.
- Modifications to plan of care.

Discharge Planning
- Long-term needs and who is responsible for actions to be taken.
- Specific referrals made.

Sample Nursing Outcomes & Interventions Classifications (NOC/NIC)

NOC—Personal Well-Being
NIC—Therapeutic Touch

Information that appears in brackets has been added by the authors to clarify and enhance the use of nursing diagnoses.

impaired Environmental Interpretation Syndrome

Taxonomy II: Perception/Cognition—Class 2 Orientation
(00127)
[Diagnostic Division: Safety]
Submitted 1994

Definition: Consistent lack of orientation to person,
place, time, or circumstances over more than 3 to 6
months necessitating a protective environment

Related Factors

Dementia (e.g., Alzheimer's disease, multi-infarct dementia,
Pick's disease, AIDS dementia)
Huntington's disease
Depression

Defining Characteristics

Objective
Consistent disorientation
Chronic confusional states
Inability to follow simple directions
Inability to reason or concentrate; slow in responding to ques-
tions
Loss of occupation, social functioning

Desired Outcomes/Evaluation Criteria—
Client Will:

• Be free of harm.

Caregiver Will:

• Identify individual client safety concerns/needs.
• Modify activities and environment to provide for safety.

Actions/Interventions

Nursing Priority No. 1.
To assess causative/precipitating factors:
Refer to NDs acute Confusion; chronic Confusion; impaired
Memory; for additional relevant assessment and interven-
tions.

Information that appears in brackets has been added by the authors to clarify
and enhance the use of nursing diagnoses.

- Determine presence of medical conditions and/or behaviors leading to client's current situation **to identify potentially useful interventions and therapies.**
- Note presence or reports of client's misinterpretation of environmental information (e.g., sensory, cognitive, or social cues).
- Discuss history and progression of condition, length of time since onset, future expectations, and incidents of injury or accidents.
- Review client's behavioral changes with SO(s) **to note differences in viewpoint, as well as to identify impairments (e.g., decreased agility, reduced range of motion of joints, loss of balance, decline in visual acuity, failure to eat, loss of interest in personal grooming, and forgetfulness resulting in unsafe actions).**
- Identify actual and/or potential environmental dangers and client's level of awareness, if any, of threat. **Highlights problems that may impact client care and safety or add to client's difficulties in interpretation of sensory input.**
- Test ability to receive and send effective communication. **Client may be nonverbal or require assistance with/ interpretation of verbalizations.**
- Review with client/SO(s) usual habits for activities, such as sleeping, eating, and self-care, **to include in plan of care.**
- Determine anxiety level in relation to situation. Note behavior that may be indicative of potential for violence.
- Evaluate responses on diagnostic examinations (e.g., memory impairments, reality orientation, attention span, and calculations). **A combination of tests (e.g., Confusion Assessment Method [CAM], Mini-Mental State Examination [MMSE], Alzheimer's Disease Assessment Scale [ADAS-cog], Brief Dementia Severity Rating Scale [BDSRS], and Neuropsychiatric Inventory [NPI]) is often needed to determine client's overall condition relating to chronic/ irreversible condition.**

Nursing Priority No. 2.

To promote safe environment:

- Collaborate in management of treatable conditions (e.g., infections, malnutrition, electrolyte imbalances, and adverse medication reactions) **that may contribute to or exacerbate confusion.**
- Provide calm environment; eliminate extraneous noise/stimuli **that may increase client's level of agitation/confusion.**

Information that appears in brackets has been added by the authors to clarify and enhance the use of nursing diagnoses.

- Keep communications simple. Use concrete terms and words that client can recognize. (Refer to ND impaired verbal Communication for additional interventions.)
- Use family/other interpreter, as needed, to comprehend client's communications.
- Provide and promote use of glasses, hearing aids, and adequate lighting **to optimize sensory input.**
- Use touch judiciously. Tell client what is being done before touching **to reduce sense of surprise or negative reaction.**
- Maintain reality-oriented environment (e.g., clocks, calendars, personal items, seasonal decorations, social events).
- Explain environmental cues to client (ongoing) **to protect safety and attempt to diminish fears.**
- Provide consistent caregivers and family-centered care as much as possible **for consistency and to decrease confusion.**
- Incorporate previous/usual patterns for activities (e.g., sleeping, eating, hygiene, desired clothing, leisure/play, or rituals) to the extent possible **to keep environment predictable and prevent client from feeling overwhelmed.**
- Limit number of visitors client interacts with at one time, if needed, **to prevent overstimulation.**
- Implement complementary therapies, as indicated and desired (e.g., music or movement therapy, massage, therapeutic touch, aromatherapy, bright-light treatment). **May help client relax, refocus attention, and stimulate memories.**
- Set limits on unsafe and/or inappropriate behavior, being alert to potential for violence.
- Provide for safety and protection against hazards, such as locking doors to unprotected areas and stairwells, prohibiting or supervising smoking, and monitoring activities of daily living (e.g., choice of clothing in relation to environment and season).
- Encourage client to use identity tags in clothes and belongings and wear a bracelet/necklace **to provide identification if he or she wanders away or becomes lost.**
- Avoid use of restraints as much as possible. Use vest (instead of wrist) restraints, when required. **Although restraints can prevent falls, they can increase client's agitation and distress.**
- Administer medications, as ordered (e.g., antidepressants, antipsychotics). Monitor for expected and/or adverse reactions and side effects and interactions. **May be used to manage symptoms of psychosis, depression, or aggressive behavior.**

Information that appears in brackets has been added by the authors to clarify and enhance the use of nursing diagnoses.

Nursing Priority No. 3.

To assist caregiver to deal with situation:

🏠• Determine family dynamics, cultural values, resources, and availability and willingness to participate in meeting client's needs.

🏠• Involve family/SO(s) in planning and care activities, as needed/desired. Maintain frequent interactions with SO(s) **in order to relay information, change care strategies, obtain feedback, and offer support.**

🏠• Evaluate SO's attention to own needs, including health status, grieving process, and respite. **Caregivers often feel guilty when taking time for themselves. Without adequate support and respite, the caregiver cannot meet the needs of the client.**

• Discuss caregiver burden, if appropriate. (Refer to NDs Caregiver Role Strain; risk for Caregiver Role Strain, for additional interventions.)

• Provide educational materials and list of available resources (help lines, Web sites, etc.) as desired, **to assist SO(s) in coping with long-term care issues.**

🌐• Identify appropriate community resources (e.g., Alzheimer's Disease and Related Disorders Association [ARDA], stroke or brain injury support group, senior support groups, clergy, social services, or respite care) **to provide client/SO with support and assist with problem-solving.**

Nursing Priority No. 4.

To promote wellness (Teaching/Discharge Considerations):

🏠• Provide specific information about disease process/prognosis and client's particular needs. **Individuals with conditions requiring ongoing monitoring of their environment usually need more social and behavioral support than medical management, although medical concerns will occur occasionally.**

🌐• Review age-appropriate ongoing treatment and social needs and appropriate resources for client and family.

💊• Instruct SO/caregivers to share information about client's condition, functional status, and medications whenever encountering new providers. **Clients often have multiple doctors, each of whom may prescribe medications, with potential for adverse effects and overmedication.**

🏠• Develop plan of care with family **to meet client's and SO's individual needs.**

Information that appears in brackets has been added by the authors to clarify and enhance the use of nursing diagnoses.

🏠• Perform home assessment, if indicated, to identify safety issues, such as securing medications and poisonous substances and locking exterior doors, **to prevent client from wandering off while SO is engaged in other household activities,** or removing matches and smoking material and knobs from the stove **to prevent client from starting fires or turning on stove burner and leaving it unattended.**

🕑• Investigate local resources; provide appropriate referrals (e.g., case managers, counselors, support groups, financial services, Meals on Wheels, adult day care, adult foster care, respite care for family, home-care agency, or nursing home placement). **Individuals are generally not capable of carrying alone the heavy burdens of caring for a relative with this problem. Caregivers need help and support (whether or not they are trying to provide total care) to deal with exhaustion and unresolved feelings.**

Documentation Focus

Assessment/Reassessment
• Assessment findings, including degree of impairment.
• Involvement and availability of family members to provide care.

Planning
• Plan of care and who is involved in planning.
• Teaching plan.

Implementation/Evaluation
• Response to treatment plan, interventions, and actions performed.
• Attainment or progress toward desired outcomes.
• Modifications to plan of care.

Discharge Planning
• Long-term needs, who is responsible for actions to be taken.
• Specific referrals made.

Sample Nursing Outcomes & Interventions Classifications (NOC/NIC)

NOC—Safe Home Environment
NIC—Surveillance: Safety

Information that appears in brackets has been added by the authors to clarify and enhance the use of nursing diagnoses.

adult Failure to Thrive

Taxonomy II: Coping/Stress Tolerance—Class 2 Coping
   Response (00101)
[Diagnostic Division: Food/Fluid]
Submitted 1998

Definition: Progressive functional deterioration of a
physical and cognitive nature. The individual's ability to
live with multisystem diseases, cope with ensuing problems, and manage his or her care is remarkably diminished.

Related Factors

Depression
[Major disease or degenerative condition]
[Aging process]

Defining Characteristics

Subjective
Reports loss of interest in pleasurable outlets
Altered mood state
Reports desire for death

Objective
Inadequate nutritional intake; consumption of minimal to no
   food at most meals (e.g., consumes less than 75% of normal
   requirements); anorexia
Unintentional weight loss (e.g., 5% in 1 month, 10% in 6
   months)
Physical decline (e.g., fatigue, dehydration, incontinence of
   bowel and bladder)
Cognitive decline; decreased perception; difficulty responding
   to environmental stimuli; demonstrated difficulty with reasoning, decision making, judgment, memory, and concentration
Apathy
Decreased participation in activities of daily living; self-care
   deficit; neglect of home environment/financial responsibilities
Decreased social skills; social withdrawal
Frequent exacerbations of chronic health problems

Information that appears in brackets has been added by the authors to clarify
and enhance the use of nursing diagnoses.

Desired Outcomes/Evaluation Criteria— Client/Caregiver Will:

- Acknowledge presence of factors affecting well-being.
- Identify corrective or adaptive measures for individual situation.
- Demonstrate behaviors and lifestyle changes necessary to enhance functional status.

Actions/Interventions

Refer to NDs Activity Intolerance; risk-prone Health Behaviors; chronic Confusion; ineffective Coping; impaired Dentition; risk for Falls; complicated Grieving; risk for Loneliness; imbalanced Nutrition: less than body requirements; Relocation Stress Syndrome; chronic low Self-Esteem; Self-Care Deficit [specify]; risk for Spiritual Distress; impaired Swallowing, as appropriate, for additional relevant interventions.

Nursing Priority No. 1.

To identify causative/contributing factors:

- Assess client's/SO's perception of factors leading to present condition, noting onset, duration, presence/absence of physical complaints, and social withdrawal **to provide comparative baseline.**
- Determine client's current medical, cognitive, emotional, and perceptual status and effect on functional abilities. **Adult failure to thrive (FTT) is characterized by malnutrition associated with consistent weight loss; loss of physical, cognitive, and social functioning; impaired immune function; and depression. Although it can occur as a result of an acute health problem, it can be associated with elder abuse.**
- Review with client previous and current life situations, including role changes and losses (e.g., death of loved ones; change in living arrangements, finances, independence) **to identify stressors affecting current situation.**
- Identify cultural beliefs and expectations regarding condition or situation and the presence of conflicts.
- Determine nutritional status. **Malnutrition (e.g., weight loss and laboratory abnormalities) and/or factors contributing to failure to eat (e.g., chronic nausea, loss of appetite, no access to food or cooking, poorly fitting dentures, no one with whom to share meals, depression, and financial**

Information that appears in brackets has been added by the authors to clarify and enhance the use of nursing diagnoses.

problems) greatly impact health status and quality of life, especially in the elderly.

• Evaluate level of adaptive behavior, knowledge, and skills about health maintenance, environment, and safety **in order to instruct, intervene, and refer appropriately.**

🏠• Ascertain safety and effectiveness of home environment and persons providing care **to identify potential for/presence of neglectful or abusive situations and need for referrals.**

Nursing Priority No. 2.

To assess degree of impairment:

✍• Collaborate in comprehensive assessment (e.g., physical, nutritional, self-care, and psychosocial) status. **Various screening criteria and assessment tools may be used to determine the extent of problem, to implement treatment, and to make appropriate referrals. Note: FTT is a recognized diagnosis for admission to hospice care.**

• Obtain current weight **to provide comparative baseline and evaluate response to interventions.**

• Active-listen client's/caregiver's perception of problem(s).

• Discuss individual concerns about feelings of loss/loneliness and relationship between these feelings and current decline in well-being. Note desire and willingness to change situation. **Motivation can impede—or facilitate—achieving desired outcomes.**

• Survey past and present availability/use of support systems.

Nursing Priority No. 3.

To assist client to achieve/maintain general well-being:

• Assist with treatment of underlying medical and psychiatric conditions **that could positively influence the current situation (e.g., resolution of infection, addressing depression).**

• Coordinate session with client/SO(s) and nutritionist **to identify specific dietary needs and creative ways to stimulate intake (e.g., offering client's favorite foods, family-style meals, participation in social events such as ice cream social, and happy hour).**

• Develop plan of action with client/caregiver **to meet immediate needs for nutrition, safety, and self-care and to facilitate implementation of actions.**

• Explore strengths/successful coping behaviors the individual has used previously. **Incorporating these into problem-**

Information that appears in brackets has been added by the authors to clarify and enhance the use of nursing diagnoses.

🌐 Cultural 🤝 Collaborative 🏠 Community/Home Care

solving builds on past successes. Refine/develop new strategies as appropriate.
- Assist client to develop goals for dealing with life or illness situation. Involve SO/family in long-range planning. **Promotes commitment to goals and plan, maximizing outcomes.**

Nursing Priority No. 4.

To promote wellness (Teaching/Discharge Considerations):
- Assist client/SO(s) to identify useful community resources (e.g., support groups, Meals on Wheels, social worker, home care or assistive care, placement services). **Enhances coping, assists with problem-solving, and may reduce risks to client and caregiver.**
- Encourage client to talk about positive aspects of life and to keep as physically active as possible **to reduce effects of dispiritedness (e.g., "feeling low," sense of being unimportant, disconnected).**
- Introduce concept of mindfulness (living in the moment). **Promotes feeling of capability and belief that this moment can be dealt with.**
- Offer opportunities to discuss life goals and support client/SO in setting and attaining new goals for this time of life to **enhance hopefulness for future.**
- Promote socialization within individual limitations. **Provides additional stimulation and reduces sense of isolation.**
- Assist client/SO/family to understand that FTT commonly occurs near the end of life and cannot always be reversed.
- Help client explore reasons for living or begin to deal with end-of-life issues and provide support for grieving. **Enhances hope and sense of control.**
- Refer to pastoral care, counseling, or psychotherapy **for grief work.**
- Discuss appropriateness of and refer to palliative services or hospice care as indicated.

Documentation Focus

Assessment/Reassessment
- Individual findings, including current weight, dietary pattern, and perceptions of self, food, and eating.
- Perception of losses and life changes.
- Ability to perform activities of daily living, participate in care, and meet own needs.
- Motivation for change, support, and feedback from SO(s).

Information that appears in brackets has been added by the authors to clarify and enhance the use of nursing diagnoses.

Planning
* Plan of care, specific interventions, and who is involved in planning.
* Teaching plan.

Implementation/Evaluation
* Responses to interventions and actions performed, general well-being, weekly weight.
* Attainment or progress toward desired outcome(s).
* Modifications to plan of care.

Discharge Planning
* Long-term needs and who is responsible for actions to be taken.
* Community resources and support groups.
* Specific referrals made.

Sample Nursing Outcomes & Interventions Classifications (NOC/NIC)

NOC—Will to Live
NIC—Mood Management

risk for Falls

Taxonomy II: Safety/Protection—Class 2 Physical Injury (00155)
[Diagnostic Division: Safety]
Submitted 2000

Definition: At risk for increased susceptibility to falling that may cause physical harm

Risk Factors

Adults
History of falls
Wheelchair use; use of assistive devices (e.g., walker, cane)
Age 65 or over; lives alone
Lower limb prosthesis

Physiological
Acute illness; postoperative conditions
Visual or hearing difficulties

Information that appears in brackets has been added by the authors to clarify and enhance the use of nursing diagnoses.

Arthritis

Orthostatic hypotension; faintness when turning or extending neck

Sleeplessness

Anemias; vascular disease

Neoplasms (i.e., fatigue/limited mobility)

Urinary urgency; incontinence; diarrhea

Postprandial blood sugar changes

Impaired physical mobility; foot problems; decreased lower extremity strength

Impaired balance; difficulty with gait; proprioceptive deficits (e.g., unilateral neglect)

Neuropathy

Cognitive

Diminished mental status

Medications

Antihypertensive agents; angiotensin-converting enzyme (ACE) inhibitors; diuretics; tricyclic antidepressants; antianxiety agents; hypnotics; tranquilizers; narcotics/opiates

Alcohol use

Environment

Restraints

Weather conditions (e.g., wet floors, ice)

Cluttered environment; throw rugs; lacks antislip material in bath/shower

Unfamiliar or dimly lit room

Children

Aged 2 or younger; male gender when less than 1 year of age

Lack of gate on stairs, window guards, and automobile restraints

Unattended infant on elevated surface (e.g., bed/changing table); bed located near window

Lack of parental supervision

> **Note:** A risk diagnosis is not evidenced by signs and symptoms, as the problem has not occurred; rather, nursing interventions are directed at prevention.

Information that appears in brackets has been added by the authors to clarify and enhance the use of nursing diagnoses.

Desired Outcomes/Evaluation Criteria— Client/Caregivers Will:

- Verbalize understanding of individual risk factors that contribute to the possibility of falls.
- Demonstrate behaviors and lifestyle changes to reduce risk factors and protect self from injury.
- Modify environment as indicated to enhance safety.
- Be free of injury.

Actions/Interventions

Nursing Priority No. 1.

To evaluate source/degree of risk:

- Observe individual's general health status, **noting multiple factors that might affect safety, such as chronic or debilitating conditions, use of multiple medications, recent trauma (especially a fall within the past year), prolonged bedrest/immobility, or a sedentary lifestyle.**
- Evaluate client's current disorders/conditions that could enhance risk potential for falls. **Acute, even short-term, situations can affect any client, such as sudden dizziness, positional blood pressures changes, new medication, change in glasses prescription, recent use of alcohol/other drugs, etc.**
- Note factors associated with age, gender, and developmental level. **Infants, young children (e.g., climbing on objects), young adults (e.g., sports activities), and elderly are at greatest risk because of developmental issues and impaired or lack of ability to self-protect.**
- Evaluate client's general and hip muscle strength, postural stability, gait and standing balance, and gross and fine motor coordination. Review history of past or current physical injuries (e.g., musculoskeletal injuries; orthopedic surgery) **altering coordination, gait, and balance.**
- Review client's medication regimen ongoing, noting number and type of drugs that could impact fall potential. **Studies have confirmed that use of multiple medications (polypharmacy) increases the risk of falls.**
- Evaluate use, misuse, or failure to use assistive aids, when indicated. **Client may have assistive device, but is at high risk for falls while adjusting to altered body state and use of unfamiliar device; or client might refuse to use devices**

Information that appears in brackets has been added by the authors to clarify and enhance the use of nursing diagnoses.

🌐 Cultural   🔵 Collaborative   🏠 Community/Home Care

for various reasons (e.g., waiting for help or perception of weakness).

- Evaluate client's cognitive status (e.g., brain injury, neurological disorders; depression). **Affects ability to perceive own limitations or recognize danger.**
- Assess mood, coping abilities, and personality styles. **Individual's temperament, typical behavior, stressors, and level of self-esteem can affect attitude toward safety issues, resulting in carelessness or increased risk taking without consideration of consequences.**
- Ascertain client's/SO's level of knowledge about and attendance to safety needs. **May reveal lack of understanding, insufficient resources, or simple disregard for personal safety (e.g., "I can't watch him every minute," "We can't hire a home assistant," "It's not manly..." etc.).**
- Consider hazards in the care setting and/or home/other environment. **Identifying needs or deficits provides opportunities for intervention and/or instruction (e.g., concerning clearing of hazards, intensifying client supervision, obtaining safety equipment, or referring for vision evaluation).**
- Review results of various fall risk assessment tools (e.g., Functional Ambulation Profile (FAP); the Johns Hopkins Hospital Fall Risk Assessment Tool; the Tinetti Balance and Gait Instrument [not a comprehensive listing]).
- Note socioeconomic status and availability and use of resources in other circumstances. **Can affect current coping abilities.**

Nursing Priority No. 2.

To assist client/caregiver to reduce or correct individual risk factors:

- Assist in treatments and provide information regarding client's disease/condition(s) **that may result in increased risk of falls.**
- Review consequences of previously determined risk factors (e.g., falls caused by failure to make provisions for previously identified impairments or safety needs) **for follow-up instruction or interventions.**
- Review medication regimen and how it affects client. Instruct in monitoring of effects and side effects. **Use of certain medications (e.g., narcotics/opiates, psychotropics, antihypertensives, diuretics) can contribute to weakness, confusion,**

Information that appears in brackets has been added by the authors to clarify and enhance the use of nursing diagnoses.

and balance and gait disturbances. Review medications with client and primary care provider **to determine if changes (e.g., different medication or dosage) could reduce client's fall risk.**

• Practice client safety. **Demonstrates behaviors for client/caregiver(s) to emulate.**

🏠• Recommend or implement needed interventions and safety devices **to manage conditions that could contribute to falling and to promote safe environment for individual and others:**

Evaluate vision and encourage use of prescription eyewear, as needed. **Note: Client with bifocals, trifocals, or implanted lenses may have difficulty perceiving steps or uneven surfaces, increasing risk for falls even when wearing glasses.**

Situate bed to enable client to exit toward his or her stronger side whenever possible.

Place bed in lowest possible position, use a raised-edge mattress, pad floor at side of bed, or place mattress on floor as appropriate.

Use half side rail instead of full side rails or upright pole **to assist individual in arising from bed.**

Provide chairs with firm, high seats and lifting mechanisms when indicated.

Provide appropriate day or night lighting.

Assist with transfers and ambulation; show client/SO ways to move safely.

Provide and instruct in use of mobility devices and safety devices, like grab bars and call light or personal assistance systems.

Clear environment of hazards (e.g., obstructing furniture, small items on the floor, electrical cords, throw rugs).

Lock wheels on movable equipment (e.g., wheelchairs, beds).

Encourage use of treaded slippers, socks, and shoes, and maintain nonskid floors and floor mats.

Provide foot and nail care.

∞• Determine caregiver's expectations of children, cognitive impairment, and/or elderly family members and compare with actual abilities. **Reality of client's abilities and needs may be different from perception or desires of caregivers.**

∞• Discuss need for and sources of supervision (e.g., babysitters, before- and after-school programs, elderly day care, personal companions).

🏠• Perform home visit when appropriate. Determine that home safety issues are addressed, including supervision, access to

---

Information that appears in brackets has been added by the authors to clarify and enhance the use of nursing diagnoses.

🌐 Cultural 🌐 Collaborative 🏠 Community/Home Care

emergency assistance, and client's ability to manage self-care in the home. **May be needed to adequately determine client's needs and available resources.**

- Refer to rehabilitation team, physical or occupational therapist, as appropriate, **to improve client's balance, strength, or mobility; to improve or relearn ambulation; and to identify and obtain appropriate assistive devices for mobility, environmental safety, or home modification.**

Nursing Priority No. 3.

To promote wellness (Teaching/Discharge Considerations):

- Refer to other resources as indicated. **Client/caregivers may need financial assistance, home modifications, referrals for counseling, home care, sources for safety equipment, or placement in extended-care facility.**
- Provide educational resources (e.g., home safety checklist, equipment directions for proper use, appropriate Web sites) **for later review and reinforcement of learning.**
- Promote community awareness about the problems of design of buildings, equipment, transportation, and workplace accidents that contribute to falls.
- Connect client/family with community resources, neighbors, and friends **to assist elderly or handicapped individuals in providing such things as structural maintenance and clearing of snow, gravel, or ice from walks and steps.**

Documentation Focus

Assessment/Reassessment
- Individual risk factors noting current physical findings (e.g., signs of injury—bruises, cuts; anemia, fatigue; use of alcohol, drugs, and prescription medications).
- Client's/caregiver's understanding of individual risks and safety concerns.

Planning
- Plan of care and who is involved in planning.
- Teaching plan.

Implementation/Evaluation
- Individual responses to interventions, teaching, and actions performed.
- Specific actions and changes that are made.

Information that appears in brackets has been added by the authors to clarify and enhance the use of nursing diagnoses.

- Attainment or progress toward desired outcomes.
- Modifications to plan of care.

Discharge Planning

- Long-term plans for discharge needs, lifestyle, and home setting and community changes, and who is responsible for actions to be taken.
- Specific referrals made.

Sample Nursing Outcomes & Interventions Classifications (NOC/NIC)

NOC—Fall Prevention Behavior
NIC—Fall Prevention

dysfunctional Family Processes

Taxonomy II: Role Relationships—Class 2 Family Relationships (00063)
[Diagnostic Division: Social Interaction]
Submitted as dysfunction Family Processes: Alcoholism 1994; name change 2008

Definition: Psychosocial, spiritual, and physiological functions of the family unit are chronically disorganized, which leads to conflict, denial of problems, resistance to change, ineffective problem-solving, and a series of self-perpetuating crises

Related Factors

Substance abuse
Family history of substance abuse/resistance to treatment
Inadequate coping skills; addictive personality; lack of problem-solving skills
Biochemical influences; genetic predisposition to substance abuse

Defining Characteristics

Subjective

Feelings

Anxiety, tension, distress; chronic low self-esteem; worthlessness; lingering resentment

---

Information that appears in brackets has been added by the authors to clarify and enhance the use of nursing diagnoses.

Anger; suppressed rage; frustration; shame; embarrassment; hurt; unhappiness; guilt

Emotional isolation; loneliness; powerlessness; insecurity; hopelessness; rejection

Responsibility for substance abuser's behavior; vulnerability; mistrust

Depression; hostility; fear; confusion; dissatisfaction; loss

Being different from other people; misunderstood

Emotional control by others; being unloved; lack of identity

Abandonment; confuses love and pity; moodiness; failure

Roles and Relationships

Family denial; deterioration in family relationships; disturbed family dynamics; ineffective spouse communication; marital problems; intimacy dysfunction

Altered role function; disrupted family roles; inconsistent parenting; low perception of parental support; chronic family problems

Lack of skills necessary for relationships; lack of cohesiveness; disrupted family rituals

Pattern of rejection; economic problems; neglected obligations

Objective

Feelings

Repressed emotions

Roles and Relationships

Closed communication systems

Triangulating family relationships; reduced ability of family members to relate to each other for mutual growth and maturation

Family does not demonstrate respect for individuality/autonomy of its members

Behavioral

Substance abuse; substance abuse other than alcohol; nicotine addiction

Enabling maintenance of substance use pattern (e.g., alcohol use); inadequate understanding of, or deficient knowledge about substance abuse

Family special occasions are substance-use centered

Rationalization; denial of problems; refusal to get help; inability to accept or receive help appropriately

Inappropriate expression of anger; blaming; criticizing; verbal abuse of children, spouse, or parent

---

Information that appears in brackets has been added by the authors to clarify and enhance the use of nursing diagnoses.

Lying; broken promises; lack of reliability; manipulation; dependency

Inability to express or accept wide range of feelings; difficulty with intimate relationships; diminished physical contact

Harsh self-judgment; difficulty having fun; self-blaming; isolation; complicated grieving; seeking approval or affirmation

Impaired communication; controlling, contradictory, or paradoxical communication; power struggles

Ineffective problem-solving skills; conflict avoidance; orientation toward tension relief rather than achievement of goals; agitation; escalating conflict; chaos

Disturbances in concentration; disturbances in academic performance in children; failure to accomplish developmental tasks; difficulty with life cycle transitions

Inability to meet the emotional, security, or spiritual needs of its members

Inability to adapt to change; immaturity; stress-related physical illnesses; inability to deal constructively with traumatic experiences

Desired Outcomes/Evaluation Criteria— Family Will:

- Verbalize understanding of dynamics of codependence.
- Participate in individual/family treatment programs.
- Identify ineffective coping behaviors and consequences of choices and actions.
- Demonstrate and plan for necessary lifestyle changes.
- Take action to change self-destructive behaviors and alter behaviors that contribute to client's drinking or substance use.
- Demonstrate improvement in parenting skills.

Actions/Interventions

Nursing Priority No. 1.

To assess contributing factors/underlying problem(s):

- Assess current level of functioning of family members.
- Ascertain family's understanding of current situation; note results of previous involvement in treatment.
- Review family history, explore roles of family members and circumstances involving substance use.
- Determine history of accidents or violent behaviors within family and safety issues.

Information that appears in brackets has been added by the authors to clarify and enhance the use of nursing diagnoses.

🌐 Cultural   ⊛ Collaborative   🏠 Community/Home Care

- Discuss current and past methods of coping. **May be able to identify methods that would be useful in the current situation.**
- Determine extent and understanding of enabling behaviors being evidenced by family members.
- Identify sabotage behaviors of family members. **Issues of secondary gain (conscious or unconscious) may impede recovery.**
- Note presence and extent of behaviors of family, client, and self that might be "too helpful," such as frequent requests for help, excuses for not following through on agreed-on behaviors, feelings of anger or irritation with others. **Enabling behaviors can complicate acceptance and resolution of problem.**

Nursing Priority No. 2.

To assist family to change destructive behaviors:

- Obtain mutual agreement on behaviors and responsibilities for nurse and client. **Maximizes understanding of what is expected of each individual.**
- Confront and examine denial and sabotage behaviors used by family members. **Helps individuals recognize and move beyond blocks to recovery.**
- Discuss use of anger, rationalization, and/or projection and ways in which these interfere with problem resolution.
- Encourage family to deal with anger **to prevent escalation to violence.** Problem-solve concerns.
- Determine family strengths, areas for growth, individual/family successes.
- Remain nonjudgmental in approach to family members and to member who uses alcohol/drugs.
- Provide information regarding effects of addiction on mood/personality of the involved person. **Helps family members understand and cope with negative behaviors without being judgmental or reacting angrily.**
- Distinguish between destructive aspects of enabling behavior and genuine motivation to aid the user.
- Identify use of manipulative behaviors and discuss ways to avoid or prevent these situations. **Manipulation has the goal of controlling others; when family members accept self-responsibility and commit to stop using it, new healthy behaviors will ensue.**

Information that appears in brackets has been added by the authors to clarify and enhance the use of nursing diagnoses.

Nursing Priority No. 3.

🏠 To promote wellness (Teaching/Discharge Considerations):

- Provide factual information to client/family about the effects of addictive behaviors on the family and what to expect after discharge.
- Provide information about enabling behavior, **an addictive disease characteristic for both user and nonuser who are codependent.**
- Discuss importance of restructuring life activities, work/leisure relationships. **Previous lifestyle/relationships supported substance use, requiring change to prevent relapse.**
- Encourage family to refocus celebrations excluding alcohol use **to reduce risk of relapse.**
- Provide support for family members; encourage participation in group work. **Involvement in a group provides information about how others are dealing with problems, provides role models, and gives individual an opportunity to practice new healthy skills.**
- Encourage involvement with, and refer to, self-help groups (e.g., Al-Anon, Alateen, Narcotics Anonymous, or family therapy groups) **to provide ongoing support and assist with problem-solving.**
- Provide bibliotherapy as appropriate.
- In addition, refer to NDs interrupted Family Processes; compromised/disabled family Coping, as appropriate.

Documentation Focus

Assessment/Reassessment

- Assessment findings, including history of substance(s) that have been used and family risk factors and safety concerns.
- Family composition and involvement.
- Results of prior treatment involvement.

Planning

- Plan of care and who is involved in planning.
- Teaching plan.

Implementation/Evaluation

- Responses of family members to treatment, teaching, and actions performed.
- Attainment or progress toward desired outcome(s).
- Modifications to plan of care.

Information that appears in brackets has been added by the authors to clarify and enhance the use of nursing diagnoses.

🌐 Cultural 🔄 Collaborative 🏠 Community/Home Care

Discharge Planning

- Long-term needs, who is responsible for actions to be taken.
- Specific referrals made.

Sample Nursing Outcomes & Interventions Classifications (NOC/NIC)

NOC—Family Functioning
NIC—Substance Use Treatment

interrupted Family Processes

Taxonomy II: Role Relationships—Class 2 Family Relationships (00060)
[Diagnostic Division: Social Interactions]
Submitted 1982; Nursing Diagnosis Extension and Classification Revision 1998

Definition: Change in family relationships and/or functioning

Related Factors

Situational transition or crises
Developmental transition or crises
Shift in health status of a family member
Shift in family roles; power shift of family members
Modification in family finances or status
Interaction with community

Defining Characteristics

Subjective

Changes in expressions of conflict within family, conflict with or isolation from community resources
Changes in satisfaction with family; intimacy changes

Objective

Changes in assigned tasks, participation in problem-solving or decision-making, communication patterns, mutual support, availability for emotional support or affective responsiveness
Changes in effectiveness in completing assigned tasks, somatic complaints
Power alliance changes; stress-reduction behavior changes

Information that appears in brackets has been added by the authors to clarify and enhance the use of nursing diagnoses.

Desired Outcomes/Evaluation Criteria— Family Will:

- Express feelings freely and appropriately.
- Demonstrate individual involvement in problem-solving processes directed at appropriate solutions for the situation or crisis.
- Direct energies in a purposeful manner to plan for resolution of the crisis.
- Verbalize understanding of condition, treatment regimen, and prognosis.
- Encourage and allow affected member to handle situation in own way, progressing toward independence.

Actions/Interventions

Nursing Priority No. 1.

To assess individual situation for causative/contributing factors:

- Determine pathophysiology, illness/trauma, or developmental crisis present.
- Identify family developmental stage (e.g., marriage, birth of a child, children leaving home). **Provides baseline for establishing plan of care.**
- Note components and availability of the family: parent(s), children, male/female, extended family.
- Observe patterns of communication in family. Are feelings expressed? Freely? Who talks to whom? Who makes decisions? For whom? Who visits? When? What is the interaction between family members? **Identifies weakness/areas of concern to be addressed as well as strengths that can be used for resolution of problem.**
- Assess boundaries of family members. Do members share family identity and have little sense of individuality? Do they seem emotionally distant and not connected with one another? **Answers to these questions help identify specific problems needing to be addressed.**
- Ascertain role expectations of family members. Who is the ill member (e.g., nurturer, provider)? How does the illness affect the roles of others?
- Identify "family rules"; e.g., how adult concerns (finances, illness, etc.) are kept from the children.
- Determine effectiveness of parenting skills and parents' expectations.
- Note energy direction. Are efforts at resolution/problem solving purposeful or scattered?

Information that appears in brackets has been added by the authors to clarify and enhance the use of nursing diagnoses.

Cultural   Collaborative   Community/Home Care

- Listen for expressions of despair or helplessness (e.g., "I don't know what to do") **to note degree of distress and inability to handle what is happening.**
- Note cultural and/or religious factors **that may affect perceptions/expectations of family members.**
- Assess availability and use of support systems outside of the family.

Nursing Priority No. 2.
To assist family to deal with situation/crisis:

- Deal with family members in a warm, caring, and respectful way.
- Acknowledge difficulties and realities of the situation. **Reinforces that some degree of conflict is to be expected and can be used to promote growth.**
- Encourage expressions of anger. Avoid taking comments personally as the client is usually angry at the situation over which he or she has little or no control. **Maintains boundaries between nurse and family.**
- Stress importance of continuous, open dialogue between family members **to facilitate ongoing problem-solving.**
- Provide information, as necessary, in verbal and written formats. Reinforce as necessary.
- Assist family to identify and encourage their use of previously successful coping behaviors.
- Recommend contact by family members on a regular, frequent basis.
- Arrange for and encourage family participation in multidisciplinary team conference or group therapy, as appropriate.
- Involve family in social support and community activities of their interest and choice.

Nursing Priority No. 3.
To promote wellness (Teaching/Discharge Considerations):

- Encourage use of stress-management techniques (e.g., appropriate expression of feelings, relaxation exercises).
- Provide educational materials and information **to assist family members in resolution of current crisis.**
- Refer to classes (e.g., parent effectiveness, specific disease/disability support groups, self-help groups, clergy, psychological counseling, family therapy), as indicated.
- Assist family with identifying situations that may lead to fear or anxiety. (Refer to NDs Fear; Anxiety.)

Information that appears in brackets has been added by the authors to clarify and enhance the use of nursing diagnoses.

- Involve family in planning for future and mutual goal setting. **Promotes commitment to goals/continuation of plan.**
- Identify community agencies (e.g., Meals on Wheels, visiting nurse, trauma support group, American Cancer Society, or Veterans Administration) for both immediate and long-term support.

Documentation Focus

Assessment/Reassessment
- Assessment findings, including family composition, developmental stage of family, and role expectations.
- Family communication patterns.

Planning
- Plan of care, specific interventions, and who is involved in planning.
- Teaching plan.

Implementation/Evaluation
- Each individual's response to interventions, teaching, and actions performed.
- Attainment or progress toward desired outcome(s).
- Modifications to plan of care.

Discharge Planning
- Long-term needs, noting who is responsible for actions to be taken.
- Specific referrals made.

Sample Nursing Outcomes & Interventions Classifications (NOC/NIC)

NOC—Family Functioning
NIC—Family Process Maintenance

---

readiness for enhanced Family Processes

Taxonomy II: Role Relationships—Class 2 Family Relationships (00159)
[Diagnostic Division: Social Interaction]
Submitted 2002

Definition: A pattern of family functioning that is sufficient to support the well-being of family members and can be strengthened

---

Information that appears in brackets has been added by the authors to clarify and enhance the use of nursing diagnoses.

Defining Characteristics

Subjective

Expresses willingness to enhance family dynamics

Communication is adequate

Relationships are generally positive; interdependent with community; family tasks are accomplished

Energy level of family supports activities of daily living

Family adapts to change

Objective

Family functioning meets needs of family members

Activities support the safety/growth of family members

Family roles are appropriate/flexible for developmental stages

Family resilience is evident

Respect for family members is evident

Boundaries of family members are maintained

Balance exists between autonomy and cohesiveness

Desired Outcomes/Evaluation Criteria— Client Will:

- Express feelings freely and appropriately.
- Verbalize understanding of desire for enhanced family dynamics.
- Demonstrate individual involvement in problem-solving to improve family communications.
- Acknowledge awareness of and respect for boundaries of family members.

Actions/Interventions

Nursing Priority No. 1.

To determine status of family:

- Determine family composition: parent(s), children, male/female, and extended family. **Many family forms exist in society today, such as biological, nuclear, single parent, step family, communal, and same-sex couple or family. A better way to determine a family may be to determine the attribute of affection, strong emotional ties, a sense of belonging, and durability of membership.**
- Identify participating members of family and how they define family. **Establishes members of family who need to be**

Information that appears in brackets has been added by the authors to clarify and enhance the use of nursing diagnoses.

directly involved/taken into consideration when developing plan of care to improve family functioning.

- Note stage of family development (e.g., single, young adult, newly married, family with young children, family with adolescents, grown children, later in life).
- Ascertain motivation and expectations for change.
- Observe patterns of communication in the family. Are feelings expressed? Freely? Who talks to whom? Who makes decisions? For whom? Who visits? When? What is the interaction between family members? **Identifies possible weaknesses to be addressed, as well as strengths that can be used for improving family communication.**
- Assess boundaries of family members. Do members share family identity and have little sense of individuality? Do they seem emotionally connected with one another? **Individuals need to respect one another and boundaries need to be clear so family members are free to be responsible for themselves.**
- Identify "family rules" that are accepted in the family. **Families interact in certain ways over time and develop patterns of behavior that are accepted as the way "we behave" in this family. "Functional family" rules are constructive and promote the needs of all family members.**
- Note energy direction. **Efforts at problem-solving and resolution of different opinions may be purposeful or may be scattered and ineffective.**
- Determine cultural and/or religious factors influencing family interactions. **Expectations related to socioeconomic beliefs may be different in various cultures. For instance, traditional views of marriage and family life may be strongly influenced by Roman Catholicism in Italian-American and Latino-American families. In some cultures, the father is considered the authority figure and the mother is the homemaker. These beliefs may change with stressors or circumstances (e.g., financial, loss or gain of a family member, personal growth).**
- Note health of married individuals. **Recent reports have determined that marriage increases life expectancy by as much as 5 years.**

Nursing Priority No. 2.

To assist the family to improve interactions:

- Establish nurse-family relationship. **Promotes a warm, caring atmosphere in which family members can share thoughts, ideas, and feelings openly and nonjudgmentally.**

Information that appears in brackets has been added by the authors to clarify and enhance the use of nursing diagnoses.

- Acknowledge realities, and possible difficulties, of individual situation. **Reinforces that some degree of conflict is to be expected in family interactions that can be used to promote growth.**
- Stress importance of continuous, open dialogue between family members. **Facilitates ongoing expression of open, honest feelings and opinions and effective problem-solving.**
- Assist family to identify and encourage use of previously successful coping behaviors. **Promotes recognition of previous successes and confidence in own abilities to learn and improve family interactions.**
- Acknowledge differences among family members with open dialogue about how these differences have occurred. **Conveys an acceptance of these differences among individuals and helps to look at how they can be used to strengthen the family.**
- Identify effective parenting skills already being used and additional ways of handling difficult behaviors. **Allows individual family members to realize that some of what has been done already has been helpful and encourages them to learn new skills to manage family interactions in a more effective manner.**

Nursing Priority No. 3.
🏠 To promote optimum well-being:
- Discuss and encourage use and participation in stress-management techniques. **Relaxation exercises, visualization, and similar skills can be useful for promoting reduction of anxiety and ability to manage stress that occurs in their lives.**
- Encourage participation in learning role-reversal activities. **Helps individuals to gain insight and understanding of other person's feelings and perspective/point of view.**
- Involve family members in setting goals and planning for the future. **When individuals are involved in the decision making, they are more committed to carrying out a plan to enhance family interactions as life goes on.**
- Provide educational materials and information. **Enhances learning to assist in developing positive relationships among family members.**
- Assist family members in identifying situations that may create problems and lead to stress/anxiety. **Thinking ahead can help individuals anticipate helpful actions to handle/prevent conflict and untoward consequences.**

Information that appears in brackets has been added by the authors to clarify and enhance the use of nursing diagnoses.

- Refer to classes/support groups, as appropriate. **Family effectiveness, self-help, psychology, and religious affiliations can provide role models and new information to enhance family interactions.**

Documentation Focus

Assessment/Reassessment
- Assessment findings, including family composition, developmental stage of family, and role expectations.
- Cultural or religious values and beliefs regarding family and family functioning.
- Family communication patterns.
- Motivation and expectations for change.

Planning
- Plan of care, specific interventions, and who is involved in planning.
- Educational plan.

Implementation/Evaluation
- Each individual's response to interventions, teaching, and actions performed.
- Attainment or progress toward desired outcome(s).
- Modifications to lifestyle.
- Changes in treatment plan.

Discharge Planning
- Long-term needs, noting who is responsible for actions to be taken.
- Specific referrals made.

Sample Nursing Outcomes & Interventions Classifications (NOC/NIC)

NOC—Family Social Climate
NIC—Family Support

Information that appears in brackets has been added by the authors to clarify and enhance the use of nursing diagnoses.

Cultural · Collaborative · Community/Home Care

Fatigue

Taxonomy II: Activity/Rest—Class 3 Energy Balance
(00093)
[Diagnostic Division: Activity/Rest]
Submitted 1988; Nursing Diagnosis Extension and Classification Revision 1998

Definition: An overwhelming sustained sense of exhaustion and decreased capacity for physical and mental
work at the usual level

Related Factors

Psychological
Stress; anxiety; depression
Reports boring lifestyle

Environmental
Noise; lights; humidity; temperature

Situational
Occupation; negative life events

Physiological
Increased physical exertion; sleep deprivation
Pregnancy; disease states; malnutrition; anemia
Poor physical condition
Altered body chemistry (e.g., medications, drug withdrawal,
chemotherapy)

Defining Characteristics

Subjective
Reports an unremitting or overwhelming lack of energy; in-
ability to maintain usual routines or usual level of physical
activity
Reports feeling tired
Perceived need for additional energy to accomplish routine
tasks; increase in rest requirements
Reports inability to restore energy even after sleep
Reports guilt over not keeping up with responsibilities
Compromised libido
Increase in physical complaints

Information that appears in brackets has been added by the authors to clarify
and enhance the use of nursing diagnoses.

Objective

Lethargic; listless; drowsy; lack of energy
Compromised concentration
Disinterest in surroundings; introspection
Decreased performance

Desired Outcomes/Evaluation Criteria—Client Will:

- Report improved sense of energy.
- Identify basis of fatigue and individual areas of control.
- Perform activities of daily living and participate in desired activities at level of ability.
- Participate in recommended treatment program.

Actions/Interventions

Nursing Priority No. 1.

To assess causative/contributing factors:

- Identify presence of physical and/or psychological conditions (e.g., pregnancy; infectious processes; blood loss, anemia; connective tissue disorders [e.g., MS, lupus]; trauma, chronic pain syndromes [e.g., arthritis]; cardiopulmonary disorders; cancer and cancer treatments; hepatitis; AIDS; major depressive disorder; anxiety states; substance use or abuse). **Important information can be obtained from knowing if fatigue is a result of an underlying condition or disease process (acute or chronic), whether an exacerbating or remitting condition is in exacerbation, and/or whether fatigue has been present over a long time without any identifiable cause.**
- Note diagnosis or possibility of chronic fatigue syndrome (CFS), also sometimes called chronic fatigue immune dysfunction syndrome (CFIDS). **Defining Characteristics listed above indicate that this fatigue far exceeds feeling tired after a busy day. Because no direct tests help in diagnosis of CFS, it is one of exclusion. CSF has been defined as a distinct disorder (affecting children and adults) characterized by chronic (often relapsing, but always debilitating) fatigue, lasting for at least 6 months (often for much longer), causing impairments in overall physical and mental functioning and without an apparent etiology.**
- ∞ Note age, gender, and developmental stage. **Some studies show a prevalence of fatigue more often in females than**

Information that appears in brackets has been added by the authors to clarify and enhance the use of nursing diagnoses.

🌐 Cultural   🔄 Collaborative   🏠 Community/Home Care

males; it most often occurs in adolescent girls and in young to middle-aged adults, but the condition may be present in any person at any age.

- Review medication regimen/use. **Certain medications, including prescription (especially beta-adrenergic blockers, chemotherapy), over-the-counter drugs, herbal supplements, and combinations of drugs and/or substances, are known to cause and/or exacerbate fatigue.**
- Ascertain client's belief about what is causing the fatigue.
- Assess vital signs **to evaluate fluid status and cardiopulmonary response to activity.**
- Determine presence/degree of sleep disturbances. **Fatigue can be a consequence of, and/or exacerbated by, sleep deprivation.**
- Note recent lifestyle changes, including conflicts (e.g., expanded responsibilities, demands of others, job-related conflicts); maturational issues (e.g., adolescent with an eating disorder); and developmental issues (e.g., new parenthood, loss of spouse/SO).
- Assess psychological and personality factors that may affect reports of fatigue level.
- Evaluate aspect of "learned helplessness" that may be manifested by giving up. **Can perpetuate a cycle of fatigue, impaired functioning, and increased anxiety and fatigue.**

Nursing Priority No. 2.
To determine degree of fatigue/impact on life:

- Obtain client/SO descriptions of fatigue (i.e., lacking energy or strength, tiredness, weakness lasting over length of time). Note presence of additional concerns (e.g., irritability, lack of concentration, difficulty making decisions, problems with leisure, relationship difficulties) **to assist in evaluating impact on client's life.**
- Ask client to rate fatigue (using a 0 to 10 or similar numerical scale) and its effects on ability to participate in desired activities. **Fatigue may vary in intensity and is often accompanied by irritability, lack of concentration, difficulty making decisions, problems with leisure, and relationship difficulties that can add to stress level and aggravate sleep problems.**
- Discuss lifestyle changes or limitations imposed by fatigue state.
- Interview parent/caregiver regarding specific changes observed in child or elder client. **These individuals may not be**

Information that appears in brackets has been added by the authors to clarify and enhance the use of nursing diagnoses.

able to verbalize feelings or relate meaningful information.

- Note daily energy patterns (i.e., peaks and valleys). **Helpful in determining pattern/timing of activity.**
- Measure physiological response to activity (e.g., changes in blood pressure or heart and respiratory rate).
- Evaluate need for individual assistance or assistive devices.
- Review availability and current use of support systems and resources.
- Perform, or review results of, testing, such as the Multidimensional Assessment of Fatigue (MAF); Piper Fatigue Scale (PFS); Global Fatigue Index (GFI), as appropriate. **Can help determine manifestation, intensity, duration, and emotional meaning of fatigue.**

Nursing Priority No. 3.

To assist client to cope with fatigue and manage within individual limits of ability:

- Accept reality of client reports of fatigue and do not underestimate effect on client's quality of life. **For example, clients with MS are prone to more frequent and severe fatigue following minimal energy expenditure and require a longer recovery period than is usual; postpolio clients often display a cumulative effect if they fail to pace themselves and rest when early signs of fatigue develop.**
- Establish realistic activity goals with client and encourage forward movement. **Enhances commitment to promoting optimal outcomes.**
- Plan interventions to allow individually adequate rest periods. Schedule activities for periods when client has the most energy **to maximize participation.**
- Involve client/SO(s) in schedule planning.
- Encourage client to do whatever possible (e.g., self-care, sit up in chair, go for walk, interact with family, play game). Increase activity level, as tolerated.
- Instruct in methods to conserve energy:

  Sit instead of stand during daily care and other activities.
  Carry several small loads instead of one large load.
  Combine and simplify activities.
  Take frequent, short breaks during activities.
  Delegate tasks.
  Ask for and accept assistance.
  Say "No" or "Later."

Information that appears in brackets has been added by the authors to clarify and enhance the use of nursing diagnoses.

Plan steps of activity before beginning so that all needed materials are at hand.

🔒• Encourage use of assistive devices (e.g., wheeled walker, handicap parking spot, elevator, backpack for carrying objects), as needed, **to extend active time/conserve energy for other tasks.**

🔒• Assist with self-care needs; keep bed in low position and travelways clear of furniture; assist with ambulation, as indicated.

🔒• Avoid or limit exposure to temperature and humidity extremes, **which can negatively impact energy level.**

🔒• Provide diversional activities. Avoid both overstimulation and understimulation (cognitive and sensory). **Participating in pleasurable activities can refocus energy and diminish feelings of unhappiness, sluggishness, and worthlessness that can accompany fatigue.**

🔒• Discuss routines to promote restful sleep. (Refer to ND Insomnia)

• Encourage nutritionally dense, easy-to-prepare-and-consume foods, and avoidance of caffeine and high-sugar foods and beverages **to promote energy.**

• Instruct in/implement stress-management skills of visualization, relaxation, and biofeedback, when appropriate.

⊕• Refer to comprehensive rehabilitation program, physical and occupational therapy for programmed daily exercises and activities **to improve stamina, strength, and muscle tone and to enhance sense of well-being.**

Nursing Priority No. 4.

🔒To promote wellness (Teaching/Discharge Considerations):

• Discuss therapy regimen relating to individual causative factors (e.g., physical and/or psychological illnesses) and help client/SO(s) to understand relationship of fatigue to illness.

• Assist client/SO(s) to develop plan for activity and exercise within individual ability. Stress necessity of allowing sufficient time to finish activities.

• Instruct client in ways to monitor responses to activity and significant signs/symptoms **that indicate the need to alter activity level.**

• Promote overall health measures (e.g., nutrition, adequate fluid intake, and appropriate vitamin and iron supplementation).

⊕• Provide supplemental oxygen, as indicated. **Presence of anemia and hypoxemia reduces oxygen available for cellular uptake and contributes to fatigue.**

Information that appears in brackets has been added by the authors to clarify and enhance the use of nursing diagnoses.

- Encourage client to develop assertiveness skills, to prioritize goals and activities, to learn to delegate duties or tasks, or to say "No." Discuss burnout syndrome, when appropriate, and actions client can take to change individual situation.
- Assist client to identify appropriate coping behaviors. **Promotes sense of control and improves self-esteem.**
- Identify support groups and community resources.
- Refer to counseling or psychotherapy, as indicated.
- Identify resources to assist with routine needs (e.g., Meals on Wheels, homemaker or housekeeper services, yard care).

Documentation Focus

Assessment/Reassessment
- Manifestations of fatigue and other assessment findings.
- Degree of impairment and effect on lifestyle.
- Expectations of client/SO(s) relative to individual abilities and specific condition.

Planning
- Plan of care, specific interventions, and who is involved in the planning.
- Teaching plan.

Implementation/Evaluation
- Client's response to interventions, teaching, and actions performed.
- Attainment or progress toward desired outcome(s).
- Modifications to plan of care.

Discharge Planning
- Discharge needs/plan, actions to be taken, and who is responsible.
- Specific referrals made.

Sample Nursing Outcomes & Interventions Classifications (NOC/NIC)

NOC—Endurance
NIC—Energy Management

Information that appears in brackets has been added by the authors to clarify and enhance the use of nursing diagnoses.

🌐 Cultural 🔄 Collaborative 🏠 Community/Home Care

Fear [specify focus]

Taxonomy II: Coping/Stress Tolerance—Class 2 Coping
 Responses (00148)
[Diagnostic Division: Ego Integrity]
Submitted 1980; Revised 2000

Definition: Response to perceived threat (real or imagined) that is consciously recognized as a danger

Related Factors

Innate origin (e.g., sudden noise, height, pain, loss of physical support); innate releasers (neurotransmitters); phobic stimulus

Learned response (e.g., conditioning, modeling from or identification with others)

Unfamiliarity with environmental experience(s)

Separation from support system in potentially stressful situation (e.g., hospitalization, hospital procedures/[treatments])

Language barrier; sensory impairment

Defining Characteristics

Subjective

Reports apprehension; excitement; being scared; alarm; panic; terror; dread; decreased self-assurance; increased tension; jitteriness

Cognitive

Identifies object of fear; stimulus believed to be a threat

Physiological

Anorexia; nausea; fatigue; dry mouth; [palpitations]

Objective

Cognitive

Diminished productivity, learning ability, or problem-solving ability

Behaviors

Increased alertness; avoidance behaviors; attack behaviors; impulsiveness; narrowed focus on the source of the fear

---

Information that appears in brackets has been added by the authors to clarify and enhance the use of nursing diagnoses.

Physiological

Increased pulse; vomiting; diarrhea; muscle tightness; increased respiratory rate; dyspnea; increased systolic blood pressure; pallor; increased perspiration; pupil dilation

Desired Outcomes/Evaluation Criteria— Client Will:

- Acknowledge and discuss fears, recognizing healthy versus unhealthy fears.
- Verbalize accurate knowledge of and sense of safety related to current situation.
- Demonstrate understanding through use of effective coping behaviors (e.g., problem-solving) and resources.
- Display lessened fear as evidenced by appropriate range of feelings and relief of signs/symptoms (specific to client).

Actions/Interventions

Nursing Priority No. 1.

To assess degree of fear and reality of threat perceived by the client:

- Ascertain client's/SO's perception of what is occurring and how this affects life. **Fear is a defensive mechanism in protecting oneself but, if left unchecked, can become disabling to the client's life.**
- Determine client's age and developmental level. **Helps in understanding usual or typical fears experienced by individuals (e.g., toddler often has different fears than adolescent or older person suffering with dementia being removed from home/usual living situation).**
- Note ability to concentrate, level of attention, degree of incapacitation (e.g., "frozen with fear," inability to engage in necessary activities). **Indicative of extent of anxiety or fear related to what is happening and need for specific interventions to reduce physiological reactions. Presence of a severe reaction (panic or phobias) requires more intensive intervention.**
- Compare verbal and nonverbal responses **to note congruencies or misperceptions of situation. Client may be able to verbalize what he/she is afraid of, if asked, providing opportunity to address actual fears.**
- Be alert to signs of denial or depression. **Depression may be associated with fear that interferes with productive life and daily activities.**

Information that appears in brackets has been added by the authors to clarify and enhance the use of nursing diagnoses.

- Identify sensory deficits that may be present, such as vision or hearing impairment. **Affects sensory reception and interpretation of environment. Inability to correctly sense and perceive stimuli leads to misunderstanding, increasing fear.**
- Investigate client's reports of subjective experiences, which could be indicative of delusions/hallucinations, **to help determine client's interpretation of surroundings and/or stimuli.**
- Be alert to and evaluate potential for violence.
- Measure vital signs and physiological responses to situation. **Fear and acute anxiety can both involve sympathetic arousal (e.g., increased heart rate, respirations, and blood pressure hyperalertness; antiduresis; dilation of skeletal blood vessels; constriction of gut blood vessels and a surge of catecholamine release).**
- Assess family dynamics. **Actions and responses of family members may exacerbate or soothe fears of client; conversely, if the client is immersed in illness, whether from crisis or fear, it can take a toll on the family/involved others.** Refer to other NDs, such as interrupted Family Processes; readiness for enhanced family Coping; compromised or disabled family Coping; Anxiety.

Nursing Priority No. 2.

To assist client/SO(s) in dealing with fear/situation:

- Stay with the client or make arrangements to have someone else be there. **Providing client with usual or desired support persons can diminish feelings of fear.**
- Discuss client's perceptions and fearful feelings. Active-listen client's concerns. **Promotes atmosphere of caring and permits explanation or correction of misperceptions.**
- Provide information in verbal and written form. Speak in simple sentences and concrete terms. **Facilitates understanding and retention of information.**
- Acknowledge normalcy of fear, pain, despair, and give "permission" to express feelings appropriately and freely. **Promotes attitude of caring, opens door for discussion about feelings and/or addressing reality of situation.**
- Provide opportunity for questions and answer honestly. **Enhances sense of trust and nurse-client relationship.**
- ∞ Provide presence and physical contact (e.g., hugging, refocusing attention, rocking a child), as appropriate, when

---

Information that appears in brackets has been added by the authors to clarify and enhance the use of nursing diagnoses.

painful procedures are anticipated **to soothe fears and provide assurance.**

- Modify procedures, if possible (e.g., substitute oral for intramuscular medications, combine blood draws, or use finger stick method) **to limit degree of stress and avoid overwhelming a fearful individual.**
- Manage environmental factors, such as loud noises, harsh lighting, changing person's location without knowledge of family/SO(s), strangers in care area, unfamiliar people, high traffic flow, **which can cause or exacerbate stress, especially to very young or to older individuals.**
- Present objective information, when available, and allow client to use it freely. Avoid arguing about client's perceptions of the situation. **Limits conflicts when fear response may impair rational thinking.**
- Promote client control, where possible, and help client identify and accept those things over which control is not possible. **Strengthens internal locus of control.**
- Provide touch, Therapeutic Touch, massage, and other adjunctive therapies as indicated. **Aids in meeting basic human need, decreasing sense of isolation, and assisting client to feel less anxious. Note: Therapeutic Touch requires the nurse to have specific knowledge and experience to use the hands to correct energy field disturbances by redirecting human energies to help or heal.** (Refer to ND disturbed Energy Field.)
- Encourage contact with a peer who has successfully dealt with a similarly fearful situation. **Provides a role model, and client is more likely to believe others who have had similar experience(s).**

Nursing Priority No. 3.

To assist client in learning to use own responses for problem-solving:

- Acknowledge usefulness of fear for taking care of self.
- Explain relationship between disease and symptoms if appropriate. **Providing accurate information promotes understanding of why the symptoms occur, allaying anxiety about them.**
- Identify client's responsibility for the solutions while reinforcing that the nurse will be available for help if desired or needed. **Enhances sense of control.**

Information that appears in brackets has been added by the authors to clarify and enhance the use of nursing diagnoses.

⊕ Cultural ⊛ Collaborative 🏠 Community/Home Care

- Determine internal and external resources for assistance (e.g., awareness and use of effective coping skills in the past; SOs who are available for support).
- Explain procedures within level of client's ability to understand and handle being aware of how much information client wants **to prevent confusion or information overload.**
- Explain relationship between disease and symptoms, if appropriate.
- Review use of antianxiety medications and reinforce use as prescribed.

Nursing Priority No. 4.
To promote wellness (Teaching/Discharge Considerations):

- Support planning for dealing with reality. **Assists in identifying areas in which control can be exercised and those in which control is not possible, thus enabling client to handle fearful situations/feelings.**
- Instruct in use of relaxation or visualization and guided imagery skills. **Promotes release of endorphins and aids in developing internal locus of control, reducing fear and anxiety. May enhance coping skills, allowing body to go about its work of healing.**
- Encourage regular physical activity within limits of ability. Refer to physical therapist to develop exercise program to meet individual needs. **Provides a healthy outlet for energy generated by fearful feelings and promotes relaxation.**
- Provide for and deal with sensory deficits in appropriate manner (e.g., speak clearly and distinctly, use touch carefully, as indicated by situation).
- Refer to pastoral care, mental health care providers, support groups, community agencies and organizations, as indicated. **Provides information, ongoing assistance to meet individual needs, and opportunity for discussing concerns and obtaining further care when indicated.**

Documentation Focus

Assessment/Reassessment
- Assessment findings, noting individual factors contributing to current situation, source of fear.
- Manifestations of fear.

Information that appears in brackets has been added by the authors to clarify and enhance the use of nursing diagnoses.

Planning
- Plan of care and who is involved in the planning.
- Teaching plan.

Implementation/Evaluation
- Client's responses to treatment plan, interventions, and actions performed.
- Attainment or progress toward desired outcome(s).
- Modifications to plan of care.

Discharge Planning
- Long-term needs and who is responsible for actions to be taken.
- Specific referrals made.

Sample Nursing Outcomes & Interventions Classifications (NOC/NIC)

NOC—Fear Self-Control
NIC—Anxiety Reduction

---

ineffective infant Feeding Pattern

Taxonomy II: Nutrition—Class 1 Ingestion (00107)
[Diagnostic Division: Food/Fluid]
Submitted 1992; Revised 2006

Definition: Impaired ability of an infant to suck or coordinate the suck/swallow response resulting in inadequate oral nutrition for metabolic needs

---

Related Factors

Prematurity
Neurological impairment or delay
Oral hypersensitivity
Prolonged nil by mouth (NPO)
Anatomic abnormality

Defining Characteristics

Subjective
[Caregiver reports infant's inability to achieve an effective suck]

Information that appears in brackets has been added by the authors to clarify and enhance the use of nursing diagnoses.

Objective

Inability to initiate or sustain an effective suck
Inability to coordinate sucking, swallowing, and breathing

Desired Outcomes/Evaluation Criteria— Client Will:

- Display adequate output as measured by sufficient number of wet diapers daily.
- Demonstrate appropriate weight gain.
- Be free of aspiration.

Actions/Interventions

Nursing Priority No. 1.

To identify contributing factors/degree of impaired function:

- Assess infant's suck, swallow, and gag reflexes. **Provides comparative baseline and is useful in determining appropriate feeding method.**
- Note developmental age, structural abnormalities (e.g., cleft lip/palate), mechanical barriers (e.g., endotrachial tube, ventilator).
- Determine level of consciousness, neurological impairment, seizure activity, presence of pain.
- Observe parent/infant interactions **to determine level of bonding and comfort that could impact stress level during feeding activity.**
- Note type and scheduling of medications, **which could cause sedative effect and impair feeding activity.**
- Compare birth and current weight and length measurements **to note progress.**
- Assess signs of stress when feeding (e.g., tachypnea, cyanosis, fatigue, or lethargy).
- Note presence of behaviors indicating continued hunger after feeding.

Nursing Priority No. 2.

To promote adequate infant intake:

- Determine appropriate method for feeding (e.g., special nipple or feeding device, gavage or enteral tube feeding) and choice of breast milk or formula to meet infant needs.
- Review early infant feeding cues (e.g., rooting, lip smacking, sucking fingers or hand) versus late cue of crying. **Early**

Information that appears in brackets has been added by the authors to clarify and enhance the use of nursing diagnoses.

recognition of infant hunger promotes timely/more rewarding feeding experience for infant and mother.

- Demonstrate techniques and procedures for feeding. Note proper positioning of infant, "latching-on" techniques, rate of delivery of feeding, frequency of burping. (Refer to ND ineffective Breastfeeding, as appropriate.)
- Limit duration of feeding to maximum of 30 minutes based on infant's response (e.g., signs of fatigue) **to balance energy expenditure with nutrient intake.**
- Monitor caregiver's efforts. Provide feedback and assistance, as indicated. **Enhances learning, encourages continuation of efforts.**
- Refer nursing mother to lactation specialist for assistance and support in dealing with unresolved issues (e.g., teaching infant to suck).
- Emphasize importance of calm, relaxed environment during feeding **to reduce detrimental stimuli and enhance mother's and infant's focus on feeding activity.**
- Adjust frequency and amount of feeding according to infant's response. **Prevents stress associated with under- or overfeeding.**
- Advance diet, adding solids or thickening agent, as appropriate for age and infant needs.
- Alternate feeding techniques (e.g., nipple and gavage) according to infant's ability and level of fatigue.
- Alter medication/feeding schedules, as indicated, **to minimize sedative effects and have infant in alert state.**

Nursing Priority No. 3.

To promote wellness (Teaching/Discharge Considerations):

- Encourage Kangaroo care, placing infant skin-to-skin upright, tummy down, on mother's or father's chest. **Skin-to-skin care increases bonding and may promote stable heart rate, temperature and respiration in infant.**
- Instruct caregiver in techniques to prevent or alleviate aspiration.
- Discuss anticipated growth and development goals for infant, corresponding caloric needs.
- Suggest monitoring infant's weight and nutrient intake periodically.
- Recommend participation in classes, as indicated (e.g., first aid, infant CPR).

Information that appears in brackets has been added by the authors to clarify and enhance the use of nursing diagnoses.

🌐 Cultural   ㉒ Collaborative   🏠 Community/Home Care

- Refer to support groups (e.g., La Leche League, parenting support groups, stress reduction, or other community resources, as indicated).
- Provide bibliotherapy and appropriate Web sites for further information.

Documentation Focus

Assessment/Reassessment
- Type and route of feeding, interferences to feeding and reactions.
- Infant's measurements.

Planning
- Plan of care, specific interventions, and who is involved in planning.
- Teaching plan.

Implementation/Evaluation
- Infant's response to interventions (e.g., amount of intake, weight gain, response to feeding) and actions performed.
- Caregiver's involvement in infant care, participation in activities, response to teaching.
- Attainment of or progress toward desired outcome(s).
- Modifications to plan of care.

Discharge Planning
- Long-term needs, referrals made, and who is responsible for follow-up actions.

Sample Nursing Outcomes & Interventions Classifications (NOC/NIC)

NOC—Swallowing Status: Oral Phase
NIC—Swallowing Therapy

readiness for enhanced Fluid Balance

Taxonomy II: Nutrition—Class 5 Hydration (00160)
[Diagnostic Division: Food/Fluid]
Submitted 2002

Definition: A pattern of equilibrium between the fluid volume and chemical composition of body fluids that is sufficient for meeting physical needs and can be strengthened

Information that appears in brackets has been added by the authors to clarify and enhance the use of nursing diagnoses.

Defining Characteristics

Subjective

Expresses willingness to enhance fluid balance
No excessive thirst

Objective

Stable weight; no evidence of edema
Moist mucous membranes
Intake adequate for daily needs
Straw-colored urine; specific gravity within normal limits; urine output appropriate for intake
Good tissue turgor; risk for deficient fluid volume

Desired Outcomes/Evaluation Criteria— Client Will:

- Maintain fluid volume at a functional level as indicated by adequate urinary output, stable vital signs, moist mucous membranes, good skin turgor.
- Demonstrate behaviors to monitor fluid balance.
- Be free of thirst.
- Be free of evidence of fluid overload (e.g., absence of edema and adventitious lung sounds).

Actions/Interventions

Nursing Priority No. 1.

To determine potential for fluid imbalance and ways that client is managing:

- Note presence of factors with potential for fluid imbalance: (1) diagnoses or disease processes (e.g., hyperglycemia, ulcerative colitis, chronic obstructive pulmonary disease [COPD], burns, cirrhosis of the liver, vomiting, diarrhea, hemorrhage), or situations (e.g., diuretic therapy, hot or humid climate, prolonged exercise, getting overheated or feverish, diuretic effect of caffeine and alcohol) that may lead to deficits; or (2) conditions or situations potentiating fluid excess (e.g., renal failure, cardiac failure, stroke, cerebral lesions, renal or adrenal insufficiency, psychogenic polydipsia, acute stress, surgical procedures, use of anesthesia, excessive or rapid infusion of IV fluids). **Body fluid balance is regulated by intake (food and fluid), output (kidney, gastrointestinal [GI] tract, skin, and lungs), and regulatory hormonal**

Information that appears in brackets has been added by the authors to clarify and enhance the use of nursing diagnoses.

🌐 Cultural   🔵 Collaborative   🏠 Community/Home Care

mechanisms. **Balance is maintained within a relatively narrow margin and can be easily disrupted by multiple factors.**

∞ • Determine potential effects of age and developmental stage. **Elderly individuals have less body water than younger adults, decreased thirst response, reduced effectiveness of compensatory mechanisms (e.g., kidneys are less efficient in conserving sodium and water), and potential for functional and environmental issues that affect their ability to manage fluid intake. Infants and children have a relatively higher percentage of total body water and metabolic rate and are often less able than adults to control their fluid intake.**

• Evaluate environmental factors that could impact fluid balance. **Persons with impaired mobility, diminished vision, or who are confined to bed cannot as easily meet their own needs and may be reluctant to ask for assistance. Persons whose work environment is restrictive or outside may also have greater challenges in meeting fluid needs.**

• Assess vital signs (e.g., temperature, blood pressure, heart rate), skin and mucous membrane moisture, and urine output. Weigh, as indicated. **Predictors of fluid balance that should be in client's usual range in a healthy state.**

Nursing Priority No. 2.
To prevent occurrence of imbalance:

• Monitor input and output (I&O) (e.g., frequency of voids or diaper changes), as appropriate, being aware of insensible losses (e.g., diaphoresis in hot environment, use of oxygen, permanent tracheostomy), and "hidden sources" of intake (e.g., foods high in water content) **to ensure accurate picture of fluid status.**

• Weigh client regularly, and compare with recent weight history. **Useful in early recognition of water retention or unexplained losses.**

∞ • Establish and review with client individual fluid needs and replacement schedule. Make sure client has access to fluids at all times. Distribute fluids over 24-hour period. Teach elderly person to drink when not thirsty and to drink small amount frequently, rather than large amounts infrequently. **Enhances likelihood of cooperation with meeting therapeutic goals while avoiding periods of thirst if fluids are restricted. Note: Thirst declines with aging, but hydration needs do not.**

Information that appears in brackets has been added by the authors to clarify and enhance the use of nursing diagnoses.

- Encourage regular oral intake (e.g., fluids between meals, additional fluids during hot weather or when exercising) **to maximize intake and maintain fluid balance.**
- Distribute fluids over 24-hour period in presence of fluid restriction. **Prevents peaks/valleys in fluid level and associated thirst.**
- Administer or discuss judicious use of medications, as indicated (e.g., antiemetics, antidiarrheals, antipyretics, diuretics). **Medications may be indicated to prevent fluid imbalance if individual becomes sick.**

Nursing Priority No. 3.
To promote optimum wellness:

- Discuss client's individual conditions and factors that could cause occurrence of fluid imbalance, as individually appropriate (such as prevention of hyperglycemic episodes) **so that client/SO can take corrective action.**
- Identify and instruct in ways to meet specific fluid needs (e.g., client could carry water bottle when going to sports events or measure specific 24-hour fluid portions if restrictions apply) **to manage fluid intake over time.**
- Instruct client/SO(s) in how to measure and record I&O, if needed for home management. **Provides means of monitoring status and adjusting therapy to meet changing needs.**
- Establish regular schedule for weighing **to help monitor changes in fluid status.**
- Identify actions (if any) client may take to correct imbalance. **Encourages responsibility for self-care.**
- Review any dietary needs or restrictions and safe substitutes for salt, as appropriate. **Helps prevent fluid retention/edema formation.**
- Review or instruct in medication regimen and administration, and discuss potential for interactions/side effects that could disrupt fluid balance.
- Instruct in signs and symptoms indicating need for immediate/further evaluation and follow-up care **to prevent complications and/or allow for early intervention.**

Documentation Focus

Assessment/Reassessment
- Individual findings, including factors affecting ability to manage (regulate) body fluids.
- I&O, fluid balance, changes in weight, and vital signs.

Information that appears in brackets has been added by the authors to clarify and enhance the use of nursing diagnoses.

Planning
- Plan of care and who is involved in the planning.
- Teaching plan.

Implementation/Evaluation
- Client's responses to treatment, teaching, and actions performed.
- Attainment or progress toward desired outcome(s).
- Modifications to plan of care.

Discharge Planning
- Long-term needs, noting who is responsible for actions to be taken.
- Specific referrals made.

Sample Nursing Outcomes & Interventions Classifications (NOC/NIC)

NOC—Fluid Balance
NIC—Fluid Monitoring

[deficient hyper/hypotonic Fluid Volume]

[Diagnostic Division: Food/Fluid]

Definition: [Decreased intravascular, interstitial, and/or intracellular fluid. This refers to dehydration with changes in sodium.]

NOTE: NANDA has restricted deficient Fluid Volume to address only isotonic dehydration. For client needs related to dehydration associated with alterations in sodium, the authors have provided this second diagnostic label.

Related Factors

[Hypertonic dehydration: uncontrolled diabetes mellitus/insipidus, hyperosmolar nonketotic diabetic coma (HHNC), increased intake of hypertonic fluids/IV therapy, inability to respond to thirst reflex, inadequate free water supplementation (high-osmolarity enteral feeding formulas), renal insufficiency or failure]

Information that appears in brackets has been added by the authors to clarify and enhance the use of nursing diagnoses.

[Hypotonic dehydration: chronic illness, malnutrition, excessive use of hypotonic IV solutions (e.g., D5W), renal insufficiency]

Defining Characteristics

Subjective
[Reports of fatigue, nervousness, exhaustion]
[Thirst]

Objective
[Increased urine output, dilute urine (initially) and/or decreased output/oliguria]
[Weight loss]
[Decreased venous filling; hypotension (postural)]
[Increased pulse rate; decreased pulse volume and pressure]
[Decreased skin turgor; dry skin/mucous membranes]
[Increased body temperature]
[Change in mental status (e.g., confusion)]
[Hemoconcentration; altered serum sodium]

Desired Outcomes/Evaluation Criteria— Client Will:

- Maintain fluid volume at a functional level, as evidenced by individually adequate urinary output, stable vital signs, moist mucous membranes, good skin turgor.
- Verbalize understanding of causative factors and purpose of individual therapeutic interventions and medications.
- Demonstrate behaviors to monitor and correct deficit, as indicated, when condition is chronic.

Actions/Interventions

Nursing Priority No. 1.
To assess causative/precipitating factors:

- Note possible conditions or processes that may lead to deficits: (1) fluid loss (e.g., diarrhea, vomiting, excessive sweating; heat stroke; diabetic ketoacidosis; burns, other draining wounds; gastrointestinal obstruction; salt-wasting diuretics; rapid breathing or mechanical ventilation; surgical drains); (2) limited intake (e.g., sore throat or mouth; client dependent on others for eating or drinking; NPO status); (3) fluid shifts (e.g., ascites, effusions, burns, sepsis); and (4) environmental fac-

---

Information that appears in brackets has been added by the authors to clarify and enhance the use of nursing diagnoses.

tors (e.g., isolation, restraints, malfunctioning air conditioning, exposure to extreme heat).

∞• Determine effects of age. Obtain weight and measure subcutaneous fat and muscle mass **to ascertain total body water [TBW], which is approximately 60% of adult's weight and 75% of infant's weight. Very young and extremely elderly individuals are quickly affected by fluid volume deficit and are least able to express need. For example, elderly people often have a decreased thirst reflex and/or may not be aware of water needs. Infants/young children and other nonverbal persons cannot describe thirst.**

• Review client's medications, including prescription, over-the-counter (OTC) drugs, herbs, and nutritional supplements **to identify medications that can alter fluid and electrolyte balance. These may include diuretics, vasodilators, beta-blockers, aldosterone inhibitors, angiotensin-converting enzyme (ACE) blockers, and medications that can cause syndrome of inappropriate secretion of antidiuretic hormone (e.g., phenothiazines, vasopressin, some antineoplastic drugs)**

• Evaluate nutritional status, noting current intake, weight changes, problems with oral intake, use of supplements/tube feedings. Measure subcutaneous fat and muscle mass.

Nursing Priority No. 2.
To evaluate degree of fluid deficit:

• Assess vital signs, including temperature (often elevated), pulse (may be elevated), and respirations. Note strength of peripheral pulses.

• Measure blood pressure (may be low) with the client lying, sitting, and standing, when possible, and monitor invasive hemodynamic parameters, as indicated (e.g., central venous pressure [CVP], pulmonary artery pressure [PAP] or pulmonary capillary wedge pressure [PCWP]).

• Note presence of physical signs (e.g., dry mucous membranes, poor skin turgor, delayed capillary refill).

• Note change in usual mentation, behavior, or functional abilities (e.g., confusion, falling, loss of ability to carry out usual activities, lethargy, dizziness). **These signs indicate sufficient dehydration to cause poor cerebral perfusion and/or electrolyte imbalance.**

• Observe urinary output and color and measure amount and specific gravity. Measure or estimate other fluid losses (e.g.,

---

Information that appears in brackets has been added by the authors to clarify and enhance the use of nursing diagnoses.

gastric, respiratory, wound losses) **to more accurately deter-mine replacement needs.**

- Review laboratory data (e.g., Hb/Hct; electrolytes [sodium, potassium, chloride, bicarbonate]; BUN; creatinine; total protein/albumin) **to evaluate body's response to fluid loss and to determine replacement needs.**

Nursing Priority No. 3.

To correct/replace fluid losses to reverse pathophysiological mechanisms:

- Assist with treatment of underlying conditions causing or contributing to dehydration and electrolyte imbalances.
- Administer fluids and electrolytes, as indicated. **Fluids used for replacement depend on (1) the type of dehydration present (e.g., hypertonic or hypotonic) and (2) the degree of deficit determined by age, weight, and type of condition causing the deficit.**
- Establish 24-hour replacement needs and routes to be used (e.g., IV, PO, enteral feedings). **Steady rehydration over time prevents peaks and valleys in fluid level.**
- Note client preferences and provide beverages and foods with high fluid content.
- Limit intake of alcohol and caffeinated beverages, **which tend to exert a diuretic effect.**
- Provide nutritious diet via appropriate route; give adequate free water with enteral feedings.
- Maintain accurate intake and output (I&O), calculate 24-hour fluid balance, and weigh daily.

Nursing Priority No. 4.

To promote comfort and safety:

- Bathe less frequently, using mild cleanser or soap, and provide optimal skin care with suitable emollients **to maintain skin integrity and prevent excessive dryness.**
- Provide frequent oral and eye care **to prevent injury from dryness.**
- Change position frequently **to reduce pressure on fragile, dehydrated skin and tissues.**
- Provide for safety measures when client is confused.
- Replace electrolytes, as ordered.
- Administer or discontinue medications, as indicated, **when disease process or medications are contributing to dehydration.**

Information that appears in brackets has been added by the authors to clarify and enhance the use of nursing diagnoses.

Nursing Priority No. 5.

🔨To promote wellness (Teaching/Discharge Considerations):

- Discuss factors related to occurrence of deficit, as individually appropriate. **Early identification of risk factors can decrease occurrence and severity of complications associated with hypovolemia.**
- Identify and instruct in ways to meet specific fluid needs.
- ∞• Instruct client/SO(s) in how to monitor color of urine (**dark urine equates with concentration and dehydration**), and/or how to measure and record I&O (**may include weighing or counting diapers in infant/toddler),** as indicated.
- Identify actions (if any) client may take to correct deficiencies.
- Review or instruct in medication regimen, administration, and interactions and side effects.
- Instruct in signs and symptoms indicating need for immediate or further evaluation and follow-up care.

Documentation Focus

Assessment/Reassessment

- Individual findings, including factors affecting ability to manage (regulate) body fluids and degree of deficit.
- I&O, fluid balance, changes in weight, urine specific gravity, and vital signs.
- Results of diagnostic testing and laboratory studies.

Planning

- Plan of care and who is involved in the planning.
- Teaching plan.

Implementation/Evaluation

- Client's responses to treatment, teaching, and actions performed.
- Attainment or progress toward desired outcome(s).
- Modifications to plan of care.

Discharge Planning

- Long-term needs, noting who is responsible for actions to be taken.
- Specific referrals made.

Information that appears in brackets has been added by the authors to clarify and enhance the use of nursing diagnoses.

Sample Nursing Outcomes & Interventions Classifications (NOC/NIC)

NOC—Fluid Balance
NIC—Fluid/Electrolyte Management

deficient [isotonic] Fluid Volume

Note: This diagnosis has been structured to address isotonic dehydration (hypovolemia) excluding states in which changes in sodium occur. For client needs related to dehydration associated with alterations in sodium, refer to [deficient hyper/hypotonic Fluid Volume].

Taxonomy II: Nutrition—Class 5 Hydration (00027)
[Diagnostic Division: Food/Fluid]
Submitted 1978; Revised 1996

Definition: Decreased intravascular, interstitial, and/or intracellular fluid. This refers to dehydration, water loss alone without a change in sodium.

Related Factors ——————————————

Active fluid volume loss (e.g., hemorrhage, gastric intubation, acute or prolonged diarrhea, wounds, abdominal cancer; burns, fistulas, ascites [third spacing]; use of hyperosmotic radiopaque contrast agents)
Failure of regulatory mechanisms (e.g., fever, thermoregulatory response, renal tubule damage)

Defining Characteristics ——————————

Subjective
Thirst
Weakness

Objective
Decreased urine output; increased urine concentration
Decreased venous filling; decreased pulse volume or pressure
Sudden weight loss (except in third spacing)
Decreased blood pressure; increased pulse rate, body temperature
Decreased skin or tongue turgor; dry skin or mucous membranes

---

Information that appears in brackets has been added by the authors to clarify and enhance the use of nursing diagnoses.

Change in mental state
Elevated hematocrit (Hct)

deficient [isotonic] FLUID VOLUME

Desired Outcomes/Evaluation Criteria— Client Will:

- Maintain fluid volume at a functional level as evidenced by individually adequate urinary output with normal specific gravity, stable vital signs, moist mucous membranes, good skin turgor and prompt capillary refill, resolution of edema (e.g., ascites).
- Verbalize understanding of causative factors and purpose of individual therapeutic interventions and medications.
- Demonstrate behaviors to monitor and correct deficit, as indicated.

Actions/Interventions

Nursing Priority No. 1.
To assess causative/precipitating factors:

- Identify relevant diagnoses **that may create a fluid volume depletion (decreased intravascular plasma volume, such as might occur with rapid blood loss or hemorrhage from trauma; or vascular, pregnancy-related, or gastrointestinal [GI] bleeding disorders); significant fluid (other than blood) loss such as might occur with severe gastroenteritis with vomiting and diarrhea; or extensive burns.**
- Note presence of other factors (e.g., laryngectomy or tracheostomy tubes, drainage from wounds and fistulas or suction devices; water deprivation or fluid restrictions; decreased level of consciousness; dialysis; hot/humid climate, prolonged exercise; increased metabolic rate secondary to fever; increased caffeine or alcohol) **that may contribute to lack of fluid intake or loss of fluid by various routes.**
- ∞• Determine effects of age. **Elderly individuals are at higher risk because of decreasing response and effectiveness of compensatory mechanisms (e.g., kidneys are less efficient in conserving sodium and water). Infants and children have a relatively high percentage of total body water, are sensitive to loss, and are less able to control their fluid intake.**
- Prepare for and assist with diagnostic evaluations (e.g., imaging studies, x-rays) **to locate source of bleeding or cause for hypovolemia.**

Information that appears in brackets has been added by the authors to clarify and enhance the use of nursing diagnoses.

Diagnostic Studies   ∞ Pediatric/Geriatric/Lifespan   Medications   **405**

Nursing Priority No. 2.

To evaluate degree of fluid deficit:

- Estimate or measure traumatic or procedural fluid losses and note possible routes of insensible fluid losses. Determine customary and current weight. **These factors are used to determine degree of dehydration and method of fluid replacement.**
- Assess vital signs, noting low blood pressure—severe hypotension, rapid heart beat, and thready peripheral pulses. **These changes in vital signs are associated with fluid volume loss and/or hypovolemia. Note: In an acute, life-threatening hemorrhage state, cold, pale, moist skin may be noted reflecting body compensatory mechanisms to profound hypovolemia.**
- Observe/measure urinary output (hourly/24-hour totals). Note color **(may be dark greenish brown because of concentration)** and specific gravity **(a number higher than 1.25 is associated with dehydration, with usual range being 1.010–1.025).**
- Note change in usual mentation, behavior, and functional abilities (e.g., confusion, falling, loss of ability to carry out usual activities, lethargy, and dizziness). **These signs indicate sufficient dehydration to cause poor cerebral perfusion or can reflect electrolyte imbalance. In a hypovolemic shock state, mentation changes rapidly and client may present in coma.**
- Note complaints and physical signs associated with dehydration (e.g., scanty, concentrated urine; lack of tears when crying [infant, child]; dry, sticky mucous membranes; lack of sweating; delayed capillary refill; poor skin turgor; confusion; sleepiness; lethargy; muscle weakness; dizziness or lightheadedness; headache).
- Measure abdominal girth when ascites or third spacing of fluid occurs. Assess for peripheral edema formation.
- Review laboratory data (e.g., hemoglobin [Hb]/Hct, prothrombin time, activated partial thromboplastin time [aPTT]; electrolytes [sodium, potassium, chloride, bicarbonate] and glucose; blood urea nitrogen [BUN], creatinine [Cr]) **to evaluate body's response to bleeding/other fluid loss and to determine replacement needs. Note: In isotonic dehydration, electrolyte levels may be lower, but concentration ratios remain near normal.**

Information that appears in brackets has been added by the authors to clarify and enhance the use of nursing diagnoses.

🌐 Cultural ☢ Collaborative 🏠 Community/Home Care

Nursing Priority No. 3.

To correct/replace losses to reverse pathophysiological mechanisms:

- Control blood loss (e.g., gastric lavage with room temperature or cool saline solution, drug administration) and prepare for surgical intervention.
- Stop fluid loss (e.g., administer medication to stop vomiting/diarrhea, fever).
- Administer fluids and electrolytes (e.g., blood, isotonic sodium chloride solution, lactated Ringer's solution, albumin, fresh frozen plasma, dextran, hetastarch).
- Establish 24-hour fluid replacement needs and routes to be used. **Prevents peaks and valleys in fluid level.**
- Note client preferences regarding fluids and foods with high fluid content.
- Keep fluids within client's reach and encourage frequent intake, as appropriate.
- Control humidity and ambient air temperature, as appropriate, especially when major burns are present; or increase or decrease in presence of fever. Reduce bedding and clothes; provide tepid sponge bath. Assist with hypothermia, when ordered, **to reduce high fever and elevated metabolic rate.** (Refer to ND Hyperthermia.)
- Maintain accurate input and output (I&O) and weigh daily. Monitor urine specific gravity.
- Monitor vital signs (lying/sitting/standing) and invasive hemodynamic parameters, as indicated (e.g., CVP, pulmonary artery pressure/pulmonary capillary wedge pressure).

Nursing Priority No. 4.

To promote comfort and safety:

- Change position frequently **to reduce pressure on fragile skin and tissues.**
- Bathe every other day, provide optimal skin care with emollients.
- Provide frequent oral as well as eye care **to prevent injury from dryness.**
- Change dressings frequently, use adjunct appliances as indicated, for draining wounds **to protect skin and monitor losses for replacement.**
- Provide for safety measures when client is confused.

Information that appears in brackets has been added by the authors to clarify and enhance the use of nursing diagnoses.

deficient [isotonic] FLUID VOLUME

- Administer medications (**e.g., antiemetics or antidiarrheals to limit gastric or intestinal losses; antipyretics to reduce fever**).
- Observe for sudden or marked elevation of blood pressure, restlessness, moist cough, dyspnea, basilar crackles, and frothy sputum. **Too rapid a correction of fluid deficit may compromise the cardiopulmonary system, causing fluid overload and edema, especially if colloids are used in initial fluid resuscitation.**
- Refer to NDs Diarrhea; Hyperthermia for additional interventions.

Nursing Priority No. 5.
To promote wellness (Teaching/Discharge Considerations):

- Discuss factors related to occurrence and ways client/SO(s) can prevent dehydration, as indicated.
- Assist client/SO(s) to learn to measure own I&O.
- Recommend restriction of caffeine, alcohol, as indicated **to reduce effects of diuresis.**
- Review medications, and interactions and side effects.
- Note signs/symptoms indicating need for emergent or further evaluation and follow-up care.

Documentation Focus

Assessment/Reassessment
- Assessment findings, including degree of deficit and current sources of fluid intake.
- I&O, fluid balance, changes in weight, presence of edema, urine specific gravity, and vital signs.
- Results of diagnostic studies.

Planning
- Plan of care and who is involved in planning.
- Teaching plan.

Implementation/Evaluation
- Client's responses to interventions, teaching, and actions performed.
- Attainment or progress toward desired outcome(s).
- Modifications to plan of care.

Information that appears in brackets has been added by the authors to clarify and enhance the use of nursing diagnoses.

Discharge Planning

- Long-term needs, plan for correction, and who is responsible for actions to be taken.
- Specific referrals made.

Sample Nursing Outcomes & Interventions Classifications (NOC/NIC)

NOC—Hydration
NIC—Hypovolemia Management

excess Fluid Volume

Taxonomy II: Nutrition—Class 5 Hydration (00026)
[Diagnostic Division: Food/Fluid]
Submitted 1982; Revised 1996

Definition: Increased isotonic fluid retention

Related Factors

Compromised regulatory mechanism [e.g., syndrome of inappropriate antidiuretic hormone (SIADH) or decreased plasma proteins as found in conditions such as malnutrition, draining fistulas, burns, organ failure]
Excess fluid intake
Excess sodium intake
Pharmaceutical agents, such as chlorpropamide, tolbutamide, vincristine, triptylines, carbamazepine

Defining Characteristics

Subjective
Orthopnea [difficulty breathing]
Anxiety

Objective
Edema; anasarca; weight gain over short period of time
Intake exceeds output; oliguria
Adventitious breath sounds [rales or crackles]; changes in respiratory pattern; dyspnea
Increased central venous pressure (CVP); jugular vein distention; positive hepatojugular reflex

---

Information that appears in brackets has been added by the authors to clarify and enhance the use of nursing diagnoses.

S3 heart sound
Pulmonary congestion; pleural effusion; pulmonary artery pressure changes; blood pressure changes
Change in mental status; restlessness
Specific gravity changes
Decreased hemoglobin (Hb)/hematocrit (Hct); azotemia; electrolyte imbalance

Desired Outcomes/Evaluation Criteria—Client Will:

- Stabilize fluid volume as evidenced by balanced input and output (I&O), vital signs within client's normal limits, stable weight, and free of signs of edema.
- Verbalize understanding of individual dietary and fluid restrictions.
- Demonstrate behaviors to monitor fluid status and reduce recurrence of fluid excess.
- List signs that require further evaluation.

Actions/Interventions

Nursing Priority No. 1.
To assess causative/precipitating factors:

- Note presence of medical conditions or situations (e.g., heart failure, chronic kidney disease, renal or adrenal insufficiency, excessive or rapid infusion of IV fluids, cerebral lesions, psychogenic polydipsia, acute stress, anesthesia, surgical procedures, decreased or loss of serum proteins) **that can contribute to excess fluid intake or retention.**
- Note amount and rate of fluid intake from all sources: oral, intravenous (IV), ventilator humidifier, and so forth.
- Review nutritional issues (e.g., intake of sodium, potassium, and protein). **Imbalances in these areas are associated with fluid imbalances.**

Nursing Priority No. 2.
To evaluate degree of excess:

- Compare current weight with admission and/or previously stated weight. Weigh daily or on a regular schedule, as indicated.
- Measure vital signs and invasive hemodynamic parameters (e.g. central venous pressure [CVP], pulmonary artery pressure [PAP], pulmonary capillary wedge pressure [PCWP]), if

---

Information that appears in brackets has been added by the authors to clarify and enhance the use of nursing diagnoses.

🌐 Cultural 🌀 Collaborative 🏠 Community/Home Care

available. **Blood pressure may be high because of excess fluid volume or low if cardiac failure is occurring.**

• Auscultate breath sounds **for presence of crackles, congestion.**
• Record occurrence of exertional breathlessness, dyspnea at rest, or paroxysmal nocturnal dyspnea. **Indication of pulmonary congestion and potential of developing pulmonary edema that can interfere with oxygen–carbon dioxide exchange at the capillary level.**
• Auscultate heart tones for S_3, ventricular gallop.
• Assess for presence of neck vein distention, hepatojugular reflux.
• Note presence of edema (puffy eyelids, dependent swelling of ankles and feet if ambulatory or up in chair; sacrum and posterior thighs when recumbent), anasarca. **Heart failure and renal failure are associated with dependent edema because of hydrostatic pressures, with dependent edema being a defining characteristic for excess fluid.**
• Measure abdominal girth **for changes that may indicate increasing fluid retention/edema.**
• Measure and record I&O accurately. Include "hidden" fluids (e.g., IV antibiotic additives, liquid medications, ice chips). Calculate 24-hour fluid balance (plus or minus). Note patterns, times, and amount of urination (e.g., nocturia, oliguria).
• Evaluate mentation for confusion, personality changes. **Signs of decreased cerebral oxygenation (e.g., cerebral edema) or electrolyte imbalance (e.g., hyponatremia).**
• Assess neuromuscular reflexes **to evaluate for presence of electrolyte imbalances such as hypernatremia.**
• Assess appetite, note presence of nausea, vomiting **to determine presence of problems associated with imbalance of electrolytes (e.g., glucose, sodium, potassium, calcium).**
• Observe skin and mucous membranes **for presence of decubitus or ulceration.**
• Review laboratory data (e.g., blood urea nitrogen/creatine [BUN/Cr], hemaglobin [Hb]/hematacrit [Hct], serum albumin, proteins, and electrolytes; urine specific gravity and osmolality, sodium excretion) and chest x-ray **to evaluate degree of fluid and electrolyte imbalance and response to therapies.**

Nursing Priority No. 3.

To promote mobilization/elimination of excess fluid:

• Restrict fluid intake as indicated (especially when sodium retention is less than water retention or when fluid retention is related to renal failure).

Information that appears in brackets has been added by the authors to clarify and enhance the use of nursing diagnoses.

- Provide for sodium restrictions if needed (as might occur in sodium retention in excess of water retention). **Restricting sodium favors renal excretion of excess fluid and may be more useful than fluid restriction.**
- Record I&O accurately; calculate 24-hour fluid balance noting plus or minus **so that adjustments can be made in the following 24-hour intake if needed.**
- Set an appropriate rate of fluid intake or infusion throughout 24-hour period **to prevent peaks and valleys in fluid level and thirst.**
- Weigh daily or on a regular schedule, as indicated. **Provides a comparative baseline and evaluates the effectiveness of diuretic therapy when used (i.e., if I&O is 1 liter negative, a weight loss of 2.2 pounds should be noted).**
- Administer medications (e.g., diuretics, cardiotonics, steroid replacement, plasma or albumin volume expanders).
- Elevate edematous extremities, change position frequently **to reduce tissue pressure and risk of skin breakdown.**
- Place in semi-Fowler's position, as appropriate, **to facilitate movement of diaphragm, thus improving respiratory effort.**
- Promote early ambulation **to reduce tissue pressure and risk of skin breakdown**.
- Use safety precautions if confused or debilitated.
- Assist with procedures, as indicated (e.g., dialysis).

Nursing Priority No. 4.
To maintain integrity of skin and oral mucous membranes:

- Refer to NDs impaired/risk for impaired Skin Integrity; impaired Oral Mucous Membrane.

Nursing Priority No. 5.
To promote wellness (Teaching/Discharge Considerations):

- Review dietary restrictions and safe substitutes for salt (e.g., lemon juice or spices such as oregano).
- Discuss importance of fluid restrictions and "hidden sources" of intake (such as foods high in water content).
- Instruct client/family in use of voiding record, I&O.
- Consult dietitian, as needed.
- Suggest interventions, such as frequent oral care, chewing gum/hard candy, use of lip balm, **to reduce discomfort of fluid restrictions.**

Information that appears in brackets has been added by the authors to clarify and enhance the use of nursing diagnoses.

Cultural   Collaborative   Community/Home Care

- Review drug regimen (and side effects) used to increase urine output and/or manage hypertension, kidney disease, or heart failure.
- Emphasize need for mobility and/or frequent position changes **to prevent stasis and reduce risk of tissue injury.**
- Identify "danger" signs requiring notification of healthcare provider **to ensure timely evaluation/intervention.**

Documentation Focus

Assessment/Reassessment

- Assessment findings, noting existing conditions contributing to and degree of fluid retention (vital signs; amount, presence, and location of edema; and weight changes).
- I&O, fluid balance.
- Results of laboratory tests and diagnostic studies.

Planning

- Plan of care and who is involved in the planning.
- Teaching plan.

Implementation/Evaluation

- Response to interventions, teaching, and actions performed.
- Attainment or progress toward desired outcome(s).
- Modifications to plan of care.

Discharge Planning

- Long-range needs, noting who is responsible for actions to be taken.

Sample Nursing Outcomes & Interventions Classifications (NOC/NIC)

NOC—Fluid Overload Severity
NIC—Hypervolemia Management

---

risk for deficient Fluid Volume

Taxonomy II: Nutrition—Class 5 Hydration (00028)
[Diagnostic Division: Food/Fluid]
Submitted 1978; Revised 2010

Definition: At risk for experiencing decreased intravascular, interstitial, and/or intracellular fluid. This refers to a risk for dehydration, water loss alone without change in sodium.

Information that appears in brackets has been added by the authors to clarify and enhance the use of nursing diagnoses.

Risk Factors

Extremes of age or weight
Loss of fluid through abnormal routes (e.g., indwelling tubes); failure of regulatory mechanisms
Deficient knowledge
Factors influencing fluid needs (e.g., hypermetabolic state)
Pharmaceutical agents (e.g., diuretics)
Active fluid loss; excessive losses through normal routes (e.g., diarrhea)
Deviations affecting access, intake, or absorption of fluids

> **NOTE:** A risk diagnosis is not evidenced by signs and symptoms as the problem has not occurred; rather, nursing interventions are directed at prevention.

Desired Outcomes/Evaluation Criteria— Client Will:

- Identify individual risk factors and appropriate interventions.
- Maintain fluid volume at a functional level as evidenced by individually adequate urinary output with normal specific gravity, stable vital signs, moist mucous membranes, good skin turgor, and prompt capillary refill.
- Demonstrate behaviors or lifestyle changes to prevent development of fluid volume deficit.

Actions/Interventions

Nursing Priority No. 1.

To assess causative/contributing factors:

- Note possible conditions or processes that may lead to deficits: (1) fluid loss (e.g., fever, diarrhea, vomiting, excessive sweating; heat stroke; diabetic ketoacidosis; burns, other draining wounds; gastrointestinal obstruction; salt-wasting diuretics; rapid breathing, mechanical ventilation; surgical drains); (2) limited intake (e.g., sore throat or mouth; client dependent on others for eating and drinking; nothing-by-mouth [NPO] status); (3) fluid shifts (e.g., ascites, effusions, burns, sepsis); and (4) environmental factors (e.g., isolation, restraints, malfunctioning air conditioning, exposure to extreme heat).
- ∞ Determine effects of age. **Very young and extremely elderly individuals are quickly affected by fluid volume deficit and**

Information that appears in brackets has been added by the authors to clarify and enhance the use of nursing diagnoses.

Cultural   Collaborative   Community/Home Care

are least able to express need. For example, elderly people often have a decreased thirst reflex and/or may not be aware of water needs. Infants, young children, and other nonverbal persons cannot describe thirst.

- Note client's level of consciousness and mentation **to evaluate ability to express needs.**
- ∞• Assess older client's "hydration habits" **to determine best approach if client has potential for dehydration. Note: A recent study identified four categories of nursing home residents: (1) Can drink (the client is functionally capable of consuming fluids, but doesn't for any number of reasons), (2) can't drink (frailty or dysphagia makes this client incapable of consuming fluids safely), (3) won't drink (client may fear incontinence or may have never in life consumed many fluids), and (4) end of life.**
- Evaluate nutritional status, noting current intake, type of diet (e.g., client is NPO or is on a restricted diet). Note problems (e.g., impaired mentation, nausea, fever, facial injuries, immobility, insufficient time for intake) **that can negatively affect fluid intake.**
- Review client's medications, including prescription, over-the-counter drugs, herbs, and nutritional supplements, **to identify medications that can alter fluid and electrolyte balance. These may include diuretics, vasodilators, beta-blockers, aldosterone inhibitors, angiotensin-converting enzyme (ACE) blockers, and medications that can cause syndrome of inappropriate secretion of antidiuretic hormone (e.g., phenothiazides, vasopressin, some antineoplastic drugs).**
- Review laboratory data (e.g., hemaglobin/hematocrit, electrolytes, blood urea nitrogen/creatine [BUN/Cr]).

Nursing Priority No. 2.
To prevent occurrence of deficit:
- Monitor I&O balance, being aware of altered intake or output **to ensure accurate picture of fluid status.**
- Weigh client and compare with recent weight history. Perform serial weights **to determine trends.**
- Assess skin turgor and oral mucous membranes **for signs of dehydration.**
- Monitor vital signs for changes (e.g., orthostatic hypotension, tachycardia, fever).
- Determine individual fluid needs and establish replacement over 24 hours **to increase client's daily intake.**

Information that appears in brackets has been added by the authors to clarify and enhance the use of nursing diagnoses.

🏠 • Encourage oral intake:

Provide water and other fluid needs to a minimum amount daily (up to 2.5 L/day or amount determined by healthcare provider for client's age, weight, and condition).

Offer fluids between meals and regularly throughout the day.

Provide fluids in manageable cup, bottle, or with drinking straw.

Allow for adequate time for eating and drinking at meals.

Ensure that immobile or restrained client is assisted.

Encourage a variety of fluids in small frequent offerings, attempting to incorporate client's preferred beverages and temperature (e.g., iced or hot).

Limit fluids that tend to exert a diuretic effect (e.g., caffeine, alcohol).

Promote intake of high-water content foods (e.g., popsicles, gelatin, soup, eggnog, watermelon) and/or electrolyte replacement drinks (e.g., Smartwater, Gatorade, Pedialyte), as appropriate.

🤝 • Provide supplemental fluids (e.g., enteral, parenteral), as indicated. **Fluids may be given in this manner if client is unable to take oral fluid, is NPO for procedures, or when rapid fluid resuscitation is required.**

💉 • Administer medications as indicated (e.g., anti-emetics, antidiarrheals, antipyretics).

Nursing Priority No. 3.

To promote wellness (Teaching/Discharge Considerations):

∞ • Discuss individual risk factors, potential problems, and specific interventions **to reduce risk of injury and dehydration (e.g., proper clothing and bedding and increased fluid intake for infants and elderly during hot weather, use of room cooler or fan for comfortable ambient environment, fluid replacement options and schedule).**

💉 • Review appropriate use of medications **that have potential for causing or exacerbating dehydration.**

🏠 • Encourage client to maintain diary of food/fluid intake; number and amount of voidings and stools; and so forth.

• Refer to NDs [deficient hyper/hypotonic Fluid Volume]; deficient [isotonic] Fluid Volume.

Documentation Focus

Assessment/Reassessment

• Individual findings, including individual factors influencing fluid needs or requirements.

Information that appears in brackets has been added by the authors to clarify and enhance the use of nursing diagnoses.

🌐 Cultural   🤝 Collaborative   🏠 Community/Home Care

- Baseline weight, vital signs.
- Results of laboratory tests.
- Specific client preferences for fluids.

Planning
- Plan of care and who is involved in planning.
- Teaching plan.

Implementation/Evaluation
- Responses to interventions, teaching, and actions performed.
- Attainment or progress toward desired outcome(s).
- Modifications to plan of care.

Discharge Planning
- Individual long-term needs, noting who is responsible for actions to be taken.
- Specific referrals made.

Sample Nursing Outcomes & Interventions Classifications (NOC/NIC)

NOC—Fluid Balance
NIC—Fluid Monitoring

risk for imbalanced Fluid Volume

Taxonomy II: Nutrition—Class 5 Hydration (00025)
[Diagnostic Division: Food/Fluid]
Submitted 1998; Revised 2008

Definition: At risk for a decrease, increase, or rapid shift from one to the other of intravascular, interstitial, and/or intracellular fluid that may compromise health. This refers to body fluid loss, gain, or both.

Risk Factors

Abdominal surgery; intestinal obstruction
Pancreatitis; ascites
Burns; sepsis
Traumatic injury (e.g., fractured hip)
Receiving apheresis

Information that appears in brackets has been added by the authors to clarify and enhance the use of nursing diagnoses.

> **NOTE:** A risk diagnosis is not evidenced by signs and symptoms, as the problem has not occurred; rather, nursing interventions are directed at prevention.

Desired Outcomes/Evaluation Criteria— Client Will:

• Demonstrate adequate fluid balance as evidenced by stable vital signs, palpable pulses of good quality, normal skin turgor, moist mucous membranes, individual appropriate urinary output, lack of excessive weight fluctuation (loss or gain), and no edema present.

Actions/Interventions

Nursing Priority No. 1.
To determine risk/contributing factors:

• Note potential sources of fluid loss and intake (e.g., presence of conditions, such as diabetes insipidus, hyperosmolar nonketotic syndrome, bowel obstruction, heart/kidney/liver failure, sepsis; major invasive procedures, such as surgery; use of anesthesia; preoperative vomiting and dehydration; draining wounds; use or overuse of certain medications, such as diuretics, laxatives, anticoagulants; use of IV fluids and delivery device; administration of total parenteral nutrition [TPN]).

∞• Note client's age, current level of hydration, and mentation. **Provides information regarding ability to tolerate fluctuations in fluid level and risk for creating or failing to respond to problem (e.g., confused client may have inadequate intake, disconnect tubings, or readjust IV flow rate).**

• Review laboratory data, chest x-ray **to determine changes indicative of electrolyte and/or fluid status.**

Nursing Priority No. 2.
To prevent fluctuations/imbalances in fluid levels:

• Measure and record intake:

  Include all sources (e.g., oral, intravenous [IV], antibiotic additives, liquids with medications).

• Measure and record output:

  Monitor urine output hourly or as needed. Report urine output less than 30 mL/hr or 0.5 mL/kg/hr **because this may in-**

Information that appears in brackets has been added by the authors to clarify and enhance the use of nursing diagnoses.

dicate deficient fluid volume or cardiac or kidney failure.

Observe color of all excretions **to evaluate for bleeding.**

Measure or estimate amount of liquid stool; weigh diapers or continence pads, when indicated.

∞ Inspect dressing(s), weigh dressings, estimate blood loss in surgical sponges, count dressings or pads saturated per hour.

Measure emesis and output from drainage devices (e.g., gastric, wound, chest).

Estimate or calculate insensible fluid losses **to include in replacement calculations.**

Calculate 24-hour fluid balance (intake more than output or output more than intake).

• Weigh daily, or as indicated, and evaluate changes as they relate to fluid status. **Provides for early detection and prompt intervention as needed.**

• Auscultate blood pressure, calculate pulse pressure. **Pulse pressure widens before systolic blood pressure drops in response to fluid loss.**

• Monitor vital sign responses to activities. **Blood pressure and heart and respiratory rate often increase initially when either fluid deficit or excess is present.**

• Assess for clinical signs of dehydration (e.g., hypotension, dry skin and mucous membranes, delayed capillary refill) or fluid excess (e.g., peripheral/dependent edema, adventitious breath sounds, distended neck veins).

• Note increased lethargy, hypotension, muscle cramping. **Electrolyte imbalances may be present.**

• Establish fluid oral intake, incorporating beverage preferences when possible.

⊛ • Maintain fluid and sodium restrictions, when needed.

⊛ • Administer IV fluids, as prescribed, using infusion pumps **to deliver fluids accurately and at desired rates to prevent either underfusion or overinfusion.**

• Tape tubing connections longitudinally **to reduce risk of disconnection and loss of fluids.**

⊛ • Assist with treatment of underlying conditions. Prepare for procedures (e.g., surgery for trauma, cold lavage for bleeding ulcer, etc.) and/or use of specific fluids or medications **to prevent dehydration, fluid volume depletion.**

Refer to NDs [deficient hyper/hypotonic Fluid Volume] and deficient [isotonic] Fluid Volume, for additional interventions.

Information that appears in brackets has been added by the authors to clarify and enhance the use of nursing diagnoses.

⊛ • Assist with treatment of underlying conditions. Prepare for procedures (e.g., dialysis, ultrafiltration, pacemaker, cardiac assist device) and/or use of specific drugs (e.g., antihypertensives, cardiotonics, diuretics) **to correct fluid overload situation.**

Refer to ND excess Fluid Volume for additional interventions.

Nursing Priority No. 3.

To promote wellness (Teaching/Discharge Considerations):

🏠 • Discuss individual risk factors, potential problems, and specific interventions **to prevent or limit occurrence of fluid deficit or excess.**

🏠 • Instruct client/SO(s) in how to measure and record input and output, if indicated.

🥄 • Review or instruct in medication or nutritional regimen (e.g., enteral/parenteral feedings) **to alert to potential complications and appropriate management.**

⊛ • Identify signs and symptoms indicating need for prompt evaluation/follow-up care.

Documentation Focus

Assessment/Reassessment
• Individual findings, including individual factors influencing fluid needs/requirements.
• Baseline weight, vital signs.
• Results of laboratory test and diagnostic studies.
• Specific client preferences for fluids.

Planning
• Plan of care and who is involved in planning.
• Teaching plan.

Implementation/Evaluation
• Responses to interventions, teaching, and actions performed.
• Attainment or progress toward desired outcome(s).
• Modifications to plan of care.

Discharge Planning
• Individual long-term needs, noting who is responsible for actions to be taken.
• Specific referrals made.

Information that appears in brackets has been added by the authors to clarify and enhance the use of nursing diagnoses.

🌐 Cultural ⊛ Collaborative 🏠 Community/Home Care

Sample Nursing Outcomes & Interventions Classifications (NOC/NIC)

NOC—Fluid Balance
NIC—Fluid Monitoring

impaired Gas Exchange

Taxonomy II: Elimination and Exchange—Class 4 Respiratory Function (00030)
[Diagnostic Division: Respiration]
Submitted 1980; Revised 1996, 1998 by Nursing Diagnosis Extension and Classification

Definition: Excess or deficit in oxygenation and/or carbon dioxide elimination at the alveolar-capillary membrane (may be an entity of its own, but it also may be an end result of other pathology with an interrelatedness between airway clearance and/or breathing pattern problems)

Related Factors

Ventilation-perfusion imbalance (as in altered blood flow, such as pulmonary embolus or increased vascular resistance; heart failure; hypovolemic shock)

Alveolar-capillary membrane changes (e.g., acute respiratory distress syndrome; chronic conditions, such as restrictive/obstructive lung disease, pneumoconiosis, asbestosis or silicosis)

[Altered oxygen supply (e.g., altitude sickness)]

[Altered oxygen-carrying capacity of blood (e.g., sickle cell or other anemia, carbon monoxide poisoning)]

Defining Characteristics

Subjective
Dyspnea
Visual disturbances
Headache upon awakening
[Sense of impending doom]

Objective
Confusion
Restlessness; irritability

Information that appears in brackets has been added by the authors to clarify and enhance the use of nursing diagnoses.

Somnolence

Abnormal arterial blood gases (ABGs)/arterial pH; hypoxia/hypoxemia; hypercapnia; decreased carbon dioxide

Cyanosis (in neonates only); abnormal skin color (e.g., pale, dusky)

Abnormal breathing (e.g., rate, rhythm, depth); nasal flaring

Tachycardia; [dysrhythmias]

Diaphoresis

[Polycythemia]

Desired Outcomes/Evaluation Criteria— Client Will:

- Demonstrate improved ventilation and adequate oxygenation of tissues by ABGs within client's usual parameters and absence of symptoms of respiratory distress (as noted in Defining Characteristics).
- Verbalize understanding of causative factors and appropriate interventions.
- Participate in treatment regimen (e.g., breathing exercises, effective coughing, use of oxygen) within level of ability or situation.

Actions/Interventions

Nursing Priority No. 1.

To assess causative/contributing factors:

- Note presence of factors listed in Related Factors. Refer to NDs ineffective Airway Clearance; ineffective Breathing Pattern, as appropriate. **Gas exchange problems can be related to multiple factors, including anemias, anesthesia, surgical procedures, high altitude, allergic response, altered level of consciousness, anxiety, fear, aspiration, decreased lung compliance, excessive or thick secretions, immobility, infection, medication and drug toxicity or overdose, neuromuscular impairment of breathing pattern, pain, and smoking.**

Nursing Priority No. 2.

To evaluate degree of compromise:

- Note respiratory rate, depth, use of accessory muscles, pursed-lip breathing; areas of pallor/cyanosis, such as peripheral (nailbeds) versus central (circumoral) or general duskiness. **Provides insight into the work of breathing and adequacy**

Information that appears in brackets has been added by the authors to clarify and enhance the use of nursing diagnoses.

🌐 Cultural 😊 Collaborative 🏠 Community/Home Care

of alveolar ventilation. **Tachypnea is usually present to some degree during illness (especially with fever or upper respiratory infections), but if tachypnea is accompanied by use of accessory muscles of inspiration (e.g. external intercostals), the client may have insufficient muscle strength to sustain the work of breathing.**

- Auscultate breath sounds, note areas of decreased/adventitious breath sounds as well as fremitus. **In this nursing diagnosis, ventilatory effort is insufficient to deliver enough oxygen or to get rid of sufficient amounts of carbon dioxide. Abnormal breath sounds are indicative of numerous problems (e.g., hypoventilation such as might occur with atelectasis or presence of secretions, improper endotracheal (ET) tube placement, collapsed lung) and must be evaluated for further intervention.**
- Note character and effectiveness of cough mechanism. **Affects ability to clear airways of secretions**.
- Assess level of consciousness and mentation changes. **Decreased level of consciousness can be an indirect measurement of impaired oxygenation, but it also impairs one's ability to protect the airway, potentially further adversely affecting oxygenation.**
- Note client reports of somnolence, restlessness, headache on arising. Assess energy level and activity tolerance, noting reports or evidence of fatigue, weakness, problems with sleep **that are associated with diminished oxygenation.**
- Monitor vital signs and cardiac rhythm. **All vital signs are impacted by changes in oxygenation.**
- Evaluate pulse oximetry and capnography **to determine oxygenation and levels of carbon dioxide retention;** evaluate lung volumes and forced vital capacity **to assess lung mechanics, capacities, and function.**
- Review other pertinent laboratory data (e.g., ABGs, complete blood count (CBC)); chest x-rays.
- Note effect of illness on self-esteem and body image.

Nursing Priority No. 3.

To correct/improve existing deficiencies:

- Elevate head of bed and position client appropriately. **Elevation or upright position facilitates respiratory function by gravity; however, client in severe distress will seek position of comfort.**
- Provide airway adjuncts and suction, as indicated, **to clear or maintain open airway, when client is unable to clear**

Information that appears in brackets has been added by the authors to clarify and enhance the use of nursing diagnoses.

secretions, or to improve gas diffusion when client is showing desaturation of oxygen by oximetry or ABGs.

- Encourage frequent position changes and deep-breathing and coughing exercises. Use incentive spirometer, chest physiotherapy, intermittent positive-pressure breathing, as indicated. **Promotes optimal chest expansion, mobilization of secretions, and oxygen diffusion.**

- Provide supplemental oxygen at lowest concentration indicated by laboratory results and client symptoms or situation.

- Monitor for carbon dioxide narcosis (e.g., change in level of consciousness, changes in O_2 and CO_2 blood gas levels, flushing, decreased respiratory rate, headaches), **which may occur in client receiving long-term oxygen therapy.**

- Maintain adequate input and output **for mobilization of secretions,** but avoid fluid overload.

- Use sedation judiciously **to avoid depressant effects on respiratory functioning.**

- Ensure availability of proper emergency equipment, including ET/tracheostomy set and suction catheters appropriate for age and size of infant, child, or adult.

- Avoid use of face mask in elderly emaciated client **as oxygen can leak out around the mask because of poor fit, and mask can increase client's agitation.**

- Encourage adequate rest and limit activities to within client tolerance. Promote calm, restful environment. **Helps limit oxygen needs and consumption.**

- Provide psychological support, Active-listen questions/concerns **to reduce anxiety.**

- Administer medications as indicated (e.g., inhaled and systemic glucocorticosteroids, antibiotics, bronchodilators, methylxanthines, antitussives/mucolytics, vasodilators). **Pharmacological agents are varied, specific to the client, but generally used to prevent and control symptoms, reduce frequency and severity of exacerbations, and improve exercise tolerance.**

- Monitor and instruct client in therapeutic and adverse effects as well as interactions of drug therapy.

- Minimize blood loss from procedures (e.g., tests, hemodialysis) **to limit adverse affects of anemia.**

- Assist with procedures as individually indicated (e.g., transfusion, phlebotomy, bronchoscopy) **to improve respiratory function/oxygen-carrying capacity.**

- Monitor and adjust ventilator settings (e.g., fractional concentration of inspired oxygen, tidal volume, inspiratory/

Information that appears in brackets has been added by the authors to clarify and enhance the use of nursing diagnoses.

🌐 Cultural 😊 Collaborative 🏠 Community/Home Care

expiratory ratio, sigh, positive end-expiratory pressure), as indicated, when mechanical support is being used.

- Keep environment allergen and pollutant free **to reduce irritant effect of dust and chemicals on airways.**

Nursing Priority No. 4.

To promote wellness (Teaching/Discharge Considerations):

- Review risk factors, particularly environmental/employment related, **to promote prevention or management of risk.**
- Discuss implications of smoking related to the illness or condition at each visit. Encourage client and SO(s) to stop smoking; recommend smoking cessation programs **to reduce health risks and/or prevent further decline in lung function.**
- Discuss reasons for allergy testing when indicated.
- Review individual drug regimen and ways of dealing with side effects.
- Instruct in the use of relaxation, stress-reduction techniques, as appropriate.
- Reinforce need for adequate rest, while encouraging activity and exercise (e.g., upper and lower extremity strength and flexibility training, and endurance) **to decrease dyspnea and improve quality of life.**
- Emphasize the importance of nutrition **in improving stamina and reducing the work of breathing.**
- Review oxygen-conserving techniques (e.g., sitting instead of standing to perform tasks; eating small meals; performing slower, purposeful movements).
- Review job description and work activities **to identify need for job modifications or vocational rehabilitation.**
- Discuss home oxygen therapy and safety measures, as indicated, when home oxygen is implemented **to ensure client's safety, especially when used in the very young, fragile elderly, or when cognitive or neuromuscular impairment is present.**
- Identify and refer to specific suppliers for supplemental oxygen/necessary respiratory devices, as well as other individually appropriate resources, such as home care agencies, Meals on Wheels, and so on, **to facilitate independence.**

Documentation Focus

Assessment/Reassessment

- Assessment findings, including respiratory rate, character of

---

Information that appears in brackets has been added by the authors to clarify and enhance the use of nursing diagnoses.

breath sounds; frequency, amount, and appearance of secretions; presence of cyanosis; laboratory findings; and mentation level.
* Conditions that may interfere with oxygen supply.

Planning
* Plan of care, specific interventions, and who is involved in the planning.
* Ventilator settings, liters of supplemental oxygen.
* Teaching plan.

Implementation/Evaluation
* Client's responses to treatment, teaching, and actions performed.
* Attainment or progress toward desired outcome(s).
* Modifications to plan of care.

Discharge Planning
* Long-term needs, identifying who is responsible for actions to be taken.
* Community resources for equipment and supplies postdischarge.
* Specific referrals made.

Sample Nursing Outcomes & Interventions Classifications (NOC/NIC)

NOC—Respiratory Status: Gas Exchange
NIC—Respiratory Monitoring

dysfunctional Gastrointestinal Motility

Taxonomy II: Elimination and Exchange—Class 2 Gastrointestinal Function (00196)
[Diagnostic Division: Elimination]
Submitted 2008

Definition: Increased, decreased, ineffective, or lack of peristaltic activity within the gastrointestinal system

Related Factors

Aging; prematurity
Surgery
Malnutrition; enteral feedings

Information that appears in brackets has been added by the authors to clarify and enhance the use of nursing diagnoses.

⊕ Cultural ⊛ Collaborative 🏠 Community/Home Care

Pharmaceutical agents (e.g., narcotics/opiates, laxatives, antibiotics, anesthesia)

Food intolerance (e.g., gluten, lactose); ingestion of contaminants (e.g., food, water)

Sedentary lifestyle; immobility

Anxiety

Defining Characteristics

Subjective
Absence of flatus

Abdominal cramping; pain

Diarrhea

Difficulty passing stool

Nausea; regurgitation

Objective
Change in bowel sounds (e.g., absent, hypoactive, hyperactive)

Abdominal distention

Accelerated gastric emptying; diarrhea

Increased gastric residual; bile-colored gastric residual

Dry/hard stool

Vomiting

Desired Outcomes/Evaluation Criteria— Client Will:

- Reestablish and maintain normal pattern of bowel functioning.
- Verbalize understanding of causative factors and rationale for treatment regimen.
- Demonstrate appropriate behaviors to assist with resolution of causative factors.

Actions/Interventions

Nursing Priority No. 1.
To assess causative/contributing factors:

- Note presence of conditions (e.g., congestive heart failure, major trauma, chronic conditions, sepsis) affecting systemic circulation/perfusion **that can result in gastrointestinal (GI) hypoperfusion, and short- and/or long-term gastrointestinal (GI) dysfunction.**

Information that appears in brackets has been added by the authors to clarify and enhance the use of nursing diagnoses.

- Determine presence of disorders causing localized or diffuse reduction in GI blood flow, such as esophageal varices, GI hemorrhage, pancreatitis, intraperitoneal hemorrhage, **to identify client at higher risk for ineffective tissue perfusion.**
- Note presence of chronic/long-term disorders, such as gastrointestinal reflux disease (GERD), hiatal hernia, inflammatory bowel (e.g., ulcerative colitis, Crohn's disease), malabsorption (e.g., dumping syndrome, celiac disease), short-bowel syndrome, as may occur after surgical removal of portions of the small intestine. **These conditions are associated with increased, decreased, or ineffective peristaltic activity.**
- Note client's age and developmental concerns. **Premature or low-birth-weight neonates are at risk for developing necrotizing enterocolitis (NEC). Children are prone to infections causing gastroenteritis manifested by vomiting and diarrhea. The elderly have problems associated with decreased motility, such as constipation.**
- Review client's medication regimen. **Medications (e.g., laxatives, antibiotics, opiates, sedatives, iron preparations) may cause or exacerbate intestinal issues. In addition, likelihood of bleeding increases from use of medications such as nonsteroidal anti-inflammatory agents (NSAIDs), Coumadin, Plavix.**
- Note lifestyle issues that can affect GI function (**e.g., people who regularly engage in competitive sports such as long-distance running, cycling; persons with poor sanitary living conditions; people who travel to areas with contaminated food or water; overeating or intake of foods associated with gastric distress or intestinal distention**).
- Ascertain whether client is experiencing anxiety; acute, extreme or chronic stress; or other psychogenic factors present in person with emotional or psychiatric disorders (including anorexia/bulimia, etc.) **that can affect GI function.**
- Review laboratory and other diagnostic studies **to evaluate for GI problems, such as bleeding, inflammation, toxicity, and infection; or to help identify masses, dilation/obstruction, abnormal stool and gas patterns, and so forth.**

Nursing Priority No. 2.
To note degree of dysfunction/organ involvement:

- Assess vital signs, noting presence of low blood pressure, elevated heart rate, fever. **May suggest hypoperfusion or**

Information that appears in brackets has been added by the authors to clarify and enhance the use of nursing diagnoses.

developing sepsis. **Fever in presence of bright red blood in stool may indicate ischemic colitis.**

- Ascertain presence and characteristics of abdominal pain. **Pain is a common symptom of GI disorders and can vary in location, duration, and intensity.**
- Investigate reports of pain out of proportion to degree of traumatic injury. **May reflect developing abdominal compartment syndrome.**
- Inspect abdomen, noting contour. **Distention of bowel may indicate accumulation of fluids (salivary, gastric, pancreatic, biliary, and intestinal) and gases formed from bacteria, swallowed air, or any food or fluid the client has consumed.**
- Auscultate abdomen. **Hypoactive bowel sounds may indicate ileus. Hyperactive bowels sounds may indicate early intestinal obstruction or irritable bowel or GI bleeding.**
- Palpate abdomen **to note masses, enlarged organs (such as spleen, liver, or portions of colon); elicitation of pain with touch; pulsation of aorta.**
- Measure abdominal girth and compare with client's customary waist size or belt length **to monitor development or progression of distention.**
- Note frequency and characteristics of bowel movements. **Bowel movements by themselves are not necessarily diagnostic, but need to be considered in total assessment as they may reveal underlying problem or effect of pathology.**
- Note presence of nausea, with or without vomiting, and relationship to food intake or other events, if indicated. **History can provide important information about cause (e.g., pregnancy, gastroenteritis, cancers, myocardial infarction, hepatitis, systemic infections, contaminated food, drug toxicity).**
- Evaluate client's current nutritional status, noting ability to ingest and digest food. **Health depends on the intake, digestion and absorption of nutrients, which both affect and are affected by GI function.**
- Measure intra-abdominal pressure as indicated. **Tissue edema or free fluid collecting in the abdominal cavity leads to intra-abdominal hypertension, which if untreated, can cause abdominal compartment syndrome with end-stage organ failure.**

Information that appears in brackets has been added by the authors to clarify and enhance the use of nursing diagnoses.

dysfunctional GASTROINTESTINAL MOTILITY

Nursing Priority No. 3.

To correct/improve existing dysfunction:

- Collaborate in treatment of underlying conditions **to correct or treat disorders associated with client's current GI dysfunction.**
- Maintain GI rest when indicated—nothing by mouth (NPO) fluids only, gastric or intestinal decompression **to reduce intestinal bloating and risk of vomiting.**
- Measure GI output periodically, and note characteristics of drainage **to manage fluid losses and replacement needs.**
- Administer fluids and electrolytes as indicated **to replace losses and to improve GI circulation and function.**
- Encourage early ambulation. **Promotes general circulation, stimulates peristalsis and intestinal function.**
- Collaborate with dietitian or nutritionist **to provide diet sufficient in nutrients by best possible route—oral, enteral, parenteral.**
- Provide small servings of easily digested food and fluids when oral intake tolerated.
- Encourage rest after meals **to maximize blood flow to digestive system.**
- Manage pain with medications as ordered, and nonpharmacological interventions such as positioning, back rub, heating pad (unless contraindicated) **to enhance muscle relaxation and reduce discomfort.**
- Encourage client to report changes in nature or intensity of pain, **as this may indicate worsening of condition, requiring more intensive interventions.**
- Collaborate with physician for medication management. **Dose modification, discontinuation of certain drugs, or alternative route of administration may be required to improve client's GI tolerance and/or function.**
- Prepare client for procedures and surgery, as indicated. **May require a variety of interventions to treat problem causing or contributing to severe GI dysfunction.**

Nursing Priority No. 4.

To promote wellness (Teaching/Discharge Considerations):

- Provide information regarding cause of GI dysfunction and treatment plans, utilizing best learning methods for client, and including written information, bibliography, and other resources **for postdischarge learning.**
- Discuss normal variations in bowel patterns **to help alleviate unnecessary concern, initiate planned interventions, or**

Information that appears in brackets has been added by the authors to clarify and enhance the use of nursing diagnoses.

seek timely medical care. **May prevent overuse of laxatives or help client understand when food, fluid, or drug modifications are needed.**

- Encourage discussion of feelings regarding prognosis and long-term effects of condition. **Major or unplanned life changes can strain coping abilities, impairing functioning and jeopardizing relationships, and may even result in depression.**
- Discuss value of relaxation and distraction techniques or counseling **if anxiety or other emotional/psychiatric issue is suspected to play a role in GI dysfunction.**
- Identify necessary changes in lifestyle and assist client to incorporate disease management into activities of daily living (ADLs). **Promotes independence and ability to manage own needs.**
- Review specific dietary changes and restrictions with client. **May need adaptations in food choices and eating habits (e.g., may need to avoid overeating in general, schedule mealtime in relation to activities and bedtime, avoid certain foods [or food element, such as wheat or gluten] and/ or alcohol).**
- Suggest healthier variations in preparation of foods, as indicated—broiled instead of fried, spices added to foods instead of salt, addition of higher fiber foods, use of lactose-free dairy products—**when these factors are affecting GI health.**
- Discuss fluid intake appropriate to individual situation. **Water is necessary to general health and GI function; client may need encouragement to increase intake or to make appropriate fluid choices if intake restricted for certain medical conditions.**
- Recommend maintenance of normal weight, or weight loss if client obese, **to decrease risk associated with GI disorders such as GERD or gallbladder disease.**
- Emphasize benefits of regular exercise in promoting normal GI function.
- Recommend smoking cessation. **Risk for acquiring or exacerbating certain GI disorders (e.g., Crohn's disease) may be increased with smoking. Also, recent review of relevant studies reveals various deleterious short- and long-term effects of smoking on the GI organs.**
- Discuss medication regimen, including reasons for and consequences of failure to take prescribed long-term maintenance. **Nonadherance can negatively affect treatment efficacy and client's quality of life.**

Information that appears in brackets has been added by the authors to clarify and enhance the use of nursing diagnoses.

- Emphasize importance of avoiding use of NSAIDs, including aspirin; corticosteroids; some over-the-counter drugs; vitamins containing potassium; mineral oil; or alcohol when taking anticoagulants. **These medications can be harmful to GI mucosa and increase risk of bleeding.**
- Refer to NDs bowel Incontinence; Constipation; Diarrhea, for additional interventions.

Documentation Focus

Assessment/Reassessment
- Individual findings, noting nature, extent, and duration of problem, effect on independence and lifestyle.
- Dietary pattern, recent intake, food intolerances.
- Frequency and characteristics of stools.
- Characteristics of abdominal tenderness or pain, precipitators, and what relieves pain.

Planning
- Plan of care and who is involved in planning.
- Teaching plan.

Implementation/Evaluation
- Response to interventions, teaching, and actions performed.
- Attainment or progress toward desired outcome(s).
- Modifications to plan of care.

Discharge Planning
- Long-term needs and who is responsible for actions to be taken.
- Available resources, specific referrals made.

Sample Nursing Outcomes & Interventions Classifications (NOC/NIC)

NOC—Gastrointestinal Function
NIC—Bowel Management

Information that appears in brackets has been added by the authors to clarify and enhance the use of nursing diagnoses.

risk for dysfunctional Gastrointestinal Motility

Taxonomy II: Elimination and Exchange—Class 2 Gastrointestinal Function (00197)
[Diagnostic Division: Elimination]
Submitted 2008

Definition: At risk for increased, decreased, ineffective, or lack of peristaltic activity within the gastrointestinal system

Risk Factors

Aging; prematurity
Abdominal surgery; decreased gastrointestinal circulation
Food intolerance (e.g., gluten, lactose); change in food or water; unsanitary food preparation
Pharmaceutical agents (e.g., antibiotics, laxatives, narcotics/opiates, proton pump inhibitors)
Gastrointestinal reflux disease (GERD)
Diabetes mellitus
Infection (e.g., bacterial, parasitic, viral)
Sedentary lifestyle; immobility
Stress; anxiety

NOTE: A risk diagnosis is not evidenced by signs and symptoms, as the problem has not occurred; rather, nursing interventions are directed at prevention.

Desired Outcomes/Evaluation Criteria—Client Will (Include Specific Time Frame):

* Maintain normal pattern of bowel functioning.
* Verbalize understanding of individual risk factors and benefits of managing condition.
* Identify preventive interventions to reduce risk and promote normal bowel pattern.

Actions/Interventions

Nursing Priority No. 1.

* Note presence of conditions affecting systemic circulation or perfusion such as congestive heart failure, major trauma with

---

Information that appears in brackets has been added by the authors to clarify and enhance the use of nursing diagnoses.

blood loss, sepsis, shock, **which can result in hypoperfusion and short- or long-term gastrointestinal (GI) dysfunction.**

- Determine presence of disorders (e.g., esophageal varices, pancreatitis), foreign body ingestion, or prior abdominal surgery with adhesions, **which can impact peristaltic activity.**
- Assess client's current situation with regard to prior GI history. **Client may have an isolated incident putting him or her at risk (e.g., blunt force trauma to abdomen, prior history of strangulated hernia) or be at higher risk for recurrent GI dysfunction associated with history of prior GI problems.**
- Auscultate abdomen **to evaluate peristaltic activity and note developing bowel disorders.**
- Palpate abdomen for masses, enlarged organs (e.g., spleen, liver, or portions of colon), elicitation of pain with touch **that could point to changes in organ size or function.**
- Note frequency and characteristics of bowel movements. **Bowel movements by themselves are not necessarily diagnostic, but they can help make a differential diagnosis.**
- Ascertain presence and characteristics of abdominal pain. **Pain is a common symptom of GI disorders, with location and type aiding in identifying underlying problems.**
- Assess vital signs for changes in blood pressure, heart rate, or body temperature. **May suggest injury or infection of the GI organs, or developing systemic infection/sepsis**.
- Evaluate client's current nutritional status, noting ability to ingest and digest food.
- ∞ Note client's age and developmental concerns. **Premature/low-birth-weight neonates are at risk for developing necrotizing enterocolitis (NEC). Children are prone to infections causing gastroenteritis manifested by vomiting and diarrhea. The elderly have problems associated with decreased motility (e.g., constipation related to slower peristalsis, lack of sufficient fiber and fluid intake, or chronic use of laxatives).**
- Note lifestyle issues **that can affect GI function (e.g., people who regularly engage in competitive sports such as long-distance running, cycling; persons with poor sanitary living conditions; people who travel to areas with contaminated food or water; overeating or intake of foods associated with gastric distress or intestinal distention; anorexia or bulimia).**
- Ascertain whether client is experiencing anxiety, stress, or other psychogenic factors.
- Review client's drug regimen. **Medications such as laxatives, antibiotics, anticholesterol agents, opiates, sedatives,**

Information that appears in brackets has been added by the authors to clarify and enhance the use of nursing diagnoses.

iron preparations, and nonsteroidal anti-inflammatory agents (NSAIDs) may cause or exacerbate intestinal issues.

- Review laboratory and other diagnostic studies **to identify factors that may affect GI function.**

Nursing Priority No. 2.

To reduce or correct individual risk factors:

- Discuss normal variations in bowel patterns **so client can initiate planned interventions, or seek timely medical care.**
- Collaborate in treatment of underlying conditions.
- Practice and promote hand hygiene and other infection precautions **to prevent transmission of infections that may cause or spread gastrointestinal illnesses.**
- Maintain GI rest when indicated (e.g., nothing by mouth [NPO], fluids only, gastric or intestinal decompression after abdominal surgery) **to reduce intestinal bloating and reduce risk of vomiting.**
- Administer fluids and electrolytes as indicated **to replace losses and to maintain GI circulation and function.**
- Administer prescribed prophylactic medications **to reduce potential for GI complications such as bleeding, ulceration of stomach mucosa, viral diarrheas.**
- Collaborate with dietitian or nutritionist **to provide diet sufficient in nutrients and provided by best possible route (e.g., oral, enteral, parenteral).**
- Emphasize importance and assist with early ambulation, especially following surgery, **to stimulate peristalsis and help reduce GI complications associated with immobility.**
- Encourage relaxation and distraction techniques if anxiety is suspected to play a role in GI dysfunction.
- Refer to NDs bowel Incontinence, Constipation; Diarrhea; dysfunctional GastroIntestinal Motility, for additional interventions.

Nursing Priority No. 3.

To promote wellness (Teaching/Discharge Considerations):

- Review measures to maintain bowel health:

  Use of dietary fiber and/or stool softeners.

  Fluid intake appropriate to individual.

  Establish or maintain regular bowel evacuation habits, incorporating privacy needs, assistance to bathroom on regular schedule, and so forth, as indicated.

  Emphasize benefits of regular exercise in promoting normal GI function.

Information that appears in brackets has been added by the authors to clarify and enhance the use of nursing diagnoses.

- Discuss dietary recommendations with client/SO. **The client may elect to make adaptations in food choices and eating habits to avoid GI complications.**
- Instruct in healthier variations in preparation of foods, as indicated **when these factors may affect GI health.**
- Recommend maintenance of normal weight, or weight loss if client obese, **to decrease risk associated with GI disorders such as GERD or gallbladder disease.**
- Collaborate with physician in medication management. **Dose modification, discontinuation of certain drugs (e.g., laxatives, opioids, antidepressants, iron supplements), or alternative route of administration may be required to reduce risk of GI dysfunction.**
- Emphasize importance of discussing with physician current and new prescribed medications, and/or planned use of certain medications (e.g., NSAIDs, including aspirin; corticosteroids, some over-the-counter (OTC) drugs, herbal supplements) **that can be harmful to GI mucosa.**
- Recommend smoking cessation. **Studies have shown various deleterious short- and long-term effects of smoking on the GI circulation and organs. Smoking is a risk factor for acquiring or exacerbating certain GI disorders such as Crohn's disease.**
- Review foodborne and waterborne illnesses, contamination and hygiene issues, as indicated, and make needed follow-up referrals.
- Refer to appropriate resources (e.g., Social Services, Public Health Services) **for follow-up if client at risk for ingestion of contaminated water or food sources or would benefit from teaching concerning food preparation and storage.**
- Recommend and/or refer to physician for vaccines as indicated. **The Centers for Disease Control and Prevention (CDC) make recommendations for travelers and/or persons in high-risk areas or situations in which person might be exposed to contaminated food or water.**

Documentation Focus

Assessment/Reassessment
- Individual findings, noting specific risk factors.
- Dietary pattern, recent intake, food intolerances.
- Frequency and characteristics of stools.

Information that appears in brackets has been added by the authors to clarify and enhance the use of nursing diagnoses.

🌐 Cultural 🔄 Collaborative 🏠 Community/Home Care

Planning
- Plan of care and who is involved in planning.
- Teaching plan.

Implementation/Evaluation
- Response to interventions, teaching, and actions performed.
- Attainment or progress toward desired outcome(s).
- Modifications to plan of care.

Discharge Planning
- Long-term needs and who is responsible for actions to be taken.
- Available resources, specific referrals made.

Sample Nursing Outcomes & Interventions Classifications (NOC/NIC)

NOC—Gastrointestinal Function
NIC—Bowel Management

risk for ineffective Gastrointestinal Perfusion

Taxonomy II: Activity/Rest Class 4: Cardiovascular/
  Pulmonary Responses (00197)
[Diagnostic Division: Circulation]
Submitted 2008

Definition: At risk for change in gastrointestinal circulation that may compromise health

Risk Factors

Acute gastrointestinal hemorrhage; [hypovolemia]

Trauma; abdominal compartment syndrome

Vascular disease (e.g., peripheral vascular disease, aortoiliac occlusive disease); abdominal aortic aneurysm

Myocardial infarction; poor left ventricular performance; hemodynamic instability

Coagulopathy (e.g., sickle cell anemia, disseminated intravascular coagulation), abnormal partial thromboplastin time, abnormal prothrombin time; [emboli]

Gastrointestinal disease (e.g., duodenal or gastric ulcer, ischemic colitis, ischemic pancreatitis); gastric paresis; gastroesophageal varices

---

Information that appears in brackets has been added by the authors to clarify and enhance the use of nursing diagnoses.

Liver dysfunction; renal failure; diabetes mellitus; stroke

Smoking

Treatment-related side effects (e.g., cardiopulmonary bypass, medication, anesthesia, gastric surgery)

Age over 60 years; female gender

NOTE: A risk diagnosis is not evidenced by signs and symptoms, as the problem has not occurred; rather, nursing interventions are directed at prevention.

Desired Outcomes/Evaluation Criteria—Client Will (Include Specific Time Frame):

- Demonstrate adequate tissue perfusion as evidenced by active bowel sounds; absence of abdominal pain, nausea, and vomiting
- Verbalize understanding of condition, therapy regimen, side effects of medication, and when to contact healthcare provider.
- Engage in behaviors and lifestyle changes to improve circulation.

Actions/Interventions

Nursing Priority No. 1.

To identify individual risk factors/needs:

- Note presence of conditions affecting systemic circulation and perfusion such as heart failure with left ventricular dysfunction, major trauma with blood loss and hypotension, septic shock, and so forth. **Blood loss and hypovolemic or hypotensive shock can result in gastrointestinal (GI) hypoperfusion and bowel ischemia.**
- Determine presence of disorders such as esophageal varices, pancreatitis; abdominal or chest trauma, increase of intra-abdominal pressure; prior history of bowel obstruction or strangulated hernia, **which could cause local or regional reduction in GI blood flow.**
- Identify client with history of bleeding or coagulation disorders, such as prior GI bleed, coagulopathies; cancer, **to identify risk for potential bleeding problems.**
- Note client's age and gender when assessing for impaired GI perfusion (**e.g., studies suggest that risk for GI bleeding increases with age in both sexes, but that risk for abdominal aortic aneurysm is higher in men than in women**).

Information that appears in brackets has been added by the authors to clarify and enhance the use of nursing diagnoses.

Premature or low-birth-weight neonates are at risk for developing necrotizing enterocolitis (NEC).

• Investigate reports of abdominal pain, noting location, intensity, and duration. **Many disorders can result in abdominal pain, some of which can include conditions affecting gastrointestinal perfusion such as postprandial abdominal angina due to occlusive mesenteric vascular disease, abdominal compartment syndrome, or other potential perforating disorders such as duodenal or gastric ulcer, or ischemic pancreatitis.**

• Review routine medication regimen (e.g., nonsteroidal anti-inflammatory drugs (NSAIDs), Coumadin, low-dose aspirin such as used for prophylaxis in certain cardiovascular conditions, corticosteroids). **Likelihood of bleeding increases from use of these medications.**

• Note history of smoking, **which can potentiate vasoconstriction; or excessive alcohol use/abuse, which can cause general inflammation of the stomach mucosa and potentiate risk of GI bleeding; or liver involvement and esophageal varices.**

• Auscultate abdomen to evaluate peristaltic activity. **Hypoactive or absent bowel sounds may indicate intraperitoneal injury, bowel perforation, and bleeding. Abdominal bruit can indicate abdominal aortic injury or aneurysm.**

• Palpate abdomen for distention, masses, enlarged organs (such as spleen, liver, or portions of colon); elicitation of pain with touch; pulsation of aorta.

• Percuss abdomen for fixed or shifting dullness over regions that normally contain air. **Can indicate accumulated blood or fluid.**

• Measure and monitor progression of abdominal girth as indicated. **Can reflect bowel problems such as obstruction, or organ failure (e.g., heart, liver, or kidney) or organ injury with intra-abdominal fluid and gas accumulation.**

• Note reports of nausea or vomiting accompanied by problems with bowel elimination. **May reflect hypoperfusion of the GI tract, which is particularly vulnerable to even small decreases in circulating volume.**

• Assess client with severe or prolonged vomiting, or forceful coughing, engaging in lifting or straining activities or childbirth, **which can result in a tear in the esophageal or stomach wall, resulting in hemorrhage.**

• Evaluate stool color and consistency. Test for occult blood, as indicated.

Information that appears in brackets has been added by the authors to clarify and enhance the use of nursing diagnoses.

- Test gastric suction contents for blood when tube is used to decompress stomach and/or manage vomiting.
- Assess vital signs, noting sustained hypotension, **which can result in hypoperfusion of abdominal organs.**
- Review laboratory and other diagnostic studies (e.g., complete blood count (CBC), bilirubin, liver enzymes, electrolytes, stool guaiac; endoscopy, abdominal ultrasound or computed tomography (CT) scan, aortic angiography, paracentesis) **to identify any conditions or disorders that may affect GI perfusion and function.**

Nursing Priority No. 2.
To reduce or correct individual risk factors:

- Collaborate in treatment of underlying conditions **to correct or treat disorders that could affect GI perfusion.**
- Administer fluids and electrolytes as indicated **to replace losses and to maintain GI circulation and cellular function.**
- Administer prescribed prophylactic medications in at-risk clients during illness and hospitalization (e.g., anti-emetics, proton pump inhibitors, antihistamines, anticholinergics, antibiotics) **to reduce potential for stress-related GI complications.**
- Maintain gastric or intestinal decompression, when indicated; measure output periodically, and note characteristics of drainage.
- Provide small, easily digested food and fluids when oral intake tolerated.
- Encourage rest after meals **to maximize blood flow to digestive system.**
- Prepare client for surgery as indicated such as gastric resection, bypass graft, mesenteric endarterectomy.
- Refer to NDs dysfunctional Gastrointestinal Motility; Nausea; imbalanced Nutrition: less than body requirements, for additional interventions.

Nursing Priority No. 3.
To promote wellness (Teaching/Discharge Considerations):

- Discuss individual risk factors (e.g., family history, obesity, age, smoking, hypertension, diabetes, clotting disorders) and potential outcomes of atherosclerosis (e.g., systemic and peripheral vascular disease conditions), as appropriate. **Information necessary for client to make informed choices about remedial risk factors and commit to lifestyle changes.**

Information that appears in brackets has been added by the authors to clarify and enhance the use of nursing diagnoses.

🌐 Cultural ☯ Collaborative 🏠 Community/Home Care

- Identify necessary changes in lifestyle and assist client to incorporate disease management into activities of daily living (ADLs).
- Encourage client to quit smoking, join Smoke-out, other smoking-cessation programs **to reduce risk of vasoconstriction compromising GI perfusion.**
- Establish regular exercise program **to enhance circulation and promote general well-being.**
- Emphasize importance of routine follow-up and laboratory monitoring as indicated. **Important for effective disease management and possible changes in therapeutic regimen.**
- Emphasize importance of discussing with primary care provider current and new prescribed medications, and/or planned use of certain medications (e.g., anticoagulants, NSAIDs including aspirin; corticosteroids, some over-the-counter drugs, herbal supplements), **which can be harmful to GI mucosa or cause bleeding.**

Documentation Focus

Assessment/Reassessment
- Individual findings, noting specific risk factors.
- Vital signs, adequacy of circulation.
- Abdominal assessment, characteristics of emesis or gastric drainage and stools.

Planning
- Plan of care and who is involved in planning.
- Teaching plan.

Implementation/Evaluation
- Response to interventions, teaching, and actions performed.
- Attainment or progress toward desired outcome(s).
- Modifications to plan of care.

Discharge Planning
- Long-term needs and who is responsible for actions to be taken.
- Available resources, specific referrals made.

Sample Nursing Outcomes & Interventions Classifications (NOC/NIC)

NOC—Tissue Perfusion: Abdominal Organs
NIC—Surveillance

Information that appears in brackets has been added by the authors to clarify and enhance the use of nursing diagnoses.

Grieving

Taxonomy II: Coping/Stress Tolerance—Class 2 Coping
  Responses (00136)
[Diagnostic Division: Ego Integrity]
Submitted as anticipatory Grieving 1980; Revised 1996,
  2006

Definition: A normal complex process that includes emotional, physical, spiritual, social, and intellectual responses and behaviors by which individuals, families, and communities incorporate an actual, anticipated, or perceived loss into their daily lives

Related Factors

Anticipatory loss or loss of significant object (e.g., possessions, job, status, home, parts and processes of body)
Anticipatory loss or loss/death of a significant other

Defining Characteristics

Subjective

Anger; pain; suffering; despair; blame
Alteration in activity level; alterations in dream patterns; disturbed sleep pattern
Making meaning of the loss; personal growth
Experiencing relief

Objective

Detachment; disorganization; psychological distress; panic behavior
Maintaining the connection to the deceased
Alterations in immune or neuroendocrine function

Desired Outcomes/Evaluation Criteria— Client/Family Will:

- Identify and express feelings (e.g., sadness, guilt, fear) freely and effectively.
- Acknowledge impact or effect of the grieving process (e.g., physical problems of eating, sleeping) and seek appropriate help.
- Look toward and plan for future, one day at a time.

Information that appears in brackets has been added by the authors to clarify and enhance the use of nursing diagnoses.

Cultural   Collaborative   Community/Home Care

Community Will:

- Recognize needs of citizens, including underserved population.
- Activate or develop plan to address identified needs.

Actions/Interventions

Nursing Priority No. 1.

To identify causative/contributing factors:

- Determine circumstances of current situation (e.g., sudden death, prolonged fatal illness, loved one kept alive by extreme medical interventions). **Grief can be anticipatory (mourning the loss of loved one's former self before actual death) or actual. Both types of grief can provoke a wide range of intense and often conflicting feelings. Grief also follows losses other than death (e.g., traumatic loss of a limb, loss of home by a tornado, loss of known self due to brain injury).**
- Evaluate client's perception of anticipated or actual loss and meaning to him or her: "What are your concerns?" "What are your fears?" "Your greatest fear?" "How do you see this affecting you or your lifestyle?"
- Identify cultural or religious beliefs that may impact sense of loss.
- Ascertain response of family/SO(s) to client's situation and concerns.
- Determine significance of loss to community (e.g., school bus accident with loss of life, major tornado damage to infrastructure, financial failure of major employer).

Nursing Priority No. 2.

To determine current response:

- Note emotional responses, such as withdrawal, angry behavior, crying.
- Observe client's body language and check out meaning with the client. Note congruency with verbalizations.
- Note cultural and religious expectations that may dictate client's responses **to assess appropriateness of client's reaction to the situation.**
- Identify problems with eating, activity level, sexual desire, role performance (e.g., work, parenting). **Indicators of severity of feelings client is experiencing and need for specific interventions to address these issues.**

Information that appears in brackets has been added by the authors to clarify and enhance the use of nursing diagnoses.

GRIEVING

- Determine impact on general well-being (e.g., increased frequency of minor illnesses, exacerbation of chronic condition).
- Note family communication and interaction patterns.
- Determine availability and use of community resources and support groups.
- Note community plans in place to deal with major loss (e.g., team of crisis counselors stationed at a school to address the loss of classmates, vocational counselors or retraining programs, outreach of services from neighboring communities).

Nursing Priority No. 3.

To assist client/community to deal with situation:

- Provide open environment and trusting relationship. **Promotes a free discussion of feelings and concerns.**
- Use therapeutic communication skills of Active-listening, silence, acknowledgment. Respect client desire/request not to talk.
- Inform children about death or anticipated loss in age-appropriate language. **Providing accurate information about impending loss or change in life situation will help child begin mourning process.**
- Provide puppets or play therapy for toddlers and young children. **May help them more readily express grief and deal with loss.**
- Permit appropriate expressions of anger, fear. Note hostility toward or feelings of abandonment by spiritual power. (Refer to appropriate NDs; e.g., Spiritual Distress.)
- Provide information about normalcy of individual grief reaction.
- Be honest when answering questions, providing information. **Enhances sense of trust and nurse-client relationship.**
- Provide assurance to child that cause for situation is not own doing, bearing in mind age and developmental level. **May lessen sense of guilt and affirm there is no need to assign blame to self or any family member.**
- Provide hope within parameters of specific situation. Refrain from giving false reassurance.
- Review past life experiences and previous loss(es), role changes, and coping skills, noting strengths and successes. **May be useful in dealing with current situation and problem solving existing needs.**
- Discuss control issues, such as what is in the power of the individual to change and what is beyond control. **Recognition**

Information that appears in brackets has been added by the authors to clarify and enhance the use of nursing diagnoses.

Cultural Collaborative Community/Home Care

of these factors helps client focus energy for maximal benefit and outcome.

- Incorporate family/SO(s) in problem solving. **Encourages family to support and assist client to deal with situation while meeting needs of family members.**
- Determine client's status and role in family (e.g., parent, sibling, child) and address loss of family member role.
- Instruct in use of visualization and relaxation techniques.
- Use sedatives or tranquilizers with caution. **May retard passage through the grief process, although short-term use may be beneficial to enhance sleep.**
- Encourage community members or groups to engage in talking about event or loss and verbalizing feelings. Seek out underserved populations to include in process.
- Encourage individuals to participate in activities to deal with loss, rebuild community.

Nursing Priority No. 4.

To promote wellness (Teaching/Discharge Considerations):

- Give information that feelings are okay and are to be expressed appropriately. **Expression of feelings can facilitate the grieving process, but destructive behavior can be damaging.**
- Provide information that on birthdays, major holidays, at times of significant personal events, or anniversary of loss, client may experience (needs to be prepared for) intense grief reactions. **If these reactions start to disrupt day-to-day functioning, client may need to seek help.** (Refer to NDs complicated Grieving; ineffective community Coping, as appropriate.)
- Encourage continuation of usual activities or schedule and involvement in appropriate exercise program.
- Identify and promote family and social support systems.
- Discuss and assist with planning for future or funeral, as appropriate.
- Refer to additional resources, such as pastoral care, counseling, psychotherapy, community or organized support groups (including hospice), as indicated, for both client and family/SO(s), **to meet ongoing needs and facilitate grief work.**
- Support community efforts to strengthen support or develop plan to foster recovery and growth.

Information that appears in brackets has been added by the authors to clarify and enhance the use of nursing diagnoses.

Documentation Focus

Assessment/Reassessment
- Assessment findings, including client's perception of anticipated loss and signs/symptoms that are being exhibited.
- Responses of family/SO(s) or community members, as indicated.
- Availability and use of resources.

Planning
- Plan of care and who is involved in planning.
- Teaching plan.

Implementation/Evaluation
- Client's response to interventions, teaching, and actions performed.
- Attainment or progress toward desired outcome(s).
- Modifications to plan of care.

Discharge Planning
- Long-term needs and who is responsible for actions to be taken.
- Specific referrals made.

Sample Nursing Outcomes & Interventions Classifications (NOC/NIC)

NOC—Grief Resolution
NIC—Grief Work Facilitation

---

complicated Grieving

Taxonomy II: Coping/Stress Tolerance—Class 2 Coping Responses (00135)
[Diagnostic Division: Ego Integrity]
Submitted as dysfunctional Grieving 1980; Revised 1996, 2004, 2006

Definition: A disorder that occurs after the death of a significant other, in which the experience of distress accompanying bereavement fails to follow normative expectations and manifests in functional impairment

---

Information that appears in brackets has been added by the authors to clarify and enhance the use of nursing diagnoses.

🌐 Cultural   ✪ Collaborative   🏠 Community/Home Care

Related Factors

Death of a significant other
Emotional instability
Lack of social support
Loss of significant object (e.g., possessions, job, status, home, parts and processes of body)

Defining Characteristics

Subjective

Reports anxiety, lack of acceptance of the death, persistent painful memories, distressful feelings about the deceased, self-blame
Reports feelings of anger, disbelief, detachment from others, mistrust
Reports feeling dazed, empty, stunned, in shock
Decreased sense of well-being; fatigue; low levels of intimacy; depression
Yearning

Objective

Decreased functioning in life roles
Persistent emotional distress; separation or traumatic distress
Preoccupation with thoughts of the deceased; longing for the deceased, searching for the deceased; self-blame
Experiencing somatic symptoms of the deceased
Rumination
Grief avoidance

Desired Outcomes/Evaluation Criteria— Client Will:

- Acknowledge presence and impact of dysfunctional situation.
- Demonstrate progress in dealing with stages of grief at own pace.
- Participate in work and self-care activities of daily living (ADLs) as able.
- Verbalize a sense of progress toward grief resolution, hope for the future.

Information that appears in brackets has been added by the authors to clarify and enhance the use of nursing diagnoses.

Actions/Interventions

Nursing Priority No. 1.

To determine causative/contributing factors:

- Identify loss that is present. Note circumstances of death, such as sudden or traumatic (e.g., fatal accident, suicide, homicide), related to socially sensitive issue (e.g., AIDS, suicide, murder) or associated with unfinished business (e.g., spouse died during time of crisis in marriage; son has not spoken to parent for years). **These situations can sometimes cause individual to become stuck in grief and unable to move forward with life.**
- Determine significance of the loss to client (e.g., presence of chronic condition leading to divorce or disruption of family unit and change in lifestyle, financial security).
- Identify cultural or religious beliefs and expectations that may impact or dictate client's response to loss.
- Ascertain response of family/SO(s) to client's situation (e.g., sympathetic or urging client to "just get over it").

Nursing Priority No. 2.

To determine degree of impairment/dysfunction:

- Observe for cues of sadness (e.g., sighing; faraway look; unkempt appearance; inattention to conversation; somatic complaints, such as exhaustion, headaches).
- Listen to words/communications indicative of renewed or intense grief (e.g., constantly bringing up death or loss even in casual conversation long after event; outbursts of anger at relatively minor events; expressing desire to die), **indicating person is possibly unable to adjust or move on from feelings of severe grief.**
- Identify stage of grief being expressed: denial, isolation, anger, bargaining, depression, acceptance.
- Determine level of functioning, ability to care for self.
- Note availability and use of support systems and community resources.
- Be aware of avoidance behaviors (e.g., anger, withdrawal, long periods of sleeping, or refusing to interact with family; sudden or radical changes in lifestyle; inability to handle everyday responsibilities at home, work, or school; conflict).
- Determine if client is engaging in reckless or self-destructive behaviors (e.g., substance abuse, heavy drinking, promiscuity, aggression) **to identify safety issues.**

Information that appears in brackets has been added by the authors to clarify and enhance the use of nursing diagnoses.

Cultural   Collaborative   Community/Home Care

- Identify cultural factors and ways individual has dealt with previous loss(es) **to put current behavior and responses in context.**
- Refer to mental health providers for specific diagnostic studies and intervention in issues associated with debilitating grief.
- Refer to ND Grieving for additional interventions, as appropriate.

Nursing Priority No. 3.

To assist client to deal appropriately with loss:

- Encourage verbalization without confrontation about realities. **Helps to begin resolution and acceptance.**
- Encourage client to talk about what he or she chooses and refrain from forcing the client to "face the facts."
- Active-listen feelings and be available for support and assistance. Speak in soft, caring tone.
- Encourage expression of anger, fear, and anxiety. Refer to appropriate NDs.
- Permit verbalization of anger with acknowledgment of feelings and setting of limits regarding destructive behavior. **Enhances client safety and promotes resolution of grief process.**
- Acknowledge reality of feelings of guilt or blame, including hostility toward spiritual power. Do not minimize loss, avoid clichés and easy answers. (Refer to ND Spiritual Distress.) Assist client to take steps toward resolution.
- Respect the client's needs and wishes for quiet, privacy, talking, or silence.
- Give "permission" to be at this point when the client is depressed.
- Provide comfort and availability as well as caring for physical needs.
- Reinforce use of previously effective coping skills. Instruct in, or encourage use of, visualization and relaxation techniques.
- Assist SO(s) to cope with client's response and include age-specific interventions. **Family/SO(s) may not understand or be intolerant of client's distress and inadvertently hamper client's progress.**
- Include family/SO(s) in setting realistic goals for meeting needs of family members.
- Encourage family members to participate in support group or family focused therapy as indicated.

Information that appears in brackets has been added by the authors to clarify and enhance the use of nursing diagnoses.

- 🖌• Use sedatives or tranquilizers with caution **to avoid retarding resolution of grief process.**

Nursing Priority No. 4.

🏠 To promote wellness (Teaching/Discharge Considerations):

- Discuss with client/SO(s) healthy ways of dealing with difficult situations.
- 🌐• Have client identify familial, religious, and cultural factors that have meaning for him or her. **May help bring loss into perspective and promote grief resolution.**
- Encourage involvement in usual activities, exercise, and socialization within limits of physical ability and psychological state.
- Advocate planning for the future, as appropriate, to individual situation (e.g., staying in own home after death of spouse, returning to sporting activities following traumatic amputation, choice to have another child or to adopt, rebuilding home following a disaster).
- 🩺• Refer to other resources (e.g., pastoral care, family counseling, psychotherapy, organized support groups). **Provides additional help, when needed, to resolve situation/continue grief work.**

Documentation Focus

Assessment/Reassessment

- Assessment findings, including meaning of loss to the client, current stage of the grieving process, and responses of family/SO(s).
- Cultural or religious beliefs and expectations.
- Availability and use of resources.

Planning

- Plan of care and who is involved in the planning.
- Teaching plan.

Implementation/Evaluation

- Client's response to interventions, teaching, and actions performed.
- Attainment or progress toward desired outcome(s).
- Modifications to plan of care.

Information that appears in brackets has been added by the authors to clarify and enhance the use of nursing diagnoses.

🌐 Cultural 🩺 Collaborative 🏠 Community/Home Care

Discharge Planning

- Long-term needs and who is responsible for actions to be taken.
- Specific referrals made.

Sample Nursing Outcomes & Interventions Classifications (NOC/NIC)

NOC—Grief Resolution
NIC—Grief Work Facilitation

risk for complicated Grieving

Taxonomy II: Coping/Stress Tolerance – Class 2 Coping Responses (00172)
[Diagnostic Division: Ego Integrity]
Submitted as risk for dysfunctional Grieving 2004; Revised 2006

Definition: At risk for a disorder that occurs after the death of a significant other, in which the experience of distress accompanying bereavement fails to follow normative expectations and manifests in functional impairment

Risk Factors

Death of a significant other
Emotional instability
Lack of social support
[Loss of significant object (e.g., possessions, job, status, home, parts and processes of body)]

NOTE: A risk diagnosis is not evidenced by signs and symptoms, as the problem has not occurred; rather, nursing interventions are directed at prevention.

Desired Outcomes/Evaluation Criteria— Client Will:

- Acknowledge awareness of individual factors affecting client in this situation. (See Risk Factors.)
- Identify emotional responses and behaviors occurring after the death or loss.

Information that appears in brackets has been added by the authors to clarify and enhance the use of nursing diagnoses.

• Participate in therapy to learn new ways of dealing with anxiety and feelings of inadequacy.
• Discuss meaning of loss to individual/family.
• Verbalize a sense of beginning to deal with grief process.

Actions/Interventions

Nursing Priority No. 1.
To identify risk/contributing factors:

• Determine loss that has occurred and meaning to client. Note whether loss was sudden or expected.
∞• Ascertain gestational age of fetus at time of loss or length of life of infant or child. **Death of child may be more difficult for parents/family to deal with based on individual values and sense of life unlived.**
• Note stage of grief client is experiencing. **Stages of grief may progress in a predictable manner or stages may be random or revisited.**
• Assess client's ability to manage activities of daily living and period of time since loss has occurred. **Periods of crying, feelings of overwhelming sadness, and loss of appetite and insomnia can occur with grieving; however, when they persist and interfere with normal activities, client may need additional assistance.**
🏠• Note availability and use of support systems, community resources.
🌐• Identify cultural or religious beliefs and expectations that may impact or dictate client's response to loss.
• Assess status of relationships, marital difficulties, and adjustments to loss.

Nursing Priority No. 2.
To assist client to deal appropriately with loss:

• Discuss meaning of loss to client. Active-listen responses without judgment.
• Encourage expression of feelings, including anger, fear, or anxiety. Let client know that all feelings are okay, while setting limits on destructive behavior.
• Respect client's desire for quiet, privacy, talking, or silence.
• Acknowledge client's sense of relief or guilt at feeling relief when death follows a long and debilitating course. **Sadness and loss are still there, but the death may be a release, or client may feel guilty about having a sense of relief.**

Information that appears in brackets has been added by the authors to clarify and enhance the use of nursing diagnoses.

🌐 Cultural   🌐 Collaborative   🏠 Community/Home Care

∞• Discuss the circumstances surrounding the death of a fetus or child. Was it sudden or expected? Have other children been lost (multiple miscarriages)? Was a congenital anomaly present? **Repeated losses increase sense of futility and compromise resolution of grieving process.**
• Meet with both members of the couple **to determine how they are dealing with the loss.**
◑• Encourage client/SOs to honor cultural practices through funerals, wakes, sitting shiva, and so forth.
• Assist SO(s)/family to understand and be tolerant of client's feelings and behavior.

Nursing Priority No. 3.
🏠To promote wellness (Teaching/Discharge Considerations):
• Encourage client/SO(s) to identify healthy coping skills they have used in the past. **These can be used in current situation to facilitate dealing with grief.**
• Assist in setting goals for meeting needs of client and family members to move beyond the grieving process.
• Suggest resuming involvement in usual activities, exercise, and socialization within physical and psychological abilities.
• Discuss planning for the future, as appropriate to individual situation (e.g., staying in own home after death of spouse, returning to sporting activities following traumatic amputation, choosing to have another child or to adopt, rebuilding home following a disaster).
🌐• Refer to other resources, as needed, such as counseling, psychotherapy, spiritual advisor, grief support group. **Depending upon meaning of the loss, individual may require ongoing support to work through grief.**

Documentation Focus

Assessment/Reassessment
• Assessment findings, including meaning of loss to the client, current stage of the grieving process, psychological status, and responses of family/SO(s).
• Availability and use of resources.

Planning
• Plan of care and who is involved in the planning.
• Teaching plan.

Information that appears in brackets has been added by the authors to clarify and enhance the use of nursing diagnoses.

Implementation/Evaluation
- Client's response to interventions, teaching, and actions performed.
- Attainment or progress toward desired outcome(s).
- Modifications to plan of care.

Discharge Planning
- Long-term needs and who is responsible for actions to be taken.
- Specific referrals made.

Sample Nursing Outcomes & Interventions Classifications (NOC/NIC)

NOC—Grief Resolution
NIC—Grief Work Facilitation

risk for disproportionate Growth

Taxonomy II: Growth/Development—Class 1 Growth (00113)
[Diagnostic Division: Teaching/Learning]
Nursing Diagnosis Extension and Classification Submission 1998

Definition: At risk for growth above the 97th percentile or below the 3rd percentile for age, crossing two percentile channels

Risk Factors

Prenatal
Maternal nutrition, infection; multiple gestation
Substance abuse; teratogen exposure
Congenital or genetic disorders

Individual
Prematurity
Malnutrition; caregiver's or individual maladaptive feeding behaviors; insatiable appetite; anorexia
Infection; chronic illness
Substance abuse [including anabolic steroids]

Information that appears in brackets has been added by the authors to clarify and enhance the use of nursing diagnoses.

🌐 Cultural   ✪ Collaborative   🏠 Community/Home Care

Environmental
Deprivation; economically disadvantaged
Violence; natural disasters
Teratogen; lead poisoning

Caregiver
Abuse
Mental illness
Learning difficulties (mental handicap); severe learning disability

> **NOTE:** A risk diagnosis is not evidenced by signs and symptoms, as the problem has not occurred; rather, nursing interventions are directed at prevention.

Desired Outcomes/Evaluation Criteria— Client Will:

- Receive appropriate nutrition as indicated by individual needs.
- Demonstrate weight and growth stabilizing or progress toward age-appropriate size.
- Participate in plan of care as appropriate for age and ability.

Caregiver Will:

- Verbalize understanding of potential for growth delay or deviation and plans for prevention.

Actions/Interventions

Nursing Priority No. 1.
To assess causative/contributing factors:

- Determine factors or condition(s) existing that could contribute to growth deviation as listed in Risk Factors, including familial history of pituitary tumors, Marfan's syndrome, genetic anomalies, use of certain drugs or substances during pregnancy, maternal diabetes or other chronic illness, poverty or inability to attend to nutritional issues, eating disorders, and so forth.
- Identify nature and effectiveness of parenting/caregiving activities (e.g., inadequate, inconsistent, unrealistic or

---

Information that appears in brackets has been added by the authors to clarify and enhance the use of nursing diagnoses.

insufficient expectations; lack of stimulation, limit setting, responsiveness).

- Note severity and pervasiveness of situation (e.g., individual showing effects of long-term physical or emotional abuse or neglect versus individual experiencing recent-onset situational disruption or inadequate resources during period of crisis or transition).

- Evaluate nutritional status. **Overfeeding or malnutrition (protein and other basic nutrients) on a constant basis prevents child from reaching healthy growth potential, even if no disorder/disease exists.** (Refer to ND imbalanced Nutrition: [specify].)

- Determine cultural, familial, and societal issues **that may impact situation (e.g., childhood obesity a risk for American children; parental concern for amount of food intake; expectations for "normal growth").**

- Assess significant stressful events, losses, separation, and environmental changes (e.g., abandonment, divorce, death of parent/sibling, aging, move).

- Assess cognition, awareness, orientation, behavior (e.g., withdrawal or aggression), reaction to environment and stimuli.

- Active-listen concerns about body size, ability to perform competitively (e.g., sports, body building) **to ascertain the potential for use of anabolic steroids or other drugs.**

Nursing Priority No. 2.

To prevent/limit deviation from growth norms:

- Determine chronological age and where child should be on growth charts **to determine growth expectations.** Note reported losses or alterations in functional level. **Provides comparative baseline.**

- Note familial factors (e.g., parent's body build and stature) **to help determine individual developmental expectations (e.g., when child should attain a certain weight and height) and how the expectations may be altered by child's condition.**

- Investigate deviations from normal (e.g., height and weight, head circumference, hand and feet size, facial features). **Deviations can be multifactorial and require varying interventions (e.g., weight deviation only [increased or decreased] may be remedied by changes in nutrition and exercise; other deviations may require in-depth evaluation and long-term treatment).**

Information that appears in brackets has been added by the authors to clarify and enhance the use of nursing diagnoses.

⬤ Cultural ⬤ Collaborative 🏠 Community/Home Care

∞• Determine if child's growth is above 97th percentile (very tall and large) for age. **Suggests need for evaluation for endocrine or other disorders or pituitary tumor (could result in gigantism). Other disorders may be characterized by excessive weight for height (e.g., hypothyroidism, Cushing's syndrome), abnormal sexual maturation, or abnormal body/limb proportions.**

∞• Determine if child's growth is below 3rd percentile (very short and small) for age. **May require evaluation for failure to thrive related to intrauterine growth retardation, prematurity or very low birth weight, small parents, poor nutrition, stress or trauma, or medical condition (e.g., intestinal disorders with malabsorption, diseases of heart, kidneys, diabetes mellitus). Treatment of underlying condition may alter or improve child's growth pattern.**

• Note reports of changes in facial features, joint pain, lethargy, sexual dysfunction, and/or progressive increase in hat, glove, ring, or shoe size in adults, especially after age 40. **Individual should be referred for further evaluation for hyperpituitarism, growth hormone imbalance, or acromegaly.**

• Review results of studies such as skull and hand x-rays, bone scans (such as computed tomography [CT] or magnetic resonance imaging [MRI]), chest or abdominal imaging **to determine bone age and extent of bone and soft tissue overgrowth; presence of pituitary or other growth hormone secreting tumor.** Note laboratory studies (e.g., growth hormone levels, glucose tolerance, thyroid and other endocrine studies, serum transferrin and prealbumin) **to identify pathology.**

• Assist with therapy to treat or correct underlying conditions (e.g., Crohn's disease, cardiac problems, renal disease); endocrine problems (e.g., hyperpituitarism, hypothyroidism, type 1 diabetes mellitus, growth hormone abnormalities); genetic or intrauterine growth retardation; infant feeding problems; nutritional deficits.

• Include nutritionist and other specialists (e.g., physical and occupational therapist) in developing plan of care. **Helpful in determining specific dietary needs for growth and weight issues as well as child's issues with foods (e.g., child who is sensory overresponsive may be bothered by food textures; child with posture problems may need to stand to eat, etc.); child may require assistive devices and appropriate exercise and rehabilitation programs.**

Information that appears in brackets has been added by the authors to clarify and enhance the use of nursing diagnoses.

- Determine need for medications (e.g., appetite stimulants or antidepressants, growth hormones).
- Monitor growth periodically. **Aids in evaluating effectiveness of interventions and promotes early identification of need for additional actions.**

Nursing Priority No. 3.

To promote wellness (Teaching/Discharge Considerations):

- Provide information regarding normal growth, as appropriate, including pertinent reference materials and credible Web sites.
- Address caregiver issues (e.g., parental abuse, learning deficiencies, environment of poverty) **that could impact client's ability to thrive.**
- Discuss appropriateness of appearance, grooming, touching, language, and other associated developmental issues. (Refer to NDs delayed Growth and Development; Self-Care Deficit [specify].)
- Recommend involvement in regular exercise or sports medicine program **to enhance muscle tone and strength and appropriate body building.**
- Promote lifestyle that prevents or limits complications (e.g., management of obesity, hypertension, sensory or perceptual impairments); regular medical follow-up; nutritionally balanced meals; socialization for age and development **to maintain functional independence and enhance quality of life.**
- Discuss consequences of substance use or abuse with girls and women of child-bearing age; provide pregnant women with information regarding known teratogenic agents. **Education can influence mother to abstain from use of drugs or agents that may cause birth defects.**
- Refer for genetic screening, as appropriate. **There are many reasons for referral, including (and not limited to) positive family history of a genetic disorder (e.g., fragile X syndrome, muscular dystrophy), woman with exposure to toxins or potential teratogenic agents, women older than 35 years at delivery, previous child born with congenital anomalies, history of intrauterine growth retardation, and so forth.**
- Emphasize importance of periodic reassessment of growth and development (e.g., periodic laboratory studies to monitor hormone levels, bone maturation, and nutritional status). **Aids in evaluating effectiveness of interventions over time, pro-**

Information that appears in brackets has been added by the authors to clarify and enhance the use of nursing diagnoses.

Cultural ⊗ Collaborative 🏠 Community/Home Care

motes early identification of need for additional actions, and helps to avoid preventable complications.

- Identify available community resources, as appropriate (e.g., public health programs, such as Women, Infants, and Children (WIC); medical equipment supplies; nutritionists; substance-abuse programs; specialists in endocrine problems/genetics).

Documentation Focus

Assessment/Reassessment
- Assessment findings, individual needs, including current growth status, and trends.
- Caregiver's understanding of situation and individual role.

Planning
- Plan of care and who is involved in the planning.
- Teaching plan.

Implementation/Evaluation
- Client's responses to interventions, teaching, and actions performed.
- Caregiver response to teaching.
- Attainment or progress toward desired outcome(s).
- Modifications to plan of care.

Discharge Planning
- Identified long-term needs and who is responsible for actions to be taken.
- Specific referrals made, sources for assistive devices, educational tools.

Sample Nursing Outcomes & Interventions Classifications (NOC/NIC)

NOC—Growth
NIC—Nutritional Monitoring

---

delayed Growth and Development

Taxonomy II: Growth/Development—Class 1 Growth/
   Class 2 Development (00111)
[Diagnostic Division: Teaching/Learning]
Submitted 1986

Definition: Deviations from age-group norms

Information that appears in brackets has been added by the authors to clarify and enhance the use of nursing diagnoses.

Related Factors

Inadequate caretaking; [physical or emotional neglect or abuse]
Indifference; inconsistent responsiveness; multiple caretakers
Separation from SOs
Environmental or stimulation deficiencies
Effects of physical disability; [chronic illness]
Prescribed dependence; [insufficient expectations for self-care]
[Substance use or abuse]

Defining Characteristics

Subjective
Inability to perform self-care or self-control activities appropriate for age

Objective
Delay or difficulty in performing skills typical of age group
    [loss of previously acquired skills]
Altered physical growth
Flat affect; listlessness; decreased responses

Desired Outcomes/Evaluation Criteria— Client Will:

- Perform motor, social, and/or expressive skills typical of age group within scope of present capabilities.
- Perform self-care and self-control activities appropriate for age.
- Demonstrate weight and growth stabilization or progress toward age-appropriate size.

Parents/Caregivers Will:

- Verbalize understanding of growth or developmental delay or deviation and plan(s) for intervention.
- (Refer to ND risk for delayed Development for additional actions or interventions.)

Actions/Interventions

Nursing Priority No. 1.
To assess causative/contributing factors:

- Determine existing condition(s), such as limited intellectual capacity, physical disabilities, chronic illness, genetic anom-

Information that appears in brackets has been added by the authors to clarify and enhance the use of nursing diagnoses.

🌐 Cultural   🅐 Collaborative   🏠 Community/Home Care

alies, substance use or abuse, multiple birth (e.g., twins), minimal length of time between pregnancies. **These conditions contribute to growth or developmental deviation, necessitating specific evaluation and interventions depending on the situation.**

- Determine nature of parenting/caretaking activities. **Presence of conflict and negative interaction between parent/caregiver and child (e.g., inadequate, inconsistent parenting, unrealistic or insufficient expectations; lack of stimulation, limit setting, and responsiveness) interferes with the development of age-appropriate skills and maturation.**
- Note severity and pervasiveness of situation (e.g., long-term physical or emotional abuse versus situational disruption or inadequate assistance during period of crisis or transition). **Problems existing over a long period may have more severe effects and require longer course of treatment.**
- Assess occurrence and frequency of significant stressful events, losses, separation, and environmental changes (e.g., abandonment; divorce; death of parent/sibling; aging; unemployment; new job; moves; new baby or sibling; marriage; new stepparent). **Lack of resolution or repetition of stressors can have a cumulative effect over time and result in regression in/or deterioration of functional level.**
- Determine presence of environmental risk factors (e.g., child of parent[s] with active substance abuse issues or who are abusive, neglectful, or mentally disabled).
- Active-listen SO's concerns about client's body size, ability to communicate or perform desired/needed activities or participate competitively (e.g., sports, body building).
- Determine use of drugs, **which may affect body growth.**
- Evaluate usual care setting (e.g., home, day care, institutional environment) **to determine adequacy of care provided, including nourishing meals, healthy sleep or rest time, stimulation, diversional or play activities.**

Nursing Priority No. 2.

To determine degree of deviation from norms:

- Note chronological age, familial factors (e.g., including body build and stature), and cultural concerns **to determine individual growth and developmental expectations.**
- Review expectations for current height and weight percentile. **Compares measurements to "standard" or normal range for children of same age and gender to determine degree of deviation.**

Information that appears in brackets has been added by the authors to clarify and enhance the use of nursing diagnoses.

- Review results of lab tests (e.g., thyroid, growth hormones) and diagnostic studies (e.g., radiographs, bone scans assessing bone growth plates and age) **to evaluate problems with growth and assist in determining interventions and treatment needs.**
- Record height and weight over time **to determine trends, identify needs, and evaluate effectiveness of therapies.**
- Identify present age and developmental stage. Note reported deficits in functional level or evidence of precocious development. **Developmental surveillance is a flexible, ongoing process that involves the use of both skilled observation of the child and concerns of parents, health professionals, teachers, and others to identify children with variations in normal growth and development.**
- Review expected skills/activities, using authoritative text (e.g., Gesell, Mussen-Conger) or assessment tools (e.g., Draw-a-Person, Denver Developmental Screening Test [DDST], Bender's Visual Motor Gestalt Test (aka Bender-Gestalt), Early Language Milestone [ELM] Scale 2, and Developmental Language Disorders [DLD]). **Provides guide for evaluation of growth and development and for comparative measurement of individual's progress.**
- Note degree of individual deviation, multiple skills affected (e.g., speech, motor activity, socialization) versus a single area of difficulty, such as toileting.
- Note whether difficulty is temporary or permanent (e.g., setback or delay versus irreversible condition, such as brain damage, stroke, dementia).
- Investigate sexual acting-out behaviors inappropriate for age. **May indicate sexual abuse.**
- Note findings of psychological evaluation of client and family **to determine factors that may impact development of client or impair psychological health of family.**

Nursing Priority No. 3.

To correct/minimize growth deviations and associated complications:

- Participate in treatment of underlying medical or psychological conditions (e.g., malnourishment, kidney failure, congenital heart disease, cystic fibrosis, inflammatory bowel disease, bone or cartilage conditions, endocrine disorders, adverse effects of medications, mental illness, substance abuse), as appropriate.

Information that appears in brackets has been added by the authors to clarify and enhance the use of nursing diagnoses.

🌐 Cultural 🤝 Collaborative 🏠 Community/Home Care

- Review medication regimen given to stimulate or suppress growth, as appropriate, or possibly to shrink pituitary tumor when present.
- Emphasize necessity of not stopping medications without approval of healthcare provider.
- Discuss appropriateness and potential complications of bone-lengthening procedures.
- Review consequences of substance use or abuse.
- Include nutritionist and other specialists (e.g., physical or occupational therapists) in developing plan of care. Encourage "early intervention services" for children birth to 3 years of age with developmental delays. **Federally funded entitlement programs for qualified child (e.g., Down syndrome or cerebral palsy; prematurity; deprived physical or social environment) is aimed at maximizing child's development. Services include nursing, occupational, physical, or speech therapy, service coordination, social work, and assistive technologies.**
- Monitor growth and development factors periodically. **Aids in evaluating effectiveness of interventions over time and promotes early identification of need for additional actions.**

Nursing Priority No. 4.

To assist client (and/or caregivers) to prevent, minimize, or overcome delay or regressed development:

- Provide anticipatory guidance for parents/caregivers regarding expectations for client's development **to clarify misconceptions and assist them in dealing with reality of situation.**
- Consult appropriate professional resources (e.g., occupational, rehabilitation, or speech therapists; special education teacher, job counselor) **to address specific individual needs.**
- Encourage recognition that certain deviations or behaviors are appropriate for a specific developmental age level (e.g., 14-year-old functioning at level of 6-year-old, is not able to anticipate the consequences of his or her actions). **Promotes acceptance of client, as presented, and helps shape expectations reflecting actual situation.**
- Avoid blame when discussing contributing factors. **Parent/caregivers usually feel inadequate and blame themselves for being "a poor parent/care provider." Adding blame further diverts the individual's focus from learning new**

Information that appears in brackets has been added by the authors to clarify and enhance the use of nursing diagnoses.

behaviors or making changes to achieve the desired outcomes.

• Maintain positive, hopeful attitude. **Supports self-actualizing nature of the individual and attempts to maintain or return to optimal level of self-control or self-care activities.**

• Refer family/client for counseling/psychotherapy **to deal with issues of abuse or neglect.**

• Encourage setting of short-term, realistic goals **for achieving developmental potential.**

• Involve client in opportunities to practice new behaviors (e.g., role playing, group activities). **Strengthens learning process.**

• Identify equipment needs (e.g., adaptive or growth-stimulating computer programs, communication devices).

• Evaluate progress on continual basis **to increase complexity of tasks and goals, as appropriate.**

• Provide positive feedback for efforts, successes, and adaptation while minimizing failures. **Encourages continuation of efforts, thus improving outcome.**

• Assist client/caregivers to accept and adjust to irreversible developmental deviations (e.g., Down syndrome).

• Provide support for caregiver during transitional crises (e.g., residential schooling, institutionalization).

Nursing Priority No. 5.

To promote wellness (Teaching/Discharge Considerations):

• Provide information regarding normal growth and development process, as appropriate. **Individuals need to know about normal process so deviations can be recognized when necessary.**

• Determine reasonable expectations for individual without restricting potential (i.e., set realistic goals that, if met, can be advanced). **Provides hope for achievement and promotes continued personal growth.**

• Discuss appropriateness of appearance, grooming, touching, language, and other associated developmental issues. (Refer to ND Self-Care Deficit [specify].)

• Recommend involvement in regular exercise or sports medicine program **to enhance muscle tone and strength, and appropriate body building.**

• Emphasize importance of periodic reassessment of growth and development (e.g., periodic laboratory studies to monitor hormone levels and nutritional status). **Aids in evaluating effectiveness of interventions over time, promotes early**

Information that appears in brackets has been added by the authors to clarify and enhance the use of nursing diagnoses.

identification of need for additional actions, and helps to avoid preventable complications.

- Recommend that client wears medical alert bracelet when taking replacement growth hormones **to alert care providers in case client is injured or ill.**
- Encourage attendance at appropriate educational programs (e.g., parenting and expectant parent classes; infant stimulation sessions; seminars on life stresses, aging process). **Can provide information for client/family to learn to manage current situation and adapt to future changes.**
- Provide pertinent reference materials including reliable Web sites regarding normal growth and development as appropriate. **Enhances learning at own pace.**
- Discuss community responsibilities (e.g., services required to be provided to school-age child). Include social worker or special education team in planning process **for meeting educational, physical, psychological, and monitoring needs of child.**
- Identify community resources, as appropriate: public health programs, such as Women, Infants, and Children (WIC); well-baby care provider; nutritionist; substance abuse programs; early-intervention programs; seniors' activity or support groups; gifted and talented programs; sheltered workshop; disabled children's services; medical equipment supplier. **Provides additional assistance to support family efforts in treatment program.**
- Refer to social services, as indicated, **to determine safety of client and consideration of placement in foster care.**
- Refer to the NDs impaired Parenting; interrupted Family Processes.

Documentation Focus

Assessment/Reassessment
- Assessment findings, individual needs, current growth status and trends, and developmental level, evidence of regression.
- Caregiver's understanding of situation and individual role.
- Safety of individual, need for placement.

Planning
- Plan of care and who is involved in the planning.
- Teaching plan.

Information that appears in brackets has been added by the authors to clarify and enhance the use of nursing diagnoses.

Implementation/Evaluation
- Client's responses to interventions, teaching, and actions performed.
- Caregiver response to teaching.
- Attainment or progress toward desired outcome(s).
- Modifications to plan of care.

Discharge Planning
- Identified long-term needs and who is responsible for actions to be taken.
- Specific referrals made; sources for assistive devices, educational tools.

Sample Nursing Outcomes & Interventions Classifications (NOC/NIC)

NOC—Child Development: [specify age group]
NIC—Developmental Enhancement: Child [or] Adolescent

deficient community Health

Taxonomy II: Health Promotion—Class 2 Health Management (00215)
[Diagnostic Division: Teaching/Learning]
Submitted 2010

Definition: Presence of one or more health problems or factors that deter wellness or increase the risk of health problems experienced by an aggregate

Related Factors

Lack of access to public healthcare providers; limited resources
Lack of community experts
Program has inadequate budget or [only] partly addresses health problem
Program has inadequate community support or consumer satisfaction
Program has inadequate evaluation plan or outcome data

Defining Characteristics

Subjective
Community members or agencies verbalize overburdening of resources or inability to meet therapeutic needs of all members

---

Information that appears in brackets has been added by the authors to clarify and enhance the use of nursing diagnoses.

🌐 Cultural   ✪ Collaborative   🏠 Community/Home Care

Objective

Incidence of risks relating to health problems or hospitalization experienced by aggregates or populations

Incidence of risks relating to physiological or psychological states experienced by aggregates or populations

No program available to enhance wellness for an aggregate or population

No program available to prevent, reduce, or eliminate one or more health problems for an aggregate or population

Desired Outcomes/Evaluation Criteria— Community Will:

• Identify both strengths and limitations affecting community treatment programs for meeting health-related goals.
• Participate in problem-solving of factors interfering with regulating and integrating community programs.
• Develop plans to address identified community health needs.

Actions/Interventions

Nursing Priority No. 1.

To identify causative/precipitating factors:

🏠• Evaluate healthcare providers' understanding, terminology, and practice policies relating to community (populations and aggregate). **Population-based practice considers the broad determinants of health, such as income/social status, housing, nutrition, employment/working conditions, social support networks, education, neighborhood safety/ violence issues, physical environment, personal health practices and coping skills, cultural customs and values, and community capacity to support family and economic growth.**

• Investigate health problems, unexpected outbreaks or acceleration of illness, and health hazards in the community. **Identifying specific problems allows for population-based interventions emphasizing primary prevention, promoting health, and preventing problems before they occur. Current available resources provide a starting point to determine needs of the community and plan for future needs.**

• Evaluate strengths and limitations of community healthcare resources for wellness, illness or sequelae of illness. **Knowledge of currently available resources and ease of access provide a starting point to determine needs of the community and plan for future needs.**

Information that appears in brackets has been added by the authors to clarify and enhance the use of nursing diagnoses.

- Note reports from members of the community regarding ineffective or inadequate community functioning.
- Determine areas of conflict among members of community. **Cultural or religious beliefs, values, social mores, and lack of a shared vision may limit dialogue or creative problem-solving if not addressed.**
- Ascertain effect of related factors on community. **Issues of safety, poor air quality, lack of education or information, and lack of sufficient healthcare facilities affect citizens and how they view their community—whether it is a healthy, positive environment in which to live or lacks adequate healthcare or safety resources.**
- Determine knowledge and understanding of treatment regimen.
- Note use of resources available to community for developing and funding programs.

Nursing Priority No. 2.

To assist community to develop strategies to improve community functioning/management:

- Foster cooperative spirit of community without negating individuality of members/groups. **As individuals feel valued and respected, they are more willing to work together with others to develop plan for identifying and improving healthcare for the community.**
- Involve community in determining and prioritizing healthcare goals **to facilitate planning process.**
- Plan together with community health and social agencies **to problem-solve solutions to identified and anticipated problems and needs.**
- Identify specific populations at risk or underserved **to actively involve them in process.**
- Create teaching plan, form speakers' bureau **to disseminate information to community members regarding value of treatment and preventive programs.**
- Network with others involved in educating healthcare providers and healthcare consumers regarding community needs. Present information in a culturally appropriate manner. **Disseminating information to community members regarding value of treatment or preventive programs helps people know and understand the importance of these actions and be willing to support the programs.**

Information that appears in brackets has been added by the authors to clarify and enhance the use of nursing diagnoses.

⊕ Cultural ⊛ Collaborative 🏠 Community/Home Care

Nursing Priority No. 3.

To promote wellness (Teaching/Discharge Considerations):

• Assist community to develop a plan for continuing assessment of community needs and the functioning and effectiveness of plan. **Promotes proactive approach in planning for the future and continuation of efforts to improve healthy behaviors and necessary services.**

• Encourage community to form partnerships within the community and between the community and the larger society **to aid in long-term planning for anticipated or projected needs and concerns.**

Documentation Focus

Assessment/Reassessment

• Assessment findings, including members' perceptions of community problems, healthcare resources.
• Community use of available resources.

Planning

• Plan of care and who is involved in planning.
• Teaching plan.

Implementation/Evaluation

• Community's response to plan, teaching, and interventions performed.
• Attainment or progress toward desired outcome(s).
• Modifications to plan of care.

Discharge Planning

• Long-term goals and who is responsible for actions to be taken.
• Specific referrals made.

Sample Nursing Outcomes & Interventions Classifications (NOC/NIC)

NOC—Community Competence
NIC—Community Health Development

Information that appears in brackets has been added by the authors to clarify and enhance the use of nursing diagnoses.

risk-prone Health Behavior

Taxonomy II: Health Promotion—Class 2 Health Management (00188)
[Diagnostic Division: Ego Integrity]
Submitted as impaired Adjustment 1986; Nursing Diagnosis Extension and Classification Revision 1998; Revised/Renamed 2006, 2009

Definition: Impaired ability to modify lifestyle/behaviors in a manner that improves health status

Related Factors

Inadequate comprehension; low self-efficacy
Multiple stressors
Smoking; excessive alcohol
Inadequate social support; low socioeconomic status
Negative attitude toward healthcare

Defining Characteristics

Subjective
Minimizes health status change
Failure to achieve optimal sense of control

Objective
Failure to take action that prevents health problems
Demonstrates nonacceptance of health status change

NOTE: A risk diagnosis is not evidenced by signs and symptoms as the problem has not occurred; rather, nursing interventions are directed at prevention.

Desired Outcomes/Evaluation Criteria—Client Will:

- Demonstrate increasing interest/participation in self-care.
- Develop ability to assume responsibility for personal needs when possible.
- Identify stress situations leading to difficulties in adapting to change in health status and specific actions for dealing with them.

Information that appears in brackets has been added by the authors to clarify and enhance the use of nursing diagnoses.

- Initiate lifestyle changes that will permit adaptation to current life situations.
- Identify and use appropriate support systems.

Actions/Interventions

Nursing Priority No. 1.
To assess degree of impaired function:

- Perform a physical and/or psychosocial assessment **to determine the extent of the limitation(s) of the current condition.**
- Listen to the client's perception of inability or reluctance to adapt to situations that are currently occurring.
- Survey (with the client) past and present significant support systems (e.g., family, church, groups, organizations) **to identify helpful resources.**
- Explore the expressions of emotions signifying impaired adjustment by client/SO(s) (e.g., overwhelming anxiety, fear, anger, worry, passive and/or active denial).
- ∞ Note child's interaction with parent/caregiver. **Development of coping behaviors is limited at this age, and primary caregivers provide support for the child and serve as role models.**
- ∞ Determine whether child displays problems with school performance, withdraws from family or peers, or demonstrates aggressive behavior toward others/self.

Nursing Priority No. 2.
To identify the causative/contributing factors relating to the change in health behavior:

- Listen to client's perception of the factors leading to the present dilemma, noting onset, duration, presence or absence of physical complaints, and social withdrawal.
- Review previous life situations and role changes with client **to determine effects of prior experiences and coping skills used.**
- Note substance use/abuse (e.g., smoking, alcohol, prescription medications, street drugs) **that may be used as a coping mechanism, exacerbate health problem, or impair client's comprehension of situation.**
- 🏠 Determine lack of/inability to use available resources.
- Review available documentation and resources to determine actual life experiences (e.g., medical records, statements by SO[s], consultants' notes). **In situations of great stress,**

Information that appears in brackets has been added by the authors to clarify and enhance the use of nursing diagnoses.

physical and/or emotional, the client may not accurately assess occurrences leading to the present situation.

Nursing Priority No. 3.

To assist client in coping/dealing with impairment:

- Organize a team conference (including client and ancillary services) **to focus on contributing factors affecting adjustment and plan for management of the situation.**
- Acknowledge client's efforts to adjust: "Have done your best." **Lessens feelings of blame, guilt, or defensive response.**
- Share information with adolescent's peers with permission as indicated when illness/injury affects body image. **Peers are primary support for this age group.**
- Explain disease process, causative factors, and prognosis, as appropriate, and promote questioning **to enhance understanding.**
- Provide an open environment encouraging communication **so that expression of feelings concerning impaired function can be dealt with realistically and openly.**
- Use therapeutic communication skills (Active-listening, acknowledgment, silence, I-statements).
- Discuss/evaluate resources that have been useful to the client in adapting to changes in other life situations (e.g., vocational rehabilitation, employment experiences, psychosocial support services).
- Develop a plan of action with client to meet immediate needs (e.g., physical safety and hygiene, emotional support of professionals and SO[s]) and assist in implementation of the plan. **Provides a starting point to deal with current situation for moving ahead with plan and for evaluation of progress.**
- Explore previously used coping skills and application to current situation. Refine or develop new strategies, as appropriate.
- Identify and problem-solve with the client frustration in daily health-related care. **Focusing on smaller factors of concern gives individual the ability to perceive impaired function from a less-threatening perspective, one-step-at-a-time concept.**
- Involve SO(s) in long-range planning for emotional, psychological, physical, and social needs.

Information that appears in brackets has been added by the authors to clarify and enhance the use of nursing diagnoses.

🌐 Cultural ✑ Collaborative 🏠 Community/Home Care

Nursing Priority No. 4.

🏠 To promote wellness (Teaching/Discharge Considerations):

- Identify strengths the client perceives in current life situation. Keep focus on the present, **as unknowns of the future may be too overwhelming.**
- Refer to other resources in the long-range plan of care (e.g., occupational therapy, vocational rehabilitation, smoking cessation program, Alcoholics Anonymous), as indicated.
- Assist client/SO(s) to see appropriate alternatives and potential changes in locus of control.
- Assist SO(s) to learn methods for managing present needs. (Refer to NDs specific to client's deficits.)
- Pace and time learning sessions **to meet client's needs.** Provide feedback during and after learning experiences (e.g., self-catheterization, range-of-motion exercises, wound care, therapeutic communication) **to enhance retention, skill, and confidence.**

Documentation Focus

Assessment/Reassessment

- Reasons for, and degree of, impaired adaptation.
- Client's/SO's perception of the situation.
- Effect of behavior on health status/condition.

Planning

- Plan for adjustments and interventions for achieving the plan and who is involved.
- Teaching plan.

Implementation/Evaluation

- Client responses to the interventions, teaching, and actions performed.
- Attainment or progress toward desired outcome(s).
- Modifications to plan of care.

Discharge Planning

- Resources that are available for the client and SO(s) and referrals that are made.

Sample Nursing Outcomes & Interventions Classifications (NOC/NIC)

NOC—Acceptance: Health Status
NIC—Coping Enhancement

Information that appears in brackets has been added by the authors to clarify and enhance the use of nursing diagnoses.

ineffective Health Maintenance

Taxonomy II: Health Promotion—Class 2 Health Management (00099)
[Diagnostic Division: Safety]
Submitted 1982

Definition: Inability to identify, manage, and/or seek out help to maintain health

This diagnosis contains components of other NDs. We suggest subsuming health maintenance interventions under the "basic" nursing diagnosis when a single causative factor is identified (e.g., deficient Knowledge [specify]; ineffective Self-Health Management; chronic Confusion; impaired verbal Communication; ineffective Coping; compromised family Coping; delayed Growth and Development).

Related Factors

Deficient communication skills
Unachieved developmental tasks
Inability to make appropriate judgments
Perceptual or cognitive impairment
Diminished or lack of gross or fine motor skills
Ineffective individual or family coping; complicated grieving; spiritual distress
Insufficient resources (e.g., equipment, finances)

Defining Characteristics

Subjective
Lack of expressed interest in improving health behaviors

Objective
Demonstrated lack of knowledge about basic health practices
Inability to take the responsibility for meeting basic health practices; history of lack of health-seeking behavior
Demonstrated lack of adaptive behaviors to environmental changes
Impairment of personal support system

Information that appears in brackets has been added by the authors to clarify and enhance the use of nursing diagnoses.

🌐 Cultural 🌐 Collaborative 🏠 Community/Home Care

Desired Outcomes/Evaluation Criteria— Client Will:

- Identify necessary health maintenance activities.
- Verbalize understanding of factors contributing to current situation.
- Assume responsibility for own healthcare needs within level of ability.
- Adopt lifestyle changes supporting individual healthcare goals.

SO/Caregiver Will:

- Verbalize ability to cope adequately with existing situation, provide support/monitoring as indicated.

Actions/Interventions

Nursing Priority No. 1.

To assess causative/contributing factors:

- Recognize differing perceptions regarding health issues between healthcare providers and clients. Explore ways to partner. **Awareness that healthcare provider's goals may not be the same as client goals can provide opportunities to explore and communicate. If left undone, the door is open for frustration on both sides, affecting client care experience and/or perceived outcome of care.**
- Identify health practices and beliefs in client's personal and family history, including health values, religious or cultural beliefs, and expectations regarding healthcare. **Clients and healthcare providers do not always view a health risk in the same way. The client may not view current situation as a problem or be unaware of routine health maintenance practices and needs.**
- Note client's age (e.g., very young or elderly); cognitive, emotional, physical, and developmental status; and level of dependence and independence. **Client's status may range from complete dependence (dysfunctional) to partial or relative independence and determines type of interventions/ support needed.**
- Determine whether impairment is an acute or sudden onset situation, progressive illness, long-term health problem, or exacerbation or complication of chronic illness. **Requires more**

Information that appears in brackets has been added by the authors to clarify and enhance the use of nursing diagnoses.

intensive or long-lasting support and interventions with progressive or chronic conditions.

- Evaluate medication regimen and also for substance use or abuse (e.g., alcohol or other drugs). **Can affect client's understanding of information or desire and ability to help self.**
- Ascertain recent changes in lifestyle (e.g., widowed man who has no skills for taking care of his own/family's health needs; loss of independence; changing support systems).
- Note setting where client lives (e.g., long-term/other residential care facility, rural versus urban setting; homebound, homeless). **Socioeconomic status, and geographic location contribute to an individual's ability to achieve or maintain good health.**
- Note desire and level of ability to meet health maintenance needs, as well as self-care activities of daily living (ADLs).
- Determine level of adaptive behavior, knowledge, and skills about health maintenance, environment, and safety. **Determines beginning point for planning and interventions to assist client in addressing needs.**
- Assess client's ability and desire to learn. Determine barriers to learning (e.g., can't read, speaks or understands different language than is used in the present setting, is overcome with grief or stress, has no interest in subject).
- Assess communication skills and ability or need for interpreter. Identify support person requesting or willing to accept information. **Ability to understand is essential to identification of needs and planning care. May need to provide the information to another individual if client is unable to comprehend.**
- Note client's use of professional services and resources (e.g., appropriate or inappropriate/nonexistent).

Nursing Priority No. 2.

To assist client/caregiver(s) to maintain and manage desired health practices:

- Discuss with client/SO(s) beliefs about health and reasons for not following prescribed plan of care. **Determines client's view about current situation and potential for change.**
- Evaluate environment **to note individual adaptation needs.**
- Develop plan with client/SO(s) for self-care. **Allows for incorporating existing disabilities with client's/SO's desires and ability to adapt and organize care activities.**

Information that appears in brackets has been added by the authors to clarify and enhance the use of nursing diagnoses.

- ⊕• Involve comprehensive specialty health teams when indicated (e.g., pulmonary, psychiatric, enterostomal, intravenous therapy, nutritional support, substance abuse counselors).
- Provide anticipatory guidance **to maintain and manage effective health practices during periods of wellness and identify ways client can adapt when progressive illness/ long-term health problems occur.**
- Encourage socialization and personal involvement **to enhance support system, provide pleasant stimuli, and prevent permanent regression.**
- ⊕• Provide for communication and coordination between the healthcare facility team and community healthcare providers **to provide continuation of care.**
- ⚗• Monitor adherence to prescribed medical regimen **to problem-solve difficulties in adherence and alter the plan of care, as needed.**

Nursing Priority No. 3.
To promote wellness (Teaching/Discharge Considerations):

- 🏠• Provide information about individual healthcare needs, using client's/SO's preferred learning style (e.g., pictures, words, video, Internet) **to assist client in understanding own situation and enhance interest/involvement in meeting own health needs.**
- ∞• Limit amount of information presented at one time, especially when dealing with the elderly or cognitively or developmentally impaired client. Present new material through self-paced instruction when possible. **Allows client time to process and store new information.**
- 🏠• Help client/SO(s) develop realistic healthcare goals. Provide a written copy to those involved in planning process **for future reference and revision, as appropriate.**
- 🏠• Assist client/SO(s) to develop stress management skills.
- Identify ways to adapt things in current circumstances **to meet client's changing needs and abilities and environmental concerns.**
- ⊕• Identify signs and symptoms requiring further medical screening, evaluation, and follow-up care.
- ⊕• Make referral, as needed, for community support services (e.g., homemaker/home attendant, Meals on Wheels, skilled nursing care, well-baby clinic, senior citizen healthcare activities). **Client may need additional assistance to maintain self-sufficiency.**

Information that appears in brackets has been added by the authors to clarify and enhance the use of nursing diagnoses.

- Refer to social services, as indicated, **for assistance with financial, housing, or legal concerns (e.g., conservatorship).**
- Refer to support groups, as appropriate (e.g., senior citizens, Salvation Army shelter, homeless clinic, Alcoholics or Narcotics Anonymous).
- Arrange for hospice service for client with terminal illness **to help client and family deal with end-of-life issues in a positive manner.**

Documentation Focus

Assessment/Reassessment
- Assessment findings, including individual abilities; family involvement; support factors, and availability of resources.
- Cultural or religious beliefs and healthcare values.

Planning
- Plan of care and who is involved in planning.
- Teaching plan.

Implementation/Evaluation
- Responses of client/SO(s) to plan, specific interventions, teaching, and actions performed.
- Attainment or progress toward desired outcome(s).
- Modifications to plan of care.

Discharge Planning
- Long-range needs and who is responsible for actions to be taken.
- Specific referrals made.

Sample Nursing Outcomes & Interventions Classifications (NOC/NIC)

NOC—Health Promoting Behavior
NIC—Health System Guidance

---

impaired Home Maintenance

Taxonomy II: Activity/Rest—Class 5 Self-Care (00098)
[Diagnostic Division: Safety]
Submitted 1980

Definition: Inability to independently maintain a safe growth-promoting immediate environment

---

Information that appears in brackets has been added by the authors to clarify and enhance the use of nursing diagnoses.

🌐 Cultural   🤝 Collaborative   🏠 Community/Home Care

Related Factors

Disease; illness; injury
Insufficient family organization or planning
Insufficient finances
Impaired functioning
Lack of role modeling
Unfamiliarity with neighborhood resources
Deficient knowledge
Inadequate support systems

Defining Characteristics

Subjective

Household members report difficulty in maintaining their home
   in a comfortable [safe] fashion
Household members request assistance with home maintenance
Household members report outstanding debts, financial crises

Objective

Disorderly or unclean surroundings; offensive odors
Inappropriate household temperature
Presence of vermin
Repeated unhygienic disorders or infections
Lack of necessary equipment; unavailable cooking equipment
Insufficient or lack of clothes or linen
Overtaxed family members

Desired Outcomes/Evaluation Criteria—Client/Caregiver Will:

- Identify individual factors related to difficulty in maintaining
  a safe environment.
- Verbalize plan to eliminate health and safety hazards.
- Adopt behaviors reflecting lifestyle changes to create and sustain a healthy, growth-promoting environment.
- Demonstrate appropriate, effective use of resources.

Actions/Interventions

Nursing Priority No. 1.

To assess causative/contributing factors:

- Identify presence of, or potential for, physical or mental conditions (e.g., advanced age, chronic illnesses, brain/other

---

Information that appears in brackets has been added by the authors to clarify
and enhance the use of nursing diagnoses.

traumatic injuries; severe depression or other mental illness; multiple persons in one home incapable of handling home tasks) **that compromise client's/SO's functional abilities in taking care of home.**

- Note presence of personal and/or environmental factors (e.g., family member with multiple care tasks; addition of family member(s) [e.g., new baby, or ill parent moving in]; substance abuse; poverty/inadequate financial resources; absence of family/ support systems; lifestyle of self-neglect; client comfortable with home environment, has no desire for change) **that can contribute to neglect of home cleanliness or repair.**
- Determine problem in household and degree of discomfort and unsafe conditions noted by client/SO(s). **Safety problems may be obvious (e.g., lack of heat or water; unsanitary rooms), while other problems may be more subtle and difficult to manage (e.g., lack of finances for home repair; or lack of knowledge about food storage or rodent control).**
- Assess client's/SO's level of cognitive, emotional, or physical functioning **to ascertain needs and capabilities in handling tasks of home management.**
- Identify lack of interest, knowledge, or misinformation **to determine need for health education/home safety program or other intervention.**
- 🏠 Discuss home environment or perform home visit, as appropriate, **to determine ability to care for self and to identify potential health and safety hazards.**
- 🤝 Identify support systems available to client/SO(s) **to determine needs and initiate referrals (e.g., companionship, daily care, household cleaning or homemaking, running errands).**
- Determine financial resources to meet needs of individual situation.

Nursing Priority No. 2.
To help client/SO(s) create/maintain a safe, growth-promoting environment:

- 🤝 Coordinate planning with multidisciplinary team, as appropriate.
- 🏠 Discuss home environment or perform home visit as indicated **to determine client's ability to care for self, to identify potential health and safety hazards, and to determine adaptations that may be needed (e.g., wheelchair-accessible doors and hallways, safety bars in bathroom, safe place for child play, clean water available, working cook stove or microwave, secured screens on windows).**

Information that appears in brackets has been added by the authors to clarify and enhance the use of nursing diagnoses.

- Assist client/SO(s) to develop plan for maintaining a clean, healthful environment (e.g., sharing of household tasks and repairs between family members, contract services, exterminators, trash removal).
- Educate and assist client/family to address lifestyle adjustments that may be required, such as personal/home hygiene practices, elimination of substance abuse or unsafe smoking habits; proper food storage, stress management; etc. **Individuals may not be aware of impact of these factors on their health or welfare or they may be overwhelmed and in need of specific assistance for varying periods of time.**
- Assist client/SO(s) to identify and acquire necessary equipment (e.g., lifts, commode chair, safety grab bars, cleaning supplies, structural adaptations) **to meet individual needs.**
- Identify resources available for appropriate assistance (e.g., visiting nurse, budget counseling, homemaker, Meals on Wheels, physical or occupational therapy, social services).
- Discuss options for financial assistance with housing needs. **Client may be able to stay in home with minimal assistance or may need significant assistance over a wide range of possibilities, including removal from the home.**

Nursing Priority No. 3.
To promote wellness (Teaching/Discharge Considerations):

- Evaluate client at each community contact or before facility discharge **to determine if home maintenance needs are ongoing in order to initiate appropriate referrals.**
- Discuss environmental hazards **that may negatively affect health or ability to perform desired activities.**
- Develop long-term plan for taking care of environmental needs (e.g., assistive personnel to clean house, do laundry; trash removal; and pest control services).
- Identify ways to access and use community resources and support systems (e.g., extended family, neighbors).
- Refer to NDs deficient Knowledge [Learning Need (specify)]; Self Care Deficit [specify]; ineffective Coping; compromised family Coping; Caregiver Role Strain; risk for Injury.

Documentation Focus

Assessment/Reassessment
- Assessment findings include individual and environmental factors.
- Availability and use of support systems.

Information that appears in brackets has been added by the authors to clarify and enhance the use of nursing diagnoses.

Planning
- Plan of care and who is involved in planning; support systems and community resources identified.
- Teaching plan.

Implementation/Evaluation
- Client's/SO's responses to interventions, teaching, and actions performed.
- Attainment or progress toward desired outcome(s).
- Modifications to plan of care.

Discharge Planning
- Long-term needs and who is responsible for actions to be taken.
- Specific referrals made, equipment needs/resources.

Sample Nursing Outcomes & Interventions Classifications (NOC/NIC)

NOC—Self-Care: Instrumental Activities of Daily Living (IADL)
NIC—Home Maintenance Assistance

---

readiness for enhanced Hope

Taxonomy II: Life Principles—Class 1 Values (00185)
[Diagnostic Division: Ego Integrity]
Submitted 2006

Definition: A pattern of expectations and desires for mobilizing energy on one's own behalf that is sufficient for well-being and can be strengthened

---

Defining Characteristics

Subjective
Expresses desire to enhance hope; belief in possibilities; congruency of expectations with desires; ability to set achievable goals; problem-solving to meet goals
Expresses desire to enhance sense of meaning to life; interconnectedness with others; spirituality

---

Information that appears in brackets has been added by the authors to clarify and enhance the use of nursing diagnoses.

🌐 Cultural   🔵 Collaborative   🏠 Community/Home Care

Desired Outcomes/Evaluation Criteria— Client Will:

- Identify and verbalize feelings related to expectations and desires.
- Verbalize belief in possibilities for the future.
- Discuss current situation and desire to enhance hope.
- Set short-term goals that will lead to behavioral changes to meet desire for enhanced hope.

Actions/Interventions

Nursing Priority No. 1.
To determine needs and desire for improvement:

- Review familial and social history to identify past situations (e.g., illness, emotional conflicts, alcoholism) that have led to decision to improve life.
- Determine current physical condition of client/SO(s). **Treatment regimen can influence ability to promote positive feelings of hope.**
- Ascertain client's perception of current state and expectations/ goals for the future (e.g., general well-being, prosperity, independence).
- Identify spiritual beliefs and cultural values that influence sense of hope and connectedness and give meaning to life.
- Note degree of involvement in activities and relationships with others. **Superficial interactions with others can limit sense of connectedness and reduce enjoyment of relationships.**
- Determine level of commitment and expectations for change and congruency of expectations with desires.

Nursing Priority No. 2.
To assist client to achieve goals and strengthen sense of hope:

- Establish a therapeutic relationship, showing positive regard and sense of hope for the client. **Enhances feelings of worth and comfort, inspiring client to continue pursuit of goals.**
- Help client recognize areas that are in his or her control versus those that are not. **To be most effective, client needs to expend energy in those areas where he or she has control/ can make changes and let the others go.**
- Assist client to develop manageable short-term goals.

Information that appears in brackets has been added by the authors to clarify and enhance the use of nursing diagnoses.

- Identify activities to achieve goals and facilitate contingency planning. **Helps client deal with situation in manageable steps, enhancing chances for success and sense of control.**
- Explore interrelatedness of unresolved emotions, anxieties, fears, and guilt. **Provides opportunity to address issues that may be limiting individual's ability to improve life situation.**
- Assist client to acknowledge current coping behaviors and defense mechanisms that are not helping client move toward goals. **Allows client to focus on coping mechanisms that are more successful in problem-solving.**
- Encourage client to concentrate on progress not perfection. **If client can accept that perfection is difficult and generally not the focus—rather, achieving the desired goal is the focus—then he or she may be able to view own accomplishments with pride.**
- Involve client in care and explain all procedures thoroughly, answering questions truthfully. **Enhances trust and relationship, promoting hope for a positive outcome.**
- Express hope to client and encourage SO(s) and other health team members to do so. **Enhances client's sense of hope and belief in possibility of a positive outcome.**
- Identify ways to strengthen sense of interconnectedness or harmony with others **to support sense of belonging and connection that promotes feelings of wholeness and hopefulness.**

Nursing Priority No. 3.

To promote optimum wellness:

- Demonstrate and encourage use of relaxation techniques, guided imagery, and meditation activities.
- Provide positive feedback for actions taken to improve problem-solving skills and for setting achievable goals. **Acknowledges client's efforts and reinforces gains.**
- Explore how beliefs give meaning and value to daily living. **As client's understanding of these issues improves, hope for the future is strengthened.**
- Encourage life-review by client **to acknowledge own successes, identify opportunity for change, and clarify meaning in life.**
- Identify ways for client to express and strengthen spirituality. **There are many options for enhancing spirituality through connectedness with self/others (e.g., volunteering,**

Information that appears in brackets has been added by the authors to clarify and enhance the use of nursing diagnoses.

⊕ Cultural ⊛ Collaborative 🏠 Community/Home Care

mentoring, involvement in religious activities). (Refer to ND readiness for enhanced Spiritual Well-Being.)

- Encourage client to join groups with similar or new interests. **Expanding knowledge and making friendships with new people will broaden horizons for the individual.**
- Refer to community resources and support groups, spiritual advisor, as indicated.

Documentation Focus

Assessment/Reassessment
- Assessment findings, including client's perceptions of current situation, relationships, sense of desire for enhancing life.
- Motivation and expectations for improvement.

Planning
- Plan of care and who is involved in planning.
- Teaching plan.

Implementation/Evaluation
- Responses to interventions, teaching, and actions performed.
- Attainment or progress toward desired outcome(s).
- Modifications to plan of care.

Discharge Planning
- Long-term needs and goals for change, and who is responsible for actions to be taken.
- Specific referrals made.

Sample Nursing Outcomes & Interventions Classifications (NOC/NIC)

NOC—Hope
NIC—Hope Inspiration

Hopelessness

Taxonomy II: Self-Perception—Class 1 Self-Concept (00124)
[Diagnostic Division: Ego Integrity]
Submitted 1986

Definition: Subjective state in which an individual sees limited or no alternatives or personal choices available and is unable to mobilize energy on own behalf

---

Information that appears in brackets has been added by the authors to clarify and enhance the use of nursing diagnoses.

Related Factors

Prolonged activity restriction
Deteriorating physiological condition
Long-term stress; abandonment
Lost belief in spiritual power or transcendent values

Defining Characteristics

Subjective

Verbal cues (e.g., despondent content, "I can't," sighing); [believes things will not change]

Objective

Passivity; decreased verbalization
Decreased affect, appetite, or response to stimuli
Lack of initiative or involvement in care
Sleep pattern disturbance
Turning away from speaker; shrugging in response to speaker; closing eyes

Desired Outcomes/Evaluation Criteria— Client Will:

- Recognize and verbalize feelings.
- Identify and use coping mechanisms to counteract feelings of hopelessness.
- Involve self in and control (within limits of the individual situation) own self-care and activities of daily living.
- Set progressive short-term goals that develop and sustain behavioral changes and foster positive outlook.
- Participate in diversional activities of own choice.

Actions/Interventions

Nursing Priority No. 1.

To identify causative/contributing factors:

- Review familial and social history and physiological history for problems, such as history of poor coping abilities, disorder of familial relating patterns, emotional problems, recent or long-term illness of client or family member, multiple social and/or physiological traumas to individual or family members.
- Note current familial, social, or physical situation of client (e.g., newly diagnosed with chronic or terminal disease, lack

---

Information that appears in brackets has been added by the authors to clarify and enhance the use of nursing diagnoses.

🌐 Cultural   Collaborative 🏠 Community/Home Care

of support system, recent job loss, loss of spiritual or religious faith, recent multiple traumas, alcoholism or other substance abuse).

⊕• Identify cultural or spiritual values **that can impact beliefs in own ability to change situation.**

• Determine coping behaviors and defense mechanisms displayed.

• Discuss problem of alcohol or drug abuse. **Client may feel hopeless, believing behavior is impossible to stop.**

• Determine suicidal thoughts and if the client has a plan. **Hopelessness is a symptom of suicidal ideation.**

Nursing Priority No. 2.
To assess level of hopelessness:

• Note behaviors indicative of hopelessness. (Refer to Defining Characteristics.)

• Determine coping behaviors previously used and client's perception of effectiveness then and now.

• Evaluate and discuss use of defense mechanisms (useful or not), such as increased sleeping, use of drugs (including alcohol), illness behaviors, eating disorders, denial, forgetfulness, daydreaming, ineffectual organizational efforts, exploiting own goal setting, regression.

Nursing Priority No. 3.
To assist client to identify feelings and to begin to cope with problems as perceived by the client:

• Establish a therapeutic and facilitative relationship showing positive regard for the client. **Client may then feel safe to disclose feelings and feel understood and listened to.**

✎• Complete Beck's Depression Scale. Explain all tests and procedures. Involve client in planning schedule for care. Answer questions truthfully. **Enhances trust and therapeutic relationship, enabling client to talk freely about concerns.**

• Discuss initial signs of hopelessness (e.g., procrastination, increasing need for sleep, decreased physical activity, and withdrawal from social or familial activities).

• Encourage client to verbalize and explore feelings and perceptions (e.g., anger, helplessness, powerlessness, confusion, despondency, isolation, grief).

∞• Provide opportunity for children to "play out" feelings (e.g., puppets or art for preschooler, peer discussions for adolescents). **Provides insight into perceptions and may give direction for coping strategies.**

Information that appears in brackets has been added by the authors to clarify and enhance the use of nursing diagnoses.

∞• Engage teens in discussions and arrange to do activities with them. **Parents can make a difference in their children's lives by being with them, discussing sensitive topics, and going different places with them.**

• Express hope to client and encourage SO(s) and other health team members to do so. **Client may not identify positives in own situation.**

• Assist client to identify short-term goals. Encourage activities to achieve goals; facilitate contingency planning. **Promotes dealing with situation in manageable steps, enhancing chances for success and sense of control.**

• Discuss current options and list actions that may be taken to gain some control of situation. Correct misconceptions expressed by the client.

• Endeavor to prevent situations that might lead to feelings of isolation or lack of control in client's perception.

• Promote client control in establishing time, place, and frequency of therapy sessions. Involve family members in the therapy situation, as appropriate.

• Help client recognize areas in which he or she has control versus those that are not within his or her control.

• Encourage risk taking in situations in which the client can succeed.

• Help client begin to develop coping mechanisms that can be learned and used effectively **to counteract hopelessness.**

• Encourage structured and controlled increase in physical activity. **Enhances sense of well-being.**

• Demonstrate and encourage use of relaxation exercises, guided imagery.

• Discuss safe use of prescribed antidepressants, including expected effects, adverse side effects, and interactions with other drugs.

Nursing Priority No. 4.
To promote wellness (Teaching/Discharge Considerations):

• Provide positive feedback for actions taken to deal with and overcome feelings of hopelessness. **Encourages continuation of desired behaviors.**

• Assist client/family to become aware of factors/situations leading to feelings of hopelessness. **Provides opportunity to avoid/modify situation.**

• Facilitate client's incorporation of personal loss. **Enhances grief work and promotes resolution of feelings.**

Information that appears in brackets has been added by the authors to clarify and enhance the use of nursing diagnoses.

- Encourage client/family to develop support systems in the immediate community.
- Help client to become aware of, nurture, and expand spiritual self. (Refer to ND Spiritual Distress.)
- Introduce the client into a support group before the individual therapy is terminated **for continuation of therapeutic process.**
- Stress need for continued monitoring of medication regimen by healthcare provider.
- Refer to other resources for assistance, as indicated (e.g., clinical nurse specialist, psychiatrist, social services, spiritual advisor, Alcoholics or Narcotics Anonymous, Al-Anon or Alateen).

Documentation Focus

Assessment/Reassessment
- Assessment findings, including degree of impairment, use of coping skills, and support systems.

Planning
- Plan of care and who is involved in planning.
- Teaching plan.

Implementation/Evaluation
- Responses to interventions, teaching, and actions performed.
- Attainment or progress toward desired outcome(s).
- Modifications to plan of care.

Discharge Planning
- Identified long-term needs, client's goals for change and who is responsible for actions to be taken.
- Specific referrals made.

Sample Nursing Outcomes & Interventions Classifications (NOC/NIC)

NOC—Depression Self-Control
NIC—Hope Inspiration

Information that appears in brackets has been added by the authors to clarify and enhance the use of nursing diagnoses.

risk for compromised Human Dignity

Taxonomy II: Self-Perception—Class 1 Self-Concept
(00174)
[Diagnostic Division: Ego Integrity]
Submitted 2006

Definition: At risk for perceived loss of respect and
honor

Risk Factors

Loss of control of body functions; exposure of the body
Perceived humiliation or invasion of privacy
Disclosure of confidential information; stigmatizing label; use
of undefined medical terms
Perceived dehumanizing treatment/intrusion by clinicians
Inadequate participation in decision making
Cultural incongruity

Desired Outcomes/Evaluation Criteria—Client Will:

- Verbalize awareness of specific problem.
- Identify positive ways to deal with situation.
- Demonstrate problem-solving skills.
- Express desire to increase participation in decision-making
  process.
- Express sense of dignity in situation.

Actions/Interventions

Nursing Priority No. 1.

To evaluate source/degree of risk:

- Determine client's perceptions and specific factors that could
  lead to sense of loss of dignity. **Human dignity is a totality
  of the individual's uniqueness—mind, body, and spirit.**
- Note labels or terms used by staff, friends/family that stig-
  matize the client. **Human dignity is threatened by insensi-
  tive, as well as inadequate healthcare and lack of client
  participation in care decisions.**
- Ascertain cultural beliefs and values and degree of importance
  to client. **Some individuals cling to their basic culture, es-**

Information that appears in brackets has been added by the authors to clarify
and enhance the use of nursing diagnoses.

⊕ Cultural ⊛ Collaborative 🏠 Community/Home Care

**pecially during times of stress, which may result in conflict
with current circumstances.**

- Identify healthcare goals and expectations.
- Note availability of family/friends for support and encouragement.
- Ascertain response of family/SO(s) to client's situation.

Nursing Priority No. 2.

To assist client/caregiver to reduce or correct individual risk
factors:

- Ask client by what name he or she would like to be called. **A
person's name is important to his or her identity and recognizes one's individuality. Many older people prefer to
be addressed in a formal manner (e.g., Mr. or Mrs.).**
- Active-listen feelings and be available for support and assistance, as desired, **so client's concerns can be addressed.**
- Provide for privacy when discussing sensitive or personal issues.
- ∞ Encourage family/SO(s) to treat client with respect and understanding, especially when the client is older and may be
irritable and difficult to deal with. **Everyone should be
treated with respect and dignity regardless of individual
ability/frailty.**
- Use understandable terms when talking to client/family about
the medical condition, procedures, and treatments. **Most lay
people do not understand medical terms and may be hesitant to ask what is meant.**
- Respect the client's needs and wishes for quiet, privacy, talking, or silence.
- Include client and family in decision making, especially regarding end-of-life issues. **Helps individuals feel respected
and valued, and that they are participants in the care process.**
- Protect client's privacy when providing personal care or during procedures. Assure client is covered adequately when care
is being given **to prevent unnecessary exposure/
embarrassment.**
- Cleanse client immediately when vomiting, bleeding, or incontinence occurs. Speak in a gentle voice and assure client
that these things cannot be helped and nurses are glad to take
care of the problem.
- ⊕ Involve facility/local ethics committee, as appropriate, **to facilitate mediation and resolution of issues.**

Information that appears in brackets has been added by the authors to clarify
and enhance the use of nursing diagnoses.

Nursing Priority No. 3.

To promote wellness (Teaching/Discharge Considerations):

🏠• Discuss client's rights as an individual. **Hospitals and other care settings have a Patient's Bill of Rights, and a broader view of human dignity is stated in the U.S. Constitution.**

🏠• Discuss and assist with planning for the future, taking into account client's desires and rights.

⊕• Incorporate identified familial, religious, and cultural factors that have meaning for client.

⊛• Refer to other resources (e.g., pastoral care, counseling, organized support groups, classes), as appropriate.

Documentation Focus

Assessment/Reassessment

* Assessment findings, including individual risk factors, client's perceptions, and concerns about involvement in care.
* Individual cultural and religious beliefs, values, healthcare goals.
* Responses and involvement of family/SO(s).

Planning

* Plan of care and who is involved in planning.
* Teaching plan.

Implementation/Evaluation

* Client's response to interventions, teaching, and actions performed.
* Attainment or progress toward desired outcome(s).
* Modifications to plan of care.

Discharge Planning

* Long-term needs and who is responsible for actions to be taken.
* Specific referrals made.

Sample Nursing Outcomes & Interventions Classifications (NOC/NIC)

NOC—Client Satisfaction: Protection of Rights
NIC—Cultural Brokerage

Information that appears in brackets has been added by the authors to clarify and enhance the use of nursing diagnoses.

Hyperthermia

Taxonomy II: Safety/Protection—Class 6 Thermoregulation (00007)
[Diagnostic Division: Safety]
Submitted 1986

Definition: Body temperature elevated above normal range

Related Factors

Exposure to hot environment; inappropriate clothing
Vigorous activity; dehydration
Decreased perspiration
Pharmaceutical agents; anesthesia
Increased metabolic rate; [febrile] illness; trauma

Defining Characteristics

Subjective
Reports headache, weakness, dizziness, nausea

Objective
Increase in body temperature above normal range
Flushed skin; skin warm to touch
Tachypnea; tachycardia; [unstable blood pressure]
Seizures; convulsions; [muscle rigidity, fasciculations]
Confusion

Desired Outcomes/Evaluation Criteria—Client Will:

- Maintain core temperature within normal range.
- Be free of complications such as irreversible brain or neurological damage, acute renal failure.
- Identify underlying cause or contributing factors and importance of treatment, as well as signs/symptoms requiring further evaluation or intervention.
- Demonstrate behaviors to monitor and promote normothermia.
- Be free of seizure activity.

Information that appears in brackets has been added by the authors to clarify and enhance the use of nursing diagnoses.

Actions/Interventions

Nursing Priority No. 1.

To assess causative/contributing factors:

- Identify underlying cause. **These factors can include (1)** *excessive heat production,* **such as occurs with strenuous exercise, fever, shivering, tremors, convulsions, hyperthyroid state, infection or sepsis; malignant hyperpyrexia, heatstroke, use of sympathomimetic drugs; (2)** *impaired heat dissipation,* **such as occurs with heatstroke, dermatological diseases, burns, inability to perspire such as occurs with spinal cord injury and certain medications (e.g., diuretics, sedatives, certain heart and blood pressure medications); (3)** *loss of thermoregulation,* **such as may occur in infections, brain lesions, drug overdose.**
- Note chronological and developmental age of client. **Children are more susceptible to heatstroke; elderly or impaired individuals may not be able to recognize and/or act on symptoms of hyperthermia.**

Nursing Priority No. 2.

To evaluate effects/degree of hyperthermia:

- Monitor core temperature by appropriate route (e.g., tympanic, rectal). Note presence of temperature elevation (>98.6° F [37° C]) or fever (100.4° F [38° C]). **Rectal and tympanic temperatures most closely approximate core temperature; however, abdominal temperature monitoring may be done in the premature neonate.**
- Assess neurological responses, noting level of consciousness and orientation, reaction to stimuli, reaction of pupils, presence of posturing or seizures.
- Monitor blood pressure and invasive hemodynamic parameters if available (e.g., mean arterial pressure [MAP], central venous pressure [CVP]; pulmonary arterial pressure [PAP], pulmonary capillary wedge pressure [PCWP]). **Central hypertension or postural hypotension can occur.**
- Monitor heart rate and rhythm. **Dysrhythmias and electrocardiogram (ECG) changes are common due to electrolyte imbalance, dehydration, specific action of catecholamines, and direct effects of hyperthermia on blood and cardiac tissue.**
- Monitor respirations. **Hyperventilation may initially be present, but ventilatory effort may eventually be impaired by seizures, hypermetabolic state (shock and acidosis).**

Information that appears in brackets has been added by the authors to clarify and enhance the use of nursing diagnoses.

🌐 Cultural 🔄 Collaborative 🏠 Community/Home Care

- Auscultate breath sounds, noting adventitious sounds such as crackles (rales).
- Monitor and record all sources of fluid loss such as urine **(oliguria and/or renal failure may occur due to hypotension, dehydration, shock, and tissue necrosis);** vomiting and diarrhea; wounds, fistulas; and insensible losses, **which can potentiate fluid and electrolyte losses.**
- Note presence or absence of sweating as body attempts to increase heat loss by evaporation, conduction, and diffusion. **Evaporation is decreased by environmental factors of high humidity and high ambient temperature, as well as body factors producing loss of ability to sweat or sweat gland dysfunction (e.g., spinal cord transection, cystic fibrosis, dehydration, vasoconstriction).**
- Monitor laboratory studies, such as arterial blood gas (ABGs), electrolytes, cardiac and liver enzymes **(may reveal tissue degeneration);** glucose; urinalysis **(myoglobinuria, proteinuria, and hemoglobinuria can occur as products of tissue necrosis);** and coagulation profile **(for presence of disseminated intravascular coagulation [DIC]).**

Nursing Priority No. 3.

To assist with measures to reduce body temperature/restore normal body/organ function:

- Administer antipyretics, orally or rectally (e.g., ibuprofen, acetaminophen), as ordered. Refrain from use of aspirin products in children **(may cause Reye's syndrome or liver failure)** or individuals with a clotting disorder or receiving anticoagulant therapy.
- Promote surface cooling by means of undressing **(heat loss by radiation and conduction);** cool environment and/or fans **(heat loss by convection);** cool, tepid sponge baths or immersion **(heat loss by evaporation and conduction);** local ice packs, especially in groin and axillae **(areas of high blood flow). Note:** In pediatric clients, tepid water is preferred. **Alcohol sponge baths are contraindicated because they increase peripheral vascular constriction and central nervous system (CNS) depression; cold water sponges or immersion can increase shivering, producing heat.**
- Monitor use of hypothermia blanket and wrap extremities with bath towels **to minimize shivering.** Turn off hypothermia blanket when core temperature is within 1 to 3 degrees of desired temperature **to allow for downward drift.**

Information that appears in brackets has been added by the authors to clarify and enhance the use of nursing diagnoses.

• Administer medications (e.g., chlorpromazine or diazepam), as ordered, **to control shivering and seizures.**

• Assist with internal cooling methods to treat malignant hyperthermia **to promote rapid core cooling.**

• Promote client safety (e.g., maintain patent airway; padded side rails; skin protection from cold, such as when hypothermia blanket is used; observation of equipment safety measures).

• Provide supplemental oxygen **to offset increased oxygen demands and consumption.**

• Administer medications, as indicated, **to treat underlying cause,** such as antibiotics **(for infection),** dantrolene **(for malignant hyperthermia),** beta-adrenergic blockers **(for thyroid storm).**

• Administer replacement fluids and electrolytes **to support circulating volume and tissue perfusion.**

• Maintain bedrest **to reduce metabolic demands and oxygen consumption.**

• Provide high-calorie diet, enteral or parenteral nutrition **to meet increased metabolic demands.**

Nursing Priority No. 4.

To promote wellness (Teaching/Discharge Considerations):

• Instruct parents in how to measure child's temperature, at what body temperature to give antipyretic medications, and what symptoms to report to physician. **Fever may be treated at home to relieve the general discomfort and lethargy associated with fever. Fever is reportable, however, especially in infants or very young children with or without other symptoms and in older children or adults if it is unresponsive to antipyretics and fluids, because it often accompanies a treatable infection (viral or bacterial).**

• Review specific risk factor or cause, such as (1) underlying conditions (hyperthyroidism, dehydration, neurological diseases, nausea, vomiting, sepsis); (2) use of certain medications (diuretics, blood pressure medications, alcohol or other drugs [cocaine, amphetamines]); (3) environmental factors (exercise or labor in hot environment, lack of air conditioning, lack of acclimatization); (4) reaction to anesthesia (malignant hyperthermia); (5) other risk factors (salt or water depletion, elderly living alone).

• Identify those factors that client can control (if any), such as (1) treating underlying disease process (e.g., thyroid control

---

Information that appears in brackets has been added by the authors to clarify and enhance the use of nursing diagnoses.

medication), (2) protecting oneself from excessive exposure to environmental heat (e.g., proper clothing, restriction of activity, scheduling outings during cooler part of day, use of fans/air-conditioning where possible), and (3) understanding of family traits (e.g., malignant hyperthermia reaction to anesthesia is often familial).

∞• Instruct families/caregivers (of young children, persons who are outdoors in very hot climate, elderly living alone) in dangers of heat exhaustion and heatstroke and ways to manage hot environments. Caution parents to avoid leaving young children in unattended car, emphasizing the extreme hazard to the child in a very short period of time **to prevent heat injury and death.**

• Discuss importance of adequate fluid intake **to prevent dehydration.**

• Review signs/symptoms of hyperthermia (e.g., flushed skin, increased body temperature, increased respiratory and heart rate, fainting, loss of consciousness, seizures). **Indicates need for prompt intervention.**

• Recommend avoidance of hot tubs and saunas, as appropriate **(e.g., clients with multiple sclerosis and cardiac conditions; during pregnancy, as the high temperature may affect fetal development or increase cardiac workload).**

∞• Identify community resources, especially for elderly clients, to address specific needs **(e.g., provision of fans for individual use, location of cooling rooms—usually in a community center—during heat waves, daily telephone contact to assess wellness).**

Documentation Focus

Assessment/Reassessment
• Temperature and other assessment findings, including vital signs and state of mentation.

Planning
• Plan of care, specific interventions, and who is involved in the planning.
• Teaching plan.

Implementation/Evaluation
• Responses to interventions, teaching, and actions performed.
• Attainment or progress toward desired outcome(s).
• Modifications to plan of care.

Information that appears in brackets has been added by the authors to clarify and enhance the use of nursing diagnoses.

Discharge Planning

• Referrals that are made, those responsible for actions to be taken.

Sample Nursing Outcomes & Interventions Classifications (NOC/NIC)

NOC—Thermoregulation
NIC—Temperature Regulation

Hypothermia

Taxonomy II: Safety/Protection—Class 6 Thermoregulation (00006)
[Diagnostic Division: Safety]
Submitted 1986; Revised 1988

Definition: Body temperature below normal range

Related Factors

Exposure to cool environment [prolonged exposure, such as homeless living on street; immersion in cold water; near drowning; medically induced hypothermia, or cardiopulmonary bypass]
Inadequate clothing
Evaporation from skin in cool environment
Decreased ability to shiver
Aging [or very young]
Illness; trauma; damage to hypothalamus
Malnutrition; decreased metabolic rate, inactivity
Consumption of alcohol; pharmaceutical agents; [drug overdose]

Defining Characteristics

Objective
Body temperature below normal range
Shivering; piloerection
Cool skin
Pallor; slow capillary refill; cyanotic nail beds
Hypertension; tachycardia
[Core temperature 95° F (35° C): increased respirations, poor judgment, shivering]

Information that appears in brackets has been added by the authors to clarify and enhance the use of nursing diagnoses.

[Core temperature 95° F to 93.2° F (35° C to 34° C): bradycardia or tachycardia, myocardial irritability and dysrhythmias, muscle rigidity, shivering, lethargy, confusion, decreased co-ordination]

[Core temperature 93.2° F to 86° F (34° C to 30° C): hypoventilation, bradycardia, generalized rigidity, metabolic acidosis, coma]

[Core temperature below 86° F (30° C): no apparent vital signs, heart rate unresponsive to drug therapy, coma, cyanosis, dilated pupils, apnea, areflexia, no shivering (appears dead)]

Desired Outcomes/Evaluation Criteria— Client Will:

- Display core temperature within normal range.
- Be free of complications, such as cardiac failure, respiratory infection or failure, thromboembolic phenomena.
- Identify underlying cause or contributing factors that are within client control.
- Verbalize understanding of specific interventions to prevent hypothermia.
- Demonstrate behaviors to monitor and promote normothermia.

Actions/Interventions

Nursing Priority No. 1.
To assess causative/contributing factors:

- Note underlying cause, for example, **(1) *decreased heat production,* such as occurs with hypopituitary, hypoadrenal and hypothyroid conditions, hypoglycemia and neuromuscular inefficiencies seen in extremes of age; (2) *increased heat loss,* such as occurs with exposure to cold weather, winter outdoor activities; cold water drenching or immersion, improper clothing, shelter, or food for conditions; vasodilation from medications, drugs, or poisons; skin-surface problems such as burns or psoriasis; fluid losses, dehydration; surgery, open wounds, exposed skin or viscera; multiple rapid infusions of cold solutions or transfusions of banked blood; overtreatment of hyperthermia; (3) *impaired thermoregulation,* such as occurs with hypothalamus failure, which might occur with central nervous system [CNS] trauma or tumor; intracranial bleeding or stroke; toxicological and metabolic disorders; Parkinson's disease, multiple sclerosis.**

Information that appears in brackets has been added by the authors to clarify and enhance the use of nursing diagnoses.

∞• Note contributing factors, such as age of client (e.g., premature neonate, child, elderly person); concurrent or coexisting medical problems (e.g., brainstem injury, CNS trauma, near drowning, sepsis, hypothyroidism); other factors (e.g., alcohol or other drug use or abuse; homelessness); living conditions; relationship status (e.g., mentally impaired client alone).

Nursing Priority No. 2.
To prevent further decrease in body temperature:
* Remove wet clothing. Wrap in warm blankets, extra clothing, as appropriate.
* Increase physical activity if possible.
∞• Place infant under radiant warmer or in isolette, and monitor temperature closely. Place knit cap on infant's head.
* Prevent pooling of antiseptic and irrigating solutions under client in operating room. Cover skin areas outside of operative field.
* Prevent drafts in room; raise ambient temperature.
* Avoid use of heat lamps or hot water bottles. **Surface rewarming can result in rewarming shock due to surface vasodilation.**
* Provide warm liquids if client can swallow.
* Provide warm, nutrient-dense food (carbohydrates, proteins, and fats) and fluids (hot sweet liquids are easily digestible and absorbable).
⊛• Warm intravenous (IV) solutions, as appropriate.

Nursing Priority No. 3.
To evaluate effects of hypothermia:
* Measure core temperature with low-register thermometer (measuring below 94° F [34° C]).
* Assess respiratory effort **(rate and tidal volume are reduced when metabolic rate decreases and respiratory acidosis occurs).**
* Auscultate lungs, noting adventitious sounds. **Pulmonary edema, respiratory infection, and pulmonary embolus are possible complications of hypothermia.**
* Monitor heart rate and rhythm. **Cold stress reduces pacemaker function and causes bradycardia unresponsive to atropine, atrial fibrillation, atrioventricular blocks, and ventricular tachycardia. Ventricular fibrillation occurs most frequently when core temperature is 82° F (28° C) or below.**

Information that appears in brackets has been added by the authors to clarify and enhance the use of nursing diagnoses.

- Monitor blood pressure, noting hypotension. **Can occur due to vasoconstriction and shunting of fluids as a result of cold injury effect on capillary permeability.**
- Measure urine output. **Oliguria and renal failure can occur due to low flow state and/or following hypothermic osmotic diuresis.**
- Note CNS effects (e.g., mood changes, sluggish thinking, amnesia, complete obtundation) and peripheral CNS effects (e.g., paralysis—87.7° F [31° C] dilated pupils—below 86° F [30° C] flat electroencephalography [EEG]—68° F [20° C]).
- Monitor laboratory studies, such as arterial blood gas (ABGs) **(respiratory and metabolic acidosis)**; electrolytes; complete blood count (CBC) **(increased hematocrit, decreased white blood cell count)**; cardiac enzymes **(myocardial infarct may occur owing to electrolyte imbalance, cold-stress catecholamine release, hypoxia, or acidosis)**; coagulation profile; glucose; pharmacological profile **(for possible cumulative drug effects).**

Nursing Priority No. 4.

To restore normal body temperature/organ function:

- Assist with measures to normalize core temperature, such as warmed IV solutions and warm solution lavage of body cavities (gastric, peritoneal, bladder) or cardiopulmonary bypass, if indicated.
- Rewarm no faster than 1 to 2 degrees per hour **to avoid sudden vasodilation, increased metabolic demands on heart, and hypotension (rewarming shock).**
- Assist with surface warming by means of heated blankets, warm environment or radiant heater, electronic heating/cooling devices. Cover head, neck, and thorax. Leave extremities uncovered, as appropriate, **to maintain peripheral vasoconstriction.** Refrain from instituting surface rewarming prior to core rewarming in severe hypothermia **as it may cause after drop of temperature by shunting cold blood back to heart in addition to rewarming shock as a result of surface vasodilation).**
- Protect skin and tissues by repositioning, applying lotion or lubricants, and avoiding direct contact with heating appliance or blanket. **Impaired circulation can result in severe tissue damage.**
- Keep client quiet; handle gently **to reduce potential for fibrillation in cold heart.**

Information that appears in brackets has been added by the authors to clarify and enhance the use of nursing diagnoses.

- Provide CPR, as necessary, with compressions initially at one-half normal heart rate **(severe hypothermia causes slowed conduction, and cold heart may be unresponsive to medications, pacing, and defibrillation).**
- Maintain patent airway. Assist with intubation, if indicated.
- Provide heated, humidified oxygen when used.
- Turn off warming blanket when temperature is within 1 to 3 degrees of desired temperature **to avoid hyperthermia situation.**
- Administer IV fluids with caution **to prevent overload as the vascular bed expands (cold heart is slow to compensate for increased volume).**
- Avoid vigorous drug therapy. **As rewarming occurs, organ function returns, correcting endocrine abnormalities, and tissues become more receptive to the effects of drugs previously administered.**
- Perform range-of-motion exercises, provide sequential compression devices (SCDs), reposition, encourage coughing and deep-breathing exercises, avoid restrictive clothing or restraints **to reduce effects of circulatory stasis.**
- Provide well-balanced, high-calorie diet or feedings **to replenish glycogen stores and nutritional balance.**

Nursing Priority No. 5.

To promote wellness (Teaching/Discharge Considerations):

- Review specific risk factors or causes of hypothermia. Note that hypothermia can be *accidental* (see Related Factors) or *intentional* (such as occurs when induced-hypothermia therapy is used after cardiac arrest or brain injury), requiring interventions to protect client from adverse effects.
- Discuss signs/symptoms of early hypothermia (e.g., changes in mentation, poor judgment, somnolence, impaired coordination, slurred speech) **to facilitate recognition of problem and timely intervention.**
- Identify factors that client can control (if any), such as protection from environment/adequate heat in home; layering clothing and blankets; minimizing heat loss from head with hat/scarf; appropriate cold weather clothing; avoidance of alcohol/other drugs if anticipating exposure to cold; potential risk for future hypersensitivity to cold, and so forth.
- Identify assistive community resources, as indicated (e.g., social services, emergency shelters, clothing suppliers, food bank, public service company, financial resources). **Individual/SO may be in need of numerous resources if hypo-**

Information that appears in brackets has been added by the authors to clarify and enhance the use of nursing diagnoses.

thermia was associated with inadequate housing, home-lessness, malnutrition.

Documentation Focus

Assessment/Reassessment
- Findings, noting degree of system involvement, respiratory rate, ECG pattern, capillary refill, and level of mentation.
- Graph temperature.

Planning
- Plan of care and who is involved in planning.
- Teaching plan.

Implementation/Evaluation
- Responses to interventions, teaching, and actions performed.
- Attainment or progress toward desired outcome(s).
- Modifications to plan of care.

Discharge Planning
- Long-term needs, identifying who is responsible for each action.

Sample Nursing Outcomes & Interventions Classifications (NOC/NIC)

NOC—Thermoregulation
NIC—Hypothermia Treatment

---

readiness for enhanced Immunization Status

Taxonomy II: Health Promotion—Class 2 Health Management (00186)
Safety/Protection—Class 1 Infection/Class 5 Defensive Protection
[Diagnostic Division: Safety]
Submitted 2006

Definition: A pattern of conforming to local, national, and/or international standards of immunization to prevent infectious disease(s) that is sufficient to protect a person, family, or community and can be strengthened

---

Information that appears in brackets has been added by the authors to clarify and enhance the use of nursing diagnoses.

Defining Characteristics

Subjective

Expresses desire to enhance:
Knowledge of immunization standards
Immunization status
Identification of providers of immunizations
Record-keeping of immunizations
Identification of possible problems associated with immunizations
Behavior to prevent infectious diseases

Desired Outcomes/Evaluation Criteria—Client/Caregiver Will:

- Express understanding of immunization recommendations.
- Develop plan to obtain appropriate immunizations.
- Identify and adopt behaviors to reduce risk of infectious disease.
- Maintain and update immunization records.

Community Will:

- Provide information to community regarding immunization requirements or recommendations.
- Identify underserved populations requiring immunization support and ways to meet their needs.
- Develop plan to provide mass immunizations in time of major threat or disease outbreak.

Actions/Interventions

Nursing Priority No. 1.

To determine current immunization status:

- Assess client's history of immunizations. **Response may vary widely depending on client's age (infant to adult), cultural influences, travel history, family beliefs about immunization (e.g., fears about combination vaccines, concerns that vaccines cause harm such as autism or seizures), and medical conditions (e.g., some vaccines should not be given to children with certain cancers, persons taking immunosuppressant drugs, or those with serious allergies to eggs).**
- Ascertain motivation and expectations for change. **Public opinions about vaccination include varied and deep-seated**

Information that appears in brackets has been added by the authors to clarify and enhance the use of nursing diagnoses.

beliefs, **a result of the tension between divergent cultural viewpoints and value systems. Motivation to improve and high expectations can encourage client to make changes that will improve his or her life.**

• Determine if adult client works in or frequents high-risk areas (e.g., doctor's office, home care, homeless or immigrant shelters or clinics, correctional facility) **to review potential exposures and determine new vaccines or boosters client may need.**

• Address client's/SO's concerns (e.g., client may wonder if annual flu shots are truly beneficial or whether adult boosters may be needed for particular immunizations received in childhood; parent may be concerned about safety of vaccine supply). **Helps to clarify plans and deal with misconceptions or myths.**

• Identify conditions that may preclude client receiving specific immunizations **such as history of prior adverse reaction, current fever illness, pregnancy, and current cancer or other immunosuppressant treatments.**

🏠• Review community plan for dealing with immunizations and disease outbreak. **Identifies community strengths and limitations.**

Nursing Priority No. 2.

To assist client/SO/community to develop/strengthen plan to meet identified needs:

• Review parents' knowledge regarding immunizations recommended or required to enter school (e.g., hepatitis B, rotavirus, *Haemophilus influenzae,* mumps/measles/rubella [MMR], varicella, and hepatitis A prior to kindergarten; diphtheria/tetanus/pertussis [DTP], human papillomavirus [HPV] by middle-school age; meningitis for college freshmen planning to live in dorm) **to document status, plan for boosters, and/or discuss appropriate intervals for follow-up.**

• Review protective benefit of each vaccine, route of administration, expected side effects, and potential adverse reactions **so that client/SO(s) can make informed decisions.**

∞• Discuss appropriate time intervals for all recommended immunizations, as well as catch-up and booster options for children birth to 18 years.

• Identify requirements for client preparing for international travel **to ascertain potential for contracting vaccine-preventable disease in geographical area of client's travel so that vaccines can be provided, if needed.**

Information that appears in brackets has been added by the authors to clarify and enhance the use of nursing diagnoses.

• Inform of exemptions when client/SO desires. **Some states permit medical, religious, personal, and philosophical exemptions when parent does not want child to participate in immunization programs.** Refer to appropriate care providers for further discussion or intervention.

• Define and discuss current needs and anticipated or projected concerns of community health promotion programs. **Agreement on scope and parameters of needs is essential for effective planning.**

• Prioritize goals **to facilitate accomplishment.**

• Identify available community resources (**e.g., persons, groups, financial, governmental, as well as other communities**).

• Seek out and involve underserved and at-risk groups within the community. **Supports communication and commitment of community as a whole.**

Nursing Priority No. 3.

To promote optimum wellness:

• Review reasons to continue immunization programs. **Viruses and bacteria that cause vaccine-preventable disease and death still exist and can be passed on to people who are not protected, thus increasing medical, social, and economic costs.**

• Provide reliable vaccine information in written form or Internet Web sites (**e.g., brochures or fact sheets from the Centers for Disease Control, American Academy of Pediatrics, National Network for Immunization Information**).

• Identify community resources for obtaining immunizations, such as Public Health Department, family physician.

• Keep abreast of new and ongoing issues about immunizations that should be addressed with clients (e.g., human papillomavirus [HPV] is at this time the most commonly sexually transmitted infection in the United States and mainly occurs in adolescents and young adults). **Allows client/SO to make informed decisions, overcome problems with communication, and promote disease prevention.**

• Discuss management of common side effects (e.g., muscle pain, rash, fever, site swelling).

• Support development of community plans for maintaining and enhancing efforts **to increase immunization level of population.**

Information that appears in brackets has been added by the authors to clarify and enhance the use of nursing diagnoses.

- Establish mechanism for self-monitoring of community needs and evaluation of efforts.
- Use multiple formats (e.g., TV, radio, print media, billboards and computer bulletin boards, speakers' bureau, reports to community leaders and groups on file and accessible to the public) **to keep community informed regarding immunization needs, disease prevention.**

Documentation Focus

Assessment/Reassessment
- Assessment findings of immunization status, potential risks, or disease exposure.
- Identified areas of concern, strengths, and limitations.
- Understanding of immunization needs, safety concerns, and disease prevention.
- Motivation and expectations for change.

Planning
- Action plan and who is involved in planning.
- Teaching plan.

Implementation/Evaluation
- Individual/family responses to interventions, teaching, and actions performed.
- Response of community entities to the actions performed.
- Attainment or progress toward desired outcome(s).
- Modifications to plan.

Discharge Planning
- Identified needs, referrals for follow-up care, support systems.
- Short- and long-term plans to deal with current, anticipated, and potential community needs and who is responsible for follow-through.
- Specific referrals made, coalitions formed.

Sample Nursing Outcomes & Interventions Classifications (NOC/NIC)

NOC—Immunization Behavior
NIC—Immunization/Vaccination Management

Information that appears in brackets has been added by the authors to clarify and enhance the use of nursing diagnoses.

ineffective Impulse Control

Taxonomy II: Perception/Cognition—Class 4 Cognition
   (00222)
[Diagnostic Division: Ego Integrity]
Submitted 2010

Definition: A pattern of performing rapid, unplanned reactions to internal or external stimuli without regard for
the negative consequences of these reactions to the impulsive individual or to others

Related Factors

Anger; denial; delusion
Insomnia; fatigue
Chronic low self-esteem; disturbed body image; hopelessness
Stress vulnerability; environment that might cause irritation,
   frustration
Ineffective coping; codependency
Smoker; substance abuse
Economically disadvantage
Social isolation; suicidal feelings
Compunction [i.e., feeling of uneasiness about rightness of ac-
   tion]; unpleasant physical symptoms
Organic brain disorders; disorder of cognition, development,
   mood, personality

Defining Characteristics

Subjective
Inability to save money or regulate finances
Asking personal questions of others despite their discomfort

Objective
Acting without thinking
Sensation seeking; sexual promiscuity
Sharing personal details inappropriately; too familiar with
   strangers
Irritability; temper outbursts; violence
Pathological gambling

Information that appears in brackets has been added by the authors to clarify
and enhance the use of nursing diagnoses.

🌐 Cultural 🤝 Collaborative 🏠 Community/Home Care

Desired Outcomes/Evaluation Criteria— Client Will:

- Acknowledge problem with impulse control.
- Identify feelings that precede desire to engage in impulsive actions.
- Verbalize desire to learn new ways of controlling impulsive behavior.
- Participate in anger management therapy.

Actions/Interventions

Nursing Priority No. 1.

To assess causative/contributing factors:

- Investigate causes/individual factors that may be involved in client's situation. **Current theory suggests unbalanced neurotransmitters in the brain may be a cause as well as hormone imbalances implicated in violent and aggressive behavior. Brain injuries/tumors may also result in poor impulse control.**
- Explore individual's inability to control actions. **Healthy people are aware of an impulse and are able to make a decision about following the urge or not. The key differentiation between healthy impulsiveness and an impulse disorder is the negative consequences that follow.**
- Note negative consequences incurred by client's impulsive actions such as repeat detentions or suspensions from school, loss of employment, financial ruin, arrests/convictions, civil litigation. **Those with lack of control engage in the behavior even if the individual knows that there will be a negative consequence.**
- Ascertain degree of anxiety client experiences when having an impulse to act on the desire. **Not acting on the impulse creates intense anxiety or arousal in the individual. Engaging in the behavior produces release of the anxiety and possibly pleasure or gratification. This may be followed by remorse, regret, or conversely, satisfaction.**
- Identify behaviors indicative of attention deficit disorder for further evaluation by therapeutic team.

Nursing Priority No. 2.

To assist client to develop strategies to manage impulsive behaviors:

Information that appears in brackets has been added by the authors to clarify and enhance the use of nursing diagnoses.

- Collaborate with treatment of underlying conditions, when possible. **Individuals with impulsive control disorders don't necessarily present for treatment. Those with kleptomania, fire starters, and compulsive gamblers usually come to the attention of court authorities and may be referred for mental health services.**
- Encourage client to make the decision to change and set personally achievable goals.
- Have client identify negative consequences of behavior by expressing own feelings and anxieties regarding the adverse impact on his/her life. **Helps individual begin to understand problems of impulsive behavior.**
- Help client take responsibility and control in situation. **Recognizing own control over impulsive behavior can help client begin to manage problems.**
- Develop a treatment plan for child with attention deficit hyperactivity disorder (ADHD) in conjunction with the parents and the physician. **Medications and behavioral therapy can be helpful, along with monitoring the child and setting goals that are realistic and achievable.**
- Organize a routine schedule for the child with Asperger's syndrome. **Deficits in cognitive functioning make it difficult for the child to see the big picture, process information, see the consequences of an action, and understand the concept of time.**
- Plan for problem with "melt-downs," tantrums, or rage in children with Asperger's syndrome. **These children do not recognize feelings and parents/caregivers need to maintain a calm manner, remove child in a nonpunitive calming fashion. The child who is acting out may need to go to a safe room where he/she can regain control.**
- Discuss issue of hypersexuality.
- Determine use of medications. **No specific medications have been approved by the FDA for use with impulse control disorders; however, some medications such as SSRI antidepressants are being used successfully.**

Nursing Priority No. 3.

To promote wellness (Teaching/Discharge Considerations):

- Involve in cognitive/behavioral therapy. **Having the client identify behavioral patterns that result in negative consequences/harmful effects allows the individual to recognize these situations and use techniques that facilitate self-restraint.**

Information that appears in brackets has been added by the authors to clarify and enhance the use of nursing diagnoses.

- Discuss the use of exposure therapy. **This helps the client build up a tolerance for the trigger situation while using self-control.**
- Encourage client to become involved in group or community activities. **Provides opportunity to earn new social skills and feel better about self.**

Documentation Focus

Assessment/Reassessment
- Individual findings, including type of situation involved in client's loss of control.
- Negative consequences incurred due to behavior.
- Client awareness of consequences of actions.

Planning
- Plan of care, specific interventions, and who is involved in planning.
- Individual teaching plan.

Implementation/Evaluation
- Responses to interventions, teaching and actions performed.
- Attainment or progress toward desired outcome(s).
- Any modifications to plan of care.

Discharge Planning
- Long-term needs and who is responsible for actions to be taken.
- Specific referrals made.

Sample Nursing Outcomes & Interventions Classifications (NOC/NIC)

NOC—Impulse Self-Control
NIC—Impulse Control Training

---

bowel Incontinence

Taxonomy II: Elimination and Exchange—Class 2 Gastrointestinal Function (00014)
[Diagnostic Division: Elimination]
Submitted 1975; Nursing Diagnosis Extension and Classification Revision 1998

Definition: Change in normal bowel habits characterized by involuntary passage of stool

---

Information that appears in brackets has been added by the authors to clarify and enhance the use of nursing diagnoses.

Related Factors

Toileting self-care deficit; environmental factors (e.g., inaccessible bathroom); impaired cognition; immobility

Dietary habits; medications; laxative abuse

Stress

Colorectal lesions; impaired reservoir capacity

Incomplete emptying of bowel; impaction; chronic diarrhea

General decline in muscle tone; abnormally high abdominal or intestinal pressure

Rectal sphincter abnormality; loss of rectal sphincter control; lower or upper motor nerve damage

Defining Characteristics

Subjective

Recognizes rectal fullness, but reports inability to expel formed stool

Urgency; inability to delay defecation

Self-report of inability to feel rectal fullness

Objective

Constant dribbling of soft stool

Fecal staining of clothing/bedding

Fecal odor

Red perianal skin

Inability to recognize/inattention to urge to defecate

Desired Outcomes/Evaluation Criteria— Client Will:

* Verbalize understanding of causative and controlling factors.
* Identify individually appropriate interventions.
* Participate in therapeutic regimen to control incontinence.
* Establish/maintain as regular a pattern of bowel functioning as possible.

Actions/Interventions

Nursing Priority No. 1.

To assess causative/contributing factors:

* Identify pathophysiological conditions present (e.g., congenital abnormalities such as spina bifida; anal surgery; degen-

---

Information that appears in brackets has been added by the authors to clarify and enhance the use of nursing diagnoses.

🌐 Cultural 🌐 Collaborative 🏠 Community/Home Care

erative disorders of the nervous system; acute or chronic cognitive impairments; inflammatory bowel disorders).

- Determine historical aspects of incontinence with preceding/precipitating events. **Common factors include (1) structural changes in the sphincter muscle (e.g., hemorrhoids, rectal prolapse, anal or gynecological surgery; vaginal delivery; inadequate repair of obstetric sphincter disruption; (2) injuries to sensory nerves (e.g., spinal cord injury, multiple sclerosis); major trauma; stroke, tumor, radiation therapy; (3) strong-urge diarrhea (e.g., ulcerative colitis, Crohn's disease, infectious diarrhea); (4) dementia (e.g., acute or chronic cognitive impairment, not necessarily related to sphincter control); (5) result of toxins (e.g., salmonella); (6) aging, particularly in menopausal women; and (7) effects of improper diet or type and rate of enteral feedings.**

∞• Note client's age and gender. **Bowel incontinence is more common in children and elderly adults (difficulty responding to urge in a timely manner, problems walking or undoing zippers, decrease of maximum squeeze pressure); more common in boys than girls, but more common in elderly women than elderly men.**

- Review medication regimen (e.g., sedatives/hypnotics, narcotics, muscle relaxants, antacids). **Many medications and their side effects or interactions can increase potential for bowel problems.**

- Review results of diagnostic studies (e.g., abdominal x-rays, colon endoscopy/other imaging, complete blood count, serum chemistries, stool for blood [guaiac]), as appropriate.

- Palpate abdomen **for distention, masses, tenderness.**

Nursing Priority No. 2.
To determine current pattern of elimination:

- Ascertain timing and characteristic aspects of incontinent occurrence, noting preceding or precipitating events. **Helps to identify patterns or worsening trends. Interventions are different for sudden acute accident than for chronic long-term incontinence problems.**

- Note stool characteristics including consistency (may be liquid, hard formed, or hard at first and then soft), amount (may be a small amount of liquid or entire solid bowel movement), and frequency. **Provides information that can help differentiate**

Information that appears in brackets has been added by the authors to clarify and enhance the use of nursing diagnoses.

type of incontinence present and provides comparative baseline for response to interventions.

- Encourage client/SO to record times at which incontinence occurs **to note relationship to meals, activity, medications, or client's behavior.**
- Auscultate abdomen **for presence, location, and characteristics of bowel sounds.**

Nursing Priority No. 3.

To promote control/management of incontinence:

- Assist in treatment of causative/contributing factors (e.g., as listed in the Related Factors and Defining Characteristics).
- Establish bowel program in client requiring constant bowel care, with predictable time for defecation efforts; use suppositories and/or digital stimulation when indicated. Maintain daily program initially. Progress to alternate days dependent on usual pattern or amount of stool.
- Establish a toileting program where possible (e.g., take client to the bathroom, or place on commode or bedpan at specified intervals, taking into consideration individual needs and incontinence patterns) **to maximize success of program and preserve client's comfort and self-esteem.**
- Encourage and instruct client/caregiver in providing diet high in bulk/fiber and adequate fluids (minimum of 2,000 to 2,400 mL/day). Encourage warm fluids after meals.
- Identify and eliminate problem foods **to avoid diarrhea, constipation, and gas formation.**
- Give stool softeners, fiber-filled agents, bulk formers as indicated.
- Adjust enteral feedings and/or change formula, as indicated, **to reduce diarrhea effect.**
- Provide pericare with frequent gentle cleansing and use of emollients **to avoid perineal excoriation.**
- Promote exercise program, as individually able, **to increase muscle tone/strength, including perineal muscles.**
- Provide incontinence aids/pads until control is obtained. **Note:** Incontinence pads should be changed frequently **to reduce incidence of skin rashes/breakdown.**
- Demonstrate techniques (e.g., contracting abdominal muscles, leaning forward on commode, manual compression) **to increase intra-abdominal pressure during defecation,** and left to right abdominal massage to stimulate peristalsis.
- Refer to ND Diarrhea if incontinence is due to uncontrolled diarrhea; Refer to ND Constipation if incontinence is due to impaction.

Information that appears in brackets has been added by the authors to clarify and enhance the use of nursing diagnoses.

Nursing Priority No. 4.

To promote wellness (Teaching/Discharge Considerations):

🏠• Review and encourage continuation of successful interventions as individually identified.

💊• Instruct in use of suppositories or stool softeners, if indicated, **to stimulate timed defecation.**

🏠• Identify foods (e.g., daily bran muffins, prunes) **that promote bowel regularity.**

🏠• Provide emotional support to client and SO(s), especially when condition is long-term or chronic. **Enhances coping with difficult situation.**

🏠• Encourage scheduling of social activities within time frame of bowel program, as indicated (e.g., avoid a 4-hour excursion if bowel program requires toileting every 3 hours and facilities will not be available), **to maximize social functioning and success of bowel program.**

🏠• Refer client/caregivers to outside resources when condition is long term or chronic **to obtain care assistance and emotional support and respite.**

Documentation Focus

Assessment/Reassessment

• Current and previous pattern of elimination, physical findings, character of stool, actions tried.

Planning

• Plan of care and who is involved in planning.
• Teaching plan.

Implementation/Evaluation

• Client's/caregiver's responses to interventions, teaching, and actions performed.
• Changes in pattern of elimination, characteristics of stool.
• Attainment or progress toward desired outcome(s).
• Modifications to plan of care.

Discharge Planning

• Identified long-term needs, noting who is responsible for each action.
• Specific bowel program at time of discharge.

Information that appears in brackets has been added by the authors to clarify and enhance the use of nursing diagnoses.

Sample Nursing Outcomes & Interventions Classifications (NOC/NIC)

NOC—Bowel Continence
NIC—Bowel Incontinence Care

functional urinary **Incontinence**

Taxonomy II: Elimination and Exchange—Class 1 Urinary System (00020)
[Diagnostic Division: Elimination]
Submitted 1986; Nursing Diagnosis Extension and Classification Revision 1998

Definition: Inability of usually continent person to reach toilet in time to avoid unintentional loss of urine

Related Factors

Altered environmental factors [e.g., poor lighting or inability to locate bathroom]
Neuromuscular limitations
Weakened supporting pelvic structures
Impaired vision or cognition
Psychological factors; [reluctance to call for assistance or use bedpan]

Defining Characteristics

Subjective
Senses need to void

Objective
Loss of urine before reaching toilet; amount of time required to reach toilet exceeds length of time between sensing urge to void and uncontrolled voiding
Able to completely empty bladder
May be incontinent only in early morning

Desired Outcomes/Evaluation Criteria—Client/Caregiver Will:

• Verbalize understanding of condition and identify interventions to prevent incontinence.

Information that appears in brackets has been added by the authors to clarify and enhance the use of nursing diagnoses.

🌐 Cultural   🤝 Collaborative   🏠 Community/Home Care

- Alter environment to accommodate individual needs.
- Report voiding in individually appropriate amounts.
- Urinate at acceptable times and places.

Actions/Interventions

Nursing Priority No. 1.

To assess causative/contributing factors:

- Identify or differentiate client with functional incontinence (e.g., bladder and urethra are functioning normally, but client either cannot get to toilet or fails to recognize need to urinate in time to get to the toilet) from other types of incontinence. **Many of these causes are transient and reversible, but can often occur in elderly hospitalized client.**
- Evaluate cognition. **Delirium or acute confusion or psychiatric illness can affect mental status, orientation to place, recognition of urge to void, and/or its significance.**
- Note presence and type of functional impairments (e.g., poor eyesight, mobility problems, dexterity problems, self-care deficits) **that can hinder ability to get to bathroom.**
- Identify environmental conditions that interfere with timely access to bathroom or successful toileting process. **Unfamiliar surroundings, poor lighting, improperly fitted chair walker, low toilet seat, absence of safety bars, and travel distance to toilet may affect self-care ability.**
- Determine if client is voluntarily postponing urination. **Often the demands of the work setting (e.g., restrictions on bathroom breaks, heavy workload and inability to find time for bathroom breaks) make it difficult for individuals to go to the bathroom when the need arises, resulting in incontinence.**
- Review medical history for conditions known to increase urine output or alter bladder tone. **For example, diabetes mellitus, prolapsed bladder, and multiple sclerosis can affect frequency of urination and ability to hold urine until individual can reach the bathroom.**
- Note use of medications or agents that can increase urine formation. **Diuretics, alcohol, caffeine are several substances that can increase amount and frequency of voiding.**
- Test urine for presence of glucose. **Hyperglycemia can cause polyuria and overdistention of the bladder, resulting in problems with continence.**

Information that appears in brackets has been added by the authors to clarify and enhance the use of nursing diagnoses.

Nursing Priority No. 2.

To assess degree of interference/disability:

- Determine frequency and timing of continent and incontinent voids. Note time of day or night when incontinence occurs, as well as timing issues (e.g., difference between the time it takes to get to bathroom and remove clothing and involuntary loss of urine).
- Ascertain effect on client's lifestyle (including socialization and sexuality) and self-esteem. **Individuals with incontinence problems are often embarrassed, withdraw from social activities and relationships, and hesitate to discuss the problem—even with their healthcare provider.**

Nursing Priority No. 3.

To assist in treating/preventing incontinence:

- Remind client to void when needed and schedule voiding times **to reduce incontinence episodes and promote comfort for client who ambulates slowly because of physical limitations or who has cognitive decline.**
- Administer prescribed diuretics in the morning **to lessen nighttime voidings.**
- Reduce or eliminate use of hypnotics, if possible, **as client may be too sedated to recognize or respond to urge to void.**
- Provide means of summoning assistance (e.g., call light or bell) and respond immediately to summons. **Enables client to obtain toileting help, as needed. Quick response to summons can promote continence.**
- Use night-lights **to mark bathroom location.**
- Provide cues, such as adequate room lighting, signs, color coding of door, **to assist client who is disoriented to find the bathroom.**
- Remove throw rugs, excess furniture in travel path to bathroom.
- Provide bedside commode, urinal, or bedpan, as indicated.
- Adapt clothes for quick removal, e.g., Velcro fasteners, full skirts, crotchless panties, suspenders or elastic waists instead of belts on pants. **Facilitates toileting once urge to void is noted.**
- Assist client to assume normal anatomic position **for ease of complete bladder emptying.**
- Schedule voiding for every 2 to 3 hours. Encourage client to resist ignoring urge to urinate or have a bowel movement. **Emptying bladder on a regular schedule or when feeling urge reduces risk for incontinence. Since urge to void may**

Information that appears in brackets has been added by the authors to clarify and enhance the use of nursing diagnoses.

🌐 Cultural   ☯ Collaborative   🏠 Community/Home Care

be difficult to differentiate from urge to defecate, advise client to respond to urge.

- Restrict fluid intake 2 to 3 hours before bedtime **to reduce nighttime voidings.**
- Include physical/occupational therapist in determining ways to alter environment and identifying appropriate assistive devices to meet client's individual needs.
- Refer to urologist or continence specialist as indicated for interventions such as pelvic floor strengthening exercises, biofeedback techniques, vaginal weight training. **May be useful/ needed to meet individual needs of client.**

Nursing Priority No. 4.

To promote wellness (Teaching/Discharge Considerations):

- Discuss with client/SO(s) need for prompted and scheduled voidings **to manage continence when client is unable to respond immediately to urge to void.**
- Suggest limiting intake of coffee, tea, and alcohol **because of diuretic effect and impact on voiding pattern.**
- Maintain positive regard **to reduce embarrassment associated with incontinence, need for assistance, use of bedpan.**
- Promote participation in developing long-term plan of care.
- Refer to NDs reflex urinary Incontinence; stress urinary Incontinence; urge urinary Incontinence.

Documentation Focus

Assessment/Reassessment

- Current elimination pattern and assessment findings.
- Effect on lifestyle and self-esteem.

Planning

- Plan of care and who is involved in planning.
- Teaching plan.

Implementation/Evaluation

- Response to interventions, teaching, and actions performed.
- Attainment or progress toward desired outcome(s).
- Modifications to plan of care.

Discharge Planning

- Long-term needs and who is responsible for actions to be taken.
- Specific referrals made.

Information that appears in brackets has been added by the authors to clarify and enhance the use of nursing diagnoses.

Sample Nursing Outcomes & Interventions Classifications (NOC/NIC)

NOC—Urinary Continence
NIC—Prompted Voiding

overflow urinary Incontinence

Taxonomy II: Elimination and Exchange—Class 1 Urinary—Function (00176)
[Diagnostic Division: Elimination]
Submitted 2006

Definition: Involuntary loss of urine associated with overdistention of the bladder

Related Factors

Bladder outlet obstruction; fecal impaction
Urethral obstruction; severe pelvic prolapse
Detrusor external sphincter dyssynergia; detrusor hypocontractility
Side effects of anticholinergic, decongestant medications, or calcium channel blockers

Defining Characteristics

Subjective
Reports involuntary leakage of small volumes of urine
Nocturia

Objective
Bladder distention
High postvoid residual volume
Observed involuntary leakage of small volumes of urine

Desired Outcomes/Evaluation Criteria—Client Will:

- Verbalize understanding of causative factors and appropriate interventions for individual situation.
- Demonstrate techniques or behaviors to alleviate or prevent overflow incontinence.

Information that appears in brackets has been added by the authors to clarify and enhance the use of nursing diagnoses.

🌐 Cultural 🌐 Collaborative 🏠 Community/Home Care

- Void in sufficient amounts with no palpable bladder distention; experience no post-void residuals greater than 50 mL; have no dribbling or overflow.

Actions/Interventions

Nursing Priority No. 1.
To assess causative/contributing factors:

- Review client's history for (1) bladder outlet obstruction (e.g., prostatic hypertrophy, urethral stricture, urinary stones or tumors); (2) nonfunctioning detrusor muscle (i.e., sensory or motor paralytic bladder due to underlying neurological disease); or (3) atonic bladder that has lost its muscular tone (i.e., chronic overdistention) **to identify potential for or presence of conditions associated with overflow incontinence.**
- ∞ Note client's age and gender. **Urinary incontinence due to overflow bladder is more common in men because of the prevalence of obstructive prostate gland enlargement. However, age and sex is not a factor in other conditions affecting overflow bladder incontinence, such as nerve damage from diseases such as diabetes, alcoholism, Parkinson's disease, multiple sclerosis, or spina bifida.**
- Review medication regimen **for drugs that can cause or exacerbate retention and overflow incontinence (e.g., anticholinergic agents, calcium channel blockers, psychotropics, anesthesia, opiates, sedatives, alpha- and beta-adrenergic blockers, antihistamines, neuroleptics).**

Nursing Priority No. 2.
To determine degree of interference/disability:

- Note client reports of symptoms common to overflow incontinence, such as:

  Feeling no need to urinate, while simultaneously losing urine; frequent leaking or dribbling

  Feeling the urge to urinate, but not being able to

  Feeling as though the bladder is never completely empty

  Passing a dribbling stream of urine, even after spending a long time at the toilet

  Frequently getting up at night to urinate
- Prepare for and assist with urodynamic testing (e.g., uroflowmetry **to assess urine speed and volume;** cystometrogram **to measure bladder pressure and volume;** bladder scan **to measure retention and/or postvoid residual;** leak point pressure).

Information that appears in brackets has been added by the authors to clarify and enhance the use of nursing diagnoses.

Nursing Priority No. 3.

To assist in treating/preventing overflow incontinence:

- Collaborate in treatment of underlying conditions (e.g., medications or surgery for prostatic hypertrophy or severe pelvic prolapse; use of medication, such as terazosin, to relax urinary sphincter; altering dose or discontinuing medications contributing to retention). **If the underlying cause of the overflow problem can be treated or eliminated, client may be able to return to normal voiding pattern.**

- Assess client for constipation and/or fecal impaction. Administer stool softeners, laxatives, enema/other treatments as indicated. **Chronic constipation is a factor in weakening muscles that control urination. Fecal impaction can be a cause of urinary retention and overflow incontinence, especially in elderly clients.**

- Demonstrate/instruct client/SO(s) in use of gentle massage over bladder (Credé's maneuver). **May facilitate bladder emptying when cause is detrusor weakness.**

- Implement intermittent or continuous catheterization. **Short-term use may be required while acute conditions are treated (e.g., infection, surgery for enlarged prostate); long-term use is required for permanent conditions (e.g., spinal cord injuries [SCI] or other neuromuscular conditions resulting in permanent bladder dysfunction).**

Nursing Priority No. 4.

To promote wellness (Teaching/Discharge Considerations):

- Establish regular schedule for bladder emptying whether voiding or using catheter.
- Stress need for adequate fluid intake, including use of acidifying fruit juices or ingestion of vitamin C **to discourage bacterial growth and stone formation.**
- Instruct client/SO(s) in clean intermittent self-catheterization (CISC) techniques.
- Review signs/symptoms of complications requiring prompt medical evaluation/intervention.

Documentation Focus

Assessment/Reassessment

- Current elimination pattern and effect on lifestyle and sleep pattern.

Information that appears in brackets has been added by the authors to clarify and enhance the use of nursing diagnoses.

Planning
- Plan of care and who is involved in planning.
- Teaching plan.

Implementation/Evaluation
- Response to interventions, teaching, and actions performed.
- Attainment or progress toward desired outcome(s).
- Modifications to plan of care.

Discharge Planning
- Long-term needs and who is responsible for actions to be taken.
- Specific referrals made.

Sample Nursing Outcomes & Interventions Classifications (NOC/NIC)

NOC—Urinary Continence
NIC—Urinary Incontinence Care

---

reflex urinary Incontinence

Taxonomy II: Elimination and Exchange—Class 1 Urinary Function (00018)
[Diagnostic Division: Elimination]
Submitted 1986; Nursing Diagnosis Extension and Classification Revision 1998

Definition: Involuntary loss of urine at somewhat predictable intervals when a specific bladder volume is reached

---

Related Factors

Tissue damage (e.g., due to radiation cystitis, inflammatory bladder conditions, radical pelvic surgery)
Neurological impairment above level of sacral or pontine micturition center

Defining Characteristics

Subjective
No sensation of bladder fullness, urge to void, or of voiding
Sensation of urgency without voluntary inhibition of bladder contraction

---

Information that appears in brackets has been added by the authors to clarify and enhance the use of nursing diagnoses.

Sensations associated with full bladder (e.g., sweating, restlessness, abdominal discomfort)

Objective

Predictable pattern of voiding

Inability to voluntarily inhibit or initiate voiding

Incomplete emptying with [brain] lesion above pontine micturition center

Incomplete emptying with [spinal cord] lesion above sacral micturition center

Desired Outcomes/Evaluation Criteria— Client Will:

- Verbalize understanding of condition or contributing factors.
- Establish bladder regimen appropriate for individual situation.
- Demonstrate behaviors or techniques to control condition and prevent complications.
- Urinate at acceptable times and places.

Actions/Interventions

Nursing Priority No. 1.

To assess degree of interference/disability:

- Note condition or disease process as listed in Related Factors (e.g., pelvic cancer, radiation, or surgery; central nervous system [CNS] disorders, stroke, multiple sclerosis [MS], Parkinson's disease, diabetes with bladder neuropathy, spinal cord injuries, and brain tumors resulting in neurogenic bladder [either hypnotic or spastic]; interstitial cystitis [IC] **affecting bladder storage, emptying, and control.**
- Note whether client experiences any sense of bladder fullness or awareness of incontinence. **Individuals with reflex incontinence have little, if any, awareness of need to void. Loss of sensation of bladder filling can result in overfilling, inadequate emptying (retention), and dribbling.** (Refer to NDs acute/chronic Urinary Retention; overflow urinary Incontinence.)
- Review voiding diary, if available, or record frequency and time of urination.
- Measure amount of each voiding **because incontinence often occurs once a specific bladder volume is achieved.**
- Determine actual bladder volume (via bladder scan) in client with incomplete emptying or on scheduled catheterization **to**

Information that appears in brackets has been added by the authors to clarify and enhance the use of nursing diagnoses.

evaluate for urinary retention when attempting toilet training, to establish schedule for intermittent catheterization, and to avoid unnecessary catheterization.

- Measure or scan postvoid residuals or catheterization volumes. **Determines frequency for emptying bladder and reduces incontinence episodes.**
- Evaluate client's ability to manipulate or use urinary collection device or catheter **to determine long-term need for assistance.**
- Refer to urologist or appropriate specialist for testing of bladder capacity and muscle fibers and sphincter control.

Nursing Priority No. 2.

To assist in managing incontinence:

- Collaborate in treatment of underlying cause or management of reflex incontinence. **Of all the types of urinary incontinence, reflex incontinence probably is the most difficult to treat; however, this condition may be treated with medications, neuromodulation (electrical stimulation of specific nerves to influence the nerve circuit that controls urination), bladder surgery, or indwelling bladder catheters.**
- Determine availability and use of resources or assistance.
- Involve client/SO/caregiver in developing plan of care to address specific needs.
- Encourage minimum of 1,500 to 2,000 mL of fluid intake daily. **Reduces risk of bladder and kidney infection/stone formation and may reduce symptoms of IC when caused by concentrated urine.**
- Instruct client or take to toilet before the expected time of incontinence **in an attempt to stimulate the reflexes for voiding.**
- Engage in bladder retraining program as appropriate. **Suppression of urgency and progressive small increases in intervals between voiding may help reduce urinary frequency in clients with IC.**
- Set alarm to awaken during night, if necessary, to maintain catheterization schedule or use external catheter or external collection device, as appropriate. **Developing a regular time to empty the bladder will prevent urinary retention or overflow incontinence during the night.**
- Implement continuous catheterization or intermittent self-catheterization using small-lumen straight catheter, if condition indicates, **to prevent chronic urinary retention due to an obstructed, weak, or nonfunctioning bladder.**

Information that appears in brackets has been added by the authors to clarify and enhance the use of nursing diagnoses.

• Evaluate effectiveness of medication when used. **Pentosan polysulfate sodium (Elmiron) has been approved by the FDA for moderate or better improvement in overall symptoms in IC; low-dose amitriptyline (Elavil) may increase bladder capacity through beta-adrenergic receptors on the bladder.**

Nursing Priority No. 3.

To promote wellness (Teaching/Discharge Considerations):

- Encourage continuation of regularly timed bladder program **to limit overdistention and related complications.**
- Suggest use of incontinence pads or briefs during day and for social contact, if appropriate, dependent on client's activity level, amount of urine loss, manual dexterity, and cognitive ability.
- Stress importance of perineal care following voiding and frequent changing of incontinence pads, if used.
- Encourage limited intake of coffee, tea, and alcohol **because of diuretic effect, which may affect predictability of voiding pattern,** or avoidance of citrus, artificial sweeteners, tomatoes, spicy foods, as well as caffeine, **which can cause flare-ups/exacerbate symptoms of IC.**
- Instruct in proper care of catheter and cleaning techniques when used **to reduce risk of infection.**
- Review signs/symptoms of urinary complications and need for timely medical follow-up care.

Documentation Focus

Assessment/Reassessment

- Individual findings including degree of disability and effect on lifestyle.
- Availability of resources or support person.

Planning

- Plan of care and who is involved in planning.
- Teaching plan.

Implementation/Evaluation

- Responses to treatment plan, interventions, and actions performed.
- Attainment or progress toward desired outcome(s).
- Modifications to plan of care.

Information that appears in brackets has been added by the authors to clarify and enhance the use of nursing diagnoses.

Discharge Planning
- Long-term needs and who is responsible for actions to be taken.
- Available resources, equipment needs and sources.

Sample Nursing Outcomes & Interventions Classifications (NOC/NIC)

NOC—Urinary Continence
NIC—Urinary Incontinence Care

stress urinary Incontinence

Taxonomy II: Elimination and Exchange—Class 1 Urinary Function (00017)
[Diagnostic Division: Elimination]
Submitted 1986; Revised 2006

Definition: Sudden leakage of urine with activities that increase intra-abdominal pressure

Related Factors

Degenerative changes in pelvic muscles; weak pelvic muscles
High intra-abdominal pressure (e.g., obesity, gravid uterus)
Intrinsic urethral sphincter deficiency

Defining Characteristics

Subjective
Reports involuntary leakage of small amounts of urine on exertion [e.g., lifting, impact aerobics]; with sneezing, laughing, or coughing; in the absence of detrusor contraction or an overdistended bladder

Objective
Observed involuntary leakage of small amounts of urine on exertion [e.g., lifting, impact aerobics]; with sneezing, laughing, or coughing; in the absence of detrusor contraction or an overdistended bladder

Desired Outcomes/Evaluation Criteria—Client Will:

- Verbalize understanding of condition and interventions for bladder conditioning.

Information that appears in brackets has been added by the authors to clarify and enhance the use of nursing diagnoses.

- Demonstrate behaviors or techniques to strengthen pelvic floor musculature.
- Remain continent even with increased intra-abdominal pressure.

Actions/Interventions

Nursing Priority No. 1.
To assess causative/contributing factors:

- Identify physiological causes of increased intra-abdominal pressure (e.g., obesity, gravid uterus, repeated heavy lifting); contributing history such as multiple births; bladder or pelvic trauma, fractures; surgery (e.g., radical prostatectomy, bladder or other pelvic surgeries that may damage sphincter muscles); and participation in high-impact athletic or military field activities (particularly women).
- Assess for urine loss (usually small amount) with coughing, sneezing, or sports activities; relaxed pelvic musculature and support, noting inability to start or stop stream while voiding, bulging of perineum when bearing down.
- Note client's sex and age. **The majority of clients with stress urinary incontinence are women, although men who undergo surgical prostatectomy may also experience it. Although pregnancy and childbirth is a known cause in younger women, stress incontinence is also common in older women, possibly related to loss of estrogen and weakened muscles in the pelvic organs.**
- Review client's medications for those that may cause or exacerbate stress incontinence (e.g., alpha-adrenergic blockers, angiotensin-converting enzyme [ACE] inhibitors, loop diuretics).

Nursing Priority No. 2.
To assess degree of interference/disability:

- Observe voiding patterns, time and amount voided, and stimulus provoking incontinence. Review voiding diary, if available.
- Prepare for, and assist with, appropriate testing. **Diagnosing urinary incontinence often requires comprehensive evaluation (e.g., measuring bladder filling and capacity, bladder scan, leak-point pressure, rate of urinary flow, pelvic ultrasound, cystogram/other scans) to differentiate stress incontinence from other types.**

Information that appears in brackets has been added by the authors to clarify and enhance the use of nursing diagnoses.

- Determine effect on lifestyle (including daily activities; participation in sports, exercise, or recreation; socialization; sexuality; and self-esteem).
- Ascertain methods of self-management (e.g., regularly timed voiding, limiting liquid intake, using undergarment protection).
- Assess for concomitant urge or functional incontinence, noting whether bladder irritability, reduced bladder capacity, or voluntary overdistention is present. (Refer to appropriate NDs.)

Nursing Priority No. 3.

To assist in treating/preventing incontinence:

- Suggest and implement self-help techniques:

  Keep a voiding diary, as indicated. **The use of a frequency/volume chart is helpful in bladder training.**

  Practice timed voidings (e.g., every 3 hours during the day) **to keep bladder relatively empty.**

  Extend time between voidings to 3- to 4-hour intervals. **May improve bladder capacity and retention time.**

  Void before physical exertion, such as exercise/sports activities, heavy lifting, **to reduce potential for incontinence.**

  Encourage weight loss, as indicated, **to reduce pressure on pelvic organs.**

  Suggest limiting use of coffee, tea, and alcohol **because of diuretic effect.**

  Recommend regular pelvic floor–strengthening exercises (Kegel exercises). **These exercises involve tightening the muscles of the pelvic floor and need to be done numerous times throughout the day.**

  Suggest starting and stopping stream two or three times during voiding **to isolate muscles involved in voiding process for exercise training.**

  Incorporate bent-knee sit-ups into exercise program **to increase abdominal muscle tone.**

- Administer medications, as indicated, such as midodrine (Pro-Amatine); oxybutynin (Ditropan); tolterodine (Detrol); solifenacin (Vesicare). **May improve bladder tone and capacity and increase effectiveness of bladder sphincter and proximal urethra contractions.**

- Assist with medical treatment of underlying urological condition, as indicated. **Stress incontinence may be treated with surgical intervention (e.g., bladder neck suspension, pubovaginal sling to reposition bladder and strengthen**

Information that appears in brackets has been added by the authors to clarify and enhance the use of nursing diagnoses.

pelvic musculature; or prostate surgery) or nonsurgical therapies (e.g., behavioral modification, pelvic muscle exercises, medications, use of pessary, vaginal cones; electrical stimulation; biofeedback).

Nursing Priority No. 4.

🏠 To promote wellness (Teaching/Discharge Considerations):

* Discuss participation in incontinence management for activities such as heavy lifting, impact aerobics **that increase intra-abdominal pressure.** Substitute swimming, bicycling, or low-impact exercise.
* Refer to weight-loss program or support group **when obesity is a contributing factor.**
* Suggest use of incontinence pads or briefs, as needed. Consider client's activity level, amount of urine loss, physical size, manual dexterity, and cognitive ability **to determine specific product choices best suited to individual situation and needs.**
🏠• Emphasize importance of perineal care following voiding and frequent changing of incontinence pads **to prevent incontinence-associated dermatitis and infection.** Recommend application of oil-based emollient **to protect skin from irritation.**

Documentation Focus

Assessment/Reassessment

* Individual findings including pattern of incontinence and physical factors present.
* Effect on lifestyle and self-esteem.
* Client understanding of condition.

Planning

* Plan of care and who is involved in the planning.
* Teaching plan.

Implementation/Evaluation

* Responses to interventions, teaching, actions performed, and changes that are identified.
* Attainment or progress toward desired outcome(s).
* Modifications to plan of care.

Information that appears in brackets has been added by the authors to clarify and enhance the use of nursing diagnoses.

Discharge Planning
* Long-term needs and who is responsible for specific actions.
* Specific referrals made.

Sample Nursing Outcomes & Interventions Classifications (NOC/NIC)

NOC—Urinary Continence
NIC—Pelvic Muscle Exercise

urge urinary Incontinence

Taxonomy II: Elimination and Exchange—Class 1 Urinary Function (00019)
[Diagnostic Division: Elimination]
Submitted 1986; Revised 2006

Definition: Involuntary passage of urine occurring soon after a strong sense of urgency to void

Related Factors

Decreased bladder capacity
Bladder infection; atrophic urethritis or vaginitis
Alcohol or caffeine intake; [increased fluid intake]
Diuretic use
Fecal impaction
Detrusor hyperactivity with impaired bladder contractility

Defining Characteristics

Subjective
Reports: urinary urgency, involuntary loss of urine with bladder contractions or spasms; inability to reach toilet in time to avoid urine loss

Objective
Observed inability to reach toilet in time to avoid urine loss

Desired Outcomes/Evaluation Criteria— Client Will:

* Verbalize understanding of condition.
* Demonstrate behaviors or techniques to control or correct situation.

Information that appears in brackets has been added by the authors to clarify and enhance the use of nursing diagnoses.

- Report increase in interval between urge and involuntary loss of urine.
- Void every 3 to 4 hours in individually appropriate amounts.

Actions/Interventions

Nursing Priority No. 1.

To assess causative/contributing factors:

- Note presence of conditions often associated with urgent voiding (e.g., urinary tract infection; pregnancy; pelvic or gynecological surgery; prostatitis or prostate surgery; obesity; bladder tumors or stones; nerve damage from conditions such as diabetes, stroke, Parkinson's disease, multiple sclerosis; certain cancers, including bladder and prostate; recent or lengthy use of indwelling urinary catheter) **affecting bladder capacity; pelvic, bladder, or urethral musculature tone; and/or innervation.**
- Ask client about urgency (more than just normal desire to void). **Urgency (also called overactive bladder [OAB]) is a sudden compelling need to void that is difficult to defer and may be accompanied by leaking or urge incontinence.**
- Note factors that may affect ability to respond to urge to void in timely manner (e.g., impaired mobility, debilitation, sensory or perceptual impairments). **Impaired mobility, use of sedation, or cognitive impairments may result in client failing to recognize need to void or moving too slowly to make it to the bathroom, with subsequent loss of urine.**
- Review client's medications and substance use (e.g., diuretics, antipsychotic agents, sedatives, caffeine, alcohol) **for agents that increase urine production or exert a bladder irritant effect.**
- Assess for signs and symptoms of bladder infection (e.g., cloudy, odorous urine; burning pain with voiding; bacteriuria) **associated with acute, painful urgency symptoms.**
- Prepare for and assist with appropriate testing (e.g., prevoid or postvoid bladder scanning; pelvic examination for strictures; impaired perineal sensation or musculature; urinalysis; uroflowmetry voiding pressures; cystoscopy; cystometrogram) **to determine anatomical and functional status of bladder and urethra.**
- Assess for concomitant stress or functional incontinence. **Older women often have a mix of stress and urge incontinence, while individuals with dementia or disabling neurological disorders tend to have urge and functional in-**

Information that appears in brackets has been added by the authors to clarify and enhance the use of nursing diagnoses.

🌐 Cultural 🌐 Collaborative 🏠 Community/Home Care

continence. (Refer to NDs stress/functional urinary Incontinence for additional interventions.)

Nursing Priority No. 2.

To assess degree of interference/disability:

- Record frequency of voiding during a typical 24-hour period.
- Discuss degree of urgency and length of warning time between initial urge and loss of urine. **Overactivity or irritability shortens the length of time between urge and urine loss and helps clarify the type of incontinence.**
- Ascertain if client experiences triggers (e.g., sound of running water, putting hands in water, seeing a restroom sign, "key-in-the-lock" syndrome).
- Measure amount of urine voided, especially noting amounts less than 100 mL or greater than 550 mL. **Bladder capacity may be impaired or bladder contractions facilitating emptying may be ineffective.** (Refer to ND [acute/chronic] Urinary Retention.)
- Ascertain effect on lifestyle (including daily activities, socialization, sexuality) and self-esteem. **There is a considerable impact on the quality of life of individuals with an incontinence problem, affecting socialization and view of themselves as sexual beings and sense of self-esteem.**

Nursing Priority No. 3.

To assist in treating/preventing incontinence:

- Collaborate in treating underlying cause and/or managing urge symptoms. **Urgency symptoms may resolve with treatment of medical problem (e.g., infection, recovery from surgery, childbirth, or pelvic trauma) or may be resistant to resolution (e.g., incontinence associated with neurogenic bladder).**
- Administer medications as indicated (e.g., antibiotic for urinary tract infection, or antimuscarinics [oxybutynin (Ditropan), tolterodine (Detrol), solifenacin (Vesicare)]) **to reduce voiding frequency and urgency by blocking overactive detrusor contractions.**
- Provide assistance or devices, as indicated, for client who is mobility impaired (e.g., provide means of summoning assistance; place bedside commode, urinal, or bedpan within client's reach).
- Offer assistance to cognitively impaired client (e.g., prompt client, or take to bathroom on regularly timed schedule) **to**

Information that appears in brackets has been added by the authors to clarify and enhance the use of nursing diagnoses.

reduce frequency of incontinence episodes and promote comfort.

🏠 • Recommend lifestyle changes:

Adjust fluid intake to 1500 to 2000 mL/day. Regulate liquid intake at prescheduled times (with and between meals) and limit fluids 2 to 3 hours prior to bedtime **to promote predictable voiding pattern and limit nocturia.**

Modify foods and fluids as indicated (e.g., reduce caffeine, citrus juices, spicy foods, etc.) **to reduce bladder irritation.**

Manage bowel elimination **to prevent urinary problems associated with constipation or fecal impaction.**

🏠 • Encourage client to participate in behavioral interventions, if able:

Establish voiding schedule (habit and bladder training) based on client's usual voiding pattern and gradually increase time interval.

Recommend consciously delaying voiding by using distraction (e.g., slow deep breaths); self-statements (e.g., "I can wait"); and contracting pelvic muscles when exposed to triggers, which are **behavioral techniques for urge suppression.**

Encourage regular pelvic floor strengthening exercises or Kegel exercises as indicated by specific condition.

Instruct client to tighten pelvic floor muscles before arising from bed. **Helps prevent loss of urine as abdominal pressure changes.**

Suggest starting and stopping stream two or more times during voiding **to isolate muscles involved in voiding process for exercise training.**

🔄 • Refer to specialists or treatment program, as indicated, for additional and specialized interventions (e.g., biofeedback, use of vaginal cones, electronic stimulation therapy, possible surgical interventions).

Nursing Priority No. 4.

🏠 To promote wellness (Teaching/Discharge Considerations):

• Encourage comfort measures (e.g., use of incontinence pads or undergarments, wearing loose-fitting or especially adapted clothing) **to prepare for and manage urge incontinence symptoms over the long term and enhance sense of security and confidence in abilities to be socially active.**

• Emphasize importance of regular perineal care **to prevent skin irritation and incontinence-related dermatitis.**

Information that appears in brackets has been added by the authors to clarify and enhance the use of nursing diagnoses.

- Identify signs/symptoms indicating urinary complications and need for timely medical follow-up care.

Documentation Focus

Assessment/Reassessment
- Individual findings, including pattern of incontinence, effect on lifestyle, and self-esteem.

Planning
- Plan of care, specific interventions, and who is involved in planning.
- Teaching plan.

Implementation/Evaluation
- Response to interventions, teaching, and actions performed.
- Attainment or progress toward desired outcome(s).
- Modifications to plan of care.

Discharge Planning
- Discharge needs and who is responsible for actions to be taken.
- Specific referrals made.

Sample Nursing Outcomes & Interventions Classifications (NOC/NIC)

NOC—Urinary Continence
NIC—Urinary Bladder Training

---

risk for urge urinary Incontinence

Taxonomy II: Elimination and Exchange—Class 1 Urinary Function (00022)
[Diagnostic Division: Elimination]
Submitted 1998 (Nursing Diagnosis Extension and Classification)

Definition: At risk for involuntary passage of urine occurring soon after a strong sensation of urgency to void

---

Risk Factors

Effects of pharmaceutical agents, caffeine, or alcohol
Detrusor hyperreflexia with impaired bladder contractility

Information that appears in brackets has been added by the authors to clarify and enhance the use of nursing diagnoses.

Atrophic urethritis or vaginitis
Impaired bladder contractility; involuntary sphincter relaxation
Ineffective toileting habits
Small bladder capacity; fecal impaction

> **NOTE:** A risk diagnosis is not evidenced by signs and symptoms as the problem has not occurred; rather, nursing interventions are directed at prevention.

Desired Outcomes/Evaluation Criteria— Client Will:

- Identify individual risk factors and appropriate interventions.
- Demonstrate behaviors or lifestyle changes to prevent development of problem.

Actions/Interventions

Nursing Priority No. 1.

To assess potential for developing incontinence:

- Identify client with potential for urge incontinence as noted in Risk Factors.
- Note presence of conditions often associated with urgent voiding (e.g., urinary tract infection; pregnancy; pelvic or gynecological surgery; prostatitis or prostate surgery; obesity; bladder tumors or stones; nerve damage from conditions such as diabetes, stroke, Parkinson's disease, multiple sclerosis; certain cancers, including the bladder and prostate; recent or lengthy use of indwelling urinary catheter) **affecting bladder capacity; pelvic, bladder, or urethral musculature tone and/or innervation.**
- Determine use or presence of bladder irritants (e.g., significant intake of alcohol or caffeine), **resulting in increased output or concentrated urine.**
- Review client's medication regimen (e.g., diuretics, antipsychotic agents, sedatives) **for use of drugs that increase urine production or that may impair client's recognition of or ability to respond to urge to void.**
- Review history for long-standing habits or medical conditions (e.g., frequent voluntary voiding, impaired mobility, use of sedatives) **that may reduce bladder capacity.**
- Note conditions (e.g., impaired sensory perception or mobility, cognitive impairment or dementia, central nervous system disorders) **that may affect ability to respond to urge to void.**

Information that appears in brackets has been added by the authors to clarify and enhance the use of nursing diagnoses.

🌐 Cultural ✪ Collaborative 🏠 Community/Home Care

- Measure amount of urine voided, especially noting amounts less than 100 mL or greater than 550 mL **to determine bladder capacity and effectiveness of bladder contractions to facilitate emptying.**
- Prepare for, and assist with, appropriate testing (e.g., urinalysis, noninvasive bladder scanning, cystometrogram) **to evaluate voiding pattern and identify potential functional concerns.**

Nursing Priority No. 2.
To prevent occurrence of problem:

- Assist in treatment of underlying conditions that may contribute to urge incontinence. **Urgency symptoms may resolve with treatment of medical problem (e.g., urinary tract infection, recovery from pelvic surgery, childbirth, or pelvic trauma; use of estrogen-based oral or topical products for atrophic vaginitis, etc.)**
- Ascertain client's awareness and concerns about developing problem and whether lifestyle might be affected (e.g., daily living activities, socialization, sexual patterns).
- Regulate liquid intake at prescheduled times (with and between meals) **to promote predictable voiding pattern.**
- Establish schedule for voiding (habit training) based on client's usual voiding pattern.
- Manage bowel elimination **to prevent continence problems associated with constipation or fecal impaction.**
- Provide assistance or devices, as indicated, for clients who are mobility impaired (e.g., providing means of summoning assistance; placing bedside commode, urinal, or bedpan within client's reach).
- Encourage regular pelvic floor strengthening exercises or Kegel exercises. **Can improve pelvic musculature tone and strength, preventing or halting incontinence.**

Nursing Priority No. 3.
To promote wellness (Teaching/Discharge Considerations):

- Provide information to client/SO(s) about potential for urge incontinence (also called overactive bladder [OAB]) and lifestyle measures to prevent or limit incontinence:

  Recommend limiting intake of coffee, tea, and alcohol **because of their irritating effect on the bladder.**

  Suggest wearing loose-fitting or especially adapted clothing **to facilitate response to voiding urge.**

Information that appears in brackets has been added by the authors to clarify and enhance the use of nursing diagnoses.

- Emphasize importance of perineal care after each voiding **to reduce risk of ascending infection and incontinence-related dermatitis.**
- Identify signs/symptoms indicating urinary complications and need for medical follow-up care.

Documentation Focus

Assessment/Reassessment
- Individual findings, including specific risk factors and pattern of voiding.

Planning
- Plan of care, specific interventions, and who is involved in planning.
- Teaching plan.

Implementation/Evaluation
- Response to interventions, teaching, and actions performed.
- Attainment or progress toward desired outcome(s).
- Modifications to plan of care.

Discharge Planning
- Discharge needs and who is responsible for actions to be taken.
- Specific referrals made.

Sample Nursing Outcomes & Interventions Classifications (NOC/NIC)

NOC—Urinary Continence
NIC—Urinary Bladder Training

---

risk for Infection

Taxonomy II: Safety/Protection—Class 1 Infection (00004)
[Diagnostic Division: Safety]
Submitted 1986; Revised 2010

Definition: At risk for being invaded by pathogenic organisms

---

Information that appears in brackets has been added by the authors to clarify and enhance the use of nursing diagnoses.

Risk Factors

Inadequate primary defenses—broken skin (e.g., intravenous catheter placement, invasive procedures), traumatized tissue (e.g., trauma, tissue destruction); smoking, decrease in ciliary action, stasis of body fluids, change in pH of secretions, altered peristalsis, premature/prolonged rupture of amniotic membranes

Inadequate secondary defenses—decreased hemoglobin, leukopenia, suppressed inflammatory response; immunosuppression (e.g., inadequate acquired immunity; pharmaceutical agents including immunosuppressants, steroids, monoclonal antibodies, immunomodulators)

Increased environmental exposure to pathogens—outbreaks; invasive procedures

Chronic disease—diabetes mellitus, obesity; malnutrition

Inadequate vaccination

[Exposure to multiple healthcare workers in multiple care settings]

> **NOTE:** A risk diagnosis is not evidenced by signs and symptoms, as the problem has not occurred; rather, nursing interventions are directed at prevention.

Desired Outcomes/Evaluation Criteria— Client Will:

- Verbalize understanding of individual causative or risk factor(s).
- Identify interventions to prevent or reduce risk of infection.
- Demonstrate techniques, lifestyle changes to promote safe environment.
- Achieve timely wound healing; be free of purulent drainage or erythema; be afebrile.

Actions/Interventions

Nursing Priority No. 1.

To assess causative/contributing factors:

- Note risk factors for occurrence of infection (e.g., extremes of age; immunocompromised host; trauma; skin/tissue wounds; poor nutritional status; communities or persons sharing close quarters and/or equipment, such as college dorm, group home, long-term care facility, day care, or correctional

---

Information that appears in brackets has been added by the authors to clarify and enhance the use of nursing diagnoses.

facility; prolonged illness or hospitalization; multiple surgeries or invasive procedures; indwelling catheters; intravenous (IV) drug use; accidental or intentional environmental exposure, such as an act of bioterrorism).

- Observe for localized signs of infection at insertion sites of invasive lines, sutures, surgical incisions, wounds.
- Assess and document skin conditions around insertions of pins, wires, and tongs, noting inflammation and drainage.
- Obtain appropriate tissue or fluid specimens for observation and culture and sensitivities testing. Note signs and symptoms of sepsis (systemic infection): fever, chills, diaphoresis, altered level of consciousness, positive blood cultures.

Nursing Priority No. 2.

To reduce/correct existing risk factors:

- Emphasize constant and proper hand hygiene by all caregivers between therapies and clients. Wear gloves when appropriate to minimize contamination of hands and discard after each client. Wash hands after glove removal. Instruct client/SO/visitors to wash hands, as indicated, as this is **a first-line defense against healthcare-associated infections (HAIs).**
- Monitor client's visitors and caregivers for respiratory illnesses. Ask sick visitors to leave client area or offer masks and tissues to client or visitors who are coughing or sneezing **to limit exposures, thus reducing cross-contamination.**
- Post visual alerts in healthcare settings instructing clients/SO(s) to inform healthcare providers if they have symptoms of respiratory infections or influenza-like symptoms.
- Encourage parents of sick children to keep them away from childcare settings and school until afebrile for 24 hours.
- Provide for isolation, as indicated (e.g., contact, droplet, and airborne precautions). Educate staff in infection control procedures. **Reduces risk of cross-contamination.**
- Emphasize proper use of personal protective equipment (PPE) by staff and visitors, as dictated by agency policy **for particular exposure risk (e.g., airborne, droplet, splash risk), including mask or respiratory filter of appropriate particulate regulator, gowns, aprons, head covers, face shields, protective eyewear.**
- Perform or instruct in daily mouth care. Include use of antiseptic mouthwash for individuals in acute or long-term care settings **at high risk for nosocomial or HAIs.**

Information that appears in brackets has been added by the authors to clarify and enhance the use of nursing diagnoses.

🌐 Cultural 🌐 Collaborative 🏠 Community/Home Care

- Recommend routine or preoperative body shower or scrubs, when indicated (e.g., orthopedic, plastic surgery), **to reduce bacterial colonization.**
- Maintain sterile technique for all invasive procedures (e.g., IV, urinary catheter, pulmonary suctioning).
- Fill bubbling humidifiers and nebulizers with *sterile* water, not distilled or tap water. Avoid use of room-air humidifiers unless unit is sterilized daily and filled with sterile water.
- Use heat and moisture exchangers instead of heated humidifier with mechanical ventilator.
- Assist with weaning from mechanical ventilator as soon as possible **to reduce risk of ventilator-associated pneumonia (VAP).**
- Choose proper vascular access device based on anticipated treatment duration and solution/medication to be infused and best available aseptic insertion techniques.
- Change surgical or other wound dressings, as indicated, using proper technique for changing/disposing of contaminated materials.
- Cleanse incisions and insertion sites per facility protocol with appropriate antimicrobial topical or solution **to reduce potential for catheter-related bloodstream infections, and to prevent growth of bacteria.**
- Separate touching surfaces when skin is excoriated, such as in herpes zoster. Use gloves when caring for open lesions **to minimize auto-inoculation or transmission of viral diseases (e.g., herpes simplex virus, hepatitis, AIDS).**
- Cover perineal and pelvic region dressings or casts with plastic when using bedpan **to prevent contamination.**
- Encourage early ambulation, deep breathing, coughing, position changes, and early removal of endotrachial (ET) tube or nasal or oral feeding tubes **for mobilization of respiratory secretions and prevention of aspiration/respiratory infections.**
- Encourage or assist with use of adjuncts (e.g., respiratory aids, such as incentive spirometry) **to prevent pneumonia.**
- Maintain adequate hydration, stand or sit to void, and catheterize, if necessary, **to avoid bladder distention and urinary stasis.**
- Provide regular urinary catheter and perineal care. **Reduces risk of ascending urinary tract infection.**

Information that appears in brackets has been added by the authors to clarify and enhance the use of nursing diagnoses.

- Assist with medical procedures (e.g., wound or joint aspiration, incision and drainage of abscess, bronchoscopy), as indicated.
- Administer/monitor medication regimen (e.g., antimicrobials, drip infusion into osteomyelitis, subeschar clysis, topical antibiotics) and note client's response **to determine effectiveness of therapy or presence of side effects.**
- Administer prophylactic antibiotics and immunizations, as indicated.

Nursing Priority No. 3.

To promote wellness (Teaching/Discharge Considerations):

- Review individual nutritional needs, appropriate exercise program, and need for rest.
- Instruct client/SO(s) in techniques to protect the integrity of skin, care for lesions, and prevention of spread of infection.
- Emphasize necessity of taking antivirals or antibiotics, as directed (e.g., dosage and length of therapy). **Premature discontinuation of treatment when client begins to feel well may result in return of infection and potentiation of drug-resistant strains.**
- Discuss importance of not taking antibiotics or using "leftover" drugs unless specifically instructed by healthcare provider. **Inappropriate use can lead to development of drug-resistant strains or secondary infections.**
- Discuss the role of smoking in respiratory infections.
- Promote safer-sex practices and report sexual contacts of infected individuals **to prevent the spread of HIV and other sexually transmitted infections (STIs).**
- Provide information and involve in appropriate community and national education programs **to increase awareness of and prevention of communicable diseases.**
- Discuss precautions with client engaged in international travel, and refer for immunizations **to reduce incidence and transmission of global infections.**
- Promote childhood immunization program. Encourage adults to obtain/update immunizations as appropriate.
- Include information in preoperative teaching about ways to reduce potential for postoperative infection (e.g., respiratory measures to prevent pneumonia, wound and dressing care, avoidance of others with infection).
- Review use of prophylactic antibiotics if appropriate (e.g., prior to dental work for clients with history of rheumatic fever or valvular heart disease).

Information that appears in brackets has been added by the authors to clarify and enhance the use of nursing diagnoses.

- Encourage contacting healthcare provider for prophylactic therapy, as indicated, following exposure to individuals with infectious disease (e.g., tuberculosis, hepatitis, influenza).
- Identify resources available to the individual (e.g., substance abuse rehabilitation or needle exchange program, as appropriate; free condoms).
- Refer to NDs readiness for enhanced Immunization Status; risk for Disuse Syndrome; impaired Home Maintenance; ineffective Health Maintenance.

Documentation Focus

Assessment/Reassessment
- Individual risk factors, including recent or current antibiotic therapy.
- Wound and/or insertion sites, character of drainage or body secretions.
- Signs and symptoms of infectious process.

Planning
- Plan of care, specific interventions, and who is involved in planning.
- Teaching plan.

Implementation/Evaluation
- Responses to interventions, teaching, and actions performed.
- Attainment or progress toward desired outcome(s).
- Modifications to plan of care.

Discharge Planning
- Discharge needs, referrals made, and who is responsible for actions to be taken.
- Specific referrals made.

Sample Nursing Outcomes & Interventions Classifications (NOC/NIC)

NOC—Knowledge: Infection Management
NIC—Infection Protection

Information that appears in brackets has been added by the authors to clarify and enhance the use of nursing diagnoses.

risk for Injury

Taxonomy II: Safety/Protection—Class 2 Physical Injury
(00035)
[Diagnostic Division: Safety]
Submitted 1978

Definition: At risk for injury as a result of environmental conditions interacting with the individual's adaptive and defensive resources

Risk Factors

Internal

Physical (e.g., broken skin, altered mobility); tissue hypoxia; malnutrition

Abnormal blood profile (e.g., leukocytosis/leukopenia, altered clotting factors, thrombocytopenia, sickle cell, thalassemia, decreased hemoglobin)

Biochemical dysfunction; sensory dysfunction

Integrative or effector dysfunction; immune/autoimmune dysfunction

Psychological (affective orientation); developmental age (physiological, psychosocial)

External

Biological (e.g., immunization level of community, microorganism)

Chemical (e.g., pollutants, poisons, drugs, pharmaceutical agents, alcohol, nicotine, preservatives, cosmetics, dyes); nutritional (e.g., vitamins, food types)

Physical (e.g., design, structure, and arrangement of community, building, and/or equipment); mode of transport

Human (e.g., nosocomial agents, staffing patterns, or cognitive, affective, psychomotor factors)

NOTE: A risk diagnosis is not evidenced by signs and symptoms, as the problem has not occurred; rather, nursing interventions are directed at prevention.

Desired Outcomes/Evaluation Criteria— Client/Caregivers Will:

• Verbalize understanding of individual factors that contribute to possibility of injury.

Information that appears in brackets has been added by the authors to clarify and enhance the use of nursing diagnoses.

- Demonstrate behaviors, lifestyle changes to reduce risk factors and protect self from injury.
- Modify environment as indicated to enhance safety.
- Be free of injury.

Actions/Interventions

In reviewing this ND, it is apparent there is much overlap with other diagnoses. We have chosen to present generalized interventions. Although there are commonalities to injury situations, we suggest that the reader refer to other primary diagnoses as indicated, such as acute or chronic Confusion; risk for Contamination; risk for Falls; impaired Environmental Interpretation Syndrome; impaired Gas Exchange; impaired Home Maintenance; impaired Mobility [specify]; impaired/risk for impaired Parenting; imbalanced Nutrition [specify]; risk for Poisoning; impaired/risk for impaired Skin Integrity; Sleep Deprivation; risk for Suffocation; risk for Infection; risk for Trauma; risk for other-directed/self-directed Violence; Wandering, for additional interventions.

Nursing Priority No. 1.

To evaluate degree/source of risk inherent in the individual situation:

- Perform thorough assessments regarding safety issues when planning for client care and/or preparing for discharge from care. **Failure to accurately assess and intervene or refer these issues can place the client at needless risk and creates negligence issues for the healthcare practitioner.**
- Ascertain knowledge of safety needs, injury prevention, and motivation to prevent injury in home, community, and work settings.
- ∞ Note client's age, gender, developmental stage, decision-making ability, level of cognition/competence. **Affects client's ability to protect self and/or others, and influences choice of interventions and teaching.**
- ∞ Review expectations caregivers have of children, cognitively impaired, and/or elderly family members.
- Assess mood, coping abilities, personality styles (e.g., temperament, aggression, impulsive behavior, level of self-esteem) **that may result in carelessness or increased risk taking without consideration of consequences.**
- Assess client's muscle strength, gross and fine motor coordination **to identify risk for falls.**

Information that appears in brackets has been added by the authors to clarify and enhance the use of nursing diagnoses.

- Note socioeconomic status and availability and use of resources.
- Evaluate individual's emotional and behavioral response to violence in environmental surroundings (e.g., home, neighborhood, peer group, media). **May affect client's view of and regard for own/others' safety.**
- Determine potential for abusive behavior by family members/SO(s)/peers.
- Observe for signs of injury and age (current, recent, and past such as old or new bruises, history of fractures, frequent absences from school or work) **to determine need for evaluation of intentional injury or abuse in client relationship or living environment.**

Nursing Priority No. 2.

To assist client/caregiver to reduce or correct individual risk factors:

- Provide healthcare within a culture of safety (e.g., adherence to nursing standards of care and facility safe-care policies) **to prevent errors resulting in client injury, promote client safety, and model safety behaviors for client/SO(s):**

  Monitor environment for potentially unsafe conditions and modify as needed.

  Orient or reorient client to environment, as needed.

  Place confused elderly client or young child near nurses' station.

  Instruct client/SO(s) to request assistance as needed; make sure call light is within reach and client knows how to operate.

  Maintain bed or chair in lowest position with wheels locked.

  Ensure that floors are clear of hazards and that pathway to bathroom is unobstructed and properly lighted.

  Provide seat raisers for chairs, use stand-assist, repositioning, or lifting devices as indicated.

  Place assistive devices (e.g., walker, cane, glasses, hearing aid) within reach and ascertain that client is using them.

  Safety lock exit and stairwell doors **when client can wander away.**

  Administer medications and infusions using "6 rights" system (right patient, right medication, right route, right dose, right time, right reason).

- Inform and educate client/SO(s) regarding all treatments and medications and so forth.
- Develop plan of care with family to meet client's and SO's individual needs.

Information that appears in brackets has been added by the authors to clarify and enhance the use of nursing diagnoses.

- Provide information regarding disease or condition(s) that may result in increased risk of injury (e.g., weakness, dementia, head injury, immunosuppression, use of multiple medications, use of alcohol or other drugs, exposure to environmental chemicals or other hazards).
- Identify interventions and safety devices **to promote safe physical environment and individual safety.**
- Refer to physical or occupational therapist, as appropriate, **to identify high-risk tasks, conduct site visits; select, create, modify equipment or assistive devices; and provide education about body mechanics and musculoskeletal injuries, in addition to providing therapies as indicated.**
- Demonstrate and encourage use of techniques to reduce or manage stress and vent emotions, such as anger, hostility.
- Review consequences of previously determined risk factors that client is reluctant to modify (e.g., oral cancer in teenager using smokeless tobacco, occurrence of spontaneous abortion, fetal alcohol syndrome or neonatal addiction in prenatal woman using drugs, fall related to failure to use assistive equipment, toddler getting into medicine cabinet, binge drinking while skiing, health and legal implications of illicit drug use, working too many hours for safe operation of machinery or vehicles).
- Discuss importance of self-monitoring of condition or emotions **that can contribute to occurrence of injury (e.g., fatigue, anger, irritability).**
- Encourage participation in self-help programs, such as assertiveness training, positive self-image, to enhance self-esteem and sense of self-worth.
- Perform home assessment and identify safety issues, such as locking up medications and poisonous substances, locking exterior doors **to prevent client from wandering off while SO is engaged in other household activities,** or removing matches and smoking material and knobs from the stove **so confused client does not start a fire or turn on burner and leave it unattended.**
- Discuss need for and sources of supervision (e.g., before- and after-school programs, elderly day care).
- Discuss concerns about childcare, discipline practices.

Nursing Priority No. 3.

To promote wellness (Teaching/Discharge Considerations):

- Identify individual needs and resources for safety education such as First Aid/CPR classes, babysitter class, water or gun

---

Information that appears in brackets has been added by the authors to clarify and enhance the use of nursing diagnoses.

safety, smoking cessation, substance abuse program, weight and exercise management, industry and community safety courses.
- Provide telephone numbers and other contact numbers, as individually indicated (e.g., doctor, 911, poison control, police, lifeline, hazardous materials handler).
- Refer to other resources, as indicated (e.g., counseling, psychotherapy, budget counseling, parenting classes).
- Provide bibliotherapy or written resources **for later review and self-paced learning.**
- Promote community education programs geared to increasing awareness of safety measures and resources available to the individual (e.g., correct use of child safety seats, bicycle helmets, home hazard information, firearm safety, fall prevention, CPR and First Aid).
- Promote community awareness about the problems of design of buildings, equipment, transportation, and workplace practices that contribute to accidents.
- Identify community resources/neighbors/friends to assist elderly/handicapped individuals in providing such things as structural maintenance and removal of snow and ice from walks and steps.

Documentation Focus

Assessment/Reassessment
- Individual risk factors, noting current physical findings (e.g., bruises, cuts).
- Client's/caregiver's understanding of individual risks and safety concerns.
- Availability and use of resources.

Planning
- Plan of care and who is involved in planning.
- Teaching plan.

Implementation/Evaluation
- Individual responses to interventions, teaching, and actions performed.
- Specific actions and changes that are made.
- Attainment or progress toward desired outcome(s).
- Modifications to plan of care.

Information that appears in brackets has been added by the authors to clarify and enhance the use of nursing diagnoses.

Discharge Planning

- Long-range plans for discharge needs, lifestyle and community changes, and who is responsible for actions to be taken.
- Specific referrals made.

Sample Nursing Outcomes & Interventions Classifications (NOC/NIC)

NOC—Safety Behavior: Personal
NIC—Surveillance: Safety

Insomnia

Taxonomy II: Activity/Rest—Class 1 Sleep/Rest (00095)
[Diagnostic Division: Activity/Rest]
Submitted 2006

Definition: A disruption in amount and quality of sleep that impairs functioning

Related Factors

Intake of stimulants or alcohol; pharmaceutical agents; gender-related hormonal shifts

Stress (e.g., ruminative pre-sleep pattern); depression; fear; anxiety; grief

Impairment of normal sleep pattern (e.g., travel, shift work); parental responsibilities; interrupted sleep; inadequate sleep hygiene (current)

Activity pattern (e.g., timing, amount); frequent daytime naps

Physical discomfort (e.g., pain, shortness of breath, cough, gastroesophageal reflux, nausea, incontinence/urgency)

Environmental factors (e.g., ambient noise, daylight/darkness exposure, ambient temperature/humidity, unfamiliar setting)

Defining Characteristics

Subjective

Reports:

Difficulty falling or staying asleep; waking up too early

Dissatisfaction with sleep (current); nonrestorative sleep

Sleep disturbances that produce next-day consequences; lack of energy; difficulty concentrating; changes in mood

---

Information that appears in brackets has been added by the authors to clarify and enhance the use of nursing diagnoses.

Decreased health status or quality of life
Increased accidents

Objective
Observed lack of energy
Observed changes in affect
Increased absenteeism (e.g., work/school)

Desired Outcomes/Evaluation Criteria— Client Will:

* Verbalize understanding of sleep impairment.
* Identify individually appropriate interventions to promote sleep.
* Adjust lifestyle to accommodate chronobiological rhythms.
* Report improvement in sleep-rest pattern.
* Report increased sense of well-being and feeling rested.

Actions/Interventions

Nursing Priority No. 1.
To identify causative/contributing factors:

* Identify presence of Related Factors such as chronic pain, arthritis, dyspnea, movement disorders, dementia, obesity, pregnancy, menopause, psychiatric disorders; metabolic diseases (e.g., hyperthyroidism, diabetes); prescribed and over-the-counter (OTC) drugs; alcohol, stimulant, or other recreational drug use; circadian rhythm disorders (e.g., shift work, jet lag); environmental factors (e.g., noise, no control over thermostat, uncomfortable bed); major life stressors (e.g., grief, loss, finances) **that can contribute to insomnia.**
* ∞ Note age **(high percentage of elderly individuals are affected by sleep problems). Two primary sleep disorders that increase with age are sleep apnea (SA) and periodic limb movements in sleep (PLMS).**
* ∞ Observe parent-infant interaction and provision of emotional support. Note mother's sleep-wake pattern. **Lack of knowledge of infant cues or problem relationships may create tension interfering with sleep. Structured sleep routines based on adult schedules may not meet child's needs.**
* Ascertain presence and frequency of enuresis, incontinence, or need for frequent nighttime voidings, **interrupting sleep.**
* Review psychological assessment, noting individual and personality characteristics **if anxiety disorders or depression could be affecting sleep.**

Information that appears in brackets has been added by the authors to clarify and enhance the use of nursing diagnoses.

🌐 Cultural   🕮 Collaborative   🏠 Community/Home Care

- Determine recent traumatic events in client's life (e.g., death in family, loss of job). **Physical and emotional trauma often affects client's sleep patterns and quality for a short period of time. This disruption can become long term and require more intensive assessment and intervention.**
- Review client's medications, including prescription drugs (e.g., beta-blockers, sedative antidepressants, sedative neuroleptics; bronchodilators, weight-loss drugs, thyroid preparations), OTC products, and herbals **to determine if adjustments may be needed (such as change in dose or time medication is taken) or if a different medication may be needed.**
- Evaluate use of caffeine and alcoholic beverages. **May interfere with falling asleep or duration and quality of sleep (overindulgence interferes with rapid eye movement [REM] sleep).**
- Assist with diagnostic testing (e.g., polysomnography; daytime multiple sleep latency testing; Actigraphy; full-night sleep studies) **to determine cause and type of sleep disturbance.**

Nursing Priority No. 2.

To evaluate sleep pattern and dysfunction(s):

- Review sleep diary (where available); observe and/or obtain feedback from client/SO(s) regarding client's sleep problems, usual bedtime, rituals and routines, number of hours of sleep, time of arising, and environmental needs **to determine usual sleep pattern and provide comparative baseline.**
- Listen to subjective reports of sleep quality (e.g., client never feels rested, or feels excessively sleepy during day).
- Identify circumstances that interrupt sleep and the frequency at which they occur.
- Determine client's/SO's expectations of adequate sleep. **Provides opportunity to address misconceptions or unrealistic expectations.**
- Investigate whether client snores and in what position(s) this occurs **to determine if further evaluation is needed to rule out obstructive SA.**
- Note alteration of habitual sleep time, such as change of work pattern, rotating shifts, change in normal bedtime (hospitalization). **Helps identify circumstances that are known to interrupt sleep patterns resulting in mental and physical fatigue, affecting concentration, interest, energy, and appetite.**

Information that appears in brackets has been added by the authors to clarify and enhance the use of nursing diagnoses.

- Observe physical signs of fatigue (e.g., restlessness, hand tremors, thick speech).
- Develop a chronological chart **to determine peak perform-ance rhythm.**

Nursing Priority No. 3.

To assist client to establish optimal sleep/rest patterns:

- Collaborate in treatment of underlying medical and psychiatric problem (e.g., obstructive SA, pain, gastroesophageal reflux disease [GERD], lower urinary tract infection [UTI]/ prostatic hypertrophy; depression, bipolar disorder; complicated grief).
- Arrange care to provide for uninterrupted periods for rest, especially allowing for longer periods of sleep at night when possible. Do as much care as possible without waking client.
- Explain necessity of disturbances for monitoring vital signs and/or other care when client is hospitalized.
- Provide quiet environment and comfort measures (e.g., back rub, washing hands/face, cleaning and straightening sheets) in preparation for sleep.
- Discuss and implement effective age-appropriate bedtime rituals (e.g., going to bed at same time each night, drinking warm milk, rocking, story reading, cuddling, favorite blanket or toy) **to enhance client's relaxation, reinforce that bed is a place to sleep, and promote sense of security for child or confused elder.**
- Recommend limiting intake of chocolate and caffeinated or alcoholic beverages, especially prior to bedtime.
- Limit fluid intake in evening if nocturia is a problem **to reduce need for nighttime elimination.**
- Explore other sleep aids (e.g., warm bath, light protein snack before bedtime; soothing music, etc.). **Nonpharmaceutical aids may enhance falling asleep free of concern of medication side effects such as morning hangover or drug dependence.**
- Administer pain medications (if required) 1 hour before sleep **to relieve discomfort and take maximum advantage of sedative effect.**
- Monitor effects of drug regimen—amphetamines or stimulants (e.g., methylphenidate [Ritalin] used in narcolepsy).
- Use barbiturates and/or other sleeping medications sparingly. **Research indicates long-term use of these medications, especially in the absence of cognitive behavioral therapy (CBT), can actually induce sleep disturbances.**

Information that appears in brackets has been added by the authors to clarify and enhance the use of nursing diagnoses.

🌐 Cultural 🔄 Collaborative 🏠 Community/Home Care

- Encourage routine use of continuous positive airway pressure (CPAP) therapy, when indicated, **to obtain optimal benefit of treatment for SA.**
- Develop behavioral program for insomnia, such as:

Establishing and maintaining a regular sleeping time and waking-up time

Thinking relaxing thoughts when in bed

Not napping in the daytime

Exercising daily, but not immediately before bedtime

Avoiding heavy meals at bedtime

Using bed only for sleeping or sex

Wearing comfortable, loose-fitting clothing to bed and participating in relaxing activity until sleepy

Not reading or watching TV in bed

Getting out of bed if not asleep in 15 to 30 minutes

Getting up the same time each day—even on weekends and days off

Getting adequate exposure to bright light during day

Individually tailoring stress reduction program, music therapy, relaxation routine

- Administer and monitor effects of prescribed medications to promote sleep (e.g., *benzodiazepines,* such as zolpiden [Ambien], zaleplon [Sonata], eszopiclone [Lunesta]; *antidepressants,* such as trazadone [Desyrel], ncfazodone [Serzone]; *melatonin agonists,* such as ramelteon [Rozrem]). **While most are effective in the short term, many lose effectiveness over time. The client may have adverse side effects or develop tolerance and misuse the drug. Many drug regimens are most effective when combined with CBT, in which the client can be weaned off medications at some point.**
- Refer to sleep specialist, as indicated or desired. **Follow-up evaluation or intervention may be needed when insomnia is seriously impacting client's quality of life, productivity, and safety (e.g., on the job, at home, on the road).**

Nursing Priority No. 4.

To promote wellness (Teaching/Discharge Considerations):

- Assure client that occasional sleeplessness should not threaten health. **Worrying about not sleeping can perpetuate or exacerbate the problem.**
- Assist client to develop individual program of relaxation. Demonstrate techniques (e.g., biofeedback, self-hypnosis, visualization, progressive muscle relaxation).

Information that appears in brackets has been added by the authors to clarify and enhance the use of nursing diagnoses.

- Encourage participation in regular exercise program during day **to aid in stress control and release of energy. Note: Exercise at bedtime may stimulate rather than relax client and actually interfere with sleep.**
- Recommend inclusion of bedtime snack (e.g., milk or mild juice, crackers, protein source such as cheese/peanut butter) in dietary program **to reduce sleep interference from hunger or hypoglycemia.**
- Provide for child's (or impaired individual's) sleep time safety (e.g., infant placed on back, bedrails or bed in low position, nonplastic sheets).
- Investigate use of aids to block out light and noise, such as sleep mask, darkening shades or curtains, earplugs, monotonous sounds such as low-level background noise (white noise).
- Participate in program to "reset" the body's sleep clock (chronotherapy) **when client has delayed-sleep-onset insomnia.**
- Assist individual to develop schedules that take advantage of peak performance times as identified in chronobiological chart.
- Recommend midmorning nap if one is required. **Napping, especially in the afternoon, can disrupt normal sleep patterns.**
- Assist client to deal with grieving process when loss has occurred. (Refer to ND Grieving.)

Documentation Focus

Assessment/Reassessment
- Assessment findings, including specifics of sleep pattern (current and past) and effects on lifestyle and level of functioning.
- Medications or interventions used, previous therapies tried.

Planning
- Plan of care and who is involved in planning.
- Teaching plan.

Implementation/Evaluation
- Client's response to interventions, teaching, and actions performed.
- Attainment or progress toward desired outcome(s).
- Modifications to plan of care.

Information that appears in brackets has been added by the authors to clarify and enhance the use of nursing diagnoses.

Cultural   Collaborative   Community/Home Care

Discharge Planning
- Long-term needs and who is responsible for actions to be taken.
- Specific referrals made.

Sample Nursing Outcomes & Interventions Classifications (NOC/NIC)

NOC—Sleep
NIC—Sleep Enhancement

decreased Intracranial Adaptive Capacity

Taxonomy II: Coping/Stress Tolerance—Class 3 Neuro-behavioral Stress (00049)
[Diagnostic Division: Circulation]
Submitted 1994

Definition: Intracranial fluid dynamic mechanisms that normally compensate for increases in intracranial volume are compromised, resulting in repeated disproportionate increases in intracranial pressure (ICP) in response to a variety of noxious and nonnoxious stimuli

Related Factors

Brain injuries
Sustained increase in ICP of 10–15 mm Hg
Decreased cerebral perfusion pressure ($\leq$50–60 mm Hg
Systemic hypotension with intracranial hypertension

Defining Characteristics

Objective
Repeated increases of ICP of >10 mm Hg for more than 5 minutes following a variety of external stimuli
Disproportionate increase in ICP following stimulus
Elevated P_2 ICP waveform
Volume pressure response test variation (volume-to-pressure ratio of 2, pressure-volume index of less than 10)
Baseline ICP >10 mm Hg
Wide amplitude ICP waveform

Information that appears in brackets has been added by the authors to clarify and enhance the use of nursing diagnoses.

Desired Outcomes/Evaluation Criteria— Client Will:

- Demonstrate stable ICP as evidenced by normalization of pressure waveforms and appropriate response to stimuli.
- Display improved neurological signs.

Actions/Interventions

Nursing Priority No. 1.

To assess causative/contributing factors:

- Determine factors related to individual situation (e.g., cause of loss of consciousness or coma [such as fall, motor vehicle crash, gunshot wound], infection such as meningitis, or encephalitis, brain tumor) and potential for increased intracranial presssure [ICP].
- Monitor and document changes in ICP; monitor waveform and corresponding event (e.g., suctioning, position change, monitor alarms, family visit). **ICP monitoring may be done in a critically ill client with a Glasgow Coma Scale (GCS) score of 8 or less. The ICP offers data that supplement the neurological examination and can be crucial in client whose examination findings are affected by sedatives, paralytics, or other factors. Elevated pressure can be caused by the injury, environmental stimuli, or treatment modalities.**

Nursing Priority No. 2.

To note degree of impairment:

- Assess and document client's eye opening, position, and movement; size, shape, equality, light reactivity of pupils; and consciousness and mental status via GCS **to determine client's baseline neurological status and monitor changes over time.**
- Note purposeful and nonpurposeful motor response (posturing, etc.), comparing right and left sides. **Posturing and abnormal flexion of extremities usually indicates diffuse cortical damage. Absence of spontaneous movement on one side indicates damage to the motor tracts in the opposite cerebral hemisphere.**
- Test for presence of reflexes (e.g., blink, cough, gag, Babinski's reflex), nuchal rigidity. **Helps identify location of injury (e.g., loss of blink reflex suggests damage to the pons**

Information that appears in brackets has been added by the authors to clarify and enhance the use of nursing diagnoses.

🌐 Cultural   🟢 Collaborative   🏠 Community/Home Care

and medulla, absence of cough and gag reflexes reflects damage to medulla).

- Monitor vital signs and cardiac rhythm before, during, after activity. **Helps determine parameters for "safe" activity. Mean arterial blood pressure should be maintained above 90 mm Hg to maintain cerebral perfusion pressure (CPP) greater than 70 mm Hg, which reflects adequate blood supply to the brain. Fever in brain injury can be associated with injury to the hypothalamus or bleeding, systemic infection (e.g., pneumonia), or drugs. Hyperthermia exacerbates cerebral ischemia. Irregular respiration patterns can suggest location of cerebral insult. Cardiac dysrhythmias can be due to brainstem injury and stimulation of the sympathetic nervous system. Bradycardia may occur with high ICP.**
- Review results of diagnostic imaging (e.g., computed tomography [CT] scans) **to note location, type, and severity of tissue injury.**

Nursing Priority No. 3.

To minimize/correct causative factors/maximize perfusion:

- Elevate head of bed, as individually appropriate. **Studies show that in most cases, 30 degrees elevation significantly decreases ICP while maintaining cerebral blood flow.**
- Maintain head and neck in neutral position, support with small towel rolls or pillows **to maximize venous return.** Avoid placing head on large pillow or causing hip flexion of 90 degrees or more.
- Decrease extraneous stimuli and provide comfort measures (e.g., quiet environment, soft voice, tapes of familiar voices played through earphones, back massage, gentle touch as tolerated) **to reduce central nervous system stimulation and promote relaxation.**
- Limit painful procedures (e.g., venipunctures, redundant neurological evaluations) to those that are absolutely necessary.
- Provide rest periods between care activities and limit duration of procedures. Lower lighting and noise level, schedule and limit activities **to provide restful environment, reduce agitation and limit spikes in ICP associated with noxious stimuli.**
- Limit or prevent activities that increase intrathoracic or abdominal pressures (e.g., coughing, vomiting, straining at stool). Avoid or limit use of restraints. **These factors markedly increase ICP.**

Information that appears in brackets has been added by the authors to clarify and enhance the use of nursing diagnoses.

- Suction with caution—only when needed—to just beyond end of endotracheal tube without touching tracheal wall or carina. Administer lidocaine intratracheally per protocol **to reduce cough reflex,** and hyperoxygenate before suctioning, as appropriate, **to minimize hypoxia.**
- Maintain patency of urinary drainage system **to reduce risk of hypertension, increased ICP, and associated dysreflexia when a spinal cord injury is also present and spinal cord shock is past.** (Refer to ND Autonomic Dysreflexia.)
- Weigh, as indicated. Calculate fluid balance every shift or daily **to determine fluid needs, maintain hydration, and prevent fluid overload.**
- Administer or restrict fluid intake, as necessary. Administer IV fluids via pump or control device **to maintain circulating volume and cerebral perfusion pressure or to prevent inadvertent fluid bolus or vascular overload with potential cerebral edema and increased ICP.**
- Regulate environmental temperature; use cooling blanket as indicated **to decrease metabolic and O_2 needs when fever present or therapeutic hypothermia therapy is used.**
- Investigate increased restlessness **to determine causative factors and initiate corrective measures as early as possible.**
- Provide appropriate safety measures and initiate treatment for seizures **to prevent injury and increased ICP or hypoxia.**
- Administer supplemental oxygen, as indicated, **to prevent cerebral ischemia;** hyperventilate (as indicated per protocol) when on mechanical ventilation. **Therapeutic hyperventilation may be used (PaCO$_2$ of 30 to 35 mm) to reduce intracranial hypertension for a short period of time, while other methods of ICP control are initiated.**
- Administer medications (e.g., antihypertensives, diuretics, analgesics, sedatives, antipyretics, vasopressors, antiseizure drugs, neuromuscular blocking agents, and corticosteroids), as appropriate, **to maintain cerebral homeostasis and manage symptoms associated with neurological injury.**
- Administer enteral or parenteral nutrition **to achieve positive nitrogen balance, reducing effects of post–brain injury metabolic and catabolic states, which can lead to complications.**
- Prepare client for surgery, as indicated (e.g., evacuation of hematoma or space-occupying lesion), **to reduce ICP and enhance circulation.**

Information that appears in brackets has been added by the authors to clarify and enhance the use of nursing diagnoses.

Nursing Priority No. 4.

To promote wellness (Teaching/Discharge Considerations):

- Identify signs/symptoms suggesting increased ICP (in client at risk without an ICP monitor), such as restlessness, deterioration in neurological responses.
- Review appropriate interventions.

Documentation Focus

Assessment/Reassessment

- Neurological findings noting right and left sides separately (such as pupils, motor response, reflexes, restlessness, nuchal rigidity); GCS.
- Response to activities and events (e.g., changes in pressure waveforms or vital signs).
- Presence and characteristics of seizure activity.

Planning

- Plan of care and who is involved in planning.
- Teaching plan.

Implementation/Evaluation

- Response to interventions and actions performed.
- Attainment or progress toward desired outcome(s).
- Modifications to plan of care.

Discharge Planning

- Future needs, plan for meeting them, and determining who is responsible for actions.
- Referrals as identified.

Sample Nursing Outcomes & Interventions Classifications (NOC/NIC)

NOC—Tissue Perfusion: Cerebral
NIC—Cerebral Edema Management

---

neonatal Jaundice

Taxonomy II: Nutrition—Class 4 Metabolism (00194)
[Diagnostic Division: Safety]
Submitted 2008; Revised 2010

Definition: The yellow-orange tint of the neonate's skin and mucous membranes that occurs after 24 hours of life as a result of unconjugated bilirubin in the circulation

---

Information that appears in brackets has been added by the authors to clarify and enhance the use of nursing diagnoses.

Related Factors

Neonate age 1 to 7 days

Feeding pattern not well established

Abnormal weight loss (more than 7% to 8% in breastfeeding newborn; 15% in term infant)

Stool (meconium) passage delayed

Infant experiences difficulty making the transition to extrauterine life

Defining Characteristics

Objective

Yellow-orange skin; yellow sclera, mucous membranes

Abnormal skin bruising

Abnormal blood profile (e.g., hemolysis; total serum bilirubin more than 2 mg/dL; total serum bilirubin in the high-risk range on age in hour-specific nomogram)

Desired Outcomes/Evaluation Criteria— Infant Will: (Include Specific Time Frame)

- Display decreasing bilirubin levels with resolution of jaundice.
- Be free of central nervous system (CNS) involvement or complications associated with therapeutic regimen.

Parent/Caregiver Will: (Include Specific Time Frame)

- Verbalize understanding of cause, treatment, and possible outcomes of hyperbilirubinemia.
- Demonstrate appropriate care of infant.

Actions/Interventions

Nursing Priority No. 1.

To assess causative/contributing factors:

- Determine infant and maternal blood groups and blood types. **ABO incompatibilities affect 20% of all pregnancies.**
- Note gender, race, and place of birth. **Risk of developing jaundice is higher in males, infants of East Asian or American Indian descent, and those living at high altitudes.**
- Review intrapartal record for specific risk factors, such as low birth weight (LBW) or intrauterine growth retardation

---

Information that appears in brackets has been added by the authors to clarify and enhance the use of nursing diagnoses.

(IUGR), prematurity, abnormal metabolic processes, vascular injuries, abnormal circulation, sepsis, or polycythemia.

- Note use of instruments or vacuum extractor for delivery. Assess infant for presence of birth trauma, cephalohematoma, and excessive ecchymosis or petechiae. **Resorption of blood trapped in fetal scalp tissue and excessive hemolysis may increase the amount of bilirubin being released.**

- Review infant's condition at birth, noting need for resuscitation or evidence of excessive ecchymosis or petechiae, cold stress, asphyxia, or acidosis. **Asphyxia and acidosis reduce affinity of bilirubin to albumin, increasing the amount of unbound circulating (indirect) bilirubin, which may cross the blood-brain barrier, causing CNS toxicity.**

- Evaluate maternal and prenatal nutritional levels; note possible neonatal hypoproteinemia, especially in preterm infant. **One gram of albumin carries 16 mg of unconjugated bilirubin; therefore, lack of sufficient albumin (hypoproteinemia) in the newborn increases risk of jaundice.**

- Assess infant for signs of hypoglycemia such as jitteriness, irritability, and lethargy. Obtain heel stick glucose levels as indicated. **Hypoglycemia necessitates use of fat stores for energy-releasing fatty acids, which compete with bilirubin for binding sites on albumin.**

- Determine successful initiation and adequacy of breastfeeding. **Poor caloric intake and dehydration associated with ineffective breastfeeding increase risk of developing hyperbilirubinemia.**

- Evaluate infant for pallor, edema, or hepatosplenomegaly. **These signs may be associated with hydrops fetalis, Rh incompatibility, and in-utero hemolysis of fetal red blood cells (RBCs).**

- Evaluate for jaundice in natural light, noting sclera and oral mucosa, yellowing of skin immediately after blanching, and specific body parts involved. Assess oral mucosa, posterior portion of hard palate, and conjunctival sacs in dark-skinned newborns.

- Note infant's age at onset of jaundice. Aids in differentiating type of jaundice (i.e., physiological, breast milk induced, or pathological). **Physiological jaundice usually appears between the second and third day of life, breast milk jaundice between the fourth and the seventh day of life, and pathological jaundice occurs within the first 24 hours of life, or when the total serum bilirubin level rises by more than 5 mg/dL per day.**

Information that appears in brackets has been added by the authors to clarify and enhance the use of nursing diagnoses.

Nursing Priority No. 2.

To evaluate degree of compromise:

- Review laboratory studies including total serum bilirubin and albumin levels, hemoglobin and hematocrit, reticulocyte count.
- Calculate plasma bilirubin-albumin binding capacity. **Aids in determining risk of kernicterus and treatment needs.**
- Assess infant for progression of signs and behavioral changes associated with bilirubin toxicity. **Early-stage toxicity involves neuro-depression-lethargy, poor feeding, high-pitched cry, diminished or absent reflexes; late-stage hypotonia, neuro-hyperreflexia-twitching, convulsions, opisthotonos, fever.**
- Evaluate appearance of skin and urine, noting brownish-black color. **An uncommon side effect of phototherapy involves exaggerated pigment changes (bronze baby syndrome) that may last for 2 to 4 months but is not associated with harmful sequelae.**

Nursing Priority No. 3.

To correct hyperbilirubinemia and prevent associated complications:

- Keep infant warm and dry; monitor skin and core temperature frequently. **Prevents cold stress and the release of fatty acids that compete for binding sites on albumin, thus increasing the level of freely circulating bilirubin.**
- Initiate early oral feedings within 4 to 6 hours following birth, especially if infant is to be breastfed. **Establishes proper intestinal flora necessary for reduction of bilirubin to urobilinogen and decreases reabsorption of bilirubin from bowel.**
- Encourage frequent breastfeeding—8 to 12 times per day. Assist mother with pumping of breasts as needed **to maintain milk production.**
- Administer small amounts of breast milk substitute (L-aspartic acid or enzymatically hydrolyzed casein [EHC]) for 24 to 48 hours if indicated. **Use of feeding additives is under investigation for inhibition of beta-glucuronidase leading to increased fecal excretion of bilirubin; results have been mixed.**
- Apply transcutaneous jaundice meter. **Provides noninvasive screening of jaundice.**

Information that appears in brackets has been added by the authors to clarify and enhance the use of nursing diagnoses.

🌐 Cultural 🕸 Collaborative 🏠 Community/Home Care

- Initiate phototherapy per protocol, using fluorescent bulbs placed above the infant or fiberoptic pad or blanket (except for newborns with Rh disease). **Primary therapy for neonates with unconjugated hyperbilirubinemia.**
- Apply eye patches, ensuring correct fit during periods of phototherapy, to prevent retinal injury. Remove eye covering during feedings or other care activities as appropriate **to provide visual stimulation and interaction with caregivers/parents.**
- Avoid application of lotion or oils to skin of infant receiving phototherapy **to prevent dermal irritation or injury.**
- Reposition infant every 2 hours **to ensure that all areas of skin are exposed to bili light when fiberoptic pad or blanket is not used.**
- Cover male groin with small pad **to protect from heat-related injury to testes.**
- Monitor infant's weight loss, urine output and specific gravity, and fecal water loss from loose stools associated with phototherapy **to determine adequacy of fluid intake.** *Note:* **Infant may sleep for longer periods in conjunction with phototherapy, increasing risk of dehydration.**
- Administer intravenous immunoglobulin (IVIG) to neonates with Rh or ABO isoimmunization. **Rate of hemolysis in Rh disease or other cases of immune hemolytic jaundice usually exceeds the rate of bilirubin reduction related to phototherapy. IVIG inhibits antibodies that cause red cell destruction, helping to limit the rise in bilirubin levels.**
- Administer enzyme induction agent (phenobarbital) as appropriate. **May be used on occasion to stimulate hepatic enzymes to enhance clearance of bilirubin.**
- Assist with preparation and administration of exchange transfusion. **Exchange transfusions are occasionally required in cases of severe hemolytic anemia unresponsive to other treatment options or in presence of acute bilirubin encephalopathy as evidenced by hypertonia, arching, retrocollis, opisthotonos, fever, high-pitched cry.**
- Document events during transfusion, carefully recording amount of blood withdrawn and injected (usually 7 to 20 mL at a time).

Nursing Priority No. 4.
To promote wellness (Teaching/Discharge Considerations):

- Provide information about types of jaundice and pathophysiological factors and future implications of hyperbilirubinemia.

Information that appears in brackets has been added by the authors to clarify and enhance the use of nursing diagnoses.

Promotes understanding, corrects misconceptions, and can reduce fear and feelings of guilt.

- Review means of assessing infant status (feedings, intake and ouptut, stools, temperature, and serial weights if scale available) and for monitoring increasing bilirubin levels (e.g., observing blanching of skin over bony prominence or behavior changes), especially if infant is to be discharged early. *Note:* **Persistence of jaundice in formula-fed infant beyond 2 weeks, or 3 weeks in breastfed infant, requires further evaluation.**
- Provide parents with 24-hour emergency telephone number and name of contact person, stressing importance of reporting increased jaundice or changes in behavior.
- Refer to lactation specialist **to enhance or reestablish breast-feeding process.**
- Arrange appropriate referral for home phototherapy program if necessary.
- Provide written explanation of home phototherapy, safety precautions, and potential problems. **Home phototherapy is recommended only for full-term infants after the first 48 hours of life, if serum bilirubin levels are between 14 and 18 mg/dL, with no increase in direct reacting bilirubin concentration.**
- Make appropriate arrangements for follow-up testing of serum bilirubin at same laboratory facility. **Treatment is discontinued once serum bilirubin concentrations fall below 14 mg/dL. Untreated or chronic hyperbilirubinemia can lead to permanent damage such as high-pitch hearing loss, cerebral palsy, or mental retardation.**
- Discuss possible long-term effects of hyperbilirubinemia and the need for continued assessment and early intervention. **Neurological damage associated with kernicterus includes cerebral palsy, mental retardation, sensory difficulties, delayed speech, poor muscle coordination, learning difficulties, death.**

Documentation Focus

Assessment/Reassessment
- Assessment findings, risk or related factors.
- Adequacy of intake—hydration level, character and number of stools.
- Laboratory results and bilirubin trends.

Information that appears in brackets has been added by the authors to clarify and enhance the use of nursing diagnoses.

Planning

- Plan of care, specific interventions, and who is involved in the planning.
- Teaching plan and resources provided.

Implementation/Evaluation

- Client's responses to treatment and actions performed.
- Parents' understanding of teaching.
- Attainment or progress toward desired outcome(s).
- Modifications to plan of care.

Discharge Planning

- Long-range needs, identifying who is responsible for actions to be taken.
- Community resources for equipment and supplies postdischarge.
- Specific referrals made.

Sample Nursing Outcomes & Interventions Classifications (NOC/NIC)

NOC—Newborn Adaptation
NIC—Phototherapy: Neonate

---

risk for neonatal Jaundice

Taxonomy II: Nutrition—Class 4 Metabolism (00230)
[Diagnostic Division: Safety]
Submitted 2008; Revised 2010

Definition: At risk for yellow-orange tint of the neonate's skin and mucous membranes that occurs after 24 hours of life as a result of unconjugated bilirubin in the circulation

---

Risk Factors

Neonate age 1 to 7 days; prematurity
Feeding pattern not well established
Abnormal weight loss (more than 7% to 8% in breastfeeding newborn; 15% in term infant)
Stool (meconium) passage delayed
Infant experiences difficulty making the transition to extrauterine life

---

Information that appears in brackets has been added by the authors to clarify and enhance the use of nursing diagnoses.

Desired Outcomes/Evaluation Criteria— Infant Will: (Include Specific Time Frame)

- Be free of signs of hyperbilirubinemia with normal bilirubin level
- Establish effective feeding pattern

Parent/Caregiver Will: (Include Specific Time Frame)

- Verbalize understanding of cause, treatment, and possible outcomes of hyperbilirubinemia.
- Demonstrate appropriate care of infant.

Actions/Interventions

Nursing Priority No. 1.

To determine individual risk factors:

- Determine infant and maternal blood group and blood type. **ABO incompatibilities affect 20% of all pregnancies, most commonly occurring in mothers with type O blood.**
- Note gender, race, and place of birth. **Risk of developing jaundice is higher in males, infants of East Asian or American Indian descent, and those living at high altitudes. Incidence is lower for African American infants.**
- Review intrapartal record for specific risk factors, such as low birth weight (LBW) or intrauterine growth retardation (IUCR), prematurity, abnormal metabolic processes, vascular injuries, abnormal circulation, sepsis, or polycythemia.
- Note use of instruments or vacuum extractor for delivery. Assess infant for presence of birth trauma, cephalhematoma, and excessive ecchymosis or petechiae. **Resorption of blood trapped in fetal scalp tissue and excessive hemolysis may increase the amount of bilirubin being released.**
- Review infant's condition at birth, noting need for resuscitation or evidence of excessive ecchymosis or petechiae, cold stress, asphyxia, or acidosis. **Asphyxia and acidosis reduce affinity of bilirubin to albumin, increasing the amount of unbound circulating (indirect) bilirubin, which may cross the blood-brain barrier, causing CNS toxicity.**
- Evaluate maternal and prenatal nutritional levels; note possible neonatal hypoproteinemia, especially in preterm infant. **One gram of albumin carries 16 mg of unconjugated bil-**

Information that appears in brackets has been added by the authors to clarify and enhance the use of nursing diagnoses.

Cultural   Collaborative   Community/Home Care

irubin; therefore, lack of sufficient albumin (hypoprotein-emia) in the newborn increases risk of jaundice.

- Assess infant for signs of hypoglycemia such as jitteriness, irritability, and lethargy. Obtain heel stick glucose levels as indicated. **Hypoglycemia necessitates use of fat stores for energy-releasing fatty acids, which compete with bilirubin for binding sites on albumin.**
- Determine successful initiation and adequacy of breastfeed-ing. **Poor caloric intake and dehydration associated with ineffective breastfeeding increase risk of developing hy-perbilirubinemia.**
- Examine infant for pallor, edema, or hepatosplenomegaly. **These signs may be associated with hydrops fetalis, Rh incompatibility, and in-utero hemolysis of fetal red blood cells.**
- Evaluate for jaundice in natural light, noting sclera and oral mucosa, yellowing of skin immediately after blanching, and specific body parts involved. Assess oral mucosa, posterior portion of hard palate, and conjunctival sacs in dark-skinned newborns.

Nursing Priority No. 2.

To prevent onset of hyperbilirubinemia:

- Review laboratory studies including total serum bilirubin and albumin levels, hemoglobin/hematocrit, reticulocyte count, as indicated.
- Keep infant warm and dry; monitor skin and core temperature frequently. **Prevents cold stress and the release of fatty ac-ids that compete for binding sites on albumin thus increas-ing the level of freely circulating bilirubin.**
- Initiate early oral feedings within 4 to 6 hours following birth, especially if infant is to be breastfed. **Establishes proper in-testinal flora necessary for reduction of bilirubin to uro-bilinogen and decreases reabsorption of bilirubin from bowel.**
- Encourage frequent breastfeeding—8 to 12 times per day. Assist mother with pumping of breasts as needed **to maintain milk production for hospitalized preterm infant.**
- Administer intravenous immunoglobulin (IVIG) to neonates with Rh or ABO isoimmunization. **IVIG inhibits Rh anti-bodies that cause red cell destruction helping to limit the rise in bilirubin levels.**

Information that appears in brackets has been added by the authors to clarify and enhance the use of nursing diagnoses.

Nursing Priority No. 3.

To promote wellness (Teaching/Discharge Considerations):

- Review means of assessing infant status (feedings, intake/output, stools, temperature, and serial weights if scale available) and for monitoring increasing bilirubin levels (e.g., observing blanching of skin over bony prominence or behavior changes), especially if infant is to be discharged early. **Enables parents to monitor infant for early signs of increasing bilirubin levels.**
- Provide parents with 24-hour emergency telephone number and name of contact person, stressing importance of reporting signs of jaundice or changes in infant's behavior.
- Refer to lactation specialist as indicated **to assist with establishing/enhancing breastfeeding process.**
- Review proper formula preparation/storage and demonstrate feeding techniques **to meet nutritional and fluid needs.**
- Make arrangements for follow-up testing of serum bilirubin at same laboratory facility.

Documentation Focus

Assessment/Reassessment

- Assessment findings, risk or related factors.
- Adequacy of intake—hydration level, character and number of stools.
- Laboratory results—bilirubin level.

Implementation/Evaluation

- Parents understanding of teaching.
- Attainment or progress toward desired outcome(s).
- Modifications to plan of care.

Discharge Planning

- Home care needs and who is responsible for actions to be taken.
- Any referrals made.

Sample Nursing Outcomes & Interventions Classifications (NOC/NIC)

NOC—Newborn Adaptation
NIC—Newborn Monitoring

Information that appears in brackets has been added by the authors to clarify and enhance the use of nursing diagnoses.

deficient Knowledge [Learning Need] (Specify)

Taxonomy II: Perception/Cognition—Class 4 Cognition (00126)
[Diagnostic Division: Teaching/Learning]
Submitted 1980

Definition: Absence or deficiency of cognitive information related to specific topic (lack of specific information necessary for client/SO to make informed choices regarding condition, treatment, and/or lifestyle changes)

Related Factors

Lack of exposure or recall
Information misinterpretation
Unfamiliarity with information resources
Cognitive limitation
Lack of interest in learning

Defining Characteristics

Subjective
Reports the problem
Request for information; statements reflecting misconceptions

Objective
Inaccurate follow-through of instruction or performance of test
Exaggerated or inappropriate behaviors (e.g., hysterical, hostile, agitated, apathetic)
Development of preventable complication

Desired Outcomes/Evaluation Criteria—Client Will:

- Participate in learning process.
- Identify interferences to learning and specific action(s) to deal with them.
- Exhibit increased interest and assume responsibility for own learning by beginning to look for information and ask questions.
- Verbalize understanding of condition, disease process, and treatment.

Information that appears in brackets has been added by the authors to clarify and enhance the use of nursing diagnoses.

- Identify relationship of signs/symptoms to the disease process and correlate symptoms with causative factors.
- Perform necessary procedures correctly and explain reasons for the actions.
- Initiate necessary lifestyle changes and participate in treatment regimen.

Actions/Interventions

Nursing Priority No. 1.
To assess readiness to learn and individual learning needs:
- Ascertain level of knowledge, including anticipatory needs.
- Determine client's ability, readiness, and barriers to learning. **Individual may not be physically, emotionally, or mentally capable at this time.**
- Be alert to signs of avoidance. **Client may need to suffer consequences of lack of knowledge before he or she is ready to accept information.**
- Identify support individuals/SO(s) requiring information (e.g., parent, caregiver, spouse).

Nursing Priority No. 2.
To determine other factors pertinent to the learning process:
- Note personal factors (e.g., age and developmental level, gender, social and cultural influences, religion, life experiences, level of education, emotional stability).
- Determine blocks to learning: language barriers (e.g., client can't read; speaks or understands a different language than healthcare provider), physical factors (e.g., cognitive impairment, aphasia, dyslexia), physical stability (e.g., acute illness, activity intolerance), difficulty of material to be learned.
- Assess the level of the client's capabilities and the possibilities of the situation. **May need to help SO(s) and/or caregivers to learn.**

Nursing Priority No. 3.
To assess the client's/SO's motivation:
- Identify motivating factors for the individual (e.g., client needs to stop smoking because of advanced lung cancer or client wants to lose weight because family member died of complications of obesity). **Motivation may be a negative stimulus (e.g., smoking caused lung cancer) or positive (e.g., client wants to promote health and prevent disease).**

Information that appears in brackets has been added by the authors to clarify and enhance the use of nursing diagnoses.

- Provide information relevant only to the situation **to prevent overload.**
- Provide positive reinforcement. **Can encourage continuation of efforts.** Avoid use of negative reinforcers (e.g., criticism, threats).

Nursing Priority No. 4.
To establish priorities in conjunction with client:

- Determine client's most urgent need from both client's and nurse's viewpoint **(which may differ and require adjustments in teaching plan).**
- Discuss client's perception of need. Relate information to client's personal desires, needs, values, and beliefs **so that client feels competent and respected.**
- Differentiate "critical" content from "desirable" content. **Identifies information that can be addressed at a later time.**

Nursing Priority No. 5.
To establish the content to be included:

- Identify information that needs to be remembered (cognitive).
- Identify information having to do with emotions, attitudes, and values (affective).
- Identify psychomotor skills that are necessary for learning.

Nursing Priority No. 6.
To develop learner's objectives:

- State objectives clearly in learner's terms **to meet learner's (not instructor's) needs.**
- Identify outcomes (results) to be achieved.
- Recognize level of achievement, time factors, and short- and long-term goals.
- Include the affective goals (e.g., reduction of stress).

Nursing Priority No. 7.
To identify teaching methods to be used:

- Determine client's method of accessing information (visual, auditory, kinesthetic, gustatory/olfactory) and include in teaching plan **to facilitate learning or recall.**
- ∞• Involve the client/SO(s) by using age-appropriate materials tailored to client's literacy skills, questions, and dialogue.

Information that appears in brackets has been added by the authors to clarify and enhance the use of nursing diagnoses.

- Involve with others who have same problems, needs, or concerns (e.g., group presentations, support groups). **Provides role model and sharing of information.**
- Provide mutual goal setting and learning contracts. **Clarifies expectations of teacher and learner.**
- Use team and group teaching as appropriate.

Nursing Priority No. 8.

To facilitate learning:

- Use short, simple sentences and concepts. Repeat and summarize as needed.
- Use gestures and facial expressions that help convey meaning of information.
- Discuss one topic at a time; avoid giving too much information in one session.
- Provide written information or guidelines and self-learning modules for client to refer to as necessary. **Reinforces learning process; allows client to proceed at own pace.**
- Pace and time learning sessions and learning activities to individual's needs. Evaluate effectiveness of learning activities with client.
- Provide an environment that is conducive to learning.
- Be aware of factors related to teacher in the situation (e.g., vocabulary, dress, style, knowledge of the subject, and ability to impart information effectively).
- Begin with information the client already knows and move to what the client does not know, progressing from simple to complex. **Can arouse interest/limit sense of being overwhelmed.**
- Deal with the client's anxiety or other strong emotions. Present information out of sequence, if necessary, dealing first with material that is most anxiety producing **when the anxiety is interfering with the client's ability to learn.**
- Provide active role for client in learning process. **Promotes sense of control over situation and is means for determining that client is assimilating and using new information.**
- Provide for feedback (positive reinforcement) and evaluation of learning and acquisition of skills.
- Be aware of informal teaching and role modeling that takes place on an ongoing basis (e.g., answering specific questions and reinforcing previous teaching during routine care).
- Assist client to use information in all applicable areas (e.g., situational, environmental, personal).

Information that appears in brackets has been added by the authors to clarify and enhance the use of nursing diagnoses.

Nursing Priority No. 9.

To promote wellness (Teaching/Discharge Considerations):

- Provide access information for contact person **to answer questions and validate information postdischarge.**
- Identify available community resources and support groups.
- Provide information about additional learning resources (e.g., bibliography, Web sites, tapes). **May assist with further learning and promote learning at own pace.**

Documentation Focus

Assessment/Reassessment

- Individual findings including learning style, identified needs, presence of learning blocks (e.g., hostility, inappropriate behavior).

Planning

- Plan for learning, methods to be used, and who is involved in the planning.
- Teaching plan.

Implementation/Evaluation

- Responses of the client/SO(s) to the learning plan and actions performed. How the learning is demonstrated.
- Attainment or progress toward desired outcome(s).
- Modifications to plan of care.

Discharge Planning

- Additional learning and referral needs.

Sample Nursing Outcomes & Interventions Classifications (NOC/NIC)

NOC— Knowledge: [specify—42 choices]
NIC—Teaching: [specify—30 choices]

---

readiness for enhanced Knowledge (specify)

Taxonomy II: Perception/Cognition—Class 4 Cognition (00161)
[Diagnostic Division: Teaching/Learning]
Submitted 2002

Definition: A pattern of cognitive information related to a specific topic, or its acquisition, that is sufficient for meeting health-related goals and can be strengthened

---

Information that appears in brackets has been added by the authors to clarify and enhance the use of nursing diagnoses.

Defining Characteristics

Subjective
Expresses an interest in learning
Explains knowledge of the topic; describes previous experiences pertaining to the topic

Objective
Behaviors congruent with expressed knowledge

Desired Outcomes/Evaluation Criteria—Client Will:

- Exhibit responsibility for own learning by seeking answers to questions.
- Verify accuracy of informational resources.
- Verbalize understanding of information gained.
- Use information to develop individual plan to meet healthcare needs and goals.

Actions/Interventions

Nursing Priority No. 1.
To develop plan for learning:

- Verify client's level of knowledge about specific topic. **Provides opportunity to ensure accuracy and completeness of knowledge base for future learning.**
- Determine motivation and expectations for learning. **Provides insight useful in developing goals and identifying information needs.**
- Assist client to identify learning goals. **Helps to frame or focus content to be learned and provides measure to evaluate learning process.**
- Ascertain preferred methods of learning (e.g., auditory, visual, interactive, or "hands-on"). **Identifies best approaches to facilitate learning process.**
- Note personal factors (e.g., age/developmental level, gender, social/cultural influences, religion, life experiences, level of education) **that may impact learning style, choice of informational resources.**
- Determine any challenges to learning: language barriers (e.g., client can't read, speaks or understands language other than that of care provider, dyslexia); physical factors (e.g., sensory deficits, such as vision or hearing deficits, aphasia); physical

---

Information that appears in brackets has been added by the authors to clarify and enhance the use of nursing diagnoses.

🌐 Cultural 🅰 Collaborative 🏠 Community/Home Care

stability (e.g., acute illness, activity intolerance); difficulty of material to be learned. **Identifies special needs to be addressed if learning is to be successful.**

Nursing Priority No. 2.

To facilitate learning:

- Identify and provide information in varied formats appropriate to client's learning style (e.g., audiotapes, print materials, videos, classes or seminars, Internet). **Use of multiple formats increases learning and retention of material.**
- Provide information about additional or outside learning resources (e.g., bibliography, pertinent Web sites). **Promotes ongoing learning at own pace.**
- Discuss ways to verify accuracy of informational resources. **Encourages independent search for learning opportunities while reducing likelihood of acting on erroneous or unproven data that could be detrimental to client's well-being.**
- Identify available community resources/support groups. **Provides additional opportunities for role modeling, skill training, anticipatory problem-solving, and so forth.**
- Be aware of informal teaching and role modeling that takes place on an ongoing basis (e.g., community and peer role models, support group feedback, print advertisements, popular music or videos). **Incongruencies may exist, creating questions and potentially undermining learning process.**

Nursing Priority No. 3.

To enhance optimum wellness:

- Assist client to identify ways to integrate and use information in all applicable areas (e.g., situational, environmental, personal). **Ability to apply or use information increases desire to learn and retain information.**
- Encourage client to journal, keep a log, or graph as appropriate. **Provides opportunity for self-evaluation of effects of learning, such as better management of chronic condition, reduction of risk factors, acquisition of new skills.**

Documentation Focus

Assessment/Reassessment

- Individual findings, including learning style and identified needs, presence of challenges to learning.
- Motivation and expectations for learning.

Information that appears in brackets has been added by the authors to clarify and enhance the use of nursing diagnoses.

Planning

- Plan for learning, methods to be used, and who is involved in the planning.
- Educational plan.

Implementation/Evaluation

- Responses of the client/SO(s) to the learning plan and actions performed.
- How the learning is demonstrated.
- Attainment or progress toward desired outcome(s).
- Modifications to lifestyle and treatment plan.

Discharge Planning

- Additional learning/referral needs.

Sample Nursing Outcomes & Interventions Classifications (NOC/NIC)

NOC—Knowledge: [specify—42 choices]
NIC—Teaching: Individual

Latex Allergy Response

Taxonomy II: Safety/Protection—Class 5 Defensive Processes (00041)
[Diagnostic Division: Safety]
Submitted 1998; Revised 2006

Definition: A hypersensitive reaction to natural latex rubber products

Related Factors

Hypersensitivity to natural latex rubber protein

Defining Characteristics

Subjective

Life-threatening reactions occurring less than 1 hour after exposure to latex proteins: Tightness in chest
Gastrointestinal characteristics: Abdominal pain; nausea
Orofacial characteristics: Itching of the eyes; nasal/facial/oral itching; nasal congestion
Generalized characteristics: Generalized discomfort; increasing complaint of total body warmth

---

Information that appears in brackets has been added by the authors to clarify and enhance the use of nursing diagnoses.

Type IV reactions occurring more than 1 hour after exposure to latex protein: Discomfort reaction to additives such as thiurams and carbamates

Objective

Life-threatening reactions occurring less than 1 hour after exposure to latex proteins:

Contact urticaria progressing to generalized symptoms

Edema of the lips, tongue, uvula, throat

Dyspnea; wheezing; bronchospasm; respiratory arrest

Hypotension; syncope; cardiac arrest

Orofacial characteristics: Edema of sclera/eyelids; erythema/tearing of the eyes; nasal/facial erythema; rhinorrhea

Generalized characteristics: Flushing; generalized edema; restlessness

Type IV reactions occurring more than 1 hour after exposure to latex protein: Eczema; irritation; redness

Desired Outcomes/Evaluation Criteria— Client Will:

• Be free of signs of hypersensitive response.
• Verbalize understanding of individual risks and responsibilities in avoiding exposure.
• Identify signs/symptoms requiring prompt intervention.

Actions/Interventions

Nursing Priority No. 1.

To assess contributing factors:

• Identify persons in high-risk categories such as (1) those with history of certain food allergies (e.g., banana, avocado, chestnut, kiwi, papaya, peach, nectarine); (2) prior allergies, asthma, and skin conditions (e.g., eczema and other dermatitis); (3) those occupationally exposed to latex products (e.g., healthcare workers, police, firefighters, EMTs, food handlers, hairdressers, cleaning staff, factory workers in plants that manufacture latex-containing products); (4) those with neural tube defects (e.g., spina bifida); or (5) those with congenital urological conditions requiring frequent surgeries and/or catheterizations (e.g., extrophy of the bladder). **The most severe reactions tend to occur with latex proteins contacting internal tissues during invasive procedures and when they touch mucous membranes of the mouth, vagina, urethra, or rectum.**

Information that appears in brackets has been added by the authors to clarify and enhance the use of nursing diagnoses.

- Question client regarding latex allergy upon admission to healthcare facility, especially when procedures are anticipated (e.g., laboratory, emergency department, operating room, wound care management, one-day surgery, dentist). **This is basic safety information to help healthcare providers prevent/prepare for safe environment for client and themselves while providing care.**
- Discuss history of recent exposure; for example, blowing up balloons or using powdered gloves (**might be an acute reaction to the powder**); use of latex diaphragm/condoms (may affect either partner).
- Note positive skin-prick test when client is skin-tested with latex extracts. **This is a sensitive, specific, and rapid test, and should be used with caution in persons with suspected sensitivity as it carries risk of anaphylaxis.**
- Perform challenge/patch test, if appropriate, **to identify specific allergens in client with known type 4 hypersensitivity.**
- Note response to radioallergosorbent test (RAST) or enzyme-linked assays (ELISA) of latex-specific IgE. **Performed to measure the quantity of IgE antibodies in serum after exposure to specific antigens and has generally replaced skin tests and provocation tests, which are inconvenient, often painful, and/or hazardous to the client.**

Nursing Priority No. 2.

To take measures to reduce/limit allergic response/avoid exposure to allergens:

- Ascertain client's current symptoms, noting presence of rash, hives, or itching; red, teary eyes; edema; diarrhea; nausea; feeling of faintness **to help identify where client is along a continuum of reactions so that appropriate treatments can be initiated.**
- Determine time since exposure (e.g., immediate or delayed onset, such as 24 to 48 hours).
- Assess skin (usually hands but may be anywhere) for dry, crusty, hard bumps, scaling, lesions, and horizontal cracks. **May be irritant contact dermatitis (the least serious and most common type of hypersensitivity reaction) or allergic contact dermatitis (a delayed-onset and more severe form of skin/other tissue reaction).**
- Assist with treatment of dermatitis/type 4 reaction (e.g., washing affected skin with mild soap and water, possible appli-

---

Information that appears in brackets has been added by the authors to clarify and enhance the use of nursing diagnoses.

cation of topical steroid ointment, avoidance of further exposure to latex).

- Monitor closely for signs of systemic reactions (e.g., difficulty breathing or swallowing, wheezing; hoarseness, stridor; hypotension, tremors, chest pain, tachycardia, dysrhythmias; edema of face, eyelids, lips, tongue, and mucous membranes). **Indicative of anaphylactic reaction and can lead to cardiac arrest.**
- Administer treatment, as appropriate. **If severe/life-threatening reaction occurs, urgent interventions may include antihistamines, epinephrine, intravenous fluids, corticosteroids, and oxygen and mechanical ventilation, if indicated.**
- Ascertain that latex-safe environment (e.g., surgery/hospital room) and products are available according to recommended guidelines and standards, including equipment and supplies (e.g., powder-free, low-protein latex products and latex-free items such as gloves, syringes, catheters, tubings, tape, thermometers, electrodes, oxygen cannulas, underpads, storage bags, diapers, feeding nipples), as appropriate.
- Educate all care providers in ways to prevent inadvertent exposure (e.g., post latex precaution signs in client's room, document allergy to latex in chart/client bracelet), and emergency treatment measures should they be needed.

Nursing Priority No. 3.
To promote wellness (Teaching/Learning):

- Instruct client/SO(s) to survey and routinely monitor environment for latex-containing products, and replace as needed.
- Provide list of suppliers of products that can replace latex (e.g., rubber grip utensils/toys/hoses, rubber-containing pads, undergarments, carpets, shoe soles, computer mouse pad, erasers, rubber bands).
- Emphasize necessity of wearing medical ID bracelet and informing all new care providers of hypersensitivity **to reduce preventable exposures.**
- Advise client to be aware of potential for related food allergies (e.g., bananas, kiwis, melons, tomatoes, avocados, nuts [among others]). **These foods can trigger a latex-like allergic reaction because the proteins in them mimic latex proteins as they break down in the body.**
- Instruct client/family/SO about signs of reaction as well as how to implement emergency treatment. **Promotes awareness of problem and facilitates timely intervention.**

Information that appears in brackets has been added by the authors to clarify and enhance the use of nursing diagnoses.

🏠 • Provide worksite review/recommendations to prevent exposure. **Latex allergy can be a disabling occupational disorder. Education about the problem promotes prevention of allergic reaction, facilitates timely intervention, and helps nurse to protect clients, latex-sensitive colleagues, and themselves.**

🏠 • Refer to resources, including but not limited to ALERT (Allergy to Latex Education & Resource Team, Inc.), Latex Allergy News, Spina Bifida Association, National Institute for Occupational Safety and Health (NIOSH), Kendall's Healthcare Products (Web site), and Hudson RCI (Web site) **for further information about common latex products in the home, latex-free products, and assistance.**

Documentation Focus

Assessment/Reassessment
- Assessment findings, pertinent history of contact with latex products, and frequency of exposure.
- Type and extent of symptomatology.

Planning
- Plan of care and interventions, and who is involved in planning.
- Teaching plan.

Implementation/Evaluation
- Response to interventions, teaching, and actions performed.
- Attainment or progress toward desired outcome(s).
- Modifications to plan of care.

Discharge Planning
- Discharge needs and referrals made, additional resources available.

Sample Nursing Outcomes & Interventions Classifications (NOC/NIC)

NOC—Allergic Response: Systemic
NIC—Latex Precautions

Information that appears in brackets has been added by the authors to clarify and enhance the use of nursing diagnoses.

🌐 Cultural 😊 Collaborative 🏠 Community/Home Care

risk for Latex Allergy Response

Taxonomy II: Safety/Protection—Class 5 Defensive Processes (00042)
[Diagnostic Division: Safety]
Submitted 1998; Revised 2006

Definition: Risk of hypersensitivity to natural latex rubber products

Risk Factors

History of reactions to latex
Allergies to bananas, avocados, tropical fruits, kiwi, chestnuts, poinsettia plants
History of allergies/asthma
Professions with daily exposure to latex
Multiple surgical procedures, especially from infancy

> **NOTE:** A risk diagnosis is not evidenced by signs and symptoms, as the problem has not occurred; rather, nursing interventions are directed at prevention.

Desired Outcomes/Evaluation Criteria—Client Will:

- Identify and correct potential risk factors in the environment.
- Demonstrate appropriate lifestyle changes to reduce risk of exposure.
- Identify resources to assist in promoting a safe environment.
- Recognize need for/seek assistance to limit response/complications.

Actions/Interventions

Nursing Priority No. 1.

To assess causative/contributing factors:

- Identify persons in high-risk categories such as (1) those with history of certain food allergies (e.g., banana, avocado, chestnut, kiwi, papaya, peach, nectarine); (2) asthma, skin conditions (e.g., eczema); (3) those occupationally exposed to latex products (e.g., healthcare workers, police, firefighters, EMTs,

---

Information that appears in brackets has been added by the authors to clarify and enhance the use of nursing diagnoses.

food handlers, hairdressers, cleaning staff, factory workers in plants that manufacture latex-containing products); (4) those with neural tube defects (e.g., spina bifida); or (5) those with congenital urological conditions requiring frequent surgeries and/or catheterizations (e.g., extrophy of the bladder). **The most severe reactions tend to occur when latex proteins contact internal tissues during invasive procedures and when they touch mucous membranes of the mouth, vagina, urethra, or rectum.**

- Ascertain if client could be exposed through catheters, intravenous tubing, dental/other procedures in a healthcare setting. **Although many healthcare facilities and providers use latex-safe equipment, latex is present in many medical supplies and/or in the healthcare environment, with possible risk to client and healthcare provider.**

Nursing Priority No. 2.
To assist in correcting factors that could lead to latex allergy:

- Question client regarding latex allergy upon admission to healthcare facility, especially when procedures are anticipated (e.g., laboratory, emergency department, operating room, wound care management, one-day surgery, dentist). **Basic safety information to help healthcare providers prevent/prepare for safe environment for client and themselves while providing care.**
- Discuss necessity of avoiding/limiting latex exposure if sensitivity is suspected.
- Recommend that client/family survey environment and remove any medical or household products containing latex.
- Create latex-safe environments (e.g., substitute nonlatex products, such as natural rubber gloves, PCV intravenous tubing, latex-free tape, thermometers, electrodes, oxygen cannulas) **to enhance client safety by reducing exposure.**
- Obtain lists of latex-free products and supplies for client/care provider if appropriate **in order to limit exposure.**
- Ascertain that facilities and/or employers have established policies and procedures **to address safety and reduce risk to workers and clients.**
- Promote good skin care when latex gloves may be preferred for barrier protection in specific disease conditions such as HIV or during surgery. Use powder-free gloves, wash hands immediately after glove removal; refrain from use of oil-based

---

Information that appears in brackets has been added by the authors to clarify and enhance the use of nursing diagnoses.

hand cream. **Reduces dermal and respiratory exposure to latex proteins that bind to the powder in gloves.**

Nursing Priority No. 3.
To promote wellness (Teaching/Discharge Considerations):

🏠• Discuss ways to avoid exposure to latex products with client/ SO/caregiver.

🏠• Instruct client and care providers about potential for sensitivity reactions, how to recognize symptoms of latex allergy (e.g., skin rash; hives; flushing; itching; nasal, eye, or sinus symptoms; asthma; and [rarely] shock).

🏠• Identify measures to take if reactions occur.

⊕• Refer to allergist/other physician **for testing, as appropriate.**

🏠• Provide worksite review/recommendations, as indicated. **Latex allergy can be a disabling occupational disorder. Education about the problem promotes prevention of allergic reaction, facilitates timely intervention, and helps nurse to protect clients, latex-sensitive colleagues, and themselves.**

Documentation Focus

Assessment/Reassessment
• Assessment findings, pertinent history of contact with latex products, and frequency of exposure.

Planning
• Plan of care, interventions, and who is involved in planning.
• Teaching plan.

Implementation/Evaluation
• Response to interventions, teaching, and actions performed.

Discharge Planning
• Discharge needs and referrals made.

Sample Nursing Outcomes & Interventions Classifications (NOC/NIC)

NOC—Allergic Response: Localized
NIC—Latex Precautions

Information that appears in brackets has been added by the authors to clarify and enhance the use of nursing diagnoses.

sedentary **Lifestyle**

Taxonomy II: Health Promotion—Class 1 Health Awareness (00168)
[Diagnostic Division: Activity/Rest]
Submitted 2004

Definition: Reports a habit of life that is characterized by a low physical activity level

Related Factors

Lack of interest, motivation, or resources (time, money, companionship, facilities)
Lack of training for accomplishment of physical exercise
Deficient knowledge of the health benefits of physical exercise

Defining Characteristics

Subjective
Reports preference for activities low in physical activity

Objective
Chooses a daily routine lacking physical exercise
Demonstrates physical deconditioning

Desired Outcomes/Evaluation Criteria—Client Will:

- Verbalize understanding of importance of regular exercise to general well-being.
- Identify necessary precautions or safety concerns and self-monitoring techniques.
- Formulate realistic exercise program with gradual increase in activity.

Nursing Priority No. 1.

To assess precipitating/etiological factors:

- Identify conditions that may contribute to immobility or the onset and continuation of inactivity or sedentary lifestyle (e.g., obesity, depression, multiple sclerosis, arthritis, Parkinson's disease, surgery, hemiplegia or paraplegia, chronic pain, brain injury) **that may contribute to immobility or the onset and continuation of inactivity or sedentary lifestyle.**

Information that appears in brackets has been added by the authors to clarify and enhance the use of nursing diagnoses.

Cultural   Collaborative   Community/Home Care

- ∞• Assess client's age, developmental level, motor skills, ease and capability of movement, posture, and gait. **Determines type and intensity of needed interventions related to activity.**
- Note emotional and behavioral responses to problems associated with self- or condition-imposed sedentary lifestyle. **Feelings of frustration and powerlessness may impede attainment of goals.**
- Determine usual exercise and dietary habits, physical limitations, work environment, family dynamics, available resources.

Nursing Priority No. 2.

To motivate and stimulate client involvement:

- Establish therapeutic relationship acknowledging reality of situation and client's feelings. **Changing a lifelong habit can be difficult, and client may be feeling discouragement with body and hopelessness (i.e., unable to turn situation around into a positive experience).**
- ⊕• Ascertain client's perception of current activity/exercise patterns, impact on life, and cultural expectations of client/others.
- Determine client's actual ability to participate in exercise or activities, noting attention span, physical limitations and tolerance, level of interest or desire, and safety needs. **Identifies barriers that need to be addressed.**
- Discuss motivation for change. **Concerns of SO(s) regarding threats to personal health and longevity or acceptance by teen peers may be sufficient to cause client to initiate change; to sustain change, however, client must want to change for himself or herself.**
- Review necessity for, and benefits of, regular exercise. **Research confirms that exercise has benefits for the whole body (e.g., can boost energy, enhance coordination, reduce muscle deterioration, improve circulation, lower blood pressure, produce healthier skin and a toned body, prolong youthful appearance). Exercise has also been found to boost cardiac fitness in both conditioned and out-of-shape individuals.**
- Involve client, SO, parent, or caregiver in developing exercise plan and goals to meet individual needs, desires, and available resources.
- Introduce activities at client's current level of functioning, progressing to more complex activities, as tolerated.
- ∞• Recommend mix of age and gender-appropriate activities or stimuli (e.g., movement classes, walking, hiking, jazzercise or other dancing, swimming, biking, skating, bowling, golf,

---

Information that appears in brackets has been added by the authors to clarify and enhance the use of nursing diagnoses.

weight training). **Activities need to be personally meaningful for client to derive the most enjoyment and to sustain motivation to continue with program.**

🏠 • Encourage change of scenery (indoors and out, where possible) and periodic changes in the personal environment when client is confined inside.

Nursing Priority No. 3.

To promote optimal level of function and prevent exercise failure:

🔄 • Assist with treatment of underlying condition impacting participation in activities **to maximize function within limitations of situation.**

🔄 • Collaborate with physical medicine specialist or occupational/ physical therapist in providing active or passive range-of-motion exercises, isotonic muscle contractions. **Techniques such as gait training, strength training, and exercise to improve balance and coordination can be helpful in rehabilitating client.**

🏠 • Schedule ample time to perform exercise activities balanced with adequate rest periods.

🏠 • Provide for safety measures as indicated by individual situation, including environmental management/fall prevention. (Refer to ND risk for Falls.)

🏠 • Reevaluate ability/commitment periodically. **Changes in strength/endurance signal readiness for progression of activities or possibly to decrease exercise if overly fatigued. Wavering commitment may require change in types of activities, addition of a workout buddy to reenergize involvement.**

🏠 • Discuss discrepancies in planned and performed activities with client aware and unaware of observation. Suggest methods for dealing with identified problems. **May be necessary when client is using avoidance or controlling behavior, or is not aware of own abilities due to anxiety/fear.**

🏠 • Review importance of adequate intake of fluids, especially during hot weather/strenuous activity.

Nursing Priority No. 4.

🏠 To promote wellness (Teaching/Discharge Considerations):

• Educate client/SO about benefits of physical activity as it relates to client's particular situation. **Many studies have**

Information that appears in brackets has been added by the authors to clarify and enhance the use of nursing diagnoses.

shown the health benefits of physical activity in the setting of chronic illness, e.g., it increases function in arthritis, improves glycemic control in type 2 diabetes, and can enhance quality of life.

- Review components of physical fitness: (1) muscle strength and endurance, (2) flexibility, (3) body composition (muscle mass, percentage of body fat), and (4) cardiovascular health. **Fitness routines need to include all elements to attain maximum benefits and prevent deconditioning.**

- Instruct in safety measures as individually indicated (e.g., warm-up and cool-down activities; taking pulse before, during, and after activity; wearing reflective clothing when jogging, reflectors on bicycle; locking wheelchair before transfers; judicious use of medications; supervision as indicated).

- Recommend keeping an activity or exercise log, including physical and psychological responses, changes in weight, endurance, body mass. **Provides visual evidence of progress or goal attainment and encouragement to continue with program.**

- Encourage client to involve self in exercise as part of wellness management for the whole person.

- Encourage parents to set a positive example for children by participating in exercise and engaging in an active lifestyle.

- Identify community resources, charity activities, support groups. **Community walking or hiking trails, sports leagues, and so on, provide free or low-cost options. Activities such as 5K walks for charity, participation in Special Olympics, or age-related competitive games provide goals to work toward.** *Note:* **Some individuals may prefer solitary activities; however, most individuals enjoy supportive companionship when exercising.**

- Discuss alternatives for exercise program in changing circumstances (e.g., walking the mall during inclement weather, using exercise facilities at hotel when traveling, water aerobics at local swimming pool, joining a gym).

- Promote individual participation in community awareness of problem and discussion of solutions. **Physical inactivity (and associated diseases) is a major public health problem that affects huge numbers of people in all regions of the world. Recognizing the problem and future consequences may empower the global community to develop effective measures to promote physical activity and improve public health.**

Information that appears in brackets has been added by the authors to clarify and enhance the use of nursing diagnoses.

- Introduce and promote established goals for increasing physical activity, such as Sports, Play, and Active Recreation for Kids (SPARK) and Physician-Based Assessment and Counseling for Exercise (PACE), **to address national concerns about obesity and major barriers to physical activity, such as time constraints, lack of training in physical activity or behavioral change methods, and lack of standard protocols.**

Documentation Focus

Assessment/Reassessment
- Individual findings, including level of function and ability to participate in specific or desired activities.
- Motivation for change.

Planning
- Plan of care and who is involved in the planning.
- Teaching plan.

Implementation/Evaluation
- Responses to interventions, teaching, and actions performed.
- Attainment or progress toward desired outcome(s).
- Modifications to plan of care.

Discharge Planning
- Discharge and long-range needs, noting who is responsible for each action to be taken.
- Specific referrals made.
- Sources of, and maintenance for, assistive devices.

Sample Nursing Outcomes & Interventions Classifications (NOC/NIC)

NOC—Knowledge: Prescribed Activity
NIC—Exercise Promotion

risk for impaired Liver Function

Taxonomy II: Nutrition—Class 4 Metabolism (0000178)
[Diagnostic Division: Food/Fluid]
Submitted 2006; Revised 2008

Definition: At risk for a decrease in liver function that may compromise health

---

Information that appears in brackets has been added by the authors to clarify and enhance the use of nursing diagnoses.

🌐 Cultural   🔵 Collaborative   🏠 Community/Home Care

Risk Factors

Viral infection (e.g., hepatitis A, hepatitis B, hepatitis C, Epstein-Barr); HIV co-infection
Hepatotoxic medications (e.g., acetaminophen, statins)
Substance abuse (e.g., alcohol, cocaine)

> **NOTE:** A risk diagnosis is not evidenced by signs and symptoms, as the problem has not occurred; rather, nursing interventions are directed at prevention.

Desired Outcomes/Evaluation Criteria— Client Will:

- Verbalize understanding of individual risk factors that contribute to possibility of liver damage/failure.
- Demonstrate behaviors, lifestyle changes to reduce risk factors and protect self from injury.
- Be free of signs of liver failure as evidenced by liver function studies within normal levels, and absence of jaundice, hepatic enlargement, or altered mental status.

Actions/Interventions

Nursing Priority No. 1.
To identify individual risk factors/needs:

- Determine presence of condition(s) as listed in Risk Factors, noting whether problem is acute (e.g., viral hepatitis, acetaminophen overdose) or chronic (e.g., alcoholic hepatitis or cirrhosis). **Influences choice of interventions.**
- Note client history of known/possible exposure to virus, bacteria, or toxins **that can damage liver:**

    Works in high-risk occupation (e.g., performs tasks that involve contact with blood, blood-contaminated body fluids, other body fluids, or sharps).
    Injects drugs, especially if client shared a needle; received tattoo or piercing with an unsterile needle.
    Received blood or blood products prior to 1989.
    Ingested contaminated food or water or experienced poor sanitation practices by food-service workers.
    Close contact (e.g., lives with or has sex with infected person or carrier; infant born to infected mother).

Information that appears in brackets has been added by the authors to clarify and enhance the use of nursing diagnoses.

Regular exposure to toxic chemicals (e.g., carbon tetrachloride cleaning agents, bug spray, paint fumes, and tobacco smoke).

Uses prescription drugs (e.g., sulfonamides, phenothiazines, isoniazid).

Ingests certain herbal remedies or mega doses of vitamins.

Uses alcohol with medications (including over-the-counter medications).

Consumes alcohol heavily and/or over long period of time.

Ingested acetaminophen (accidentally, as may occur when client takes too large a dose or has several medications containing acetaminophen over time; or intentionally, as may occur with suicide attempt).

Travels internationally to or immigrates from areas/countries such as Africa, Southeast Asia, Korea, China, Vietnam, Eastern Europe, Mediterranean countries, or the Caribbean.

- Review results of laboratory tests (e.g., abnormal liver function studies, drug toxicity, HVB positive) and other diagnostic studies (e.g., ultrasonography, computed tomography [CT] scanning; magnetic resonance [MRI] imaging) **that indicate presence of hepatotoxic condition and need for medical treatment.**

Nursing Priority No. 2.

To assist client to reduce or correct individual risk factors:

- Educate client on way(s) to prevent exposure to/incidence of hepatitis infections and limit damage to liver:

Practice safer sex (e.g., avoid multiple-partner sex, wear condoms, avoid sex with partners known to be infected).

Wash hands well after using the bathroom or changing soiled diapers/briefs.

Avoid injecting drugs or sharing needles.

Avoid sharing razors, toothbrushes, or nail clippers.

Make sure needles and inks are sterile for tattooing and body piercing.

Use proper precautions and appropriate protective equipment when working in high-risk occupations, such as healthcare, police and fire departments, emergency services, daycare services, and chemical manufacturing, **where one is most at risk for inhalation of toxins, needle sticks, or body fluid exposure.**

Information that appears in brackets has been added by the authors to clarify and enhance the use of nursing diagnoses.

Avoid tap water and practice good hygiene and sanitation when traveling internationally.

Use harsh cleansers and aerosol products in well-ventilated room; wear mask and gloves, cover skin, and wash well afterward. **Insecticides and other chemicals can reach the liver through skin and destroy liver cells.**

Obtain vaccinations when appropriate. **Some hepatitis strains (e.g., A & B) are preventable, thus minimizing risk of liver damage.**

- Assist with medical treatment of underlying condition **to support organ function and minimize liver damage.**

- Emphasize importance of responsible drinking or avoiding alcohol, when indicated, **to reduce incidence of cirrhosis or severity of liver damage or failure.**

- Encourage client with liver dysfunction to avoid fatty foods. **Fat interferes with normal function of liver cells and can cause additional damage and permanent scarring to liver cells when they can no longer regenerate.**

- Encourage smoking cessation. **The additives in cigarettes pose a challenge to the liver by reducing the liver's ability to eliminate toxins.**

- Refer to nutritionist, as indicated, for dietary needs, including intake of calories, proteins, vitamins, and trace minerals, **to promote healing and limit effects of deficiencies.**

- Discuss safe use and concerns about client's medication regimen (e.g., acetaminophen; nonsteroidal anti-inflammatory agents; herbal or vitamin supplements; phenobarbitol; cholesterol-lowering drugs, such as "statins"; some antibiotics [e.g., sulfonamides, INH]; certain cardiovascular drugs [e.g., amiodarone, hydralazine]; antidepressants [e.g., tricyclics]) **known to cause hepatotoxicity, either alone or in combination, or in overdose situation.**

- Identify signs/symptoms that warrant prompt notification of healthcare provider (e.g., increased abdominal girth; rapid weight loss or gain; increased peripheral edema; dyspnea, fever; blood in stool or urine; excess bleeding of any kind; jaundice). **Indicators of severe liver dysfunction, possible organ failure.**

- Refer to specialist or liver treatment center, as indicated. **May be beneficial for person with chronic liver disease when decompensating, or client with hepatitis and other coexisting disease condition (e.g., HIV) or intolerance to treatment due to side effects.**

Information that appears in brackets has been added by the authors to clarify and enhance the use of nursing diagnoses.

Nursing Priority No. 3.

🏠 To promote wellness (Teaching/Discharge Considerations):

💊• Encourage client routinely taking acetaminophen for pain management to read labels, determine strength of medication, note safe number of doses over 24 hours, become familiar with "hidden" sources of acetaminophen (e.g., Nyquil, Vicodin), limit alcohol intake **to avoid/limit risk of liver damage.**

• Emphasize importance of hand hygiene and avoidance of fresh produce, use of bottled water and avoidance of raw meat and seafood **if client is traveling to area where hepatitis A is endemic or food or waterborne illness is a risk.**

• Instruct in measures including protection from blood and other body fluids, sharps safety, safer sex practices, avoiding needle sharing and body tattoos or piercings **to prevent occupational and nonoccupational exposures to hepatitis.**

💊• Discuss need and refer for vaccination, as indicated (e.g., healthcare and public safety worker, children under 18, international traveler, recreational drug user, men who have sexual relationships with other men, client with clotting disorders or liver disease, anyone sharing household with an infected person), **to prevent exposure and transmission of blood or body fluid hepatitis and limit risk of liver injury.**

💊• Discuss appropriateness of prophylactic immunizations. **Although the best way to protect against hepatitis B and C infections is to prevent exposure to viruses, postexposure prophylaxis should be initiated promptly to prevent or limit severity of infection.**

💊• Provide information regarding availability of gamma globulin, immune serum globulin, HepB immunoglobulin, HepB vaccine (Recombivax HB, Engerix-B) through health department or family physician.

🌐• Emphasize necessity of follow-up care (in client with chronic liver disease) and adherence to therapeutic regimen.

🌐• Refer to community resources, drug and alcohol treatment program, as indicated.

Documentation Focus

Assessment/Reassessment
• Assessment findings, including individual risk factors.
• Results of laboratory tests and diagnostic studies.

Planning
• Plan of care and who is involved in planning.
• Teaching plan.

Information that appears in brackets has been added by the authors to clarify and enhance the use of nursing diagnoses.

🌐 Cultural 🌐 Collaborative 🏠 Community/Home Care

Implementation/Evaluation

- Response to interventions, teaching, and actions performed.
- Attainment or progress toward desired outcome(s).
- Modifications to plan of care.

Discharge Planning

- Long-term needs, plan for follow-up, and who is responsible for actions to be taken.
- Specific referrals made.

Sample Nursing Outcomes & Interventions Classifications (NOC/NIC)

NOC—Knowledge: Disease Process
NIC—Substance Use Treatment

risk for Loneliness

Taxonomy II: Self-Perception—Class 1 Self-Concept (00054)
[Diagnostic Division: Social Interaction]
Submitted 1994; Revised 2006

Definition: At risk for experiencing discomfort associated with a desire or need for more contact with others

Risk Factors

Affectional deprivation
Physical or social isolation
Cathectic deprivation

NOTE: A risk diagnosis is not evidenced by signs and symptoms, as the problem has not occurred; rather, nursing interventions are directed at prevention.

Desired Outcomes/Evaluation Criteria— Client Will:

- Identify individual difficulties and ways to address them.
- Engage in social activities.
- Report involvement in interactions and relationship client views as meaningful.

Information that appears in brackets has been added by the authors to clarify and enhance the use of nursing diagnoses.

Parent/Caregiver Will:

- Provide infant with consistent and loving caregiving.
- Participate in programs for adolescents and families.

Actions/Interventions

Nursing Priority No. 1.
To identify causative/precipitating factors:

- Differentiate between ordinary loneliness and a state or constant sense of dysphoria. **Influences type of and intensity of interventions.**
- ∞• Note client's age and duration of problem; that is, situational (such as leaving home for college) or chronic. **Adolescents may experience lonely feelings related to the changes that are happening as they become adults. Elderly individuals incur multiple losses associated with aging, loss of spouse, decline in physical health, and changes in roles that intensify feelings of loneliness.**
- Determine degree of distress, tension, anxiety, restlessness present. Note history of frequent illnesses, accidents, crises. **Most people feel lonely at some time in their lives related to situational occurrences that engender these feelings, which are normal in the circumstances.**
- Note presence and proximity of family, SO(s), and whether they are helpful or not.
- Discuss with client whether there is a person or persons in his or her life who can be trustworthy and who will listen with empathy to the feelings that are expressed.
- Determine how individual perceives and deals with solitude. **A person may feel alone in a crowd or may choose to be alone and enjoy the quiet.**
- Review issues of separation from parents as a child, loss of SO(s)/spouse.
- Assess sleep and appetite disturbances, ability to concentrate. **Indicators of distress related to feelings of loneliness and low self-esteem.**
- Note expressions of "yearning" for an emotional partnership.

Nursing Priority No. 2.
To assist client to identify feelings and situations in which he or she experiences loneliness:

- Establish nurse-client relationship. **Client may feel free to talk about feelings in context of an empathetic relationship.**

Information that appears in brackets has been added by the authors to clarify and enhance the use of nursing diagnoses.

- Discuss individual concerns about feelings of loneliness and relationship between loneliness and lack of SO(s). Note desire and willingness to change situation. **Motivation can impede—or facilitate—achieving desired outcomes.**
- Support expression of negative perceptions of others and note whether client agrees. **Provides opportunity for client to clarify reality of situation, recognize own denial.**
- Accept client's expressions of loneliness as a primary condition and not necessarily as a symptom of some underlying condition.

Nursing Priority No. 3.

To assist client to become involved:

- Discuss reality versus perceptions of situation.
- Discuss importance of emotional bonding (attachment) between infants or young children and parents/caregivers when appropriate.
- Involve in classes, such as assertiveness, language and communication, social skills, **to address individual needs and potential for enhanced socialization.**
- Role-play situations **to develop interpersonal skills.**
- Discuss positive health habits, including personal hygiene, exercise activity of client's choosing.
- Identify individual strengths, areas of interest **that provide opportunities for involvement with others.**
- Encourage attendance at support group activities to meet individual needs (e.g., therapy, separation/grief, religious).
- Help client establish plan for progressive involvement, beginning with a simple activity (e.g., call an old friend, speak to a neighbor) and leading to more complicated interactions and activities.
- Provide opportunities for interactions in a supportive environment (e.g., have client accompanied, as in a "buddy system") during initial attempts to socialize. **Helps reduce stress, provides positive reinforcement, and facilitates successful outcome.**

Nursing Priority No. 4.

To promote wellness (Teaching/Discharge Considerations):

- Inform client that loneliness can be overcome. **It is up to the individual to build self-esteem and learn to feel good about self.**
- Encourage involvement in special-interest groups (e.g., computers, gardening club, reading circles, bird watchers);

Information that appears in brackets has been added by the authors to clarify and enhance the use of nursing diagnoses.

charitable services (e.g., serving in a soup kitchen, youth groups, animal shelter).

🏠• Suggest volunteering for church committee or choir; attending community events with friends and family; becoming involved in political issues or campaigns; enrolling in classes at local college or continuing education programs.

🤝• Refer to appropriate counselors for help with relationships and so on.

• Refer to NDs Hopelessness; Anxiety; Social Isolation.

Documentation Focus

Assessment/Reassessment
• Assessment findings, including client's perception of problem, availability of resources and support systems.
• Client's desire and commitment to change.

Planning
• Plan of care and who is involved in planning.
• Teaching plan.

Implementation/Evaluation
• Response to interventions, teaching, and actions performed.
• Attainment or progress toward desired outcome(s).
• Modifications to plan of care.

Discharge Planning
• Long-term needs, plan for follow-up, and who is responsible for actions to be taken.
• Specific referrals made.

Sample Nursing Outcomes & Interventions Classifications (NOC/NIC)

NOC—Loneliness
NIC—Socialization Enhancement

---

risk for disturbed **Maternal-Fetal Dyad**

Taxonomy II: Sexuality—Class 3 Reproduction (00209)
[Diagnostic Division: Safety]
Submitted 2008

Definition: At risk for disruption of the symbiotic maternal-fetal dyad as a result of comorbid or pregnancy-related conditions

---

Information that appears in brackets has been added by the authors to clarify and enhance the use of nursing diagnoses.

🌐 Cultural 🤝 Collaborative 🏠 Community/Home Care

Risk Factors

Complications of pregnancy (e.g., premature rupture of membranes, placenta previa or abruption, late prenatal care, multiple gestation)

Compromised oxygen transport (e.g., anemia, [sickle cell anemia], cardiac disease, asthma, hypertension, seizures, premature labor, hemorrhage)

Impaired glucose metabolism (e.g., diabetes, steroid use)

Physical abuse

Substance abuse (e.g., tobacco, alcohol, drugs)

Treatment-related side effects (e.g., pharmaceutical agents, surgery)

> **NOTE:** A risk diagnosis is not evidenced by signs and symptoms, as the problem has not occurred; rather, nursing interventions are directed at prevention.

Desired Outcomes/Evaluation Criteria— Client Will: (Include Specific Time Frame)

- Verbalize understanding of individual risk factors or condition(s) that may impact pregnancy.
- Engage in necessary alterations in lifestyle and daily activities to manage risks.
- Participate in screening procedures as indicated.
- Identify signs/symptoms requiring medical evaluation or intervention.
- Display fetal growth within normal limits and carry pregnancy to term.

Actions/Interventions

Nursing Priority No. 1.
To identify individual risk/contributing factors:

- Review history of previous pregnancies for presence of complications, such as premature rupture of membranes (PROM), placenta previa, miscarriage or pregnancy losses due to premature dilation of the cervix, preterm labor or deliveries, previous birth defects, hyperemesis gravidarum, or repeated urinary tract or vaginal infections.
- Obtain history about prenatal screening and amount and timing of care. **Lack of prenatal care can place both mother and fetus at risk.**

Information that appears in brackets has been added by the authors to clarify and enhance the use of nursing diagnoses.

- Note conditions potentiating vascular changes/reduced placental circulation (e.g., diabetes, gestational hypertension, cardiac problems, smoking) or those that alter oxygen-carrying capacity (e.g., asthma, anemia, Rh incompatibility, hemorrhage). **Extent of maternal vascular involvement and reduction of oxygen-carrying capacity have a direct influence on uteroplacental circulation and gas exchange.**
- Note maternal age. **Maternal age above 35 years is associated with increased risk of spontaneous abortions, preterm delivery or stillbirths, fetal chromosomal abnormalities and malformations, and intrauterine growth retardation (IUGR). In pregnant adolescents (younger than 15), the most common high-risk conditions include gestational hypertension, anemia, labor dysfunction, cephalopelvic disproportion and low birth weight, and preterm delivery.**
- Ascertain current/past dietary patterns and practices. **Client may be malnourished, obese, or underweight (weight less than 100 lb or over 200 lb).**
- Assess for severe, unremitting nausea and vomiting, especially when it persists after the first trimester (hyperemesis gravidarum).
- Note history of exposure to teratogenic agents, infectious diseases (e.g., tuberculosis, influenza, measles); high-risk occupations; exposure to toxic substances such as lead, organic solvents, carbon monoxide; use of certain over-the-counter or prescription medications; substance use or abuse (including illicit drugs and alcohol).
- Identify family or cultural influences in pregnancy. **Family history may include multiple births or congenital diseases, or generational abuse or lack of support or finances. Cultural background may identify health risks associated with nationality (e.g., sickle cell in people of African descent or Tay-Sachs disease in people of eastern European Jewish ancestry); or religious practices (e.g., exclusion of dairy products, or no maternal immunizations for rubella) that can impact health of mother or fetal development.**
- Review laboratory studies. **Low hemoglobin suggests anemia, which is associated with hypoxia. Blood type and Rh group may reveal incompatibility risks; elevated serum glucose may be seen in gestational diabetes mellitus (GDM); elevated liver function studies suggest hypertensive liver involvement; drop in platelet count may be associated with gestational hypertension and HELLP (he-**

Information that appears in brackets has been added by the authors to clarify and enhance the use of nursing diagnoses.

molysis, elevated liver enzymes, and low platelet) syndrome. **Nutritional studies may reveal decreased levels of serum proteins, electrolytes, minerals, or vitamins essential to maternal health and fetal development.**

- Review vaginal, cervical, or rectal cultures and serology results. **May reveal presence of sexually transmitted infections (STIs) or identify active or carrier state of hepatitis, HIV, AIDS.**
- Assist in screening for and identifying genetic or chromosomal disorders. **Disorders such as phenylketonuria (PKU) or sickle cell disease necessitate special treatment to prevent negative effects on fetal growth.**
- Investigate current home situation. **May have history of unstable relationship, or inadequate/lack of housing that affects safety as well as general well-being.**

Nursing Priority No. 2.

To monitor maternal/fetal status:

- Weigh client and compare current weight with pregravid weight. Have client record weight between visits. **Underweight clients are at risk for anemia, inadequate protein and calorie intake, vitamin or mineral deficiencies, and gestational hypertension. Overweight women are at increased risk for development of gestational hypertension, gestational diabetes, and hyperinsulinemia of the fetus.**
- Assess fetal heart rate (FHR), noting rate and regularity. Have client monitor fetal movement daily as indicated. Tachycardia in a term infant may indicate a compensatory mechanism to reduced oxygen levels and/or presence of sepsis. A reduction in fetal activity occurs before bradycardia.
- Test urine for presence of ketones. **Indicates inadequate glucose utilization and breakdown of fats for metabolic processes.**
- Provide information and assist with procedures as indicated, for example:

  Amniocentesis: **May be performed for genetic purposes or to assess fetal lung maturity. Spectrophotometric analysis of the fluid may be done to detect bilirubin after 26 weeks gestation.**

  Ultrasonography: **Assesses gestational age of fetus, detects presence of multiples, or fetal abnormalities. Locates placenta (and amniotic fluid pockets before amniocentesis, if performed), monitors clients at risk for reduced or inadequate placental perfusion (such as adolescents,**

Information that appears in brackets has been added by the authors to clarify and enhance the use of nursing diagnoses.

clients older than 35 years, and clients with diabetes, gestational hypertension, cardiac or kidney disease, anemia, or respiratory disorders).

Biophysical profile: Assesses fetal well-being through ultrasound evaluation to measure amniotic fluid index (AFI), FHR, nonstress test (NST) reactivity, fetal breathing movement, body movement (large limbs), and muscle tone (flexion and extension).

Contraction stress test (CST): A positive CST with late decelerations indicates a high-risk client and fetus with possible reduced uteroplacental reserves.

- Screen for abuse during pregnancy. Prenatal abuse is correlated with a low maternal weight gain, infections, anemia, delay in seeking prenatal care until the third trimester, and preterm delivery.
- Screen for preterm uterine contractions, which may or may not be accompanied by cervical dilatation.

Nursing Priority No. 3.
To correct/improve maternal/fetal well-being:

- Instruct client in reportable symptoms and monitor for unusual symptoms at each prenatal visit (e.g., vaginal bleeding, headache along with blurred vision and ankle swelling, faintness, persistent vomiting). Provides opportunity for early intervention in event of developing complications.
- Assist in treatment of underlying medical condition(s) that have potential for causing maternal or fetal harm.
- Assess perceived impact of complication on client and family members. Encourage verbalization of concerns. Family stress is amplified in a high-risk pregnancy, where concerns focus on the health of both the client and the fetus.
- Facilitate positive adaptation to situation, through Active-listening, acceptance, and problem-solving. Helps in successful accomplishment of the psychological tasks of pregnancy.
- Develop dietary plan with client that provides necessary nutrients (calories, protein, vitamins, and minerals).
- Promote fluid intake of at least two quarts of noncaffeinated fluid per day to prevent dehydration, which may compromise optimal uterine and placental functioning and increase uterine irritability.
- Encourage client to participate in individually appropriate adaptations and self-care techniques, such as scheduling rest periods two to three times a day, avoiding overexertion or heavy

---

Information that appears in brackets has been added by the authors to clarify and enhance the use of nursing diagnoses.

🌐 Cultural 🔄 Collaborative 🏠 Community/Home Care

lifting, or maintaining contact with family and daily life if bedrest is required.

_🥄_• Review medication regimen. **Prepregnancy treatment for chronic conditions may require alteration for maternal and fetal safety.**

• Review availability and use of resources.

_🥄_• Administer Rh immunoglobulin (RhIgG) to client at 28 weeks gestation in Rh-negative clients with Rh-positive partners, or following amniocentesis, if indicated.

• Encourage modified or complete bedrest as indicated. **Activity level may need modification, depending on symptoms of uterine activity, cervical changes, or bleeding. Side-lying position increases renal and placental perfusion, which is effective in preventing supine hypotensive syndrome.**

_💊_• Provide supplemental oxygen as appropriate. **Increases the oxygen available for fetal uptake, especially in presence of severe anemia or sickle cell crisis.**

_💊_• Prepare for and assist with intrauterine fetal exchange transfusion as indicated by titers (Kleihauer-Betke test).

Nursing Priority No. 4.

🏠 To promote wellness (Teaching/Discharge Considerations):

• Emphasize the normalcy of pregnancy, focus on pregnancy milestones, "countdown to birth." **Avoids or limits perception of "sick role"; promotes sense of hope that modifications or restrictions serve a worthwhile purpose.**

• Discuss implications of preexisting condition and possible impact on pregnancy. **Pregnancy may have no effect or may reduce or exacerbate severity of symptoms of chronic conditions.**

• Provide information about risks of weight reduction during pregnancy and about nourishment needs of client and fetus. **Prenatal calorie restriction and resultant weight loss may result in nutrient deficiency or ketonemia, with negative effects on fetal central nervous system and possible IUGR.**

_💊_• Encourage smoking cessation, refer to community program or support group as indicated. **Severe adverse effects of smoking on the fetus may be reduced if mother quits smoking early in pregnancy, and pregnancy outcomes can still be improved if mother stops smoking as late as 32 weeks gestation.**

• Help client/couple plan restructuring of roles and activities necessitated by complication of pregnancy.

Information that appears in brackets has been added by the authors to clarify and enhance the use of nursing diagnoses.

- Have client demonstrate new behaviors and therapeutic techniques. **During pregnancy, control of condition may require specific modified or new behaviors.**
- Recommend client assess uterine tone and contractions for 1 hour, once or twice a day as indicated **to monitor uterine irritability or early indication of premature labor.**
- Encourage close monitoring of blood glucose levels, as appropriate. **Type I or insulin-dependent diabetes mellitus clients generally need to check blood glucose levels 4 to 12 times/day because insulin needs may increase 2 to 3 times above pregravid baseline.**
- Demonstrate technique and specific equipment used when FHR monitoring is done in the home setting.
- Identify danger signals requiring immediate notification of healthcare provider (e.g., PROM, preterm labor, vaginal drainage or bleeding).
- Review availability and use of resources. **Presence or absence of supportive resources can make the difference for the client and family in being able to manage the situation.**
- Refer to community service agencies (e.g., visiting nurse, social service) or resources, such as Sidelines. **Community supports may be needed for ongoing assessment of medical problem, family status, coping behaviors, and financial stressors.** *Note:* **Sidelines is a national telephone support group for pregnant women on bedrest.**
- Refer for counseling if family does not sustain positive coping and growth. **May be necessary to promote growth and to prevent family disintegration.**

Documentation Focus

Assessment/Reassessment
- Assessment findings, including weight, signs of pregnancy, safety concerns.
- Specific risk factors, comorbidities, and treatment regimen.
- Results of screening laboratory tests and diagnostic studies.
- Participation in prenatal care.
- Cultural beliefs and practices.

Planning
- Plan of care, specific interventions, and who is involved in the planning.
- Community resources for equipment and supplies.

Information that appears in brackets has been added by the authors to clarify and enhance the use of nursing diagnoses.

- Specific referrals made.
- Teaching plan.

Implementation/Evaluation
- Client/fetal response to treatment and actions performed.
- Client's response to teaching provided.
- Attainment or progress toward desired outcome(s).
- Modifications to plan of care.

Sample Nursing Outcomes & Interventions Classifications (NOC/NIC)

NOC—Prenatal Health Behavior
NIC—High-Risk Pregnancy Care

impaired Memory

Taxonomy II: Perception/Cognition—Class 4 Cognition (00131)
[Diagnostic Division: Neurosensory]
Submitted 1994

Definition: Inability to remember or recall bits of information or behavioral skills

Related Factors

Hypoxia; anemia
Fluid or electrolyte imbalance; decreased cardiac output
Neurological disturbances
Excessive environmental disturbances
[Substance abuse; effects of medications]
[Age]

Defining Characteristics

Subjective
Reports experiences of forgetting
Inability to recall events or factual information

Objective
Inability to recall if a behavior was performed
Inability to learn/retain new skills or information
Inability to perform a previously learned skill
Forgets to perform a behavior at a scheduled time

Information that appears in brackets has been added by the authors to clarify and enhance the use of nursing diagnoses.

Desired Outcomes/Evaluation Criteria— Client Will:

- Verbalize awareness of memory problems.
- Establish methods to help in remembering essential things when possible.
- Accept limitations of condition and use resources effectively.

Actions/Interventions

Nursing Priority No. 1.

To assess causative factor(s)/degree of impairment:

- Determine physical, biochemical, and environmental factors (e.g., systemic infections; brain injury; pulmonary disease with hypoxia; use of multiple medications; exposure to toxic substances; use or abuse of alcohol or other drugs; traumatic event; removal from known environment) **that may be associated with confusion and loss of memory.**
- Note client's age and potential for depression. **Depressive disorders affecting memory and concentration are particularly prevalent in older adults; however, impairments can occur in depressed persons of any age.**
- Note presence of stressful situation(s) and degree of anxiety. **Can increase client's confusion and disorganization and further interfere with attempts at recall. Stress may also speed up memory decline in person whose cognitive function is already impaired.** (Refer to ND Anxiety for additional interventions as indicated.)
- Collaborate with medical and psychiatric providers in evaluating orientation, attention span, ability to follow directions, send/receive communication, appropriateness of response **to determine presence and/or severity of impairment.**
- Perform or review results of cognitive testing (e.g., Blessed Information-Memory-Concentration [BIMC] test, Mini-Mental Status Examination [MMSE]). **A combination of tests may be needed to obtain a complete picture of the client's overall condition and prognosis.**
- Evaluate skill proficiency levels. **Evaluation may include many self-care activities (e.g., daily grooming, steps in preparing a meal, participating in a lifelong hobby, balancing a checkbook, and driving ability) to determine level of independence or needed assistance.**
- Ascertain how client/family view the problem (e.g., practical problems of forgetting and/or role and responsibility impair-

---

Information that appears in brackets has been added by the authors to clarify and enhance the use of nursing diagnoses.

⊕ Cultural ⊛ Collaborative 🏠 Community/Home Care

ments related to loss of memory and concentration) **to determine significance and impact of problem.**

Nursing Priority No. 2.

To maximize level of function:

- Assist with treatment of underlying conditions (e.g., electrolyte imbalances, infection, anemia, drug interactions/reaction to medications; alcohol or other drug intoxication; malnutrition, vitamin deficiencies; pain) **where treatment can improve memory processes.**
- Orient/reorient client as needed. Introduce self with each client contact **to meet client's safety and comfort needs.** (Refer to NDs acute/chronic Confusion, for additional interventions.)
- Implement appropriate memory-retraining techniques (e.g., keeping calendars, writing lists, memory cue games, mnemonic devices, using computers).
- Assist with and instruct client and family in associate-learning tasks, such as practice sessions recalling personal information, reminiscing, locating a geographic location (Stimulation Therapy). **Practice may improve performance and integrate new behaviors into the client's coping strategies.**
- Encourage ventilation of feelings of frustration and helplessness. Refocus attention to areas of control and progress **to diminish feelings of powerlessness/hopelessness.**
- Provide for and emphasize importance of pacing learning activities and getting sufficient rest **to avoid fatigue and frustration that may further impair cognitive abilities.**
- Monitor client's behavior and assist in use of stress-management techniques (e.g., music therapy, reading, television, games, socialization) **to reduce boredom and enhance enjoyment of life.**
- Structure teaching methods and interventions to client's level of functioning and/or potential for improvement.
- Determine client's response to and effects of medications prescribed to improve attention, concentration, memory processes and to lift spirits or modify emotional responses. **Medication for cognitive enhancement can be effective, but benefits need to be weighed against whether quality of life is improved after side effects and cost of drugs are considered.**

Nursing Priority No. 3.

To promote wellness (Teaching/Discharge Considerations):

- Assist client/SO(s) to establish compensation strategies (e.g., menu planning with a shopping list, timely completion of

---

Information that appears in brackets has been added by the authors to clarify and enhance the use of nursing diagnoses.

tasks on a daily planner, checklists at the front door to ascertain that lights and stove are off before leaving) **to improve functional lifestyle and safety.** (Refer to NDs acute/chronic Confusion for additional interventions.)

- Refer for follow-up with counselors, rehabilitation programs, job coaches, social or financial support systems **to help deal with persistent or difficult problems.**
- Refer to rehabilitation services **that are matched to the needs, strengths, and capacities of individual and modified as needs change over time.**
- Discuss and encourage safety interventions, as indicated (e.g., assistance with meal preparation, evaluation of driving abilities, cessation of tobacco use or its use only under supervision, removal of guns and other weapons) **to prevent injury to client/others.**
- Assist client to deal with functional limitations (such as loss of driving privileges) and identify resources **to meet individual needs, maximizing independence.**

Documentation Focus

Assessment/Reassessment
- Individual findings, testing results, and perceptions of significance of problem.
- Actual impact on lifestyle and independence.

Planning
- Plan of care and who is involved in planning process.
- Teaching plan.

Implementation/Evaluation
- Responses to interventions, teaching, and actions performed.
- Attainment or progress toward desired outcome(s).
- Modifications to plan of care.

Discharge Planning
- Long-term needs and who is responsible for actions to be taken.
- Specific referrals made.

Sample Nursing Outcomes & Interventions Classifications (NOC/NIC)

NOC—Memory
NIC—Memory Training

Information that appears in brackets has been added by the authors to clarify and enhance the use of nursing diagnoses.

⊕ Cultural Collaborative 🏠 Community/Home Care

impaired bed Mobility

Taxonomy II: Activity/Rest—Class 2 Activity/Exercise
(00091)
[Diagnostic Division: Safety]
Submitted 1998; Revised 2006

Definition: Limitation of independent movement from
one bed position to another

Related Factors

Neuromuscular or musculoskeletal impairment
Insufficient muscle strength; deconditioning; obesity
Environmental constraints (e.g., bed size or type, treatment
equipment, restraints)
Pain; sedating pharmaceutical agents
Deficient knowledge
Cognitive impairment

Defining Characteristics

Objective

Impaired ability to turn from side to side; move from supine to
sitting, sitting to supine; reposition self in bed; move from
supine to prone, prone to supine; move from supine to long-
sitting, long-sitting to supine

Desired Outcomes/Evaluation Criteria— Client/Caregiver Will:

- Verbalize willingness to participate in repositioning program.
- Verbalize understanding of situation and risk factors, individual therapeutic regimen, and safety measures.
- Demonstrate techniques and behaviors that enable safe repositioning.
- Maintain position of function and skin integrity as evidenced
  by absence of contractures, footdrop, decubitus, and so forth.
- Maintain or increase strength and function of affected and/or
  compensatory body part.

Information that appears in brackets has been added by the authors to clarify
and enhance the use of nursing diagnoses.

Actions/Interventions

Nursing Priority No. 1.
To identify causative/contributing factors:

* Determine diagnoses that contribute to immobility (e.g., multiple sclerosis, arthritis, Parkinson's disease, hemi-/para-/tetraplegia, fractures [especially hip joint and long bone fractures], multiple trauma, burns, head injury, depression, dementia).
* Note individual risk factors and current situation, such as surgery, casts, amputation, traction, pain, age, general weakness or debilitation **that can contribute to problems related to bed rest.**
* Determine degree of perceptual or cognitive impairment and/or ability to follow directions. **Impairments related to age, acute, or chronic conditions (including severe depression, dementia); trauma; surgery; or medications require alternative interventions or changes in plan of care.**

Nursing Priority No. 2.
To assess functional ability:

* Determine functional level classification 0 to 4 **(The client at level 0 is completely independent; 1 = requires use of equipment or device; 2 = requires help from another person for assistance; 3 = requires help from another person and equipment device; 4 = dependent, does not participate in activity).**
* Note emotional and behavioral responses to problems of immobility. **Can negatively affect self-concept and self-esteem, autonomy, and independence.**
* Note presence of complications related to immobility. **The effects of immobility are rarely confined to one body system and can include decline in cognition, muscle wasting, contractures, pressure sores, constipation, aspiration pneumonia, etc.** (Refer to ND Disuse Syndrome.)

Nursing Priority No. 3.
To promote optimal level of function and prevent complications:

* Assist with treatment of underlying condition(s) **to maximize potential for mobility and optimal function.**
* Ascertain that dependent client is placed in best bed for situation (e.g., correct size, support surface, and mobility func-

---

Information that appears in brackets has been added by the authors to clarify and enhance the use of nursing diagnoses.

Cultural   Collaborative   Community/Home Care

tions) **to promote mobility and enhance environmental safety.**

🏠• Change client's position frequently, moving individual parts of the body (e.g., legs, arms, head) using appropriate support and proper body alignment. Encourage periodic changes in head of bed (if not contraindicated by conditions such as an acute spinal cord injury), with client in supine and prone positions at intervals **to improve circulation, reduce tightening of muscles and joints, normalize body tone, and more closely simulate body positions an individual would normally use.**

• Turn dependent client frequently, utilizing bed and mattress positioning settings to assist movements; reposition in good body alignment, using appropriate supports.

• Instruct client and caregivers in methods of moving client relative to specific situations (e.g., turning side to side, prone, or sitting) **to provide support for the client's body and to prevent injury to the lifter.**

🏠• Perform and encourage regular skin examination for reddened or excoriated areas. Use a pressure-risk assessment scale (e.g. Braden, Norton) as appropriate. Provide frequent skin care (e.g., cleansing, moisturizing, gentle massage) **to reduce pressure on sensitive areas and prevent development of problems with skin or tissue integrity.** (Refer to NDs impaired Skin Integrity; impaired Tissue Integrity.)

🏠• Provide or assist with daily range-of-motion interventions (active and passive) **to maintain joint mobility, improve circulation, and prevent contractures.**

🏠• Assist with activities of hygiene, feeding, and toileting, as indicated. Assist on and off bedpan and into sitting position (or use cardioposition bed or foot-egress bed) to facilitate elimination.

💊• Administer medication prior to activity as needed for pain relief **to permit maximal effort and involvement in activity.**

• Observe for change in strength to do more or less self-care **to adjust care as indicated.**

• Provide diversional activities (e.g., television, books, games, music, visiting), as appropriate, **to decrease boredom and potential for depression.**

• Ensure telephone and call bell is within reach **to promote safety and timely response.**

• Provide individually appropriate methods to communicate adequately with client.

Information that appears in brackets has been added by the authors to clarify and enhance the use of nursing diagnoses.

- Provide extremity protection (padding, exercises, etc.). (Refer to NDs impaired Skin Integrity; risk for Peripheral Neurovascular Dysfunction, for additional interventions.)
- Collaborate with rehabilitation team, physical or occupational therapists to create exercise and adaptive program designed specifically for client, identifying assistive devices (e.g., splints, braces, boots) and equipment (e.g., transfer board, sling, trapeze, hydraulic lift, specialty beds).
- Refer to NDs Activity Intolerance; impaired physical Mobility; impaired wheelchair Mobility; risk for Disuse Syndrome; impaired Transfer Ability; impaired Walking, for additional interventions.

Nursing Priority No. 4.

To promote wellness (Teaching/Discharge Considerations):

- Involve client/SO(s) in determining activity schedule. **Promotes commitment to plan, maximizing outcomes.**
- Encourage continuation of regular exercise regimen **to maintain and enhance gains in strength and muscle control.**
- Obtain, or identify sources for, assistive devices. Demonstrate safe use and proper maintenance.

Documentation Focus

Assessment/Reassessment
- Individual findings, including level of function, ability to participate in specific or desired activities.

Planning
- Plan of care and who is involved in the planning.

Implementation/Evaluation
- Responses to interventions, teaching, and actions performed.
- Attainment or progress toward desired outcome(s).
- Modification to plan of care.

Discharge Planning
- Discharge and long-term needs, noting who is responsible for each action to be taken.
- Specific referrals made.
- Sources for, and maintenance of, assistive devices.

Information that appears in brackets has been added by the authors to clarify and enhance the use of nursing diagnoses.

🌐 Cultural 🔄 Collaborative 🏠 Community/Home Care

Sample Nursing Outcomes & Interventions Classifications (NOC/NIC)

NOC—Body Position: Self-Initiated
NIC—Bed Rest Care

impaired physical **Mobility**

Taxonomy II: Activity/Rest—Class 2 Activity/Exercise (00085)
[Diagnostic Division: Safety]
Submitted 1973; Nursing Diagnosis Extension and Classification Revision 1998

Definition: Limitation in independent, purposeful physical movement of the body or of one or more extremities

Related Factors

Sedentary lifestyle; activity intolerance; disuse; deconditioning; decreased endurance; limited cardiovascular endurance

Decreased muscle mass, strength, or control; joint stiffness; contractures; loss of integrity of bone structures

Pain; discomfort

Neuromuscular or musculoskeletal impairment

Sensoriperceptual or cognitive impairment; developmental delay

Depressive mood state; anxiety

Malnutrition; altered cellular metabolism; body mass index above 75th age-appropriate percentile

Deficient knowledge regarding value of physical activity; cultural beliefs regarding age-appropriate activity; lack of environmental supports (e.g., physical or social)

Prescribed movement restrictions; reluctance to initiate movement

Pharmaceutical agents

Defining Characteristics

Subjective

[Report of pain or discomfort on movement; unwillingness to move]

Objective

Limited range of motion; limited ability to perform gross or fine motor skills; difficulty turning

---

Information that appears in brackets has been added by the authors to clarify and enhance the use of nursing diagnoses.

Exertional dyspnea

Slowed movement; uncoordinated or jerky movements; movement-induced tremor; decreased [slower] reaction time

Postural instability; gait changes

Engages in substitutions for movement (e.g., increased attention to other's activity, controlling behavior, focus on pre-illness disability/activity)

Specify level of independence using a standardized functional scale [such as]

[0—Full self-care

I—Requires use of equipment or device

II—Requires assistance or supervision of another person

III—Requires assistance or supervision of another person and equipment or device

IV—Is dependent and does not participate]

Desired Outcomes/Evaluation Criteria—Client Will:

* Verbalize understanding of situation and individual treatment regimen and safety measures.
* Demonstrate techniques or behaviors that enable resumption of activities.
* Participate in activities of daily living (ADLs) and desired activities.
* Maintain position of function and skin integrity as evidenced by absence of contractures, footdrop, decubitus, and so forth.
* Maintain or increase strength and function of affected and/or compensatory body part.

Actions/Interventions

Nursing Priority No. 1.

To identify causative/contributing factors:

* Determine diagnosis that contributes to immobility (e.g., multiple sclerosis, arthritis, Parkinson's disease, cardiopulmonary disorders, hemi- or paraplegia, depression).
* Note factors affecting current situation (e.g., surgery, fractures, amputation, tubings [chest tube, Foley catheter, intravenous tubes, pumps] and potential time involved (e.g., few hours in bed after surgery versus serious trauma requiring long-term bedrest or debilitating disease limiting movement). **Identifies potential impairments and determines type of interventions needed to provide for client's safety.**

Information that appears in brackets has been added by the authors to clarify and enhance the use of nursing diagnoses.

- Assess client's developmental level, motor skills, ease and capability of movement, posture and gait **to determine presence of characteristics of client's unique impairment and to guide choice of interventions.**
- ∞ Note older client's general health status. **While aging, per se, does not cause impaired mobility, several predisposing factors in addition to age-related changes can lead to immobility (e.g., diminished body reserves of musculoskeletal system, chronic diseases, sedentary lifestyle, decreased ability to quickly and adequately correct movements affecting center of gravity).**
- Assess degree of pain, listening to client's description about manner in which pain limits mobility.
- Ascertain client's perception of activity and exercise needs and impact of current situation. Identify cultural beliefs and expectations affecting recovery or response to long-term limitations. **Helps to determine client's expectations and beliefs related to activity and potential long-term effect of current immobility. Also identifies barriers that may be addressed (e.g., lack of safe place to exercise, focus on pre-illness or disability activity, controlling behavior, depression, cultural expectations, distorted body image).**
- ∞ Note decreased motor agility or essential tremor related to age.
- Determine history of falls and relatedness to current situation. **Client may be restricting activity because of weakness or debilitation, actual injury during a fall, or from psychological distress (i.e., fear and anxiety) that can persist after a fall.** (Refer to ND risk for Falls for additional interventions.)
- Assess nutritional status and client's report of energy level. **Deficiencies in nutrients and water, electrolytes, and minerals can negatively affect energy and activity tolerance.**

Nursing Priority No. 2.
To assess functional ability:

- Determine degree of immobility in relation to previously suggested scale.
- Determine degree of perceptual or cognitive impairment and ability to follow directions. **Impairments related to age, chronic or acute disease condition, trauma, surgery, or medications require alternative interventions or changes in plan of care.**
- Observe movement when client is unaware of observation **to note any incongruencies with reports of abilities.**

Information that appears in brackets has been added by the authors to clarify and enhance the use of nursing diagnoses.

- Note emotional/behavioral responses to problems of immobility. **Feelings of frustration or powerlessness may impede attainment of goals.**
- Determine presence of complications related to immobility (e.g., pneumonia, elimination problems, contractures, decubitus, anxiety). (Refer to ND risk for Disuse Syndrome.)

Nursing Priority No. 3.

To promote optimal level of function and prevent complications:

- Assist with treatment of underlying condition causing pain and/or dysfunction.
- Assist or have client reposition self on a regular schedule as dictated by individual situation (including frequent shifting of weight when client is wheelchair bound).
- Instruct in use of siderails, overhead trapeze, roller pads, walker, cane, **for position changes, transfers, and ambulation.**
- Support affected body parts or joints using pillows, rolls, foot supports or shoes, gel pads, foam, etc., **to maintain position of function and reduce risk of pressure ulcers.**
- Provide regular skin care to include pressure area management.
- Provide or recommend pressure-reducing mattress, such as egg crate, or pressure-relieving mattress, such as alternating air pressure or water. **Reduces tissue pressure and aids in maximizing cellular perfusion to prevent dermal injury.**
- Encourage adequate intake of fluids and nutritious foods. **Promotes well-being and maximizes energy production.**
- Administer medications prior to activity as needed for pain relief **to permit maximal effort and involvement in activity.**
- Schedule activities with adequate rest periods during the day **to reduce fatigue.**
- Provide client with ample time to perform mobility-related tasks.
- Identify energy-conserving techniques for ADLs. **Limits fatigue, maximizing participation.**
- Encourage participation in self-care; occupational, diversional, or recreational activities. **Enhances self-concept and sense of independence.**
- Discuss discrepancies in movement when client aware and unaware of observation and methods for dealing with identified problems.

Information that appears in brackets has been added by the authors to clarify and enhance the use of nursing diagnoses.

🌐 Cultural 🤝 Collaborative 🏠 Community/Home Care

- Provide for safety measures as indicated by individual situation, including environmental management and fall prevention.
- Collaborate with physical medicine specialist and occupational or physical therapists in providing range-of-motion exercise (active or passive), isotonic muscle contractions (e.g., flexion of ankles, push-and-pull exercises), assistive devices, and activities (e.g., early ambulation, transfers, stairs) **to develop individual exercise and mobility program, to identify appropriate mobility devices, and to limit or reduce effects and complications of immobility.**

Nursing Priority No. 4.

To promote wellness (Teaching/Discharge Considerations):

- Encourage client's/SO's involvement in decision making as much as possible. **Enhances commitment to plan, optimizing outcomes.**
- Review safety measures as individually indicated (e.g., use of heating pads, locking wheelchair before transfers, removal or securing of scatter/area rugs).
- Involve client and SO(s) in care, assisting them to learn ways of managing problems of immobility.
- Demonstrate use of standing aids and mobility devices (e.g., walkers, strollers, scooters, braces, prosthetics) and have client/care provider demonstrate knowledge about, and safe use of device. Identify appropriate resources for obtaining and maintaining appliances and equipment. **Promotes independence and enhances safety.**
- Review individual dietary needs. Identify appropriate vitamin or herbal supplements.

Documentation Focus

Assessment/Reassessment
- Individual findings, including level of function, ability to participate in specific or desired activities.

Planning
- Plan of care and who is involved in the planning.
- Teaching plan.

Implementation/Evaluation
- Responses to interventions, teaching, and actions performed.
- Attainment or progress toward desired outcome(s).
- Modifications to plan of care.

Information that appears in brackets has been added by the authors to clarify and enhance the use of nursing diagnoses.

Discharge Planning

- Discharge and long-term needs, noting who is responsible for each action to be taken.
- Specific referrals made.
- Sources for, and maintenance of, assistive devices.

Sample Nursing Outcomes & Interventions Classifications (NOC/NIC)

NOC—Mobility Level
NIC—Exercise Therapy: [specify]

---

impaired wheelchair Mobility

Taxonomy II: Activity/Rest—Class 2 Activity/Exercise (00089)
[Diagnostic Division: Safety]
Submitted 1998; Revised 2006

Definition: Limitation of independent operation of wheelchair within environment

---

Related Factors

Neuromuscular or musculoskeletal impairments (e.g., contractures)
Insufficient muscle strength; limited endurance; deconditioning; obesity
Impaired vision
Pain
Depressed mood; cognitive impairment
Deficient knowledge
Environmental constraints (e.g., stairs, inclines, uneven surfaces, unsafe obstacles, distances, lack of assistive devices or person, wheelchair type)

Defining Characteristics

Impaired ability to operate manual or power wheelchair on even or uneven surface, an incline or decline, or curbs

NOTE: Specify level of independence using a standardized functional scale. (Refer to ND impaired physical Mobility.)

Information that appears in brackets has been added by the authors to clarify and enhance the use of nursing diagnoses.

🌐 Cultural ✑ Collaborative 🏠 Community/Home Care

Desired Outcomes/Evaluation Criteria— Client Will:

- Move safely within environment, maximizing independence.
- Identify and use resources appropriately.

Caregiver Will:

- Provide safe mobility within environment and community.

Actions/Interventions

Nursing Priority No. 1.
To identify causative/contributing factors:

- Determine diagnosis that contributes to immobility (e.g., amyotrophic lateral sclerosis, spinal cord injury, spastic cerebral palsy, brain injury) and client's functional level and individual abilities.
- Identify factors in environments frequented by the client that contribute to inaccessibility (e.g., uneven floors or surfaces, lack of ramps, steep incline or decline, narrow doorways or spaces).
- Ascertain access to and appropriateness of public and/or private transportation.

Nursing Priority No. 2.
To promote optimal level of function and prevent complications:

- Determine that client's underlying physical, cognitive, and emotional impairment(s) (e.g., brain or spinal cord injury, fractures/other trauma, pain, depression, vision deficits) are treated or being managed **to maximize ability, desire, and motivation to participate in wheelchair activities.**
- Ascertain that wheelchair provides the base mobility to maximize function. **Proper seating and support for people in wheelchairs is critical to their ability to travel, work, learn at school, play, and interact socially. If a family member will be assisting the person using the wheelchair, their needs may also need to be considered in the wheelchair selection.**
- Provide for, and instruct client in, safety while in a wheelchair (e.g., adaptive cushions, supports for all body parts, repositioning and transfer assistive devices, and height adjustment).

Information that appears in brackets has been added by the authors to clarify and enhance the use of nursing diagnoses.

- Note evenness of surfaces client would need to negotiate and refer to appropriate sources for modifications. Clear pathways of obstructions.
- Recommend or refer for modifications to home, work, or school and recreational settings frequented by client **to provide safe and suitable environments.**
- Determine need for and capabilities of assistive persons. Provide training and support as indicated.
- Monitor client's use of joystick, sip and puff, sensitive mechanical switches, and so forth, **to provide necessary equipment if condition or capabilities change.**
- Collaborate with physical medicine, physical or occupational therapists in planning activities to improve client's ability to independently operate wheelchair within limits of tolerance and adjustment to various environments. **May require individual instruction and encouragement, strengthening exercises, assistance with various tasks and close supervision.**
- Monitor client for adverse effects of immobility (e.g., contractures, muscle atrophy, deep venous thrombosis, pressure ulcers). (Refer to NDs Disuse Syndrome; risk for Peripheral Neurovascular Dysfunction, for additional interventions.)

Nursing Priority No. 3.

To promote wellness (Teaching/Discharge Considerations):

- Identify or refer to medical equipment suppliers **to customize client's wheelchair and accessories (e.g., side guards, head rests, heel loops, brake extensions, tool packs) and electronics suited to client's ability (e.g., sip and puff, head movement, sensitive switches).**
- Encourage client's/SO's involvement in decision making as much as possible. **Enhances commitment to plan, optimizing outcomes.**
- Involve client/SO(s) in care, assisting them in managing immobility problems. **Promotes independence.**
- Demonstrate, discuss, and provide information regarding wheelchair safety as individually appropriate, including safe transfers, dealing with uneven surfaces, ramps and curbs; programming speed on power chairs, etc. Include information and refer for wheelchair preventative maintenance measures

---

Information that appears in brackets has been added by the authors to clarify and enhance the use of nursing diagnoses.

(e.g., for wheelchair locks, tires, axles, casters, metal parts, batteries), as indicated. **Wheelchair safety involves people and equipment. This includes not only acquiring the best chair, but also provision for obtaining relief when chair malfunctions.**

- Refer to support groups relative to specific medical condition or disability; independence or political action groups. **Provides role modeling, assistance with problem-solving and social change.**
- Identify community resources **to provide ongoing support.**

Documentation Focus

Assessment/Reassessment
- Individual findings, including level of function, ability to participate in specific or desired activities.
- Type of wheelchair and equipment needs.

Planning
- Plan of care and who is involved in the planning.
- Teaching plan.

Implementation/Evaluation
- Responses to interventions, teaching, and actions performed.
- Attainment or progress toward desired outcome(s).
- Modifications to plan of care.

Discharge Planning
- Discharge and long-term needs, noting who is responsible for each action to be taken.
- Specific referrals made.
- Sources for, and maintenance of, assistive devices.

Sample Nursing Outcomes & Interventions Classifications (NOC/NIC)

NOC—Ambulation: Wheelchair
NIC—Positioning: Wheelchair

Information that appears in brackets has been added by the authors to clarify and enhance the use of nursing diagnoses.

Moral Distress

Taxonomy II: Life Principles—Class 3 Value/Belief/Action
   Congruence (00175)
[Diagnostic Division: Ego Integrity]
Submitted 2006

Definition: Response to the inability to carry out one's
chosen ethical/moral decision/action

Related Factors

Conflict among decision makers (e.g., family, healthcare providers, insurance payers)
Conflicting information guiding moral or ethical decision making; cultural conflicts
Treatment decisions; end-of-life decisions; loss of autonomy
Time constraints for decision making; physical distance of decision maker

Defining Characteristics

Subjective
Expresses anguish (e.g., powerlessness, guilt, frustration, anxiety, self-doubt, fear) over difficulty of acting on one's
moral choice

Desired Outcomes/Evaluation Criteria— Client Will:

- Verbalize understanding of causes for conflict in own situation.
- Be aware of own moral values conflicting with desired/
  required course of action.
- Identify positive ways or actions necessary to deal with situation.
- Express sense of satisfaction with or acceptance of resolution.

Actions/Interventions

Nursing Priority No. 1.
To identify cause/situation in which moral distress is occurring:
- Determine client's perceptions and specific factors resulting
  in a sense of distress and all parties involved in situation.

Information that appears in brackets has been added by the authors to clarify
and enhance the use of nursing diagnoses.

🌐 Cultural 🔄 Collaborative 🏠 Community/Home Care

Moral conflict centers around diminishing the harm suffered, with the involved individuals usually struggling with decisions about what "can be done" to prevent, improve, or cure a medical condition or what "ought to be done" in a specific situation, often within financial constraints or scarcity of resources.

- Note use of sarcasm, avoidance, apathy, crying, or reports of depression or loss of meaning. **Individuals may not understand their feelings of uneasiness/distress or know that the emotional basis for moral distress is anger.**

- Ascertain response of family/SO(s) to client's situation or healthcare choices.

- Identify healthcare goals and expectations. **New treatment options or technology can prolong life or postpone death based on the individual's personal viewpoint, increasing the possibility of conflict with others, including healthcare providers.**

- Ascertain cultural beliefs and values, and degree of importance to client. **Cultural diversity may lead to disparate views or expectations between clients, SO/family members, and healthcare providers. When tensions between conflicting values cannot be resolved, persons experience moral distress.**

- Note attitudes and expressions of dissatisfaction of caregivers/staff. **Client may feel pressure or disapproval if own views are not congruent with expectations of those perceived to be more knowledgeable or in "authority." Furthermore, healthcare providers may themselves feel moral distress in carrying out requested actions/interventions.**

- Determine degree of emotional and physical distress (e.g., fatigue, headaches, forgetfulness, anger, guilt, resentment) individual(s) are experiencing and impact on ability to function. **Moral distress can be very destructive, affecting one's ability to carry out daily tasks or care for self or others, and may lead to a crisis of faith.**

- Assess sleep habits of involved parties. **Evidence suggests that sleep deprivation can harm a person's physical health and emotional well-being, hindering the ability to integrate emotion and cognition to guide moral judgments.**

- Use a moral distress tool, such as the Moral Distress Assessment Questionnaire (MDAQ) **to help measure degree of involvement and identify possible actions to improve situation.**

Information that appears in brackets has been added by the authors to clarify and enhance the use of nursing diagnoses.

• Note availability of family/friends for support and encouragement.

Nursing Priority No. 2.

To assist client/involved individuals to develop/effectively use problem-solving skills:

• Encourage involved individuals to recognize and name the experience resulting in moral sensitivity. **Brings concerns out in the open so they can be dealt with.**
• Use skills, such as Active-listening, I-messages, and problem-solving to assist individual(s) **to clarify feelings of anxiety and conflict.**
• Make time available for support and provide information as desired **to help individuals understand the ethical dilemma that led to moral distress.**
• Provide for privacy when discussing sensitive or personal issues.
• Ascertain coping behaviors client has used successfully in the past that may be helpful in dealing with current situation.
• Provide time for nonjudgmental discussion of philosophic issues/questions about impact of conflict leading to moral questioning of current situation.
• Identify role models (e.g., other individuals who have experienced similar problems in their lives). **Sharing of experiences, identifying options can be helpful to deal with current situation.**
• Involve facility/local ethics committee or ethicist as appropriate **to educate, make recommendations, and facilitate mediation/resolution of issues.**

Nursing Priority No. 3.

To promote wellness (Teaching/Discharge Considerations):

• Engage all parties, as appropriate, in developing plan to address conflict. **Resolving one's moral distress requires making changes or compromises while preserving one's integrity and authenticity.**
• Incorporate identified familial, religious, and cultural factors that have meaning for client.
• Refer to appropriate resources for support and guidance (e.g., pastoral care, counseling, organized support groups, classes), as indicated.

Information that appears in brackets has been added by the authors to clarify and enhance the use of nursing diagnoses.

🌐 Cultural 🔵 Collaborative 🏠 Community/Home Care

⊛ • Assist individuals to recognize that if they follow their moral decisions, they may clash with the legal system. Suggest referral to appropriate resource for legal opinion/options.

Documentation Focus

Assessment/Reassessment
- Individual findings, including nature of moral conflict, individuals involved in conflict.
- Physical and emotional responses to conflict.
- Individual cultural or religious beliefs and values, healthcare goals.
- Responses and involvement of family/SOs.

Planning
- Plan of care and who is involved in planning.
- Teaching plan.

Implementation/Evaluation
- Responses to interventions, teaching.
- Attainment or progress toward desired outcome(s).
- Modifications to plan of care.

Discharge Planning
- Long-term needs and who is responsible for actions to be taken.
- Available resources.
- Specific referrals made.

Sample Nursing Outcomes & Interventions Classifications (NOC/NIC)

NOC—Decision Making
NIC—Decision-Making Support

Nausea

Taxonomy II: Comfort—Class 1 Physical Comfort (00134)
[Diagnostic Division: Food/Fluid]
Submitted 1998; Revised 2002, 2010

Definition: A subjective phenomenon of an unpleasant feeling in the back of the throat and stomach that may or may not result in vomiting

---

Information that appears in brackets has been added by the authors to clarify and enhance the use of nursing diagnoses.

Related Factors

Treatment
Gastric irritation
Gastric distention
Pharmaceutical agents
Radiation therapy or exposure

Biophysical
Biochemical disorders (e.g., uremia, diabetic ketoacidosis); pregnancy
Localized tumors (e.g., acoustic neuroma, primary or secondary brain tumors, bone metastases at base of the skull); intra-abdominal tumors
Toxins (e.g., tumor-produced peptides, abdominal metabolites due to cancer)
Esophageal or pancreatic disease; liver or splenetic capsule stretch
Gastric distention
Gastric irritation
Motion sickness; Ménière's disease; labyrinthitis
Increased intracranial pressure; meningitis
Pain

Situational
Noxious odors or taste; unpleasant visual stimulation
Pain
Psychological factors; anxiety; fear

Defining Characteristics

Subjective
Reports nausea; sour taste in mouth

Objective
Aversion toward food
Increased salivation
Increased swallowing; gagging sensation

Desired Outcomes/Evaluation Criteria—Client Will:

- Be free of nausea.
- Manage chronic nausea, as evidenced by acceptable level of dietary intake.
- Maintain or regain weight as appropriate.

Information that appears in brackets has been added by the authors to clarify and enhance the use of nursing diagnoses.

Nursing Priority No. 1.

To determine causative/contributing factors:

- Assess for presence of conditions of the gastrointestinal (GI) tract (e.g., peptic ulcer disease, bleeding into the stomach; cholecystitis, appendicitis, gastritis, constipation, intestinal blockage, ingestion of "problem" foods; food poisoning; excessive alcohol intake) **that may cause or exacerbate nausea.**
- Note systemic conditions that may result in nausea (e.g., pregnancy, cancer treatment, myocardial infarction, hepatitis, systemic infections, toxins, drug toxicity, presence of neurogenic causes [stimulation of the vestibular system], central nervous system trauma/tumor). **Helps in determining appropriate interventions or need for treatment of underlying condition.**
- Identify situations that client perceives as anxiety inducing, threatening, or distasteful (e.g., "This is nauseating"). **May be able to limit or control exposure to situations or take medication prophylactically.**
- Note psychological factors, including those that are culturally determined (e.g., eating certain foods considered repulsive in one's own culture; seeing or smelling something "gross"; anorexia and bulimia).
- Determine if nausea is potentially self-limiting and/or mild (e.g., first trimester of pregnancy, 24-hour GI viral infection) or is severe and prolonged (e.g., advanced cancer with multiple medications accompanied by anorexia, constipation, imbalances of calcium/other blood salts; certain cancer treatments; hyperemesis gravidarum). **Suggests severity of effect on fluid and electrolyte balance and nutritional status.**
- Note client age and developmental level. **Vomiting may occur along with nausea, especially in children (usually part of a short-lived viral infection). Nausea can occur with food intolerances, inner ear problems, pain, or medication reactions in any age client. Nausea in the elderly (in the absence of acute disease condition) may be associated with GI motility dysfunction, or medications, pain, or end-of-life issues. Nausea in a girl/woman of childbearing age may indicate pregnancy or hormonal influences associated with menstruation, anorexia, or migraine headaches.**

Information that appears in brackets has been added by the authors to clarify and enhance the use of nursing diagnoses.

- Review medication regimen, especially in elderly client on multiple drugs. **Polypharmacy with drug interactions and side effects may cause or exacerbate nausea.**
- Review results of diagnostic studies.

Nursing Priority No. 2.

To promote comfort and enhance intake:

- Administer and monitor response to medications used to treat underlying cause of nausea (e.g., vestibular, bowel obstruction, dysmotility of upper gut, infection, inflammation, toxins) **to determine effectiveness of treatment and to monitor for adverse effects of added medication (e.g., oversedation with risk of aspiration).**
- Select route of medication administration best suited to client's needs (i.e., oral, sublingual, injectable, rectal, transdermal).
- Review pain control regimen. **Converting to long-acting opioids or combination drugs may decrease stimulation of the chemotactic trigger zone, reducing the occurrence of opioid-related nausea.**
- Have client try dry foods such as toast, crackers, dry cereal before arising when nausea occurs in the morning or throughout the day, as appropriate.
- Encourage client to begin with ice chips or sips/small amounts of fluids—4 to 8 ounces for adult; 1 ounce or less for child.
- Advise client to drink liquids 30 minutes before or after meals, instead of with meals.
- Provide diet and snacks of preferred or bland foods (including skinless chicken, rise, toast, pasta, potatoes) and fluids (including caffeine-free nondiet carbonated beverages, clear soup broth, nonacidic fruit juice, gelatin, sherbet or ices) **to reduce gastric acidity and improve nutrient intake.**
- Avoid milk/dairy products, overly sweet or fried and fatty foods, gas-forming vegetables (e.g., broccoli, cauliflower, cucumbers) **that may increase nausea or be more difficult to digest.**
- Encourage client to eat small meals spaced throughout the day instead of large meals **so stomach does not feel excessively full.**
- Instruct client to eat slowly, chewing food well **to enhance digestion.**
- Recommend client remain seated after meal or with head well elevated above feet if in bed.

Information that appears in brackets has been added by the authors to clarify and enhance the use of nursing diagnoses.

- Provide clean, peaceful environment and fresh air with fan or open window. Avoid offending odors, such as cooking smells, smoke, perfumes, mechanical emissions when possible, **as they may stimulate or worsen nausea.**
- Provide frequent oral care (especially after vomiting) **to cleanse mouth and minimize "bad tastes."**
- Encourage deep, slow breathing **to promote relaxation and refocus attention away from nausea.**
- Use distraction with music, chatting with family/friends, watching TV **to refocus attention away from unpleasant sensations.**
- Administer antiemetic on regular schedule before, during, and after administration of antineoplastic agents **to prevent or control side effects of medication.**
- Time chemotherapy doses **for least interference with food intake.**
- Avoid sudden changes in position or excessive motion; move to aisle seat on plane, or front seat or car. Focus on distance, face forward when riding. **The actions may help prevent or limit severity of nausea associated with motion sickness.**
- Investigate use of accupressure point therapy (e.g., elastic band worn around wrist with small, hard bump that presses against accupressure point). **Some individuals with chronic nausea or history of motion sickness report this to be helpful; without sedative effect of medication.**

Nursing Priority No. 3.

To promote wellness (Teaching/Discharge Considerations):

- Review individual factors or triggers causing nausea and ways to avoid problem. **Provides necessary information for client to manage own care. Some individuals develop anticipatory nausea (a conditioned reflex) that recurs each time he or she encounters the situation that triggers the reflex.**
- Instruct in proper use, side effects, and adverse reactions of antiemetic medications. **Enhances client safety and effective management of condition.**
- Discuss appropriate use of over-the-counter medications and herbal products (e.g., Dramamine, antacids, antiflatulents, ginger), or the use of THC (Marinol).
- Encourage use of nonpharmacological interventions. **Activities such as self-hypnosis, progressive muscle relaxation, biofeedback, guided imagery, and systemic desensitization promote relaxation, refocus client's attention, increase sense of control, and decrease feelings of helplessness.**

Information that appears in brackets has been added by the authors to clarify and enhance the use of nursing diagnoses.

- Advise client to prepare and freeze meals in advance, have someone else cook, or use microwave or oven instead of stove-top cooking **for days when nausea is severe or cooking is impossible.**
- Suggest wearing loose-fitting clothing **to reduce external pressure on abdomen.**
- Recommend recording weight weekly, if appropriate, **to help monitor fluid and nutritional status.**
- Discuss potential complications and possible need for medical follow-up or alternative therapies. **Timely recognition and intervention may limit severity of complications (e.g., dehydration).**
- Review signs of dehydration and emphasize importance of replacing fluids and/or electrolytes (with products such as Gatorade or other electrolyte drinks for adults or Pedialyte for children). **Increases likelihood of preventing potentially serious electrolyte depletion.**
- Identify signs (e.g., emesis appears bloody, black, or like coffee grounds; feeling faint) requiring immediate notification of healthcare provider.

Documentation Focus

Assessment/Reassessment
- Individual findings, including individual factors causing nausea.
- Baseline and periodic weight, vital signs.
- Specific client preferences for nutritional intake.
- Response to medication.

Planning
- Plan of care and who is involved in planning.
- Teaching plan.

Implementation/Evaluation
- Response to interventions, teaching, and actions performed.
- Attainment or progress toward desired outcome(s).
- Modifications to plan of care.

Discharge Planning
- Individual long-term needs, noting who is responsible for actions to be taken.
- Specific referrals made.

Information that appears in brackets has been added by the authors to clarify and enhance the use of nursing diagnoses.

Sample Nursing Outcomes & Interventions Classifications (NOC/NIC)

NOC—Nausea & Vomiting Control
NIC—Nausea Management

Noncompliance [ineffective Adherence] [Specify]

Taxonomy II: Life Principles—Class 3 Value/Belief/Action Congruence (00079)
[Diagnostic Division: Teaching/Learning]
Submitted 1973; Revised 1996, 1998

Definition: Behavior of person and/or caregiver that fails to coincide with a health-promoting or therapeutic plan agreed on by the person (and/or family and/or community) and healthcare professional. In the presence of an agreed-on health-promoting, or therapeutic plan, person's or caregiver's behavior is fully or partially non-adherent and may lead to clinically ineffective or partially ineffective outcomes.

NOTE: When the plan of care is reviewed with client/SO, use of the term *noncompliance* may create a negative response and sense of conflict between healthcare providers and client. Labeling the client noncompliant may also lead to problems with third-party reimbursement. Where possible, use of the ND ineffective Self-Health Management is recommended.

Related Factors

Healthcare Plan
Duration; intensity; complexity
Cost; financial flexibility of plan

Individual
Personal or developmental abilities; deficient knowledge or skill relevant to the regimen behavior; motivational forces
Individual's value system; health beliefs; cultural influences; spiritual values
SO(s)
Denial; issues of secondary gain

Information that appears in brackets has been added by the authors to clarify and enhance the use of nursing diagnoses.

Health System

Individual health coverage

Credibility of provider; difficulty in client-provider relationship; provider continuity or regular follow-up; provider reimbursement; communication skills/teaching skills of the provider

Access or convenience of care; satisfaction with care

Network

Involvement of members in health plan; social value regarding plan

Perceived beliefs of significant others

Defining Characteristics

Subjective

[Reports of failure to adhere, does not believe in efficacy of therapy, unwilling to follow treatment regimen]

Objective

Behavior indicative of failure to adhere

Objective tests provide evidence of failure to adhere (e.g., physiological measures, detection of physiological markers)

Failure to progress

Evidence of development of complications or exacerbation of symptoms

Failure to keep appointments

Desired Outcomes/Evaluation Criteria— Client Will:

- Verbalize accurate knowledge of condition and understanding of treatment regimen.
- Make choices at level of readiness based on accurate information.
- Verbalize commitment to mutually agreed upon goals and treatment plan.
- Access resources appropriately.
- Demonstrate progress toward health goals.

Actions/Interventions

Nursing Priority No. 1.

To determine reason for alteration/disregard of therapeutic regimen/instructions:

Information that appears in brackets has been added by the authors to clarify and enhance the use of nursing diagnoses.

- Determine client's/SO's perception and understanding of the situation (illness, treatment).
- Listen to/Active-listen client's complaints/comments. **Helps to identify client's thinking about the treatment regimen (e.g., may be concerned about side effects of medications or success of procedures/transplantation).**
- Note language spoken, read, and understood.
- Be aware of developmental level as well as chronological age of client.
- Assess level of anxiety, locus of control, sense of powerlessness, and so forth.
- Determine who (e.g., client, SO, other) manages the medication regimen and whether individual knows what the medications are and why they are prescribed.
- Ascertain how client remembers to take medications and how many doses have been missed in the last 72 hours, last week, last 2 weeks, and last month.
- Identify factors that interfere with taking medications or lead to lack of adherence (e.g., depression, active alcohol or other drug use, low literacy, lack of support, lack of belief in treatment efficacy). **Forgetfulness is the most common reason given for not complying with the treatment plan.**
- Note length of illness. **Individuals tend to become passive and dependent in long-term, debilitating illnesses.**
- Clarify value system: cultural and religious values, health and illness beliefs of the client/SO(s).
- Determine social characteristics, demographic and educational factors, as well as personality of the client.
- Verify psychological meaning of the behavior (e.g., may be denial). Note issues of secondary gain—**family dynamics, school or workplace issues, involvement in legal system may unconsciously affect client's decision making.**
- Assess availability and use of support systems and resources.
- Be aware of nurses'/healthcare providers' attitudes and behaviors toward the client. (Do they have an investment in the client's compliance or recovery? What is the behavior of the client and nurse when client is labeled "noncompliant"?) **Some care providers may be enabling client, whereas others' judgmental attitudes may impede treatment progress.**

Nursing Priority No. 2.

To assist client/SO(s) to develop strategies for dealing effectively with the situation:

- Develop therapeutic nurse-client relationship. **Promotes trust, provides atmosphere in which client/SO(s) can**

Information that appears in brackets has been added by the authors to clarify and enhance the use of nursing diagnoses.

freely express views and concerns. **Adherence assessment is most successful when conducted in a positive, nonjudgmental atmosphere.**

- Explore client involvement in or lack of mutual goal setting. **Client will be more likely to follow-through on goals he or she participated in developing.**
- Review treatment strategies. Identify which interventions in the plan of care are most important in meeting therapeutic goals and which are least amenable to compliance. **Sets priorities and encourages problem solving areas of conflict.**
- Contract with the client for participation in care. **Enhances commitment to follow-through.**
- Encourage client to maintain self-care, providing for assistance when necessary. Accept client's evaluation of own strengths and limitations while working with client to improve abilities.
- Provide for continuity of care in and out of the hospital or care setting, including long-range plans. **Supports trust, facilitates progress toward goals.**
- Provide information and help client to know where and how to find it on own. **Promotes independence and encourages informed decision making.**
- Give information in manageable amounts, using verbal, written, and audiovisual modes at level of client's ability. **Using client's style of learning facilitates learning, enabling client to understand diagnosis and treatment regimen.**
- Have client paraphrase instructions and information heard. **Helps validate client's understanding and reveals misconceptions.**
- Accept the client's choice or point of view, even if it appears to be self-destructive. Avoid confrontation regarding beliefs **to maintain open communication.**
- Establish graduated goals or modified regimen, as necessary (e.g., client with chronic obstructive pulmonary disease who smokes a pack of cigarettes a day may be willing to reduce that amount). **May improve quality of life, encouraging progression to more advanced goals.**

Nursing Priority No. 3.

🏠 To promote wellness (Teaching/Discharge Considerations):

- Stress importance of the client's knowledge and understanding of the need for treatment or medication, as well as consequences of actions and choices.

Information that appears in brackets has been added by the authors to clarify and enhance the use of nursing diagnoses.

- Develop a system for self-monitoring **to provide a sense of control and enable client to follow own progress and assist with making choices.**
- Suggest using a medication reminder system. **These have been shown to improve client adherence by a significant percentage.**
- Provide support systems **to reinforce negotiated behaviors.** Encourage client to continue positive behaviors, especially if client is beginning to see benefit.
- Refer to counseling, therapy and/or other appropriate resources.
- Refer to NDs ineffective Coping; compromised family Coping; deficient Knowledge [Learning Need (specify)]; Anxiety; ineffective Self-Health Management.

Documentation Focus

Assessment/Reassessment
- Individual findings including deviation from prescribed treatment plan and client's reasons in own words.
- Consequences of actions to date.

Planning
- Plan of care and who is involved in planning.
- Teaching plan.

Implementation/Evaluation
- Response to interventions, teaching, and actions performed.
- Attainment or progress toward desired outcome(s).
- Modifications to plan of care.

Discharge Planning
- Long-term needs and who is responsible for actions to be taken.
- Specific referrals made.

Sample Nursing Outcomes & Interventions Classifications (NOC/NIC)

NOC—Compliance Behavior
NIC—Mutual Goal Setting

Information that appears in brackets has been added by the authors to clarify and enhance the use of nursing diagnoses.

imbalanced Nutrition: less than body requirements

Taxonomy II: Nutrition—Class 1 Ingestion (00002)
[Diagnostic Division: Food/Fluid]
Submitted 1975; Revised 2000

Definition: Intake of nutrients insufficient to meet metabolic needs

Related Factors

Inability to ingest or digest food; inability to absorb nutrients
Biological/psychological factors; insufficient finances
[Increased metabolic demands (e.g., burns)]

Defining Characteristics

Subjective

Reports food intake less than recommended daily allowances;
  lack of food
Lack of interest in food; aversion to eating; reported altered taste
  sensation; perceived inability to digest food
Satiety immediately after ingesting food
Abdominal pain or cramping
Lack of information; misinformation; misconceptions

Objective

Body weight 20% or more below ideal range; [decreased subcutaneous fat or muscle mass]
Loss of weight with adequate food intake
Hyperactive bowel sounds; diarrhea; steatorrhea
Weakness of muscles required for mastication or swallowing;
  poor muscle tone
Sore buccal cavity; pale mucous membranes; capillary fragility
Excessive hair loss [or increased growth of hair on body (lanugo)]; [cessation of menses]
Abnormal laboratory studies (e.g., decreased albumin, total proteins; iron deficiency; electrolyte imbalances)

Desired Outcomes/Evaluation Criteria— Client Will:

- Demonstrate progressive weight gain toward goal.
- Display normalization of laboratory values and be free of signs of malnutrition as reflected in Defining Characteristics.

Information that appears in brackets has been added by the authors to clarify and enhance the use of nursing diagnoses.

- Verbalize understanding of causative factors when known and necessary interventions.
- Demonstrate behaviors, lifestyle changes to regain and/or maintain appropriate weight.

Actions/Interventions

Nursing Priority No. 1.
To assess causative/contributing factors:

∞• Identify client at risk for malnutrition (e.g., institutionalized elderly; client with chronic illness; child or adult living in poverty/low-income area; client with jaw or facial injuries; intestinal surgery, postmalabsorptive or restrictive surgical interventions for weight loss; hypermetabolic states [e.g., burns, hyperthyroidism]; malabsorption syndromes, lactose intolerance; cystic fibrosis; pancreatic disease; prolonged time of restricted intake; prior nutritional deficiencies).

∞• Assess pediatric concerns (e.g., changes in nutritional needs related to growth phase; congenital anomalies, including tracheoesophageal fistula, cleft lip/palate; metabolic or malabsorption problems, such as diabetes, phenylketonuria, cerebral palsy; chronic infections).

- Determine client's ability to chew, swallow, and taste food. Evaluate teeth and gums for poor oral health, and note denture fit, as indicated. **All factors that affect ingestion and/or digestion of nutrients.**

- Ascertain understanding of individual nutritional needs **to determine informational needs of client/SO.**

- Determine lifestyle factors that may affect weight. **Socioeconomic resources, amount of money available for purchasing food, proximity of grocery store, and available storage space for food are all factors that may impact food choices and intake.**

- Explore specific eating habits, the meaning of food to client (e.g., never eats breakfast, snacks throughout entire day, fasts for weight control, no time to eat properly), and individual food preferences and intolerances/aversions. **Identifies eating practices that may need to be corrected and provides insight into dietary interventions that may appeal to client.**

- Assess drug interactions, disease effects, allergies, use of laxatives, diuretics **that may be affecting appetite, food intake, or absorption.**

- Evaluate impact of cultural, ethnic, or religious desires and influences **that may affect food choices or to identify**

Information that appears in brackets has been added by the authors to clarify and enhance the use of nursing diagnoses.

factors (e.g., dementia, severe depression) that may be interfering with client's appetite and food intake.

• Determine psychological factors, perform psychological assessment, as indicated, **to assess body image and congruency with reality.**

• Note occurrence of amenorrhea, tooth decay, swollen salivary glands, and report of constant sore throat, **suggesting bulimia and affecting ability to eat.**

• Review usual activities and exercise program noting repetitive activities (e.g., constant pacing) or inappropriate exercise (e.g., prolonged jogging). **May reveal obsessive nature of weight-control measures.**

Nursing Priority No. 2.

To evaluate degree of deficit:

• Assess weight; measure muscle mass or calculate body fat by means of anthropometric measurements and growth scales **to identify deviations from the norm and to establish baseline parameters.**

• Observe for absence of subcutaneous fat and muscle wasting, loss of hair, fissuring of nails, delayed healing, gum bleeding, swollen abdomen, and so on, **which indicate protein-energy malnutrition.**

• Auscultate bowel sounds. Note characteristics of stool (color, amount, frequency, etc.).

• Assist in nutritional status assessment, using screening tools (e.g., Mini Nutritional Assessment [MNA], the Malnutrition Universal Screening Tool [MUST], or similar tool).

• Review indicated laboratory data (e.g., serum albumin/prealbumin, transferrin, amino acid profile, iron, BUN, nitrogen balance studies, glucose, liver function, electrolytes, total lymphocyte count, indirect calorimetry).

Nursing Priority No. 3.

To establish a nutritional plan that meets individual needs:

• Note age, body build, strength, activity level, and current condition or treatment needs. **Helps determine nutritional needs.**

• Evaluate total daily food intake. Obtain diary of calorie intake, patterns, and times of eating, **to reveal possible cause of malnutrition and changes that could be made in client's intake.**

Information that appears in brackets has been added by the authors to clarify and enhance the use of nursing diagnoses.

🌐 Cultural   🟢 Collaborative   🏠 Community/Home Care

- Calculate basal energy expenditure (BEE) using Harris-Benedict (or similar) formula and estimate energy and protein requirements.
- Assist in treating or managing underlying causative factors (e.g., cancer, malabsorption syndrome, impaired cognition, depression, medications that decrease appetite, fad diets, anorexia).
- Collaborate with interdisciplinary team **to set nutritional goals when client has specific dietary needs, malnutrition is profound, or long-term feeding problems exist.**
- Provide diet modifications, as indicated. For example:

  Optimize client's intake of protein, carbohydrates, fats, calories within eating style and needs

  Several small meals and snacks daily

  Mechanical soft or blenderized tube feedings

  Appetite stimulants (e.g., wine), if indicated

  High-calorie, nutrient-rich dietary supplements, such as meal-replacement shake

  Formula tube feedings; parenteral nutrition infusion
- Administer pharmaceutical agents, as indicated:

  Digestive drugs or enzymes

  Vitamin and mineral (iron) supplements, including chewable multivitamin

  Medications (e.g., antacids, anticholinergics, antiemetics, antidiarrheals)
- Determine whether client prefers or tolerates more calories in a particular meal.
- Use flavoring agents (e.g., lemon and herbs) if salt is restricted **to enhance food satisfaction and stimulate appetite.**
- Encourage use of sugar or honey in beverages if carbohydrates are tolerated well.
- Encourage client to choose foods or have family member bring foods that seem appealing **to stimulate appetite.**
- Avoid foods that cause intolerances or increase gastric motility (e.g., foods that are gas forming, hot/cold, or spicy; caffeinated beverages; milk products), according to individual needs.
- Limit fiber or bulk, if indicated, **because it may lead to early satiety.**
- Promote pleasant, relaxing environment, including socialization when possible **to enhance intake.**
- Prevent or minimize unpleasant odors or sights. **May have a negative effect on appetite and eating.**

Information that appears in brackets has been added by the authors to clarify and enhance the use of nursing diagnoses.

- Assist with or provide oral care before and after meals and at bedtime.
- Encourage use of lozenges and so forth **to stimulate salivation when dryness is a factor.**
- Promote adequate and timely fluid intake. Limit fluids 1 hour prior to meal **to reduce possibility of early satiety.**
- Weigh regularly and graph results **to monitor effectiveness of efforts.**
- Develop individual strategies when problem is mechanical (e.g., wired jaws or paralysis following stroke). Consult occupational therapist **to identify appropriate assistive devices,** or speech therapist **to enhance swallowing ability.** (Refer to ND impaired Swallowing.)
- Refer to structured (behavioral) program of nutrition therapy (e.g., documented time and length of eating period, blenderized food or tube feeding, administered parenteral nutritional therapy) per protocol, **particularly when problem is anorexia nervosa or bulimia.**
- Recommend and support hospitalization **for controlled environment in severe malnutrition or life-threatening situations.**
- Refer to social services or other community resources **for possible assistance with client's limitations in buying and preparing foods.**

Nursing Priority No. 4.
To promote wellness (Teaching/Discharge Considerations):

- Emphasize importance of well-balanced, nutritious intake. Provide information regarding individual nutritional needs and ways to meet these needs within financial constraints.
- Provide positive regard, love, and acknowledgment of "voice within" guiding client with eating disorder.
- Develop consistent, realistic weight goal with client.
- Weigh at regular intervals and document results **to monitor effectiveness of dietary plan.**
- Consult with dietitian or nutritional support team, as necessary, **for long-term needs.**
- Develop regular exercise and stress reduction program.
- Review drug regimen, side effects, and potential interactions with other medications and over-the-counter drugs.
- Review medical regimen and provide information and assistance, as necessary.
- Assist client to identify and access resources, such as way to obtain nutrient-dense, low-budget foods, Supplemental

---

Information that appears in brackets has been added by the authors to clarify and enhance the use of nursing diagnoses.

Nutrition Assistance Program (SNAP), Meals on Wheels, community food banks, and/or other appropriate assistance programs.

⊕• Refer for dental hygiene or other professional care, including counseling or psychiatric care, family therapy, as indicated.

• Provide and reinforce client teaching regarding preoperative and postoperative dietary needs when surgery is planned.

• Assist client/SO(s) to learn how to blenderize food and/or perform tube feeding.

⊕• Refer to home health resources **for initiation and supervision of home nutrition therapy when used.**

Documentation Focus

Assessment/Reassessment
• Baseline and subsequent assessment findings to include signs/symptoms as noted in Defining Characteristics and laboratory diagnostic findings.
• Caloric intake.
• Individual cultural or religious restrictions, personal preferences.
• Availability and use of resources.
• Personal understanding or perception of problem.

Planning
• Plan of care and who is involved in planning.
• Teaching plan.

Implementation/Evaluation
• Client's responses to interventions, teaching, and actions performed.
• Results of periodic weigh-in.
• Attainment or progress toward desired outcome(s).
• Modifications to plan of care.

Discharge Planning
• Long-term needs, and who is responsible for actions to be taken.
• Specific referrals made.

Sample Nursing Outcomes & Interventions Classifications (NOC/NIC)

NOC—Nutritional Status
NIC—Nutrition Management

Information that appears in brackets has been added by the authors to clarify and enhance the use of nursing diagnoses.

imbalanced Nutrition: more than body requirements

Taxonomy II: Nutrition—Class 1 Ingestion (00001)
[Diagnostic Division: Food/Fluid]
Submitted 1975; Revised 2000

Definition: Intake of nutrients that exceeds metabolic needs

Related Factors

Excessive intake in relationship to metabolic need
Excessive intake in relationship to physical activity (caloric expenditure)

Defining Characteristics

Subjective

Dysfunctional eating patterns (e.g., pairing food with other activities)
Eating in response to external cues (e.g., time of day, social situation)
Concentrating food intake at end of day
Eating in response to internal cues other than hunger (e.g., anxiety)
Sedentary lifestyle

Objective

Weight 20% over ideal for height and frame
Triceps skin fold more than 25 mm in women, more than 15 mm in men

Desired Outcomes/Evaluation Criteria— Client Will:

• Verbalize a realistic self-concept and body image (congruent mental and physical picture of self).
• Demonstrate acceptance of self as is rather than an idealized image.
• Demonstrate appropriate changes in lifestyle and behaviors, including eating patterns, food quantity/quality, and exercise program.
• Attain desirable body weight with optimal maintenance of health.

Information that appears in brackets has been added by the authors to clarify and enhance the use of nursing diagnoses.

🌐 Cultural 🐾 Collaborative 🏠 Community/Home Care

Nursing Priority No. 1.

To identify causative/contributing factors:

- Assess risk or presence of conditions associated with obesity (e.g., familial pattern of obesity; slow metabolism, hypothyroidism; type 2 diabetes; high blood pressure; high cholesterol; or history of stroke, heart attack, gallstones, gout, arthritis, sleep apnea) **to ascertain treatments or interventions that may be needed in addition to weight management.**

∞• Obtain weight history, noting if client has weight gain out of character for self or family, is or was obese child, or used to be much more physically active than is now **to identify trends.**

- Review daily activity and regular exercise program. **Sedentary lifestyle is frequently associated with obesity and is a primary focus for modification.**

- Ascertain how client perceives food and the act of eating. **Individual beliefs, values, and types of foods available influence what people eat, avoid, or alter.**

- Review diary of foods and fluids ingested; times and patterns of eating; activities, place; whether alone or with other(s); and feelings before, during, and after eating. **Provides opportunity for individual to focus on and internalize realistic picture of the amount and type of food ingested and corresponding eating habits and feelings.**

- Calculate total calorie intake, using client's 24-hour recall or weekly food diary. Evaluate usual intake of different food groups.

- Ascertain previous dieting history.

- Discuss client's view of self, including what being heavy does for the client. **Familial traits, cultural beliefs, or life goals may place high importance on food and intake as well as large body size (e.g., Samoan, wrestler/football lineman).**

- Note negative and positive monologues (self-talk) of the individual.

- Obtain comparative body drawing by having client draw self on wall with chalk, then standing against it and having actual body outline drawn. **Determines whether client's view of self-body image is congruent with reality.**

- Ascertain occurrence of negative feedback from SO(s). **May reveal control issues, impact motivation for change.**

- Review results of body fat measurement (e.g., skin calipers, bioelectric impedance analysis [BIA], dual-energy x-ray

---

Information that appears in brackets has been added by the authors to clarify and enhance the use of nursing diagnoses.

absorptiometry [DEXA] scanning, hydrostatic weighing) **to determine presence and severity of obesity.**

Nursing Priority No. 2.

To establish weight reduction program:

- Discuss client's motivation for weight loss (e.g., for own satisfaction or self-esteem or to gain approval from another person). **Helps client determine realistic motivating factors for individual situation (e.g., acceptance of self "as is," improvement of health status).**
- Obtain commitment or contract for weight loss.
- Record height, weight, body build, gender, and age. **Provides comparative baseline and helps determine nutritional needs.**
- Calculate calorie requirements based on physical factors (including age, body type, current activity factors, and illness condition).
- Provide information regarding specific nutritional needs. **Obese individual may be deficient in needed nutrients (e.g., proteins, vitamins, or minerals) or may eat too much of one food group (e.g., fats or carbohydrates). Depending on client's desires and needs, many weight-management programs are available that focus on particular factors (e.g., low carbohydrates, low fat, low calories). Reducing portion size and following a balanced diet along with increasing exercise is often what is needed to improve health.**
- Set realistic goals for weekly weight loss.
- Discuss eating behaviors (e.g., eating over sink, "nibbling," kinds of activities associated with eating) and identify necessary modifications.
- Encourage client to start with small changes (e.g., adding one more vegetable/day, introducing healthier versions of favorite foods, learning to read/understand nutrition labels) **to slowly change eating habits.**
- Develop carbohydrate and fat portion control and appetite-reduction plan **to support continuation of behavioral changes.**
- Emphasize need for adequate fluid intake and taking fluids between meals rather than with meals **to meet fluid requirements and reduce possibility of early satiety, followed quickly by recurrent hunger.**
- Discuss smart snacks (e.g., low-fat yogurt with fruit, nuts, apple slices with peanut butter, low-fat string cheese) **to assist client in finding healthy options.**

Information that appears in brackets has been added by the authors to clarify and enhance the use of nursing diagnoses.

🌐 Cultural   🔄 Collaborative   🏠 Community/Home Care

- Collaborate with physician and dietitian or nutrition team **in creating and evaluating effective nutritional program.**
- Encourage involvement in planned exercise program of client's choice and within physical abilities.
- Monitor individual drug regimen (e.g., appetite suppressants, hormone therapy, vitamin and mineral supplements).
- Provide positive reinforcement and encouragement for efforts as well as actual weight loss. **Enhances commitment to program and person's sense of self-worth.**
- Refer to bariatric specialist for additional interventions (e.g., extremely low calorie diet, surgical weight loss procedures).

Nursing Priority No. 3.

To promote wellness (Teaching/Discharge Considerations):

- Discuss reality of obesity and health consequences as well as myths client/SO(s) may believe about weight and weight loss.
- Assist client to choose nutritious foods that reflect personal likes, meet individual needs, and are within financial budget.
- Encourage parent to model good nutritional choices (e.g., offer vegetables, fruits, and low-fat foods at daily meals and snacks) **to assist child in adopting healthy eating habits.**
- Identify ways to manage stress or tension during meals. **Promotes relaxation to permit focus on act of eating and awareness of satiety.**
- Review and discuss strategies to deal appropriately with stressful events/feelings **instead of overeating.**
- Encourage variety and moderation in dietary plan **to decrease boredom.**
- Advise client to plan for special occasions (birthday/holidays) by reducing intake before event and/or eating "smart" **to redistribute or reduce calories and allow for participation in food events.**
- Discuss importance of an occasional treat by planning for inclusion in diet **to avoid feelings of deprivation arising from self-denial.**
- Recommend client weigh only once per week, same time and clothes, and graph on chart. Measure body fat when possible **(more accurate measure).**
- Discuss normalcy of ups and downs of weight loss: plateauing, set point (at which weight is not being lost), hormonal influences, and so forth. **Prevents discouragement when progress stalls.**
- Encourage buying personal items/clothing as a reward for weight loss or other accomplishments. Suggest disposing of

---

Information that appears in brackets has been added by the authors to clarify and enhance the use of nursing diagnoses.

"fat clothes" **to encourage positive attitude of permanent change and remove "safety valve" of having wardrobe available "just in case" weight is regained.**

🏠 • Involve SO(s) in treatment plan as much as possible **to provide ongoing support and increase likelihood of success.**

⊛ • Refer to community support groups, psychotherapy, as indicated.

⊛ • Provide contact number for dietitian and bibliography and Web sites for resources **to address ongoing nutrition concerns/dietary needs.**

• Refer to NDs disturbed Body Image; ineffective Coping, for additional interventions, as appropriate.

Documentation Focus

Assessment/Reassessment
• Individual findings, including current weight, dietary pattern; perceptions of self, food, and eating; motivation for loss, support and feedback from SO(s).
• Results of laboratory and diagnostic testing.
• Results of weekly weigh-in.

Planning
• Plan of care, specific interventions, and who is involved in planning.
• Teaching plan.

Implementation/Evaluation
• Responses to interventions, weekly weight, and actions performed.
• Attainment or progress toward desired outcome(s).
• Modifications to plan of care.

Discharge Planning
• Long-term needs and who is responsible for actions to be taken.
• Specific referrals made.

Sample Nursing Outcomes & Interventions Classifications (NOC/NIC)
NOC—Weight Loss Behavior
NIC—Weight Reduction Assistance

Information that appears in brackets has been added by the authors to clarify and enhance the use of nursing diagnoses.

🌐 Cultural ⊛ Collaborative 🏠 Community/Home Care

risk for imbalanced Nutrition: more than body requirements

Taxonomy II: Nutrition—Class 1 Ingestion (00003)
[Diagnostic Division: Food/Fluid]
Submitted 1980; Revised 2000

Definition: At risk for an intake of nutrients that exceeds metabolic needs

Risk Factors

Dysfunctional eating patterns; pairing food with other activities; eating in response to external cues (e.g., time of day, social situation) or internal cues other than hunger (e.g., anxiety); concentrating food intake at the end of the day

Parental obesity

Rapid transition across growth percentiles in children; reports use of solid food as major food source before 5 months of age

Higher baseline weight at beginning of each pregnancy

Observed use of food as reward or comfort measure

Sedentary lifestyle

[Majority of foods consumed are concentrated, high-caloric, or fat]

> **NOTE:** A risk diagnosis is not evidenced by signs and symptoms, as the problem has not occurred; rather, nursing interventions are directed at prevention.

Desired Outcomes/Evaluation Criteria— Client Will:

- Verbalize understanding of body and energy needs.
- Identify lifestyle and cultural factors that predispose to obesity.
- Demonstrate behaviors, lifestyle changes to reduce risk factors.
- Acknowledge responsibility for own actions and need to "act, not react" to stressful situations.
- Maintain weight at a satisfactory level for height, body build, age, and gender.

Information that appears in brackets has been added by the authors to clarify and enhance the use of nursing diagnoses.

Actions/Interventions

Nursing Priority No. 1.

To assess potential factors for undesired weight gain:

- Note presence of factors as listed in Risk Factors. **A high correlation exists between obesity in parents and their children. When one parent is obese, 40% of the children may be overweight; when both are obese, the occurrence may be as high as 80%.**
- ∞ Determine age, activity level, and exercise patterns **to identify areas where changes might be useful to prevent obesity and promote health. For example, older adults need same nutrients as younger adults but in smaller amounts and with attention to certain components, such as calcium, fiber, vitamins, protein, and water.**
- ∞ Calculate growth percentiles in infants/children using growth chart **to identify deviations from the norm.**
- Review laboratory data **for indicators of endocrine or metabolic disorders.**
- Identify cultural factors or lifestyle that may predispose to weight gain. **Socioeconomic group, familial eating patterns, amount of money available for purchasing food, proximity of grocery store, and available storage space for food are all factors that may impact food choices and intake.**
- Assess eating patterns in relation to risk factors. Note patterns of hunger and satiety. **Patterns differ in those who are predisposed to weight gain (e.g., client is skipping meals to reduce total calories, but is unaware that this practice decreases the metabolic rate).**
- Determine weight change patterns, history of dieting and kinds of diets used. Determine whether yo-yo dieting or bulimia is a factor.
- Identify personality characteristics that may indicate potential for obesity (e.g., rigid thinking patterns, external locus of control, negative body image or self-concept, negative monologues [self-talk], dissatisfaction with life).
- Determine psychological significance of food to the client (e.g., derives love and comfort from food, uses food to escape deep unhappiness, eats when stressed or anxious).
- Listen to concerns and assess motivation to prevent weight gain. **If client's concern regarding weight control is motivated by reasons other than personal well-being (e.g.,**

Information that appears in brackets has been added by the authors to clarify and enhance the use of nursing diagnoses.

🌐 Cultural 🔁 Collaborative 🏠 Community/Home Care

partner's expectations or demands), the likelihood of success is decreased.

Nursing Priority No. 2.

To assist client to develop preventive program to avoid weight gain:

∞• Provide information, as indicated, on nutrition, taking into account client's age and developmental stage (e.g., toddler, teenager, pregnant woman, elderly person with chronic disease), physical health and activity tolerance, financial and socioeconomic factors, and client's/SO's potential for management of risk factors.
• Review guidelines for achieving and maintaining healthy body weight:
  Eat from each food group (fruits, vegetables, whole grains, lean meats, dairy and fats).
  Choose "nutrient-dense" forms of foods that provide substantial amounts of fiber, vitamins, electrolytes, and minerals.
  Avoid saturated fats, trans fats, cholesterol, salt (sodium), and added sugars.
  Focus on portion sizes: calorie-dense foods (high in fat and/or sugar) should be eaten in smaller quantities, whereas high-fiber foods can be eaten in larger quantities.
  Discuss smart snacks (e.g., low-fat yogurt with fruit, nuts, apple slices with peanut butter, low-fat string cheese)
• Help client develop new eating patterns and habits (e.g., eating slowly, eating only when hungry, controlling portion size, stopping when full, not skipping meals).
• Discuss importance and help client develop a program of exercise and relaxation techniques. **Encourages client to incorporate plan into lifestyle.**
• Assist client to develop strategies for reducing stressful thinking or actions. **Promotes relaxation, reduces likelihood of stress and comfort eating.**

Nursing Priority No. 3.

🏠 To promote wellness (Teaching/Discharge Considerations):

• Review individual risk factors and provide information **to assist the client with motivation and decision making.**
⚗• Consult with dietitian or nutritionist about specific nutrition and dietary issues.
∞• Provide information to new mothers about nutrition for developing babies.

Information that appears in brackets has been added by the authors to clarify and enhance the use of nursing diagnoses.

- Encourage client to make a decision to lead an active life and control food habits.
- Assist client in learning to be in touch with own body and to identify feelings that may provoke "comfort eating," such as anger, anxiety, boredom, sadness.
- Develop a system for self-monitoring **to provide a sense of control and enable the client to follow own progress and assist with making choices.**
- Provide bibliography, including reliable Internet sites for resources **to reinforce learning, address ongoing nutrition needs, support informed decision making.**
- Refer to support groups and appropriate community resources for education/behavior modification, as indicated.

Documentation Focus

Assessment/Reassessment
- Findings related to individual situation, risk factors, current caloric intake and dietary pattern, activity level.
- Baseline height and weight, growth percentile.
- Results of laboratory tests.
- Motivation to reduce risks and prevent weight problems.

Planning
- Plan of care and who is involved in the planning.
- Teaching plan.

Implementation/Evaluation
- Response to interventions, teaching, and actions performed.
- Attainment or progress toward desired outcome(s).
- Modifications to plan of care.

Discharge Planning
- Long-term needs, noting who is responsible for actions to be taken.
- Specific referrals made.

Sample Nursing Outcomes & Interventions Classifications (NOC/NIC)

NOC—Weight Maintenance Behavior
NIC—Weight Management

Information that appears in brackets has been added by the authors to clarify and enhance the use of nursing diagnoses.

⊕ Cultural ⊛ Collaborative 🏠 Community/Home Care

readiness for enhanced **Nutrition**

Taxonomy II: Nutrition—Class 1 Ingestion (00163)
[Diagnostic Division: Food/Fluid]
Submitted 2002

Definition: A pattern of nutrient intake that is sufficient for meeting metabolic needs and can be strengthened

Defining Characteristics

Subjective

Expresses knowledge of healthy food or fluid choices; expresses willingness to enhance nutrition
Eats regularly
Attitude toward eating or drinking is congruent with health goals

Objective

Consumes adequate food or fluid
Follows an appropriate standard for intake (e.g., the food pyramid or American Diabetic Association guidelines)
Safe preparation or storage for food/fluids

Desired Outcomes/Evaluation Criteria— Client Will:

- Demonstrate behaviors to attain or maintain appropriate weight.
- Be free of signs of malnutrition.
- Be able to safely prepare and store foods.

Actions/Interventions

Nursing Priority No. 1.

To determine current nutritional status and eating patterns:

- Review client's knowledge of current nutritional needs and ways client is meeting these needs. **Provides baseline for further teaching and interventions.**
- Assess eating patterns and food and fluid choices in relation to any health risk factors and health goals. **Helps to identify specific strengths and weaknesses that can be addressed.**
- ∞• Verify that age-related and developmental needs are met. **These factors are constantly presented throughout the life**

Information that appears in brackets has been added by the authors to clarify and enhance the use of nursing diagnoses.

span, although differing for each age group. For example, older adults need same nutrients as younger adults, but in smaller amounts, and with attention to certain components, such as calcium, fiber, vitamins, protein, and water. Infants/children require small meals and constant attention to needed nutrients for proper growth and development while dealing with child's food preferences and eating habits.

• Evaluate influence of cultural or religious factors **to determine what client considers to be normal dietary practices, as well as to identify food preferences and restrictions, and eating patterns that can be strengthened and/or altered, if indicated.**

• Assess how client perceives food, food preparation, and the act of eating **to determine client's feelings and emotions regarding food and self-image.**

• Ascertain occurrence of, or potential for, negative feedback from SO(s). **May reveal control issues that could impact client's commitment to change.**

• Determine patterns of hunger and satiety. **Helps identify strengths and weaknesses in eating patterns and potential for change (e.g., person predisposed to weight gain may need a different time for a big meal than evening or need to learn what foods reinforce feelings of satisfaction).**

• Assess client's ability to safely store and prepare foods **to determine if health information or resources might be needed.**

Nursing Priority No. 2.
To assist client/SO(s) to develop plan to meet individual needs:

• Determine motivation and expectation for change.

• Assist in obtaining and review results of individual testing (e.g., weight/height, body fat percent, lipids, glucose, complete blood count, total protein) **to determine that client is healthy and/or identify dietary changes that may be helpful in attaining health goals.**

• Encourage client's beneficial eating patterns/habits (e.g., controlling portion size, eating regular meals, reducing high-fat or fast-food intake, following specific dietary program, drinking water and healthy beverages). **Positive feedback promotes continuation of healthy lifestyle habits and new behaviors.**

• Discuss use of nonfood rewards.

Information that appears in brackets has been added by the authors to clarify and enhance the use of nursing diagnoses.

🌐 Cultural 😊 Collaborative 🏠 Community/Home Care

- Provide instruction and reinforce information regarding special needs. **Enhances decision-making process and promotes responsibility for meeting own needs.**
- Encourage reading of food labels and instruct in meaning of labeling, as indicated, **to assist client/SO(s) in making healthful choices.**
- Consult with, or refer to, dietitian, or physician, as indicated. **Client/SO(s) may benefit from advice regarding specific nutrition and dietary issues or may require regular follow-up to determine that needs are being met when a medically prescribed program is to be followed.**
- Develop a system for self-monitoring **to provide a sense of control and enable the client to follow own progress and assist in making choices.**

Nursing Priority No. 3.

To promote optimum wellness:

- Review individual risk factors and provide additional information and response to concerns. **Assists the client with motivation and decision making.**
- Provide bibliotherapy and help client/SO(s) identify and evaluate resources they can access on their own. **When referencing the Internet or nontraditional, unproven resources, the individual must exercise some restraint and determine the reliability of the source/information before acting on it.**
- Encourage variety and moderation in dietary plan **to decrease boredom and encourage client in efforts to make healthy choices about eating and food.**
- Discuss use of nutritional supplements, over-the-counter and herbal products. **Confusion may exist regarding the need for and use of these products in a balanced dietary regimen.**
- Assist client to identify and access community resources when indicated. **May benefit from assistance such as Supplemental Nutrition Assistance Program (SNAP), WIC, budget counseling, Meals on Wheels, community food banks, and/or other assistance programs.**

Documentation Focus

Assessment/Reassessment

- Assessment findings, including client perception of needs and desire/expectations for improvement.

Information that appears in brackets has been added by the authors to clarify and enhance the use of nursing diagnoses.

- Individual cultural or religious restrictions, personal preferences.
- Availability and use of resources.

Planning
- Individual goals for enhancement.
- Plan for growth and who is involved in planning.

Implementation/Evaluation
- Response to activities and learning, and actions performed.
- Attainment or progress toward desired outcome(s).
- Modifications to plan.

Discharge Planning
- Long-term needs, expectations, and plan of action.
- Available resources and specific referrals made.

Sample Nursing Outcomes & Interventions Classifications (NOC/NIC)

NOC—Knowledge: Diet
NIC—Nutritional Counseling

impaired Oral Mucous Membrane

Taxonomy II: Safety/Protection—Class 2 Physical Injury (00045)
[Diagnostic Division: Food/Fluid]
Submitted 1982; Nursing Diagnosis Extension and Classification Revision 1998

Definition: Disruption of the lips and/or soft tissue of the oral cavity

Related Factors

Dehydration; nil by mouth (NPO) for more than 24 hours; malnutrition

Decreased salivation; medication side effects; diminished hormone levels (women); mouth breathing

Deficient knowledge of appropriate oral hygiene

Ineffective oral hygiene; barriers to oral self-care or professional care

---

Information that appears in brackets has been added by the authors to clarify and enhance the use of nursing diagnoses.

Mechanical factors (e.g., ill-fitting dentures, braces, tubes [endotracheal/nasogastric], surgery in oral cavity); loss of supportive structures; trauma; cleft lip or palate

Chemical irritants (e.g., alcohol, tobacco, acidic foods, drugs, regular use of inhalers or other noxious agents)

Treatment-related side effects (e.g., chemotherapy, pharmaceutical agents, radiation therapy); immunosuppressed immunocompromised; decreased platelets; infection

Stress; depression

Defining Characteristics

Subjective

Xerostomia (dry mouth)

Oral pain, discomfort

Reports bad taste in mouth; diminished taste; difficulty eating or swallowing

Objective

Coated tongue; smooth atrophic tongue; geographic tongue

Gingival or mucosal pallor

Stomatitis; hyperemia; gingival hyperplasia; macroplasia; vesicles; nodules; papules

White patches or plaques; spongy patches; white, curd-like exudate

Oral lesions or ulcers; fissures; bleeding; cheilitis; desquamation; mucosal denudation

Purulent drainage or exudates; presence of pathogens; enlarged tonsils

Edema

Halitosis; [carious teeth]

Gingival recession, pocketing deeper than 4 mm

Red or bluish masses (e.g., hemangiomas)

Difficult speech

Desired Outcomes/Evaluation Criteria— Client Will:

- Verbalize understanding of causative factors.
- Identify specific interventions to promote healthy oral mucosa.
- Demonstrate techniques to restore/maintain integrity of oral mucosa.
- Report or demonstrate a decrease in symptoms as noted in Defining Characteristics.

Information that appears in brackets has been added by the authors to clarify and enhance the use of nursing diagnoses.

Actions/Interventions ———————————————

Nursing Priority No. 1.

To identify causative/contributing factors affecting oral health:

- Note presence of illness, disease, or trauma (e.g., gingivitis, periodontal disease; presence of oral ulcerations; bacterial, viral, fungal, or oral infections; facial fractures; cancer or cancer therapies; generalized debilitating conditions) **that affect health of oral tissues.**
- Determine type of oral mucous membrane problem (e.g., severe or chronic dry mouth [xerostomia] associated with lack of saliva; abnormal tongue surfaces; gingivitis or periodontal disease; ulcerations or other lesions) **that may cause inflammation affecting ability to eat or more serious complications.**
- Collaborate in evaluating abnormal lesions of mouth, tongue, and cheeks (e.g., white or red patches, ulcers). **White ulcerated spots may be canker sores, especially in children; white curd patches (thrush) are common in infants. Reddened, swollen bleeding gums may indicate infection, poor nutrition, or poor oral hygiene. A red tongue may be related to vitamin deficiencies. Malignant lesions are more common in elderly than younger persons (especially if there is a history of smoking or alcohol use) or in persons who rarely visit a dentist.**
- Observe for chipped, sharp-edged teeth, or malpositioned teeth. Note fit of dentures or other prosthetic devices when used.
- Note use of tobacco (including smokeless) and alcohol/other drugs (e.g., methamphetamines), **which may predispose mucosa to effects of nutritional deficiencies, infection, cell damage, and cancer.**
- Determine nutrition and fluid intake and reported changes (e.g., avoiding eating, change in taste, chews painstakingly, swallows numerous times for even small bites, unexplained weight loss) **that can indicate problems with oral mucosa.**
- Assess medication use and possibility of side effects **affecting health or integrity of oral mucous membranes.**
- Determine allergies to food, drugs, other substances **that may result in irritation or disruption of oral mucosa.**
- Evaluate client's ability to provide self-care and availability of necessary equipment or assistance. **Client's age, as well as current health status, affects ability to provide self-care.**

———————————————

Information that appears in brackets has been added by the authors to clarify and enhance the use of nursing diagnoses.

- Review oral hygiene practices: frequency and type (e.g., brushing, flossing, WaterPik); professional dental care.

Nursing Priority No. 2.

To correct identified/developing problems:

- Collaborate in treatment of underlying conditions (e.g., structural defects, infections) **that may correct or limit problem with oral tissues.**
- Routinely inspect oral cavity and throat for inflammation, sores, lesions, and/or bleeding. **Can help with early identification and management of mucous membrane concerns.**
- Encourage adequate fluids **to prevent dry mouth and dehydration.**
- Encourage use of tart, sour, and citrus foods and drinks; chewing gum; or hard candy **to stimulate saliva.**
- Lubricate lips and provide commercially prepared oral lubricant solution.
- Provide for increased humidity, if indicated, by vaporizer or room humidifier if client is mouth-breather.
- Provide dietary modifications (e.g., food of comfortable texture, temperature, density) **to reduce discomfort and improve intake,** and adequate nutrients and vitamins **to promote healing.**
- Avoid irritating foods and fluids, temperature extremes. Provide soft or pureed diet as required.
- Use lemon/glycerin swabs with caution; **may be irritating if mucosa is injured.**
- Assist with oral care, as indicated **for irrigation and treatment of mouth, gums, and mucous membrane surfaces:**

  Offer tap water or saline rinses, diluted alcohol-free mouthwashes, mucosal coating agents, lubricating agents, topical anesthetics.

  Provide gentle gum massage and tongue brushing with soft toothbrush or sponge/cotton-tip applicators.

  Assist with or encourage brushing and flossing **when client is unable to do self-care.**

  Review safe use of electric or battery-powered mouth care devices (e.g., toothbrush, plaque remover), as indicated.

  Assist with or provide denture care when indicated (e.g., remove and clean after meals and at bedtime).

- Provide anesthetic lozenges or analgesics such as Stanford solution, viscous lidocaine (Xylocaine), sucralfate slurry, as

---

Information that appears in brackets has been added by the authors to clarify and enhance the use of nursing diagnoses.

indicated, **to provide protection or reduce oral discomfort and pain.**

🥄• Administer antibiotics, as ordered, **when infection is present.**

• Reposition endotrachial tubes and airway adjuncts routinely, carefully padding teeth or prosthetics **to minimize pressure on tissues.**

• Emphasize avoiding alcohol, smoking, or chewing tobacco especially if periodontal disease present or if client has xerostomia or other oral discomforts, **which may further irritate and damage mucosa.**

🔵• Refer for evaluation of dentures or other prosthetics, structural defects **when impairments are affecting oral health.**

Nursing Priority No. 3.

🏠To promote wellness (Teaching/Discharge Considerations):

• Review current oral hygiene patterns and provide information about oral health as required or desired **to correct deficiencies and encourage proper care.**

🔵• Recommend regular dental checkups and care, and episodic evaluation of oral health prior to certain medical treatments (e.g., chemotherapy, radiation) **to maintain oral health and reduce risks associated with impaired tissues.**

∞• Instruct parents in oral hygiene techniques and proper dental care for infants/children (e.g., safe use of pacifier, brushing of teeth and gums, avoidance of sweet drinks and candy, recognition and treatment of thrush). **Encourages early initiation of good oral health practices and timely intervention for treatable problems.**

• Discuss special mouth care required during and after illness or trauma or following surgical repair (e.g., cleft lip or palate) **to facilitate healing.**

• Identify need for and demonstrate use of special "appliances" **to perform own oral care.**

• Listen to concerns about appearance and provide accurate information about possible treatments and outcomes. Discuss effect of condition on self-esteem and body image, noting withdrawal from usual social activities or relationships, and/or expressions of powerlessness.

🥄• Review information regarding drug regimen, use of local anesthetics.

• Promote good general health and mental health habits including stress management. **(Altered immune response can affect the oral mucosa.)**

Information that appears in brackets has been added by the authors to clarify and enhance the use of nursing diagnoses.

- Provide nutritional information **to correct deficiencies, reduce gum irritation or disease, prevent dental caries.**
- Recommend regular dental checkups and professional care.
- Identify community resources (e.g., low-cost dental clinics, smoking cessation resources, cancer information services and support group, Meals on Wheels, Supplemental Nutrition Assistance Program (SNAP), home care aide).

Documentation Focus

Assessment/Reassessment
- Condition of oral mucous membranes, routine oral care habits and interferences.
- Availability of oral care equipment and products.
- Knowledge of proper oral hygiene and care.
- Availability and use of resources.

Planning
- Plan of care and who is involved in planning.
- Teaching plan.

Implementation/Evaluation
- Responses to interventions, teaching, and actions performed.
- Attainment or progress toward desired outcome(s).
- Modifications to plan of care.

Discharge Planning
- Long-term needs and who is responsible for actions to be taken.
- Specific referrals made, resources for special appliances.

Sample Nursing Outcomes & Interventions Classifications (NOC/NIC)

NOC—Oral Hygiene
NIC—Oral Health Restoration

Information that appears in brackets has been added by the authors to clarify and enhance the use of nursing diagnoses.

acute Pain

Taxonomy II: Comfort—Class 1 Physical Comfort (00132)
[Diagnostic Division: Pain/Comfort]
Submitted 1996

Definition: Unpleasant sensory and emotional experience arising from actual or potential tissue damage or
described in terms of such damage (International Association for the Study of Pain); sudden or slow onset of any
intensity from mild to severe with an anticipated or predictable end and a duration of less than 6 months

Related Factors

Injuring agents (biological, chemical, physical, psychological)

Defining Characteristics

Subjective
Reports pain; coded report (e.g., use of pain scale)
Changes in appetite; sleep pattern disturbance

Objective
Observed evidence of pain
Guarding behavior; protective gestures; positioning to avoid
pain
Facial mask (e.g., eyes lack luster, beaten look, fixed or scattered movement, grimace)
Expressive behavior (e.g., restlessness, moaning, crying, vigilance, irritability, sighing)
Distraction behavior (e.g., pacing, seeking out other people and/
or activities, repetitive activities)
Diaphoresis; changes in blood pressure, heart rate, respiratory
rate; pupillary dilation
Self-focus; narrowed focus (e.g., altered time perception, impaired thought process, reduced interaction with people and
environment)

Desired Outcomes/Evaluation Criteria—
Client Will:

- Report pain is relieved or controlled.
- Follow prescribed pharmacological regimen.
- Verbalize nonpharmacological methods that provide relief.

Information that appears in brackets has been added by the authors to clarify
and enhance the use of nursing diagnoses.

- Demonstrate use of relaxation skills and diversional activities, as indicated, for individual situation.
- Verbalize sense of control of response to acute situation and positive outlook for the future.

Actions/Interventions

Nursing Priority No. 1.
To assess etiology/precipitating contributory factors:

- Note client's age and developmental level and current condition (e.g., infant/child, critically ill, ventilated, sedated, or cognitively impaired client) **affecting ability to report pain parameters**.
- Determine and document presence of possible pathophysiological and psychological causes of pain (e.g., inflammation; tissue trauma, fractures; surgery; infections; heart attack or angina; abdominal conditions [e.g., appendicitis, cholecystitis]; burns; grief; fear, anxiety; depression; and personality disorders).
- Note location of surgical procedures, **as this can influence the amount of postoperative pain experienced; for example, vertical or diagonal incisions are more painful than transverse or S-shaped. Presence of known or unknown complication(s) may make the pain more severe than anticipated.**
- Assess for referred pain, as appropriate, **to help determine possibility of underlying condition or organ dysfunction requiring treatment.**
- Note client's attitude toward pain and use of pain medications, including any history of substance abuse.
- Note client's locus of control (internal or external). **Individuals with external locus of control may take little or no responsibility for pain management.**
- Assist in thorough evaluation, including neurological and psychological factors (pain inventory, psychological interview), as appropriate, when pain persists.

Nursing Priority No. 2.
To evaluate client's response to pain:

- Obtain client's/SO's assessment of pain to include location, characteristics, onset, duration, frequency, quality, intensity. Identify precipitating or aggravating and relieving factors **in order to fully understand client's pain symptoms.** *Note: Experts agree that attempts should always be made to*

Information that appears in brackets has been added by the authors to clarify and enhance the use of nursing diagnoses.

obtain self-reports of pain. When that is not possible, credible information can be received from another person who
knows the client well (e.g., parent, spouse, caregiver).

∞• Use pain rating scale appropriate for age and cognition (e.g.,
0 to 10 scale, facial expression or Wong-Baker faces pain
scale [pediatric, nonverbal], adolescent pediatric pain tool,
pain assessment scale for seniors with limited ability to communicate; behavioral pain scale; checklist of nonverbal pain
indicators, etc.).

• Accept client's description of pain. Acknowledge the pain
experience and convey acceptance of client's response to pain.
**Pain is a subjective experience and cannot be felt by
others.**

• Observe nonverbal cues and pain behaviors (e.g., how client
walks, holds body, sits; facial expression; cool fingertips/toes,
which can mean constricted blood vessels) and other objective
Defining Characteristics, as noted, especially in persons who
cannot communicate verbally. **Observations may not be
congruent with verbal reports or may be only indicator
present when client is unable to verbalize.**

⊕• Note cultural and developmental influences affecting pain response. **Verbal and/or behavioral cues may have no direct
relationship to the degree of pain perceived (e.g., client
may deny pain even when feeling uncomfortable, or reactions can be stoic or exaggerated, reflecting cultural or
familial norms).**

• Monitor skin color and temperature and vital signs (e.g., heart
rate, blood pressure, respirations), **which are usually altered
in acute pain.**

• Ascertain client's knowledge of and expectations about pain
management.

• Review client's previous experiences with pain and methods
found either helpful or unhelpful for pain control in the past.

Nursing Priority No. 3.
To assist client to explore methods for alleviation/control of
pain:

• Determine client's acceptable level of pain and pain control
goals. **One client may not be 100% pain free but may feel
that a "3" is a manageable level of discomfort, while another may require medication for pain at the same level,
because the experience is subjective.**

Information that appears in brackets has been added by the authors to clarify
and enhance the use of nursing diagnoses.

- **Determine factors in client's lifestyle (e.g., alcohol or other drug use or abuse)** that can affect responses to analgesics and/or choice of interventions for pain management.
- Note when pain occurs (e.g., only with ambulation, every evening) **to medicate prophylactically, as appropriate.**
- Collaborate in treatment of underlying condition or disease processes causing pain and proactive management of pain (e.g., epidural analgesia, nerve blockade for postoperative pain).
- Provide comfort measures (e.g., touch, repositioning, use of heat or cold packs, nurse's presence), quiet environment, and calm activities **to promote nonpharmacological pain management.**
- Instruct in and encourage use of relaxation techniques, such as focused breathing, imaging, CDs/tapes (e.g., "white" noise, music, instructional) **to distract attention and reduce tension.**
- Encourage diversional activities (e.g., TV/radio, socialization with others).
- Review procedures and expectations including when treatment may cause pain **to reduce concern of the unknown and associated muscle tension.**
- Encourage verbalization of feelings about the pain such as concern about tolerating pain, anxiety, pessimistic thoughts **to evaluate coping abilities and to identify areas of additional concern.**
- Use puppets to demonstrate procedure for child **to enhance understanding and reduce level of anxiety and fear.**
- Suggest parent be present during procedures **to comfort child.**
- Identify ways of avoiding or minimizing pain (e.g., splinting incision during cough; using firm mattress and proper supporting shoes for low back pain; good body mechanics).
- Work with client to prevent pain. Use flow sheet to document pain, therapeutic interventions, response, and length of time before pain recurs. Instruct client to report pain as soon as it begins **as timely intervention is more likely to be successful in alleviating pain.**
- Establish collaborative approach for pain management based on client's understanding about and acceptance of available treatment options. **Pain medications may include pills/ liquids or suckers, skin patch, or suppository forms; injections, intravenous dosing; or patient-controlled**

Information that appears in brackets has been added by the authors to clarify and enhance the use of nursing diagnoses.

analgesia (PCA) or regional analgesia (e.g., epidural and spinal blocking) based on client's symptomatology and mechanism of pain as well as tolerance for pain and various analgesics.

- Administer analgesics, as indicated, to maximum dosage, as needed, **to maintain "acceptable" level of pain. Notify physician if regimen is inadequate to meet pain control goal. Combinations of medications may be used on prescribed intervals.**
- Demonstrate and monitor use of self-administration/PCA for management of severe, persistent pain.
- Evaluate and document client's response to analgesia and assist in transitioning or altering drug regimen, based on individual needs and protocols. **Increasing or decreasing dosage, stepped program (switching from injection to oral route, increased time span as pain lessens) helps in self-management of pain.**
- Instruct client in use of transcutaneous electrical stimulation (TENS) unit, when ordered.

Nursing Priority No. 4.

To promote wellness (Teaching/Discharge Considerations):

- Acknowledge the pain experience and convey acceptance of client's response to pain. **Reduces defensive responses, promotes trust, and enhances cooperation with regimen.**
- Encourage adequate rest periods **to prevent fatigue that can impair ability to manage or cope with pain.**
- Review ways to lessen pain, including techniques such as Therapeutic Touch (TT), biofeedback, self-hypnosis, and relaxation skills.
- Discuss impact of pain on lifestyle/independence and ways to maximize level of functioning.
- Provide for individualized physical therapy or exercise program that can be continued by the client after discharge. **Promotes active, rather than passive, role and enhances sense of control.**
- Discuss with SO(s) ways in which they can assist client and reduce precipitating factors that may cause or increase pain (e.g., participating in household tasks following abdominal surgery).
- Identify specific signs/symptoms and changes in pain characteristics requiring medical follow-up.

Information that appears in brackets has been added by the authors to clarify and enhance the use of nursing diagnoses.

Documentation Focus

Assessment/Reassessment
- Individual assessment findings, including client's description of response to pain, specifics of pain inventory, expectations of pain management, and acceptable level of pain.
- Prior medication use; substance abuse.

Planning
- Plan of care and who is involved in planning.
- Teaching plan.

Implementation/Evaluation
- Response to interventions, teaching, and actions performed.
- Attainment or progress toward desired outcome(s).
- Modifications to plan of care.

Discharge Planning
- Long-term needs, noting who is responsible for actions to be taken.
- Specific referrals made.

Sample Nursing Outcomes & Interventions Classifications (NOC/NIC)

NOC—Pain Level
NIC—Pain Management

chronic Pain

Taxonomy II: Comfort—Class 1 Physical Comfort (00133)
[Diagnostic Division: Pain/Discomfort]
Submitted 1986; Revised 1996

Definition: Unpleasant sensory and emotional experience arising from actual or potential tissue damage or described in terms of such damage (International Association for the Study of Pain); sudden or slow onset of any intensity from mild to severe, constant or recurring without an anticipated or predictable end and a duration of greater than 6 months

---

Information that appears in brackets has been added by the authors to clarify and enhance the use of nursing diagnoses.

> **NOTE:** Pain is a signal that something is wrong. Chronic pain can be recurrent and periodically disabling (e.g., migraine headaches) or may be unremitting. While chronic pain syndrome includes various learned behaviors, psychological factors become the primary contribution to impairment. It is a complex entity, combining elements from other NDs, such as Powerlessness; deficient Diversional Activity; interrupted Family Processes; Self-Care Deficit; and risk for Disuse Syndrome.

Related Factors

Chronic physical or psychosocial disability

Defining Characteristics

Subjective

Reports pain; coded report (e.g., use of pain scale)
Fear of re-injury
Altered ability to continue previous activities
Changes in sleep pattern; fatigue; anorexia
[Preoccupation with pain]
[Desperately seeks alternative solutions or therapies for relief or control of pain]

Objective

Guarding or observed protective behavior; irritability; restlessness
Facial mask (e.g., eyes lack luster, beaten look, fixed or scattered movement, grimace); self-focusing
Reduced interaction with people; depression
Atrophy of involved muscle group
Sympathetic mediated responses (e.g., temperature, cold, changes of body position, hypersensitivity)

Desired Outcomes/Evaluation Criteria—Client Will:

- Verbalize and demonstrate (nonverbal cues) relief and/or control of pain or discomfort.
- Verbalize recognition of interpersonal and family dynamics and reactions that affect the pain situation.

Information that appears in brackets has been added by the authors to clarify and enhance the use of nursing diagnoses.

- Demonstrate and initiate behavioral modifications of lifestyle and appropriate use of therapeutic interventions.
- Verbalize increased sense of control and enhanced enjoyment of life.

Family/SO(s) Will:

- Cooperate in pain management program. (Refer to ND readiness for enhanced family Coping.)

Actions/Interventions

Nursing Priority No. 1.

To assess etiology/precipitating factors:

- Assess for conditions associated with long-term pain (e.g., low back pain, arthritis, fibromyalgia, neuropathies, multiple or slow-healing, traumatic musculoskeletal injuries, amputation [phantom limb pain]) **to identify client with potential for pain lasting beyond normal healing period.**
- Assist in thorough diagnosis, including physical, neurological and psychological evaluation (Minnesota Multiphasic Personality Inventory [MMPI], pain inventory, psychological interview), as indicated. **The pathophysiology of chronic pain is multifactorial. Some believe that response to it is a learned behavioral syndrome that begins with a noxious stimulus causing pain that is then somehow reinforced internally or externally.**
- Evaluate emotional components of individual situation. **Many painful conditions cause or exacerbate emotional responses (e.g., depression, withdrawal, agitation, anger) that worsen over time. Individuals with certain psycho logical syndromes (e.g., major depression, somatization disorder, hypochondriasis) may be prone to develop chronic pain syndrome.**
- Determine cultural factors for the individual situation. **Pain is perceived and expressed in different ways (e.g., moaning aloud or enduring in stoic silence); some may magnify symptoms to convince others of reality of pain.**
- Note gender and age of client. **There may be differences between how women and men perceive and/or respond to pain. Recent studies reveal large numbers of pediatric clients with chronic pain issues affecting academic attendance and function. While the prevalence of chronically**

Information that appears in brackets has been added by the authors to clarify and enhance the use of nursing diagnoses.

painful conditions (e.g., arthritis) and illnesses (e.g., cancers) is common in the elderly, they may be reluctant to report pain.

- Evaluate current and past analgesic, opioid, other drug use (including alcohol). **Provides clues to options to try or to avoid; identifies need for changes in medication regimen as well as possible need for detoxification program.**
- Make home visit when possible, observing such factors as safety equipment, adequate room, colors, plants, family interactions. Note impact of home environment on the client.

Nursing Priority No. 2.

To determine client response to chronic pain situation:

- Acknowledge and assess pain matter-of-factly, avoiding undue expressions of concern while conveying compassionate regard for client's feelings and situation of living with pain and coping with an often ill-defined disability.
- Evaluate pain behaviors. **May be exaggerated because client's perception of pain is not believed or because client believes caregivers are discounting reports of pain.**
- Determine individual client threshold for pain (physical examination, pain profile, etc.).
- Ascertain duration of pain problem, who has been consulted, and what drugs and therapies (including alternative and complementary) have been used **to determine that additional interventions might be beneficial or that current interventions should be discontinued (either not effective or no longer needed).**
- Note lifestyle effects of pain (e.g., decreased activity or deconditioning, severe fatigue, weight loss or gain, sleep difficulties, depression).
- Assess degree of personal maladjustment of the client, such as isolationism, anger, irritability, loss of work time or employment.
- Note codependent components, enabling behaviors of caregivers/family members **that support continuation of the status quo and may interfere with progress in pain management or resolution of situation.**
- Determine issues of secondary gain for the client/SO(s) (e.g., financial, marital, legal family concerns, work issues). **May interfere with progress in pain management and resolution of situation.**
- Note availability and use of personal and community resources. **Client/SO may need many things (e.g., equipment,**

Information that appears in brackets has been added by the authors to clarify and enhance the use of nursing diagnoses.

🌐 Cultural 🅒 Collaborative 🏠 Community/Home Care

financial resources, vocational training, respite services, or placement in rehabilitation facility) in order to manage painful conditions and/or concerns or difficulties associated with condition.

Nursing Priority No. 3.

To assist client to deal with pain:

- Review client pain management goals and expectations versus reality. **Pain may not be completely resolved, but may be significantly lessened to "acceptable level" or managed to the degree that client can participate in desired or needed life activities.**
- Apply pain management interventions, as appropriate (e.g., extended-relief oral pain medications and patches, nerve-blocking injection, implanted pump, electrical stimulation or transcutaneous electrical nerve stimulation unit) **to medically intervene, as indicated, in all aspects of long-term pain.**
- Encourage use of nonpharmacological methods of pain control (e.g., heat or cold applications, splinting or exercises, hydrotherapy, deep breathing, meditation, visualization, guided imagery, Therapeutic Touch [TT], posture correction and muscle-strengthening exercises, progressive muscle relaxation, biofeedback, massage).
- Assist client to learn breathing techniques (e.g., diaphragmatic breathing) **to assist in muscle and generalized relaxation.**
- Discuss the physiological dynamics of tension and anxiety and how these affect pain.
- Include client and SO(s) in establishing pattern of discussing pain for specified length of time **to limit focusing on pain.**
- Encourage client to use positive affirmations: "I am healing," "I am relaxed," "I love this life," etc. Have client be aware of internal-external dialogue, e.g., say "Cancel" when negative thoughts develop.
- Administer or encourage client use of analgesics, as indicated. **Medications may be available in pills, liquids, or suckers to take by mouth, and in injection, skin patch, and suppository form. Different medications or combinations of drugs may be used to manage persistent pain so that client may find relief and increase level of function.**
- Provide consistent and sufficient medication for pain relief, tailored to the individual, especially in one who tends to be undermedicated (e.g., elderly, cognitively impaired, person with lifelong pain, those with terminal cancer). **Medications may need to be scheduled around the clock, (not just**

Information that appears in brackets has been added by the authors to clarify and enhance the use of nursing diagnoses.

administered "as needed"), doses titrated either up or down, and dose maximized to optimize pain relief while managing side effects.

🖋️• Use tranquilizers, opioids, and analgesics sparingly where possible. **These drugs can be physically and psychologically addicting and promote sleep disturbances—especially interfering with deep REM sleep. Client may need to be detoxified if many medications are currently used.**

🖋️• Address medication misuse with client/SO and refer for appropriate counseling or interventions **when addiction is known or suspected to be interfering with client's well-being.**

• Encourage right-brain stimulation with activities such as love, laughter, and music **to release endorphins, enhancing sense of well-being.**

• Suggest use of subliminal tapes **to bypass logical part of the brain by saying "I am becoming a more relaxed person," "It is all right for me to relax," etc.**

• Assist family in developing a program of coping strategies (e.g., staying active even when modified activities are required, living a healthy lifestyle, implementing positive reinforcement for all persons, encouraging client to use own control, and diminishing attention given to pain behavior).

• Be alert to changes in pain **that may indicate a new physical problem or developing complications.**

Nursing Priority No. 4.
🏠 To promote wellness (Teaching/Discharge Considerations):

• Provide anticipatory guidance to client with condition in which pain is common and educate about when, where, and how to seek intervention or treatments.

• Assist client and SO(s) to learn how to heal by developing sense of internal control, by being responsible for own treatment, and by obtaining the information and tools to accomplish this.

∞• Discuss potential for developmental delays in child with chronic pain. Identify current level of function and review appropriate expectations for individual child.

🖋️• Review safe use of medications, management of minor side effects, and adverse effects requiring medical intervention.

• Assist client to learn to change pain behavior to wellness behavior: "Act as if you are well."

• Encourage and assist family member/SO(s) to learn home-care interventions. **Massage and other nonpharmacological**

Information that appears in brackets has been added by the authors to clarify and enhance the use of nursing diagnoses.

techniques benefit the client through reduction of pain level and sense that client is not alone/has support of SO.

🏠• Recommend that client and SO(s) take time for themselves. **Provides opportunity to reenergize and refocus on tasks at hand.**

💊• Identify and discuss potential hazards of unproved and/or nonmedical therapies and remedies.

⊕• Identify community support groups and other resources to meet individual needs (e.g., Back Pain Support Group, www.chronicpain.org; yard care, home maintenance, alternative transportation). **Proper use of resources may reduce negative pattern of "overdoing" heavy activities, then spending several days in bed recuperating.**

⊕• Refer for individual or other therapies (e.g., family counseling, marital therapy, parent effectiveness classes), as needed. **Presence of chronic pain affects all relationships and family dynamics.**

• Refer to NDs ineffective Coping; compromised family Coping.

Documentation Focus

Assessment/Reassessment
• Individual findings, including duration of problem, specific contributing factors, previously and currently used interventions.
• Perception of pain, effects on lifestyle, and expectations of therapeutic regimen.
• Family's/SO's response to client, and support for change.

Planning
• Plan of care and who is involved in planning.
• Teaching plan.

Implementation/Evaluation
• Responses to interventions, teaching, and actions performed.
• Attainment or progress toward desired outcome(s).
• Modifications to plan of care.

Discharge Planning
• Long-term needs and who is responsible for actions to be taken.
• Specific referrals made.

Information that appears in brackets has been added by the authors to clarify and enhance the use of nursing diagnoses.

Sample Nursing Outcomes & Interventions Classifications (NOC/NIC)

NOC—Pain Control
NIC—Pain Management

impaired **Parenting**

Taxonomy II: Role Relationships—Class 1 Caregiving
  Roles (00056)
[Diagnostic Division: Social Interaction]
Submitted 1998; Nursing Diagnosis Extension and Clas-
  sification Revision 1998

Definition: Inability of the primary caretaker to create,
maintain, or regain an environment that promotes the
optimum growth and development of the child

Related Factors

Infant or Child
Premature birth; multiple births; not desired gender
Illness; separation from parent
Difficult temperament; temperamental conflicts with parental
  expectations
Handicapping condition; developmental delay; altered percep-
  tual abilities; attention deficit hyperactivity disorder

Knowledge
Deficient knowledge about child development/health mainte-
  nance or parenting skills; inability to respond to infant cues
Unrealistic expectations (for self, infant, partner)
Lack of education; limited cognitive functioning; lack of cog-
  nitive readiness for parenthood
Poor communication skills
Preference for physical punishment

Physiological
Physical illness

Psychological
Young parental age
Lack of prenatal care; difficult birthing process; high number
  of/closely spaced pregnancies

Information that appears in brackets has been added by the authors to clarify
and enhance the use of nursing diagnoses.

● Cultural ② Collaborative 🏠 Community/Home Care

Disturbed sleep pattern; sleep deprivation; depression
History of mental illness or substance abuse
Disability

Social

Presence of stress (e.g., financial, legal, recent crisis, cultural move [from another country/cultural group within same country]); job problems; unemployment; financial difficulties; relocations; poor home environment
Situational or chronic low self-esteem
Lack of family cohesiveness; marital conflict; change in family unit; inadequate childcare arrangements
Role strain; single parent; father or mother of child not involved
Lack of or poor parental role model; lack of valuing of parenthood; inability to put child's needs before own
Unplanned or unwanted pregnancy
Economically disadvantaged; lack of resources; lack of transportation
Poor problem-solving skills; maladaptive coping strategies
Lack of social support networks; social isolation
History of being abusive or being abused; legal difficulties

Defining Characteristics

Subjective

Parental
Statements of inability to meet child's needs; reports inability to control child
Negative statements about child
Reports frustration or role inadequacy

Objective

Infant or Child
Frequent accidents or illness; failure to thrive
Poor academic performance or cognitive development
Poor social competence; behavioral disorders
Incidence of trauma (e.g., physical and psychological)/abuse
Lack of attachment or separation anxiety; runaway

Parental
Maternal-child interaction deficit; parental-child interaction deficit; little cuddling; inadequate attachment

---

Information that appears in brackets has been added by the authors to clarify and enhance the use of nursing diagnoses.

Inadequate child health maintenance; unsafe home environment; inappropriate childcare arrangements; inappropriate stimulation (e.g., visual, tactile, auditory)

Inappropriate caretaking skills; inconsistent care/behavior management

Inflexibility in meeting needs of child

Frequently punitive; rejection of or hostility to child; child abuse or neglect; abandonment

Desired Outcomes/Evaluation Criteria— Parents Will:

- Verbalize realistic information and expectations of parenting role.
- Verbalize acceptance of the individual situation.
- Participate in appropriate classes (e.g., parenting class).
- Identify own strengths, individual needs, and methods and resources to meet them.
- Demonstrate appropriate attachment and parenting behaviors.

Actions/Interventions

Nursing Priority No. 1.

To assess causative/contributing factors:

- Note family constellation; for example, two-parent, single, extended family, or child living with other relative, such as grandparent.
- Determine developmental stage of the family (e.g., new baby, adolescent, child leaving or returning home).
- Assess family relationships between individual members and with others.
- Assess parenting skill level, taking into account the individual's intellectual, emotional, and physical strengths and weaknesses. **Parents with significant impairments may need more education and support.**
- Observe attachment behaviors between parental figure and child. Determine cultural significance of behaviors. (Refer to ND risk for impaired Attachment.)
- Note presence of factors in the child (e.g., birth defects, hyperactivity) **that may affect attachment and caretaking needs.**
- Identify physical challenges or limitations of the parents (e.g., visual or hearing impairment, quadriplegia, severe depression). **May affect ability to care for child and suggest individual needs for assistance and support.**

Information that appears in brackets has been added by the authors to clarify and enhance the use of nursing diagnoses.

🌐 Cultural 😊 Collaborative 🏠 Community/Home Care

- Determine presence and effectiveness of support systems, role models, extended family, and community resources available to the parent(s).
- Note absence from home setting or lack of child supervision by parent (e.g., working long hours or out of town; multiple responsibilities, such as working and attending educational classes).

Nursing Priority No. 2.
To foster development of parenting skills:

- Create an environment in which relationships can be developed and needs of each individual met. **Learning is more effective when individuals feel safe.**
- Make time for listening to concerns of the parent(s).
- Emphasize positive aspects of the situation, maintaining a hopeful attitude toward the parent's capabilities and potential for improving the situation.
- Note staff attitudes toward parent/child and specific problem or disability; for example, needs of disabled parent(s) to be seen as an individual and to be evaluated apart from a stereotype. **Negative attitudes are detrimental to promoting positive outcomes.**
- Encourage expression of feelings, such as helplessness, anger, frustration. Set limits on unacceptable behaviors. **Individuals who lose control develop feelings of low self-esteem.**
- Acknowledge difficulty of situation and normalcy of feelings. **Enhances feelings of acceptance.**
- Recognize stages of grieving process when the child is disabled or other than anticipated (e.g., girl instead of boy, misshapen head, prominent birthmark). Allow time for parents to express feelings and deal with the "loss."
- Encourage attendance at skill classes (e.g., parent effectiveness). **Assists in improving parenting skills by developing communication and problem-solving techniques.**
- Emphasize parenting functions rather than mothering/fathering skills. **By virtue of gender, each person brings something to the parenting role; however, nurturing tasks can be done by both parents.**

Nursing Priority No. 3.
To promote wellness (Teaching/Discharge Considerations):

- Involve all available members of the family in learning.
- Provide information appropriate to the situation, including time management, limit setting, and stress-reduction techniques.

Information that appears in brackets has been added by the authors to clarify and enhance the use of nursing diagnoses.

Facilitates satisfactory implementation of plan and new behaviors.

- Discuss parental beliefs about childrearing, punishment and rewards, teaching. **Identifying these beliefs allows opportunity to provide new information regarding not using spanking and/or yelling and what actions can be substituted for more effective parenting.**
- Develop support systems appropriate to the situation (e.g., extended family, friends, social worker, home-care services).
- Assist parent to plan time and conserve energy in positive ways. **Enables individual to cope more effectively with difficulties as they arise.**
- Encourage parents to identify positive outlets for meeting their own needs (e.g., going out for dinner, making time for their own interests and each other, dating). **Promotes general well-being, helps parents to be more effective and reduces burnout.**
- Refer to appropriate support or therapy groups, as indicated.
- Identify community resources (e.g., childcare services, respite house) **to assist with individual needs, provide respite and support.**
- Report and take necessary actions, as legally and professionally indicated, if child's safety is a concern. **Parents/caregivers who engage in corporal punishment as a technique to ensure desired behavior of child are at increased risk for abusive behavior and possibility of childhood depression.**
- Refer to NDs ineffective Coping; compromised family Coping; risk for Violence [specify]; Self-Esteem [specify]; and interrupted Family Processes, for additional interventions as appropriate.

Documentation Focus

Assessment/Reassessment
- Individual findings, including parenting skill level, deviations from normal parenting expectations, family makeup, and developmental stages.
- Availability and use of support systems and community resources.

Planning
- Plan of care and who is involved in planning.
- Teaching plan.

Information that appears in brackets has been added by the authors to clarify and enhance the use of nursing diagnoses.

🌐 Cultural   🅒 Collaborative   🏠 Community/Home Care

Implementation/Evaluation

- Responses by parent(s)/child to interventions, teaching, and actions performed.
- Attainment or progress toward desired outcome(s).
- Modification to plan of care.

Discharge Planning

- Long-term needs and who is responsible for actions to be taken.
- Specific referrals made.

Sample Nursing Outcomes & Interventions Classifications (NOC/NIC)

NOC—Parenting Performance
NIC—Parenting Promotion

readiness for enhanced Parenting

Taxonomy II: Role Relationships—Class 1 Caregiving Roles (00164)
[Diagnostic Division: Social Interaction]
Submitted 2002

Definition: A pattern of providing an environment for children or other dependent person(s) that is sufficient to nurture growth and development, and can be strengthened

Defining Characteristics

Subjective

Expresses willingness to enhance parenting
Children report or other dependent person(s) express(es) satisfaction with home environment

Objective

Emotional support of children or dependent person(s); evidence of attachment
Needs of children or dependent person(s) is/are met (e.g., physical and emotional)
Exhibits realistic expectations of children or dependent person(s)

Information that appears in brackets has been added by the authors to clarify and enhance the use of nursing diagnoses.

Desired Outcomes/Evaluation Criteria— Parents Will:

- Verbalize realistic information and expectations of parenting role.
- Identify own strengths, individual needs, and methods and resources to meet them.
- Participate in activities to enhance parenting skills.
- Demonstrate improved parenting behaviors.

Actions/Interventions

Nursing Priority No. 1.
To determine need/motivation for improvement:

- Ascertain motivation and expectation for change.
- Note family constellation: two-parent; single parent; extended family; child living with other relative, such as grandparent; or relationship of dependent person. **Understanding makeup of the family provides information about needs to assist individuals in improving their family connections.**
- Determine developmental stage of the family (e.g., new child, adolescent, child leaving/returning home, retirement). **These maturational crises bring changes in the family, which can provide opportunity for enhancing parenting skills and improving family interactions.**
- Assess family relationships and identify needs of individual members, noting any special concerns that exist, such as birth defects, illness, hyperactivity. **The family is a system, and when members make decisions to improve parenting skills, the changes affect all parts of the system. Identifying needs, special situations, and relationships can help in the development of a plan to bring about effective change.**
- Assess parenting skill level, taking into account the individual's intellectual, emotional, and physical strengths and weaknesses. **Identifies areas of need for education, skill training, and information on which to base plan for enhancing parenting skills.**
- Observe attachment behaviors between parent(s) and child(ren), recognizing cultural backgrounds that may influence expected behaviors. **Behaviors such as eye-to-eye contact, use of en face position, talking to infant in high-pitched voice, are indicative of attachment behaviors in American culture, but may not be appropriate in another**

Information that appears in brackets has been added by the authors to clarify and enhance the use of nursing diagnoses.

Cultural   Collaborative   Community/Home Care

culture. **Failure to bond is thought to affect subsequent parent-child interactions.**

• Determine presence and effectiveness of support systems, role models, extended family, and community resources available to the parent(s). **Parents desiring to enhance abilities and improve family life can benefit by role models that help them develop their own style of parenting.**

• Note cultural or religious influences on parenting, expectations of self and child, sense of success or failure. **Expectations may vary with different cultures (e.g., Arab Americans hold children to be sacred, but childrearing is based on negative rather than positive reinforcements and parents are more strict with girls than with boys). These beliefs may interfere with desire to improve parenting skills when there is conflict between the two.**

Nursing Priority No. 2.

To foster improvement of parenting skills:

• Create an environment in which relationships can be strengthened. **A safe environment in which individuals can freely express their thoughts and feelings optimizes learning and positive interactions among family members, thus enhancing relationships.**

• Make time for listening to concerns of the parent(s). **Promotes sense of importance and of being heard and identifies accurate information regarding needs of the family for enhancing relationships.**

• Encourage expression of feelings, such as frustration or anger, while setting limits on unacceptable behaviors. **Identification of feelings promotes understanding of self and enhances connections with others in the family. Unacceptable behaviors result in diminished self-esteem and can lead to problems in the family relationships.**

• Emphasize parenting functions rather than mothering/fathering skills. **By virtue of gender, each person brings something to the parenting role; however, nurturing tasks can be done by both parents, enhancing family relationships.**

• Encourage attendance at skill classes, such as Parent or Family Effectiveness Training. **Assists in developing communication skills of Active-listening, I-messages, and problem-solving techniques to improve family relationships and promote a win-win environment.**

Information that appears in brackets has been added by the authors to clarify and enhance the use of nursing diagnoses.

Nursing Priority No. 3.

🏠 To promote optimal wellness:

* Involve all members of the family in learning. **The family system benefits from all members participating in learning new skills to enhance family relationships.**
* Encourage parents to identify positive outlets for meeting their own needs. **Activities, such as going out for dinner or dating, making time for their own interests and each other, promote general well-being and can enhance family relationships and improve family functioning.**
* Provide information, as indicated, including time management, stress-reduction techniques. **Learning about positive parenting skills, understanding growth and developmental expectations, and discovering ways to reduce stress and anxiety promote the individual's ability to deal with problems that may arise in the course of family relationships.**
* Discuss current "family rules," identifying areas of needed change. **Rules may be imposed by adults, rather than through a democratic process involving all family members, leading to conflict and angry confrontations. Setting positive family rules with all family members participating can promote an effective, functional family.**
* Discuss need for long-term planning and ways in which family can maintain desired positive relationships. **Each stage of life brings its own challenges and understanding, and preparing for each stage enables family members to move through them in positive ways, promoting family unity and resolving inevitable conflicts with win-win solutions.**

Documentation Focus

Assessment/Reassessment

* Individual findings, including parenting skill level, parenting expectations, family makeup, and developmental stages.
* Availability and use of support systems and community resources.
* Motivation and expectations for change.

Planning

* Plan for enhancement, who is involved in planning.
* Teaching plan.

Information that appears in brackets has been added by the authors to clarify and enhance the use of nursing diagnoses.

🌐 Cultural 🅒 Collaborative 🏠 Community/Home Care

Implementation/Evaluation
- Family members' responses to interventions, teaching, and actions performed.
- Attainment or progress toward desired outcome(s).
- Modifications to plan.

Discharge Planning
- Long-term needs and who is responsible for actions to be taken.
- Modification to plan.

Sample Nursing Outcomes & Interventions Classifications (NOC/NIC)

NOC—Parenting Performance
NIC—Parent Education: Childrearing Family

risk for impaired **Parenting**

Taxonomy II: Role Relationships—Class 1 Caregiving Roles (00057)
[Diagnostic Division: Social Interaction]
Submitted 1978; Nursing Diagnosis Extension and Classification Revision 1998

Definition: At risk for inability of the primary caretaker to create, maintain, or regain an environment that promotes the optimum growth and development of the child

Risk Factors

Infant or Child
Altered perceptual abilities; attention deficit hyperactivity disorder
Difficult temperament; temperamental conflicts with parental expectation
Premature birth; multiple births; not desired gender
Handicapping condition; developmental delay
Illness; prolonged separation from parent

Knowledge
Unrealistic expectations of child; deficient knowledge about child development/health maintenance or parenting skills

---

Information that appears in brackets has been added by the authors to clarify and enhance the use of nursing diagnoses.

Low educational level; lack of cognitive readiness for parent-hood; low cognitive functioning

Poor communication skills

Inability to respond to infant cues

Preference for physical punishment

Physiological

Physical illness

Psychological

Young parental age

Closely spaced pregnancies; high number of pregnancies; difficult birthing process

Sleep disruption or deprivation

Depression; history of mental illness or substance abuse

Disability

Social

Stress; job problems; unemployment; financial difficulties; poor home environment; relocation

Situational or chronic low self-esteem

Lack of family cohesiveness; marital conflict; change in family unit; inadequate childcare arrangements

Role strain; single parent; father or mother of child not involved; parent-child separation

Poor or lack of parental role model; lack of valuing of parent-hood

Unplanned or unwanted pregnancy; late or lack of prenatal care

Economically disadvantaged; lack of resources or access to resources; lack of transportation

Poor problem-solving skills; maladaptive coping strategies

Lack of social support network; social isolation

History of being abused or being abusive; legal difficulties

> **NOTE:** A risk diagnosis is not evidenced by signs and symptoms, as the problem has not occurred; rather, nursing interventions are directed at prevention.

Desired Outcomes/Evaluation Criteria—Parents Will:

• Verbalize awareness of individual risk factors.
• Identify own strengths, individual needs, and methods and resources to meet them.

Information that appears in brackets has been added by the authors to clarify and enhance the use of nursing diagnoses.

- Demonstrate behavior and lifestyle changes to reduce potential for development of problem or reduce or eliminate effects of risk factors.
- Participate in activities, classes to promote growth.

Actions/Interventions

Refer to NDs impaired Parenting; risk for impaired Attachment for interventions and documentation focus.

Documentation Focus

Refer to NDs impaired Parenting; risk for impaired Attachment for interventions and documentation focus.

Sample Nursing Outcomes & Interventions Classifications (NOC/NIC)

NOC—Parenting Performance
NIC—Parenting Promotion

---

risk for Perioperative Positioning Injury

Taxonomy II: Safety/Protection—Class 2 Physical Injury (00087)
[Diagnostic Division: Safety]
Submitted 1994; Revised 2006

Definition: At risk for inadvertent anatomical and physical changes as a result of posture or equipment used during an invasive/surgical procedure

---

Risk Factors

Disorientation; sensory/perceptual disturbances due to anesthesia
Immobilization; muscle weakness; [preexisting musculoskeletal conditions]
Obesity; emaciation; edema

> **NOTE:** A risk diagnosis is not evidenced by signs and symptoms, as the problem has not occurred; rather, nursing interventions are directed at prevention.

Information that appears in brackets has been added by the authors to clarify and enhance the use of nursing diagnoses.

Desired Outcomes/Evaluation Criteria— Client Will:

- Be free of injury related to perioperative disorientation.
- Be free of untoward skin and tissue injury or changes lasting beyond 24 to 48 hours postprocedure.
- Report resolution of localized numbness, tingling, or changes in sensation related to positioning within 24 to 48 hours, as appropriate.

Actions/Interventions

Nursing Priority No. 1.
To identify individual risk factors/needs:

∞• Review client's history, noting age, weight and height, nutritional status, physical limitations or preexisting conditions (e.g., elderly person with arthritis; extremes of weight; diabetes or other conditions affecting peripheral vascular health; nutrition and hydration impairments). **Affects choice of perioperative positioning and affects skin and tissue integrity during surgery.**
- Evaluate and document client's preoperative reports of neurological, sensory, or motor deficits **for comparative baseline of perioperative and postoperative sensations.**
- Note anticipated length of procedure and customary position **to increase awareness of potential postoperative complications (e.g., supine position may cause low back pain and skin pressure at heels, elbows, and sacrum; lateral chest position can cause shoulder and neck pain, or eye and ear injury on the client's downside).**
- Assess the individual's responses to preoperative sedation/ medication, noting level of sedation and/or adverse effects (e.g., drop in blood pressure) and report to surgeon, as indicated.
- Evaluate environmental conditions and safety issues surrounding the sedated client (e.g., client holding area, side rails up on bed or cart, someone staying with or close observation of client).

Nursing Priority No. 2.
To position client to provide protection for anatomical structures and to prevent client injury:

- Stabilize and lock cart or bed in place; support client's body and limbs; use adequate number of personnel during transfer **to prevent shear and friction injuries.**

Information that appears in brackets has been added by the authors to clarify and enhance the use of nursing diagnoses.

· Cultural · Collaborative · Community/Home Care

- Place safety strap strategically to secure client for specific procedure **to prevent unintended movement.**
- Maintain body alignment as much as possible using pillows, padding, and safety straps **to reduce potential for neurovascular complications associated with compression, overstretching, or ischemia of nerve(s).**
- Apply and reposition padding of pressure points and bony prominences (e.g., arms, elbows, sacrum, ankles, heels) and neurovascular pressure points (e.g., breasts, knees) **to maintain position of safety, especially when repositioning client and/or table attachments.**
- Check peripheral pulses and skin color and temperature periodically **to monitor circulation.**
- Protect body from contact with metal parts of the operating table, **which could produce burns or electric shock injury.**
- Reposition slowly at transfer and in bed (especially halothane-anesthetized client) **to prevent severe drop in blood pressure, dizziness, or unsafe transfer.**
- Protect airway and facilitate respiratory effort following extubation.
- Determine specific position reflecting procedure guidelines (e.g., head of bed elevated following spinal anesthesia, turn to unoperated side following pneumonectomy).
- Identify potential hazards in the surgical suite and implement corrections, as appropriate.

Nursing Priority No. 3.

To promote wellness (Teaching/Discharge Considerations):

- Maintain equipment in good working order **to identify potential hazards in the surgical suite and implement corrections as appropriate.**
- Provide perioperative teaching relative to client safety issues, including not crossing legs during procedures performed under local or light anesthesia, postoperative needs and limitations, and signs/symptoms requiring medical evaluation.
- Inform client and postoperative caregivers of expected/transient reactions (such as low backache, localized numbness, and reddening or skin indentations, all of which should disappear in 24 hours).
- Assist with therapies and perform routine nursing actions, including skin care measures, application of elastic stockings, early mobilization **to enhance circulation and promote skin and tissue integrity.**

Information that appears in brackets has been added by the authors to clarify and enhance the use of nursing diagnoses.

- Encourage and assist with frequent range-of-motion exercises, especially when joint stiffness occurs.
- Refer to appropriate resources, as needed.

Documentation Focus

Assessment/Reassessment
- Findings, including individual risk factors for problems in the perioperative setting or need to modify routine activities or positions.
- Periodic evaluation of monitoring activities.

Planning
- Plan of care and who is involved in planning.
- Teaching plan.

Implementation/Evaluation
- Response to interventions and actions performed.
- Attainment or progress toward desired outcome(s).
- Modifications to plan of care.

Discharge Planning
- Long-term needs and who is responsible for actions to be taken.

Sample Nursing Outcomes & Interventions Classifications (NOC/NIC)

NOC—Risk Control
NIC—Positioning: Intraoperative

---

risk for Peripheral Neurovascular Dysfunction

Taxonomy II: Safety/Protection—Class 2 Physical Injury (00086)
[Diagnostic Division: Neurosensory]
Submitted 1992

Definition: At risk for disruption in circulation, sensation, or motion of an extremity

---

Information that appears in brackets has been added by the authors to clarify and enhance the use of nursing diagnoses.

⬥ Cultural   ✿ Collaborative   🏠 Community/Home Care

Risk Factors

Fractures; trauma; vascular obstruction

Mechanical compression (e.g., tourniquet, cane, cast, brace, dressing, restraint)

Orthopedic surgery; immobilization

Burns

NOTE: A risk diagnosis is not evidenced by signs and symptoms, as the problem has not occurred; rather, nursing interventions are directed at prevention.

Desired Outcomes/Evaluation Criteria— Client Will:

* Maintain function as evidenced by sensation and movement within normal range for the individual.
* Identify individual risk factors.
* Demonstrate and participate in behaviors and activities to prevent complications.
* Relate signs/symptoms that require medical reevaluation.

Actions/Interventions

Nursing Priority No. 1.

To determine significance/degree of potential for compromise:

* Assess for individual risk factors: (1) trauma to extremity(ies) that cause internal tissue damage (e.g., high-velocity and penetrating trauma); fractures (especially long-bone fractures) with hemorrhage, or external pressures from burn eschar; (2) immobility (e.g., long-term bedrest, tight dressings, splints, or casting); (3) presence of conditions affecting peripheral circulation, such as atherosclerosis, Raynaud's disease, or diabetes; (4) smoking, obesity, and sedentary lifestyle; and (5) presence of conditions affecting peripheral circulation, such as atherosclerosis, cardiovascular or cerebrovascular disease; diabetes, sickle cell disease, deep vein thrombosis (DVT), coagulation disorders or use of anticoagulants, **which potentiate risk of circulation insufficiency and occlusion.**
* Monitor for tissue bleeding and spread of hematoma formation, **which can compress blood vessels and raise compartment pressures.**

Information that appears in brackets has been added by the authors to clarify and enhance the use of nursing diagnoses.

- Note position and location of casts, braces, traction apparatus **to ascertain potential for pressure on tissues.**
- Review recent and current drug regimen, noting use of anti-coagulants and vasoactive agents.

Nursing Priority No. 2.

To prevent deterioration/maximize circulation of affected limb(s):

- Conduct a comprehensive upper or lower extremity assessment in at-risk client, including color, sensation, and functional ability. **Early detection of circulatory issues may prevent the onset or severity of functional impairments associated with arterial or venous disorders of the extremities.**
- Perform neurovascular assessment in person immobilized for any reason (e.g., surgery, diabetic neuropathy, fractures) or individuals with suspected neurovascular problems. **Provides baseline for future comparisons.**
- Evaluate for differences between affected extremity and un-affected extremity, noting pain, pulses, pallor, paresthesia, paralysis, changes in motor and sensory function.
- Ask client to localize pain or discomfort and to report numbness and tingling or presence of pain with exercise or rest (atherosclerotic changes). (Refer to ND ineffective peripheral Tissue Perfusion, as appropriate.)
- Monitor presence and quality of peripheral pulse distal to injury or impairment via palpation or Doppler. **Intact pulse usually indicates adequate circulation. Occasionally, a pulse may be palpated even though circulation is blocked by a soft clot through which pulsations may be felt; or perfusion through larger arteries may continue after increased compartment pressure has collapsed the arteriole/venule circulation in the muscle.**
- Assess capillary return, skin color, and warmth in the limb(s) at risk and compare with unaffected extremities.
- Test sensation of peroneal nerve by pinch or pinprick in the dorsal web between first and second toe, and assess ability to dorsiflex toes if indicated (e.g., presence of leg fracture). **Changes in sensation cover a wide continuum and may include feeling of tingling, numbness, "pins and needles," burning, or diminished or absent sensation. Changes that might not be apparent to client could include loss of protective sensation in feet as determined by screening with tuning fork or percussion hammer.**

Information that appears in brackets has been added by the authors to clarify and enhance the use of nursing diagnoses.

 Cultural   Collaborative   Community/Home Care

- Evaluate extremity range-of-motion. **Movement may be limited or absent because of tissue edema and nerve compression or because of nerve impingement such as would occur with spinal nerve compression.**
- Monitor for tissue edema and/or tightness. **Swelling or tightness may indicate obstruction, such as might occur with DVT, or compartment syndrome.**
- Collaborate in interventions to minimize edema formation and elevated tissue pressure:

  Maintain elevation of injured extremity(ies).

  Apply cold packs around injury/fracture site as indicated.

  Remove jewelry from affected limb.

  Avoid or limit use of restraints. Pad limb and evaluate status frequently if restraints are required.

  Observe position and location of supporting ring of orthopedic splints or sling. Readjust, as indicated.
- Maximize circulation:

  Use techniques such as repositioning and padding **to relieve pressure.**

  Encourage client to routinely exercise digits or joints distal to injury.

  Encourage ambulation as soon as possible.

  Apply antiembolic hose or sequential pressure device, as indicated.

  Administer intravenous fluids, blood products, as needed, **to maintain circulating volume and tissue perfusion.**

  Administer anticoagulants or antithrombic agents, as indicated, **to prevent DVT or treat thrombotic vascular obstructions.**

  Split or bivalve cast, or reposition traction or restraints, as appropriate, **to quickly release pressure.**

  Prepare for surgical intervention (e.g., fibulectomy, fasciotomy), as indicated, **to relieve pressure and restore circulation.**
- Monitor for development of complications:

  Inspect tissues around cast edges for rough places, and pressure points. Investigate reports of "burning sensation" under cast.

  Evaluate for tenderness, swelling, pain on dorsiflexion of foot (positive Homans' sign).

  Monitor hemaglobin/hematocrit, coagulation studies (e.g., prothrombin time).

  Investigate sudden signs of limb ischemia (e.g., decreased skin temperature, pallor, increased pain), reports of pain

---

Information that appears in brackets has been added by the authors to clarify and enhance the use of nursing diagnoses.

that are extreme for type of injury, increased pain on passive movement of extremity, development of paresthesia, muscle tension or tenderness with erythema, change in pulse quality distal to injury. Place limb in neutral position, avoiding elevation. Report symptoms to physician at once **to provide for timely intervention/limit severity of problem.**

⊛ Assist with measurements of intracompartmental pressures, as indicated. **Provides for early intervention and evaluates effectiveness of therapy.**

Nursing Priority No. 3.

🏠 To promote wellness (Teaching/Discharge Considerations):

- Review proper body alignment, elevation of limbs, as appropriate.
- Keep linens off affected extremity with bed cradle or cut-out box, as indicated.
- Discuss necessity of avoiding constrictive clothing, sharp angulation of legs or crossing legs.
- Demonstrate proper application of antiembolic hose.
- Review safe use of heat or cold therapy, as indicated.
- Instruct client/SO(s) to check shoes and socks for proper fit and/or wrinkles.
- Demonstrate and recommend continuation of exercises **to maintain function and circulation of limbs.**

Documentation Focus

Assessment/Reassessment

- Specific risk factors, nature of injury to limb.
- Assessment findings, including comparison of affected and unaffected limb, characteristics of pain in involved area.

Planning

- Plan of care and who is involved in the planning.
- Teaching plan.

Implementation/Evaluation

- Response to interventions, teaching, and actions performed.
- Attainment or progress toward desired outcome(s).
- Modification of plan of care.

Information that appears in brackets has been added by the authors to clarify and enhance the use of nursing diagnoses.

Discharge Planning
- Long-term needs, referrals made, and who is responsible for actions to be taken.
- Specific referrals made.

Sample Nursing Outcomes & Interventions Classifications (NOC/NIC)

NOC—Neurological Status: Peripheral
NIC—Peripheral Sensation Management

---

disturbed Personal Identity

Taxonomy II: Self-Perception—Class 1 Self-Concept (00121)
[Diagnostic Division: Ego Integrity]
Submitted 1978; Revised 2008

Definition: Inability to maintain an integrated and complete perception of self

---

Related Factors

Situational or chronic low self-esteem; dysfunctional family processes
Situational crises; stages of growth or development; social role change
Ingestion or inhalation of toxic chemicals; use of psychoactive pharmaceutical agents
Cultural discontinuity; discrimination; perceived prejudice
Manic states; multiple personality disorder; psychiatric disorders (e.g., psychoses, depression, dissociative disorder); organic brain syndromes
Cult indoctrination

Defining Characteristics

Subjective

Disturbed body image; delusional description of self
Reports fluctuating feelings about self; feelings of strangeness, emptiness
Uncertainty about goals, cultural, or ideological values (e.g., beliefs, religious and moral questions)

Information that appears in brackets has been added by the authors to clarify and enhance the use of nursing diagnoses.

Gender confusion

Unable to distinguish between inner and outer stimuli

Objective

Contradictory personal traits

Ineffective relationships

Ineffective coping or role performance

Desired Outcomes/Evaluation Criteria— Client Will:

* Acknowledge threat to personal identity.
* Integrate threat in a healthy, positive manner (e.g., states anxiety is reduced, makes plans for the future).
* Verbalize acceptance of changes that have occurred.
* State ability to identify and accept self (long-term outcome).

Actions/Interventions

Nursing Priority No. 1.

To assess causative/contributing factors:

* Ascertain client's perception of the extent of the threat to self and how client is handling the situation.
* Determine speed of occurrence of threat. **An event that has happened quickly may be more threatening (e.g., a traumatic event resulting in change in body image).**
* Have client define own body image. **Body image is the basis of personal identity, and client's perception will affect how changes are viewed, may prevent achievement of ideals and expectations, and have a negative effect.**
* Identify physical signs of panic state such as palpitations, diaphoresis, trembling, chest or abdominal pain, nausea. (Refer to ND Anxiety.)
∞• Note age of client. **An adolescent may struggle with the developmental task of personal or sexual identity, whereas an older person may have more difficulty accepting or dealing with a threat to identity, such as progressive loss of memory.**
* Assess availability and use of support systems. Note response of family/SO(s).
∞• Note withdrawn or automatic behavior, regression to earlier developmental stage, general behavioral disorganization, or display of self-mutilation behaviors in adolescent or adult;

Information that appears in brackets has been added by the authors to clarify and enhance the use of nursing diagnoses.

🌐 Cultural ✪ Collaborative 🏠 Community/Home Care

delayed development, preference for solitary play, unusual display of self-stimulation in child.
- Determine presence of hallucinations, delusions, distortions of reality.

Nursing Priority No. 2.
To assist client to manage/deal with threat:
- Make time to listen/Active-listen client, encouraging appropriate expression of feelings, including anger and hostility.
- Provide calm environment. **Helps client to remain calm and able to discuss important issues related to the identity crisis.**
- Use crisis intervention principles **to restore equilibrium when possible.**
- Discuss client's commitment to an identity. **Those who have made a strong commitment to an identity tend to be more comfortable with self and happier than those who have not.**
- Assist client to develop strategies to cope with threat to identity. **Helps reduce anxiety and promotes self-awareness and self-esteem.**
- Engage client in activities to help in identifying self as an individual (e.g., use of mirror for visual feedback, tactile stimulation).
- Provide for simple decisions, concrete tasks, calming activities.
- Allow client to deal with situation in small steps. **May be unable to cope with larger picture when in stress overload.**
- Encourage client to develop and participate in an individualized exercise program (walking is an excellent beginning).
- Provide concrete assistance, as needed (e.g., help with activities of daily living, preparing food).
- Take advantage of opportunities to promote growth. Realize that client will have difficulty learning while in a dissociative state.
- Maintain reality orientation without confronting client's irrational beliefs. **Client may become defensive, blocking opportunity to look at other possibilities.**
- Use humor judiciously, when appropriate.
- Discuss options for dealing with issues of sexual gender (e.g., therapy, gender-change surgery when client is a transsexual).
- Refer to NDs disturbed Body Image; Self-Esteem [specify]; Spiritual Distress.

Information that appears in brackets has been added by the authors to clarify and enhance the use of nursing diagnoses.

Nursing Priority No. 3.

🏠 To promote wellness (Teaching/Discharge Considerations):

* Provide accurate information about threat to and potential consequences for individual. **Helps client to make positive decisions for future.**
* Assist client and SO(s) to acknowledge and integrate threat into future planning (e.g., wearing ID bracelet when prone to mental confusion; change of lifestyle to accommodate change of gender for transsexual client).
* Refer to appropriate support groups (e.g., day-care program, counseling/psychotherapy, gender identity).

Documentation Focus

Assessment/Reassessment

* Findings, noting degree of impairment.
* Nature of and client's perception of the threat.
* Degree of commitment to own identity.

Planning

* Plan of care and who is involved in the planning.
* Teaching plan.

Implementation/Evaluation

* Client's response to interventions/teaching and actions performed.
* Attainment or progress toward desired outcome(s).
* Modifications to plan of care.

Discharge Planning

* Long-term needs and who is responsible for actions to be taken.
* Specific referrals made.

Sample Nursing Outcomes & Interventions Classifications (NOC/NIC)

NOC—Identity
NIC—Self-Esteem Enhancement

Information that appears in brackets has been added by the authors to clarify and enhance the use of nursing diagnoses.

risk for disturbed Personal Identity

Taxonomy II: Self-Perception—Class 1 Self-Concept
  (00225)
[Diagnostic Division: Ego Identity]
Submitted 2010

Definition: Risk for the inability to maintain an integrated
and complete perception of self

Risk Factors

Situational/chronic low self-esteem; dysfunctional family processes

Situational crises; stages of development/growth; social role
change

Ingestion/inhalation of toxic chemicals; use of psychoactive
pharmaceutical agents

Cultural discontinuity; discrimination; perceived prejudice

Manic states; multiple personality disorder; psychiatric disorders (e.g., psychoses, depression, dissociative disorder); organic brain syndromes

Cult indoctrination

NOTE: A risk diagnosis is not evidenced by signs and
symptoms as the problem has not occurred; rather,
nursing actions are directed at prevention.

Desired Outcomes/Evaluation Criteria—
Client Will:

• Acknowledge concern about potential threat to identity.
• Exhibit reality-based thinking with appropriate thought con-
tent.
• Integrate perceived threat in a healthy manner (e.g., accepts
self in current situation, looks to the future).
• Use effective coping strategies to deal with situation/stressors.

Nursing Priority No. 1.

To assess risk/contributing factors:

• Ascertain client's perception of threat to self and how it is
being dealt with.

Information that appears in brackets has been added by the authors to clarify
and enhance the use of nursing diagnoses.

- Have client define own body image. **The basis of personal identity is body image, and perception of changes may affect client's view in a negative or positive manner.**
- Determine whether issues of gender identity are a concern. **Client may have conflicting feelings about how to deal with realization they are homosexual or transsexual.**
- ∞• Note age of individual. **Changes affect persons differently depending on their stage of life.**
- ⊕• Identify cultural affiliations/discontinuity. **Individuals belonging to subcultures or cults tend to come into conflict with the greater societal views, affecting one's perception of self and perception of reality.**
- Determine type and speed of changes that are imminent. **The diagnosis of a chronic illness versus a terminal illness, or a traumatic injury or disfiguring surgery that will change how life is lived, may be threatening as the thought of how different life will be affects the individual.**
- Note availability and use of support systems, including attitude of family/SOs.
- Assess behaviors such as withdrawal, general behavioral disorganization, delayed development. **Poor coping skills will affect how client deals with possibility of disturbance in personal identity.**
- 🔖• Discuss use of alcohol, other drugs. **Individuals often use these substances to avoid painful stressors.**
- Note signs of anxiety. **Use of inadequate coping strategies to deal with changes affecting lifestyle may result in exacerbation of symptoms in anxious person.** (Refer to ND Anxiety [specify level].)
- ✑• Determine distortions of reality/symptoms of mental illness. **Requires more in-depth psychological counseling/medication to help client distinguish between self and non-self.**

Nursing Priority No. 2.
To assist client to manage/deal with stressors:

- Listen/Active-listen, making time to encourage client to express feelings, including anger and hostility.
- Discuss client's concerns without confronting unreal ideas. **Irrational beliefs may interfere with ability to manage situation and maintain reality-based perception of self.**
- Encourage client and family to maintain a calm environment and positive attitude. **Anxiety is contagious and can inter-**

Information that appears in brackets has been added by the authors to clarify and enhance the use of nursing diagnoses.

fere with client's efforts to maintain control and deal with the situation.

- Help client to identify strategies to cope with current situation/possibility of threat.
- Use humor when appropriate. **Humor can be useful to help client look at reality of situation.**
- Provide activities applicable for client's situation. **For example, viewing body part for visual feedback or tactile stimulation to reconnect with affected parts of the body or participation in monitored social interactions helps client to confront fear and see self as an individual who is still worthwhile.**
- Support client in making decisions, plans for the future.
- Develop individualized exercise program. **Releases endorphins, reducing stress and promoting a sense of well-being.**
- Refer to NDs disturbed Body Image; Self-Esteem [specify]; Spiritual Distress, for additional interventions as appropriate.

Nursing Priority No. 3.

To promote wellness (Teaching/Discharge Considerations):

- Provide accurate information/resources for issues client is concerned about.
- Discuss potential changes in lifestyle that may occur with major diagnosis/accident. **Planning for these possibilities can enhance self-confidence and allow client to move forward with life.**
- Refer to appropriate support groups. **Sharing concerns with others in group settings may help client to be realistic regarding concerns about effects of anticipated changes/life challenges.**
- Explore community resources as appropriate. **Additional assistance such as day programs, individual/family counseling, drug/alcohol cessation programs can strengthen client's coping abilities and sense of control.**

Documentation Focus

Assessment/Reassessment

- Findings, noting concerns about possible changes in lifestyle, future expectations.
- Reality of potential threat.

Information that appears in brackets has been added by the authors to clarify and enhance the use of nursing diagnoses.

Planning
- Plan of care and who is involved in the planning.
- Teaching plan.

Implementation/Evaluation
- Client's response to interventions, teaching, and actions performed.

Discharge Planning
- Long-term needs, and who is responsible for actions to be taken.
- Specific referrals made.

Sample Nursing Outcomes & Interventions Classifications (NOC/NIC)

NOC—Identity
NIC—Self-Awareness Enhancement

---

risk for Poisoning

Taxonomy II: Safety/Protection—Class 4 Environmental Hazards (00037)
[Diagnostic Division: Safety]
Submitted 1980; Revised 2006

Definition: At risk of accidental exposure to, or ingestion of, drugs or dangerous products in sufficient doses that may compromise health

---

Risk Factors

Internal
Reduced vision

Deficient knowledge regarding pharmaceutical agents or poisoning prevention

Lack of proper precaution; [unsafe habits, disregard for safety measures, lack of supervision]

Reports occupational setting is without adequate safeguards

Cognitive or emotional difficulties; [chronic disease]

Cultural or religious beliefs or practices

Information that appears in brackets has been added by the authors to clarify and enhance the use of nursing diagnoses.

🌐 Cultural 🔵 Collaborative 🏠 Community/Home Care

External

Large supplies of pharmaceutical agents in house

Pharmaceutical agents stored in unlocked cabinets accessible to children or confused individuals

Availability of illicit drugs potentially contaminated by poisonous additives

Dangerous products placed within reach of children or confused individuals

[Narrow therapeutic margin of safety of specific pharmaceutical agents (e.g., therapeutic versus toxic level, half-life, method of uptake and degradation in body, adequacy of organ function)]

[Use of multiple herbal supplements or megadosing]

> **NOTE:** A risk diagnosis is not evidenced by signs and symptoms, as the problem has not occurred; rather, nursing interventions are directed at prevention.

Desired Outcomes/Evaluation Criteria— Client Will:

- Verbalize understanding of dangers of poisoning.
- Identify hazards that could lead to accidental poisoning.
- Correct external hazards as identified.
- Demonstrate necessary actions/lifestyle changes to promote safe environment.
- Refer to NDs Contamination; risk for Contamination, for additional interventions related to poisoning associated with environmental contaminants.

Actions/Interventions

Nursing Priority No. 1.

To assess causative/contributing factors:

- Identify internal and external risk factors in client's environment, including presence of infants, young children, or frail elderly **(who are at risk for accidental poisoning)** and teenagers or young adults **(who are at risk for medication experimentation);** confused or chronically ill person on multiple medications; person with potential for suicidal action; person who partakes in illicit drug use/

Information that appears in brackets has been added by the authors to clarify and enhance the use of nursing diagnoses.

dealing (e.g., marijuana, cocaine, heroin); person who manufactures drugs in home (e.g., methamphetamines).

• Note client's age, gender, socioeconomic status, developmental stage, decision-making ability, level of cognition and competence. **Affects client's ability to protect self/others and influences choice of interventions/teaching.**

• Assess mood, coping abilities, personality styles (e.g., temperament, impulsive behavior, level of self-esteem) **that may result in carelessness/increased risk taking without consideration of consequences.**

• Assess client's knowledge of safe use of drugs/herbal supplements, safety hazards in the environment, and ability to respond to potential threat. **People may believe "if a little is good, a lot is better," placing them at risk for overdose, adverse drug effects, or interactions. Knowledge and use also affects the client's storage (e.g., may not use labeled bottles) and/ or taking of medications that look alike (potentiating risk of overdose or adverse drug interactions). The elderly may unintentionally take the wrong medication at the wrong time or "double up," forgetting that they already took their daily dose of a prescription medicine.**

• Evaluate for alcohol/other drug use/abuse (e.g., cocaine, methamphetamine, lysergic acid diethylamide [LSD], methadone). **These substances have potential for adverse reactions, cumulative affects with other substances, and risk for intentional and accidental overdose.**

• Review results of laboratory tests and toxicology screening, as indicated.

• Identify environmental hazards:

Storage of household chemicals (e.g., oven, toilet bowl, or drain cleaners; dishwasher products; bleach; hydrogen peroxide; fluoride preparations; essential oils; furniture polish; lighter fluid; lamp oil; kerosene; paints; turpentine; rust remover; lubricant oils; bug sprays or powders; fertilizers). **These are all readily available toxins in various forms that are often improperly stored.**

Review client's home, employment, or work environment **for exposure to chemicals, including vapors and fumes.**

Refer to ND risk for Contamination for environmental issues.

Nursing Priority No. 2.
To assist in correcting factors that can lead to accidental poisoning:

Information that appears in brackets has been added by the authors to clarify and enhance the use of nursing diagnoses.

⬤ Cultural   ◯ Collaborative   🏠 Community/Home Care

🏠 • Discuss medication safety with client/SO(s) **to prevent accidental ingestion.**

∞ Stress importance of supervising infant, child, frail elderly, or individuals with cognitive limitations.

∞ Keep medicines and vitamins out of sight or reach of children or cognitively impaired persons.

∞ Use child-resistant or tamper-resistant caps and lock medication cabinets.

💊 Recap medication containers immediately after obtaining current dosage. Do not leave open container out.

💊 Code medicines for the visually impaired.

∞ Administer children's medications as drugs, not candy.

• Prevent duplication or possible overdose:

💊 Keep updated list of all medications (prescription, over the counter [OTC], herbals, supplements) and review with healthcare providers when medications are changed, new ones added, or new healthcare providers are consulted.

💊 Keep prescription medication in original bottle with label. Do not mix with other medication/place in unmarked containers.

∞ Have responsible SO(s)/home health nurse supervise medi-
💊 cation regimen/prepare medications for the cognitively or visually impaired or obtain prefilled medication box from pharmacy.

💊 Take prescription medications, as prescribed on label.

💊 Do not adjust medication dosage.

💊 Retain and read safety information that accompanies prescriptions about expected effects, minor side effects, reportable or adverse affects that require medical intervention, and how to manage forgotten dose.

💊 • Prevent taking medications that interact with one another or OTC, herbals, or other supplements in an undesired or dangerous manner.

💊 Keep list of and reveal medication allergies, including type of reaction, to healthcare providers/pharmacist.

💊 Wear medical alert bracelet or necklace, as appropriate.

💊 Do not take outdated or expired medications. Do not save partial prescriptions to use another time.

💊 Encourage discarding outdated or unused drug safely (disposing in hazardous waste collection areas, not down drain or toilet).

💊 Do not take medications prescribed for another person.

⊕ Coordinate care when multiple healthcare providers are involved to limit number of prescriptions and dosage levels.

Information that appears in brackets has been added by the authors to clarify and enhance the use of nursing diagnoses.

Nursing Priority No. 3.

🏠 To promote wellness (Teaching/Discharge Considerations):

- Discuss general poison prevention measures:
- ∞• Encourage parent/caregiver to place safety stickers on dangerous products (drugs and chemicals) **to warn children of harmful contents.**
- ∞• Teach children about hazards of poisonous substances and to "ask first" before eating or drinking anything.
- 🥄• Review drug side effects, potential interactions, and possibilities of misuse or overdosing (as with vitamin megadosing, etc.).
- ∞• Discuss issues regarding drug use in home (e.g., alcohol, marijuana, heroin) **to provide opportunity to address potential for client's/SO's accidental overdose or accidental ingestion by children when drugs or drug paraphernalia are in the home.**
- 🌐• Refer substance abuser to detoxification programs, inpatient/outpatient rehabilitation, counseling, support groups, psychotherapy.
- 🌐• Provide list of emergency numbers (i.e., local or national poison control numbers, physician's office) to be placed by telephone **for use if poisoning occurs.**
- 🧪• Encourage client to obtain regular screening tests at prescribed intervals (e.g., prothrombin time/international normalized ratio [INR] for Coumadin; drug levels for Dilantin, digoxin; liver function studies when lipid-lowering agents [statins] are prescribed; or renal and thyroid function and serum glucose levels for antimanics [lithium] use) **to ascertain that circulating blood levels are within therapeutic range and absence of adverse effects.**
- Encourage participation in community awareness and education programs (e.g., CPR and First Aid class, home and workplace safety, hazardous materials disposal, access to emergency medical personnel) **to assist individuals to identify and correct risk factors in environment and be prepared for emergency situation.**
- 🥄• Discuss vitamins (especially those containing iron) that can be poisonous or lethal to children.
- 🥄• Review common analgesic safety (e.g., acetaminophen is an ingredient in many OTC medications, and unintentional overdose can occur).
- 🥄• Discuss use of ipecac syrup in home. **The use of ipecac is controversial, as it may delay appropriate medical treatment (e.g., reduce the effectiveness of activated charcoal**

Information that appears in brackets has been added by the authors to clarify and enhance the use of nursing diagnoses.

🌐 Cultural 🌐 Collaborative 🏠 Community/Home Care

or oral antidotes) or be used inappropriately with adverse effects. Therefore, use in the home without direct advice from poison control professionals is not recommended.

- Encourage emergency measures, awareness, and education (e.g., CPR/First Aid class, community safety programs, ways to access emergency medical personnel) **to assist individuals to identify and correct risk factors in environment and be prepared for emergency situation.**

Documentation Focus

Assessment/Reassessment
- Identified risk factors noting internal and external concerns.
- Drug allergies or sensitivities.
- Current medications prescribed or available to individual, use of OTC medications, herbals or supplements, illicit drug use.

Planning
- Plan of care and who is involved in the planning.
- Teaching plan.

Implementation/Evaluation
- Response to interventions, teaching, and actions performed.
- Attainment or progress toward desired outcome(s).
- Modification to plan of care.

Discharge Planning
- Long-term needs and who is responsible for actions to be taken.
- Specific referrals made.

Sample Nursing Outcomes & Interventions Classifications (NOC/NIC)

NOC—Knowledge: Medication
NIC—Medication Management

Information that appears in brackets has been added by the authors to clarify and enhance the use of nursing diagnoses.

Post-Trauma Syndrome [specify stage]

Taxonomy II: Coping/Stress Tolerance—Class 1 Post-Trauma Responses (00141)
[Diagnostic Division: Ego Integrity]
Submitted 1986; Nursing Diagnosis Extension and Classification Revision 1998, 2010

Definition: Sustained maladaptive response to a traumatic, overwhelming event

Related Factors

Events outside the range of usual human experience
Serious threat to self or loved ones
Serious injury to self or loved ones; serious accidents (e.g., industrial, motor vehicle)
Physical or psychological abuse; criminal victimization
Witnessing mutilation or violent death; tragic occurrence involving multiple deaths
Disasters; sudden destruction of one's home or community; epidemics
War; being held prisoner of war; torture

Defining Characteristics

Subjective

Intrusive thoughts or dreams; nightmares; flashbacks; [excessive verbalization of the traumatic event]
Palpitations; headaches; [loss of interest in usual activities, loss of feeling of intimacy or sexuality]
Hopelessness; shame; guilt; [verbalization of survival guilt or guilt about behavior required for survival]
Anxiety; fear; grieving; depression; horror
Reports feeling numb
Gastric irritability; [change in appetite/sleep; easy fatigability]
Difficulty in concentrating

Objective

Hypervigilance; exaggerated startle response; irritability; neurosensory irritability
Anger; rage; aggression
Avoidance; repression; alienation; denial; detachment; psychogenic amnesia

---

Information that appears in brackets has been added by the authors to clarify and enhance the use of nursing diagnoses.

🌐 Cultural   😊 Collaborative   🏠 Community/Home Care

Altered mood states; [poor impulse control/explosiveness]; panic attacks

Substance abuse; compulsive behavior

Enuresis (in children)

[Difficulty with interpersonal relationships; dependence on others; work or school failure]

[Stages:

ACUTE: Begins within 6 months and does not last longer than 6 months.

CHRONIC: Lasts more than 6 months.

DELAYED ONSET: Period of latency of 6 months or more before onset of symptoms.]

Desired Outcomes/Evaluation Criteria— Client Will:

- Express own feelings or reactions, avoiding projection.
- Verbalize a positive self-image.
- Report reduced anxiety or fear when memories occur.
- Demonstrate ability to deal with emotional reactions in an individually appropriate manner.
- Demonstrate appropriate changes in behavior and lifestyle (e.g., share experiences with others, seek or get support from SO[s] as needed, change in job or residence).
- Report absence of physical manifestations (e.g., pain, chronic fatigue).

Actions/Interventions

Nursing Priority No. 1.

To assess causative factor(s) and individual reaction:

Acute

- Note occupation (e.g., police, fire, rescue, emergency department staff; corrections officer; mental health worker; disaster responders; soldier or support personnel in combat zone; as well as family members). **These occupations carry a high risk for constantly being involved in traumatic events and the potential for exacerbation of stress response and block to recovery.**
- Observe for and elicit information about physical or psychological injury and note associated stress-related symptoms (e.g., "numbness," headache, tightness in chest, nausea, pounding heart). **Anxiety is viewed as a normal reaction to a realistic danger or threat, and noting these factors can**

Information that appears in brackets has been added by the authors to clarify and enhance the use of nursing diagnoses.

identify the severity of the anxiety the client is experiencing in the circumstances. In post-traumatic stress disorder (PTSD), this anxiety reaction is changed or damaged.

- Identify psychological responses: anger, shock, acute anxiety, confusion, denial. Note laughter, crying, calm or agitated or excited (hysterical) behavior, expressions of disbelief, guilt or self-blame, labile emotions. **Indicators of severe response to trauma that client has experienced and need for specific interventions.**

- Assess client's knowledge of and anxiety related to the situation. Note ongoing threat to self (e.g., contact with perpetrator and/or associates).

- Identify social aspects of trauma or incident (e.g., disfigurement, chronic conditions or permanent disabilities, loss of home or community).

- Ascertain ethnic background and cultural or religious perceptions and beliefs about the occurrence. **Client (or significant others) may believe occurrence is retribution from God or result of some indiscretion on client's part. Individual's perception of event is influenced by cultural and community background, religious beliefs, and family influence.**

- Determine degree of disorganization (e.g., task-oriented activity is not goal directed, organized, or effective; individual is overwhelmed by emotion most of the time).

- Identify whether incident has reactivated preexisting or coexisting situations (physical or psychological). **Affects how the client views the current trauma.**

- Determine disruptions in relationships (e.g., family, friends, coworkers, SOs). **Support persons may not know how to deal with client/situation (e.g., may be oversolicitous or withdraw).**

- Note withdrawn behavior, use of denial, and use of chemical substances or impulsive behaviors (e.g., chain smoking, overeating).

- Be aware of signs of increasing anxiety (e.g., silence, stuttering, inability to sit still). **Increasing anxiety may indicate risk for violence.**

- Note verbal and nonverbal expressions of guilt or self-blame when client has survived trauma in which others died. Validate congruency of observations with verbalizations.

- Assess signs and stage of grieving for self and others.

- Identify development of phobic reactions to ordinary articles (e.g., knives); situations (e.g., walking in groups of people,

---

Information that appears in brackets has been added by the authors to clarify and enhance the use of nursing diagnoses.

🌐 Cultural　🤝 Collaborative　🏠 Community/Home Care

strangers ringing doorbell). **These may trigger feelings from original trauma and need to be dealt with sensitively, accepting reality of feelings and stressing ability of client to deal with them.**

Chronic (In Addition to Above)

- Evaluate continued somatic complaints (e.g., gastric irritation, anorexia, insomnia, muscle tension, headache). Investigate reports of new or changes in symptoms.
- Note manifestations of chronic pain or pain symptoms in excess of degree of physical injury. **Psychological responses may magnify or exacerbate physical symptoms, indicating need for interventions to help client deal with pain.**
- Be aware of signs of severe or prolonged depression. Note presence of flashbacks, intrusive memories, nightmares; panic attacks; poor impulse control; problems with memory or concentration, thoughts, and perceptions; conflict, aggression, or rage.
- Assess degree of dysfunctional coping (e.g., use or abuse of alcohol or other drugs; suicidal or homicidal ideation) and consequences. **Individuals display different levels of dysfunctional behavior in response to stress, and often the choice of chemical substances or substance abuse is a way of deadening psychic pain.**

Nursing Priority No. 2.

To assist client to deal with situation that exists:

Acute

- Provide a calm, safe environment. **Promotes sense of trust and safety.**
- Assist with documentation for police report, as indicated, and stay with the client.
- Listen to and investigate physical complaints, and take note of lack of physical complaints when injury may have occurred. **Emotional reactions may limit client's ability to recognize or verbalize physical injury.**
- Identify supportive persons for the individual (e.g., loved ones, counselor, spiritual advisor or pastor).
- Remain with client, listen as client recounts incident or concerns—possibly repeatedly. (If client does not want to talk, accept silence.) **Provides psychological support.**
- Provide environment in which client can talk freely about feelings and fears (including concerns about relationship with

---

Information that appears in brackets has been added by the authors to clarify and enhance the use of nursing diagnoses.

and response of SO) and trauma experiences and sensations (e.g., loss of control, "near-death experience").

∞• Help child express feelings about event using techniques appropriate to developmental level (e.g., play for young child, stories or puppets for preschooler, peer group for adolescent). **Children are more likely to express in play what they may not be able to verbalize directly. Adolescents may benefit from groups that help them gain knowledge, support, and a decreased sense of isolation.**

🏠• Assist in dealing with practical concerns and effects of the incident, such as court appearances, altered relationships with SO(s), employment problems. **In the period immediately following the traumatic incident, thinking becomes difficult, and assistance with practical matters will help manage necessary activities for the person to move through this time.**

• Be aware of and assist client to use ego strengths in a positive way by acknowledging ability to handle what is happening. **Enhances self-concept, supports self-esteem, and reduces sense of helplessness.**

• Allow client to work through own kind of adjustment. If the client is withdrawn or unwilling to talk, do not force the issue.

• Listen for expressions of fear of crowds and/or people.

💊• Administer anti-anxiety, sedative, or hypnotic medications with caution.

Chronic

• Continue listening to expressions of concern. **May have recurring thoughts, thus necessitating the need to continue talking about the incident.**

• Permit free expression of feelings (may continue from the crisis phase). Avoid rushing client through expressions of feelings too quickly and refrain from providing reassurance inappropriately. **Client may believe pain and/or anguish is misunderstood and may be depressed. Statements such as "You don't understand" or "You weren't there" are a defense, a way of pushing others away.**

• Encourage client to talk out experience when ready, expressing feelings of fear, anger, loss, or grief. (Refer to ND complicated Grieving.)

∞• Ascertain and monitor sleep pattern of children as well as adults. **Sleep disturbances and/or nightmares may develop, delaying resolution and/or impairing coping abilities.**

Information that appears in brackets has been added by the authors to clarify and enhance the use of nursing diagnoses.

🌐 Cultural   🐾 Collaborative   🏠 Community/Home Care

- Encourage client to become aware of and accept own feelings and reactions as being normal reactions in an abnormal situation.
- Acknowledge reality of loss of self that existed before the incident. Help client to move toward a state of acceptance as to the potential for growth that still exists within client. **Recognition that individual can never go back to being the person he or she was before the incident allows progress toward life as a different person.**
- Continue to allow client to progress at own pace.
- Give "permission" to express and deal with anger at the assailant or situation in acceptable ways.
- Avoid prompting discussion of issues that cannot be resolved. Keep discussion on practical and emotional level rather than intellectualizing the experience, **which allows client to deal with reality while taking time to work out feelings.**
- Provide for sensitive, trained counselors/therapists and engage in therapies, such as psychotherapy, Implosive Therapy (flooding), hypnosis, relaxation, Rolfing, memory work, cognitive restructuring, Eye Movement Desensitization and Reprocessing (EMDR), physical and occupational therapies.
- Administer psychotropic medications, as indicated.

Nursing Priority No. 3.

To promote wellness (Teaching/Discharge Considerations):

- Assist client to identify and monitor feelings while therapy is occurring.
- Provide information about what reactions client may expect during each phase. Let client know these are common reactions. Be sure to phrase in neutral terms of "You may or you may not . . . ." **Helps reduce fear of the unknown**
- Assist client to identify factors that may have created a vulnerable situation and that he or she may have power to change **to protect self in the future.**
- Avoid making value judgments.
- Discuss lifestyle changes client is contemplating and how they may contribute to recovery. **Helps client evaluate appropriateness of plans and identify shortcomings (e.g., moving away from effective support group).**
- Assist client to learn stress-management techniques.
- Discuss drug regimen, potential side effects of prescribed medications, and necessity of prompt reporting of untoward effects.

Information that appears in brackets has been added by the authors to clarify and enhance the use of nursing diagnoses.

- Discuss recognition of, and ways to manage, "anniversary reactions," reinforcing normalcy of recurrence of thoughts and feelings at this time.
- Suggest support group for SO(s) **to assist with understanding and ways to deal with client.**
- Encourage psychiatric consultation, especially if client is unable to maintain control, is violent, is inconsolable, or does not seem to be making an adjustment.
- Refer for long-term individual/family/marital counseling, if indicated.
- Refer to NDs Powerlessness; ineffective Coping; Grieving; complicated Grieving.

Documentation Focus

Assessment/Reassessment
- Individual findings, noting current dysfunction and behavioral and emotional responses to the incident.
- Specifics of traumatic event.
- Reactions of family/SO(s).
- Availability and use of resources.

Planning
- Plan of care and who is involved in the planning.
- Teaching plan.

Implementation/Evaluation
- Responses to interventions, teaching, and actions performed.
- Emotional changes.
- Attainment or progress toward desired outcome(s).
- Modifications to plan of care.

Discharge Planning
- Long-term needs and who is responsible for actions to be taken.
- Specific referrals made.

Sample Nursing Outcomes & Interventions Classifications (NOC/NIC)

NOC—Comfort Status: Psychospiritual
NIC—Crisis Intervention

Information that appears in brackets has been added by the authors to clarify and enhance the use of nursing diagnoses.

risk for **Post-Trauma Syndrome**

Taxonomy II: Coping/Stress Tolerance—Class 1 Post-
Trauma Responses (00145)
[Diagnostic Division: Ego Integrity]
Submitted 1998

Definition: At risk for sustained maladaptive response to
a traumatic, overwhelming event

Risk Factors

Occupation (e.g., police, fire, rescue, corrections, emergency
room staff; mental health worker; and their family members)
Perception of event; exaggerated sense of responsibility; dimin-
ished ego strength
Survivor's role in the event
Inadequate social support; unsupportive environment; displace-
ment from home
Duration of the event

NOTE: A risk diagnosis is not evidenced by signs and
symptoms, as the problem has not occurred; rather,
nursing interventions are directed at prevention.

Desired Outcomes/Evaluation Criteria—
Client Will:

- Verbalize absence of severe anxiety.
- Demonstrate ability to deal with emotional reactions in an
  individually appropriate manner.
- Report relief or absence of physical manifestations (pain,
  nightmares or flashbacks, fatigue) associated with event.

Actions/Interventions

Nursing Priority No. 1.
To assess contributing factors and individual reaction:

- Identify client who survived or witnessed traumatic event
  (e.g., airplane or motor vehicle crash, mass shooting, fire de-
  stroying home and lands, robbery at gunpoint, other violent
  act) **to recognize individual at high risk for post-trauma
  syndrome.**

Information that appears in brackets has been added by the authors to clarify
and enhance the use of nursing diagnoses.

- Note occupation (e.g., police, fire, emergency services personnel or rescue workers; soldiers and support personnel in combat areas), as listed in Risk Factors. **Studies reveal a moderate to high percentage of post-traumatic stress disorders (PTSDs) develop in these populations when they have been exposed to one or more traumatic incidents.**
- Assess client risk for developing PTSD using a screening (e.g., Breslau Short Screening Scale, or similar) tool should client report experiencing a traumatic event. **Short self-report questionnaire or other screening tool with simple "yes" or "no" responses may help with early identification of client at risk for post-trauma response.**
- Ascertain ethnic background and cultural or religious perceptions and beliefs about the occurrence. **Individual's view of how he or she is coping may be influenced by cultural background, religious beliefs, and family influence.**
- Assess client's knowledge of and anxiety related to potential for work-related trauma (e.g., shooting in line of duty or viewing body of murdered child); and number, duration, and intensity of recurring situations (e.g., EMT personnel exposed to numerous on-the-job traumatic incidents; rescuers searching for victims of natural or man-made disasters).
- Identify how client's past experiences may affect current situation. **Individual who has had previous experiences with traumatic events may be more susceptible to PTSD and ineffective coping abilities.**
- Listen for comments of guilt, humiliation, shame, or taking on responsibility (e.g., "I should have been more careful/gone back to get her"; "Don't call me a hero, I couldn't save my partner"; "My kids are the same age as the ones that died").
- Evaluate for life factors or stressors currently or recently occurring, such as displacement from home due to catastrophic event (e.g., fire, flood, violent storm) happening to individual whose child is dying with cancer or who suffered abuse as a child. **This individual is at greater risk for developing traumatic symptoms (acute added to delayed-onset reactions).**
- Identify client's general health and coping mechanisms. **Resolution of the post-trauma response is largely dependent on the coping skills the client has developed throughout own life and is able to bring to bear on current situation.**
- Determine availability and effectiveness of client's support systems, family, social, community, and so forth. (*Note:* Family members can also be at risk.)

Information that appears in brackets has been added by the authors to clarify and enhance the use of nursing diagnoses.

Nursing Priority No. 2.

To assist client to deal with situation that exists:

- Provide a calm, safe environment **in which client can deal with disruption of life.**
- Identify and discuss client's strengths (e.g., very supportive family, usually copes well with stress) as well as vulnerabilities (e.g., client tends toward alcohol or other drugs for coping, client has witnessed a murder).
- Discuss how individual coping mechanisms have worked in past traumatic events. **Client/SO(s) may be able to employ previously successful strategies to deal with current incident.**
- Evaluate client's perceptions of events and personal significance (e.g., police officer—who is also a parent—investigating death of a child).
- Provide emotional and physical presence **to strengthen client's coping abilities.**
- Encourage expression of feelings and reinforce that feelings and reactions to trauma are common and not indicators of weakness or failure. Note whether feelings expressed appear congruent with events the client experienced. **Incongruency may indicate deeper conflict and can impede resolution.**
- Help child to express feelings about event using techniques appropriate to developmental level. **Children are more likely to express in play what they may not be able to verbalize directly. Adolescents may benefit from groups, gaining knowledge, support, decreased sense of isolation, and improved coping skills.**
- Observe for signs and symptoms of stress responses, such as nightmares, reliving an incident, poor appetite, irritability, numbness and crying, family or relationship disruption. **These responses are normal in the early postincident time frame. If prolonged and persistent, the client may be experiencing PTSD.**

Nursing Priority No. 3.

To promote wellness (Teaching/Discharge Considerations):

- Educate high-risk persons and families about signs/symptoms of post-trauma response, especially if it is likely to occur in their occupation/life.
- Encourage client to identify and monitor feelings on an ongoing basis. **Promotes awareness of changes in ability to deal with stressors.**

Information that appears in brackets has been added by the authors to clarify and enhance the use of nursing diagnoses.

- Identify and discuss client's strengths (e.g., very supportive family, usually copes well with stress) as well as vulnerabilities (e.g., client tends toward alcohol or other drugs for coping, client has witnessed a murder). **Knowing one's strengths and weaknesses helps client know what actions to take to cope with and prevent anxiety from becoming overwhelming.**
- Encourage learning stress-management techniques, such as deep breathing, meditation, relaxation, exercise. **Reduces stress, enhancing coping skills, and helping to resolve situation.**
- Recommend participation in debriefing sessions that may be provided following major events. **Dealing with the stressor promptly may facilitate recovery from event or prevent exacerbation, although issues about best timing of debriefing continue to be debated.**
- Explain that post-traumatic symptoms can emerge months or sometimes years after a traumatic experience and that help and support can be obtained when needed or desired if client begins to experience intrusive memories or other symptoms.
- Identify employment, community resource groups (e.g., Assistance Support and Self Help in Surviving Trauma [ASSIST], employee peer-assistance programs, Red Cross or other survivor support services, Compassionate Friends). **Provides opportunity for ongoing support to deal with recurrent stressors.**
- Refer for individual or family counseling, as indicated.

Documentation Focus

Assessment/Reassessment
- Identified risk factors noting internal and external concerns.
- Client's perception of event and personal significance.

Planning
- Plan of care and who is involved in the planning.
- Teaching plan.

Implementation/Evaluation
- Response to interventions, teaching, and actions performed.
- Attainment or progress toward desired outcome(s).

Discharge Planning
- Long-term needs and who is responsible for actions to be taken.
- Specific referrals made.

Information that appears in brackets has been added by the authors to clarify and enhance the use of nursing diagnoses.

Sample Nursing Outcomes & Interventions Classifications (NOC/NIC)

NOC—Comfort Status: Psychospiritual
NIC—Support System Enhancement

readiness for enhanced Power

Taxonomy II: Coping/Stress Tolerance—Class 2 Coping
    Responses (00187)
[Diagnostic Division: Ego Integrity]
Submitted 2006

Definition: A pattern of participating knowingly in
change that is sufficient for well-being and can be
strengthened

Defining Characteristics

Subjective

Expresses readiness to enhance power; knowledge for partici-
    pation in change; awareness of possible changes to be made;
    identification of choices that can be made for change

Expresses readiness to enhance freedom to perform actions for
    change; involvement in creating change; participation in
    choices for daily living and health

> **NOTE:** Even though power (a response) and
> empowerment (an intervention approach) are different
> concepts, the literature related to both concepts supports
> the defining characteristics of this diagnosis.

Desired Outcomes/Evaluation Criteria— Client Will:

- Verbalize knowledge of what changes he or she wants to
  make.
- Express awareness of own ability to be in charge of changes
  to be made.
- Participate in classes or group activities to learn new skills.
- State readiness to take power over own life.

Information that appears in brackets has been added by the authors to clarify
and enhance the use of nursing diagnoses.

Actions/Interventions

Nursing Priority No. 1.

To determine need/motivation for improvement:

- Determine current situation and circumstances that client is experiencing, leading to desire to improve life.
- Ascertain motivation and expectations for change.
- Identify emotional climate in which client and relationships live and work. **The emotional climate has a great impact between people. When a power differential exists in relationships, the atmosphere is largely determined by the person or people who have the power.**
- Identify client's locus of control: internal (expressions of responsibility for self and ability to control outcomes) or external (expressions of lack of control over self and environment). **Understanding locus of control can help client work toward positive, internal control as he or she develops ability to freely recognize and choose own actions.**
- Determine cultural factors/religious beliefs influencing client's self-view.
- Assess degree of mastery client has exhibited in his or her life. **Helps client understand how he or she has functioned in the past and what is needed to improve.**
- Note presence of family/SO(s) that can, or do, act as support systems for client.
- Determine whether client knows and/or uses assertiveness skills.

Nursing Priority No. 2.

To assist client to clarify needs relative to ability to improve feelings of power:

- Discuss needs and how client is meeting them at this time.
- Listen/Active-listen client's perceptions and beliefs about how power can be gained in his or her life.
- Identify strengths, assets, and past coping strategies that were successful and can be built on **to enhance feelings of control.**
- Discuss the importance of assuming personal responsibility for life and relationships. **This skill requires one to be open to new ideas and experiences and different values and beliefs and to be inquisitive.**
- Identify things client can and cannot control. **Avoids wasting time on things that are not in the control of the client.**
- Treat expressed desires and decisions with respect. Avoid critical parenting expressions.

Information that appears in brackets has been added by the authors to clarify and enhance the use of nursing diagnoses.

Nursing Priority No. 3.

▶ To promote optimum wellness, enhancing power (Teaching/ Discharge Considerations):

- Assist client to set realistic goals for the future.
- Provide accurate verbal and written information about what is happening and discuss with client. **Reinforces learning and promotes self-paced review.**
- Assist client to learn and use assertive communication skills. **These techniques require practice, but as the client becomes more proficient, they will help client to develop more effective relationships.**
- Use I-messages instead of You-messages. **I-messages acknowledge ownership of what is said, while You-messages suggest that the other person is wrong or bad, fostering resentment and resistance instead of understanding and cooperation.**
- Discuss importance of client paying attention to nonverbal communication. **Messages are often confusing or misinterpreted when verbal and nonverbal communications are not congruent.**
- Help client learn to problem-solve differences. **Promotes win-win solutions.**
- Instruct and encourage use of stress-reduction techniques.
- Refer to support groups or classes, as indicated (e.g., assertiveness training, effectiveness for women, "Be your best").

Documentation Focus

Assessment/Reassessment
- Individual findings, noting determination to improve sense of power, locus of control.
- Motivation and expectations for change.

Planning
- Plan of care, specific interventions, and who is involved in planning.
- Teaching plan.

Implementation/Evaluation
- Client's responses to interventions, teaching, and actions performed.
- Attainment or progress toward desired outcome(s).
- Modifications to plan of care.

Information that appears in brackets has been added by the authors to clarify and enhance the use of nursing diagnoses.

Discharge Planning
* Long-term needs and who is responsible for actions to be taken.
* Specific referrals made.

Sample Nursing Outcomes & Interventions Classifications (NOC/NIC)

NOC—Personal Autonomy
NIC—Self-Modification Assistance

Powerlessness

Taxonomy II: Coping/Stress Tolerance—Class 2 Coping Responses (00125)
[Diagnostic Division: Ego Integrity]
Submitted 1982

Definition: The lived experience of lack of control over a situation, including a perception that one's own actions do not significantly affect an outcome

---

Related Factors

Institutional environment
Unsatisfactory interpersonal interaction
Illness-related regimen (e.g., chronic/debilitating conditions)

Defining Characteristics

Subjective

Moderate
Reports frustration over inability to perform previous activities
Reports doubt regarding role performance
Reports shame; alienation

Severe
Reports lack of control
Depression over physical deterioration

Objective
Dependence on others
Nonparticipation in care

Information that appears in brackets has been added by the authors to clarify and enhance the use of nursing diagnoses.

Desired Outcomes/Evaluation Criteria— Client Will:

- Express sense of control over the present situation and future outcome.
- Make choices related to and be involved in care.
- Identify areas over which individual has control.
- Acknowledge reality that some areas are beyond individual's control.

Actions/Interventions

Nursing Priority No. 1.

To assess causative/contributing factors:

- Identify situational circumstances (e.g., unfamiliar environment, immobility, diagnosis of terminal or chronic illness, lack of support system, lack of knowledge about situation).
- Determine client's perception and knowledge of condition and treatment plan.
- Ascertain client's response to treatment regimen. Does client see reason(s) and understand regimen is in the client's best interest, or is client compliant and helpless?
- Identify client's locus of control: internal (expressions of responsibility for self and ability to control outcomes—"I didn't quit smoking") or external (expressions of lack of control over self and environment—"Nothing ever works out"; "What bad luck to get lung cancer").
- Note cultural factors or religious beliefs that may contribute to how client is handling the situation.
- Assess degree of mastery client has exhibited in life. **Passive individual may have more difficulty being assertive and standing up for rights.**
- Determine if there has been a change in relationships with SO(s). **Conflict in the family, loss of a family member, or divorce can contribute to feelings of powerlessness and lack of ability to manage situation.**
- Note availability and use of resources.
- Investigate caregiver practices. Do they support client control or responsibility?

Nursing Priority No. 2.

To assess degree of powerlessness experienced by client:

- Listen to statements client makes: "They don't care"; "It won't make any difference"; "Are you kidding?"

Information that appears in brackets has been added by the authors to clarify and enhance the use of nursing diagnoses.

- Note expressions that indicate "giving up," such as "It won't do any good."
- Note behavioral responses (verbal and nonverbal) including expressions of fear, interest or apathy, agitation, withdrawal.
- Note lack of communication, flat affect, and lack of eye contact.
- Identify the use of manipulative behavior and reactions of client and caregivers. **Manipulation is used for management of powerlessness because of distrust of others, fear of intimacy, search for approval, and validation of sexuality.**

Nursing Priority No. 3.
To assist client to clarify needs relative to ability to meet them:
- Show concern for client as a person.
- Make time to listen to client's perceptions and concerns and encourage questions.
- Accept expressions of feelings, including anger and hopelessness.
- Avoid arguing or using logic with hopeless client. **Client will not believe it can make a difference.**
- Deal with manipulative behavior by being straightforward and honest with your communication and letting client know that this is a better way to get needs met.
- Express hope for the client. (**There is always hope of something.**)
- Identify strengths and assets, and past coping strategies that were successful. **Helps client to recognize own ability to deal with difficult situation.**
- Assist client to identify what he or she can do for self. Identify things the client can and cannot control.
- Encourage client to maintain a sense of perspective about the situation.

Nursing Priority No. 4.
To promote independence:
- Use client's locus of control to develop individual plan of care (e.g., for client with internal control, encourage client to take control of own care; for those with external control, begin with small tasks and add, as tolerated).
- Develop contract with client specifying goals agreed on. **Enhances commitment to plan, optimizing outcomes.**
- Treat expressed decisions and desires with respect. Avoid criticizing parenting behaviors and communications.

Information that appears in brackets has been added by the authors to clarify and enhance the use of nursing diagnoses.

- Provide client opportunities to control as many events as energy and restrictions of care permit.
- Discuss needs openly with client and set up agreed-on routines for meeting identified needs. **Minimizes use of manipulation.**
- Minimize rules and limit continuous observation to the degree that safety permits **to provide sense of control for the client.**
- Support client efforts to develop realistic steps to put plan into action, reach goals, and maintain expectations.
- Provide positive reinforcement for desired behaviors.
- Direct client's thoughts beyond present state to future when appropriate.
- Schedule frequent brief visits **to check on client, deal with client needs, and let client know someone is available.**
- Involve SO(s) in client care as appropriate.

Nursing Priority No. 5.

To promote wellness (Teaching/Discharge Considerations):

- Instruct in and encourage use of anxiety and stress-reduction techniques.
- Provide accurate verbal and written information about what is happening and discuss with client/SO(s). Repeat as often as necessary.
- Assist client to set realistic goals for the future.
- Assist client to learn and use assertive communication skills. **Use of I-messages, Active-listening, and problem-solving encourages client to be more in control of own life.**
- Refer to occupational therapist or vocational counselor, as indicated. **Facilitates return to a productive role in whatever capacity possible for the individual.**
- Encourage client to think productively and positively and take responsibility for choosing own thoughts.
- Model problem-solving process with client/SO(s). **Outcome is more likely to be accepted when arrived at by all parties involved, and participating in win-win solutions promotes sense of self-worth.**
- Suggest periodic review of own needs and goals.
- Refer to support groups, counseling or therapy, and so forth, as indicated.

Documentation Focus

Assessment/Reassessment
- Individual findings, noting degree of powerlessness, locus of control, individual's perception of the situation.

Information that appears in brackets has been added by the authors to clarify and enhance the use of nursing diagnoses.

- Specific cultural or religious factors.
- Availability and use of support system and resources.

Planning
- Plan of care and who is involved in the planning.
- Teaching plan.

Implementation/Evaluation
- Responses to interventions, teaching, and actions performed.
- Specific goals and expectations.
- Attainment or progress toward desired outcome(s).
- Modifications to plan of care.

Discharge Planning
- Long-term needs and who is responsible for actions to be taken.
- Specific referrals made.

Sample Nursing Outcomes & Interventions Classifications (NOC/NIC)

NOC—Personal Autonomy
NIC—Self-Responsibility Facilitation

risk for **Powerlessness**

Taxonomy II: Coping/Stress Tolerance—Class 2 Coping Responses (00125)
[Diagnostic Division: Ego Integrity]
Submitted 2000; Revised 2010

Definition: At risk for the lived experience of lack of control over a situation, including a perception that one's actions do not significantly affect an outcome

Risk Factors

Illness; [hospitalization]; unpredictable course of illness
Progressive debilitating disease process
Stigmatized condition or disease
Deficient knowledge
Pain; anxiety
Ineffective coping patterns
Situational or chronic low self-esteem

Information that appears in brackets has been added by the authors to clarify and enhance the use of nursing diagnoses.

Lack of social support; social marginalization; economically
   disadvantaged
Caregiving

> **NOTE:** A risk diagnosis is not evidenced by signs and
> symptoms, as the problem has not occurred; rather,
> nursing interventions are directed at prevention.

Desired Outcomes/Evaluation Criteria— Client Will:

- Express sense of control over the present situation and hope-
   fulness about future outcomes.
- Verbalize positive self-appraisal in current situation.
- Make choices related to and be involved in care.
- Identify areas over which individual has control.
- Acknowledge reality that some areas are beyond individual's
   control.

Actions/Interventions

Nursing Priority No. 1.
To assess causative/contributing factors:

- Identify situational circumstances (e.g., acute illness, sudden
   hospitalization; diagnosis of terminal or debilitating, chronic
   illness; very young or aged individual with decreased physical
   strength and mobility; lack of knowledge about illness or
   healthcare system).
- Determine client's perception and knowledge of condition
   and proposed treatment plan.
- Identify client's locus of control: internal (expressions of responsibility for self and environment) or external (expressions
   of lack of control over self and environment). **May affect
   willingness to accept responsibility to manage situation.**
- Assess client's self-esteem and degree of mastery client has
   exhibited in life situations. **Passive individual may have
   more difficulty being assertive and standing up for rights.**
- Determine cultural values or religious beliefs impacting self-
   view.
- Note availability and use of resources.
- Listen to statements client makes (e.g., "They can't really help";
   "It probably won't make a difference"). **Suggests concerns re-
   garding own power and ability to control situation.**

Information that appears in brackets has been added by the authors to clarify
and enhance the use of nursing diagnoses.

- Determine congruency of responses (verbal and nonverbal) and note expressions of fear, disinterest or apathy, or withdrawal.
- Be alert for signs of manipulative behavior and note reactions of client and caregivers. **Manipulation may be used for management of powerlessness because of fear and distrust.**

Nursing Priority No. 2.

To assist client to clarify needs and ability to meet them:

- Make time to listen to client's perceptions of the situation. **Shows concern for client as a person.**
- Encourage questions.
- Accept expressions of feelings, including anger and reluctance, to try to work things out. **Being able to express feelings freely enables client to sort out what is happening and come to a positive and realistic conclusion.**
- Express hope for client and encourage review of past experiences with successful strategies.
- Assist client to identify what he or she can do to help self and what situations can and cannot be controlled.

Nursing Priority No. 3.

🏠 To promote wellness (Teaching/Discharge Considerations):

- Encourage client to think productively and positively and to take responsibility for choosing own thoughts and reactions. **Can enhance feelings of power and sense of positive self-esteem.**
- Provide accurate verbal and written instructions about what is happening and what realistically might happen. **Reinforces learning and promotes self-paced review.**
- Involve client/SO(s) in planning process and problem-solving, using client's locus of control (e.g., for client with internal control, encourage client to take control of own care; for those with external control, begin with small tasks and add, as tolerated).
- Support client efforts to develop realistic steps to put plan into action, reach goals, and maintain expectations.
- Identify resource books or classes for assertiveness training and stress reduction, as appropriate.
- Encourage client to be active in long-term healthcare management and to engage in periodic review of own needs and goals.

Information that appears in brackets has been added by the authors to clarify and enhance the use of nursing diagnoses.

@ • Refer to support groups for chronic conditions or disability (e.g., MS Society, Easter Seals, Alzheimer's Association, Al-Anon) or counseling or therapy, as appropriate.

Documentation Focus

Assessment/Reassessment
- Individual findings, noting potential for powerlessness, locus of control, individual's perception of the situation.
- Cultural values or religious beliefs.
- Availability and use of resources.

Planning
- Plan of care and who is involved in the planning.
- Teaching plan.

Implementation/Evaluation
- Responses to interventions, teaching, and actions performed.
- Specific goals and expectations.
- Modifications to plan of care.

Discharge Planning
- Long-term needs and who is responsible for actions to be taken.
- Specific referrals made.

Sample Nursing Outcomes & Interventions Classifications (NOC/NIC)

NOC—Personal Autonomy
NIC—Self-Responsibility Facilitation

---

ineffective Protection

Taxonomy II: Health Promotion—Class 2 Health Management (00043)
[Diagnostic Division: Safety]
Submitted 1990

Definition: Decrease in the ability to guard self from internal or external threats such as illness or injury

---

Related Factors

Extremes of age
Inadequate nutrition

Information that appears in brackets has been added by the authors to clarify and enhance the use of nursing diagnoses.

Substance abuse

Abnormal blood profiles (e.g., leukopenia, thrombocytopenia, anemia, coagulation)

Pharmaceutical agents (e.g., antineoplastic, corticosteroid, immune, anticoagulant, thrombolytic)

Treatment-related side effects (e.g., surgery, radiation)

Cancer; immune disorders

Defining Characteristics

Subjective
Neurosensory alterations

Chilling

Itching

Insomnia; fatigue; weakness

Anorexia

Objective
Deficient immunity

Impaired healing; altered clotting

Maladaptive stress response

Perspiring (inappropriately)

Dyspnea; cough

Restlessness; immobility

Disorientation

Pressure ulcers

NOTE: The purpose of this diagnosis seems to combine multiple NDs under a single heading for ease of planning care when a number of variables may be present. Outcomes/evaluation criteria and interventions are specifically tied to individual related factors that are present, such as:

Extremes of age: Concerns may include body temperature or thermoregulation; memory or sensory-perceptual alterations, as well as impaired mobility, risk for falls, sedentary lifestyle, self-care deficits; risk for trauma, suffocation, or poisoning; problems with skin or tissue integrity; and fluid volume imbalances.

Inadequate nutrition: Brings up issues of nutrition, unstable blood glucose; infection, delayed surgical recovery; swallowing difficulties; impaired skin or tissue integrity; trauma, problems with coping, and family processes.

Information that appears in brackets has been added by the authors to clarify and enhance the use of nursing diagnoses.

Substance abuse: May be situational or chronic, with problems ranging from impaired respiration, decreased cardiac output, impaired liver function, and fluid volume deficits, to nutritional concerns, infection, trauma, risk for violence, and coping or family process difficulties.

Abnormal blood profile: Suggests possibility of fluid volume imbalances, decreased tissue perfusion, problems with oxygenation, activity intolerance, or risk for infection or injury.

Pharmaceutical agents and treatment-related side effects or concerns: Would include ineffective tissue perfusion, activity intolerance; cardiovascular, respiratory, and elimination concerns; risk for infection, fluid volume imbalances, impaired skin or tissue integrity, impaired liver function; pain, nutritional problems, fatigue or sleep difficulties; ineffective health management; and emotional responses (e.g., anxiety, sorrow, grieving, coping difficulties).

It is suggested that the user refer to specific NDs based on identified related factors and individual concerns for this client to find appropriate outcomes and interventions, as well as for Documentation Focus.

Sample Nursing Outcomes & Interventions Classifications (NOC/NIC)

NOC/NICs also depend on the specifics of the client's situation such as:

NOC—Symptom Control

NIC—Bleeding Precautions; Infection Protection; Postanesthesia Care

Information that appears in brackets has been added by the authors to clarify and enhance the use of nursing diagnoses.

Rape-Trauma Syndrome

Taxonomy II: Coping/Stress Tolerance—Class 1 Post-Trauma Responses (000142)
[Diagnostic Division: Ego Integrity]
Submitted 1980; Nursing Diagnosis Extension and Classification Revision 1998

Definition: Sustained maladaptive response to a forced, violent sexual penetration against the victim's will and consent [Rape is not a sexual crime, but a crime of violence, and it is identified as sexual assault. Although attacks are most often directed toward women, men also may be victims.]

Related Factors

Rape [actual or attempted forced sexual penetration]

Defining Characteristics

Subjective
Embarrassment; humiliation; shame; guilt; self-blame
Helplessness; powerlessness
Shock; fear; anxiety; anger; revenge
Nightmares; disturbed sleep pattern
Change in relationships; sexual dysfunction

Objective
Physical trauma; muscle tension or spasms
Confusion; disorganization; impaired decision making
Agitation; hyperalertness; aggression
Mood swings; vulnerability; dependence; chronic self-esteem; depression
Substance abuse; suicide attempts
Denial; phobias; paranoia; dissociative disorders

Desired Outcomes/Evaluation Criteria—Client Will:

- Deal appropriately with emotional reactions as evidenced by behavior and expression of feelings.
- Report absence of physical complications, pain, and discomfort.

Information that appears in brackets has been added by the authors to clarify and enhance the use of nursing diagnoses.

- Verbalize a positive self-image.
- Verbalize recognition that incident was not of own doing.
- Identify behaviors or situations within own control that may enhance sense of safety, reduce risk of recurrence.
- Deal with practical aspects (e.g., court appearances).
- Demonstrate appropriate changes in lifestyle (e.g., change in job, residence) as necessary and seek or obtain support from SO(s) as needed.
- Interact with individuals and groups in desired and acceptable manner.

Actions/Interventions

Nursing Priority No. 1.

To assess trauma and individual reaction, noting length of time since occurrence of event:

- Observe for and elicit information about physical injury and assess stress-related symptoms, such as numbness, headache, tightness in chest, nausea, and pounding heart.
- Identify psychological responses: anger, shock, acute anxiety, confusion, denial. Note laughter, crying, calm or agitated state, excited (hysterical) behavior, expressions of disbelief, and/or self-blame.
- Note signs of increasing anxiety (e.g., silence, stuttering, inability to sit still). **Indicates need for immediate interventions to prevent panic reaction.**
- Determine degree of disorganization. **(May need help to manage activities of daily living and other aspects of life.)**
- Identify whether incident has reactivated preexisting or co-existing situations (physical/psychological). **Can affect how the client views the current trauma and exacerbate pre-existing problems.**
- Ascertain cultural values or religious beliefs that may affect how client views incident, self, and expectations of SO/family reaction.
- Determine sexual orientation of the survivor. **Heterosexual men/boys may believe that they are now gay and need to be assured that is not true.**
- Determine disruptions in relationships with men and with others (e.g., family, friends, coworkers, SO[s]). **Many women find that they react to men in general in a different way, seeing them as reminders of the assault. Male survivors may withdraw entirely from sexual relations.**

Information that appears in brackets has been added by the authors to clarify and enhance the use of nursing diagnoses.

- Identify development of phobic reactions to ordinary articles (e.g., knives, buildings) and situations (e.g., walking in groups of people, strangers ringing doorbell).
- Note degree of intrusive repetitive thoughts, sleep disturbances.
- Assess degree of dysfunctional coping (e.g., use of alcohol, other drugs, suicidal/homicidal ideation, marked change in sexual behavior).

Nursing Priority No. 2.

To assist client to deal with situation that exists:

- Explore own feelings (nurse/caregiver) regarding rape or incest issue prior to interacting with the client. **Need to recognize own biases to prevent imposing them on the client.**

Acute Phase

- Stay with the client, do not leave child unattended. **Provides reassurance and sense of safety.**
- Involve rape response team where available. Provide same-sex examiner when appropriate.
- Evaluate infant, child, or adolescent as dictated by age, sex, and developmental level. **Age of the victim is an important consideration in deciding plan of care and appropriate interventions.** *Note:* **While underreported, it is believed that 1 in 10 men are sexually assaulted and 1 in 6 boys will be sexually assaulted or abused before the age of 18.**
- Assist with documentation of incident for police or child protective services reports, maintain sequencing and collection of evidence (chain of evidence), label each specimen, and store and package properly. **Protecting evidence is important to the judicial process when offender goes to trial.**
- Provide environment in which client can talk freely about feelings and fears, including concerns about relationship with and response of SO(s), pregnancy, sexually transmitted infections.
- Provide psychological support by listening and remaining with client. If client does not want to talk, accept silence. **May indicate Silent Reaction.**
- Listen to and investigate physical complaints. Assist with medical treatments, as indicated. **Emotional reactions may limit client's ability to recognize physical injury.**
- Assist with practical realities (e.g., safe temporary housing, money, or other needs).

Information that appears in brackets has been added by the authors to clarify and enhance the use of nursing diagnoses.

- Determine client's ego strengths and assist client to use them in a positive way by acknowledging client's ability to handle what is happening.
- Identify support persons for this individual. **The client's partner can be important to her or his recovery by being patient and comforting. When partners talk through the incident, the relationship can be strengthened.**

Postacute Phase

- Allow the client to work through own kind of adjustment (may be withdrawn or unwilling to talk); do not force the issue, but be available, if needed.
- Listen for expressions of fear of crowds, men, being alone in home, and so forth. **May reveal developing phobias.**
- Discuss specific concerns and fears. Identify appropriate actions (e.g., diagnostic testing for pregnancy, sexually transmitted infections) and provide information, as indicated.
- Include written instructions that are concise and clear regarding medical treatments, crisis support services, and so forth. **Reinforces teaching, provides opportunity to deal with information at own pace.**

Long-Term Phase

- Continue listening to expressions of concern. May need to continue to talk about the assault. Note persistence of somatic complaints (e.g., nausea, anorexia, insomnia, muscle tension, headache).
- Permit free expression of feelings (may continue from the crisis phase). Refrain from rushing client through expressions of feelings and avoid reassuring inappropriately. **Client may believe pain and/or anguish is misunderstood and depression may limit responses.**
- Acknowledge reality of loss of self that existed before the incident. Assist client to move toward an acceptance of the potential for growth that exists within individual.
- Continue to allow client to progress at own pace.
- Give "permission" to express/deal with anger at the perpetrator and situation in acceptable ways. Set limits on destructive behaviors. **Facilitates resolution of feelings without diminishing self-concept.**
- Keep discussion on practical and emotional level rather than intellectualizing the experience, **which allows client to avoid dealing with feelings.**
- Assist in dealing with ongoing concerns about and effects of the incident, such as court appearance, pregnancy, sexually transmitted infection, and relationship with SO(s).

Information that appears in brackets has been added by the authors to clarify and enhance the use of nursing diagnoses.

- Provide for sensitive, trained counselors, considering individual needs. (**Male or female counselors may be best determined on an individual basis as counselor's gender may be an issue for some clients, affecting ability to disclose.**)

Nursing Priority No. 3.

🏠 To promote wellness (Teaching/Discharge Considerations):

- Provide information about what reactions client may expect during each phase. Let client know these are common reactions and phrase in neutral terms of "You may or may not . . . ." (Be aware that although male rape perpetrators are usually heterosexual, the male victim may be concerned about his own sexuality and may exhibit a homophobic response.)
- Assist client to identify factors that may have created a vulnerable situation and that she or he may have power to change **to protect self in the future.**
- Avoid making value judgments.
- Discuss lifestyle changes client is contemplating and how they will contribute to recovery. **Helps client evaluate appropriateness of plans and make decisions that will be helpful to eventual recovery.**
- Encourage psychiatric consultation if client is violent, inconsolable, or does not seem to be making an adjustment. **Participation in a group may be helpful.**
- Refer to family/marital counseling, as indicated.
- Refer to NDs Powerlessness; ineffective Coping; Grieving; complicated Grieving; Anxiety; Fear.

Documentation Focus

Assessment/Reassessment

- Individual findings, including nature of incident, individual reactions and fears, degree of trauma (physical and emotional), effects on lifestyle.
- Cultural or religious factors.
- Reactions of family/SO(s).
- Samples gathered for evidence, disposition, and storage (chain of evidence).

Planning

- Plan of action and who is involved in planning.
- Teaching plan.

Information that appears in brackets has been added by the authors to clarify and enhance the use of nursing diagnoses.

🌐 Cultural   ⊛ Collaborative   🏠 Community/Home Care

Implementation/Evaluation
- Responses to interventions, teaching, and actions performed.
- Attainment or progress toward desired outcome(s).
- Modifications to plan of care.

Discharge Planning
- Long-term needs and who is responsible for actions to be taken.
- Specific referrals made.

Sample Nursing Outcomes & Interventions Classifications (NOC/NIC)

NOC—Abuse Recovery: Sexual
NIC—Rape-Trauma Treatment

ineffective Relationship

Taxonomy II: Role Relationships—Class 3 Role Performance (00223)
[Diagnostic Division: Ego Integrity]
Submitted 2010

Definition: A pattern of mutual partnership that is insufficient to provide for each other's needs

Related Factors

Stressful life events; developmental crises
Substance abuse
Unrealistic expectations
Poor communication skills
History of domestic violence
Cognitive changes in one partner
Incarceration of one partner

Defining Characteristics

Subjective
Reports dissatisfaction with complementary relation between partners
Reports dissatisfaction with fulfilling physical or emotional needs between partners

---

Information that appears in brackets has been added by the authors to clarify and enhance the use of nursing diagnoses.

Reports dissatisfaction with sharing of information or ideas between partners

Objective

Inability to communicate in a satisfying manner between partners

No demonstration of well-balanced autonomy or collaboration between partners

No demonstration of mutual respect between partners

No demonstration of mutual support in daily activities between partners

No demonstration of understanding of partner's insufficient (physical, social, psychological) functioning

Does not meet developmental goals appropriate for family life-cycle stage

Does not identify partner as a key person

Desired Outcomes/Evaluation Criteria— Client Will:

- Verbalize a desire to improve relationship with partner.
- Acknowledge worth and value of partner as a key person.
- Seek information regarding physical and emotional needs of partner.
- Engage in effective communication skills for both partners.
- Participate in marital therapy sessions to learn ways to develop a satisfactory relationship.

Actions/Interventions

Nursing Priority No. 1.

To assess current situation and determine needs:

∞• Determine make-up of family, length of relationship, financial situation—parents/children, older/younger, other members of household. **Stressors of family relationships within a household, difficulties with child rearing, older adult needing care, and financial difficulties can strain the relationship between partners.**

- Discuss individual's perception of own and other's needs and how partner sees own needs.
- Determine each person's self-image and locus of control. **View of self as a positive or negative individual who is in control or controlled by others influences behavior and how partners react to each other.**

Information that appears in brackets has been added by the authors to clarify and enhance the use of nursing diagnoses.

⬤ Cultural ◎ Collaborative 🏠 Community/Home Care

- Assess emotional intelligence skills of each individual. **This is the ability to recognize and control one's own emotions and recognize the emotions of the other.**
- Investigate cultural factors that may be affecting relationship and contributing to conflict. **Roles from family of origin for each person may promote conflict when beliefs clash and neither is willing to change or even discuss their thinking.**
- Determine style of communication used by partners. **Poor communication is unclear and indirect, leading to conflict, ineffective problem-solving, and poor emotional bonding in families with problems.**
- Determine how family as a whole functions. **Situational dynamics can create conflict as individuals take sides in disagreements, escalating the situation.**
- Ascertain ways in which family members deal with conflict.
- Identify concerns about sexual aspects of relationship from both partners' viewpoints. **Intimacy is an important part of a relationship.**
- Note medical problems that may be affecting sexual relationship. **Conditions, such as hysterectomy, prostatitis, breast cancer, erectile dysfunction may cause partners to withdraw from one another.**

Nursing Priority No. 2.

To assist partners to resolve existing conflict:

- Maintain positive attitude toward partners and family members. **Safe environment allows individuals to speak freely, knowing they will not be judged for comments and opinions.**
- Discuss surface symptoms of dysfunctional relationships and the fact that these are not the problems that need to be dealt with. **Individuals are often not aware of underlying emotions that are influencing their behavior and continue to focus on surface issues.**
- Explore each partner's emotional needs. **Unconscious desires to gain acceptance, recognition, sense of being cared about or valued are often motivators for relationships.**
- Discuss and clarify nonverbal communication. **Partners need to be aware of and ask about the meaning of body language, tone of voice, and subtle movements that convey positive or negative messages.**
- Assist partners/family to learn effective conflict resolution skills such as the win-win method. **Resolving to listen to each other's needs and agree on a mutually acceptable solution**

Information that appears in brackets has been added by the authors to clarify and enhance the use of nursing diagnoses.

provides new ways to resolve problems and enhances relationship.

- Provide information about Active-listening techniques. **Avoids giving advice and encourages other person to find own solution, enhancing self-esteem.**
- Have partners identify thoughts and feelings when starting a discussion with each other.
- Recommend individuals verify what they believe the other has said. **Allows speaker to correct misperception and respond more effectively.**
- Have partners role play a specific conflict that is a frequent issue. **Practicing how to defuse arguments and repair hurt feelings helps to identify other's feelings and use new skills for resolution.**
- Encourage partners to maintain a calm demeanor. **Staying focused enables individuals to think more rationally and come to a desired solution.**
- Discuss sexual concerns and provide opportunity for questions.
- Promote nonblameful self-disclosure when having a discussion. **Not placing blame results in a more considerate and respectful resolution.**

Nursing Priority No. 3.

To promote optimal functioning (Teaching/Discharge Considerations):

- Have partners acknowledge beliefs they have become aware of during therapy.
- Encourage use of relaxation, mindfulness techniques. **Helps individuals to ease anxiety and learn to relate to each other in a calm manner.**
- Discuss the appropriate use of humor and laughter in daily lives. **Helps to break the tension and lighten difficult moments.**
- Recommend books, Web sites to provide additional information.
- Refer to support groups, classes as indicated. **Parenting, assertiveness, financial assistance will help partners learn new skills as needed.**
- Include all family members in discussions, as indicated. **Promotes involvement, provides opportunities for communication and clarification of family dynamics and enhances commitment to achieving goals.**

Information that appears in brackets has been added by the authors to clarify and enhance the use of nursing diagnoses.

Cultural   Collaborative   Community/Home Care

- Refer to other physical/psychological resources, as needed. **May need further treatment to address pathology and help partners understand other's needs.**

Documentation Focus

Assessment/Reassessment
- Individual's perception of situation and self.
- Partner's views and expectations.
- How partners communicate and deal with conflict.

Planning
- Plan of care and who is involved in planning.
- Teaching plan.

Implementation/Evaluation
- Response of partners to plan, interventions and actions performed.
- Attainment or progress toward desired outcomes.

Discharge Planning
- Long-range plan and who is responsible for actions to be taken.
- Referrals made.

Sample Nursing Outcomes & Interventions Classifications (NOC/NIC)

NOC—Role Performance
NIC—Conflict Mediation

---

readiness for enhanced Relationship

Taxonomy II: Role Relationships—Class 3 Role Performance (00207)
[Diagnostic Division: Ego Integrity]
Submitted 2006

Definition: A pattern of mutual partnership that is sufficient to provide each other's needs and can be strengthened

---

Information that appears in brackets has been added by the authors to clarify and enhance the use of nursing diagnoses.

Defining Characteristics

Subjective

Reports:

Desire to enhance communication between partners

Satisfaction with sharing of information or ideas between partners

Satisfaction with fulfilling physical or emotional needs by one's partner

Satisfaction with complementary relation between partners

Identifies each other as a key person

Objective

Demonstrates:

Mutual respect between partners

Well-balanced autonomy or collaboration between partners

Mutual support in daily activities between partners

Understanding of partner's insufficient (physical, social, psychological) function

Meets developmental goals appropriate for family life cycle stage

Desired Outcomes/Evaluation Criteria— Client Will (Include Specific Time Frames):

- Verbalize a desire to learn more effective communication skills.
- Verbalize understanding of current relationship with partner.
- Seek information to improve emotional and physical needs of both partners.
- Talk with partner about circumstances that can be improved.
- Develop realistic plans to strengthen relationship.

Actions/Interventions

Nursing Priority No. 1.

To assess current situation and determine needs:

- Determine makeup of family (e.g., includes couple only, parents and children, older and younger members). **Life changes, such as developmental, situational, health-illness, can affect relationship between partners and require readjustment and thinking of ways to enhance situation.**

Information that appears in brackets has been added by the authors to clarify and enhance the use of nursing diagnoses.

🌐 Cultural   🤝 Collaborative   🏠 Community/Home Care

- Discuss client's perception of needs and how partner sees desire to improve relationship.
- Identify use of effective communication skills. **May need to improve understanding of words partners use in discussion of sensitive subjects.**
- Help client identify thoughts and feelings when starting a discussion with partner. **A system of thinking (referred to as a paradigm) forms the basis for how we look at and experience life and determines how we perceive our world, forms the basis for our reality, and exists below our level of consciousness.**
- Ask partners how they deal with conflict.
- Ascertain client's view of sexual aspects of relationship. **Changes that occur with aging or medical conditions, such as a hysterectomy or erectile dysfunction, can affect the relationship and need specific interventions to resolve.**
- Identify cultural factors relating to individual's view of role in relationship.
- Discuss how family as a whole functions. **Interrelationships with members of the family, personal and family history, and situational dynamics can improve the functioning of the whole family.**

Nursing Priority No. 2.
To assist the client to enhance existing situation:

- Maintain positive attitude toward client. **Promotes safe relationship in which client can feel free to speak openly and plan for a positive future.**
- Have couple discuss paradigms that they have become aware of in own thinking that interfere with relationship.
- Determine how each person views themselves as a positive or negative person. **One's self-image influences behavior and how they relate to others. When emotional needs are met, individuals relate to others in positive ways, while unmet needs result in low self-image and insecurity.**
- Discuss the skills of emotional intelligence that are important for maintaining positive relationships. **This is the ability to recognize and effectively control our own emotions and to recognize the emotions of others.**
- Help couple to recognize that surface symptoms of dysfunctional relationships are not the problems that need to be dealt with. **Underlying emotions influence our behaviors, and**

Information that appears in brackets has been added by the authors to clarify and enhance the use of nursing diagnoses.

individuals often are not aware of them and continue to deal with the superficial conflicts.

- Explore individual's emotional needs. **Relationships are often motivated by unconscious desires to gain acceptance, recognition, sense of being cared about or valued.**
- Note client's awareness of nonverbal communications. **Body language, tone of voice, a roll of the eyes, or subtle movements convey strong messages, positive or negative, that need to be discussed and clarified.**
- Discuss effective conflict-resolution skills.
- Encourage client to remain calm and focused regardless of circumstances. **Maintaining a calm demeanor helps individual to be able to think more clearly and be more rational in dealing with situation.**
- Recommend cross-checking or verifying what listener believes speaker said. **Clarifies communication and allows speaker to respond or correct perception of listener as needed.**
- Help partners to learn win-win method of conflict resolution.
- Role-play ways to defuse arguments and repair injured feelings. **Provides a realistic situation where each person can identify own and partner's view and practice new ways of interacting.**
- Provide open environment for partners to discuss sexual concerns and questions.
- Discuss nonblameful self-disclosure when having a dialogue. **Partners take turns talking about own needs and feelings without blaming the other, resulting in being able to find a solution in a climate of mutual consideration and respect.**

Nursing Priority No. 3.
To promote optimal functioning (Teaching/Discharge Considerations):

- Provide information for partners, using bibliotherapy and appropriate Web sites.
- Encourage couple to use humor and playfulness in their relationship. **Sharing laughter and enjoying life helps weather difficult times.**
- Discuss the importance of being an empathic, understanding, and nonjudgmental listener when either partner has a problem.
- Help individuals to learn to use the skill of Active-listening. **This avoids giving advice and helps other person to find own solution, enhancing self-esteem.**

Information that appears in brackets has been added by the authors to clarify and enhance the use of nursing diagnoses.

   Cultural Collaborative Community/Home Care

- Refer to support groups, classes on assertiveness, parenting, as indicated by individual needs.
- Include family members in discussions as needed.
- Refer for care as indicated by psychological or physical concerns of either individual.

Documentation Focus

Assessment/Reassessment
- Baseline information, individuals' perception of situation and self.
- Reasons for desire to improve relationship.
- Motivation and expectations for change.

Planning
- Plan of care and who is involved in planning.
- Teaching Plan.

Implementation/Evaluation
- Response of partners to plan, interventions, and actions performed.
- Attainment or progress toward desired outcomes(s).

Discharge Planning
- Long-range plan and who is responsible for actions to be taken.

Sample Nursing Outcomes & Interventions Classifications (NOC/NIC)

NOC—Social Interaction Skills
NIC—Role Enhancement

risk for ineffective Relationship

Taxonomy II: Role Relationships—Class 3 Role Performance (00229)
[Diagnostic Division: Ego Integrity]
Submitted 2010

Definition: Risk for a pattern of mutual partnership that is insufficient to provide for each other's needs

---

Information that appears in brackets has been added by the authors to clarify and enhance the use of nursing diagnoses.

Risk Factors

Stressful life events; developmental crises
Substance abuse
Unrealistic expectations
Poor communication skills
History of domestic violence; incarceration of one partner
Cognitive changes in one partner

Desired Outcomes/Evaluation Criteria— Client Will (Include Specific Time Frames):

- Verbalize desire to make changes to meet each other's needs as appropriate.
- Express a desire to improve communication skills.
- Develop realistic plans to improve relationship.

Actions/Interventions

Nursing Priority No. 1.

To assess current situation and determine needs:

∞ • Determine make-up of family, length of relationship, and specific stressors. **Stressors of family, such as developmental issues, elderly parents needing assistance, financial difficulties, and domestic violence, strain relationships between partners.**

- Identify how each partner sees own self-image and locus of control. **View of self as a positive or negative person who is in control or controlled by others influences how each relates to the other.**

- Discuss needs of each partner and how each views the other's needs. **Identifies misperceptions and areas of disagreement.**

- Identify style of communication and understanding of nonverbal cues used by family members. **Poor communication and lack of understanding of what the other is saying, or inferring, leads to conflicts and lack of problem-solving.**

- Determine how partners deal with conflict. **Many individuals try to avoid conflict instead of working to resolve it.**

⊕ • Identify cultural beliefs that affect how each person deals with daily activities in family.

- Identify medical problems/sexual concerns and how couple deals with issues. **Conditions such as prostate problems, breast cancer, hysterectomy, erectile dysfunction can af-**

Information that appears in brackets has been added by the authors to clarify and enhance the use of nursing diagnoses.

⊕ Cultural ⊛ Collaborative 🏠 Community/Home Care

fect interactions between partners and interfere with intimacy, causing couple to distance themselves from one another.

- Note how family as a whole functions. **Interactions among family members and situational dynamics provide information about need to improve relationships.**

Nursing Priority No. 2.

To assist couple to improve relationship:

- Maintain positive attitude in interactions with couple. **Provides an environment in which individuals feel comfortable and safe to discuss problems openly.**
- Promote awareness of individuals' beliefs and thoughts that may strain relationship. **Enables individuals to begin to discuss potential problem areas.**
- Discuss the skills of emotional intelligence. **The ability to acknowledge and control own emotions and recognize emotions of others is important to maintain healthy relationships.**
- Explore each person's emotional needs. **Understanding that unconscious needs underlie desire to gain acceptance, recognition, sense of being cared about or valued helps client to deal more openly with these issues.**
- Assist partners to understand effects of nonverbal language. **Lack of awareness of body language, tone of voice, subtle movements can be misinterpreted and need to be discussed and clarified.**
- Encourage couple to learn/reinforce effective conflict resolution skills.
- Role-play a specific problem couple argues about, using win-win method of resolution. **Practicing listening to each other's needs helps to arrive at a mutually agreeable solution.**
- Encourage partners to practice remaining calm and focused regardless of circumstances. **Remaining calm can help individuals think more clearly and be more rational in dealing with situation, avoiding further conflict.**
- Have each person verify what they heard the other person say. **Provides opportunity for the speaker to correct or acknowledge what was said.**
- Discuss issues/provide information about sexual relationship. **Conflict inevitably affects intimacy, and couple may need to resolve issues around this part of their life.**

Information that appears in brackets has been added by the authors to clarify and enhance the use of nursing diagnoses.

- Discuss use of nonblameful self-disclosure during discussions with partner. **Promotes an atmosphere of respect and mutual consideration.**

Nursing Priority No. 3.
To promote optimal functioning of couple/family (Teaching/ Discharge Considerations):

- Involve all family members in discussions, as indicated. **Encourages input from each member so he/she feels heard and views self as part of the solution.**
- Help family members learn skill of Active-listening. **Avoids giving advice and allows others to find their own solution, enhancing self-esteem.**
- Discuss appropriate use of humor and playfulness in daily interactions.
- Encourage use of relaxation, mindfulness techniques. **Promotes calm manner and ability to deal with difficult issues more effectively.**
- Recommend information sources, books, and Web sites as appropriate. **Provides additional resources to access information to assist couple in learning to deal with relationship/family issues.**
- Identify community resources/support groups as appropriate. **Individuals who have successfully dealt with similar issues can provide role model for change and effective use of problem-solving skills.**
- Refer to therapy as indicated. **May need further in-depth care to deal with individual physical/psychological problems.**

Documentation Focus

Assessment/Reassessment
- Individual's perception of situation and self.
- Partner's views and expectations.
- How partners communicate and deal with conflict.

Planning
- Plan of care and who is involved in planning.
- Teaching plan.

Implementation/Evaluation
- Response of partners to plan, interventions and actions performed.
- Attainment or progress toward desired outcomes.

Information that appears in brackets has been added by the authors to clarify and enhance the use of nursing diagnoses.

🌐 Cultural   ㉒ Collaborative   🏠 Community/Home Care

Discharge Planning
- Long-range plan and who is responsible for actions to be taken.
- Any referrals made.

Sample Nursing Outcomes & Interventions Classifications (NOC/NIC)

NOC—Role Performance
NIC—Conflict Mediation

---

impaired Religiosity

Taxonomy II: Life Principles—Class 3 Value/Belief/Action Congruence (00169)
[Diagnostic Division: Ego Integrity]
Submitted 2004

Definition: Impaired ability to exercise reliance on beliefs and/or participate in rituals of a particular faith tradition

---

NOTE: NANDA recognizes that the term "religiosity" may be culture specific; however, the term is useful in the United States and is well supported in the U.S. literature.

Related Factors

Developmental and Situational
Life transitions; aging; end-stage life crises

Physical
Illness; pain

Psychological Factors
Ineffective support, coping
Anxiety; fear of death
Personal crisis; lack of security
Use of religion to manipulate

Sociocultural
Cultural or environmental barriers to practicing religion
Lack of social integration; lack of sociocultural interaction

---

Information that appears in brackets has been added by the authors to clarify and enhance the use of nursing diagnoses.

Spiritual

Spiritual crises; suffering

Defining Characteristics

Subjective

Reports emotional distress because of separation from faith community

Reports a need to reconnect with previous belief patterns/customs

Questions religious belief patterns/customs

Difficulty adhering to prescribed religious beliefs or rituals (e.g., religious ceremonies, dietary regulations, clothing, prayer, worship/religious services, private religious behaviors/reading religious materials/media, holiday observances, meetings with religious leaders)

Desired Outcomes/Evaluation Criteria—Client Will:

- Express ability to once again participate in beliefs and rituals of desired religion.
- Discuss beliefs and values about spiritual or religious issues.
- Attend religious or worship services of choice as desired.
- Verbalize concerns about end-of-life issues and fear of death.

Actions/Interventions

Nursing Priority No. 1.

To assess causative/contributing factors:

- Determine client's usual religious or spiritual beliefs, values, past spiritual commitment. **Provides a baseline for understanding current problem or need.**
- Note client's/SO's reports and expressions of anger, alienation from God, sense of guilt or retribution. **Perception of guilt may cause spiritual crisis and suffering, resulting in rejection of religious symbols.**
- Determine sense of futility, feelings of hopelessness, lack of motivation to help self. **Indicators that client may see no, or only limited, options, alternatives or personal choices.**
- Assess extent of depression client may be experiencing. **Some studies suggest that a focus on religion may protect against depression.**

Information that appears in brackets has been added by the authors to clarify and enhance the use of nursing diagnoses.

  Cultural Collaborative Community/Home Care

- Note recent changes in behavior (e.g., withdrawal from others or religious activities; dependence on alcohol or medications). **Lack of connectedness with self/others impairs ability to trust others or feel worthy of trust from others or God.**

Nursing Priority No. 2.
To assist client/SO(s) to deal with feelings/situation:

- Use therapeutic communication skills of reflection and active-listening. **Communicates acceptance and enables client to find own solutions to concerns.**
- Encourage expression of feelings about illness, condition, death.
- Suggest use of journaling and reminiscence. **Promotes life review and can assist in clarifying values and ideas, recognizing and resolving feelings or situation.**
- Discuss differences between grief and guilt and help client to identify and deal with each. Point out consequences of actions based on guilt.
- Encourage client to identify individuals (e.g., spiritual advisor, parish nurse) who can provide needed support.
- Review client's religious affiliation, associated rituals, and beliefs. **Helps client examine what has been important in the past.**
- Provide opportunity for nonjudgmental discussion of philosophical issues related to religious belief patterns and customs. **Open communication can assist client to check reality of perceptions and identify personal options and willingness to resume desired activities.**
- Discuss desire to continue or reconnect with previous belief patterns, customs, and current barriers.
- Involve client in refining healthcare goals and therapeutic regimen, as appropriate. **Identifies role illness is playing in current concerns about ability to participate or appropriateness of participating in desired religious activities.**

Nursing Priority No. 3.
To promote spiritual wellness (Teaching/Discharge Considerations):

- Assist client to identify spiritual resources that could be helpful (e.g., contacting spiritual advisor who has qualifications and experience in dealing with specific problems individual is concerned about). **Provides answers to spiritual questions, assists in the journey of self-discovery, and can help client learn to accept and forgive self.**

Information that appears in brackets has been added by the authors to clarify and enhance the use of nursing diagnoses.

- Provide privacy for meditation, prayer, or performance of rituals, as appropriate.
- Explore alternatives or modifications of ritual based on setting and individual needs and limitations.

Documentation Focus

Assessment/Reassessment
- Individual findings, including nature of spiritual conflict, effects of participation in treatment regimen.
- Physical and emotional responses to conflict.

Planning
- Plan of care and who is involved in planning.
- Teaching plan.

Implementation/Evaluation
- Responses to interventions, teaching, and actions performed.
- Attainment or progress toward desired outcome(s).
- Modifications to plan of care.

Discharge Planning
- Long-term needs and who is responsible for actions to be taken.
- Available resources, specific referrals made.

Sample Nursing Outcomes & Interventions Classifications (NOC/NIC)

NOC—Spiritual Health
NIC—Spiritual Support

---

readiness for enhanced Religiosity

Taxonomy II: Life Principles—Class 3 Value/Belief/Action Congruence (00171)
[Diagnostic Division: Ego Integrity]
Submitted 2004

Definition: A pattern of reliance on religious beliefs and/or participation in rituals of a particular faith tradition that is sufficient for well-being and can be strengthened

---

Information that appears in brackets has been added by the authors to clarify and enhance the use of nursing diagnoses.

🌐 Cultural   🔄 Collaborative   🏠 Community/Home Care

Defining Characteristics

Subjective

Expresses desire to strengthen religious belief patterns or customs that have provided comfort or religion in the past

Requests assistance to increase participation in prescribed religious beliefs (e.g., religious ceremonies, dietary regulations/rituals, clothing, prayer, worship/religious services, private religious behaviors, reading religious materials/media, holiday observances)

Requests assistance to expand religious options; requests religious materials/experiences

Requests meeting with religious leaders/facilitators

Requests forgiveness, reconciliation

Questions or rejects belief patterns or customs that are harmful

Desired Outcomes/Evaluation Criteria— Client Will:

- Acknowledge need to strengthen religious affiliations and continue or resume previously comforting rituals.
- Verbalize willingness to seek help to enhance desired religious beliefs.
- Become involved in spiritually based programs of own choice.
- Recognize the difference between belief patterns and customs that are helpful and those that may be harmful.

Actions/Interventions

Nursing Priority No. 1.

To determine spiritual state/motivation for growth:

- Determine client's current thinking about desire to learn more about religious beliefs and actions.
- Ascertain religious beliefs of family of origin and climate in which client grew up. **Early religious training deeply affects children and is carried on into adulthood. Conflict between family's beliefs and client's current learning may need to be addressed.**
- Discuss client's spiritual commitment, beliefs, and values. **Enables examination of these issues and helps client learn more about self and what he or she desires/believes.**
- Explore how spirituality and religious practices have affected client's life.
- Ascertain motivation and expectations for change.

Information that appears in brackets has been added by the authors to clarify and enhance the use of nursing diagnoses.

Nursing Priority No. 2.

To assist client to integrate values and beliefs to strengthen sense of wholeness and achieve optimum balance in daily living:

- Establish nurse-client relationship in which dialogue can occur. **Client can feel safe to say anything and know it will be accepted.**
- Identify barriers and beliefs that might hinder growth and/or self-discovery. **Previous practices and beliefs may need to be considered and accepted or discarded in new search for religious beliefs.**
- Discuss cultural beliefs of family of origin and how they have influenced client's religious practices. **As client expands options for learning new or other religious beliefs and practices, these influences will provide information for comparing and contrasting new information.**
- Explore connection of desire to strengthen belief patterns and customs to daily life. **Becoming aware of how these issues affect the individual's daily life can enhance ability to incorporate them into everything he or she does.**
- Identify ways in which individual can develop a sense of harmony with self and others.

Nursing Priority No. 3.

To enhance optimum spiritual wellness:

- Encourage client to seek out and experience different religious beliefs, services, and ceremonies. **Trying out different religions will give client more information to contrast and compare what will fit his or her belief system.**
- Provide bibliotherapy or reading materials pertaining to spiritual issues client is interested in learning about.
- Help client learn about stress-reducing activities (e.g., meditation, relaxation exercises, mindfulness). **Promotes general well-being and sense of control over self and ability to choose religious activities desired. Mindfulness is a method of being in the moment.**
- Encourage participation in religious activities, worship or religious services, reading religious materials or reviewing multimedia sources, study groups, volunteering in choir, or undertaking other needed duties.
- Refer to community resources (e.g., parish nurse, religion classes, other support groups).

Information that appears in brackets has been added by the authors to clarify and enhance the use of nursing diagnoses.

Documentation Focus

Assessment/Reassessment
* Assessment findings, including client's religious beliefs and practices, perception of need.
* Motivation and expectations for growth or enhancement.

Planning
* Plan for growth and who is involved in planning.

Implementation/Evaluation
* Response to activities, learning, and actions performed.
* Attainment or progress toward desired outcome(s).
* Modifications to plan.

Discharge Planning
* Long-term needs/expectations and plan of action.
* Specific referrals made.

Sample Nursing Outcomes & Interventions Classifications (NOC/NIC)

NOC—Spiritual Health
NIC—Spiritual Growth Facilitation

risk for impaired **Religiosity**

Taxonomy II: Life Principles—Class 3 Value/Belief/Action Congruence (00170)
[Diagnostic Division: Ego Integrity]
Submitted 2004

Definition: At risk for an impaired ability to exercise reliance on religious beliefs and/or participate in rituals of a particular faith tradition

Risk Factors

Developmental
Life transitions

Environmental
Lack of transportation
Barriers to practicing religion

Information that appears in brackets has been added by the authors to clarify and enhance the use of nursing diagnoses.

Physical
Illness; hospitalization; pain

Psychological
Ineffective support, coping, or caregiving
Depression
Lack of security

Sociocultural
Lack of social interaction; social isolation
Cultural barrier to practicing religion

Spiritual
Suffering

> **NOTE:** A risk diagnosis is not evidenced by signs and symptoms, as the problem has not occurred; rather, nursing interventions are directed at prevention.

Desired Outcomes/Evaluation Criteria— Client Will:

- Express understanding of relation of situation/health status to thoughts and feelings of concern about ability to participate in desired religious activities.
- Seek solutions to individual factors that may interfere with reliance on religious beliefs/participation in religious rituals.
- Identify and use resources appropriately.

Actions/Interventions

Nursing Priority No. 1.
To assess causative/contributing factors:

- Ascertain current situation (e.g., illness, hospitalization, prognosis of death, depression, lack of support systems, financial concerns). **Identifies problems client is dealing with in the moment that may be affecting desire to be involved with religious activities.**
- Note client's concerns or expressions of anger, belief that illness or situation is result of lack of faith. **Individual may blame himself or herself for what has happened and could reject religious beliefs and/or God.**

Information that appears in brackets has been added by the authors to clarify and enhance the use of nursing diagnoses.

🌐 Cultural 🔵 Collaborative 🏠 Community/Home Care

- Determine client's usual religious or spiritual beliefs, past or current involvement in specific church activities.
- Identify cultural values and expectations regarding religious beliefs and/or practices.
- Note quality of relationships with SO(s) and friends. **Individual may withdraw from others in relation to the stress of illness, pain, and suffering. Others may be encouraging client to rely on religious beliefs at a time when individual is questioning own beliefs in the current situation.**
- Assess for barriers (e.g., lack of transportation, lack of family involvement) to participation in desired religious activities.
- Ascertain substance use or abuse. **Individuals often turn to use of various substances in distress, and this can affect the ability to deal with problems in a positive manner.**

Nursing Priority No. 2.
To assist client to deal with feelings/situation:

- Develop nurse-client relationship. **Individual can express feelings and concerns freely when he or she feels safe to do so.**
- Use therapeutic communications skills of Active-listening, reflection, and I-messages. **Helps client find own solutions to problems and concerns and promotes sense of control.**
- Have client identify and prioritize current or immediate needs. **Dealing with current needs is easier than trying to predict the future.**
- Provide time for nonjudgmental discussion of individual's spiritual beliefs and fears about impact of current illness and/or treatment regimen. **Helps clarify thoughts and promote ability to deal with stresses of what is happening.**
- Review with client past difficulties in life and coping skills that were used at those times.
- Encourage client to discuss feelings about death and end-of-life issues when illness or prognosis is grave.

Nursing Priority No. 3.
To promote spiritual wellness (Teaching/Discharge Considerations):

- Have client identify support systems available.
- Help client learn relaxation techniques, meditation, guided imagery, and mindfulness/living in the moment and enjoying it.
- Take the lead from the client in initiating participation in religious activities, prayer, other activities. **Client may be**

Information that appears in brackets has been added by the authors to clarify and enhance the use of nursing diagnoses.

vulnerable in current situation and must be allowed to decide own participation in these actions.

⊕ • Refer to appropriate resources (e.g., crisis counselor, governmental agencies, spiritual advisor) who has qualifications or experience dealing with specific problems, such as death/dying, relationship problems, substance abuse, suicide, hospice, psychotherapy, Alcoholics or Narcotics Anonymous.

Documentation Focus

Assessment/Reassessment
• Individual findings, including risk factors, nature of current distress.
• Physical and emotional response to distress.
• Availability and use of resources.

Planning
• Plan of care and who is involved in planning.
• Teaching plan.

Implementation/Evaluation
• Responses to interventions, teaching, and actions performed.
• Attainment or progress toward desired outcome(s).
• Modifications to plan of care.

Discharge Planning
• Long-term needs and who is responsible for actions to be taken.
• Available resources, specific referrals made.

Sample Nursing Outcomes & Interventions Classifications (NOC/NIC)

NOC—Spiritual Health
NIC—Religious Ritual Enhancement

Relocation Stress Syndrome

Taxonomy II: Coping/Stress Tolerance—Class 1 Post-Trauma Responses (00114)
[Diagnostic Division: Ego Integrity]
Submitted 1992; Revised 2000

Definition: Physiological and/or psychosocial disturbance following transfer from one environment to another

---

Information that appears in brackets has been added by the authors to clarify and enhance the use of nursing diagnoses.

Related Factors

Move from one environment to another
Losses; reports feeling of powerlessness
Lack of adequate support system; lack of predeparture counseling; unpredictability of experience
Isolation; language barrier
Impaired psychosocial health; passive coping
Decreased health status

Defining Characteristics

Subjective

Anxiety (e.g., separation); anger
Insecurity; worry; fear
Loneliness; depression
Reports unwillingness to move; concern over relocation
Sleep pattern disturbance

Objective

Increased verbalization of needs
Pessimism; frustration
Increased physical symptoms or illness
Withdrawal; aloneness; alienation; [hostile behavior or outbursts]
Loss of identity, self-worth; situational or chronic low self-esteem; dependency
Increased confusion or cognitive impairment

Desired Outcomes/Evaluation Criteria—Client Will:

- Verbalize understanding of reason(s) for change.
- Demonstrate appropriate range of feelings and lessened fear.
- Participate in routine and special or social events as able.
- Verbalize acceptance of situation.
- Experience no catastrophic event.

Actions/Interventions

Nursing Priority No. 1.

To assess degree of stress as perceived/experienced by client and determine issues of safety:

- Determine situation or cause for relocation (e.g., planned move for new job; deployment or returning from military

---

Information that appears in brackets has been added by the authors to clarify and enhance the use of nursing diagnoses.

duty; loss of home or community due to natural or man-made disaster such as fire, earthquake, flood, war or act of terror; older adult unable to care for self, caregiver burnout; change in marital or health status). **Influences needs and choice of interventions.**

- Ascertain if client participated in the decision to relocate and perceptions about change(s) and expectations for the future. **Decision may have been made without client's input or understanding of event or consequences, which can impact adjustment.**

- Note client's age, developmental level, role in family. **Age and position in life cycle makes a difference in the impact of issues involved in relocating. For example, child can be traumatized by transfer to new school or loss of peers, especially a military adolescent who is subjected to multiple, often frequently occurring, moves; elderly person may be affected by loss of long-term home, neighborhood setting, and support persons.**

- Identify cultural and/or religious concerns or conflicts **that may affect client's coping or impact social interactions and expectations.**

- Note ethnic ties and primary language spoken and read. Obtain interpreter where appropriate. **Affects client, SO(s), and healthcare providers who must try to reduce the client's feelings of alienation, while communicating with client of another primary language, or client who is displaced from cultural attachments.**

- Monitor behavior, noting presence of anxiety, suspiciousness or paranoia, irritability, defensiveness. Compare with SO's/staff's description of customary responses. **Move may temporarily exacerbate mental deterioration (cognitive inaccessibility) and impair communication (social inaccessibility).**

- Note signs of increased stress in recently relocated client. **Client may report or demonstrate irritability, withdrawal, crying, moodiness, problems sleeping, or fatigue; "new" physical discomfort or pain (e.g., stomachaches, headaches, back pain); change in appetite; increased use of alcohol or other drugs; or greater susceptibility to colds.**

- Determine involvement of family/SO(s). Note availability and use of support systems and resources.

- Identify issues of safety that may be involved.

Nursing Priority No. 2.
To assist client to deal with situation/changes:

Information that appears in brackets has been added by the authors to clarify and enhance the use of nursing diagnoses.

- Collaborate in treatment of underlying conditions (e.g., chronic confusional states, brain injury, post-trauma rehabilitation) and physical stress symptoms **that are potentially exacerbating relocation stress or that may affect the length of time that relocation is required.**
- Begin relocation planning with client and SO(s) as early as possible. Provide support and advocate for client who is unable to participate in decisions. **Having a well-organized plan for move with support and advocacy may reduce anxiety.**
- Encourage visit to new community, surroundings, school prior to transfer when possible. **Provides opportunity to "get acquainted" with new situation, reducing fear of unknown.**
- Encourage free expression of feelings about reason for relocation, including venting of anger; grief; loss of personal space, belongings, or friends; financial strains; powerlessness; and so forth. Acknowledge reality of situation and maintain hopeful attitude regarding move/change. Refer to NDs relating to client's particular situation (e.g., Grieving; ineffective Coping) for additional interventions.
- Identify strengths and successful coping behaviors the individual has used previously. **Incorporating these into problem-solving builds on past successes.**
- Encourage client to maintain contact with friends (e.g., telephone, e-mail, video or audio tapes, arranged visits) **to reduce sense of isolation.**
- Orient to surroundings and schedules. Introduce to neighbors, staff members, roommate, or residents. Provide clear, honest information about actions and events.
- Encourage individual/family to personalize area with pictures, own belongings, as possible and appropriate. **Enhances sense of belonging and creates personal space.**
- Determine client's usual schedule of activities and incorporate into routine as possible. **Reinforces sense of importance of individual.**
- Introduce planned diversional activities, such as movies, meals with new acquaintances, art therapy, music, religious activities. **Involvement increases opportunity to interact with others, decreasing isolation.**
- Place in private facility room, if appropriate, and include SO(s)/family into care activities, mealtimes, and so forth. **Keeping client secluded may be needed under some circumstances (e.g., advanced Alzheimer's disease with fear**

Information that appears in brackets has been added by the authors to clarify and enhance the use of nursing diagnoses.

or aggressive reactions) **to decrease the client's stress reactions to new environment.**

* Encourage hugging and use of touch unless client prefers to abstain from hugging, is paranoid, or agitated at the moment. **Human connection reaffirms acceptance of individual.**

* Deal with aggressive behavior by imposing calm, firm limits. Control environment and protect others from client's disruptive behavior. **Promotes safety for client and others.**

* Remain calm, place in a quiet environment, providing time out, as indicated, **to prevent escalation into panic state and violent behavior.**

* Collaborate in treatment of underlying conditions (e.g., chronic confusional states/brain injury, post-trauma rehabilitation) and physical stress symptoms **that are potentially exacerbating relocation stress.**

* Anticipate and address feelings of distress and grieving in family/caregivers when placing loved one in a different environment (e.g., nursing home, foster care).

* Refer to social worker, financial resources, mental healthcare provider, minister/spiritual advisor for additional assessment and interventions, as indicated. **May be needed if client has special needs and/or persistent problems with adaptation.**

Nursing Priority No. 3.

🏠 To promote wellness (Teaching/Discharge Considerations):

* Involve client in formulating goals and plan of care when possible. **Supports independence and commitment to achieving outcomes.**

* Encourage communication between client/family/SO **to provide mutual support and problem-solving opportunities.**

* Discuss benefits of adequate nutrition, rest, and exercise **to maintain physical well-being.**

* Involve in anxiety- and stress-reduction activities (e.g., meditation, progressive muscle relaxation, group socialization), as able, to enhance psychological well-being.

* Encourage participation in activities, hobbies, and personal interactions as appropriate. **Promotes creative endeavors, stimulating the mind.**

* Identify community supports, cultural or ethnic groups client can access.

* Support self-responsibility and coping strategies. **Fosters sense of control and self-worth.**

Information that appears in brackets has been added by the authors to clarify and enhance the use of nursing diagnoses.

Documentation Focus

Assessment/Reassessment
- Assessment findings, individual's perception of the situation and changes, sense of loss, specific behaviors.
- Cultural or religious concerns.
- Safety issues.

Planning
- Note plan of care, who is involved in planning, and who is responsible for proposed actions.
- Teaching plan.

Implementation/Evaluation
- Response to interventions (especially time out or seclusion), teaching, and actions performed.
- Sentinel events.
- Attainment or progress toward desired outcome(s).
- Modifications to plan of care.

Discharge Planning
- Long-term needs and who is responsible for actions to be taken.
- Specific referrals made.

Sample Nursing Outcomes & Interventions Classifications (NOC/NIC)

NOC—Psychosocial Adjustment: Life Change
NIC—Relocation Stress Reduction

---

risk for Relocation Stress Syndrome

Taxonomy II: Coping/Stress Tolerance—Class 1 Post-Trauma Responses (00149)
[Diagnostic Division: Ego Integrity]
Submitted 2000

Definition: At risk for physiological and/or psychosocial disturbance following transfer from one environment to another

---

Information that appears in brackets has been added by the authors to clarify and enhance the use of nursing diagnoses.

Risk Factors

Move from one environment to another
Moderate to high degree of environmental change
Lack of adequate support system; lack of predeparture counseling
Passive coping; reports powerlessness; losses
Decreased health status; moderate mental competence
Unpredictability of experiences

> **NOTE:** A risk diagnosis is not evidenced by signs and symptoms, as the problem has not occurred; rather, nursing interventions are directed at prevention.

Desired Outcomes/Evaluation Criteria— Client Will:

- Verbalize understanding of reason(s) for change.
- Express feelings and concerns openly and appropriately.
- Experience no catastrophic event.

Actions/Interventions

Nursing Priority No. 1.

To assess causative/contributing factors:

- Determine situation or cause for relocation (e.g., planned move for new job; deployment or returning from military duty; loss of home or community due to natural or man-made disaster such as fire, earthquake, war; older adult unable to care for self, caregiver burnout; change in marital or health status). **Influences needs and choice of interventions.**
- Identify cultural and/or religious concerns or conflicts. **Cultural norm may be that elders are cared for by family— not placed in a facility—causing client to feel abandoned; or individual may be required to defer to family decision maker and feel powerless in determining own destiny.**
- Ascertain if client participated in decision to relocate and perceptions about change(s) and expectations for the future. **Decision can be made without client's input or understanding of event or consequences, which can impact adjustment and sense of control over life.**
- Note client's age, developmental level, role in family. **Age and position in life cycle makes a difference in the impact**

Information that appears in brackets has been added by the authors to clarify and enhance the use of nursing diagnoses.

🌐 Cultural   🔬 Collaborative   🏠 Community/Home Care

of issues involved in relocating. For example, a child can be traumatized by transfer to new school/loss of peers; elderly persons may be affected by loss of long-term home, neighborhood setting, and support persons.

- Determine physical and emotional health status. **Stress associated with a move, even if desired, can cause or exacerbate health problems.**
- Note whether relocation will be temporary (e.g., extended care for rehabilitation therapies, moving in with family while house is being repaired after fire) or long term or permanent (e.g., move from home of many years; placement in retirement center or long-term care facility). **Client may be willing to relocate on temporary basis, seeing it as step to health and independence, but may view long-term placement as unbearable loss.**
- Determine involvement of family/SO(s). Note availability and use of support systems and resources. Ascertain presence or absence of comprehensive information and planning (e.g., when and how move will take place, if the environment for the client will be similar or greatly changed). **These factors can greatly affect client's ability to cope with change.**
- Identify issues of safety that may be involved.

Nursing Priority No. 2.

To prevent/minimize adverse response to change:

- Collaborate in treatment of underlying conditions (e.g., chronic confusional states, brain injury, post-trauma rehabilitation) and physical stress symptoms **that could exacerbate relocation stress or that affects length of time that relocation may be needed.**
- Allow as much time as possible for move preparation and provide information and support in planning.
- Discuss relocation or move with child providing information aimed at level of understanding and interest. **Child lacks ability to put problem into perspective, so minor mishap may seem catastrophic and child is more vulnerable to stress because he or she has less control over environment than most adults.**
- Avoid moving adolescent in middle of school year when possible. **Adolescent is vulnerable to emotional, social, and cognitive dysfunction because of the great importance of peer group and loss of friends and social standing caused by relocation.**

Information that appears in brackets has been added by the authors to clarify and enhance the use of nursing diagnoses.

- Support self-responsibility and coping strategies **to foster sense of control and self-worth.**
- Suggest contact with someone (friend, family, business associate) who has been to or lived in new area where move is being planned **to absorb some of their experience and knowledge.**
🏠 - Encourage visit to new community or surroundings prior to transfer when possible. **Provides opportunity to "get acquainted" with new situation, thus reducing fear of unknown.**

Nursing Priority No. 3
🏠 To promote wellness (Teaching/Discharge Considerations):

- Involve client in formulating goals and plan of care when possible. **Fosters sense of control and self-worth, supports independence and commitment to achieving outcomes.**
- Encourage client/SO to accept that relocation is an adjustment and that it takes time to adapt to new circumstances or environment.
- Instruct in anxiety- and stress-reduction activities (e.g., meditation, other relaxation techniques, exercise program, group socialization) as able **to enhance psychological well-being and coping abilities.**
- Provide client with information and list of organizations or community services (e.g., Welcome Wagon, senior citizens or teen clubs, churches, singles' groups, sports leagues) **to provide contacts for client to develop new relationships and learn more about the new setting.**
- Discuss safety issues regarding new environment (e.g., how to navigate streets or choose correct bus; locate dining hall or bathroom in facility), concerns of elopement or running away.
- Anticipate variety of emotions and reactions. **May vary from insomnia and loss of appetite to becoming involved with alcohol or other drugs or exacerbation of health problems, onset of serious illness, or behavioral problems. Awareness provides opportunity for timely intervention.**
- Refer to ND Relocation Stress Syndrome for additional interventions.

Documentation Focus ─────────────

Assessment/Reassessment
- Assessment findings, individual's perception of the situation/changes, specific behaviors.

Information that appears in brackets has been added by the authors to clarify and enhance the use of nursing diagnoses.

- Cultural or religious concerns.
- Safety issues.

Planning
- Note plan of care, who is involved in planning, and who is responsible for proposed actions.
- Teaching plan.

Implementation/Evaluation
- Response to interventions (especially time out/seclusion), teaching, and actions performed.
- Sentinel events.
- Attainment or progress toward desired outcome(s).
- Modifications to plan of care.

Discharge Planning
- Long-term needs and who is responsible for actions to be taken.
- Specific referrals made.

Sample Nursing Outcomes & Interventions Classifications (NOC/NIC)

NOC—Psychosocial Adjustment: Life Change
NIC—Relocation Stress Reduction

risk for ineffective Renal Perfusion

Taxonomy II: Activity/Rest—Class 4 Cardiovascular/
   Pulmonary Responses (00203)
[Diagnostic Division: Circulatory]
Submitted 2008

Definition: At risk for a decrease in blood circulation to the kidney that may compromise health

Risk Factors

Hypovolemia; [interruption of blood flow]; vascular embolism vasculitis

Hypertension; malignant hypertension; hyperlipidemia

Renal disease (polycystic kidney); polynephritis; exposure to nephrotoxins; glomerulonephritis, interstitial nephritis, bilateral cortical necrosis; renal artery stenosis

---

Information that appears in brackets has been added by the authors to clarify and enhance the use of nursing diagnoses.

Diabetes mellitus; malignancy

Cardiac surgery; cardiopulmonary bypass

Hypoxemia, hypoxia; metabolic acidosis

Multitrauma; abdominal compartment syndrome; burns; infection (e.g. sepsis, localized infection); systemic inflammatory response syndrome

Treatment-related side effects (e.g., pharmaceutical agents; surgery)

Advanced age; female gender

Smoking; substance abuse

> **NOTE:** A risk diagnosis is not evidenced by signs and symptoms, as the problem has not occurred; rather, nursing interventions are directed at prevention.

Desired Outcomes/Evaluation Criteria— Client Will:

- Demonstrate adequate renal perfusion as evidenced by urine output appropriate for individual, balanced intake and output, absence of edema formation or inappropriate weight gain.
- Verbalize understanding of condition, therapy regimen, side effects of medication, and when to contact healthcare provider.
- Engage in behaviors/lifestyle changes to improve circulation (e.g., smoking cessation, diabetic glucose control, medication management)

Actions/Interventions

Nursing Priority No. 1.

To assess causative/contributing factors:

- Determine history or presence of severe hypotension and hypoxemia or shock (may be cardiogenic, hypovolemia, obstructive, or septic shock), blunt or penetrating trauma, surgery with excess bleeding or fluid loss, prolonged dehydration, poorly controlled diabetes, and so forth. **Conditions associated with decreased systemic circulation and kidney ischemia.**
- Note history or presence of abrupt onset or severe hypertension, persistent hypertension (>160/100) over time, or hypertension resistant to appropriately dosed antihypertensive

---

Information that appears in brackets has been added by the authors to clarify and enhance the use of nursing diagnoses.

⊕ Cultural ⊛ Collaborative 🏠 Community/Home Care

therapy, **any of which places client at high risk for kidney damage associated with renovascular hypertension.**

- Assess hydration status. **Dehydration reduces glomerular filtration rate.**
- Ascultate for bruit over each renal artery in abdomen at mid-clavicular line, **suggesting renal artery stenosis, which is associated with renal insufficiency.**
- Determine usual voiding pattern and investigate reported deviations, such as low output or need for diuretics, **which may indicate problems with kidney perfusion.**
- Note urine color—pale (dilute) or dark (concentrated)—and measure specific gravity, as indicated, **to evaluate hydration status and kidney's ability to concentrate the urine.**
- Monitor fluid intake, urine output, and weight on a regular schedule **to provide noninvasive assessment of cardiovascular and renal function.**
- Monitor for edema. **May be present with increased fluid retention due to impaired renal function related to decreased renal perfusion.**
- Note mentation and behavior. **Adverse changes may be the consequence of fluid shifts, accumulation of toxins, acid-based and/or electrolyte imbalances when kidney dysfunction is occurring.**
- Review medication regimen, observing for certain antimicrobials, antivirals, chemotherapy agents, analgesics, immuno suppressives, herbals and diagnostic agents. Monitor peak and trough blood levels when client receiving nephrotoxic agents such as aminoglycocides (e.g.,Vancomycin), **known for potential side or toxic effects that may substantially alter kidney perfusion.**
- Discuss client's history of and current alcohol and illicit substance use/abuse. **Most street drugs, including heroin, cocaine, and ecstasy can cause high blood pressure, a risk factor for impaired renal function. Alcohol (when used heavily), cocaine, heroin, and amphetamines also can cause kidney damage.**
- Review laboratory studies (e.g., complete blood count, blood urea nitrogen/creatinine levels, protein, specific gravity, 24-hour creatinine clearance, glucose, electrolytes) **to evaluate kidney function.**
- Review diagnostic studies, as indicated, including Doppler ultrasonography, computed tomography, renogram, intraveous pyleogram; contrast or magnetic resonance angiography, **to evaluate kidney size, perfusion, and function.**

Information that appears in brackets has been added by the authors to clarify and enhance the use of nursing diagnoses.

Nursing Priority No. 2.

To reduce or correct individual risk factors:

- Collaborate in treatment of underlying conditions (e.g., angioplasty with stent placement, surgical revascularization procedures, fluids, electrolytes, nutrients, antibiotics, thrombolytics, oxygen) **to improve tissue perfusion/organ function.**

- Administer medications (e.g., vasoactive medications, including antihypertensive agents, insulin) as indicated **to treat underlying condition and improve renal blood flow and function.**

- Exercise caution when administering nephrotoxic agents, particularly when dehydration is present, **to reduce risk for acute or chronic renal failure.**

- Provide for fluid and diet restrictions as indicated, while providing adequate calories and hydration **to meet the body's needs without overtaxing kidney function.**

- Refer to NDs deficient or excess Fluid Volume, impaired Urinary Elimination for additional interventions.

Nursing Priority No. 3.

To promote wellness (Teaching/Discharge Considerations):

- Discuss individual risk factors (e.g., family history, obesity, age, smoking, hypertension, diabetes, clotting disorders) and potential outcomes of atherosclerosis such as systemic and peripheral vascular disease. **Information necessary for client to make informed choices about remedial risk factors and consider lifestyle changes to prevent onset of complications or manage symptoms when condition present.**

- Identify necessary changes in lifestyle and assist client to incorporate disease management into activities of daily living. **Promotes independence; enhances self-concept regarding ability to deal with change and manage own needs.**

- Emphasize need to manage blood pressure when client is hypertensive. Instruct about individual's antihypertensive medications (e.g., angiotensin-converting enzyme inhibitors, diuretics, beta-adrenergic blockers), and necessity for taking them as prescribed and with physician follow-up **to reduce cardiovascular complications and slow progression of renal dysfunction.**

- Instruct in home blood pressure monitoring; advise purchase of appropriate equipment; refer to community resources as indicated. **Facilitates management of hypertension, which is a major risk factor for damage to blood vessels and organ function.**

Information that appears in brackets has been added by the authors to clarify and enhance the use of nursing diagnoses.

risk for ineffective RENAL PERFUSION

- ▲ Encourage client to quit smoking, join Smoke-out or other smoking-cessation programs. **Smoking causes vasoconstriction, compromising renal perfusion.**
- ▲ Review specific fluid and dietary requirements with client/SO (e.g., reduction of cholesterol, carbohydrates, or sodium) as indicated by individual situation **to promote circulatory health and kidney function.**
- ▲ Establish regular exercise program **to enhance circulation and promote general well-being.**
- ②· Encourage regular medical and laboratory follow-up **to provide monitoring and earlier intervention for underlying conditions and to evaluate effectiveness of therapeutic interventions.**
- ②· Refer to specific support groups, counseling as appropriate **to assist with problem-solving, provide role model, enhance coping ability.**

Documentation Focus

Assessment/Reassessment
- Individual physical findings; identified risk factors.
- Baseline kidney function.
- Input and output and weight as indicated.

Planning
- Plan of care and who is involved in planning.
- Teaching plan.

Implementation/Evaluation
- Response to interventions, teaching, and actions performed.
- Attainment or progress toward desired outcome(s).
- Modifications to plan of care.

Discharge Planning
- Long-term needs and who is responsible for actions to be taken.
- Available resources, specific referrals made.

Sample Nursing Outcomes & Interventions Classifications (NOC/NIC)

NOC—Kidney Function
NIC—Fluid/Electrolyte Management

Information that appears in brackets has been added by the authors to clarify and enhance the use of nursing diagnoses.

impaired individual Resilience

Taxonomy II: Coping/Stress Tolerance—Class 2 Coping
  Responses (00210)
[Diagnostic Division: Ego Integrity]
Submitted 2008

Definition: Decreased ability to sustain a pattern of positive responses to an adverse situation or crisis

Related Factors

Demographics that increase chance of maladjustment; large
  family size; minority status; poverty; gender
Vulnerability factors that encompass indices that exacerbate the
  negative effects of the risk condition; substance abuse; poor
  impulse control; neighborhood violence
Low intelligence; low maternal education
Inconsistent parenting; parental mental illness
Psychological disorders; violence

Defining Characteristics

Subjective
Depression; guilt; isolation; social isolation; low self-esteem;
  shame
Lower perceived health status
Renewed elevation of distress
Decreased interest in academic or vocational activities

Objective
Using maladaptive coping skills (i.e., drug use, violence, etc.)

Desired Outcomes/Evaluation Criteria— Client Will (Include Specific Time Frame):

- Acknowledge reality of current situation or crisis.
- Express positive feelings about self and situation.
- Seek appropriate resources to change circumstances that affect adaptation and resilience.
- Be involved in programs to address problems presenting in life (e.g., substance abuse, low self-esteem, poverty).

Information that appears in brackets has been added by the authors to clarify
and enhance the use of nursing diagnoses.

🌐 Cultural 🌐 Collaborative 🏠 Community/Home Care

Actions/Interventions

Nursing Priority No. 1.

To assess causative/contributing factors:

- Determine individuals, family, children involved and ages and current circumstances. **Understanding the family makeup provides information that will guide choice of interventions.**
- Note underlying stressors, health concerns, debilitating conditions, mental health or behavioral issues such as unemployment, poverty, diabetes, obesity, chronic obstructive pulmonary disease, Alzheimer's disease, parental mental illness.
- Identify locus of control. **Individuals with external locus of control are less likely to feel in control or to rely on their own abilities or judgment to manage a situation.**
- Determine client's education level, family dynamics, and parenting styles, if relevant. **Drug use, violence, and poor impulse control affect individual's ability to develop resilience in adverse situations or crisis. Individual may see self as a victim rather than a survivor.**
- Note communication patterns within the family. **Skills learned within the family can determine whether the individual develops low self-esteem or positive feelings about self.**
- Identify maladaptive coping skills used by individual and in the family. **Focusing on negative in situations impairs one's ability to adjust positively and learn attributes of resiliency.**
- Note parental status including age and maturity. **Young parents may lack ability to deal with family responsibilities, financial concerns, factors associated with low socioeconomic status.**
- Ascertain stability of relationship, presence of separation or divorce. **Family members are vulnerable to break up of the family unit and may see it as causing long-term harm.**
- Determine availability and use of resources, family, support groups, financial aid.
- Note cultural factors and religious beliefs that may affect interpretation of, or response to, situation. **Helps determine individual needs and possible options.**

Nursing Priority No. 2.

To assist client to improve skills to deal with adverse situations or crises:

Information that appears in brackets has been added by the authors to clarify and enhance the use of nursing diagnoses.

- Encourage free expressions of feelings, including feelings of anger and hostility, setting limits on unacceptable behavior. **Unacceptable behavior leads to feelings of shame and guilt if not controlled.**
- Listen to client's concerns and acknowledge difficulty of adversity and making changes in situation. **Being listened to provides opportunity for client to feel valued, capable, and like a survivor rather than a victim.**
- Help client assume responsibility for own life, look at situation as a challenge rather than an obstacle, and refrain from viewing crisis as insurmountable. **People learn and develop resilience as they deal with adversities of life.**
- Provide information at client's level of comprehension, being honest in explanations. **Provides data to assist in decision-making process.**
- Have client paraphrase information provided during teaching session to **ensure understanding and to provide opportunity to correct misunderstandings.**
- Promote parent involvement in developing a positive mindset for fostering resilience in their children.
- Facilitate communication skills between client and family. **Sometimes, individuals who find themselves in difficult situations withdraw because they do not know what to do or say.**
- Focus on strengths of the individual as the problems are being assessed and diagnosed.
- Teach client/parents to practice empathy with family members.
- Discuss individual issues, such as obesity, substance use, poor impulse control, violent behavior; provide information about the risks and help client/parent understand how they can help family members develop habits that will promote physical and mental well-being.

Nursing Priority No. 3.
To promote wellness (Teaching/Discharge Considerations):

- Reinforce that client is responsible for self, for choices made, and actions taken. **The road to resilience is developed by the individual accepting that change is a part of living and then beginning to live life more fully.**
- ⊕ Provide or identify learning opportunities specific to individual needs. **Activities such as assertiveness, regular exercise, parenting classes can enhance knowledge and help develop a resilient mindset.**

Information that appears in brackets has been added by the authors to clarify and enhance the use of nursing diagnoses.

⊕ Cultural ⊕ Collaborative 🏠 Community/Home Care

- Discuss use of the problem-solving method to set mutually agreed-on goals.
- Provide anticipatory guidance relevant to current situation and long-term expectations. **Client may have many issues to resolve, and planning ahead can help individuals make changes, have hope for the future, and have a sense of control over their lives.**
- Encourage client/parents to take time for themselves. **Provides opportunity for personal growth; respite allows individuals to pursue own interests and return to tasks of life/parenting with renewed vigor.**
- Refer to community resources as appropriate, such as social services, financial, domestic violence/elder abuse program, family therapy, divorce counseling, special needs support services.

Documentation Focus

Assessment/Reassessment
- Findings, including specifics of individual situations, parental concerns, perceptions, expectations.
- Locus of control and cultural beliefs.

Planning
- Plan of care and who is involved in the planning.
- Teaching plan.

Implementation/Evaluation
- Response to interventions, teaching, and actions performed.
- Attainment or progress toward desired outcome(s).
- Modifications to plan of care.

Discharge Planning
- Long-term needs and who is responsible for actions to be taken.
- Specific referrals made.

Sample Nursing Outcomes & Interventions Classifications (NOC/NIC)

NOC—Personal Resiliency
NIC—Resiliency Promotion

Information that appears in brackets has been added by the authors to clarify and enhance the use of nursing diagnoses.

readiness for enhanced Resilience

Taxonomy II: Coping/Stress Tolerance—Class 2 Coping
   Responses (00212)
[Diagnostic Division: Ego Integrity]
Submitted 2008

Definition: A pattern of positive responses to an adverse
situation or crisis that is sufficient for optimizing human
potential and can be strengthened

Defining Characteristics

Subjective
Presence of a crisis
Reports enhanced sense of control; reports self-esteem; takes
   responsibilities for actions
Expressed desire to enhance resilience
Sets goals; makes progress toward goals
Identifies available resources or support systems
Involvement in activities

Objective
Demonstrates positive outlook
Enhances personal coping skills; use of effective communica-
   tion skills; effective use of conflict management strategies
Increases positive relationships with others
Access to resources

Desired Outcomes/Evaluation Criteria— Client Will (Include Specific Time Frames):

- Describe current situation accurately.
- Identify positive responses currently being used.
- Verbalize feelings congruent with behavior.
- Express desire to strengthen ability to deal with current situ-
  ation or crisis.

Actions/Interventions

Nursing Priority No. 1.
To determine needs and desires for improvement:

- Evaluate client's perception and ability to provide a realistic
  view of the situation. **Provides information about how cli-**

Information that appears in brackets has been added by the authors to clarify
and enhance the use of nursing diagnoses.

🌐 Cultural   ⚙ Collaborative   🏠 Community/Home Care

ent views the situation and specific expectations to aid in formulating plan of care.

- Determine client's coping abilities in current situation and expectations for change. **Motivation to improve and high expectations can encourage client to make changes that will improve his or her life. However, unrealistic expectations may hamper efforts.**
- Note client's verbal expressions indicating belief that he or she owns the responsibility for how to deal with adverse situation. **When client has internal locus of control, he or she accepts that life has its adversities and one needs to deal with them.**
- Discuss religious and cultural beliefs held by the individual.
- Identify support systems available to client.

Nursing Priority No. 2.

To assist client to enhance resilience to adverse situation:

- Active-listen and identify client's concerns about situation. **Reflecting client's statements helps to clarify what he or she is thinking and promotes accurate interpretation of reality.**
- Determine previous methods of dealing with adversity. **Helps client to remember successful skills used in the past, and see what might be helpful in current situation.**
- Discuss desire to improve ability to handle adverse situations that arise throughout life. **Willingness to be open to change requires a curiosity, listening to others' ideas and beliefs, looking at new ways to do things.**
- Discuss concept of what can be changed versus what cannot be changed.
- Determine how client is dealing with activities of daily living **While client may have some transient problems with sleeping or managing daily affairs, most people have the ability to function in a healthy manner over time.**
- Help client to learn how to empathize with others. **Understanding own emotions as well as feelings of others enhances one's resiliency during stressful times.**

Nursing Priority No. 3.

To promote optimum growth and resiliency:

- Provide factual information and anticipatory guidance relevant to current situation and long-term expectations. **Planning ahead allows for problem-solving and review of**

Information that appears in brackets has been added by the authors to clarify and enhance the use of nursing diagnoses.

options in a relaxed atmosphere, reinforcing sense of control and hope for the future.

- Review factors that might impact individual's response to stress.
- Encourage client to maintain or establish good relationships with family and friends.
- Help client avoid seeing situation as insurmountable. **While one cannot change the fact of the circumstances, how individual interprets and responds is within one's control.**
- Recommend setting realistic goals and doing something regularly, even if it is small.
- Encourage client to maintain a hopeful outlook, nurture a positive view of self, and take care of self. **Keeping a long-term perspective and paying attention to own needs help maintain and build resilience.**
- Refer to classes and/or reading materials as appropriate.

Documentation Focus

Assessment/Reassessment

- Baseline information, including client's perception of situation, view of own ability to be resilient, and support systems available.
- Ways of dealing with previous life problems.
- Motivation and expectations for change.
- Cultural or religious influences.

Planning

- Plan of care and who is involved in planning.
- Educational plan.

Implementation/Evaluation

- Responses to interventions, teaching, and actions performed.
- Attainment or progress toward desired outcomes(s).
- Modifications to plan.

Discharge Planning

- Long-term needs and who is responsible for actions to be taken.
- Specific referrals made.

Information that appears in brackets has been added by the authors to clarify and enhance the use of nursing diagnoses.

🌐 Cultural   🤝 Collaborative   🏠 Community/Home Care

Sample Nursing Outcomes & Interventions Classifications (NOC/NIC)

NOC—Personal Resiliency
NIC—Resiliency Promotion

risk for compromised Resilience

Taxonomy II: Coping/Stress Tolerance—Class 2 Coping
Responses (00211)
[Diagnostic Division: Ego Integrity]
Submitted 2008

Definition: At risk for decreased ability to sustain a pattern of positive responses to an adverse situation or crisis

Risk Factors

Chronicity of existing crises
Multiple coexisting adverse situations
Presence of an additional new crisis (e.g., unplanned pregnancy, death of a spouse or family member, loss of job, illness, loss of housing)

> **NOTE:** A risk diagnosis is not evidenced by signs and symptoms, as the problem has not occurred; rather, nursing interventions are directed at prevention.

Desired Outcomes/Evaluation Criteria—Client Will (Include Specific Time Frame):

* Acknowledge reality of individual situation or crisis.
* Verbalize feelings associated with chronic situation.
* Verbalize awareness of own ability to deal with problems.
* Identify resources for assisting with chronic and new adverse occurrence.

Actions/Interventions

Nursing Priority No. 1.
To determine individual stressors/potential challenges:

* Note underlying stressors, health concerns, debilitating conditions, mental health or behavioral issues such as

---

Information that appears in brackets has been added by the authors to clarify and enhance the use of nursing diagnoses.

unemployment, pregnancy, diabetes, Alzheimer's disease, anxiety disorder.

- Determine alcohol or other drug use, smoking, sleeping and eating habits, **which can affect ability to cope with added stress of crises effectively and in a healthy manner.**
- Assess functional capacity and how it affects client's ability to manage daily needs.
- Evaluate client's ability to verbalize and understand current situation and impact of new crisis. **Informed choice cannot be made without a good understanding of reality of situation.**
- Note speech and communication patterns. **Provides information about level of education, ability to understand situation and to relate problems to caregiver(s).**
- Determine locus of control. **Individuals with external locus of control are less likely to feel in control or to rely on their own abilities or judgment to manage a situation.**
- Evaluate client's current decision-making ability. **Crises affect individual's ability to think clearly and trust own ability to deal with situation.**
- Ascertain stability of relationship, presence of separation or divorce, deteriorating health, or recent death of family member. **Family members are vulnerable to breakup of the family unit and may see it as causing long-term liability.**

Nursing Priority No. 2.
To assess coping skills and degree of resilience:

- Active-listen and identify client's perceptions of what has occurred, as well as previous concerns.
- Determine how adverse situation is affecting client's ability to deal with what is happening now. **When an unplanned situation occurs in addition to existing problems, it often results in decreased ability to maintain optimism.**
- Determine how individual has dealt with problems in the past. **Having client remember these skills helps in thinking about what can be used to enhance current response or address future challenges.**
- Note cultural factors and religious beliefs that may affect interpretation of, or response to, the situation. **Helps determine individual needs and possible options.**
- Determine availability and use of resources, family, support groups, financial aid. **Appropriate use can help the individual continue to manage problems in their lives and plan for future needs.**

Information that appears in brackets has been added by the authors to clarify and enhance the use of nursing diagnoses.

Cultural   Collaborative   Community/Home Care

Nursing Priority No. 3.

To assist client to deal with current/future situation:

- Ask client what name he or she prefers. **Acknowledging how the individual wants to be addressed provides sense of self, promoting self-esteem.**
- Encourage free expressions of feelings, including feelings of anger and hostility, setting limits on unacceptable behavior. **Unacceptable behavior leads to feelings of shame and guilt if not controlled.**
- Allow client to react in own way without judgment by caregivers. Provide support and diversion as indicated. **Unconditional positive regard and support promote acceptance and help client to realize own ability to deal with situation.**
- Listen to client's concerns and acknowledge difficulty of adversity and possible need to make changes. **Often individuals who are feeling that life is difficult begin to doubt their ability to deal with circumstances. Being listened to provides opportunity for client to feel valued, capable, and like a survivor rather than a victim.**
- Encourage communication with caregivers and significant other(s).
- Provide reality orientation when necessary. **Depending on nature of crisis, client may be disoriented by change in environment, serious diagnosis or treatment regimen, loss of family member.**
- Provide client with factual information and expected course of situation or crisis if known. **Knowledge helps to allay anxiety, enabling client to manage more effectively and to begin to consider possible resolution of the current situation.**
- Focus on strengths of the individual as problems are being assessed and diagnosed. Improving future for client is based on strengthening the capacity to deal successfully with obstacles one meets in life.

Nursing Priority No. 4.

To promote wellness (Teaching/Discharge Considerations):

- Provide or identify learning opportunities specific to individual needs. **Activities such as assertiveness, regular exercise, parenting classes can enhance knowledge and help develop a resilient mindset.**
- Encourage an attitude of realistic hope. **Client can accept that change is a part of living and, while some plans cannot**

Information that appears in brackets has been added by the authors to clarify and enhance the use of nursing diagnoses.

be obtained because of crisis or new circumstances, new goals can be developed and life can move forward.

* Support client in evaluating current lifestyle and changes that need to be made.
* Provide anticipatory guidance relevant to current situation and long-term expectations.
* Determine need or desire for religious or spiritual counselor and make arrangements for visit. **Providing client an opportunity to discuss concerns about what has happened helps to build resilience to face future stressors.**
* Reinforce importance of client/SO taking time for self. **Provides opportunity for personal growth; respite allows individuals to pursue own interests and return to tasks of life with renewed vigor.**
* Refer to community resources as appropriate. **May need professional counseling, assistance with financial concerns, special needs support services, child or parenting care to move forward.**

Documentation Focus

Assessment/Reassessment
* Assessment findings, including details of this client's situation or crisis, expectations.
* Client's degree of resiliency.

Planning
* Plan of care, and who is involved in planning.
* Teaching plan.

Implementation/Evaluation
* Response to interventions, teaching, and actions performed.
* Attainment or progress toward desired outcome(s).
* Modifications to plan of care.

Discharge Planning
* Long-term needs and who is responsible for actions to be taken.
* Support systems available, specific referrals made.

Sample Nursing Outcomes & Interventions Classifications (NOC/NIC)

NOC—Personal Resiliency
NIC—Resiliency Promotion

Information that appears in brackets has been added by the authors to clarify and enhance the use of nursing diagnoses.

parental Role Conflict

Taxonomy II: Role Relationships—Class 1 Role Performance (00064)
[Diagnostic Division: Social Interaction]
Submitted 1988

Definition: Parent experience of role confusion and conflict in response to crisis

Related Factors

Parent-child separation due to chronic illness

Intimidation by invasive modalities (e.g., intubation); by restrictive modalities (e.g., isolation); specialized care center

Home care of a child with special needs

Change in marital status; [conflicts of the role of the single parent]

Interruptions of family life due to home-care regimen (e.g., treatments, caregivers, lack of respite)

Defining Characteristics

Subjective

Reports feeling of inadequacy to provide for child's needs (e.g., physical, emotional)

Reports concerns about changes in parental role; about family (e.g., functioning, communication, health)

Reports concern about perceived loss of control over decisions relating to child

Reports feelings of guilt/frustration; anxiety; fear

Objective

Demonstrates disruption in caretaking routines

Reluctant to participate in usual caretaking activities

Desired Outcomes/Evaluation Criteria—Parent(s) Will:

* Verbalize understanding of situation and expected parent's/child's role.
* Express feelings about child's illness or situation and effect on family life.
* Demonstrate appropriate behaviors in regard to parenting role.

Information that appears in brackets has been added by the authors to clarify and enhance the use of nursing diagnoses.

parental ROLE CONFLICT

- Assume caretaking activities as appropriate.
- Handle family disruptions effectively.

Actions/Interventions

Nursing Priority No. 1.
To assess causative/contributory factors:

- Assess individual situation and parent's perception of/concern about what is happening and expectations of self as caregiver.
- Note parental status, including age and maturity, stability of relationship, single parent, other responsibilities. **For example, increasing numbers of elderly individuals are providing full-time care for young grandchildren whose parents are unavailable or unable to provide care.**
- Ascertain parent's understanding of child's developmental stage and expectations for the future **to identify misconceptions and strengths.**
- Note coping skills currently being used by each individual as well as how problems have been dealt with in the past. **Provides basis for comparison and reference for client's coping abilities.**
- Determine use of substances (e.g., alcohol, other drugs, including prescription medications). **May interfere with individual's ability to cope and problem-solve.**
- Assess availability and use of resources, including extended family, support groups, and financial.
- Perform testing, such as Parent-Child Relationship Inventory, for further evaluation as indicated.

Nursing Priority No. 2.
To assist parents to deal with current crisis:

- Encourage free verbal expression of feelings (including negative feelings of anger and hostility), setting limits on inappropriate behavior.
- Acknowledge difficulty of situation and normalcy of feeling overwhelmed and helpless. Encourage contact with parents who experienced similar situation with child and had positive outcome.
- Provide information, including technical information when appropriate, **to meet individual needs and correct misconceptions.**
- Promote parental involvement in decision making and care as much as possible/desired. **Enhances sense of control.**

Information that appears in brackets has been added by the authors to clarify and enhance the use of nursing diagnoses.

Cultural Collaborative Community/Home Care

- Encourage interaction/facilitate communication between parent(s) and children.
- Promote use of assertiveness, relaxation skills **to help individuals deal with situation/crisis.**
- Assist parent(s) to learn proper administration of medications and treatments, as indicated.
- Provide for, or encourage use of, respite care, parental time off **to enhance emotional well-being.**
- Help single parent distinguish between parent love and partner love. **Love is constant, but attention can be given to one or the other, as appropriate.**

Nursing Priority No. 3.

To promote wellness (Teaching/Discharge Considerations):

- Provide anticipatory guidance **to encourage making plans for future needs.**
- Encourage parents to set realistic and mutually agreed-on goals.
- Discuss attachment behaviors such as breastfeeding on cue, cosleeping, baby-wearing (carrying baby around on chest/back), and playing. **Dealing with ill child/home-care pressures can strain the bond between parent and child. Activities such as these encourage secure relationships.**
- Provide and identify learning opportunities specific to needs (e.g., parenting classes, healthcare equipment use/troubleshooting).
- Refer to community resources, as appropriate (e.g., visiting nurse, respite care, social services, psychiatric care or family therapy, well-baby clinics, special needs support services).
- Refer to ND impaired Parenting for additional interventions.

Documentation Focus

Assessment/Reassessment
- Findings, including specifics of individual situation/parental concerns, perceptions, expectations.

Planning
- Plan of care and who is involved in the planning.
- Teaching plan.

Implementation/Evaluation
- Parent's responses to interventions, teaching, and actions performed.

Information that appears in brackets has been added by the authors to clarify and enhance the use of nursing diagnoses.

- Attainment or progress toward desired outcome(s).
- Modifications to plan of care.

Discharge Planning
- Long-term needs and who is responsible for each action to be taken.
- Specific referrals made.

Sample Nursing Outcomes & Interventions Classifications (NOC/NIC)

NOC—Parenting Performance
NIC—Parenting Promotion

---

ineffective **Role Performance**

Taxonomy II: Role Relationships—Class 3 Role Performance (00055)
[Diagnostic Division: Social Interaction]
Submitted 1978; Revised 1996, 1998

Definition: Patterns of behavior and self-expression that do not match the environmental context, norms, and expectations

---

NOTE: There is a typology of roles (e.g., sociopersonal [friendship, family, marital, parenting, community]; home management; intimacy [sexuality, relationship building]; leisure, exercise, or recreation; self-management; socialization [developmental transitions], community contributor; and religious) that can help to understand ineffective Role Performance.

Related Factors

Knowledge
Inadequate or lack of role model
Inadequate role preparation (e.g., role transition, skill rehearsal, validation)
Lack of education
Unrealistic role expectations

Information that appears in brackets has been added by the authors to clarify and enhance the use of nursing diagnoses.

⊕ Cultural ⊕ Collaborative 🏠 Community/Home Care

Physiological

Body image alteration; cognitive deficits; neurological deficits; physical illness; mental illness; depression; situational/chronic low self-esteem

Fatigue; pain; substance abuse

Social

Inadequate role socialization (e.g., role model, expectations, responsibilities)

Young age, developmental level

Lack of resources

Stress; conflict; job schedule demands

[Family conflict]; domestic violence

Inadequate support system; lack of rewards

Inappropriate linkage with the healthcare system

Defining Characteristics

Subjective

Altered role perceptions; change in self-/other's perception of role

Change in usual patterns of responsibility or capacity to resume role

Inadequate opportunities for role enactment

Role dissatisfaction, overload, or denial

Discrimination [by others]; powerlessness

Objective

Deficient knowledge

Inadequate adaptation to change; inappropriate developmental expectations

Inadequate confidence, motivation, self-management, or skills

Ineffective coping or role performance

Inadequate external support for role enactment

Role strain, conflict, confusion, or ambivalence; [failure to assume role]

Uncertainty; anxiety; depression; pessimism

Domestic violence; harassment; system conflict

Desired Outcomes/Evaluation Criteria—Client Will:

- Verbalize understanding of role expectations and obligations.
- Verbalize realistic perception and acceptance of self in changed role.

Information that appears in brackets has been added by the authors to clarify and enhance the use of nursing diagnoses.

- Talk with family/SO(s) about situation and changes that have occurred and limitations imposed.
- Develop realistic plans for adapting to new role or role changes.

Actions/Interventions

Nursing Priority No. 1.

To assess causative/contributing factors:

- Identify type of role dysfunction: for example, developmental (adolescent to adult); situational (husband to father, gender identity); transitions from health to illness.
- Determine client role in family constellation.
- Identify how client sees self as a man or woman in usual lifestyle or role functioning.
- Ascertain client's view of sexual functioning (e.g., loss of childbearing ability following hysterectomy).
- Identify cultural factors relating to individual's sexual roles. **Cultures define male and female roles differently (e.g., Muslim culture demands that the woman adopt a subservient role, whereas the man is seen as the powerful one in the relationship).**
- Determine client's perceptions or concerns about current situation. **May believe current role is more appropriate for the opposite sex (e.g., passive role of the patient may be somewhat less threatening for women).**
- Interview SO(s) regarding their perceptions and expectations. **Influences client's view of self.**

Nursing Priority No. 2.

To assist client to deal with existing situation:

- Discuss perceptions and significance of the situation as seen by client.
- Maintain positive attitude toward the client.
- Provide opportunities for client to exercise control over as many decisions as possible. **Enhances self-concept and promotes commitment to goals.**
- Offer realistic assessment of situation while communicating sense of hope.
- Discuss and assist client/SO(s) to develop strategies for dealing with changes in role related to past transitions, cultural expectations, and value or belief challenges. **Helps those involved deal with differences between individuals (e.g., adolescent task of separation in which parents clash with**

Information that appears in brackets has been added by the authors to clarify and enhance the use of nursing diagnoses.

● Cultural   ● Collaborative   🏠 Community/Home Care

child's choices; individual's decision to change religious affiliation).

- Acknowledge reality of situation related to role change and help client express feelings of anger, sadness, and grief. Encourage celebration of positive aspects of change and expressions of feelings.
- Provide open environment for client to discuss concerns about sexuality. **Embarrassment can block discussion of sensitive subject.** (Refer to NDs Sexual Dysfunction; ineffective Sexuality Pattern.)
- Identify role model for client. Educate about role expectations using written and audiovisual materials.
- Use the techniques of role rehearsal to help client develop new skills **to cope with changes.**

Nursing Priority No. 3.

To promote wellness (Teaching/Discharge Considerations):

- Make information available for client to learn about role expectations or demands that may occur. **Provides opportunity to be proactive in dealing with changes.**
- Accept client in changed role. Encourage and give positive feedback for changes and goals achieved. **Provides reinforcement and facilitates continuation of efforts.**
- Refer to support groups, employment counselors, parent effectiveness classes, counseling/psychotherapy, as indicated by individual need(s). **Provides ongoing support to sustain progress.**
- Refer to NDs Self-Esteem [specify]; impaired, risk for impaired, or readiness for enhanced Parenting.

Documentation Focus

Assessment/Reassessment

- Individual findings, including specifics of predisposing crises or situation, perception of role change.
- Expectations of SO(s).

Planning

- Plan of care and who is involved in planning.
- Teaching plan.

Implementation/Evaluation

- Responses to interventions, teaching, and actions performed.

Information that appears in brackets has been added by the authors to clarify and enhance the use of nursing diagnoses.

- Attainment or progress toward desired outcome(s).
- Modifications to plan of care.

Discharge Planning

- Long-term needs and who is responsible for actions to be taken.
- Specific referrals made.

Sample Nursing Outcomes & Interventions Classifications (NOC/NIC)

NOC—Role Performance
NIC—Role Enhancement

---

readiness for enhanced Self-Care

Taxonomy II: Activity/Rest—Class 5 Self-Care (00182)
[Diagnostic Division: Teaching/Learning]
Submitted 2006

Definition: A pattern of performing activities for oneself that helps to meet health-related goals and can be strengthened

Defining Characteristics

Subjective

Expresses desire to enhance independence in maintaining life, health, personal development, or well-being

Expresses desire to enhance self-care, knowledge for strategies for self-care, or responsibility for self-care

---

[NOTE: Based on the definition and defining characteristics of this ND, the focus appears to be broader than simply meeting routine basic activities of daily living and addresses independence in maintaining overall health, personal development, and general well-being.]

Desired Outcomes/Evaluation Criteria—Client Will:

- Maintain responsibility for planning and achieving self-care goals and general well-being.

Information that appears in brackets has been added by the authors to clarify and enhance the use of nursing diagnoses.

- Demonstrate proactive management of chronic conditions, potential complications or changes in capabilities.
- Identify and use resources appropriately.
- Remain free of preventable complications.

Actions/Interventions

Nursing Priority No. 1.

To determine current self-care status and motivation for growth:

- Determine individual strengths and skills of the client. **Establishes comparative baseline for potential growth and/or modifications in current strategies.** *Note:* **Assessment might include use of an instrument to evaluate client's current functional status, in addition to client's self-report.**
- Ascertain motivation and expectations for change.
- Note availability and use of resources, supportive person(s), assistive devices **to ascertain that client has means for sharing common concerns, needs, and wishes as well as has access to social support and approval (e.g., support group participants, family members, professionals).**
- ∞ Determine age and developmental issues, presence of medical conditions **that could impact potential for growth or interrupt client's ability to meet own needs.**
- Assess for potential barriers to enhanced participation in self-care (e.g., lack of information, insufficient time for discussion, sudden or progressive change in health status, catastrophic events).

Nursing Priority No. 2.

To assist client's/SO's plan to meet individual needs:

- Discuss client's understanding of current situation **to determine areas that can be clarified or strengthened**.
- Provide accurate and relevant information regarding current and future needs **so that client can incorporate into self-care plans, while minimizing problems associated with change.**
- Review coping skills (e.g., assertiveness, interpersonal relations, decision making, problem-solving, stigma management, time management) **that are useful in managing a wide range of stressful conditions.** Encourage client to ask for assistance, as needed or desired.

Information that appears in brackets has been added by the authors to clarify and enhance the use of nursing diagnoses.

- Promote client's/SO's participation in problem identification and decision making. **Optimizes outcomes and supports health promotion.**
- Active-listen client's/SO's concerns **to exhibit regard for client's values and beliefs, to support positive responses, and to address questions or concerns.**
- Encourage communication among those who are involved in the client's health promotion. **Periodic review allows for clarification of issues, reinforcement of successful interventions, and possibility for early intervention (where needed) to manage chronic conditions.**

Nursing Priority No. 3.

To promote optimum functioning (Teaching/Discharge Considerations):

- Assist client to set realistic goals for the future.
- Support client in making health-related decisions and pursuit of self-care practices that promote health **to foster self-esteem and support positive self-concept.**
- Identify reliable reference sources regarding individual needs and strategies for self-care. **Reinforces learning and promotes self-paced review.**
- Provide for ongoing evaluation of self-care program **to identify progress and needed changes for continuation of health, adaptation in management of limiting conditions.**
- Review safety concerns and modification of medical therapies or activities and environment, as needed, **to prevent injury and enhance successful functioning.**
- Refer to home care provider, social services, physical or occupational therapy, rehabilitation, and counseling resources, as indicated or requested, **for education, assistance, adaptive devices, and modifications that may be desired.**
- Identify additional community resources (e.g., senior services, handicap transportation van for appointments, accessible and safe locations for social or sports activities, Meals on Wheels).

Documentation Focus

Assessment/Reassessment

- Individual findings including strengths, health status, and any limitation(s).

Information that appears in brackets has been added by the authors to clarify and enhance the use of nursing diagnoses.

- Availability and use of community resources, support person(s), assistive devices.
- Motivation and expectations for change.

Planning
- Plan of care, specific interventions, and who is involved in planning.
- Teaching plan.

Implementation/Evaluation
- Client's responses to interventions, teaching, and actions performed.
- Attainment or progress toward desired outcome(s).
- Modifications to plan.

Discharge Planning
- Long-term needs and who is responsible for actions to be taken.
- Type of and source for assistive devices.
- Specific referrals made.

Sample Nursing Outcomes & Interventions Classifications (NOC/NIC)

NOC—Self-Care Status
NIC—Self-Modification Assistance

---

bathing, dressing, feeding, toileting Self-Care Deficit

Taxonomy II: Activity/Rest—Class 5 Self-Care (Bathing 00108, Dressing 00109, Feeding 00102, Toileting 00110) [Diagnostic Division: Hygiene]
Submitted 1980; Nursing Diagnosis Extension and Classification Revision 1998

Definition: Impaired ability to perform or complete bathing, dressing, feeding, or toileting activities for self.
Note: Specify level of independence using a standardized functional scale.

Information that appears in brackets has been added by the authors to clarify and enhance the use of nursing diagnoses.

NOTE: Self-care also may be expanded to include the practices used by the client to promote health, the individual responsibility for self, a way of thinking. Refer to NDs impaired Home Maintenance; ineffective Health Maintenance.

Related Factors

Cognitive or perceptual impairment
Weakness; fatigue; decreased motivation
Neuromuscular or musculoskeletal impairment
Environmental barriers; [mechanical restrictions such as cast, splint, traction, ventilator]
Severe anxiety
Pain; discomfort
Inability to perceive body part or spatial relationship [bathing]
Impaired mobility or transfer ability [self-toileting]

Defining Characteristics

bathing Self-Care Deficit

Inability to access bathroom [tub], get bath supplies, obtain water source, regulate bath water, wash or dry body

dressing Self-Care Deficit

Impaired ability to obtain clothing, put on/take off necessary items of clothing, fasten clothing, put on/take off socks or shoes

Inability to choose clothing, pick up clothing, put clothing on upper or lower body, remove clothes, put on or remove socks/shoes

Inability to use zippers or assistive devices, maintain appearance at a satisfactory level

feeding Self-Care Deficit

Inability to prepare food for ingestion, open containers

Inability to handle utensils, get food onto utensil, bring food from a receptacle to the mouth, use assistive device, pick up cup or glass

Inability to ingest food safely or in a socially acceptable manner, manipulate food in mouth, chew or swallow food, ingest sufficient food, complete a meal

---

Information that appears in brackets has been added by the authors to clarify and enhance the use of nursing diagnoses.

🌐 Cultural   🅒 Collaborative   🏠 Community/Home Care

toileting Self-Care Deficit

Inability to get to toilet or commode, manipulate clothing for toileting, sit on or rise from toilet or commode, carry out proper toilet hygiene, flush toilet or [empty] commode

Desired Outcomes/Evaluation Criteria— Client Will:

- Identify individual areas of weakness or needs.
- Verbalize knowledge of healthcare practices.
- Demonstrate techniques and lifestyle changes to meet self-care needs.
- Perform self-care activities within level of own ability.
- Identify personal and community resources that can provide assistance.

Actions/Interventions

Nursing Priority No. 1.

To identify causative/contributing factors:

- Determine age and developmental issues **affecting ability of individual to participate in own care.**
- Note concomitant medical problems or existing conditions that may be factors for care (e.g., recent trauma or surgery, heart disease, renal failure, spinal cord injury, cerebral vascular accident, multiple sclerosis, malnutrition, pain, Alzheimer's disease).
- Review medication regimen **for possible effects on alertness/ mentation, energy level, balance, perception.**
- Note other etiological factors present, including language barriers, speech impairment, visual acuity or hearing problem, emotional stability/ability. (Refer to NDs impaired verbal Communication; impaired Environmental Interpretation; risk for Unilateral Neglect; [disturbed Sensory Perception specify], for related interventions.)
- Assess barriers to participation in regimen **that can limit use of resources or choice of options (e.g., lack of information, insufficient time for discussion, psychological or intimate family problems that may be difficult to share, fear of appearing stupid or ignorant, social or economic limitations, work or home environment problems).**

Information that appears in brackets has been added by the authors to clarify and enhance the use of nursing diagnoses.

bathing, dressing, feeding, toileting SELF-CARE DEFICIT

Nursing Priority No. 2.

To assess degree of disability:

- Identify degree of individual impairment and functional level according to scale (as listed in ND impaired physical Mobility).
- Assess memory and intellectual functioning. Note developmental level to which client has regressed or progressed.
- Determine individual strengths and skills of the client.
- Note whether deficit is temporary or permanent, should decrease or increase with time.

Nursing Priority No. 3.

To assist in correcting/dealing with situation:

- Collaborate in treatment of underlying conditions **to enhance client's capabilities, maximize rehabilitation potential.**
- Provide accurate and relevant information regarding current and future needs **so that client can incorporate into self-care plans while minimizing problems (e.g., heightened anxiety, depression, resistance) often associated with change.**
- Perform or assist with meeting client's needs (e.g., personal care assistance is part of nursing care and should not be neglected while self-care independence is promoted and integrated).
- Promote client's/SO's participation in problem identification and desired goals and decision making. **Enhances commitment to plan, optimizing outcomes, and supporting recovery and/or health promotion.**
- Develop plan of care appropriate to individual situation, scheduling activities to conform to client's usual or desired schedule.
- Active-listen client's/SO(s)' concerns. **Exhibits regard for client's values and beliefs, clarifies barriers to participation in self-care, provides opportunity to work on problem-solving solutions and to provide encouragement and support.**
- Practice and promote short-term goal setting and achievement **to recognize that today's success is as important as any long-term goal, accepting ability to do one thing at a time and conceptualization of self-care in a broader sense.**
- Provide for communication among those who are involved in caring for or assisting the client. **Enhances coordination and continuity of care.**

Information that appears in brackets has been added by the authors to clarify and enhance the use of nursing diagnoses.

∞• Instruct in or review appropriate skills necessary for self-care, using terms understandable to client (e.g., child, adult, cognitively impaired person) and with sensitivity to developmental needs for practice, repetition, or reluctance. **Individualized teaching best affords reinforcement of learning. Sensitivity to special needs attaches value to the client's needs.**

• Establish remotivation or resocialization programs when indicated.

• Establish "contractual" partnership with client/SO(s), if appropriate, **for motivation or behavioral modification.**

②• Refer to and assist with rehabilitation program **to enhance client's capabilities and promote independence.**

• Provide privacy and equipment within easy reach during personal care activities.

🏠• Allow sufficient time for client to accomplish tasks to fullest extent of ability. Avoid unnecessary conversation or interruptions.

• Assist with necessary adaptations to accomplish activities of daily living. Begin with familiar, easily accomplished tasks **to encourage client and build on successes.**

②• Collaborate with rehabilitation professionals to identify and obtain assistive devices, mobility aids, and home modification as necessary (e.g., adequate lighting, visual aids; bedside commode; raised toilet seat and grab bars for bathroom; modified clothing; modified eating utensils).

• Identify energy-saving behaviors (e.g., sitting instead of standing when possible). (Refer to NDs Activity Intolerance; Fatigue, for additional interventions.)

🏠• Implement bowel or bladder training program, as indicated. (Refer to NDs Constipation; bowel Incontinence; impaired Urinary Elimination, for appropriate interventions.)

• Encourage food and fluid choices reflecting individual likes and abilities that meet nutritional needs. Provide assistive devices or alternate feeding methods, as appropriate. (Refer to ND impaired Swallowing for related interventions.)

⚖• Assist with medication regimen as necessary, encouraging timely use of medications (e.g., taking diuretics in morning when client is more awake and able to manage toileting, use of pain relievers prior to activity to facilitate movement, postponing intake of medications that cause sedation until self-care activities completed).

🏠• Make home visit, as indicated **to assess environmental and discharge needs.**

Information that appears in brackets has been added by the authors to clarify and enhance the use of nursing diagnoses.

Nursing Priority No. 4.

To meet specific self-care needs:

Bathing deficit

🏠 • Ask client/SO for input on bathing habits or cultural bathing
⊕   preferences. **Creates opportunities for client to (1) keep
    long-standing routines (e.g., bathing at bedtime to im-
    prove sleep) and (2) exercise control over situation. This
    enhances self-esteem, while respecting personal and cul-
    tural preferences.**

• Bathe or assist client in bathing, providing for any or all hygiene needs as indicated. **Type (e.g., bed bath, towel bath,
  tub bath, shower) and purpose (e.g., cleansing, removing
  odor, or simply soothing agitation) of bath is determined
  by individual need.**

• Obtain hygiene supplies (e.g., soap, toothpaste, toothbrush,
  mouthwash, lotion, shampoo, razor, towels) for specific activity to be performed and place in client's easy reach **to provide visual cues and facilitate completion of activity.**

• Ascertain that all safety equipment is in place and properly
  installed (e.g., grab bars, antislip strips, shower chair, hydraulic lift) and that client/caregiver(s) can safely operate equipment.

• Instruct client to request assistance when needed and place
  call device within easy reach, or stay with client as dictated
  by safety needs.

∞ • Provide for adequate warmth (e.g., covering client during bed
  bath or warming bathroom). **Certain individuals (especially
  infants, the elderly, and very thin or debilitated persons)
  are prone to hypothermia and can experience evaporative
  cooling during and after bathing.**

• Determine that client can perceive water temperature, adjust
  water temperature safely, or that water is correct temperature
  for client's bath or shower **to prevent chilling or burns. This
  step requires that client is cognitively and physically able
  to perceive hot and cold and to adjust faucets safely.**

• Assist client in and out of shower or tub as indicated.

• Provide for or assist with grooming activities (e.g., shaving,
  hair care, cleaning and clipping nails, makeup) on a routine,
  consistent basis. Encourage participation, guiding client's
  hand through tasks, as indicated. **Experiencing the normal
  process of a task through established routine and guided
  practice facilitates optimal relearning.**

Information that appears in brackets has been added by the authors to clarify
and enhance the use of nursing diagnoses.

⊕ Cultural ⊛ Collaborative 🏠 Community/Home Care

Dressing deficit

🏠• Ascertain that appropriate clothing is available. **Clothing may need to be modified for client's particular medical condition or physical limitations.**

• Assist client in choosing clothing or lay out clothing as indicated.

• Dress client or assist with dressing, as indicated. **Client may need assistance in putting on or taking off items of clothing (e.g., shoes and socks, or over-the-head shirt) or may require partial or complete assistance with fasteners (e.g., buttons, snaps, zippers, shoelaces).**

• Allow sufficient time for dressing and undressing.

• Use adaptive clothing as indicated (e.g., clothing with front closure, wide sleeves and pant legs, Velcro or zipper closures). **These may be helpful for client with limited arm or leg movement or impaired fine motor skills or cognitively impaired person who desires to dress self but cannot do so with regular clothing fasteners.**

• Teach client to dress affected side first, then unaffected side (when client has paralysis or injury to one side of body).

Feeding deficit

🏠• Assess client's need and ability to prepare food as indicated (including shopping, cooking, cutting food, opening containers, etc.).

• Encourage food and fluid choices reflecting individual likes and abilities and that meet nutritional needs **to maximize food intake.**

• Ascertain that client can swallow safely, checking gag and swallow reflexes, as indicated. (Refer to ND impaired Swallowing for related interventions.)

• Provide food and fluid of appropriate consistency **to facilitate swallowing.** Cut food into bite-size pieces **to prevent overfilling mouth and reduce risk of choking.**

• Assist client to handle utensils or in guiding utensils to mouth. **May require specialized equipment (e.g., rocker knife, plate guard, built-up handles) to increase independence or assistance with movement of arms and hands.**

• Assist client with small cup, glass, or bottle for liquids, using straw or adaptive lids as indicated **to enhance fluid intake while reducing spills.**

• Allow client time for intake of sufficient food **for feeling satisfied or completing a meal.**

Information that appears in brackets has been added by the authors to clarify and enhance the use of nursing diagnoses.

- Assist client with social graces when eating with others; provide privacy when manners might be offensive to others or client could be embarrassed.
- Collaborate with nutritionist, speech-language pathologist, occupational therapist, or physician **for special diets or feeding methods necessary to provide adequate nutrition.**
- Feed client, allowing adequate time for chewing and swallowing, **when client is not able to obtain nutrition by self-feeding.** Avoid providing fluids until client has swallowed food and mouth is clear. **Prevents "washing down" foods, reducing risk of choking.**

Toileting deficit
- Provide mobility assistance to bathroom or commode or place on bedpan or offer urinal, as indicated.
- Direct or accompany cognitively impaired client to bathroom, as needed.
- Observe for behaviors such as pacing, fidgeting, holding crotch **that may be indicative of need for prompt toileting.**
- Provide privacy **that may be indicative of need for prompt toileting.**
- Assist with manipulation of clothing, if needed, **to decrease incidence of functional incontinence caused by difficulty removing clothing/underwear.**
- Observe need for and assist in obtaining modified clothing or fasteners **to assist client in manipulation of clothing, fostering independence in self-toileting.**
- Provide or assist with use of assistive equipment (e.g., raised toilet seat, support rails, spill-proof urinals, fracture pans, bedside commode) **to promote independence and safety in sitting down or arising from toilet or for aiding elimination when client is unable to go to bathroom.**
- Keep toilet paper or wipes and hand-washing items within client's easy reach.
- Implement bowel or bladder training/retraining programs as indicated.

Nursing Priority No. 5.
To promote wellness (Teaching/Discharge Considerations):
- Assist the client to become aware of rights and responsibilities in health and healthcare and to assess own health strengths— physical, emotional, and intellectual.
- Support client in making health-related decisions and assist in developing self-care practices and goals that promote health.

Information that appears in brackets has been added by the authors to clarify and enhance the use of nursing diagnoses.

- Provide for ongoing evaluation of self-care program, identifying progress and needed changes.
- Review and modify program periodically to accommodate changes in client's abilities. **Assists client to adhere to plan of care to fullest extent.**
- Encourage keeping a journal of progress and practicing of independent living skills **to foster self-care and self-determination.**
- Review safety concerns. Modify activities or environment **to reduce risk of injury and promote successful community functioning.**
- Refer to home care provider, social services, physical or occupational therapy, rehabilitation, and counseling resources, as indicated.
- Identify additional community resources (e.g., senior services, Meals on Wheels).
- Review instructions from other members of healthcare team and provide written copy. **Provides clarification, reinforcement; allows periodic review by client/caregivers.**
- Give family information about respite or other care options. **Allows them free time away from the care situation to renew themselves.** (Refer to ND Caregiver Role Strain for additional interventions.)
- Assist and support family with alternative placements as necessary. **Enhances likelihood of finding individually appropriate situation to meet client's needs.**
- Be available for discussion of feelings about situation (e.g., grieving, anger) **Provides opportunity for client/family to get feelings out in the open and begin to problem-solve solutions as indicated.**
- Refer to NDs risk for Falls; risk for Injury; ineffective Coping; compromised family Coping; risk for Disuse Syndrome; situational low Self-Esteem; impaired physical Mobility; Powerlessness, as appropriate.

Documentation Focus

Assessment/Reassessment

- Individual findings, functional level, and specifics of limitation(s).
- Needed resources and adaptive devices.
- Availability and use of community resources.
- Who is involved in care or provides assistance.

Information that appears in brackets has been added by the authors to clarify and enhance the use of nursing diagnoses.

Planning
* Plan of care and who is involved in planning.
* Teaching plan.

Implementation/Evaluation
* Response to interventions, teaching, and actions performed.
* Attainment or progress toward desired outcome(s).
* Modifications of plan of care.

Discharge Planning
* Long-term needs and who is responsible for actions to be taken.
* Type of and source for assistive devices.
* Specific referrals made.

Sample Nursing Outcomes & Interventions Classifications (NOC/NIC)

Bathing Deficit
NOC—Self-Care: Bathing
NIC—Self-Care Assistance: Bathing/Hygiene

Dressing Deficit
NOC—Self-Care: Dressing
NIC—Self-Care Assistance: Dressing/Grooming

Feeding Deficit
NOC—Self-Care: Eating
NIC—Self-Care Assistance: Feeding

Toileting Deficit
NOC—Self-Care: Toileting
NIC—Self-Care Assistance: Toileting

---

readiness for enhanced Self-Concept

Taxonomy II: Self-Perception—Class 1 Self-Concept (00167)
[Diagnostic Division: Ego Integrity]
Submitted 2002

Definition: A pattern of perceptions or ideas about the self that is sufficient for well-being and can be strengthened

---

Information that appears in brackets has been added by the authors to clarify and enhance the use of nursing diagnoses.

Defining Characteristics

Subjective

Expresses willingness to enhance self-concept
Accepts strengths, limitations
Expresses confidence in abilities
Expresses satisfaction with thoughts about self, sense of worthiness
Expresses satisfaction with body image, personal identity, role performance

Objective

Actions are congruent with verbal expressions

Desired Outcomes/Evaluation Criteria—Client Will:

- Verbalize understanding of own sense of self-concept.
- Participate in programs and activities to enhance self-esteem.
- Demonstrate behaviors and lifestyle changes to promote positive self-esteem.
- Participate in family, group, or community activities to enhance self-concept.

Actions/Interventions

Nursing Priority No. 1.

To assess current situation and desire for improvement:

- Determine current status of individual's belief about self. **Self-concept consists of the physical self (body image), the personal self (identity), and self-esteem. Information about client's current thinking about self provides a beginning for making changes to improve self.**
- Determine availability and quality of family/SO(s) support. **Presence of supportive people who reflect positive attitudes regarding the individual promotes a positive sense of self.**
- Identify family dynamics—present and past. **Self-esteem begins in early childhood and is influenced by perceptions of how the individual is viewed by SOs. Provides information about family functioning that will help to develop plan of care for enhancing client's self-concept.**
- Note willingness to seek assistance and motivation for change. **Individuals who have a sense of their own**

Information that appears in brackets has been added by the authors to clarify and enhance the use of nursing diagnoses.

self-image and are willing to look at themselves realistically will be able to progress in the desire to improve.

- Determine client's concept of self in relation to cultural or religious ideals and beliefs. **Cultural characteristics are learned in the family of origin and shape how the individual views self.**

- Observe nonverbal behaviors and note congruence with verbal expressions. Discuss cultural meanings of nonverbal communication. **Incongruencies between verbal and nonverbal communication require clarification. Interpretation of nonverbal expressions is culturally determined and needs to be clarified to avoid misinterpretation.**

Nursing Priority No. 2.

To facilitate personal growth:

- Develop therapeutic relationship. Be attentive, maintain open communication, use skills of Active-listening and I-messages. **Promotes trusting situation in which client is free to be open and honest with self and others.**

- Validate client's communication, provide encouragement for efforts.

- Accept client's perceptions or view of current status. **Provides opportunity for client to develop realistic plan for improving self-concept, while feeling safe in existing view of self.**

- Be aware that people are not programmed to be rational. **Individuals must seek information, choosing to learn, and to think rather than merely to accept or react in order to have respect for self, facts, and honesty and to develop positive self-esteem.**

- Discuss client perception of self, confronting misconceptions and identifying negative self-talk. Address distortions in thinking, such as self-referencing (beliefs that others are focusing on individual's weaknesses or limitations); filtering (focusing on negative and ignoring positive); catastrophizing (expecting the worst outcomes). **Addressing these issues openly allows client to identify things that may negatively affect self-esteem and provides opportunity for change.**

- Have client list current and past successes and strengths. **Emphasizes fact that client is and has been successful in many actions taken.**

- Use positive I-messages rather than praise. **Praise is a form of external control, coming from outside sources, whereas**

Information that appears in brackets has been added by the authors to clarify and enhance the use of nursing diagnoses.

readiness for enhanced SELF-CONCEPT

Cultural Collaborative Community/Home Care

I-messages allow the client to develop internal sense of self-esteem.

- Discuss what behavior does for client (positive intention). Ask what options are available to the client/SO(s). **Encourages thinking about what inner motivations are and what actions can be taken to enhance self-esteem.**

- Give reinforcement for progress noted. **Positive words of encouragement support development of effective coping behaviors.**

- Encourage client to progress at own rate. **Adaptation to a change in self-concept depends on its significance to the individual and disruption to lifestyle.**

- Involve in activities or exercise program of choice, promote socialization. **Enhances sense of well-being and can help to energize client.**

Nursing Priority No. 3.

To promote optimum sense of self-worth and happiness:

- Assist client to identify goals that are personally achievable. Provide positive feedback for verbal and behavioral indications of improved self-view. **Increases likelihood of success and commitment to change.**

- Refer to vocational or employment counselor, educational resources, as appropriate. **Assists with improving development of social or vocational skills.**

- Encourage participation in classes, activities, or hobbies that client enjoys or would like to experience. **Provides opportunity for learning new information and skills that can enhance feelings of success, improving self-esteem.**

- Reinforce that current decision to improve self-concept is ongoing. **Continued work and support are necessary to sustain behavior changes and personal growth.**

- Discuss ways to develop optimism. **Optimism is a key ingredient in happiness and can be learned.**

- Suggest assertiveness training classes. **Enhances ability to interact with others and develop more effective relationships, enhancing one's self-concept.**

- Emphasize importance of grooming and personal hygiene and assist in developing skills to improve appearance and dress for success as needed. **Looking one's best improves sense of self-esteem, and presenting a positive appearance enhances how others see one.**

Information that appears in brackets has been added by the authors to clarify and enhance the use of nursing diagnoses.

Documentation Focus

Assessment/Reassessment
- Individual findings, including evaluations of self and others, current and past successes.
- Interactions with others, lifestyle.
- Motivation for and willingness to change.

Planning
- Plan of care and who is involved in planning.
- Educational plan.

Implementation/Evaluation
- Responses to interventions, teaching, and actions performed.
- Attainment or progress toward desired outcome(s).
- Modifications to plan of care.

Discharge Planning
- Long-term needs and who is responsible for actions to be taken.
- Specific referrals made.

Sample Nursing Outcomes & Interventions Classifications (NOC/NIC)

NOC—Self-Esteem
NIC—Self-Modification Assistance

chronic low Self-Esteem

Taxonomy II: Self-Perception—Class 2 Self-Esteem (00119)
[Diagnostic Division: Ego Integrity]
Submitted 1988; Revised 1996, 2008

Definition: Long-standing negative self-evaluation/feelings about self or self-capabilities

Related Factors

Repeated negative reinforcement, failures
Lack of affection, approval, or membership in group
Perceived lack of belonging or respect from others
Perceived discrepancy between self and cultural or spiritual norms

---

Information that appears in brackets has been added by the authors to clarify and enhance the use of nursing diagnoses.

🔵 Cultural   🌀 Collaborative   🏠 Community/Home Care

Traumatic event or situation
Ineffective adaptation to loss
Psychiatric disorders

Defining Characteristics

Subjective
Reports feelings of shame or guilt
Evaluation of self as unable to deal with events
Rejects positive or exaggerates negative feedback about self

Objective
Hesitant to try new things or situations
Frequent lack of success in life events
Exaggerates negative feedback about self
Overly conforming; dependent on others' opinions
Lack of eye contact
Nonassertive or indecisive behavior; passive
Excessively seeks reassurance

Desired Outcomes/Evaluation Criteria— Client Will:

- Verbalize understanding of negative evaluation of self and reasons for this problem.
- Participate in treatment program to promote change in self-evaluation.
- Demonstrate behaviors and lifestyle changes to promote positive self-image.
- Verbalize increased sense of self-worth in relation to current situation.
- Participate in family, group, or community activities to enhance change.

Actions/Interventions

Nursing Priority No. 1.
To assess causative/contributing factors:

- Determine factors of low self-esteem related to current situation (e.g., family crises, physical disfigurement, social isolation), noting age and developmental level of individual. **Current crises may exacerbate long-standing feelings and perception of self-evaluation as not being worthwhile.**

Information that appears in brackets has been added by the authors to clarify and enhance the use of nursing diagnoses.

- Assess content of negative self-talk. Note client's perceptions of how others view him or her.
- Determine availability and quality of family/SO(s) support.
- Identify family dynamics—present and past—and cultural influences. **Family may engage in "put-downs" or "teasing" in ways that give client the message that he or she is worthless.**
- Be alert to client's concept of self in relation to cultural/religious ideal(s).
- Note nonverbal behavior (e.g., nervous movements, lack of eye contact). **Incongruencies between verbal/nonverbal communication require clarification.**
- Determine degree of participation and cooperation with therapeutic regimen (e.g., maintaining scheduled medications such as antidepressants/antipsychotics).
- Ascertain willingness to seek assistance, desire for change.

Nursing Priority No. 2.

To promote client sense of self-esteem in dealing with current situation:

- Develop therapeutic relationship. Be attentive, validate client's communication, provide encouragement for efforts, maintain open communication, use skills of Active-listening and I-messages. **Promotes trusting situation in which client is free to be open and honest with self and therapist.**
- Address presenting medical/safety issues.
- Accept client's perceptions or view of situation. Avoid threatening existing self-esteem.
- Be aware that people are not programmed to be rational. **To have respect for self, facts, honesty, and to develop positive self-esteem, one must seek information, choosing to learn, and to think, rather than merely accepting/reacting.**
- Discuss client perceptions of self related to what is happening; confront misconceptions and negative self-talk. Address distortions in thinking, such as self-referencing (belief that others are focusing on individual's weaknesses/limitations), filtering (focusing on negative and ignoring positive), catastrophizing (expecting the worst outcomes). **Addressing these issues openly provides opportunity for change.**
- Emphasize need to avoid comparing self with others. Encourage client to focus on aspects of self that can be valued.
- Have client review past successes and strengths. **May help client see that he or she can develop an internal locus of**

Information that appears in brackets has been added by the authors to clarify and enhance the use of nursing diagnoses.

control (a belief that one's successes and failures are the result of one's efforts).

- Use positive I-messages rather than praise. **Assists client to develop internal sense of self-esteem.**
- Discuss what a given behavior does for client (positive intention). What options are available to the client/SO(s)?
- Assist client to deal with sense of powerlessness. (Refer to ND Powerlessness.)
- Set limits on aggressive or problem behaviors such as acting out, suicide preoccupation, or rumination. Put self in client's place (empathy not sympathy). **These negative behaviors diminish sense of self-concept.**
- Give reinforcement for progress noted. **Positive words of encouragement promote continuation of efforts, supporting development of coping behaviors.**
- Encourage client to progress at own rate. **Adaptation to a change in self-concept depends on its significance to individual, disruption to lifestyle, and length of illness/debilitation.**
- Assist client to recognize and cope with events, alterations, and sense of loss of control by incorporating changes accurately into self-concept.
- Involve in activities or exercise program, promote socialization. **Enhances sense of well-being/can help energize client.**

Nursing Priority No. 3.
🏠 To promote wellness (Teaching/Discharge Considerations):

- Discuss inaccuracies in self-perception with client/SO(s).
- Model behaviors being taught, involving client in goal setting and decision making. **Facilitates client's developing trust in own unique strengths.**
- Prepare client for events/changes that are expected, when possible **to provide opportunity for client to prepare self, or reduce negative reactions associated with the unknown.**
- Provide structure in daily routine/care activities.
- Emphasize importance of grooming and personal hygiene. Assist in developing skills as indicated (e.g., makeup classes, dressing for success). **People feel better about themselves when they present a positive outer appearance.**
- Assist client to identify goals that are personally achievable. **Increases likelihood of success and commitment to change.**
- Provide positive feedback for verbal and behavioral indications of improved self-view.

Information that appears in brackets has been added by the authors to clarify and enhance the use of nursing diagnoses.

- Refer to vocational or employment counselor, educational resources, as appropriate. **Assists with development of social or vocational skills, enhancing sense of self-concept and inner locus of control.**
- Encourage participation in class, activities, or hobbies that client enjoys or would like to experience.
- Reinforce that this therapy is a brief encounter in overall life of the client/SO(s), with continued work and ongoing support being necessary **to sustain behavior changes and personal growth.**
- Refer to classes (e.g., assertiveness training, positive self-image, communication skills) **to assist with learning new skills to promote self-esteem.**
- Refer to counseling, therapy, mental health, or special-needs support groups, as indicated.

Documentation Focus

Assessment/Reassessment

- Individual findings, including early memories of negative evaluations (self and others), subsequent or precipitating failure events.
- Effects on interactions with others, lifestyle.
- Specific medical and safety issues.
- Motivation for and willingness to change.

Planning

- Plan of care and who is involved in planning.
- Teaching plan.

Implementation/Evaluation

- Responses to interventions, teaching, and actions performed.
- Attainment or progress toward desired outcome(s).
- Modifications to plan of care.

Discharge Planning

- Long-term needs and who is responsible for actions to be taken.
- Specific referrals made.

Sample Nursing Outcomes & Interventions Classifications (NOC/NIC)

NOC—Self-Esteem
NIC—Self-Esteem Enhancement

Information that appears in brackets has been added by the authors to clarify and enhance the use of nursing diagnoses.

● Cultural ● Collaborative ▲ Community/Home Care

situational low Self-Esteem

Taxonomy II: Self-Perception—Class 2 Self-Esteem
(00120)
[Diagnostic Division: Ego Integrity]
Submitted 1988; Revised 1996, 2000

Definition: Development of a negative perception of self-worth in response to a current situation

Related Factors

Developmental changes
Functional impairment; disturbed body image
Loss
Social role changes
Failures; rejections; lack of recognition
Behavior inconsistent with values

Defining Characteristics

Subjective

Reports current situational challenge to self-worth
Reports helplessness or uselessness
Evaluation of self as unable to deal with situations or events

Objective

Self-negating verbalizations
Indecisive or nonassertive behavior

Desired Outcomes/Evaluation Criteria— Client Will:

- Verbalize understanding of individual factors that precipitated current situation.
- Identify feelings and underlying dynamics for negative perception of self.
- Express positive self-appraisal.
- Demonstrate behaviors to restore positive self-esteem.
- Participate in treatment regimen or activities to correct factors that precipitated crisis.

Information that appears in brackets has been added by the authors to clarify and enhance the use of nursing diagnoses.

Nursing Priority No. 1.

To assess causative/contributing factors:

- Determine individual situation (e.g., family crisis, termination of a relationship, loss of employment, physical disfigurement) related to low self-esteem in the present circumstances.
- Identify client's basic sense of self-esteem and image client has of self: existential, physical, psychological.
- Assess degree of threat and perception of client in regard to crisis. **One individual views a serious situation as manageable, while another individual may be overly concerned about a minor problem.**
- Ascertain sense of control client has (or perceives self to have) over self and situation. Note client's locus of control (internal or external). **Important in determining whether the client believes he or she has control over the situation or whether one is at the mercy of fate or luck.**
- Determine client's awareness of own responsibility for dealing with situation, personal growth, and so forth. **When client is aware of and accepts own responsibility, may indicate internal locus of control.**
- Verify client's concept of self in relation to cultural/religious ideals. **May provide client with support or reinforce negative self-evaluation.**
- Review past coping skills in relation to current episode.
- Assess negative attitudes and/or self-talk.
- Note nonverbal body language. **Incongruencies between verbal and nonverbal communication require clarification.**
- Assess for self-destructive or suicidal behavior. (Refer to ND risk for Suicide, as appropriate.)
- Identify previous adaptations to illness or disruptive events in life. **May be predictive of current outcome.**
- Assess family/SO(s) dynamics and support of client.
- Note availability and use of resources.

Nursing Priority No. 2.

To assist client to deal with loss/change and recapture sense of positive self-esteem:

- Assist with treatment of underlying condition when possible. **For example, cognitive restructuring and improved con-**

───────────

Information that appears in brackets has been added by the authors to clarify and enhance the use of nursing diagnoses.

⊕ Cultural ⊛ Collaborative 🏠 Community/Home Care

centration in mild brain injury often result in restoration of positive self-esteem.

- Encourage expression of feelings, anxieties. **Facilitates grieving the loss.**
- Active-listen client's concerns and negative verbalizations without comment or judgment.
- Identify individual strengths and assets and aspects of self that remain intact and can be valued. Reinforce positive traits, abilities, self-view.
- Help client identify own responsibility and control or lack of control in situation. **When able to acknowledge what is out of his or her control, client can focus attention on area of own responsibility.**
- Assist client to problem-solve situation, developing plan of action and setting goals to achieve desired outcome. **Enhances commitment to plan, optimizing outcomes.**
- Convey confidence in client's ability to cope with current situation.
- Mobilize support systems.
- Provide opportunity for client to practice alternative coping strategies, including progressive socialization opportunities.
- Encourage use of visualization, guided imagery, and relaxation **to promote positive sense of self.**
- Provide feedback of client's self-negating remarks or behavior, using I-messages, **to allow the client to experience a different view.**
- Encourage involvement in decisions about care when possible.

Nursing Priority No. 3.
To promote wellness (Teaching/Discharge Considerations):

- Encourage client to set long-range goals for achieving necessary lifestyle changes. **Supports view that this is an ongoing process.**
- Support independence in activities of daily living or mastery of therapeutic regimen. **Confident individual is more secure and positive in self-appraisal.**
- Promote attendance in therapy or support group, as indicated.
- Involve extended family/SO(s) in treatment plan. **Increases likelihood they will provide appropriate support to client.**
- Provide information to assist client in making desired changes. **Appropriate books, DVDs, or other resources allow client to learn at own pace.**

Information that appears in brackets has been added by the authors to clarify and enhance the use of nursing diagnoses.

- Suggest participation in group or community activities (e.g., assertiveness classes, volunteer work, support groups).

Documentation Focus

Assessment/Reassessment

- Individual findings, noting precipitating crisis, client's perceptions, effects on desired lifestyle/interaction with others.
- Cultural values or religious beliefs, locus of control.
- Family support, availability and use of resources.

Planning

- Plan of care and who is involved in planning.
- Teaching plan.

Implementation/Evaluation

- Responses to interventions, teaching, actions performed, and changes that may be indicated.
- Attainment or progress toward desired outcome(s).
- Modifications to plan of care.

Discharge Planning

- Long-term needs and goals and who is responsible for actions to be taken.
- Specific referrals made.

Sample Nursing Outcomes & Interventions Classifications (NOC/NIC)

NOC—Self-Esteem
NIC—Self-Esteem Enhancement

---

risk for chronic low **Self-Esteem**

Taxonomy II: Self-Perception—Class 2 Self-Esteem (00224)
[Diagnostic Division: Ego Integrity]
Submitted 2010

Definition: At risk for long-standing negative self-evaluating/feelings about self or self-capabilities

---

Information that appears in brackets has been added by the authors to clarify and enhance the use of nursing diagnoses.

Risk Factors

Traumatic event/situation
Repeated failures/negative reinforcement
Ineffective adaptation to loss
Perceived lack of belonging or respect from others
Lack of affection
Lack of membership in group
Perceived discrepancy between self and cultural or spiritual
    norms
Psychiatric disorder

Desired Outcomes/Evaluation Criteria— Client Will (Include Specific Time Frame):

- Acknowledge understanding of discrepancy between self and cultural/spiritual norms.
- Participate in therapy program to improve self-esteem.
- Demonstrate behaviors to change negative self-evaluation.
- Verbalize understanding of reason for failures and how to make changes for success.
- Participate in family, group, or community activities to enhance change.

Actions/Interventions

Nursing Priority No. 1.

To assess causative/contributing factors:

- ∞ Note age and developmental level of client and circumstances surrounding current situation. **Younger people may not have learned skills to deal with negative occurrences and/or rejection from others.**
- Elicit client's perceptions of current situation.
- Determine client's awareness of self-destructive behavior, acting out, aggression, suicidal thoughts. **Choices individual makes result from low self-esteem and pleasing others and lead to feelings of worthlessness.**
- Determine content of negative self-talk and client's perception of how others see him or her. **As negative thoughts are repeated in one's head, they become the basis for believing that the individual is indeed worthless and others must agree with that conclusion.**
- Observe nonverbal behavior (e.g., nervous movements, lack of eye contact) and how it relates to verbal statements.

Information that appears in brackets has been added by the authors to clarify and enhance the use of nursing diagnoses.

Incongruence between verbal and nonverbal needs to be clarified to be sure perceived meaning of communication is accurate.

- Note religious and cultural factors that have influenced client. **Family of origin affects how one views self in relation to family members and others in society. For instance, Islamic families tend to be patriarchal, with the father exercising unmitigated power over female family members and making all decisions for them.**

- Determine family makeup and whether they are available and supportive. **Support of family is essential to client's self-esteem. Individual's predominant worldview (positive or negative) is determined by the time he/she is 5 years of age.**

- Note family dynamics and how client interacts within the family. **Crucial to individual's development and self-esteem in a positive or negative way.**

- Evaluate current medication regimen noting client adherence. **Maintaining therapeutic regimen requires ongoing evaluation to determine efficacy or need for change.**

Nursing Priority No. 2.

To promote client's sense of self-esteem in dealing with changes in life:

- Establish therapeutic nurse/client relationship, maintaining open communication and using Active-listening and I-messages. **Promotes a trusting environment in which client is free to talk about potential problems that may arise.**

- Determine willingness to improve attitudes and sense of self. **Negative perceptions, sense of alienation, and lack of involvement in positive activities lead to sense of worthlessness. Making a commitment to change provides an opportunity to learn new ways to interact with others and choose activities that promote individual successes.**

- Address possible situations that client may be facing. **Sense of loss, lack of involvement in group, traumatic event, repeated failures in attempts to change situation may discourage client from wanting to try to make life better.**

- Avoid challenging client's perception of events. **May threaten sense of self-esteem, limiting client's ability to check out perceptions and make own corrections.**

- Reinforce that people are not programmed to be rational. **They must seek information, choosing to learn and think, rather than merely accepting or reacting, in order to have respect for self and develop positive self-esteem.**

Information that appears in brackets has been added by the authors to clarify and enhance the use of nursing diagnoses.

🌐 Cultural   ✪ Collaborative   🏠 Community/Home Care

- Discuss misperceptions and negative self-talk as well as distortions in thinking, such as self-referencing (belief that others are focusing on person's weaknesses or limitations, filtering (focusing on negative and ignoring positive), or catastrophizing (believing the worst will happen). **These issues keep individual believing in a negative, worthless view of self and need to be addressed before person can move on and improve life.**
- Discuss the problem of comparing self to others. Encourage client to focus on own positive aspects. **These actions will help individual to change negative thinking.**
- List current and previous successes. **Focusing on these can help the client realize that failures can be overcome.**
- Provide positive feedback, for verbal and behavioral indications of improved self-view, using I-messages instead of praise. **Praise can be interpreted as insincere and manipulative and be rejected. Positive I-messages convey a sense of acceptance and let the individual feel good about self, enhancing self-esteem and encouraging individual to continue efforts.**
- Ask client to think about what behavior does (positive intention) in relation to low self-esteem, reluctance to join groups, and seeing self as less than others. **As individual thinks about this aspect of behavior, awareness of having a choice to change life may help to make positive changes.**
- Discuss feelings of powerlessness. Refer to ND Powerlessness [specify level].
- Contract with client/set limits on acting out, aggressive or self-destructive behaviors. Refer to NDs risk for other-/self-directed Violence; risk for Suicide, for additional interventions.
- Encourage client to progress at own pace, providing reinforcement as progress is made. **Helps individual to value self and believe life changes can be made.**
- Promote socialization, involving in exercise and activity programs. **Helps to realize involvement with others can lead to positive feelings about self.**

Nursing Priority No. 3.

To promote wellness (Teaching/Discharge Considerations):

- Involve client in goal setting and decision making. **Facilitates trust and belief that change can be made and life can improve.**

Information that appears in brackets has been added by the authors to clarify and enhance the use of nursing diagnoses.

- Encourage client to structure daily activities so routine becomes manageable. **Promotes a sense of control and belief in own abilities.**
- Discuss importance of grooming and personal hygiene, being involved in classes (i.e., Dress for Success). **Others often judge an individual by the outward appearance presented, as well as individual's own positive appraisal and sense of confidence.**
- Refer to educational resources, vocational or employment counselor, as indicated.
- Identify support groups and classes, such as assertiveness, parenting as appropriate.

Documentation Focus

Assessment/Reassessment
- Individual findings, noting risk factors, client's perceptions, and interaction with others.
- Cultural values or religious beliefs, locus of control.
- Family support, availability and use of resources.

Planning
- Plan of care and who is involved in planning.
- Individual teaching plan.

Implementation/Evaluation
- Response to interventions, teaching, actions performed, and changes that may be indicated.
- Attainment or progress toward desired outcomes.
- Modification to plan of care.

Discharge Planning
- Long-term needs and goals and who is responsible for actions to be taken.
- Specific referrals made.

Sample Nursing Outcomes & Interventions Classifications (NOC/NIC)

NOC—Self-Esteem
NIC—Self-Esteem Enhancement

Information that appears in brackets has been added by the authors to clarify and enhance the use of nursing diagnoses.

🌐 Cultural   ♲ Collaborative   🏠 Community/Home Care

risk for situational low Self-Esteem

Taxonomy II: Self-Perception—Class 2 Self-Esteem
(00153)
[Diagnostic Division: Ego Integrity]
Submitted 2000

Definition: At risk for developing a negative perception
of self-worth in response to a current situation

Risk Factors

Developmental changes
Disturbed body image; functional impairment
Loss
Social role changes
Unrealistic self-expectations; history of learned helplessness
History of neglect, abuse, abandonment
Behavior inconsistent with values
Lack of recognition; failures; rejections
Decreased control over environment
Physical illness

> **NOTE:** A risk diagnosis is not evidenced by signs and
> symptoms, as the problem has not occurred; rather,
> nursing interventions are directed at prevention.

Desired Outcomes/Evaluation Criteria—Client Will:

- Acknowledge factors that lead to possibility of feelings of low
  self-esteem.
- Verbalize view of self as a worthwhile, important person who
  functions well both interpersonally and occupationally.
- Demonstrate self-confidence by setting realistic goals and actively participating in life situation.

Actions/Interventions

Nursing Priority No. 1.

To assess causative/contributing factors:

- Determine individual factors that could contribute to diminished self-esteem.

Information that appears in brackets has been added by the authors to clarify
and enhance the use of nursing diagnoses.

- Identify client's basic sense of self-worth and image client has of self: existential, physical, psychological.
- Note client's perception of threat to self in current situation.
- Ascertain sense of control client has (or perceives to have) over self and situation.
- Determine client awareness of own responsibility for dealing with situation, personal growth, and so forth.
- Verify client's concept of self in relation to cultural or religious ideals. **Conflict between current situation and these ideals may contribute to risk of low self-esteem.**
- Assess negative attitudes and/or self-talk. **Contributes to view of situation as hopeless, difficult.**
- Note nonverbal body language. **Incongruencies between verbal and nonverbal communication require clarification.**
- Listen for self-destructive/suicidal verbalizations, noting behaviors that indicate these thoughts. **Necessitates intervention to prevent client following through on thoughts.**
- Identify previous adaptations to illness/disruptive events in life. **May be predictive of current outcome.**
- Assess family/SO(s) dynamics and support of client.
- Note availability and use of resources.

Nursing Priority No. 2.

To assist client to deal with loss/change and maintain sense of positive self-esteem:

- Encourage expression of feelings, anxieties. **Facilitates grieving the loss.**
- Active-listen client's concerns without comment or judgment.
- Help client identify individual strengths and assets, reinforcing positive traits and self-view.
- Assist client to problem-solve situation and develop plan of action.
- Convey confidence in client's ability to cope with current situation.
- Mobilize appropriate support systems.

Nursing Priority No. 3.

To promote wellness (Teaching/Discharge Considerations):

- Provide information to assist client in making desired changes. **Appropriate books, DVDs, or Internet resources allow client to learn at own pace.**

Information that appears in brackets has been added by the authors to clarify and enhance the use of nursing diagnoses.

🌐 Cultural   ✪ Collaborative   🏠 Community/Home Care

- Suggest participation in group or community activities, volunteer work **that can provide opportunity for success and positive feedback for accomplishments.**
- Involve SOs/extended family in treatment plan. **Increases likelihood they will provide appropriate support to client.**
- Promote attendance in therapy or support groups as indicated.

Documentation Focus

Assessment/Reassessment
- Individual findings, including individual expressions of lack of self-esteem, effects on interactions with others or lifestyle.
- Underlying dynamics and duration of current situation.
- Past history of self-esteem issues.
- Cultural values or religious beliefs, locus of control.
- Family support, availability and use of resources.

Planning
- Plan of care and who is involved in planning.
- Teaching plan.

Implementation/Evaluation
- Responses to interventions, teaching, actions performed, and changes that may be indicated.
- Attainment or progress toward desired outcome(s).
- Modifications to plan of care.

Discharge Planning
- Long-term needs, goals, and who is responsible for actions to be taken.
- Specific referrals made.

Sample Nursing Outcomes & Interventions Classifications (NOC/NIC)

NOC—Self-Esteem
NIC—Self-Esteem Enhancement

Information that appears in brackets has been added by the authors to clarify and enhance the use of nursing diagnoses.

ineffective Self-Health Management

Taxonomy II: Health Promotion—Class 2 Health Management (00078)
[Diagnostic Division: Teaching/Learning]
Submitted 1994; Revised 2008

Definition: Pattern of regulating and integrating into daily living a therapeutic regimen for treatment of illness and its sequelae that is unsatisfactory for meeting specific health goals

Related Factors

Complexity of healthcare system or therapeutic regimen
Decisional conflicts
Economic difficulties
Excessive demands made (e.g., individual, family); family conflict
Family patterns of healthcare
Inadequate number of cues to action
Deficient knowledge
Regimen; perceived seriousness, susceptibility, benefits, or barriers
Powerlessness
Social support deficit

Defining Characteristics

Subjective
Reports desire to manage the illness
Reports difficulty with prescribed regimens

Objective
Failure to include treatment regimens in daily living or to take action to reduce risk factors
Ineffective choices in daily living for meeting health goals
Unexpected acceleration of illness symptoms

Desired Outcomes/Evaluation Criteria—Client Will:

- Verbalize acceptance of need and desire to change actions to achieve agreed-on health goals.
- Verbalize understanding of factors or blocks involved in individual situation.

Information that appears in brackets has been added by the authors to clarify and enhance the use of nursing diagnoses.

- Participate in problem-solving of factors interfering with integration of therapeutic regimen.
- Demonstrate behaviors and changes in lifestyle necessary to maintain therapeutic regimen.
- Identify and use available resources.

Actions/Interventions

Nursing Priority No. 1.

To identify causative/contributing factors:

- Determine whether client has acute or chronic illness; if chronic, note whether more than one condition is present at the same time and assess the complexity of care needs. **These factors affect how client views and manages self care. Client may be overwhelmed, in denial, depressed, or have complications exacerbating care needs.**
- Ascertain client's knowledge and understanding of condition and treatment needs **so that he or she can make informed decisions about managing self-care. Provides a baseline so planning care can begin where the client is in relation to condition or illness and current regimen.**
- Determine client's/family's health goals and patterns of healthcare.
- Identify health practices and beliefs in client's personal and family history, including health values, religious or cultural beliefs, and expectations regarding healthcare. **The client may not view current situation as a problem or be unaware of health management needs. Expectations of others may dictate client's adaptation to situation and willingness to modify life.**
- Identify client locus of control. **Those with an internal locus of control (e.g., expressions of responsibility for self and ability to control outcomes, such as "I didn't quit smoking") are more likely to take charge of situation; individuals with an external locus of control (e.g., expressions of lack of control over self and environment, such as "What bad luck to get lung cancer") may perceive difficulties as beyond his or her control and will look to others to solve his or her problems.**
- Identify individual perceptions and expectations of treatment regimen. **May reveal misinformation, unrealistic expectations, or other factors that may be interfering with client's willingness to follow therapeutic regimen.**

Information that appears in brackets has been added by the authors to clarify and enhance the use of nursing diagnoses.

• Review complexity of treatment regimen (e.g., number of expected tasks, such as taking medication several times/day; visiting multiple healthcare providers with treatment or follow-up appointments; abundant, often conflicting, information sources). Evaluate how difficult tasks might be for client (e.g., must stop smoking or must follow strict dialysis diet even when feeling well and manage limitations while remaining active in life roles). **These factors are often involved in lack of participation in treatment plan.**

• Note availability and use of resources for assistance, caregiving, and respite care. **Client may not have, be aware of, or know how to access resources that may be available.**

Nursing Priority No. 2.

To assist client/SO(s) to develop strategies to improve management of therapeutic regimen:

• Use therapeutic communication skills **to assist client to problem-solve solution(s).**

• Explore client involvement in or lack of mutual goal setting.

• Use client's locus of control to develop individual plan to adapt regimen. **Encourage client with internal control to take control of own care; for those with external control, begin with small tasks and add, as tolerated.**

• Identify steps necessary to reach desired goal(s). **Specifying steps to take requires discussion and the use of critical thinking skills to determine how to best reach the agreed-on goals.**

• Contract with the client for participation in care.

• Accept client's evaluation of own strengths and limitations while working together to improve abilities. State belief in client's ability to cope and/or adapt to situation. **Individuals may minimize own strengths and exaggerate limitations when faced with the difficulties of a chronic illness. Stating your belief in positive terms lets client hear someone else's evaluation and begin to accept that he or she can manage the situation.**

• Provide positive reinforcement for efforts **to encourage continuation of desired behaviors.**

• Provide information and encourage client to seek out resources on own. Reinforce previous instructions and rationale, using a variety of learning modalities, including role playing, demonstration, and written materials. **Incorporating multiple modalities promotes retention of information. Devel-**

Information that appears in brackets has been added by the authors to clarify and enhance the use of nursing diagnoses.

🌐 Cultural   🎓 Collaborative   🏠 Community/Home Care

oping client's skill at finding own information encourages self-sufficiency and sense of self-worth.

Nursing Priority No. 3.

🔒To promote wellness (Teaching/Discharge Considerations):

- Emphasize importance of client knowledge and understanding of the need for treatment or medication as well as consequences of actions and choices.
- Promote client/caregiver/SO(s) participation in planning and evaluating process. **Enhances commitment to plan, promotes competent self-management, optimizing outcomes.**
- Assist client to develop strategies for monitoring symptoms and response to therapeutic regimen. **Promotes early recognition of changes, allowing proactive response.**
- Mobilize support systems, including family/SO(s), social services, and financial assistance. **Success of therapeutic regimen is enhanced by using support systems effectively, avoiding or reducing stress and worry of dealing with unresolved problems.**
- Refer to counseling or therapy (group and individual), as indicated.
- Identify home- and community-based nursing services **for assessment, follow-up care, and education in client's home.**

Documentation Focus

Assessment/Reassessment

- Findings, including underlying dynamics of individual situation, client's perception of problem or needs, locus of control.
- Cultural values, religious beliefs.
- Family involvement and needs.
- Individual strengths and limitations.
- Availability and use of resources.

Planning

- Plan of care and who is involved in planning.
- Teaching plan.

Implementation/Evaluation

- Response to interventions, teaching, and actions performed.
- Attainment or progress toward desired outcome(s).
- Modifications to plan of care.

Information that appears in brackets has been added by the authors to clarify and enhance the use of nursing diagnoses.

Discharge Planning

- Long-term needs and who is responsible for actions to be taken.
- Available resources, specific referrals made.

Sample Nursing Outcomes & Interventions Classifications (NOC/NIC)

NOC—Treatment Behavior: Illness or Injury
NIC—Self-Modification Assistance

readiness for enhanced Self-Health Management

Taxonomy II: Health Promotion—Class 2 Health Management (00162)
[Diagnostic Division: Teaching/Learning]
Submitted 2002; Name Change 2008

Definition: A pattern of regulating and integrating into daily living a therapeutic regimen for treatment of illness and its sequelae that is sufficient for meeting health-related goals and can be strengthened

Defining Characteristics

Subjective

Expresses desire to manage the illness (e.g., treatment, prevention of sequelae)
Expresses little difficulty with prescribed regimens
Describes reduction of risk factors

Objective

Choices of daily living are appropriate for meeting goals (e.g., treatment, prevention)
No unexpected acceleration of illness symptoms

Desired Outcomes/Evaluation Criteria— Client Will:

- Assume responsibility for managing treatment regimen.
- Demonstrate proactive management by anticipating and planning for eventualities of condition or potential complications.
- Identify and use additional resources as appropriate.
- Remain free of preventable complications, progression of illness and sequelae.

Information that appears in brackets has been added by the authors to clarify and enhance the use of nursing diagnoses.

🌐 Cultural   😊 Collaborative   🏠 Community/Home Care

Actions/Interventions

Nursing Priority No. 1.

To determine motivation for continued growth:

- Ascertain client's beliefs about health and his/her ability to maintain health. **Belief in ability to accomplish desired action is predictive of performance.**
- Determine client's current health status and perception of possible threats to health.
- Verify client's level of knowledge and understanding of therapeutic regimen. Note specific health goals and what measures client has been using to achieve his/her goals. **Provides opportunity to ensure accuracy and completeness of knowledge base for future learning.**
- Determine source(s) client uses when seeking health information and what is done with this information (e.g., incorporated into self-management or used as basis for seeking health care). **The manner in which people access and use healthcare information varies widely, with variables including age, race/culture, location, literacy, and computer use.**
- Active-listen concerns to identify underlying issues (e.g., physical or emotional stressors, external factors such as environmental pollutants or other hazards) **that could impact client's ability to control own health.**
- Determine influence of cultural beliefs on client/caregiver(s) participation in regimen. **These factors influence the way people view health issues and management.**
- Identify individual's expectations of long-term treatment needs and anticipated changes.
- Determine present resources used by client **to note whether changes can be arranged (e.g., increased hours of home care assistance; access to case manager to support complex or long-term program).**

Nursing Priority No. 2.

To assist client/SO(s) to develop plan to meet individual needs:

- Acknowledge client's strengths in present health management and build on in planning for future.
- Identify steps necessary to reach desired health goal(s). **Understanding the process enhances commitment and the likelihood of achieving the goals.**
- Explore with client/SO(s) areas of health over which each individual has control and discuss barriers to healthy practices

---

Information that appears in brackets has been added by the authors to clarify and enhance the use of nursing diagnoses.

(e.g., chooses fast food instead of cooking for one; lack of time or access to convenient facility or safe environment in which to exercise). **Identifies actions individual can take to plan for improving health practices.**

* Accept client's evaluation of own strengths and limitations while working together to improve abilities. **Promotes sense of self-esteem and confidence to continue efforts.**

• Incorporate client's cultural values or religious beliefs that support attainment of health goals.

* Provide information and bibliotherapy. Help client/SO(s) identify and evaluate resources they can access on their own. **When referencing the Internet or nontraditional, unproven resources, the individual must exercise some restraint and determine the reliability of the source and information provided before acting on it.**

* Acknowledge individual efforts and capabilities to reinforce movement toward attainment of desired outcomes. **Provides positive reinforcement encouraging continued progress toward desired goals.**

Nursing Priority No. 3.
🏠 To promote optimum wellness:

* Promote client/caregiver choices and involvement in planning for and implementing added tasks and responsibilities. **Knowing that he or she can make own choices promotes commitment to program and enhances probability that client will follow through with change.**

* Encourage use of exercise, relaxation skills, yoga, meditation, visualization, and guided imagery **to assist in management of stress and promote general health and well-being.**

* Assist in implementing strategies for monitoring progress and responses to therapeutic regimen. **Promotes proactive problem-solving.**

* Identify additional community resources/support groups (e.g., nutritionist/weight control program, smoking cessation program). **Provides further opportunities for role modeling, skill training, anticipatory problem-solving, and so forth.**

* Instruct in individually appropriate wellness behaviors such as breast self-examination and mammogram, testicular self-examination and prostate examination, immunizations and flu shots, regular medical and dental examinations.

Information that appears in brackets has been added by the authors to clarify and enhance the use of nursing diagnoses.

🌐 Cultural ✖ Collaborative 🏠 Community/Home Care

Documentation Focus

Assessment/Reassessment
- Findings, including dynamics of individual situation.
- Individual strengths, additional needs.
- Cultural values, religious beliefs.

Planning
- Plan of care and who is involved in planning.
- Teaching plan.

Implementation/Evaluation
- Response to interventions, teaching, and actions performed.
- Attainment or progress toward desired outcome(s).
- Modifications to plan of care.

Discharge Planning
- Short- and long-term needs and who is responsible for actions.
- Available resources, specific referrals made.

Sample Nursing Outcomes & Interventions Classifications (NOC/NIC)

NOC—Adherence Behavior
NIC—Health System Guidance

Self-Mutilation

Taxonomy II: Safety/Protection—Class 3 Violence (00151)
[Diagnostic Division: Safety]
Submitted 2000

Definition: Deliberate self-injurious behavior causing tissue damage with the intent of causing nonfatal injury to attain relief of tension

Related Factors

Adolescence; peers who self-mutilate; isolation from peers
Dissociation; depersonalization; psychotic state (e.g., command hallucinations); character disorder; borderline personality disorder; emotional disorder; developmentally delayed individual; autistic individual

Information that appears in brackets has been added by the authors to clarify and enhance the use of nursing diagnoses.

History of self-directed violence, inability to plan solutions, inability to see long-term consequences

Childhood illness, surgery, or sexual abuse; battered child

Disturbed body image; eating disorders

Ineffective coping; perfectionism

Reports negative feelings (e.g., depression, rejection, self-hatred, separation anxiety, guilt, depersonalization); low self-esteem; unstable self-esteem/body image

Poor communication between parent and adolescent; lack of family confidant

Feels threatened with loss of significant relationship

Disturbed interpersonal relationships; use of manipulation to obtain nurturing relationship with others

Family substance abuse, divorce; violence between parental figures; family history of self-destructive behaviors

Living in nontraditional settings (e.g., foster, group, or institutional care); incarceration

Inability to express tension verbally; mounting tension that is intolerable; need for quick reduction of stress

Irresistible urge to cut self/for self-directed violence; impulsivity; labile behavior

Sexual identity crisis

Substance abuse

Defining Characteristics

Subjective
Self-inflicted burns (e.g., eraser, cigarette)
Ingestion or inhalation of harmful substances

Objective
Cuts or scratches on body
Picking at wounds
Biting; abrading; severing
Insertion of object into body orifice
Hitting
Constricting a body part

Desired Outcomes/Evaluation Criteria—Client Will:

- Verbalize understanding of reasons for occurrence of behavior.
- Identify precipitating factors or awareness of arousal state that occurs prior to incident.

Information that appears in brackets has been added by the authors to clarify and enhance the use of nursing diagnoses.

- Express increased self-concept or self-esteem.
- Seek help when feeling anxious and having thoughts of harming self.

Actions/Interventions

Nursing Priority No. 1.

To assess causative/contributing factors:

- Determine underlying dynamics of individual situation as listed in Related Factors. Note presence of inflexible, maladaptive personality traits that reflect personality or character disorder (e.g., impulsive, unpredictable, inappropriate behaviors, intense anger, lack of control of anger).
- Evaluate history of mental illness (e.g., borderline personality, identity disorder, bipolar disorder).
- Identify previous episodes of self-mutilation behavior. **Some body piercing (e.g., ears) is generally accepted as decorative; piercing of multiple sites often is an attempt to establish individuality, addressing issues of separation and belonging, but is not considered self-injury behavior.**
- Determine relationship of previous self-mutilating behavior to stressful events. **Self-injury is considered to be an attempt to alter a mood state.**
- Note use or abuse of addicting substances.
- Review laboratory findings (e.g., blood alcohol, polydrug screen, glucose, and electrolyte levels). **Drug use may affect self-injury behavior.**

Nursing Priority No. 2.

To structure environment to maintain client safety:

- Assist client to identify feelings leading up to desire for self-mutilation. **Early recognition of recurring feelings provides opportunity to seek and learn other ways of coping.**
- Provide external controls/limit setting. **May decrease the opportunity to self-mutilate.**
- Include client in development of plan of care. **Commitment to plan increases likelihood of adherence.**
- Encourage appropriate expression of feelings. **Identifies feelings and promotes understanding of what leads to development of tension.**
- Note feelings of healthcare providers and family, such as frustration, anger, defensiveness, need to rescue. **Client may be manipulative, evoking defensiveness and conflict. These**

Information that appears in brackets has been added by the authors to clarify and enhance the use of nursing diagnoses.

feelings need to be identified, recognized, and dealt with openly with staff/family and client.

⊕• Provide care for client's wounds when self-mutilation occurs in a matter-of-fact manner **that conveys empathy and concern.** Refrain from offering sympathy or additional attention **that could provide reinforcement for maladaptive behavior and may encourage its repetition.**

Nursing Priority No. 3.
To promote movement toward positive changes:

- Involve client in developing goals for stopping behavior. **Enhances commitment, optimizing outcomes.**
- Develop a contract between client and counselor **to enable the client to stay physically safe, such as "I will not cut or harm myself for the next 24 hours."** Renew contract on a regular basis and have both parties sign and date each contract.
- Provide avenues of communication **for times when client needs to talk to avoid cutting or damaging self.**
- Assist client to learn assertive behavior. Include the use of effective communication skills, focusing on developing self-esteem by replacing negative self-talk with positive comments.
- Use interventions that help the client to reclaim power in own life (e.g., experiential and cognitive).

Nursing Priority No. 4.
🏠 To promote wellness (Teaching/Discharge Considerations):

- Discuss commitment to safety and ways in which client will deal with precursors to undesired behavior. **Provides opportunity for client to assume responsibility for self.**
- Promote the use of healthy behaviors, identifying consequences and outcomes of current actions.
- Identify support systems.
- Discuss living arrangements when client is discharged/relocated. **May need assistance with transition to changes required to avoid recurrence of self-mutilating behaviors.**
⊕• Involve family/SO(s) in planning for discharge and in group therapies, as appropriate. **Promotes coordination and continuation of plan, commitment to goals.**
- Discuss information about the role neurotransmitters play in predisposing an individual to beginning this behavior. **It is believed that problems in the serotonin system may make**

Information that appears in brackets has been added by the authors to clarify and enhance the use of nursing diagnoses.

the person more aggressive and impulsive, especially when combined with an environment where he or she learned that feelings are bad or wrong, leading client to turn aggression on self.

- Provide information and discuss the use of medication, as appropriate. **Antidepressant medications may be useful, but they need to be weighed against the potential for overdosing.**
- Refer to NDs Anxiety; impaired Social Interaction; Self-Esteem [specify].

Documentation Focus

Assessment/Reassessment
- Individual findings, including risk factors present, underlying dynamics, prior episodes.
- Cultural or religious practices.
- Laboratory test results.
- Substance use or abuse.

Planning
- Plan of care and who is involved in planning.
- Teaching plan.

Implementation/Evaluation
- Response to interventions, teaching, and actions performed.
- Attainment or progress toward desired outcome(s).
- Modifications to plan of care.

Discharge Planning
- Long-term needs and who is responsible for actions to be taken.
- Community resources, referrals made.

Sample Nursing Outcomes & Interventions Classifications (NOC/NIC)

NOC—Self-Mutilation Restraint
NIC—Behavior Management: Self-Harm

Information that appears in brackets has been added by the authors to clarify and enhance the use of nursing diagnoses.

risk for Self-Mutilation

Taxonomy II: Safety/Protection—Class 3 Violence
(00139)
[Diagnostic Division: Safety]
Submitted 1992; Revised 2000

Definition: At risk for deliberate self-injurious behavior causing tissue damage with the intent of causing nonfatal injury to attain relief of tension

Risk Factors

Adolescence; peers who self-mutilate; isolation from peers

Dissociation; depersonalization; psychotic state (e.g., command hallucinations); character disorder; borderline personality disorder; emotional disorder; developmentally delayed individual; autistic individual

History of self-directed violence, inability to plan solutions, inability to see long-term consequences

Childhood illness, surgery, or sexual abuse; battered child

Disturbed body image; eating disorders

Inadequate coping; loss of control over problem-solving situations; perfectionism

Reports negative feelings (e.g., depression, rejection, self-hatred, separation anxiety, guilt); low or unstable self-esteem

Feels threatened with loss of significant relationship; loss of significant relationship(s)

Disturbed interpersonal relationships; use of manipulation to obtain nurturing relationship with others

Family substance abuse, divorce; violence between parental figures; family history of self-directed violence

Living in nontraditional settings (e.g., foster, group, or institutional care); incarceration

Inability to express tension verbally; mounting tension that is intolerable; need for quick reduction of stress; irresistable urge for self-directed violence; impulsivity

Sexual identity crisis

Substance abuse

NOTE: A risk diagnosis is not evidenced by signs and symptoms, as the problem has not occurred; rather, nursing interventions are directed at prevention.

Information that appears in brackets has been added by the authors to clarify and enhance the use of nursing diagnoses.

🌐 Cultural 😊 Collaborative 🏠 Community/Home Care

Desired Outcomes/Evaluation Criteria— Client Will:

- Verbalize understanding of reasons for wanting to cut or harm self.
- Identify precipitating factors or awareness of arousal state that occurs prior to incident.
- Express increased self-concept or self-esteem.
- Demonstrate self-control as evidenced by lessened (or absence of) episodes of self-injury.
- Engage in use of alternative methods for managing feelings and individuality.

Actions/Interventions

Nursing Priority No. 1.

To assess causative/contributing factors:

- Determine underlying dynamics of individual situation as listed in Risk Factors. Note presence of inflexible, maladaptive personality traits (e.g., impulsive, unpredictable, inappropriate behaviors; intense anger or lack of control of anger) **reflecting personality or character disorder, mental illness (e.g., bipolar disorder)**, or conditions that may interfere with ability to control own behavior (e.g., psychotic state, mental retardation, autism).
- Identify previous episodes of self-mutilating behavior (e.g., cutting, scratching, bruising). **Some body piercing (e.g., ears) is generally accepted as decorative; piercing of multiple sites often is an attempt to establish individuality, addressing issues of separation and belonging, but is not considered self-injury behavior.**
- Note beliefs, cultural and religious practices that may be involved in choice of behavior. **Growing up in a family that did not allow feelings to be expressed, individuals learn that feelings are bad or wrong. Family dynamics may come out of religious or cultural expectations that believe in strict punishment for transgressions.**
- Determine use or abuse of addictive substances. **May be trying to resist impulse to self-injure by turning to drugs.**
- Review laboratory findings (e.g., blood alcohol, polydrug screen, glucose, electrolyte levels).
- Note degree of impairment in social and occupational functioning. **May dictate treatment setting (e.g., specific outpatient program, short-stay inpatient).**

Information that appears in brackets has been added by the authors to clarify and enhance the use of nursing diagnoses.

Nursing Priority No. 2.

To structure environment to maintain client safety:

- Assist client to identify feelings and behaviors that precede desire for mutilation. **Early recognition of recurring feelings provides client opportunity to seek other ways of coping.**
- Provide external controls and limit setting **to decrease the need to mutilate self.**
- Include client in development of plan of care. **Being involved in own decisions can help reestablish ego boundaries and strengthen commitment to goals and participation in therapy.**
- Encourage client to recognize and appropriately express feelings verbally.
- Keep client in continuous staff view and provide special observation checks during inpatient therapy **to promote safety.**
- Structure inpatient milieu to maintain positive, clear, open communication among staff and clients, with an understanding that "secrets are not tolerated" and failure to maintain openness will be confronted.
- Develop schedule of alternative, healthy, success-oriented activities, including involvement in such groups as Overeaters Anonymous or similar 12-step program based on individual needs; self-esteem activities include positive affirmations, visiting with friends, and exercise.
- Note feelings of healthcare providers and family, such as frustration, anger, defensiveness, distraction, despair and powerlessness, and need to rescue. **Client may be manipulative, evoking defensiveness and conflict. These feelings need to be identified, recognized, and dealt with openly with staff, family, and client.**

Nursing Priority No. 3.

To promote movement toward positive actions:

- Involve client in developing goals for preventing undesired behavior. **Enhances commitment, optimizing outcomes.**
- Assist client to learn assertive behavior. Include the use of effective communication skills, focusing on developing self-esteem by replacing negative self-talk with positive comments.
- Develop a contract between client and counselor **to enable the client to stay physically safe, such as "I will not cut or harm myself for the next 24 hours."** Renew contract on a regular basis and have both parties sign and date each con-

---

Information that appears in brackets has been added by the authors to clarify and enhance the use of nursing diagnoses.

🌐 Cultural   🌀 Collaborative   🏠 Community/Home Care

tract. Make contingency arrangements **so client can talk to counselor, as needed.**

∞• Discuss with client/family normalcy of adolescent task of separation and ways of achieving.
• Promote the use of healthy behaviors, identifying the consequences and outcomes of current actions: "Does this get you what you want?" "How does this behavior help you achieve your goals?" **Dialectical Behavior Therapy is an effective therapy in reducing self-injurious behavior along with appropriate medication.**
• Provide reinforcement for use of assertive behavior rather than nonassertive or aggressive behavior.
• Use interventions that help the client to reclaim power in own life (e.g., experiential and cognitive).
• Involve client/family in group therapies as appropriate.

Nursing Priority No. 4.

To promote wellness (Teaching/Discharge Considerations):
• Discuss commitment to safety and ways in which client will deal with precursors to undesired behavior.
• Mobilize support systems.
• Involve family/SO(s) in planning for discharge, as appropriate. **Promotes coordination and continuation of plan, commitment to goals.**
• Identify living circumstances client will be going to once discharged/relocated. **May need assistance with transition to changes required to reduce risk or avoid recurrence of self-mutilating behaviors.**
• Arrange for continued involvement in group therapy(ies).
• Discuss and provide information about the use of medication, as appropriate. **Antidepressant medications may be useful, but use needs to be weighed against potential for overdosing or adverse side effects (e.g., the antidepressant Effexor can cause hostility, suicidal ideas, and self-harm). Medications that stabilize moods, ease depression, and calm anxiety may be tried to reduce the urge to self-harm.**
• Refer to NDs Anxiety; impaired Social Interaction; Self-Esteem [specify].

Documentation Focus

Assessment/Reassessment
• Individual findings, including risk factors present, underlying dynamics, prior episodes.

Information that appears in brackets has been added by the authors to clarify and enhance the use of nursing diagnoses.

- Cultural or religious practices.
- Laboratory test results.
- Substance use or abuse.

Planning

- Plan of care and who is involved in planning.
- Teaching plan.

Implementation/Evaluation

- Response to interventions, teaching, and actions performed.
- Attainment or progress toward desired outcome(s).
- Modifications to plan of care.

Discharge Planning

- Long-term needs and who is responsible for actions to be taken.
- Community resources, referrals made.

Sample Nursing Outcomes & Interventions Classifications (NOC/NIC)

NOC—Self-Mutilation Restraint
NIC—Behavior Management: Self-Harm

Self-Neglect

Taxonomy II: Activity/Rest—Class 5 Self-Care (00193)
[Diagnostic Division: Hygiene]
Submitted 2008

Definition: A constellation of culturally framed behaviors involving one or more self-care activities in which there is a failure to maintain a socially accepted standard of health and well-being (Gibbons, Lauder, & Ludwick, 2006)

Related Factors

Major life stressor; depression
Obsessive-compulsive disorder; schizotypal or paranoid personality disorders
Frontal lobe dysfunction; executive processing ability; cognitive impairment (e.g. dementia); Capgras syndrome
Functional impairment; learning disability

Information that appears in brackets has been added by the authors to clarify and enhance the use of nursing diagnoses.

🌐 Cultural   🔵 Collaborative   🏠 Community/Home Care

Lifestyle/choice; substance abuse; malingering
Maintaining control; fear of institutionalization

Defining Characteristics

Objective
Inadequate personal or environmental hygiene
Nonadherence to health activities

Desired Outcomes/Evaluation Criteria—Client Will (Include Specific Time Frame):

- Acknowledge difficulty maintaining hygiene practices.
- Demonstrate ability to manage lifestyle changes and medication regimen.
- Perform activities of daily living within level of own ability.

Caregiver Will:

- Assist individual with personal and environmental hygiene as needed.
- Identify and assist client with medical, dental, and other healthcare appointments as indicated.

Actions/Interventions

Nursing Priority No. 1.
To identify causative or precipitating factors:

- Determine existing health problems, age, developmental level, and cognitive psychological factors, including presence of delusions affecting ability to care for own needs. **A wide variety of impairments can cause a person to neglect hygiene needs, particularly aging, homelessness, and dementia.**
- Use an appropriate screening instrument, such as the Elder Assessment Instrument. **Neglect and elder abuse is underreported, and the use of a good tool can help identify presence.**
- Identify other problems that may interfere with ability to care for self such as visual or hearing impairment, language barrier, emotional instability or lability.
- Note recent life events or changes in circumstances. **Losses such as of a loved one, financial security, or physical independence can trigger or exacerbate self-neglect behaviors.**

Information that appears in brackets has been added by the authors to clarify and enhance the use of nursing diagnoses.

- Review circumstances of client illness, possible monetary re-wards, sympathy or attention from family. **On occasion self-neglect may be malingering as an attempt to gain some-thing from others or relinquish unwanted responsibilities.**
- Perform mental status examination. **Mental illness (e.g., psy-chosis, depression, dementia) can affect individual's abil-ity or desire to maintain self-care activities or care for home surroundings.**
- Evaluate for frontal lobe dysfunction, possibility of Diogenes syndrome.
- Assess economic factors and living arrangements. **May live alone or with family members who are not helpful or may be homeless; may have little or no financial resources, re-sulting in inability to achieve or lack of concern about personal well-being.**
- Determine availability and use of resources.
- Interview SO/family members to determine level of involve-ment and support. **Client may be exhibiting acting-out/ paranoid behaviors, stressing caregivers, who may not re-alize that cognitive impairment prevents individual from exercising self-control.**

Nursing Priority No. 2.
To determine degree of impairment:

- Perform head-to-toe assessment inspecting scalp and skin, noting personal hygiene, body odor, rashes, bruising, skin tears, lesions, burns, presence of vermin; inspecting oral cav-ity for gum disease, inflammation, lesions, loose or broken teeth, fit of dentures. **Identifies specific needs and may re-veal signs of trauma or abuse.**
- Perform nutritional assessment as indicated. **Neglecting one-self often includes not eating meals regularly or not eating nutritionally balanced foods, especially when alcoholism or drug abuse is present.**
- Review medication regimen. **In addition to neglecting self-care activities, client will likely not pay attention to taking prescriptions as ordered, resulting in exacerbation of med-ical problem. Some psychotropic medications may cause individual to "feel different" or not in control of self, re-sulting in reluctance to take drug.**
- Determine client's willingness to change situation.

Nursing Priority No. 3.
To assist in correcting/dealing with situation:

Information that appears in brackets has been added by the authors to clarify and enhance the use of nursing diagnoses.

🌐 Cultural 🤝 Collaborative 🏠 Community/Home Care

- Develop multidisciplinary team specific to individual needs, such as case manager, physician, dietitian, physical or occupational therapist, rehabilitation specialist. **To develop a plan appropriate to the individual situation, making use of client's capabilities and maximizing potential.**
- Establish therapeutic relationship with client and with family, if available and willing to be involved.
- Identify specific priorities and goals of client/SOs. **Helps client to look at possibilities for dealing with difficult situation of no longer being able to maintain lifestyle and moving on to a new way of managing.**
- Promote client's/SO's participation in problem identification and decision making.
- Evaluate need for safety, balancing client's need for autonomy. **The ethical challenge of providing individual safety within the current laws for client's right to refuse care in face of self-neglect and self-destructive behaviors, which can impact others as well as the client, is difficult to manage.**
- Perform home assessment **to determine safety issues, cleanliness, compulsive hoarding, neglected property concerns.**
- Demonstrate or review skills necessary for caring for self, using terms appropriate to client's level of understanding.
- Plan time for listening to client's/SO's concerns. **Provides opportunity to determine whether plan is being followed and identify the barriers to participation.**
- Refer to NDs Self-Care Deficit; ineffective Health Maintenance; impaired Home Maintenance; [disturbed Sensory Perception], for additional interventions as appropriate.

Nursing Priority No. 4.
To promote wellness (Discharge/Evaluation Criteria):

- Establish remotivation or resocialization program when indicated. **Depending on where the client is residing, isolation may become a problem as individual withdraws from contact with others.**
- Assist with setting up medication regimen as indicated.
- Discuss dietary needs and client's ability to provide nutritious meals. **May require support such as food assistance, community pantry, elder meal program, Meals on Wheels.**
- Provide for ongoing evaluation of self-care program. **Helps to identify whether client is managing effectively or whether cognitive functioning is deteriorating and a new plan needs to be developed.**

Information that appears in brackets has been added by the authors to clarify and enhance the use of nursing diagnoses.

- Evaluate for appropriateness of providing a companion animal. **Taking responsibility for another life and sharing unconditional love can provide purpose and motivation for client to take more interest in own situation.**
- Refer to support services such as home care, day-care program, social services, food assistance, community clinic, physical/occupational therapy, senior services, as indicated.
- Investigate alternative placements as indicated.
- Discuss need for respite for family members. **Care of cognitively impaired member can be wearing, and time away allows for renewing oneself and enhancing ability to cope with continued care responsibilities.**
- Refer for counseling as indicated.

Documentation Focus

Assessment/Reassessment
- Individual findings, functional level and limitations, mental status.
- Personal safety issues.
- Needed resources, possible need for placement.

Planning
- Plan of care and who is involved in planning.
- Teaching plan.

Implementation/Evaluation
- Response to interventions, teaching, and actions performed.
- Attainment or progress toward desired outcomes.
- Modifications of plan of care.

Discharge Planning
- Long-term needs and who is responsible for actions to be taken.
- Type of assistance and resources needed.
- Specific referrals made.

Sample Nursing Outcomes & Interventions Classifications (NOC/NIC)

NOC—Self-Care Status
NIC—Self-Responsibility Facilitation

Information that appears in brackets has been added by the authors to clarify and enhance the use of nursing diagnoses.

> **[disturbed Sensory Perception** (specify: visual, auditory, kinesthetic, gustatory, tactile, olfactory])
>
> Taxonomy II: Perception/Cognition—Class 3 Sensation/ Perception (00122)
> [Diagnostic Division: Neurosensory]
> Submitted 1978; Revised 1980, 1998 (by small group work 1996); Retired 2012
>
> **Definition:** Change in the amount or patterning of incoming stimuli accompanied by a diminished, exaggerated, distorted, or impaired response to such stimuli

Related Factors

Insufficient environmental stimuli (therapeutically restricted environments [e.g., isolation, intensive care, bedrest, traction, confining illnesses, incubator]; socially restricted environment [e.g., institutionalization, homebound, aging, chronic or terminal illness, infant deprivation]; stigmatized [e.g., mentally ill, developmentally delayed, handicapped])

Excessive environmental stimuli

Altered sensory reception, transmission, or integration

Biochemical imbalances (e.g., elevated blood urea nitrogen, ammonia; hypoxia); electrolyte imbalance; [drugs (e.g., stimulants or depressants, mind-altering drugs)]

Psychological stress; [sleep deprivation]

Defining Characteristics

Subjective

[Reported] change in sensory acuity (e.g., photosensitivity, hypoesthesias or hyperesthesias, diminished or altered sense of taste, inability to tell position of body parts [proprioception])

Sensory distortions

Objective

[Measured] change in sensory acuity

Change in usual response to stimuli

Change in behavior pattern; restlessness; irritability

Change in problem-solving abilities; poor concentration

Disorientation; hallucinations; [illusions]

Impaired communication

Information that appears in brackets has been added by the authors to clarify and enhance the use of nursing diagnoses.

[disturbed SENSORY PERCEPTION (specify: visual, auditory, kinesthetic, gustatory, tactile, olfactory])

Motor incoordination, altered sense of balance/falls (e.g., Ménière's syndrome)

Desired Outcomes/Evaluation Criteria— Client Will:

- Regain or maintain usual level of cognition.
- Recognize and correct or compensate for sensory impairments.
- Verbalize awareness of sensory needs and presence of overload and/or deprivation.
- Identify and modify external factors that contribute to alterations in sensory or perceptual abilities.
- Use resources effectively and appropriately.
- Be free of injury.

Actions/Interventions

Nursing Priority No. 1.

To assess causative/contributing factors and degree of impairment:

- Identify client with condition that can affect sensing, interpreting, and communicating stimuli. **Specific clinical concerns (e.g., neurological disease or trauma, intensive care unit confinement, surgery, pain, biochemical imbalances, psychosis, substance abuse, toxemia) have the potential for altering one or more of the senses, with resultant change in the reception, sensitivity, or interpretation of sensory input.**
- ∞· Note age and developmental stage. **Problems with sensory perception may be known to client/caregiver (e.g., child wearing hearing aid, elderly adult with known macular degeneration), where compensatory interventions are in place. Screening or evaluation may be required if sensory impairments are suspected, but not obvious.**
- Review results of sensory and motor neurological testing and laboratory studies (e.g., cognitive testing or laboratory values, such as electrolytes, chemical profile, arterial blood gases, serum drug levels) **to note presence or possible cause of changes in response to sensory stimuli.**
- Monitor drug regimen **to identify prescription/drugs with effects, side effects, or drug interactions that may cause or exacerbate sensory or perceptual problems.**

Information that appears in brackets has been added by the authors to clarify and enhance the use of nursing diagnoses.

🌐 Cultural 🌀 Collaborative 🏠 Community/Home Care

- Assess ability to speak, hear, interpret, and respond to simple commands **to obtain an overview of client's mental and cognitive status and ability to interpret stimuli.**
- ⊛ Evaluate sensory awareness: stimulus of hot and cold, dull or sharp; smell, taste, visual acuity, and hearing; gait, mobility; location and function of body parts.
- Determine response to painful stimuli **to note whether response is appropriate to stimulus and is immediate or delayed.**
- Observe for behavioral responses (e.g., illusions, hallucinations, delusions, withdrawal, hostility, crying, inappropriate affect, confusion or disorientation) **that may indicate mental or emotional problems or chemical toxicity (as might occur with digoxin or other drug overdose or reaction) or be associated with brain or neurological trauma or infection.**
- Note inattention to body parts, segments of environment; lack of recognition of familiar objects or persons. **Loss of comprehension of auditory, visual, or other sensations may be indicative of unilateral neglect or inability to recognize and respond to environmental cues.**
- Ascertain client's/SO's perception of problem/changes in activities of daily living. Listen to and respect client's expressions of deprivation and take these into consideration in planning care.

Nursing Priority No. 2.

To promote normalization of response to stimuli:

- Address client by name and have personnel wear name tags and reintroduce self, as needed, **to preserve client's sense of identity and orientation.**
- Reorient to person, place, time, and events, as necessary **to reduce confusion and provide sense of normalcy to client's daily life.**
- Explain procedures and activities, expected sensations, and outcomes.
- Provide means of communication, as indicated by client's current situation.
- Encourage use of listening devices (e.g., hearing aid, audiovisual amplifier, closed-caption TV, signing interpreter) **to assist in managing auditory impairment.**
- Interpret stimuli and offer feedback **to assist client to separate reality from fantasy or altered perception.**

[disturbed SENSORY PERCEPTION (specify: visual, auditory, kinesthetic, gustatory, tactile, olfactory)]

Information that appears in brackets has been added by the authors to clarify and enhance the use of nursing diagnoses.

- Avoid isolation of client, physically or emotionally, **to prevent sensory deprivation and limit confusion.**
- Promote a stable environment with continuity of care by same personnel as much as possible.
- Eliminate extraneous noise and stimuli, including nonessential equipment, alarms or audible monitor signals when possible.
- Provide undisturbed rest and sleep periods.
- Speak to visually impaired or unresponsive client during care **to provide auditory stimulation and prevent startle reflex.**
- Provide tactile stimulation as care is given. **Touching is an important part of caring and a deep psychological need communicating presence and connection with another human being.**
- Provide sensory stimulation, including familiar smells and sounds, tactile stimulation with a variety of objects, changing of light intensity and other cues (e.g., clocks, calendars).
- Encourage SO(s) to bring in familiar objects, talk to, and touch the client frequently.
- Minimize discussion of negatives (e.g., client and personnel problems) within client's hearing. **Client may misinterpret and believe references are to himself or herself.**
- Provide diversional activities, as able (e.g., TV, radio, conversation, large-print or talking books). (Refer to ND deficient Diversional Activity.)
- Promote meaningful socialization. (Refer to ND Social Isolation.)
- Collaborate with other health team members in providing rehabilitative therapies and stimulating modalities (e.g., music therapy, sensory training, remotivation therapy) **to achieve maximal gains in function and psychosocial well-being.**
- Identify and encourage use of resources and prosthetic devices (e.g., hearing aids, computerized visual aid, glasses with a level plumbline for balance). **Useful for augmenting senses.**

Nursing Priority No. 3.
To prevent injury/complications:

- Record perceptual deficit on chart **so that caregivers are aware.**
- Place call bell or other communication device within reach and be sure client knows where it is and how to use it.
- Provide safety measures, as needed (e.g., siderails, bed in low position, adequate lighting; assistance with walking; use of vision or hearing devices).

Information that appears in brackets has been added by the authors to clarify and enhance the use of nursing diagnoses.

🌐 Cultural 🔁 Collaborative 🏠 Community/Home Care

- Review basic and specific safety information (e.g., "I am on your right side"; "This water is hot"; "Swallow now"; "Stand up"; "You cannot drive").
- Position doors and furniture so they are out of travel path for client with impaired vision or strategically place items or grab bars **to aid in maintaining balance.**
- Ambulate with assistance and devices **to enhance balance.**
- Describe where affected areas of body are when moving client.
- Limit and carefully monitor use of sedation, especially in the elderly **who are more sensitive to side effects and drug interactions affecting sensory perception and interpretation.**
- Monitor use of heating pads or ice packs; use thermometer to measure temperature of bath water **to protect from thermal injury.**
- Refer to NDs risk for Thermal Injury; risk for Trauma; risk for Falls.

Nursing Priority No. 4.

To promote wellness (Teaching/Discharge Considerations):

- Review ways to prevent or limit exposure to conditions affecting sensory functions (e.g., how exposure to loud noise and toxins can impair hearing; early childhood screening for speech and language disorders; vaccines to prevent measles, mumps, meningitis, **once known to be major causes of hearing loss).**
- Assist client/SO(s) to learn effective ways of coping with and managing sensory disturbances, anticipating safety needs according to client's sensory deficits and developmental level.
- Identify alternative ways of dealing with perceptual deficits (e.g., vision and hearing aids; augmentative communication devices; computer technologies; specific deficit-compensation techniques).
- Provide explanations of and plan care with client, involving SO(s) as much as possible. **Enhances commitment to and continuation of plan, optimizing outcomes.**
- Review home safety measures pertinent to deficits.
- Discuss drug regimen, noting possible toxic side effects of both prescription and over-the-counter drugs. **Prompt recognition of side effects allows for timely intervention/ change in drug regimen.**

Information that appears in brackets has been added by the authors to clarify and enhance the use of nursing diagnoses.

- Demonstrate use and care of sensory prosthetic devices (e.g., assistive vision or listening devices, etc.).
- Identify resources and community programs for acquiring and maintaining assistive devices.
- Refer to appropriate helping resources, such as Society for the Blind, Self-Help for the Hard of Hearing, or local support groups, screening programs, and so forth.
- Refer to additional NDs Anxiety; acute/chronic Confusion; Unilateral Neglect, as appropriate.

Documentation Focus

Assessment/Reassessment
- Individual findings, noting specific deficit and associated symptoms, perceptions of client/SO(s).
- Assistive device needs.

Planning
- Plan of care, including who is involved in planning.
- Teaching plan.

Implementation/Evaluation
- Responses to interventions, teaching, and actions performed.
- Attainment or progress toward desired outcome(s).
- Modifications to plan of care.

Discharge Planning
- Long-term needs and who is responsible for actions to be taken.
- Available resources; specific referrals made.

Sample Nursing Outcomes & Interventions Classifications (NOC/NIC)

Auditory
NOC—Sensory Function: Hearing
NIC—Communication Enhancement: Hearing Deficit

Visual
NOC—Sensory Function: Vision
NIC—Communication Enhancement: Visual Deficit

Information that appears in brackets has been added by the authors to clarify and enhance the use of nursing diagnoses.

Cultural   Collaborative   Community/Home Care

Gustatory/Olfactory
NOC—Sensory Function: Taste & Smell
NIC—Nutrition Management

Kinesthetic
NOC—Sensory Function: Proprioception
NIC—Body Mechanics Promotion

Tactile
NOC—Sensory Function: Cutaneous
NIC—Peripheral Sensation Management

Sexual Dysfunction

Taxonomy II: Sexuality—Class 2 Sexual Function (00059)
[Diagnostic Division: Sexuality]
Submitted 1980; Revised 2006

Definition: The state in which an individual experiences a change in sexual function during the sexual response phases of desire, excitation, and/or orgasm, which is viewed as unsatisfying, unrewarding, or inadequate

Related Factors

Ineffectual or absent role models; lack of SO
Lack of privacy
Misinformation; deficient knowledge
Vulnerability
Physical abuse; psychosocial abuse (e.g., harmful relationships)
Altered body function or structure (e.g., pregnancy, recent childbirth, drugs, surgery, anomalies, disease process, trauma, radiation, [effects of aging])
Biopsychosocial alteration of sexuality
Values conflict

Defining Characteristics

Subjective
Verbalization of problem; alterations in achieving perceived sex role
Actual or perceived limitations imposed by disease or therapy
Alterations in achieving sexual satisfaction; inability to achieve desired satisfaction

Information that appears in brackets has been added by the authors to clarify and enhance the use of nursing diagnoses.

Perceived deficiency of sexual desire or alteration in sexual excitation

Seeking confirmation of desirability

Change of interest in self/others

Desired Outcomes/Evaluation Criteria— Client Will:

- Verbalize understanding of sexual anatomy and function and alterations that may affect function.
- Verbalize understanding of individual reasons for sexual problems.
- Identify stressors in lifestyle that may contribute to the dysfunction.
- Identify satisfying and acceptable sexual practices and alternative ways of dealing with sexual expression.
- Discuss concerns about body image, sex role, desirability as a sexual partner with partner/SO.

Actions/Interventions

Nursing Priority No. 1.

To assess causative/contributing factors:

- Do a complete history and physical, including a sexual history, which would include usual pattern of functioning and level of desire. Note vocabulary used by the individual to maximize communication/understanding.
- Have client describe problem in own words.
- Determine importance of sex to individual/partner and client's motivation for change. **Interpersonal problems (marital and relationship), lack of trust or open communication between partners can contribute to client's concern.**
- Be alert to comments of client, **as sexual concerns are often disguised as humor, sarcasm, and/or offhand remarks.**
- Assess knowledge of client/SO regarding sexual anatomy and function and effects of current situation or condition. **Individuals are often ignorant of anatomy of sexual system and how it works, impacting client's understanding of situation and expectations.**
- Determine preexisting problems that may be factors in current situation (e.g., marital or job stress, role conflicts).
- Identify current stress factors in individual situation. **These factors may be producing enough anxiety to cause depression or other psychological reaction(s) leading to physiological symptoms.**

Information that appears in brackets has been added by the authors to clarify and enhance the use of nursing diagnoses.

🌐 Cultural 🔵 Collaborative 🏠 Community/Home Care

- • Discuss cultural values, religious beliefs, or conflicts present. **Client may have anxiety and guilt as a result of family beliefs about sex and genital area of the body because of how sexuality was communicated to the client as he or she was growing up.**
- • Determine pathophysiology, illness, surgery, or trauma involved and impact on (perception of) individual/SO. **The client may be more concerned about these issues when the sexual parts of the body are involved (e.g., mastectomy, hysterectomy, prostatectomy).**
- • Review medication regimen and drug use (prescriptions, over the counter, illegal, alcohol) and cigarette use. **Antihypertensives may cause erectile dysfunction; monoamine oxidase inhibitors and tricyclics can cause erection or ejaculation problems and anorgasmia in women; narcotics and alcohol can produce impotence and inhibit orgasm; smoking creates vasoconstriction and may be a factor in erectile dysfunction.**
- • Observe behavior and stage of grieving when related to body changes or loss of a body part (e.g., pregnancy, obesity, amputation, mastectomy).
- • Discuss client's view of body, concern about penis size, failure with performance.
- • Assist with diagnostic studies to determine cause of erectile dysfunction. **More than half of the cases have a physical cause such as diabetes, vascular problems.** Monitor penile tumescence during REM sleep **to assist in determining physical ability.**
- • Explore with client the meaning of client's behavior. (**Masturbation, for instance, may have many meanings or purposes, such as for relief of anxiety, sexual deprivation, pleasure, a nonverbal expression of need to talk, way of alienating.**) (*Note:* Nurse needs to be aware of and be in control of own feelings and response to client expressions or self-revelation.)
- • Avoid making value judgments, **as they do not help the client to cope with the situation.**

Nursing Priority No. 2.
To assist client/SO to deal with individual situation:

- • Establish therapeutic nurse-client relationship **to promote treatment and facilitate sharing of sensitive information and feelings.**

Information that appears in brackets has been added by the authors to clarify and enhance the use of nursing diagnoses.

- Assist with treatment of underlying medical conditions, including changes in medication regimen, weight management, and cessation of smoking.
- Provide factual information about individual condition involved. **Promotes informed decision making.**
- Determine what client wants to know **to tailor information to client needs.** *Note:* Information affecting client safety or consequences of actions may need to be reviewed and reinforced.
- Encourage and accept expressions of concern, anger, grief, fear. **Client needs to talk about these feelings to begin resolution.**
- Assist client to be aware of and deal with stages of grieving for loss or change.
- Encourage client to share thoughts and concerns with partner and to clarify values and impact of condition on relationship.
- Provide for or identify ways to obtain privacy **to allow for sexual expression for individual and/or between partners without embarrassment and/or objections of others.**
- Assist client/SO to problem-solve alternative ways of sexual expression. **When client is unable to perform in usual manner, there are many ways the couple can learn to satisfy sexual needs.**
- Provide information about availability of corrective measures such as medication (e.g., papaverine or sildenafil [Viagra] for erectile dysfunction) or reconstructive surgery (e.g., penile/breast implants) when indicated.
- Refer to appropriate resources, as needed (e.g., healthcare co-worker with greater comfort level and/or knowledgeable clinical nurse specialist or professional sex therapist, family counseling).

Nursing Priority No. 3.

To promote wellness (Teaching/Discharge Considerations):

- Provide sex education, explanation of normal sexual functioning when necessary.
- Provide written material appropriate to individual needs (include list of books related to client's concerns) **for reinforcement at client's leisure and readiness to deal with sensitive materials.**
- Encourage ongoing dialogue and take advantage of teachable moments that occur. **Nurse needs to become comfortable with talking about sexual issue so he or she can recognize**

Information that appears in brackets has been added by the authors to clarify and enhance the use of nursing diagnoses.

these moments and be willing to discuss the client's concerns.

- Demonstrate and assist client to learn relaxation and/or visualization techniques.
- Encourage client to engage in regular self-examination, as indicated (e.g., breast/testicular examinations).
- Identify community resources for further assistance (e.g., Reach for Recovery, CanSurmount, Ostomy Association, family or sex therapist).
- Refer for further professional assistance concerning relationship difficulties, low sexual desire, and other sexual concerns (e.g., premature ejaculation, vaginismus, painful intercourse).
- Identify resources for assistive devices or sexual "aids."

Documentation Focus

Assessment/Reassessment

- Individual findings including nature of dysfunction, predisposing factors, perceived effect on sexuality and relationships.
- Cultural or religious factors, conflicts.
- Response of SO.
- Motivation for change.

Planning

- Plan of care and who is involved in planning.
- Teaching plan.

Implementation/Evaluation

- Response to interventions, teaching, and actions performed.
- Attainment or progress toward desired outcome(s).
- Modifications to plan of care.

Discharge Planning

- Long-term needs, referrals made, and who is responsible for actions to be taken.
- Community resources, specific referrals made.

Sample Nursing Outcomes & Interventions Classifications (NOC/NIC)

NOC—Sexual Functioning
NIC—Sexual Counseling

Information that appears in brackets has been added by the authors to clarify and enhance the use of nursing diagnoses.

ineffective Sexuality Pattern

Taxonomy II: Sexuality—Class 2 Sexual Function (00065)
[Diagnostic Division: Sexuality]
Submitted 1986; Revised 2006

Definition: Expressions of concern regarding own sexuality

Related Factors

Deficient knowledge or skill deficit about alternative responses to health-related transitions, altered body function or structure, illness, or medical treatment
Lack of privacy
Impaired relationship with an SO; lack of SO
Ineffective or absent role models
Conflicts with sexual orientation or variant preferences
Fear of pregnancy or acquiring a sexually transmitted disease

Defining Characteristics

Subjective
Reported difficulties, limitations, or changes in sexual behaviors or activities
Alteration in relationship with SO
Alterations in achieving perceived sex role
Values conflicts

Desired Outcomes/Evaluation Criteria— Client Will:

* Verbalize understanding of sexual anatomy and function.
* Verbalize knowledge and understanding of sexual limitations, difficulties, or changes that have occurred.
* Verbalize acceptance of self in current (altered) condition.
* Demonstrate improved communication and relationship skills.
* Identify individually appropriate method of contraception.

Actions/Interventions

Nursing Priority No. 1.
To assess causative/contributing factors:
* Obtain complete physical and sexual history, as indicated, including perception of normal function. **Sexuality is multi-**

Information that appears in brackets has been added by the authors to clarify and enhance the use of nursing diagnoses.

  ● Cultural   Ⓞ Collaborative   🏠 Community/Home Care

faceted, beginning with one's body, biological sex, and gender (biological, social, and legal status as girls or boys, women or men).

- Note use of vocabulary (assessing basic knowledge) and comments or concerns about sexual identity. **Components of sexual identity include one's gender identity (how one feels about his or her gender) as well as one's sexual orientation (straight, lesbian, gay, bisexual, transgendered).**
- Determine importance of sex and a description of the problem in the client's own words. Be alert to comments of client/SO (e.g., discounting overt or covert sexual expressions such as "He's just a dirty old man"). **Sexual concerns are often disguised as sarcasm, humor, or in offhand remarks.**
- Elicit impact of perceived problem on SO/family. **One's values about life, love, and the people in one's life are also components of one's sexuality.**
- Note cultural values or religious beliefs and conflicts that may exist. **Individuals are enculturated as they grow up and, depending on particular family views and taboos, may harbor feelings of shame and guilt about their sexual feelings.**
- Assess stress factors in client's environment that might cause anxiety or psychological reactions (e.g., power issues involving SO, adult children, aging, employment, loss of prowess).
- Explore knowledge of effects of altered body function/limitations precipitated by illness (e.g., multiple sclerosis, arthritis, mutilating cancer surgery) or medical treatment of alternative sexual responses and expressions (e.g., undescended testicle in young male, gender change or reassignment procedure).
- Review history of substance use (prescription medications, over-the-counter drugs, alcohol, illicit drugs). **May be used by client to handle underlying feelings or anxiety.**
- Explore issues and fears associated with sex (pregnancy, sexually transmitted diseases, trust and control issues, inflexible beliefs, preference confusion, altered performance).
- Determine client's interpretation of the altered sexual activity or behavior (e.g., a way of controlling, relief of anxiety, pleasure, lack of partner). **These behaviors (when related to body changes, including pregnancy, weight loss or gain, or loss of body part) may reflect a stage of grieving.**
- Assess life cycle issues, such as adolescence, young adulthood, menopause, aging. **All people are sexual beings from birth to death. Each transition has its own concerns and**

Information that appears in brackets has been added by the authors to clarify and enhance the use of nursing diagnoses.

needs specific education to help the client deal with it in a healthy manner.

Nursing Priority No. 2.

To assist client/SO to deal with individual situation:

- Provide atmosphere in which discussion of sexual problems is encouraged and permitted. **Sense of trust or comfort enhances ability to discuss sensitive matters.**
- Avoid value judgments—**they do not help the client cope with the situation.**
- Provide information about individual situation, determining client needs and desires.
- Encourage discussion of individual situation, with opportunity for expression of feelings without judgment. **Sexuality also includes feelings, attitudes, relationships, self-image, ideals, and behaviors, and influences how one experiences the world.** (*Note:* Nurse needs to be aware of and in control of own feelings and responses to the client's expressions and/ or concerns.)
- Provide specific information and suggestions about interventions directed toward the identified problems.
- Identify alternative forms of sexual expression that might be acceptable to both partners. **When illness or trauma (e.g., rheumatoid arthritis, paraplegia, long-term chronic condition) interferes with usual sexual expression, there are many different methods that can be used to obtain sexual satisfaction.**
- Discuss ways to manage individual devices or appliances (e.g., ostomy bag, breast prostheses, urinary collection device) **when change in body image or medical condition is involved.**
- Provide anticipatory guidance about losses that are to be expected (e.g., loss of known self when transsexual surgery is planned).
- Introduce client to individuals who have successfully managed a similar problem. **Provides positive role model and support for problem-solving.**

Nursing Priority No. 3.

🏠 To promote wellness (Teaching/Discharge Considerations):

- Provide factual information about problem(s), as identified by the client.

Information that appears in brackets has been added by the authors to clarify and enhance the use of nursing diagnoses.

- Engage in ongoing dialogue with the client and SO(s), as situation permits.
- Discuss methods, effectiveness and side effects of contraceptives, if indicated. **Assists individual/couple to make an informed decision on a method that meets own values or religious beliefs.**
- Refer to community resources (e.g., Planned Parenthood; gender identity clinic; social services; Parents, Families and Friends of Lesbians and Gays), as indicated.
- Refer for intensive individual or group psychotherapy, which may be combined with couple or family and/or sex therapy, as appropriate.
- Refer to NDs Sexual Dysfunction; disturbed Body Image; Self-Esteem [specify].

Documentation Focus

Assessment/Reassessment
- Individual findings, including nature of concern, perceived difficulties, limitations or changes, specific needs and desires.
- Cultural or religious beliefs, conflicts.
- Response of SO(s).

Planning
- Plan of care and who is involved in the planning.
- Teaching plan.

Implementation/Evaluation
- Response to interventions, teaching, and actions performed.
- Attainment or progress toward desired outcome(s).
- Modifications to plan of care.

Discharge Planning
- Long-term needs, teaching, and referrals made, and who is responsible for actions to be taken.
- Community resources, specific referrals made.

Sample Nursing Outcomes & Interventions Classifications (NOC/NIC)

NOC—Sexual Identity
NIC—Sexual Counseling

Information that appears in brackets has been added by the authors to clarify and enhance the use of nursing diagnoses.

risk for **Shock**

Taxonomy II: Safety/Protection—Class 2 Physical Injury
   (00205)
[Diagnostic Division: Circulation]
Submitted 2008

Definition: At risk for an inadequate blood flow to the body's tissues, which may lead to life-threatening cellular dysfunction

Risk Factors

Hypotension
Hypovolemia
Hypoxemia, hypoxia
Infection, sepsis; systemic inflammatory response syndrome

NOTE: A risk diagnosis is not evidenced by signs and symptoms, as the problem has not occurred; rather, nursing interventions are directed at prevention.

Desired Outcomes/Evaluation Criteria— Client Will:

- Display hemodynamic stability as evidenced by vital signs within normal range for client; prompt capillary refill; adequate urinary output with normal specific gravity; usual level of mentation.
- Be afebrile and free of other signs of infection, achieve timely wound healing.
- Verbalize understanding of disease process, risk factors, and treatment plan.

Actions/Interventions

Nursing Priority No. 1.
To assess causative/contributing factors:

- Note possible medical diagnoses or disease processes that can result in one or more types of shock, such as major trauma with heavy internal or external bleeding; heart failure; head or spinal cord injury; allergic reactions; pregnancy-related

---

Information that appears in brackets has been added by the authors to clarify and enhance the use of nursing diagnoses.

🌐 Cultural   ✪ Collaborative   🏠 Community/Home Care

complications; intra-abdomimal infections, open wounds, or other conditions associated with sepsis.

- Assess for history or presence of conditions leading to hypovolemic shock, such as trauma, surgery, inadequate clotting, anticoagulant therapy; gastrointestinal or other organ hemorrhage; prolonged vomiting and diarrhea; diabetes insipidus; misuse of diuretics. **These conditions deplete the body's circulating blood volume and ability to maintain organ perfusion and function.**
- Assess for conditions associated with *cardiogenic shock,* including myocardial infarction, cardiac arrest, lethal ventricular dysrhythmias, severe valvular dysfunction, cardiomyopathies, malignant hypertension. **These conditions directly impair the heart muscle and ability to pump.**
- Assess for conditions associated with *obstructive shock,* including pulmonary embolus, aortic stenosis, cardiac tamponade, tension pneumothorax. **In these conditions, the heart itself may be healthy but cannot pump because of conditions outside the heart that prevent normal filling or adequate outflow.**
- Assess for conditions associated with *distributive shock—neural-induced,* including pain, anesthesia, spinal cord or head injury; or *chemical-induced,* including peritonitis, sepsis, burns, anaphylaxis, hyperglycemia. **These situations result in loss of sympathetic tone, blood vessel dilation, pooling of venous blood and increased capillary permeability with shifting of fluids.**
- Monitor for persistent or heavy fluid loss, including wounds, drains, vomiting, gastrointestinal tube, chest tube. Check all secretions and excretions for occult blood. Refer to NDs risk for Bleeding; risk for imbalanced Fluid Volume, for additional interventions.
- Inspect skin, noting presence of traumatic or surgical wounds, erythema, edema, tenderness, petechiae; rashes or hives **for evidence of hemorrhage, localized infections, or hypersensitivity reaction.**
- Investigate reports of increased or sudden pain in wounds or body parts, **which could indicate ischemia or infection.**
- Be aware of invasive devices such as urinary and intravascular cathethers, endotrachial tube, implanted prosthetic devices **that potentiate risk for localized and systemic infections.**
- Assess vital signs and tissue and organ perfusion **for changes associated with shock states:**

Information that appears in brackets has been added by the authors to clarify and enhance the use of nursing diagnoses.

Heart rate and rhythm—noting progressive changes in heart rate **(reflecting an attempt to increase cardiac output)** and development of dysrhythmias, **suggesting electrolyte imbalances, hypoxia.**

Respirations—noting rapid, shallow breathing, use of accessory muscles **(in an attempt to increase vital capacity and compensate for metabolic acidosis associated with poor tissue perfusion and anaerobic metabolism),** which can progress to respiratory failure.

Blood pressure—noting hypotension, postural hypotension, and narrowed pulse pressure. **May indicate hypovolemia and/or failure of cardiac pumping or compensatory mechanisms.**

Pulses and neck veins—noting rapid, weak, thready peripheral pulses; congested or flat neck veins. **Signs associated with changes in circulating volume, cardiac ouput, and progressive changes in vascular tone and/or capillary permeability.**

Temperature—higher than 100.4°F (38°C) or lower than 96.8°F (36°C) may indicate infectious process. **Temperature changes in presence of elevated heart and respiratory rate, along with mildly elevated white blood cell (WBC) count in absence of documented infection, is suggestive of systemic inflammatory response syndrome (SIRS).**

State of consciousness and mentation—noting anxiety, restlessness, confusion, lethargy, or unresponsiveness. **Can occur because of changes in oxygenation, acid-base imbalances, and toxins associated with hypoperfusion.**

Skin color and moisture—noting overall flushing or pallor; bluish lips and fingernails, slow capillary refill; or cool, clammy skin.

Urine output—noting substantially decreased ouput. **One of the most sensitive indicators of change in circulating volume or poor perfusion.**

Urine characteristics—noting color and odor **suggestive of infection source.**

Bowel sounds—noting diminished or absent bowel sounds; other changes in gastrointestinal function such as vomiting; or change in color, amount, or frequency of stools, **reflecting hypoperfusion of gastrointestinal tract.**

⊛• Measure invasive hemodynamic parameters when available—central venous pressure (CVP), mean arterial pressure

---

Information that appears in brackets has been added by the authors to clarify and enhance the use of nursing diagnoses.

(MAP), cardiac output (CO)—**to determine if intravascular fluid deficit or cardiac dysfunction exists.**

- Obtain specimens of wounds, drains, central lines, blood for culture and sensitivity.
- Review laboratory data such as complete blood count with WBCs and differential; platelet numbers and function; other coagulation factors; tests for cardiac, renal, and hepatic function; pulse oximetry/arterial blood gas; serum lactate, blood urine cultures **to identify potential sources of shock and degree of organ involvement.**
- Review diagnostic studies such as x-rays, electrocardiogram, echocardiogram, angiography with ejection fraction; computed tomography or magnetic resonance imaging scans, ultrasound **to determine presence of injuries or disorders that could cause or lead to shock conditions.**
- Refer to NDs ineffective peripheral Tissue Perfusion; risk for decreased cardiac Tissue Perfusion; risk for ineffective cerebral Tissue Perfusion; risk for ineffective Gastrointestinal Perfusion; risk for ineffective Renal Perfusion, for additional interventions and rationales.

Nursing Priority No. 2.

To prevent/correct potential causes of shock:

- Collaborate in prompt treatment of underlying conditions such as trauma, heart failure, infections, and prepare for/assist with medical and surgical interventions **to maximize systemic circulation and tissue and organ perfusion.**
- Administer oxygen by appropriate route (e.g., nasal prongs, mask, ventilator) **to maximize oxygenation of tissues.**
- Administer fluids, electrolytes, colloids, blood or blood products, as indicated, **to rapidly restore or sustain circulating volume, electrolyte balance, and prevent shock state.**
- Administer medications as indicated (e.g., vasoactive drugs, cardiac glycosides, thrombolytics, anticoagulants, antimicrobials, analgesics).
- Provide client care with infection prevention interventions, such as diligent attention to hand hygiene, aseptic wound care or dressing changes, isolation precautions, early intervention in potential infectious condition.
- Provide nutrition by best means—oral, enteral, or parenteral feeding. Refer to nutritionist or dietitian **to provide foods rich in nutrients, vitamins, and minerals needed to promote healing and support immune system health.**

Information that appears in brackets has been added by the authors to clarify and enhance the use of nursing diagnoses.

Nursing Priority No. 3.

🏠 Promote wellness (Teaching/Discharge Considerations):

- Instruct client/SO in ways to prevent and/or manage underlying conditions that cause shock, including heart disease, injuries, dehydration, infection.
- 🌐 Identify reportable signs and symptoms, including unrelieved pain, unresolved bleeding, excessive fluid loss, persistent fever and chills, change in skin color accompanied by chest pain **for timely evaluation and intervention.**
- Emphasize need for recognition of substances that cause hypersensitivity or allergic reactions (e.g., insects, medicines, foods, latex) **to reduce risk of anaphylactic shock state**.
- 💊 Teach client purpose, dosage, schedule, precautions, and potential side effects of medications given to treat underlying conditions. **Enhances compliance with drug regimen, reducing individual risk.**
- Instruct in wound and skin care as indicated **to prevent infection and promote healing.**
- Teach client/caregivers importance of good hand hygiene, clean environment, and avoiding crowds when ill, especially if client is immunocompromised.
- 💊 Reinforce importance of immunization against infections such as influenza and pneumonia, especially in client with chronic conditions.
- Encourage consumption of healthy diet, participation in regular exercise, and adequate rest **for healing and immune system support.**
- 💊 Recommend that client at risk for hypersensitivity reactions wear medical alert bracelet, maintain readily accessible emergency medication (e.g., Benadryl and/or Epi-pen).

Documentation Focus

Assessment/Reassessment

- Individual risk factors such as blood loss, presence of infection.
- Assessment findings, including respiratory rate, character of breath sounds; heart rate and rhythm; temperature; frequency, amount, and appearance of secretions; presence of cyanosis; and mentation level.
- Results of laboratory tests and diagnostic studies.

Information that appears in brackets has been added by the authors to clarify and enhance the use of nursing diagnoses.

🌐 Cultural 😊 Collaborative 🏠 Community/Home Care

Planning
- Plan of care, specific interventions, and who is involved in the planning.
- Teaching plan.

Implementation/Evaluation
- Client's responses to treatment, teaching, and actions performed.
- Attainment or progress toward desired outcome(s).
- Modifications to plan of care.

Discharge Planning
- Long-term needs, identifying who is responsible for actions to be taken.
- Community resources for equipment and supplies post-discharge.
- Specific referrals made.

Sample Nursing Outcomes & Interventions Classifications (NOC/NIC)

NOC—Circulation Status
NIC—Shock Management

---

impaired Skin Integrity

Taxonomy II: Safety/Protection—Class 2 Physical Injury (00046)
[Diagnostic Division: Safety]
Submitted 1975; Revised 1998 (by small group work 1996)

Definition: Altered epidermis and/or dermis

Related Factors

External
Hyperthermia; hypothermia
Chemical substance; radiation; pharmaceutical agents
Physical immobilization
Humidity; moisture; [excretions or secretions]
Mechanical factors (e.g., shearing forces, pressure, restraint); [trauma: injury, surgery]
Extremes in age

Information that appears in brackets has been added by the authors to clarify and enhance the use of nursing diagnoses.

Internal

Imbalanced nutritional state (e.g., obesity, emaciation); impaired metabolic state; changes in fluid status

Skeletal prominence; changes in turgor; [presence of edema]

Impaired circulation or sensation; changes in pigmentation

Developmental factors

Immunological deficit

Psychogenetic factors

Defining Characteristics

Subjective

Reports of itching, pain, numbness of affected or surrounding area

Objective

Disruption of skin surface (epidermis)

Destruction of skin layers (dermis)

Invasion of body structures

Desired Outcomes/Evaluation Criteria— Client Will:

- Display timely healing of skin lesions, wounds, or pressure sores without complication.
- Maintain optimal nutrition and physical well-being.
- Participate in prevention measures and treatment program.
- Verbalize feelings of increased self-esteem and ability to manage situation.

Actions/Interventions

Nursing Priority No. 1.

To assess causative/contributing factors:

- Identify underlying condition or pathology involved. **Skin integrity problems can be the result of (1) disease processes that affect circulation and perfusion of tissues (e.g., arteriosclerosis, venous insufficiency, hypertension, obesity, diabetes, malignant neoplasms); (2) medications (e.g., anticoagulants, corticosteroids, immunosuppressives, antineoplastics) that adversely affect or impair healing; (3) burns or radiation (can break down internal tissues as well as skin); and (4) nutrition and hydration (e.g., malnutrition deprives the body of protein and calories required for**

Information that appears in brackets has been added by the authors to clarify and enhance the use of nursing diagnoses.

cell growth and repair, and dehydration impairs transport of oxygen and nutrients). Disruption in skin integrity can be intentional (e.g., surgical incision) or unintentional (e.g., accidental trauma, drug effect, allergic reaction) and closed (e.g., contusion, abrasion, rash) or open (e.g., laceration, skin tears, penetrating wound, ulcerations).

∞• Determine client's age and developmental factors or ability to care for self. **Newborn/infant's skin is thin and provides ineffective thermal regulation, and nails are thin. Babies and children are prone to skin rashes associated with viral, bacterial, and fungal infections and allergic reactions. In adolescence, hormones stimulate hair growth and sebaceous gland activity. In adults, it takes longer to replenish epidermis cells, resulting in increased risk of skin cancers and infection. In older adults, there is decreased epidermal regeneration, fewer sweat glands, less subcutaneous fat, elastin, and collagen, causing skin to become thinner, drier, and less responsive to pain sensations.**

• Evaluate client's skin care practices and hygiene issues. **Individual's skin may be oily, dry and scaly, or sensitive and is affected by bathing frequency (or lack of bathing), temperature of water, types of soap and other cleansing agents. Incontinence (urinary or bowel) and ineffective hygiene can result in serious skin impairment and discomfort.**

• Determine nutritional status and potential for delayed healing or tissue injury exacerbated by malnutrition (e.g., pressure points on emaciated and/or elderly client).

💊• Review medication and therapy regimen (e.g., steroid use, chemotherapy, radiation).

• Evaluate client with impaired cognition, developmental delay, need for or use of restraints, long-term immobility **to identify risk for injury and safety requirements.**

• Note presence of compromised mobility, sensation, vision, hearing, or speech **that may impact client's self-care as relates to skin care (e.g., diabetic with impaired vision probably cannot satisfactorily examine own feet).**

• Assess blood supply (e.g., capillary return time, color, and warmth) and sensation of skin surfaces and affected area on a regular basis **to provide comparative baseline and opportunity for timely intervention when problems are noted.**

⊕• Calculate ankle-brachial index (ABI) **to evaluate actual/ potential for impairment of circulation to lower extremities.** *Note:* **Result less than 0.9 indicates need for close**

Information that appears in brackets has been added by the authors to clarify and enhance the use of nursing diagnoses.

monitoring or more aggressive intervention (e.g., tighter blood glucose and weight control in diabetic client).

• Review laboratory results pertinent to causative factors (e.g., studies such as hemaglobin/hematocrit, blood glucose, infectious agents [viral, bacterial, fungal], albumin and protein). (*Note:***Albumin less than 3.5 correlates to decreased wound healing and increased frequency of pressure ulcers.**)

• Obtain specimen from draining wounds when appropriate for culture and sensitivities or Gram's stain **to determine appropriate therapy.**

Nursing Priority No. 2.

To assess extent of involvement/injury:

∞• Obtain a complete history of current skin condition(s) (especially in children where recurrent rash or lesions are common), including age at onset, date of first episode, duration, original site, characteristics of lesions, and any changes that have occurred. **Common skin manifestations of sensitivity or allergies are hives, eczema, and contact dermatitis. Contagious rashes include measles, rubella, roseola, chicken pox, and scarlet fever. Bacterial, viral, and fungal infections can also cause skin problems (e.g., impetigo, cellulitis, cold sores, shingles, athlete's foot, *candidiasis* diaper rashes).**

• Perform routine skin inspections describing observed changes. Note skin color, texture, and turgor. Assess areas of least pigmentation for color changes (e.g., sclera, conjunctiva, nailbeds, buccal mucosa, tongue, palms, and soles of feet).

• Palpate skin lesions for size, shape, consistency, texture, temperature, and hydration.

• Determine degree and depth of injury or damage to integumentary system (i.e., involves epidermis, dermis, and/or underlying tissues).

• Measure length, width, depth of ulcer or wound. Note extent of tunneling or undermining, if present.

• Inspect surrounding skin for erythema, induration, maceration.

• Photograph lesion(s)/burns, as appropriate, **to document status and provide visual baseline for future comparisons.**

• Note odors emitted from the skin, lesion, or wound.

• Classify ulcer using tool such as Wagner Ulcer Classification System. **Provides consistent terminology for documentation.**

Information that appears in brackets has been added by the authors to clarify and enhance the use of nursing diagnoses.

🌐 Cultural   ㊰ Collaborative   🏠 Community/Home Care

Nursing Priority No. 3.

To determine impact of condition:

- Determine if wound is acute (e.g., injury from surgery or trauma) or chronic (e.g., venous or arterial insufficiency), **which affects healing time and the client's emotional and physical responses.**
- Determine client's level of discomfort (e.g., can vary widely from minor itching or aching, to deep pain with burns, or excoriation associated with drainage) **to clarify intervention needs and priorities.**
- Ascertain attitudes of individual/SO(s) about condition (e.g., cultural values, stigma). Note misconceptions. **Identifies areas to be addressed in teaching plan and potential referral needs.**
- Determine impact on life (e.g., work, leisure, increased caregiver requirements).
- Obtain psychological assessment of client's emotional status, as indicated, noting potential for sexual problems arising from presence of condition.
- Note presence of compromised vision, hearing, or speech. **Touch is a particularly important avenue of communication for this population, and when skin is compromised, communication may be affected.**

Nursing Priority No. 4.

To assist client with correcting/minimizing condition and promote optimal healing:

- Inspect skin on a daily basis, describing wound or lesion characteristics and changes observed.
- Periodically remeasure and photograph wound and observe for complications (e.g., infection, dehiscence) **to monitor progress of wound healing.**
- Keep the area clean and dry, carefully dress wounds, support incision (e.g., use of Steri-Strips, splinting when coughing), prevent infection, manage incontinence, and stimulate circulation to surrounding areas **to assist body's natural process of repair.**
- Assist with débridement or enzymatic therapy, as indicated (e.g., burns, severe pressure sores), **to remove nonviable, contaminated, or infected tissue.**
- Use appropriate barrier dressings, wound coverings, drainage appliances, vacuum-assisted closure device (wound vac), and

---

Information that appears in brackets has been added by the authors to clarify and enhance the use of nursing diagnoses.

skin-protective agents for open, draining wounds and stomas **to protect the wound and/or surrounding tissues.**

- Apply appropriate dressing (e.g., adhesive or nonadhesive film, hydrofiber or gel, acrylics, hydropolymers) **for wound healing and to best meet needs of client and caregiver or care setting.**
- Maintain appropriate moisture environment for particular wound (e.g., expose lesion or ulcer to air and light **if excess moisture is impeding healing** or use occlusive dressings **to maintain a moist environment for autolytic débridement of wound**), as indicated.
- Avoid or limit use of plastic material (e.g., plastic-backed linen savers). Remove wet and wrinkled linens promptly. **Moisture potentiates skin breakdown.**
- Use paper tape or nonadherent dressing on frail skin and remove gently. Use stockinette, gauze wrap, or any other similar type of wrap instead of tape to secure dressings and drains.
- Reposition client on regular schedule, involving client in reasons for and decisions about times and positions **to enhance understanding and cooperation.**
- Use appropriate padding devices (e.g., air or water mattress, gel pad, waffle boots), when indicated, **to reduce pressure on, and enhance circulation to, compromised tissues.** Avoid use of sheepskin, **which may retain heat and moisture.**
- Encourage early ambulation or mobilization. **Promotes circulation and reduces risks associated with immobility.**
- Provide optimum nutrition, including vitamins (e.g., A, C, D, E) and protein, **to provide a positive nitrogen balance to aid in skin and tissue healing and to maintain general good health.**
- Monitor periodic laboratory studies relative to general well-being and status of specific problem.
- Consult with wound or stoma specialist, as indicated, **to assist with developing plan of care for problematic or potentially serious wounds.**

Nursing Priority No. 5.
To promote wellness (Teaching/Discharge Considerations):

- Review importance of health, intact skin, as well as measures to maintain proper skin functioning. **The integumentary system is the largest multifunctional organ of the body.**
- Discuss importance of early detection of skin changes and/or complications.

Information that appears in brackets has been added by the authors to clarify and enhance the use of nursing diagnoses.

- Assist the client/SO(s) in understanding and following medical regimen and developing program of preventive care and daily maintenance. **Enhances commitment to plan, optimizing outcomes.**
- Review measures to avoid spread of communicable disease or reinfection.
- Emphasize importance of proper fit of clothing and shoes, use of specially lined shock-absorbing socks or pressure-reducing insoles for shoes **in presence of reduced sensation/circulation.**
- Identify safety factors for use of equipment or appliances (e.g., heating pad, ostomy appliances, padding straps of braces).
- Encourage client to verbalize feelings and discuss how or if condition affects self-concept or self-esteem. (Refer to NDs disturbed Body Image; situational low Self-Esteem.)
- Assist client to work through stages of grief and feelings associated with individual condition.
- Lend psychological support and acceptance of client, using touch, facial expressions, and tone of voice.
- Assist client to learn stress-reduction and alternate therapy techniques **to control feelings of helplessness and deal with situation.**
- Refer to dietitian or certified diabetes educator, as appropriate, **to enhance healing, reduce risk of recurrence of diabetic ulcers.**

Documentation Focus

Assessment/Reassessment
- Characteristics of lesion(s) or condition, ulcer classification.
- Causative and contributing factors.
- Impact of condition on personal image and lifestyle.

Planning
- Plan of care and who is involved in planning.
- Teaching plan.

Implementation/Evaluation
- Responses to interventions, teaching, and actions performed.
- Attainment or progress toward desired outcome(s).
- Modifications to plan of care.

Information that appears in brackets has been added by the authors to clarify and enhance the use of nursing diagnoses.

Discharge Planning
- Long-term needs and who is responsible for actions to be taken.
- Specific referrals made.

Sample Nursing Outcomes & Interventions Classifications (NOC/NIC)

NOC—Tissue Integrity: Skin & Mucous Membranes
NIC—Pressure Ulcer Care

risk for impaired Skin Integrity

Taxonomy II: Safety/Protection—Class 2 Physical Injury (00047)
[Diagnostic Division: Safety]
Submitted 1975; Revised 1998 (by small group work 1996)

Definition: At risk for alteration in epidermis and/or dermis

NOTE: Risk should be determined by use of a standardized risk assessment tool (e.g., Braden, Norton [or similar] Scale).

Risk Factors

External
Chemical substance; radiation
Hypothermia; hyperthermia
Physical immobilization
Excretions; secretions; humidity; moisture
Mechanical factors (e.g., shearing forces, pressure, restraint)
Extremes of age

Internal
Medications
Imbalanced nutritional state (e.g., obesity, emaciation); impaired metabolic state
Skeletal prominence; changes in skin turgor; [presence of edema]

Information that appears in brackets has been added by the authors to clarify and enhance the use of nursing diagnoses.

Impaired circulation or sensation; changes in pigmentation
Developmental factors
Psychogenetic factors
Immunological factors

> **NOTE:** A risk diagnosis is not evidenced by signs and symptoms as the problem has not occurred; rather, nursing interventions are directed at prevention.

Desired Outcomes/Evaluation Criteria— Client Will:

- Identify individual risk factors.
- Verbalize understanding of treatment/therapy regimen.
- Demonstrate behaviors and techniques to prevent skin breakdown.

Actions/Interventions

Nursing Priority No. 1.
To assess causative/contributing factors:

- Identify underlying conditions or problems **that have potential for skin integrity problems such as (1) disease processes that affect circulation and perfusion of tissues; (2) medications that adversely affect or impair healing; (3) radiation; and (4) nutrition and hydration. Disruption in skin integrity can be intentional (e.g., surgical incision) or unintentional (e.g., accidental trauma, drug effect, allergic reaction) and closed (e.g., contusion, abrasion, rash) or open (e.g., laceration, skin tears, penetrating wound, ulcerations).**

∞• Determine client's age and developmental factors or ability to care for self. **Newborn/infant's skin is thin. Babies and children are prone to skin rashes associated with viral, bacterial, and fungal infections and allergic reactions. In adolescence, hormones stimulate hair growth and sebaceous gland activity. In adults, it takes longer to replenish epidermis cells, resulting in increased risk of skin cancers and infection. In older adults, there is decreased epidermal regeneration, fewer sweat glands, and less subcutaneous fat and elastin and collagen, causing skin to become thinner, drier, and less responsive to pain sensations.**

Information that appears in brackets has been added by the authors to clarify and enhance the use of nursing diagnoses.

- Assess skin, noting moisture, color, and elasticity.
- Review with client/SO history of past skin problems (e.g., allergic reactions, rashes, easy bruising or skin tears) **that may indicate particular vulnerability.**
- Ascertain allergy history. **Individual may be sensitive or allergic to substances (e.g., insects, grasses, medications, lotions, soaps, foods) that can adversely affect the skin.**
- Assess blood supply (e.g., capillary return time, color, warmth) and sensation of skin surfaces or extremities on a regular basis **to provide comparative baseline and opportunity for timely intervention when problems are noted.**
- Evaluate client's skin care practices and hygiene issues. **Skin may be oily, dry and scaly, or sensitive, and is affected by bathing frequency (or lack of bathing), temperature of water, and types of soap and other cleansing agents. Incontinence (urinary or bowel) and ineffective hygiene can result in serious skin impairment and discomfort.**
- Note presence of compromised vision, sensation, hearing, or speech **that may impact client's self-care as relates to skin care (e.g., diabetic with impaired vision probably cannot satisfactorily examine own feet).**
- Assess for diminished circulation in lower extremities. Calculate ankle-brachial index (ABI), as appropriate (diabetic clients or others with impaired circulation to lower extremities). **Result less than 0.9 indicates need for more aggressive preventive interventions (e.g., stricter blood glucose and weight control).**
- Review laboratory results (e.g., hemoglobin/hematocrit, blood glucose, albumin, protein) **to evaluate causative factors or ability to heal.** *Note:* **Albumin <3.5 correlates to decreased wound healing and increased incidence of pressure ulcers.**

Nursing Priority No. 2.

To maintain skin integrity at optimal level:

- Perform routine skin inspections, assessing color, temperature, surface changes, texture, and contours. Evaluate color changes in areas of least pigmentation (e.g., sclera, conjunctiva, nailbeds, buccal mucosa, tongue, palms, soles of feet). Report potential problem areas (e.g., reddened/blanched areas or rashes) promptly. **Systematic inspection can identify developing problems and promotes early intervention, thus reducing likelihood of progression to skin breakdown.**

Information that appears in brackets has been added by the authors to clarify and enhance the use of nursing diagnoses.

🌐 Cultural 🅒 Collaborative 🏠 Community/Home Care

∞• Handle client gently (particularly infant, young child, elderly). **Epidermis of infants and very young children is thin and lacks subcutaneous depth that will develop with age. Skin of the older client is also thin, less elastic, and prone to injury, such as bruising and skin tears.**

• Inspect skin surfaces and pressure points routinely, especially in mobility-impaired client.

• Observe for reddened or blanched areas or skin rashes, and institute treatment immediately. **Reduces likelihood of progression to skin breakdown.**

• Maintain and instruct in good skin hygiene (e.g., shower instead of bath, washing thoroughly, using mild nondetergent soap, drying gently and lubricating with lotion or emollient, as indicated) **to reduce risk of dermal trauma, improve circulation, and promote comfort.**

• Massage bony prominences and use proper positioning, turning, lifting, and transferring techniques when moving client **to prevent friction or shear injury.**

🏠• Develop regularly timed repositioning schedule for client with mobility and sensation impairments, using turn sheet, as needed; encourage or assist with periodic weight shifts for client in chair **to reduce stress on pressure points and to promote circulation to tissues.**

• Encourage client participation in early ambulation, active and assistive range-of-motion exercises.

• Provide adequate clothing or covers; protect from drafts **to prevent vasoconstriction.**

• Keep bedclothes dry and wrinkle free; use nonirritating linens.

🏠• Use appropriate padding or pressure reducing devices (e.g., egg crate, gel pads, heel rolls or foam boots) or pressure relieving devices (e.g., air or water mattress), when indicated, **to reduce pressure on sensitive areas and enhance circulation to compromised tissues.**

• Use paper tape or a nonadherent dressing on frail skin and remove it gently or use stockinette, gauze wrap, or any other similar type of wrap instead of tape to secure dressings and drains.

• Avoid use of latex products **when client has known or suspected sensitivity.** (Refer to ND Latex Allergy Response.)

• Apply hot and cold applications judiciously **to reduce risk of dermal injury in persons with circulatory and neurosensory impairments.**

• Provide for safety measures during ambulation and other therapies that might cause dermal injury (e.g., use of properly

---

Information that appears in brackets has been added by the authors to clarify and enhance the use of nursing diagnoses.

fitting hose and footwear, safe use of heating pads or lamps, restraints).

- Provide preventive skin care to incontinent client. Change continence pads or diapers frequently; cleanse perineal skin daily; and after each incontinence episode, apply skin protectant ointment **to minimize contact with irritants (urine, stool, excessive moisture).**

Nursing Priority No. 3.

🏠 To promote wellness (Teaching/Discharge Considerations):

- Provide information to client/SO(s) about the importance of regular observation and effective skin care in preventing problems.
- Emphasize importance of adequate nutritional and fluid intake **to maintain general good health and skin turgor.**
- Encourage continuation of regular exercise program (active or assistive) **to enhance circulation.**
- Recommend elevation of lower extremities when sitting **to enhance venous return and reduce edema formation.**
- Encourage abstinence from smoking, **which causes vasoconstriction.**
- Suggest use of ice, colloidal bath, lotions **to decrease irritable itching.**
- Recommend keeping nails short or wearing gloves **to reduce risk of dermal injury when severe itching is present.**
- Discuss importance of avoiding exposure to sunlight in specific conditions (e.g., systemic lupus, tetracycline or psychotropic drug use, radiation therapy) as well as potential for development of skin cancer.
- Advise regular use of sunscreen, particularly on young child, client with fair skin (prone to burn), or client using multiple medications, and so forth, **to limit skin damage (immediate and over time) associated with sun exposure.**
- Counsel diabetic and neurologically impaired clients about importance of skin care, especially of lower extremities.
- Perform periodic assessment using a tool such as the Braden Scale **to determine changes in risk status and need for alterations in the plan of care.**
- 🔗 Refer to dietitian or certified diabetes educator, as appropriate, **to identify nutritional needs/maintain proper diabetic control.**

Information that appears in brackets has been added by the authors to clarify and enhance the use of nursing diagnoses.

Documentation Focus

Assessment/Reassessment
- Individual findings, including individual risk factors.

Planning
- Plan of care and who is involved in planning.
- Teaching plan.

Implementation/Evaluation
- Responses to interventions, teaching, and actions performed.
- Attainment or progress toward desired outcome(s).
- Modifications to plan of care.

Discharge Planning
- Long-term needs and who is responsible for actions to be taken.

Sample Nursing Outcomes & Interventions Classifications (NOC/NIC)

NOC—Risk Control
NIC—Skin Surveillance

---

readiness for enhanced Sleep

Taxonomy II: Activity/Rest—Class 1 Sleep/Rest (00165)
[Diagnostic Division: Activity/Rest]
Submitted 2002

Definition: A pattern of natural, periodic suspension of consciousness that provides adequate rest, sustains a desired lifestyle, and can be strengthened

Defining Characteristics

Subjective
Expresses willingness to enhance sleep
Reports being rested after sleep
Follows sleep routines that promote sleep habits

Objective
Amount of sleep is congruent with developmental needs
Occasional use of pharmaceutical agents to induce sleep

Information that appears in brackets has been added by the authors to clarify and enhance the use of nursing diagnoses.

Desired Outcomes/Evaluation Criteria— Client Will:

- Identify individually appropriate interventions to promote sleep.
- Verbalize feeling rested after sleep.
- Adjust lifestyle to accommodate routines that promote sleep.

Actions/Interventions

Nursing Priority No. 1.
To determine motivation for continued growth:

- Listen to client's reports of sleep quantity and quality. Determine client's/SO's perception of adequate sleep. **Reveals client's experience and expectations. Provides opportunity to address misconceptions or unrealistic expectations and plan for interventions.**
- Observe and/or obtain feedback from client/SO(s) regarding usual bedtime, desired rituals and routines, number of hours of sleep, time of arising, and environmental needs **to determine usual sleep pattern and provide comparative baseline for improvements.**
- Ascertain motivation and expectation for change.
- Note client report of potential for alteration of habitual sleep time (e.g., change of work pattern, rotating shifts) or change in normal bedtime (e.g., hospitalization). **Helps identify circumstances that are known to interrupt sleep patterns and that could disrupt the person's biological rhythms.**

Nursing Priority No. 2.
To assist client to enhance sleep/rest:

- Review client's usual bedtime rituals, routines, and sleep environment needs. **Provides information on client's management of the situation and identifies areas that might be modified when the need arises.**
- ∞• Implement effective age-appropriate bedtime rituals for infant/child (e.g., soothing bath, rocking, story reading, cuddling, favorite blanket or toy). **Rituals can enhance ability to fall asleep, reinforce that bed is a place to sleep, and promote sense of security for child.**
- Provide quiet environment and comfort measures (e.g., back rub, washing hands and face, cleaning and straight-

---

Information that appears in brackets has been added by the authors to clarify and enhance the use of nursing diagnoses.

🌐 Cultural ⊛ Collaborative 🏠 Community/Home Care

ening sheets). **Promotes relaxation and readiness for sleep.**

- Arrange care **to provide for uninterrupted periods for rest.** Explain necessity of disturbances for monitoring vital signs and/or other care when client is hospitalized. Do as much care as possible without waking client during night. **Allows for longer periods of uninterrupted sleep, especially during night.**

- Discuss dietary matters, such as limiting intake of chocolate and caffeine or alcoholic beverages (especially prior to bedtime), **which are substances known to impair falling or staying asleep.** *Note:* **Use of alcohol at bedtime may help individual initially fall asleep, but ensuing sleep is then fragmented.**

- Limit fluid intake in evening if nocturia or bedwetting is a problem **to reduce need for nighttime elimination.**

- Recommend appropriate changes to usual bedtime rituals. Explore use of warm bath, comfortable room temperature, use of soothing music, favorite calming TV show. **Nonpharmaceutical aids can enhance falling asleep.**

- Assist client in use of necessary equipment, instructing as necessary. **Client may use oxygen or continuous positive airway pressure system to improve sleep/rest if hypoxia or sleep apnea is diagnosed.**

- Investigate use of sleep mask, darkening shades or curtains, earplugs, low-level background ("white") noise. **Aids in blocking out light and disturbing noise.**

🏠 • Recommend continuing same schedule for sleep throughout week—including days off. **Maintaining same sleep—wake pattern helps sustain biological rhythms.**

Nursing Priority No. 3.
🏠 To promote optimum wellness:

- Assure client that occasional sleeplessness should not threaten health. **Knowledge that occasional insomnia is universal and usually not harmful may promote relaxation and relief from worry.**

- Encourage regular exercise during the day **to aid in stress control and release of energy.** *Note:* **Exercise at bedtime may stimulate rather than relax client and actually interfere with sleep.**

- Address sleep management techniques that may be useful during stressful conditions or lifestyle changes (e.g., pregnancy,

---

Information that appears in brackets has been added by the authors to clarify and enhance the use of nursing diagnoses.

new baby, menopause, medical procedures, new job, moving, change in relationship, grief).

 • Advise using barbiturates and/or other sleeping medications sparingly. **These medications, while useful for promoting sleep in the short term, can interfere with REM sleep.**

Documentation Focus

Assessment/Reassessment

* Assessment findings, including specifics of current and past sleep pattern, and effects on lifestyle and level of functioning.
* Medications, interventions, and previous therapies used.
* Motivation and expectations for change.

Planning

* Plan of care and who is involved in planning.
* Teaching plan.

Implementation/Evaluation

* Client's response to interventions, teaching, and actions performed.
* Attainment or progress toward desired outcome(s).
* Modifications to plan of care.

Discharge Planning

* Long-term needs and who is responsible for actions to be taken.
* Specific referrals made.

Sample Nursing Outcomes & Interventions Classifications (NOC/NIC)

NOC—Sleep
NIC—Sleep Enhancement

Information that appears in brackets has been added by the authors to clarify and enhance the use of nursing diagnoses.

Sleep Deprivation

Taxonomy II: Activity/Rest—Class 1 Sleep/Rest (00096)
[Diagnostic Division: Activity/Rest]
Submitted: Nursing Diagnosis Extension and Classification 1998

Definition: Prolonged periods of time without sleep (sustained natural, periodic suspension of relative consciousness)

Related Factors

Sustained environmental stimulation or uncomfortable sleep environment

Inadequate daytime activity; sustained circadian asynchrony; aging-related sleep stage shifts; nonsleep-inducing parenting practices

Sustained inadequate sleep hygiene; prolonged use of pharmacological agents or dietary antisoporifics

Prolonged discomfort (e.g., physical, psychological); periodic limb movement (e.g., restless leg syndrome, nocturnal myoclonus); sleep-related enuresis/painful erections

Nightmares; sleepwalking; sleep terror

Sleep apnea

Sundowner's syndrome; dementia

Idiopathic central nervous system hypersomnolence; narcolepsy; familial sleep paralysis

Defining Characteristics

Subjective

Daytime drowsiness; decreased ability to function

Malaise; lethargy; fatigue

Anxiety

Perceptual disorders (e.g., disturbed body sensation, delusions, feeling afloat); heightened pain sensitivity

Objective

Restlessness; irritability

Inability to concentrate; slowed reaction

Listlessness; apathy

Fleeting nystagmus; hand tremors

Acute confusion; transient paranoia; agitation; combativeness; hallucinations

---

Information that appears in brackets has been added by the authors to clarify and enhance the use of nursing diagnoses.

Desired Outcomes/Evaluation Criteria— Client Will:

- Identify individually appropriate interventions to promote sleep.
- Verbalize understanding of sleep disorder.
- Adjust lifestyle to accommodate chronobiological rhythms.
- Report improvement in sleep and rest pattern.

Family Will:

- Deal appropriately with parasomnias.

Actions/Interventions

Nursing Priority No. 1.

To assess causative/contributing factors:

∞• Note client's age and developmental stage. **The average adult requires 7 to 8 hours sleep; teenagers about 9 hours, infants about 16 hours. Pregnant women and new mothers, while needing more sleep, are usually sleep deprived; adolescents and young adults don't get enough sleep, have irregular sleep patterns, and are at risk for problem sleepiness; menopausal women often report interrupted sleep because of hot flashes or hormonal influences; elderly persons sleep fewer hours, report less restful sleep and need for more sleep.**

- Determine presence of physical or psychological stressors, including night-shift working hours or rotating shifts, pain, current or recent illness, death of a spouse.
- Note medical diagnoses that affect sleep (e.g., dementia, encephalitis, brain injury, narcolepsy, depression, asthma, nocturnal myoclonus [jerking of legs causing repeated awakening]).
- Review results of studies that may be done to assess for sleep-induced respiratory disorders or obstructive sleep apnea.
- Evaluate for use of medications and/or other drugs affecting sleep. **Diet pills or other stimulants, sedatives, antidepressants, antihypertensives, diuretics, narcotics, agents with anticholinergic effects, and need for medications requiring nighttime dosing can inhibit getting to sleep or remaining asleep.**
- Note environmental factors affecting sleep (e.g., unfamiliar or uncomfortable sleep environment, excessive noise and light, uncomfortable temperature, roommate actions [e.g., snoring, watching TV late at night]).

Information that appears in brackets has been added by the authors to clarify and enhance the use of nursing diagnoses.

- Determine presence of parasomnias: nightmares, terrors, or somnambulism (e.g., sitting, sleepwalking, or other complex behavior during sleep).
- Note reports of terror, brief periods of paralysis, sense of body being disconnected from the brain. **Occurrence of sleep paralysis (although not widely recognized in the United States, has been well documented elsewhere) may result in feelings of fear and reluctance to go to sleep.**

Nursing Priority No. 2.

To assess degree of impairment:

- Determine client's usual sleep pattern and expectations. **Provides comparative baseline.**
- Ascertain duration of current problem and effect on life and functional ability.
- Listen to client's/SO's subjective reports of client's sleep quality and family concerns.
- Observe for physical signs of fatigue (e.g., frequent yawning, restlessness, irritability; inability to tolerate stress; disorientation; problems with concentration or memory; behavioral, learning, or social problems).
- Determine interventions client has tried in the past. **Helps identify appropriate options.**
- Distinguish client's beneficial bedtime habits from detrimental ones (e.g., drinking late-evening milk versus drinking late-evening coffee).
- Instruct client and/or bed partner to keep a sleep-wake log **to document symptoms and identify factors that are interfering with sleep.**
- Do a chronological chart **to determine peak performance rhythms**

Nursing Priority No. 3.

To assist client to establish optimal sleep pattern:

- Review medications being taken and their effect on sleep, suggesting modifications in regimen, **if medications are found to be interfering.**
- Encourage client to restrict late afternoon or evening intake of caffeine, alcohol, and other stimulating substances and to avoid eating large evening or late-night meals. **These factors are known to disrupt sleep patterns.**
- Recommend light bedtime snack (protein, simple carbohydrate, and low fat) for individuals who feel hungry 15 to 30

Information that appears in brackets has been added by the authors to clarify and enhance the use of nursing diagnoses.

minutes before retiring. **Sense of fullness and satiety promotes sleep and reduces likelihood of gastric upset.**

- Promote adequate physical exercise activity during day. **Enhances expenditure of energy and release of tension so that client feels ready for sleep or rest.**
- Suggest abstaining from daytime naps **because they may impair ability to sleep at night.**
- Investigate anxious feelings **to help determine basis and appropriate anxiety-reduction techniques.**
- Recommend quiet activities, such as reading or listening to soothing music in the evening, **to reduce stimulation so client can relax.**
- Instruct in relaxation techniques, music therapy, meditation, and so forth, **to decrease tension, prepare for rest or sleep.**
- Limit evening fluid intake if nocturia is present **to reduce need for nighttime elimination.**
- ∞ Discuss and implement effective age-appropriate bedtime rituals (e.g., going to bed at same time each night, drinking warm milk, soothing bath, rocking, story reading, cuddling, favorite blanket or toy) **to enhance client's ability to fall asleep; reinforce that bed is a place to sleep and promote sense of security for child.**
- Provide calm, quiet environment and manage controllable sleep-disrupting factors (e.g., noise, light, room temperature).
- Administer sedatives or other sleep medications, when indicated, noting client's response. Time pain medications for peak effect and duration **to reduce need for redosing during prime sleep hours.**
- Instruct client to get out of bed **if unable to fall asleep**, leave bedroom, engage in relaxing activities and not return to bed until feeling sleepy.
- Review with client the physician's recommendations for medications or surgery (alteration of facial structures, tracheotomy) and/or apneic oxygenation therapy—continuous positive airway pressure, such as Respironics—**when sleep apnea is the cause for sleep disturbance, as documented by sleep disorder studies.**

Nursing Priority No. 4.

🔒 To promote wellness (Teaching/Discharge Considerations):

- Review possibility of next-day drowsiness or "rebound" insomnia and temporary memory loss **that may be associated with prescription sleep medications.**

Information that appears in brackets has been added by the authors to clarify and enhance the use of nursing diagnoses.

🌐 Cultural 🔵 Collaborative 🏠 Community/Home Care

- 🔬 Discuss use and appropriateness of over-the-counter sleep medications or herbal supplements. Note possible side effects and drug interactions.
- ⚕️ Refer to support group or counselor **to help deal with psychological stressors (e.g., grief, sorrow, chronic pain).** (Refer to NDs Grieving; chronic Sorrow; chronic Pain.)
- ⚕️ Encourage family counseling **to help deal with concerns arising from parasomnias.**
- ∞ Identify appropriate safety precautions (e.g., securing doors, windows, and stairways; placing client bedroom on first floor), and attach audible alarm to bedroom door **to alert parents when child is sleepwalking.**
- ⚕️ Refer to sleep specialist or sleep laboratory **when problem is unresponsive to customary interventions.**

Documentation Focus

Assessment/Reassessment
- Assessment findings, including specifics of current and past sleep pattern and effects on lifestyle and level of functioning.
- Medications, interventions tried, previous therapies.
- Family history of similar problem.

Planning
- Plan of care and who is involved in planning.
- Teaching plan.

Implementation/Evaluation
- Client's response to interventions, teaching, and actions performed.
- Attainment or progress toward desired outcome(s).
- Modifications to plan of care.

Discharge Planning
- Long-term needs and who is responsible for actions to be taken.
- Specific referrals made.

Sample Nursing Outcomes & Interventions Classifications (NOC/NIC)

NOC—Sleep
NIC—Sleep Enhancement

Information that appears in brackets has been added by the authors to clarify and enhance the use of nursing diagnoses.

disturbed Sleep Pattern

Taxonomy II: Activity/Rest—Class 1 Sleep/Rest (00198)
[Diagnostic Division: Activity/Rest]
Submitted 1980; Revised 1998
Resubmitted 2006

Definition: Time-limited interruptions of sleep amount and quality due to external factors

Related Factors

Ambient temperature, humidity; lighting; noise; noxious odors; physical restraint
Change in daylight-darkness exposure
Caregiving responsibilities
Lack of sleep privacy or control; sleep partner
Unfamiliar sleep furnishings
Interruptions (e.g., for therapeutics, monitoring, lab tests)

Defining Characteristics

Subjective
Reports no difficulty falling asleep; reports being awakened
Reports not feeling well rested; dissatisfaction with sleep

Objective
Change in normal sleep pattern
Decreased ability to function

Desired Outcomes/Evaluation Criteria—Client Will (Include Specific Time Frame):

Report improved sleep.
Report increased sense of well-being and feeling rested.
Identify individually appropriate interventions to promote sleep.

Actions/Interventions

Nursing Priority No. 1.
To assess causative/contributing factors:
• Identify presence of factors known to interfere with sleep, including current illness, hospitalization; new baby or sick family member in home. **Sleep problems can arise from**

Information that appears in brackets has been added by the authors to clarify and enhance the use of nursing diagnoses.

⊕ Cultural   Ⓒ Collaborative   🏠 Community/Home Care

internal and external factors and may require assessment over time to differentiate specific cause(s).

- Ascertain presence of short-term alteration in sleep patterns, such as can occur with travel (jet lag), sharing bed with new sleep partner, fighting with family member, crisis at work, loss of job, death in family. **Helps identify circumstances that are known to interrupt sleep acutely, but not necessarily long term.**
- Note environmental factors, such as unfamiliar or uncomfortable room; excessive noise and light, uncomfortable temperature; frequent medical and monitoring interventions; and roommate actions—snoring, watching television late at night, wanting to talk. **These factors can reduce client's ability to rest and sleep at a time when more rest is needed.** *Note:* **Clients in critical care units are known to experience lack of sleep or frequent disruptions, often compounding their illness.**

Nursing Priority No. 2.
To evaluate sleep and degree of dysfunction:

- Assess client's usual sleep patterns and compare with current sleep disturbance, relying on client/SO report of problem **to ascertain intensity and duration of problems.**
- Listen to reports of sleep quality (e.g., "short," "interrupted") and response from lack of good sleep (feeling foggy, sleepy, and woozy; fighting sleep; fatigue). **Helps clarify client's perception of sleep quantity and quality and response to inadequate sleep.**
- Determine client's sleep expectations. **Individual may have faulty beliefs or attitudes about sleep and/or unrealistic sleep expectations (e.g., "I must get 8 hours of sleep every night or I can't accomplish anything").**
- Observe for physical signs of fatigue (e.g., restlessness, hand tremors, thick speech, drooping eyes, inattention, lack of interest in activities).
- Incorporate screening information into in-depth sleep diary or testing if needed **to evaluate the type and etiology of sleep disturbance and to identify useful treatment options.**

Nursing Priority No. 3.
To assist client to establish optimal sleep/rest pattern:

- Manage environment for hospitalized client:
  Adjust ambient lighting **to maintain daytime light and nighttime dark.**

Information that appears in brackets has been added by the authors to clarify and enhance the use of nursing diagnoses.

Request visitors to leave, close room door, post "Quiet, patient sleeping" sign, as indicated, **to provide privacy.**

Encourage usual bedtime routines such as washing face and hands and brushing teeth.

Provide bedtime care such as straightening bed sheets, changing damp linens or gown, back massage **to promote physical comfort.**

Turn on soft music, calm TV program, or quiet environment, as client prefers **to enhance relaxation.**

Minimize sleep-disrupting factors (e.g., shut room door, adjust room temperature as needed, reduce talking and other disturbing noises such as phones, beepers, alarms) **to promote readiness for sleep and improve sleep duration and quality.**

Perform monitoring and care activities without waking client whenever possible. **Allows for longer periods of uninterrupted sleep, especially during night.**

Avoid or limit use of physical restraints in accordance with client's needs and facility policy.

⊕• Refer to physician or sleep specialist as indicated **for specific interventions and/or therapies, including medications, biofeedback.**

• Refer to NDs Insomnia and Sleep Deprivation for related interventions and rationale.

Nursing Priority No. 4.

🏠 To promote wellness (Teaching/Discharge Considerations):

• Assure client that occasional sleeplessness should not threaten health and that resolving time-limited situation can restore healthful sleep. **Knowledge that occasional insomnia is universal and usually not harmful may promote relaxation and relief from worry, which can perpetuate the problem.**

• Problem-solve immediate needs. **Short-term solutions (e.g., sleeping in different rooms if partner's illness is keeping client awake, acquiring a fan if sleeping quarters too warm or lacks ventilation) may be needed until client adjusts to situation or crisis is resolved, with resulting return to more usual sleep pattern.**

• Encourage appropriate indoor light settings during day and night, especially exposure to bright light or sunlight in the morning, avoidance of daytime napping as appropriate for age and situation, being active during day and more passive in evening. **Helps in promotion of normal sleep-wake patterns.**

Information that appears in brackets has been added by the authors to clarify and enhance the use of nursing diagnoses.

- Investigate use of aids to block out light and sound, such as sleep mask, room-darkening shades, earplugs, "white noise."
- Discuss use and appropriateness of over-the-counter sleep medications or herbal supplements **to provide assistance in falling and staying asleep.**

Documentation Focus

Assessment/Reassessment

- Assessment findings, including specifics of current and past sleep pattern, and effects on lifestyle and level of functioning.
- Specific interventions, medications, or previously tried therapies.

Planning

- Plan of care and who is involved in planning.
- Teaching plan.

Implementation/Evaluation

- Response to interventions, teaching, and actions performed.
- Attainment or progress toward desired outcome(s).
- Modifications to plan of care.

Discharge Planning

- Long-term needs and who is responsible for actions to be taken.
- Available resources, specific referrals made.

Sample Nursing Outcomes & Interventions Classifications (NOC/NIC)

NOC—Sleep
NIC—Sleep Enhancement

---

impaired Social Interaction

Taxonomy II: Role Relationship—Class 3 Role Performance (00052)
[Diagnostic Division: Social Interaction]
Submitted 1986

Definition: Insufficient or excessive quantity or ineffective quality of social exchange

---

Information that appears in brackets has been added by the authors to clarify and enhance the use of nursing diagnoses.

Related Factors

Deficit about ways to enhance mutuality (e.g., knowledge, skills)
Communication barriers
Self-concept disturbance
Absence of SOs
Limited physical mobility
Therapeutic isolation
Sociocultural dissonance
Environmental barriers
Disturbed thought processes

Defining Characteristics

Subjective
Discomfort in social situations
Inability to communicate/receive a satisfying sense of social engagement (e.g., belonging, caring, interest, shared history)
Family reports of changes in interaction (e.g., style, pattern)

Objective
Use of unsuccessful social interaction behaviors
Dysfunctional interaction with others

Desired Outcomes/Evaluation Criteria—Client Will:

- Verbalize awareness of factors causing or promoting impaired social interactions.
- Identify feelings that lead to poor social interactions.
- Express desire for, and be involved in, achieving positive changes in social behaviors and interpersonal relationships.
- Give self positive reinforcement for changes that are achieved.
- Develop effective social support system; use available resources appropriately.

Actions/Interventions

Nursing Priority No. 1.
To assess causative/contributing factors:

- Review social history with client/SO(s) going back far enough in time to note when changes in social behavior or patterns of relating occurred or began: for example, loss or long-term

---

Information that appears in brackets has been added by the authors to clarify and enhance the use of nursing diagnoses.

illness of loved one; failed relationships; loss of occupation, financial, or social or political (power) position; change in status in family hierarchy (job loss, aging, illness); poor coping or adjustment to developmental stage of life, as with marriage, birth or adoption of child, or children leaving home.

- Ascertain ethnic, cultural, or religious implications for the client **because these impact choice of behaviors and may even script interactions with others.**
- Review medical history, noting stressors of physical or long-term illness (e.g., stroke, cancer, multiple sclerosis, head injury, Alzheimer's disease); mental illness (e.g., schizophrenia); medications or drugs, debilitating accidents, learning disabilities (e.g., sensory integration difficulties, Asperger's disorder/autism spectrum disorder); and emotional disabilities.
- Determine family patterns of relating and social behaviors. Explore possible family scripting of behavioral expectations in the children and how the client was affected. **May result in conforming or rebellious behaviors. Parents are important in teaching their children social skills (e.g., sharing, taking turns, and allowing others to talk without interrupting).**
- Observe client while relating to family/SO(s) **to note prevalent interaction patterns.**
- Encourage client to verbalize feeling of discomfort about social situations. Identify causative factors, if any, recurring precipitating patterns, and barriers to using support systems.

Nursing Priority No. 2.
To assess degree of impairment:

- Encourage client to verbalize perceptions of problem and causes. Active-listen, noting indications of hopelessness, powerlessness, fear, anxiety, grief, anger, feeling unloved or unlovable, problems with sexual identity, hate (directed or not).
- Observe and describe social and interpersonal behaviors in objective terms, noting speech patterns, body language—in the therapeutic setting and in normal areas of daily functioning (if possible)—such as in family, job, social or entertainment settings. **Helps identify the kinds and extent of problems client is exhibiting.**
- Determine client's use of coping skills and defense mechanisms. **Affects ability to be involved in social situations.**

Information that appears in brackets has been added by the authors to clarify and enhance the use of nursing diagnoses.

- Evaluate possibility of client being the victim of or using destructive behaviors against self or others. (Refer to NDs risk for other-/self-directed Violence.) **Problems with communication lead to frustration and anger, leaving the individual with few coping skills, and may result in destructive behaviors.**
- Interview family, SO(s), friends, spiritual leaders, coworkers, as appropriate, **to obtain observations of client's behavioral changes and effect on others.**
- Note effects of changes on socioeconomic level, ethnic and religious practices.

Nursing Priority No. 3.

To assist client/SO(s) to recognize/make positive changes in impaired social and interpersonal interactions:

- Establish therapeutic relationship using positive regard for the client, Active-listening, and providing safe environment for self-disclosure.
- Have client list behaviors that cause discomfort. **Once recognized, client can choose to change as he or she learns to listen and communicate in socially acceptable ways.**
- Have family/SO(s) list client's behaviors that are causing discomfort for them. **Family needs to understand that the client is unable to use social skills that have not been learned.**
- Review/list negative behaviors observed previously by caregivers, coworkers, and so forth.
- Compare lists and validate reality of perceptions. Help client prioritize those behaviors needing change.
- Explore with client and role-play means of making agreed-on changes in social interactions and behaviors.
- Role-play random social situations in therapeutically controlled environment with "safe" therapy group. Have group note behaviors, both positive and negative, and discuss these and any changes needed.
- Role-play changes and discuss impact. Include family/SO(s), as indicated. **Enhances comfort with new behaviors.**
- Provide positive reinforcement for improvement in social behaviors and interactions. **Encourages continuation of desired behaviors and efforts for change.**
- Participate in multidisciplinary client-centered conferences to evaluate progress. Involve everyone associated with client's care, family members, SO(s), and therapy group.

Information that appears in brackets has been added by the authors to clarify and enhance the use of nursing diagnoses.

- Work with client to alleviate underlying negative self-concepts **because they often impede positive social interactions. Attempts at trying to connect with another can become devastating to self-esteem and emotional well-being.**
- Involve neurologically impaired client in individual and/or group interactions or special classes, as situation allows.
- Refer for family therapy, as indicated, **because social behaviors and interpersonal relationships involve more than the individual.**

Nursing Priority No. 4.

To promote wellness (Teaching/Discharge Considerations):

- Encourage client to keep a daily journal in which social interactions of each day can be reviewed and the comfort/discomfort experienced noted with possible causes or precipitating factors. **Helps client identify responsibility for own behavior(s) and learn new skills that can be used to enhance social interactions.**
- Assist the client to develop positive social skills through practice of skills in real social situations accompanied by a support person. Provide positive feedback during interactions with client.
- Seek community programs for client involvement that promote positive behaviors the client is striving to achieve.
- Encourage classes, reading materials, community support groups, and lectures for self-help in alleviating negative self-concepts that lead to impaired social interactions.
- Involve client in a music-based program, if available (e.g., The Listening Program). **There is a direct correlation between the musical portion of the brain and the language area, and the use of these programs may result in better communication skills.**
- Encourage ongoing family or individual therapy as long as it is promoting growth and positive change. (However, be alert to possibility of therapy being used as a crutch.)
- Provide for occasional follow-up, as appropriate, **for reinforcement of positive behaviors after professional relationship has ended.**
- Refer to psychiatric clinical nurse specialist for additional assistance when indicated.

Information that appears in brackets has been added by the authors to clarify and enhance the use of nursing diagnoses.

Documentation Focus

Assessment/Reassessment
- Individual findings, including factors affecting interactions, nature of social exchanges, specifics of individual behaviors, type of learning disability present.
- Cultural or religious beliefs and expectations.
- Perceptions and response of others.

Planning
- Plan of care and who is involved in the planning.
- Teaching plan.

Implementation/Evaluation
- Responses to interventions, teaching, and actions performed.
- Attainment or progress toward desired outcome(s).
- Modifications to plan of care.

Discharge Planning
- Long-term needs and who is responsible for actions to be taken.
- Community resources, specific referrals made.

Sample Nursing Outcomes & Interventions Classifications (NOC/NIC)

NOC—Social Interaction Skills
NIC—Socialization Enhancement

Social Isolation

Taxonomy II: Comfort—Class 3 Social Comfort (00053)
[Diagnostic Division: Social Interaction]
Submitted 1982

Definition: Aloneness experienced by the individual and perceived as imposed by others and as a negative or threatened state

Related Factors

Factors contributing to the absence of satisfying personal relationships (e.g., delay in accomplishing developmental tasks); immature interests

Information that appears in brackets has been added by the authors to clarify and enhance the use of nursing diagnoses.

Alterations in physical appearance or mental status
Altered state of wellness
Unaccepted social behavior or values
Inadequate personal resources
Inability to engage in satisfying personal relationships

Defining Characteristics

Subjective

Reports feelings of aloneness imposed by others, rejection; experiences feelings of difference from others
Reports inadequate purpose in life; values unacceptable to the dominant cultural group
Inability to meet expectations of others
Developmentally inappropriate interests
Insecurity in public

Objective

Absence of supportive SO(s)
Sad or dull affect
Developmentally inappropriate behaviors
Projects hostility
Evidence of handicap (e.g., physical/mental); illness
Uncommunicative; withdrawn; no eye contact
Preoccupation with own thoughts; repetitive or meaningless actions
Seeks to be alone; exists in a subculture
Shows behavior unaccepted by dominant cultural group

Desired Outcomes/Evaluation Criteria— Client Will:

- Identify causes and actions to correct isolation.
- Verbalize willingness to be involved with others.
- Participate in activities or programs at level of ability and desire.
- Express increased sense of self-worth.

Actions/Interventions

Nursing Priority No. 1.
To assess causative/contributing factors:
- Determine presence of factors as listed in Related Factors and other concerns (e.g., elderly, female, adolescent, ethnic or racial minority, economically/educationally disadvantaged).

Information that appears in brackets has been added by the authors to clarify and enhance the use of nursing diagnoses.

- Note onset of physical or mental illness and whether recovery is anticipated or condition is chronic or progressive. **May affect client's desire to isolate self.**
- Do physical exam, paying particular attention to any illnesses that are identified. **Individuals who are isolated appear to be susceptible to health problems, especially coronary heart disease, although little is understood about why this is true.**
- Identify blocks to social contacts (e.g., physical immobility, sensory deficits, housebound, incontinence). **Client may be unable to go out, embarrassed to be with others, and reluctant to solve these problems.**
- Ascertain implications of cultural values or religious beliefs for the client **because these impact choice of behaviors and may even script interactions with others.**
- Assess factors in client's life that may contribute to sense of helplessness (e.g., loss of spouse/parent). **Client may withdraw and fail to seek out friends who may have previously been in his or her life.**
- Ascertain client's perception regarding sense of isolation. Differentiate isolation from solitude and loneliness, **which may be acceptable or by choice.**
- Assess client's feelings about self, sense of ability to control situation, sense of hope.
- Note use and effectiveness of coping skills.
- Identify support systems available to the client, including presence of and relationship with extended family.
- Determine drug use (legal and illicit). **Possibility of a relationship between unhealthy behaviors and social isolation or the influence others have on the individual.**
- Identify behavior response of isolation (e.g., excessive sleeping or daydreaming, substance use), **which also may potentiate isolation.**
- Review history and elicit information about traumatic events that may have occurred. (Refer to ND Post-Trauma Syndrome.)

Nursing Priority No. 2.

To alleviate conditions contributing to client's sense of isolation:

- Establish therapeutic nurse-client relationship. **Promotes trust, allowing client to feel free to discuss sensitive matters.**

Information that appears in brackets has been added by the authors to clarify and enhance the use of nursing diagnoses.

- Spend time visiting with client and identify other resources available (e.g., volunteer, social worker, chaplain).
- Develop plan of action with client: Look at available resources, support risk-taking behaviors to engage in social interactions, management of personal resources, appropriate medical care or self-care, and so forth. **Learning to manage issues of daily living can increase self-confidence and promote comfort in social settings.**
- Introduce client to those with similar or shared interests and other supportive people. **Provides role models, encourages problem-solving, and possibly making friends that will relieve client's sense of isolation.**
- Provide positive reinforcement when client makes move(s) toward others. **Encourages continuation of efforts.**
- Provide for placement in sheltered community when necessary.
- Assist client to problem-solve solutions to short-term or imposed isolation (e.g., communicable disease measures, including compromised host).
- Encourage open visitation when possible and/or telephone contacts **to maintain involvement with others.**
- Provide environmental stimuli (e.g., open curtains, pictures, TV, and radio).
- Promote participation in recreational or special interest activities in setting that client views as safe.
- Identify foreign language resources, such as interpreter, newspaper, radio programming, as appropriate.

Nursing Priority No. 3.

To promote wellness (Teaching/Discharge Considerations):

- Assist client to learn or enhance skills (e.g., problem-solving, communication, social skills, self-esteem, activities of daily living).
- Encourage or assist client to enroll in classes, as desired (e.g., assertiveness, vocational, sex education).
- Involve children and adolescents in age-appropriate programs and activities **to promote socialization skills and peer contact.**
- Help client differentiate between isolation and loneliness or aloneness and about ways to prevent slipping into an undesired state.
- Involve client in programs directed at correction and prevention of identified causes of problem (e.g., senior citizen

---

Information that appears in brackets has been added by the authors to clarify and enhance the use of nursing diagnoses.

services, daily telephone contact, house sharing, pets, day-care centers, religious or spiritual resources). **Social isolation seems to be growing and may be related to time stressors, watching TV, prolonged Internet use, or fatigue, resulting in individuals' finding they don't have a close friend they can share intimate thoughts with.**

- Refer to therapists, as appropriate, **to facilitate grief work, relationship building, and so forth.**

Documentation Focus

Assessment/Reassessment
- Individual findings, including precipitating factors, effect on lifestyle and relationships, and functioning.
- Client's perception of situation.
- Cultural or religious factors.
- Availability and use of resources and support systems.

Planning
- Plan of care and who is involved in planning.
- Teaching plan.

Implementation/Evaluation
- Responses to interventions, teaching, and actions performed.
- Attainment or progress toward desired outcome(s).
- Modifications to plan of care.

Discharge Planning
- Long-term needs, referrals made, and who is responsible for actions to be taken.
- Available resources, specific referrals made.

Sample Nursing Outcomes & Interventions Classifications (NOC/NIC)

NOC—Social Involvement
NIC—Social Enhancement

Information that appears in brackets has been added by the authors to clarify and enhance the use of nursing diagnoses.

chronic Sorrow

Taxonomy II: Coping/Stress Tolerance—Class 2 Coping
   Responses (00137)
[Diagnostic Division: Ego Integrity]
Submitted 1998

Definition: Cyclical, recurring, and potentially progressive pattern of pervasive sadness experienced (by a parent, caregiver, individual with chronic illness or disability) in response to continual loss, throughout the trajectory of an illness or disability

Related Factors

Death of a loved one
Experiences chronic illness or disability (e.g., physical or mental); crises in management of the illness or disability
Crises related to developmental stages; missed opportunities or milestones
Unending caregiving

Defining Characteristics

Subjective

Reports negative feelings (e.g., anger, being misunderstood, confusion, depression, disappointment, emptiness, fear, frustration, guilt, self-blame, helplessness, hopelessness, loneliness, low self-esteem, recurring loss, overwhelmed)
Reports feelings of sadness (e.g., periodic, recurrent)
Reports feelings that interfere with ability to reach highest level of personal or social well-being

Desired Outcomes/Evaluation Criteria— Client Will:

- Acknowledge presence and impact of sorrow.
- Demonstrate progress in dealing with grief.
- Participate in work and/or self-care activities of daily living as able.
- Verbalize a sense of progress toward resolution of sorrow and hope for the future.

Information that appears in brackets has been added by the authors to clarify and enhance the use of nursing diagnoses.

Actions/Interventions

Nursing Priority No. 1.

To assess causative/contributing factors:

- Determine current and recent events or conditions contributing to client's state of mind, as listed in Related Factors (e.g., death of loved one, chronic physical or mental illness, disability).
- Look for cues of sadness (e.g., sighing, faraway look, unkempt appearance, inattention to conversation, refusing food). **Chronic sorrow has a cyclical effect, ranging from times of deepening sorrow to times of feeling somewhat better.**
- Determine level of functioning, ability to care for self.
- Note avoidance behaviors (e.g., anger, withdrawal, denial).
- Identify cultural factors or religious conflicts. **Family may experience conflict between the feelings of sorrow and anger because of change in expectation that has occurred (e.g., newborn with a disability when the expectation was for a perfect child, while religious belief is that all children are gifts from God and that the individual/parent is never "given" more than he or she can handle).**
- Ascertain response of family/SO(s) to client's situation. Assess needs of family/SO. **Family may have difficulty dealing with child/ill person because of their own feelings of sorrow and loss, and will do better when their needs are met.**
- Refer to complicated Grieving; Caregiver Role Strain; ineffective Coping, as appropriate.

Nursing Priority No. 2.

To assist client to move through sorrow:

- Encourage verbalization about situation (**helpful in beginning resolution and acceptance**). Active-listen feelings and be available for support/assistance.
- Encourage expression of anger, fear, and anxiety. (Refer to appropriate NDs.)
- Acknowledge reality of feelings of guilt/blame, including hostility toward spiritual power. (Refer to ND Spiritual Distress.) **When feelings are validated, client is free to take steps toward acceptance.**
- Provide comfort and availability as well as caring for physical needs.
- Discuss ways individual has dealt with previous losses. Reinforce use of previously effective coping skills.

Information that appears in brackets has been added by the authors to clarify and enhance the use of nursing diagnoses.

🌐 Cultural 🔄 Collaborative 🏠 Community/Home Care

- Instruct in, and encourage use of, visualization and relaxation skills.
- Discuss use of medication when depression is interfering with ability to manage life. **Client may benefit from the short-term use of an antidepressant medication to help with dealing with situation.**
- Assist SO to cope with client response. **Family/SO may not be dysfunctional but may be intolerant.**
- Include family/SO in setting realistic goals for meeting individual needs.

Nursing Priority No. 3.

To promote wellness (Teaching/Discharge Considerations):

- Discuss healthy ways of dealing with difficult situations.
- Have client identify familial, religious, and cultural factors that have meaning for him or her. **May help bring loss or distressing situation into perspective and facilitate resolution of grief and sorrow.**
- Encourage involvement in usual activities, exercise, and socialization within limits of physical and psychological state. **Maintaining usual activities may keep individuals from deepening sorrow and depression.**
- Introduce concept of mindfulness (living in the moment). **Promotes feelings of capability and belief that this moment can be dealt with.**
- Refer to other resources (e.g., pastoral care, counseling, psychotherapy, respite-care providers, support groups). **Provides additional help when needed to resolve situation, continue grief work.**

Documentation Focus

Assessment/Reassessment

- Physical and emotional response to conflict, expressions of sadness.
- Cultural issues or religious conflicts.
- Reactions of family/SO.

Planning

- Plan of care and who is involved in planning.
- Teaching plan.

Implementation/Evaluation

- Response to interventions, teaching, and actions performed.

Information that appears in brackets has been added by the authors to clarify and enhance the use of nursing diagnoses.

- Attainment or progress toward desired outcome(s).
- Modifications to plan of care.

Discharge Planning
- Long-term needs and who is responsible for actions to be taken.
- Available resources, specific referrals made.

Sample Nursing Outcomes & Interventions Classifications (NOC/NIC)

NOC—Depression Level
NIC—Hope Inspiration

Spiritual Distress

Taxonomy II: Life Principles—Class 3 Value/Belief/Action Congruence (00066)
[Diagnostic Division: Ego Integrity]
Submitted 1978; Revised 2002

Definition: Impaired ability to experience and integrate meaning and purpose in life through connectedness with self, others, art, music, literature, nature, and/or a power greater than oneself

Related Factors

Active dying
Loneliness; social alienation; self-alienation; sociocultural deprivation
Anxiety; pain
Life change
Chronic illness [of self or others]; death
Challenged belief or value system (e.g., moral or ethical implications of therapy)

Defining Characteristics

Subjective

Connections to Self
Expresses lack of hope, meaning or purpose in life, serenity (e.g., peace), love, acceptance, courage
[Expresses] anger, guilt

Information that appears in brackets has been added by the authors to clarify and enhance the use of nursing diagnoses.

● Cultural ● Collaborative 🏠 Community/Home Care

Connections With Others

Refuses interactions with SO(s) or spiritual leaders
Verbalizes being separated from support system
Expresses alienation

Connections With Art, Music, Literature, Nature

Inability to express previous state of creativity (e.g., singing/ listening to music/writing)
Disinterested in nature or reading spiritual literature

Connections With Power Greater Than Self

Sudden changes in spiritual practices
Inability to pray or participate in religious activities or to experience the transcendent
Expresses hopelessness, suffering, anger toward power greater than self
Expresses being abandoned
Requests to see a spiritual leader

Objective

Connections to Self

Ineffective coping

Connections With Power Greater Than Self

Inability to be introspective

Desired Outcomes/Evaluation Criteria— Client Will:

- Verbalize increased sense of connectedness and hope for future.
- Demonstrate ability to help self and participate in care.
- Participate in activities with others, actively seek relationships.
- Discuss beliefs and values about spiritual issues.
- Verbalize acceptance of self as not deserving illness or situation; "No one is to blame."

Actions/Interventions

Nursing Priority No. 1.

To assess causative/contributing factors:

- Determine client's religious or spiritual orientation, current involvement, presence of conflicts. **Individual spiritual**

Information that appears in brackets has been added by the authors to clarify and enhance the use of nursing diagnoses.

practices or restrictions may affect client care or create conflict between spiritual beliefs and treatment.

- Listen to client's/SO's reports or expressions of concern, anger, alienation from God, belief that illness or situation is a punishment for wrongdoing, and so forth. **Suggests need for spiritual advisor to address client's belief system, if desired.**

- Determine sense of futility, feelings of hopelessness and helplessness, lack of motivation to help self. **Indicators that client may see no, or only limited, options, alternatives, or personal choices available and lacks energy to deal with situation.**

- Note expressions of inability to find meaning in life, reason for living. Evaluate suicidal ideation. **Crisis of the spirit or loss of will to live places client at increased risk for inattention to personal well-being or harm to self.**

- Note recent changes in behavior (e.g., withdrawal from others and creative or religious activities, dependence on alcohol or medications). **Helpful in determining severity and duration of situation and possible need for additional referrals, such as substance withdrawal.**

- Assess sense of self-concept, worth, ability to enter into loving relationships. **Lack of connectedness with self and others impairs client's ability to trust others or feel worthy of trust from others.**

- Observe behavior indicative of poor relationships with others (e.g., manipulative, nontrusting, demanding). **Manipulation is used for management of client's sense of powerlessness because of distrust of others.**

- Determine support systems available to client/SO(s) and how they are used. **Provides insight to client's willingness to pursue outside resources.**

- Be aware of influence of care provider's belief system. **(It is still possible to be helpful to client while remaining neutral and refraining from promoting own beliefs.)**

Nursing Priority No. 2.

To assist client/SO(s) to deal with feelings/situation:

- Develop therapeutic nurse-client relationship. Ascertain client's views as to how care provider(s) can be most helpful. Convey acceptance of client's spiritual beliefs and concerns. **Promotes trust and comfort, encouraging client to be open about sensitive matters.**

Information that appears in brackets has been added by the authors to clarify and enhance the use of nursing diagnoses.

🌐 Cultural 😊 Collaborative 🏠 Community/Home Care

- Establish environment that promotes free expression of feelings and concerns.
- Suggest use of journaling. **Can assist in clarifying values and ideas or recognizing and resolving feelings or situation.**
- Encourage client/family to ask questions. **Demonstrates support for individual's willingness to learn.**
- Identify inappropriate coping behaviors currently being used and associated consequences. **Recognizing negative consequences of actions may enhance desire to change.**
- Ascertain past coping behaviors **to determine approaches used previously that may be more effective in dealing with current situation.**
- Problem-solve solutions and identify areas for compromise **that may be useful in resolving possible conflicts.**
- Provide calm, peaceful setting when possible. **Promotes relaxation and enhances opportunity for reflection on situation, discussions with others, meditation.**
- Set limits on acting-out behavior that is inappropriate or destructive. **Promotes safety for client/others and helps prevent loss of self-esteem.**
- Make time for nonjudgmental discussion of philosophical issues or questions about spiritual impact of illness or situation and/or treatment regimen. **Open communication can assist client in reality checks of perceptions and identifying personal options.**

Nursing Priority No. 3.

To facilitate setting goals and moving forward:

- Involve client in refining healthcare goals and therapeutic regimen, as appropriate. **Enhances commitment to plan, optimizing outcomes.**
- Discuss difference between grief and guilt and help client to identify and deal with each. Point out consequences of actions based on guilt. **Aids client in assuming responsibility for own actions and avoiding acting out of false guilt.**
- Use therapeutic communication skills of reflection and Active-listening. **Helps client find own solutions to concerns.**
- Identify role models (e.g., nurse, individual experiencing similar situation). **Provides opportunities for sharing of experiences, finding hope, and identifying options to deal with situation.**
- Assist client to learn use of meditation, prayer, and forgiveness **to heal past hurts.**

Information that appears in brackets has been added by the authors to clarify and enhance the use of nursing diagnoses.

- Provide information that anger with God is a normal part of the grieving process. **Realizing these feelings are not unusual can reduce sense of guilt, encourage open expression, and facilitate resolution of conflict.**
- Provide time and privacy to engage in spiritual growth and religious activities (e.g., prayer, meditation, scripture reading, listening to music). **Allows client to focus on self and seek connectedness.**
- Encourage and facilitate outings to neighborhood park, nature walks, or similar outings when able. **Sunshine, fresh air, and activity can stimulate release of endorphins, promoting sense of well-being.**
- ∞ Provide play therapy for child that encompasses spiritual data. **Interactive pleasurable activity promotes open discussion and enhances retention of information. Also provides opportunity for child to practice what has been learned.**
- ∞ Abide by parents' wishes in discussing and implementing child's spiritual support. **Limits confusion for child and prevents conflict of values or beliefs.**
- 🏠 Refer to appropriate resources (e.g., pastoral or parish nurse, religious counselor, crisis counselor, hospice; psychotherapy; Alcoholics or Narcotics Anonymous). **Useful in dealing with immediate situation and identifying long-term resources for support to help foster sense of connectedness.**
- Refer to NDs ineffective Coping; Powerlessness; Self-Esteem [specify]; Social Isolation; risk for Suicide.

Nursing Priority No. 4.
To promote wellness (Teaching/Discharge Considerations):

- Assist client to develop goals for dealing with life/illness situation. **Enhances commitment to goal, optimizing outcomes.**
- Encourage life-review by client. Help client find a reason for living. **Promotes sense of hope and willingness to continue efforts to improve situation.**
- Assist in developing coping skills **to deal with stressors of illness or necessary changes in lifestyle.**
- Assist client to identify SO(s) and people who could provide support as needed. **Ongoing support is required to enhance sense of connectedness and continue progress toward goals.**
- Encourage family to provide a quiet, calm atmosphere. Be willing to just "be" there and not have a need to "do" some-

---

Information that appears in brackets has been added by the authors to clarify and enhance the use of nursing diagnoses.

thing. **Helps client to think about self in the context of current situation.**

⊛• Assist client to identify spiritual resources that could be helpful (e.g., contact spiritual advisor who has qualifications or experience in dealing with specific problems, such as death and dying, relationship problems, substance abuse, suicide). **Provides answers to spiritual questions, assists in the journey of self-discovery, and can help client learn to accept and forgive self.**

Documentation Focus

Assessment/Reassessment
- Individual findings, including nature of spiritual conflict, effects of participation in treatment regimen.
- Physical and emotional responses to conflict.

Planning
- Plan of care and who is involved in planning.
- Teaching plan.

Implementation/Evaluation
- Responses to interventions, teaching, and actions performed.
- Attainment or progress toward desired outcome(s).
- Modifications to plan of care.

Discharge Planning
- Long-term needs and who is responsible for actions to be taken.
- Available resources, specific referrals made.

Sample Nursing Outcomes & Interventions Classifications (NOC/NIC)

NOC—Spiritual Health
NIC—Spiritual Support

Information that appears in brackets has been added by the authors to clarify and enhance the use of nursing diagnoses.

risk for **Spiritual Distress**

Taxonomy II: Life Principles—Class 3 Value/Belief/Action
  Congruence (00067)
[Diagnostic Division: Ego Integrity]
Nursing Diagnosis Extension and Classification Submis-
  sion 1998; Revised 2004

Definition: At risk for an impaired ability to experience
and integrate meaning and purpose in life through connectedness with self, others, art, music, literature, nature, and/or a power greater than oneself

Risk Factors

Physical
Physical or chronic illness; substance abuse

Psychosocial
Stress; anxiety; depression
Low self-esteem; poor relationships; blocks to experiencing
  love; inability to forgive; loss; separated support systems;
  racial or cultural conflict
Change in religious rituals or spiritual practices

Developmental
Life changes

Environmental
Environmental changes; natural disasters

NOTE: A risk diagnosis is not evidenced by signs and
symptoms, as the problem has not occurred; rather,
nursing interventions are directed at prevention.

Desired Outcomes/Evaluation Criteria— Client Will:

- Identify meaning and purpose in own life that reinforces hope,
  peace, and contentment.
- Verbalize acceptance of self as being worthy, not deserving
  of illness or situation, and so forth.
- Identify and use resources appropriately.

Information that appears in brackets has been added by the authors to clarify
and enhance the use of nursing diagnoses.

Actions/Interventions

Nursing Priority No. 1.

To assess causative/contributing factors:

- Ascertain current situation (e.g., natural disaster, death of a spouse, personal injustice).
- Listen to client's/SO's expressions of anger or concern, belief that illness or situation is a punishment for wrongdoing, and so forth. **May indicate possibility of becoming distressed about spiritual and religious beliefs.**
- Note client's reason for living and whether it is directly related to situation (e.g., home and business washed away in a flood, parent whose only child is terminally ill). **Questioning meaning or purpose of life may indicate inner conflict about religious beliefs.**
- Determine client's religious or spiritual orientation, current involvement, presence of conflicts, especially in current circumstances.
- Assess sense of self-concept, worth, ability to enter into loving relationships. **Feelings of abandonment may accompany sense of "not being good enough" in face of illness, disaster.**
- Observe behavior indicative of poor relationships with others (e.g., manipulative, nontrusting, demanding).
- Determine support systems available to and used by client/SO(s).
- Ascertain substance use or abuse. **Affects ability to deal with problems in a positive manner.**

Nursing Priority No. 2.

To assist client/SO(s) to deal with feelings/situation:

- Establish environment that promotes free expression of feelings and concerns. **Listening, and a quiet demeanor can convey acceptance to the client.**
- Have client identify and prioritize current or immediate needs. **Helps client focus on what needs to be done and identify manageable steps to take.**
- Make time for nonjudgmental discussion of philosophical issues or questions about spiritual impact of illness or situation and/or treatment regimen. **Client may believe that illness is the result of being sinful, bad, or that God has abandoned him or her.**
- Discuss difference between grief and guilt and help client to identify and deal with each, assuming responsibility for own

---

Information that appears in brackets has been added by the authors to clarify and enhance the use of nursing diagnoses.

actions, expressing awareness of the consequences of acting out of false guilt. **Client needs to decide whether guilt is deserved or not. Cultural and religious beliefs may lead client to feel guilty when in fact nothing has been done to feel guilty about.**

- Use therapeutic communication skills of reflection and Active-listening. **Helps client find own solutions to concerns.**
- Review coping skills used and their effectiveness in current situation. **Identifies strengths to incorporate into plan and techniques needing revision.**
- Provide role model (e.g., nurse, individual experiencing similar situation or disease). **Sharing of experiences and hope assists client to deal with reality.**
- Suggest use of journaling. **Can assist in clarifying values and ideas, recognizing and resolving feelings or situation.**
- Discuss client's interest in the arts, music, literature. **Provides insight into meaning of these issues and how they are integrated into the individual's life.**
- Refer to appropriate resources for help (e.g., crisis counselor, governmental agencies; pastoral or parish nurse, or spiritual advisor who has qualifications or experience dealing with specific problems [e.g., death and dying, relationships, substance abuse, suicide]; hospice, psychotherapy, Alcoholics or Narcotics Anonymous).

Nursing Priority No. 3.
To promote wellness (Teaching/Discharge Considerations):

- Role-play new coping techniques **to enhance integration of new skills or necessary changes in lifestyle.**
- Encourage individual to become involved in cultural activities of his or her choosing. **Art, music, plays, and other cultural activities provide a means of connecting with self and others.**
- Discuss possibilities of taking classes, being involved in discussion groups or community programs.
- Assist client to identify SO(s) and individuals or support groups that could provide ongoing support **because this is a daily need, requiring lifelong commitment.**
- Abide by parents' wishes in discussing and implementing child's spiritual support.
- Discuss benefit of family counseling, as appropriate. **Issues of this nature (e.g., situational losses, natural disasters, difficult relationships) affect family dynamics.**

Information that appears in brackets has been added by the authors to clarify and enhance the use of nursing diagnoses.

🌐 Cultural   🅐 Collaborative   🏠 Community/Home Care

Documentation Focus

Assessment/Reassessment
- Individual findings, including risk factors, nature of current distress.
- Physical and emotional responses to distress.
- Access to and use of resources.

Planning
- Plan of care and who is involved in planning.
- Teaching plan.

Implementation/Evaluation
- Responses to interventions, teaching, and actions performed.
- Attainment or progress toward desired outcome(s).
- Modifications to plan of care.

Discharge Planning
- Long-term needs and who is responsible for actions to be taken.
- Available resources, specific referrals made.

Sample Nursing Outcomes & Interventions Classifications (NOC/NIC)

NOC—Spiritual Health
NIC—Spiritual Support

---

readiness for enhanced Spiritual Well-Being

Taxonomy II: Life Principles—Class 2 Beliefs (00068)
[Diagnostic Division: Ego Integrity]
Submitted 1994; Revised 2002

Definition: A pattern of experiencing and integrating meaning and purpose in life through connectedness with self, others, art, music, literature, nature, and/or a power greater than oneself that is sufficient for well-being and can be strengthened

---

Information that appears in brackets has been added by the authors to clarify and enhance the use of nursing diagnoses.

Defining Characteristics

Subjective

Connections to Self
Expresses desire for enhanced acceptance, coping, courage, self-forgiveness, hope, joy, love, serenity (e.g., peace), meaning or purpose in life, satisfying philosophy of life, surrender
Meditation

Connections With Others
Requests interactions with significant others or spiritual leaders
Requests forgiveness of others

Connections With Powers Greater Than Self
Expresses reverence or awe; reports mystical experiences

Objective

Connections With Others
Provides service to others

Connections With Art, Music, Literature, Nature
Displays creative energy (e.g., writing poetry, singing); listens to music; reads spiritual literature; spends time outdoors

Connections With Powers Greater Than Self
Participates in religious activities; prays

Desired Outcomes/Evaluation Criteria— Client Will:

- Acknowledge the stabilizing and strengthening forces in own life needed for balance and well-being of the whole person.
- Identify meaning and purpose in own life that reinforces hope, peace, and contentment.
- Verbalize a sense of peace or contentment and comfort of spirit.
- Demonstrate behavior congruent with verbalizations that lend support and strength for daily living.

Actions/Interventions

Nursing Priority No. 1.
To determine spiritual state/motivation for growth:
- Ascertain client's perception of current state and degree of connectedness and expectations. **Provides insight into where**

Information that appears in brackets has been added by the authors to clarify and enhance the use of nursing diagnoses.

    Cultural   😇 Collaborative   🏠 Community/Home Care

client is currently and what his or her hopes for the future may be.

- Identify motivation and expectations for change.
- Review spiritual and religious history, activities, rituals, and frequency of participation. **Provides basis to build on for growth or change.**
- Determine relational values of support systems to one's spiritual centeredness. **The client's family of origin may have differing beliefs from those espoused by the individual that may be a source of conflict for the client. Comfort can be gained when family and friends share client's beliefs and support search for spiritual knowledge.**
- Explore meaning or interpretation and relationship of spirituality, life, death, and illness to life's journey. **Identifying the meaning of these issues is helpful for the client to use the information in forming a belief system that will enable him or her to move forward and live life to the fullest.**
- Clarify the meaning of one's spiritual beliefs or religious practice and rituals to daily living. **Discussing these issues allows client to explore spiritual needs and decide what fits own view of the world to enhance life.**
- Explore ways that spirituality or religious practices have affected one's life and given meaning and value to daily living. Note consequences as well as benefits. **Understanding that there is a difference between spirituality and religion and how each can be useful will help client begin to view the information in a new way.**
- Discuss life's or God's plan for the individual, if client desires. **Helpful in determining individual goals and choosing specific options.**

Nursing Priority No. 2.

To assist client to integrate values and beliefs to achieve a sense of wholeness and optimum balance in daily living:

- Explore ways beliefs give meaning and value to daily living. **As client develops understanding of these issues, the beliefs will provide support for dealing with current and future concerns.**
- Clarify reality and appropriateness of client's self-perceptions and expectations. **Necessary to provide firm foundation for growth.**
- Determine influence of cultural beliefs and values. **Most individuals are strongly influenced by the spiritual or religious orientation of their family of origin, which can be a**

Information that appears in brackets has been added by the authors to clarify and enhance the use of nursing diagnoses.

very strong determinant for client's choice of activities
and receptiveness to various options.
- Discuss the importance and value of connections to one's
daily life. **The contact that one has with others maintains
a feeling of belonging and connection and promotes feelings of wholeness and well-being.**
- Identify ways to achieve connectedness or harmony with self,
others, nature, higher power (e.g., meditation, prayer, talking
or sharing oneself with others; being out in nature, gardening,
walking; attending religious activities). **This is a highly individual and personal decision, and no action is too trivial
to be considered.**

Nursing Priority No. 3.

To enhance optimum wellness:

- Encourage client to take time to be introspective in the search
for peace and harmony. **Finding peace within oneself will
carry over to relationships with others and own outlook
on life.**
- Discuss use of relaxation or meditative activities (e.g., yoga,
tai chi, prayer). **Helpful in promoting general well-being
and sense of connectedness with self, nature, or spiritual
power.**
- Suggest attendance or involvement in dream-sharing group **to
develop and enhance learning of the characteristics of
spiritual awareness and facilitate the individual's growth.**
- Identify ways for spiritual or religious expression. **There are
multiple options for enhancing spirituality through connectedness with self/others (e.g., volunteering time to community projects, mentoring, singing in the choir, painting,
spiritual writings).**
- Encourage participation in desired religious activities, contact
with minister or spiritual advisor. **Validating own beliefs in
an external way can provide support and strengthen the
inner self.**
- Discuss and role-play, as necessary, ways to deal with alternative view or conflict that may occur with family/SO(s), society or cultural group. **Provides opportunity to try out different behaviors in a safe environment and be prepared
for potential eventualities.**
- Provide bibliotherapy, list of relevant resources (e.g., study
groups, parish nurse, poetry society), and possible Web sites
**for later reference or self-paced learning and ongoing sup-
port.**

Information that appears in brackets has been added by the authors to clarify
and enhance the use of nursing diagnoses.

Documentation Focus

Assessment/Reassessment
* Assessment findings, including client perception of needs and desire for growth or enhancement.
* Motivation and expectations for change.

Planning
* Plan for growth and who is involved in planning.

Implementation/Evaluation
* Response to activities, learning, and actions performed.
* Attainment or progress toward desired outcome(s).
* Modifications to plan.

Discharge Planning
* Long-term needs, expectations, and plan of action.
* Specific referrals made.

Sample Nursing Outcomes & Interventions Classifications (NOC/NIC)

NOC—Spiritual Health
NIC—Spiritual Growth Facilitation

Stress Overload

Taxonomy II: Coping/Stress Tolerance—Class 2 Coping Responses (00177)
[Diagnostic Division: Ego Integrity]
Submitted 2006

Definition: Excessive amounts and types of demands that require action

Related Factors

Inadequate resources (e.g., financial, social, education/knowledge level)
Intense or repeated stressors (e.g., family violence, chronic illness, terminal illness)
Multiple coexisting stressors (e.g., environmental threats/demands, physical threats/demands, social threats/demands)

Information that appears in brackets has been added by the authors to clarify and enhance the use of nursing diagnoses.

Defining Characteristics

Subjective

Reports difficulty in functioning or problems with decision making

Reports a feeling of pressure, tension, increased feelings of impatience, anger

Reports negative impact from stress (e.g., physical symptoms, psychological distress, feeling of being sick or of going to get sick)

Reports excessive situational stress (e.g., rates stress level as a 7 or above on a 10-point scale)

Objective

Demonstrates increased feelings of impatience/anger

Desired Outcomes/Evaluation Criteria—Client Will:

- Assess current situation accurately.
- Identify ineffective stress-management behaviors and consequences.
- Meet psychological needs as evidenced by appropriate expression of feelings, identification of options, and use of resources.
- Verbalize or demonstrate reduced stress reaction.

Actions/Interventions

Nursing Priority No. 1.

To identify causative/precipitating factors and degree of impairment:

- Ascertain what tragic/difficult events have occurred (e.g., family violence, death of loved one, chronic or terminal illness, workplace stress or loss of job, catastrophic natural or man-made event) over remote and recent past **to assist in determining number, duration, and intensity of events causing perception of overwhelming stress.**
- Ascertain other life events that have recently occurred (e.g., job promotion, moving to different home, change in getting married, having a new baby or adding other new family member, traveling, spending holidays with relatives) over recent

---

Information that appears in brackets has been added by the authors to clarify and enhance the use of nursing diagnoses.

months. **All such changes, even when desired, can be stressful, and can evoke stress reactions.**

- Evaluate client's report of physical or emotional problems (e.g., fatigue, aches and pains, irritable bowel, skin rashes, frequent colds, sleeplessness, crying spells, anger, feeling overwhelmed or numb, compulsive behaviors) **that can be representing body's response to stress.**
- Determine client's/SO's understanding of events, noting differences in viewpoints.

∞• Note client's gender, age, and developmental level of functioning. **Although everyone experiences stress and stressors, women, children, young adults, divorced and separated persons, and persons in roles or occupations requiring constant multitasking tend to have higher stress-related symptoms. Multiple stressors can weaken the immune system and tax physical and emotional coping mechanisms in persons of any age, but particularly the elderly.**

🌐• Note cultural values or religious beliefs that may affect client's expectation for self in dealing with situation and expectations placed on client by SO(s)/family. **It is important to look at how they define family (can be nuclear, extended, or clan), who are the primary caregivers, and what are their social goals.**

- Identify client locus of control: internal (expressions of responsibility for self and ability to control outcomes: "I didn't quit smoking") or external (expressions of lack of control over self and environment: "Nothing ever works out"). **Knowing client's locus of control will help in developing a plan of care reflecting client's ability to realistically make changes that will help to manage stress better.**
- Assess emotional responses and coping mechanisms being used.
- Determine stress feelings and self-talk client is engaging in. **Negative self-talk, all-or-nothing or pessimistic thinking, exaggeration, or unrealistic expectations all contribute to stress overload.**
- Assess degree of mastery client has exhibited in life. **Passive individual may have more difficulty being assertive and standing up for rights.**
- Determine presence or absence and nature of resources (e.g., whether family/SO(s) are supportive, lack of money, problems with relationship or social functioning).

Information that appears in brackets has been added by the authors to clarify and enhance the use of nursing diagnoses.

- Note change in relationships with SO(s). **Conflict in the family, loss of a family member, divorce can result in a change in support client is accustomed to and impair ability to manage situation.**
- Evaluate stress level, using appropriate tool (e.g., Stress & Depression, Self-Assessment Tool) to help identify areas of most distress. **While most stress seems to come from disastrous events in individual's life, positive events can also be stressful.**

Nursing Priority No. 2.

To assist client to deal with current situation:

- Active-listen to concerns and provide empathetic presence, using talk and silence as needed.
- Provide for or encourage restful environment where possible.
- Discuss situation or condition in simple, concise manner. Devote time for listening. **May help client express emotions, grasp situation, and feel more in control.**
- Deal with the immediate issues first (e.g., treatment of acute physical or psychological illness, meet safety needs, removal from traumatic or violent environment).
- Assist client in determining whether he or she can change stressor or response. **May help client to sort out things over which he or she has control and/or determine responses that can be modified.**
- Allow client to react in own way without judgment. Provide support and diversion as indicated.
- Help client to focus on strengths, to set limits on acting-out behaviors, and to learn ways to express emotions in an acceptable manner. **Promotes internal locus of control, enabling client to maintain self-concept and feel more positive about self.**
- Discuss benefits of a "Stop Doing" in place of a "To Do" list. **May help client identify and take action regarding energy drainers (e.g., internalizing others' criticism, fragmented boundaries, power struggles, unprotected personal time) in order to make room for what energizes and brings him/her closer to achieving goals.**
- Address use of ineffective or dangerous coping mechanisms (e.g., substance use or abuse, self-/other-directed violence) and refer for counseling as indicated.
- Collaborate in treatment of underlying conditions (e.g., physical injury, depression, anger management).

Information that appears in brackets has been added by the authors to clarify and enhance the use of nursing diagnoses.

🌐 Cultural ♨ Collaborative 🏠 Community/Home Care

STRESS OVERLOAD

♟ To promote wellness (Teaching/Discharge Considerations):

- Use client's locus of control to develop individual plan of care **(e.g., for client with internal control, encourage client to take control of own care; for those with external control, begin with small tasks and add as tolerated).**
- Incorporate strengths, assets, and past coping strategies that were successful for client. **Reinforces that client is able to deal with difficult situations.**
- Provide information about stress and exhaustion phase, which occurs when person is experiencing chronic or unresolved stress. **Release of cortisol can contribute to reduction in immune function, resulting in physical illness, mental disability, and life dysfunction.**
- Review stress management and coping skills that client can use:

  Practice behaviors that may help reduce negative consequences—change thinking by focusing on positives, reframing thoughts, changing lifestyle.

  Take a step back, simplify life; learn to say "no" **to reduce sense of being overwhelmed.**

  Learn to control and redirect anger.

  Develop and practice positive self-esteem skills.

  Rest, sleep, and exercise **to recuperate and rejuvenate self.**

  Participate in self-help actions (e.g., deep breathing and other relaxation exercises, find time to be alone, get involved in recreation or desired activity, plan something fun, develop humor) **to actively relax.**

  Eat right; avoid junk food, excessive caffeine, alcohol, and nicotine **to support general health.**

  Develop spiritual self (e.g., meditate or pray; block negative thoughts; learn to give and take, speak and listen, forgive and move on).

  Interact socially, reach out, nurture self and others **to reduce loneliness or sense of isolation.**

- Review proper medication use to manage exacerbating conditions (e.g., depression, mood disorders).
- Identify community resources (e.g., vocational counseling; educational programs; child/elder care, Women, Infants, or Children [WIC] or food assistance; home or respite care) **that can help client manage lifestyle and environmental stress.**
- Refer for therapy as indicated (e.g., medical treatment, psychological counseling, hypnosis, massage, biofeedback).

Information that appears in brackets has been added by the authors to clarify and enhance the use of nursing diagnoses.

Documentation Focus

Assessment/Reassessment
- Individual findings, noting specific stressors, individual's perception of the situation, locus of control.
- Specific cultural or religious factors.
- Availability and use of support systems and resources.

Planning
- Plan of care and who is involved in planning.
- Teaching plan.

Implementation/Evaluation
- Responses to interventions, teaching, and actions performed.
- Attainment or progress toward desired outcome(s).
- Modifications to plan of care.

Discharge Planning
- Long-term needs and who is responsible for actions to be taken.
- Specific referrals made.

Sample Nursing Outcomes & Interventions Classifications (NOC/NIC)

NOC—Stress Level
NIC—Coping Enhancement

risk for Sudden Infant Death Syndrome

Taxonomy II: Safety/Protection—Class 2 Physical Injury (00156)
[Diagnostic Division: Safety]
Submitted 2002

Definition: At risk for sudden death of an infant under 1 year of age

[Sudden infant death syndrome (SIDS) is the sudden death of an infant under 1 year of age, which remains unexplained after a thorough case investigation, including performance of a complete autopsy, examination of the death scene, and review of the clinical history. SIDS is a subset of sudden unexpected death in infancy (SUDI), which is the sudden and

---

Information that appears in brackets has been added by the authors to clarify and enhance the use of nursing diagnoses.

🌐 Cultural 🅒 Collaborative 🏠 Community/Home Care

unexpected death of an infant due to natural or unnatural causes.]

Risk Factors

Modifiable
Delayed or lack of prenatal care
Infants placed in the prone or side-lying position to sleep
Soft underlayment (loose articles in the sleep environment)
Infant overheating or overwrapping
Prenatal or postnatal infant smoke exposure

Potentially Modifiable
Young maternal age
Low birth weight; prematurity

Nonmodifiable
Male gender
Ethnicity (e.g., African American or Native American)
Seasonality of SIDS deaths (higher in winter and fall months)
Infant age of 2 to 4 months

> **NOTE:** A risk diagnosis is not evidenced by signs and symptoms as the problem has not occurred; rather, nursing interventions are directed at prevention.

Desired Outcomes/Evaluation Criteria— Parent/Caregiver Will:

- Verbalize understanding of modifiable factors.
- Make changes in environment to reduce risk of death occurring from other factors.
- Follow medically recommended prenatal and postnatal care.

Actions/Interventions

Nursing Priority No. 1.
To assess causative/contributing factors:

- Identify individual risk factors pertaining to situation. **Determines modifiable or potentially modifiable factors that can be addressed.** *Note:* **SIDS is the most common cause of sudden unexpected death in infancy (SUDI) between 1**

Information that appears in brackets has been added by the authors to clarify and enhance the use of nursing diagnoses.

month and 1 year of age, with peak incidence occurring between the second and fourth months. True SIDS has shown a progressive decline since 1992, while SUDI deaths have increased. It is postulated that some deaths previously classified as SIDS are now being more correctly categorized.

- Determine ethnic/cultural background of family. **Although the overall rate of SIDS in the United States has declined since 1992, disparities in risk factors and SIDS rates remain. African American infants are more than twice as likely to die of SIDS as white infants. American Indian/ Alaska Native infants are nearly three times as likely to die of SIDS as white infants. Hispanic and Asian-Pacific Islander infants have the lowest SIDS rates of any racial or ethnic group in the country.**

- Note whether mother smoked during pregnancy or is currently smoking. **Smoking is known to negatively affect the fetus prenatally as well as after birth. Some reports indicate an increased risk of SIDS in babies of smoking mothers.**

- Assess extent of prenatal care and extent to which mother followed recommended care measures. **Prenatal care is important for all pregnancies to afford the optimal opportunity for all infants to have a healthy start to life.**

- Note use of alcohol or other drugs/medications during and after pregnancy **that may have a negative impact on the developing fetus or place the infant at risk for death. Enables management to minimize any damaging effects.**

Nursing Priority No. 2.

To promote use of activities to minimize risk of SIDS:

- Recommend that infant be placed on his or her back to sleep, both at nighttime and naptime. **Research confirms that fewer infants die of SIDS when they sleep on their backs and that a side-lying position is not to be used.**

- Advise all caregivers of the infant regarding the importance of maintaining correct sleep position. **Anyone who will have responsibility for the care of the child during sleep needs to be reminded of the importance of the back to sleep position.**

- Encourage parents to schedule "tummy time" only while infant is awake. **This activity promotes strengthening of back and neck muscles while parents are close and baby is not sleeping.**

Information that appears in brackets has been added by the authors to clarify and enhance the use of nursing diagnoses.

🌐 Cultural   🌐 Collaborative   🏠 Community/Home Care

- Encourage early and medically recommended prenatal care and continue with well-baby checkups and immunizations after birth. Include information about signs of premature labor and actions to be taken to avoid problems if possible. **Prematurity presents many problems for the newborn, and keeping babies healthy prevents problems that could put the infant at risk for SIDS. Immunizing infants prevents many illnesses that can also be life threatening.**
- Encourage breastfeeding, if possible. Recommend sitting up in chair when nursing at night. **Breastfeeding has many advantages (e.g., immunological, nutritional, and psychosocial), promoting a healthy infant. Although this does not preclude the occurrence of SIDS, healthy babies are less prone to many illnesses/problems. The risk of the mother falling asleep while feeding infant in bed with resultant accidental suffocation could be of concern, but studies do not support an actual link with SIDS.**
- Discuss issues of bedsharing and the concerns regarding sudden unexpected infant deaths from accidental entrapment under a sleeping adult or suffocation by becoming wedged in a couch or cushioned chair. **While bedsharing among infants and family members is common in many cultures, there are concerns about accidental death from suffocation, especially when the mother smokes, has recently consumed alcohol, the infant's head is covered by a blanket or quilt, or there are multiple bedsharers. Also, studies show that the odds of SIDS is greater if babies who bedshare are also exposed to second-hand smoke.**
- Note cultural beliefs about bedsharing. **Bedsharing is more common among breastfed infants, young unmarried mothers; low-income families where multiple people share a bed; or those from a minority group. Additional study is needed to better understand bedsharing practices and associated risks and benefits.**

Nursing Priority No. 3.

To promote wellness (Teaching/Discharge Considerations):
- Discuss known facts about SIDS with parents. **Corrects misconceptions and helps reduce level of anxiety.**
- Avoid overdressing or overheating infants during sleep. **Infants dressed in two or more layers of clothes as they sleep have six times the risk of SIDS as those dressed in fewer layers.**

Information that appears in brackets has been added by the authors to clarify and enhance the use of nursing diagnoses.

- Place the baby on a firm mattress in an approved crib. **Avoiding soft mattresses, sofas, cushions, water beds, and other soft surfaces, while not known to prevent SIDS, will minimize chance of suffocation/SUDI.**
- Remove fluffy and loose bedding from sleep area, making sure baby's head and face are not covered during sleep. **Minimizes possibility of suffocation.**
- Discuss the use of apnea monitors. **Apnea monitors have not proved helpful in preventing SIDS, but may be used to monitor other medical problems.**
- Recommend public health nurse or similar resource visit new mothers at least once or twice following discharge. **Researchers found that Native American infants whose mothers received such visits were 80% less likely to die from SIDS than those who were never visited.**
- Ascertain that day-care center/provider(s) are trained in observation and modifying risk factors (e.g., sleeping position) **to reduce risk of death while infant is in their care.**
- Refer parents to local SIDS programs/other resources for learning (e.g., National SIDS/Infant Death Resource Center and similar Web sites) and encourage consultation with healthcare provider if baby shows any signs of illness or behaviors that concern them. **Can provide information and support for risk reduction and correction of treatable problems.**

Documentation Focus

Assessment/Reassessment
- Baseline findings, degree of parental anxiety/concern.
- Individual risk factors.

Planning
- Plan of care, interventions, and who is involved in planning.
- Teaching plan.

Implementation/Evaluation
- Parent's responses to interventions, teaching, and actions performed.
- Attainment or progress toward desired outcome(s).
- Modifications to plan of care.

Information that appears in brackets has been added by the authors to clarify and enhance the use of nursing diagnoses.

Discharge Planning

- Long-term needs and actions to be taken.
- Support systems available, specific referrals made, and who is responsible for actions to be taken.

Sample Nursing Outcomes & Interventions Classifications (NOC/NIC)

NOC—Risk Detection
NIC—Risk Identification

risk for **Suffocation**

Taxonomy II: Safety/Protection—Class 2 Physical Injury (00036)
[Diagnostic Division: Safety]
Submitted 1980

Definition: At risk of accidental suffocation (inadequate air available for inhalation)

Risk Factors

Internal
Reduced olfactory sensation
Reduced motor abilities
Deficient knowledge regarding safe situations or safety precautions
Cognitive or emotional difficulties (e.g., altered consciousness)
Disease or injury process

External
Pillow or propped bottle in an infant's crib
Hanging a pacifier around infant's neck
Playing with plastic bags; inserting small objects into airway
Children unattended in water
Discarding refrigerators without removing doors
Vehicle warming in closed garage [or faulty exhaust system]; fuel-burning heaters not vented to outside
Household gas leaks; smoking in bed
Low-strung clothesline
Eating large mouthfuls [or pieces] of food

Information that appears in brackets has been added by the authors to clarify and enhance the use of nursing diagnoses.

> **NOTE:** A risk diagnosis is not evidenced by signs and symptoms, as the problem has not occurred; rather, nursing interventions are directed at prevention.

Desired Outcomes/Evaluation Criteria— Client/Caregiver Will:

- Verbalize knowledge of hazards in the environment.
- Identify interventions appropriate to situation.
- Correct hazardous situations to prevent or reduce risk of suffocation.
- Demonstrate CPR skills and how to access emergency assistance.

Actions/Interventions

Nursing Priority No. 1.

To assess causative/contributing factors:

∞• Determine age, developmental level, and mentation (e.g., infant/young child, frail elder, person with developmental delay, altered level of consciousness, or cognitive impairments or dementia) **to identify individuals unable to be responsible for or protect self.**

- Determine client's/SO's knowledge of safety factors or hazards present in the environment **to identify misconceptions and educational needs. Suffocation can be caused by (1) spasm of airway (e.g., food or water going down wrong way, irritant gases, asthma); (2) airway obstruction (e.g., foreign body, tongue falling back in unconscious person, swelling of tissues from burn injury or allergic reaction); (3) airway compression (e.g., tying rope or band tightly around neck, hanging, throttling, smothering); (4) conditions affecting the respiratory mechanism (e.g., epilepsy, tetanus, rabies, nerve diseases causing paralysis of chest wall or diaphragm); (5) conditions affecting respiratory center in brain (e.g., electric shock; stroke or other brain trauma; medications such as morphine, barbiturates); and (6) compression of the chest (e.g., crushing as might occur with cave-in, motor vehicle crash, pressure in a massive crowd).**

- Identify level of concern or awareness and motivation of client/SO(s) to correct safety hazards and improve individual situation. **Lack of commitment may limit growth or will-**

Information that appears in brackets has been added by the authors to clarify and enhance the use of nursing diagnoses.

🌐 Cultural 🆂 Collaborative 🏠 Community/Home Care

ingness to make changes, placing dependent individuals at risk.

- Assess neurological status and note history/presence of conditions (e.g., stroke, cerebral palsy, multiple sclerosis, amyotrophic lateral sclerosis) **that have potential to compromise airway or affect ability to swallow.**
- Determine use of antiepileptics and how well epilepsy is controlled. **Seizure activity (and especially status epilepticus) is a major risk factor for respiratory inhibition or arrest, particularly when consciousness is impaired.**
- Review medication regimen **to note potential for oversedation and respiratory failure (e.g., central nervous system depressants, analgesics, sedatives, antidepressants).**
- Note reports of sleep disturbance and fatigue; **may be indicative of sleep apnea (airway obstruction).**
- Assess for allergies (e.g., medications, foods, environmental) **to which individual could have severe/anaphylactic reaction resulting in respiratory arrest.**
- Be alert to and carefully monitor those individuals who are severely depressed, mentally ill, or aggressive. **These individuals could be at risk for suicide by suffocation (e.g., inhaled carbon monoxide or death by strangling or hanging).** (Refer to ND risk for Suicide.)
- Note signs of respiratory distress (e.g., cough, stridor, wheezing, increased work of breathing) **that could indicate swelling or obstruction of airways.** Refer to NDs ineffective Airway Clearance; risk for Aspiration; ineffective Breathing Pattern; impaired spontaneous Ventilation, as appropriate, for additional interventions.

Nursing Priority No. 2,
To reverse/correct contributing factors:

- Identify and encourage relevant safety measures (e.g., seizure precautions; close supervision of toddler; avoid propping up baby bottle; and do not leave automobile engine running in closed garage) **to prevent or minimize risk of injury.**
- Recommend storing small toys, coins, cords or drawstrings, and plastic bags out of reach of infants and young children. Avoid use of plastic mattress or crib covers, comforter, or fluffy pillows in cribs **to reduce risk of accidental suffocation.** (Refer to ND risk for Sudden Infant Death Syndrome.)
- Refrain from smoking in bed; supervise smoking materials (use, disposal, storage) for impaired individuals. Keep smoking materials out of reach of children.

Information that appears in brackets has been added by the authors to clarify and enhance the use of nursing diagnoses.

- Use proper positioning, suctioning; use airway adjuncts, as indicated, for comatose individual or client with swallowing impairment or obstructive sleep apnea **to protect and maintain airway.**
- Provide diet modifications as indicated by specific needs (e.g., developmental level, presence and degree of swallowing disability, impaired cognition) **to reduce risk of aspiration.**
- Monitor medication regimen (e.g., anticonvulsants, analgesics, sedatives), noting potential for oversedation.
- Administer medications when client is sitting or standing upright and can swallow without difficulty.
- Discuss with client/SO(s) identified environmental or work-related safety hazards and problem-solve methods for resolution.
- Emphasize importance of periodic evaluation and repair of gas appliances, furnace, automobile exhaust system **to prevent exposure to carbon monoxide.**

Nursing Priority No. 3.
To promote wellness (Teaching/Discharge Considerations):

- Review safety factors identified in individual situation and methods for remediation.
- Develop plan with client/caregiver for long-range management of situation to avoid injuries. **Enhances commitment to plan, optimizing outcomes.**
- Review importance of chewing carefully, taking small amounts of food, using caution when talking or drinking while eating. Discuss possibility of choking **because of impaired swallowing or throat muscle relaxation and impaired judgment when drinking alcohol and eating.**
- Emphasize the importance of getting help when beginning to choke; instead of leaving table, remain calm and make gesture across throat, making sure someone recognizes the emergency.
- Promote public education in techniques for clearing blocked airways, back blows, Heimlich maneuver, CPR.
- Collaborate in community public health education regarding hazards for children (e.g., appropriate toy size for young child) discussing dangers of "huffing" (inhalants) and playing choking or hanging games with preteens; fire safety drills; bathtub rules; how to spot potential for depression and risk of suicidal gestures in adolescents **to reduce potential for accidental or intentional suffocation.**

Information that appears in brackets has been added by the authors to clarify and enhance the use of nursing diagnoses.

🌐 Cultural   🔵 Collaborative   🏠 Community/Home Care

- Assist individuals to learn to read package labels and identify safety hazards.
- ∞ Promote pool safety, use of approved flotation devices, proper fencing enclosure or alarm system for home pools.
- Discuss safety measures regarding use of heaters, household gas appliances, old or discarded appliances.
- Refer to NDs ineffective Airway Clearance; risk for Aspiration; ineffective Breathing Pattern; impaired Parenting.

Documentation Focus

Assessment/Reassessment
- Individual risk factors, including individual's cognitive status and level of knowledge.
- Level of concern and motivation for change.
- Equipment or airway adjunct needs.

Planning
- Plan of care and who is involved in planning.
- Teaching plan.

Implementation/Evaluation
- Responses to interventions, teaching, and actions performed.
- Attainment or progress toward desired outcome(s).
- Modifications to plan of care.

Discharge Planning
- Long-term needs, appropriate preventive measures, and who is responsible for actions to be taken.
- Specific referrals made.

Sample Nursing Outcomes & Interventions Classifications (NOC/NIC)

NOC—Risk Control
NIC—Airway Management

---

risk for Suicide

Taxonomy II: Safety/Protection—Class 3 Violence (00150)
[Diagnostic Division: Safety]
Submitted 2000

Definition: At risk for self-inflicted, life-threatening injury

---

Information that appears in brackets has been added by the authors to clarify and enhance the use of nursing diagnoses.

Risk Factors

Behavioral
History of prior suicide attempt
Buying a gun; stockpiling medicines
Making or changing a will; giving away possessions
Sudden euphoric recovery from major depression
Impulsiveness; marked changes in behavior, attitude, or school
    performance

Verbal
Threats of killing oneself; states desire to die

Situational
Living alone; retired; economically disadvantaged; relocation;
    institutionalization
Loss of autonomy or independence
Presence of gun in home
Adolescents living in nontraditional settings (e.g., juvenile de-
    tention center, prison, half-way house, group home)

Psychological
Family history of suicide; childhood abuse
Substance abuse
Psychiatric illness or disorder
Guilt
Homosexual youth

Demographic
Age (e.g., elderly people, young adult males, adolescents)
Race (e.g., Caucasian, Native American)
Male gender
Divorced; widowed

Physical
Physical or terminal illness; chronic pain

Social
Loss of important relationship; disrupted family life; poor sup-
    port systems; social isolation
Grieving; loneliness
Hopelessness; helplessness
Legal or disciplinary problem
Cluster suicides

Information that appears in brackets has been added by the authors to clarify
and enhance the use of nursing diagnoses.

🌐 Cultural   🌀 Collaborative   🏠 Community/Home Care

> **NOTE:** A risk diagnosis is not evidenced by signs and symptoms, as the problem has not occurred; rather, nursing interventions are directed at prevention.

Desired Outcomes/Evaluation Criteria— Client Will:

- Acknowledge difficulties perceived in current situation.
- Identify current factors that can be dealt with.
- Be involved in planning course of action to correct existing problems.
- Make decision that suicide is not the answer to the perceived problems.

Actions/Interventions

Nursing Priority No. 1.

To assess causative/contributing factors:

- Identify degree of risk or potential for suicide and seriousness of threat. Use a scale of 1 to 10 and prioritize according to severity of threat, availability of means.
- Note behaviors indicative of intent (e.g., gestures; presence of means, such as guns; threats; giving away possessions; previous attempts; and presence of hallucinations or delusions). **Many people signal their intent, particularly to healthcare providers.**
- Ask directly if person is thinking of acting on thoughts or feelings. **Determines intent. Most people will answer honestly because they actually want help.**
- ∞ Note age and gender. **Risk of suicide is greater in males, teens, and the elderly, but there is a rising awareness of risk in early childhood.**
- Review family history for suicidal behavior. **Individual risk is increased, especially when the person who committed suicide was close to the client.**
- Identify conditions, such as acute or chronic brain syndrome, panic state, hormonal imbalance (e.g., premenstrual syndrome, postpartum psychosis, drug induced) **that may interfere with ability to control own behavior and will require specific interventions to promote safety.**
- Review laboratory findings (e.g., blood alcohol, blood glucose, arterial blood gas, electrolytes, renal function tests), **to identify factors that may affect reasoning ability.**

Information that appears in brackets has been added by the authors to clarify and enhance the use of nursing diagnoses.

- Note withdrawal from usual activities, lack of social interactions.
- Assess physical complaints (e.g., sleeping difficulties, lack of appetite).
- Determine drug use or "self" medication.
- Note history of disciplinary problems or involvement with judicial system.
- Assess coping behaviors presently used. *Note:* Client may believe there is no alternative except suicide.
- Determine presence of SO(s)/friends who are available for support.

Nursing Priority No. 2.

To assist clients to accept responsibility for own behavior and prevent suicide:

- Develop therapeutic nurse-client relationship, providing consistent caregiver. **Promotes sense of trust, allowing individual to discuss feelings openly.**
- Maintain straightforward communication **to avoid reinforcing manipulative behavior.**
- Explain concern for safety and willingness to help client stay safe.
- Encourage expression of feelings and make time to listen to concerns. **Acknowledges reality of feelings and that they are okay. Helps individual sort out thinking and begin to develop understanding of situation and look at other alternatives.**
- Give permission to express angry feelings in acceptable ways and let client know someone will be available to assist in maintaining control. **Promotes acceptance and sense of safety.**
- Acknowledge reality of suicide as an option. Discuss consequences of actions if they follow through on intent. Ask how it will help individual to resolve problems. **Helps to focus on consequences of actions and possibility of other options.**
- Maintain observation of client and check environment for hazards that could be used to commit suicide **to increase client safety or reduce risk of impulsive behavior.**
- Help client identify more appropriate solutions/behaviors (e.g., motor activities/exercise) **to lessen sense of anxiety and associated physical manifestations.**
- Provide directions for actions client can take, avoiding negative statements, such as "Do Nots." **Promotes a positive attitude.**

Information that appears in brackets has been added by the authors to clarify and enhance the use of nursing diagnoses.

- Discuss use of psychotropic medication, positive and negative aspects. **There has been concern about the increased risk of suicide from these drugs, and research is ongoing to determine whether they help or harm.**
- Reevaluate potential for suicide periodically at key times (e.g., mood changes, increasing withdrawal), as well as when client is feeling better and discharge planning becomes active. **The highest risk exists when the client has both suicidal ideation and sufficient energy with which to act.**

Nursing Priority No. 3.

To assist client to plan course of action to correct/deal with existing situation:

- Gear interventions to individual involved (e.g., age, relationship, current situation).
- Negotiate contract with client regarding willingness not to do anything lethal for a stated period of time. Specify what caregiver will be responsible for and what client responsibilities are.
- Specify alternative actions necessary if client is unwilling to negotiate contract. **May need hospitalization to provide safety.**
- Discuss losses client has experienced and meaning of those losses. **Unresolved issues may be contributing to thoughts of hopelessness.**

Nursing Priority No. 4.

To promote wellness (Teaching/Discharge Considerations):

- Promote development of internal control by helping client look at new ways to deal with problems.
- Assist with learning problem-solving, assertiveness training, and social skills.
- Engage in physical activity programs. Releases endorphins, **promoting feelings of self-worth and improving sense of well-being.**
- Determine nutritional needs and help client to plan for meeting them.
- Involve family/SO(s) in planning **to improve understanding and support.**
- Refer to formal resources as indicated (e.g., individual/group/marital psychotherapy, substance abuse treatment program, and social services).

Information that appears in brackets has been added by the authors to clarify and enhance the use of nursing diagnoses.

Documentation Focus

Assessment/Reassessment
- Individual findings, including nature of concern (e.g., suicidal/behavioral risk factors and level of impulse control, plan of action and means to carry out plan).
- Client's perception of situation, motivation for change.

Planning
- Plan of care and who is involved in the planning.
- Details of contract regarding suicidal ideation or plans.
- Teaching plan.

Implementation/Evaluation
- Actions taken to promote safety.
- Response to interventions, teaching, and actions performed.
- Attainment or progress toward desired outcome(s).
- Modifications to plan of care.

Discharge Planning
- Long-term needs and who is responsible for actions to be taken.
- Available resources, specific referrals made.

Sample Nursing Outcomes & Interventions Classifications (NOC/NIC)

NOC—Suicide Self-Restraint
NIC—Suicide Prevention

delayed Surgical Recovery

Taxonomy II: Safety/Protection—Class 2 Physical Injury (00100)
[Diagnostic Division: Safety]
Submitted 1998; Revised 2006

Definition: Extension of the number of postoperative days required to initiate and perform activities that maintain life, health, and well-being

Related Factors

Extensive or prolonged surgical procedure
Pain

Information that appears in brackets has been added by the authors to clarify and enhance the use of nursing diagnoses.

 Cultural   Collaborative   Community/Home Care

Obesity
Preoperative expectations
Postoperative surgical site infection

Defining Characteristics

Subjective
Perception that more time is needed to recover
Report of pain or discomfort; fatigue
Loss of appetite with or without nausea
Postpones resumption of work/employment activities

Objective
Evidence of interrupted healing of surgical area (e.g., red, indurated, draining, immobilized)
Difficulty in moving about; requires help to complete self-care

Desired Outcomes/Evaluation Criteria— Client Will:

- Display complete healing of surgical area.
- Be able to perform desired self-care activities.
- Report increased energy, able to participate in usual (work or employment) activities.

Actions/Interventions

Nursing Priority No. 1.
To assess causative/contributing factors:

- Identify vulnerable client (e.g., low socioeconomic status, lack of resources, challenges related to poverty, lack of insurance or transportation, severe trauma or prolonged hospitalization with multiple complicating factors) **who is at higher risk for adverse outcomes.**
- ∞ Determine extent of surgical involvement of organs or tissues, noting age and developmental level, and general state of health **to help determine time that may be required for client to resume activities of daily living (ADLs) and other activities, or expectation of time needed for healing.**
- Identify underlying condition/pathology (e.g., cancers, burns, diabetes, obesity, multiple trauma, infections, cardiopulmonary disorders, debilitating illness) **that can adversely affect healing and prolong recuperation time.**

Information that appears in brackets has been added by the authors to clarify and enhance the use of nursing diagnoses.

- Determine the length of operative procedure or time under anesthesia (e.g., typical or lengthy); type and severity of perioperative complications (e.g., trauma or other conditions requiring multiple surgeries; heavy bleeding during procedure); type of surgical wound (e.g., clean, clean-contaminated, or grossly contaminated, acutely infected); and development of postoperative complications (e.g., surgical site infection, suture reactions, dehiscence, ventilator-associated pneumonia, deep vein thrombosis) **that can affect the pace of healing or prolong recovery.**

- Determine cultural expectations regarding recovery process and participation of client/others (e.g., client is expected to be inactive and cared for by others). **Family beliefs and cultural values, stress and fear related to surgery (and the reason for it), possible stigma about relative condition or disease, or change in body image; or motivation to return to usual role and activities all impact rate and expectations for sick role and recovery.**

- Assess nutritional status and current intake **to determine if nutrition is adequate to support healing.**

- Review current medication regimen and determine dosages and use of multiple drugs with potential for adverse side effects and interactions **affecting cognition, organ function, and tissue healing.**

- Perform pain assessment **to ascertain whether pain management is adequate to meet client's needs during recovery.**

- Evaluate client's cognitive and emotional state, noting presence of postoperative changes, including confusion, depression, apathy, expressions of helplessness **to determine possible psychological interferences.**

- Review results of laboratory tests (e.g., complete blood count, blood or wound cultures, glucose) **to assess for presence and type of infections, metabolic or endocrine dysfunction, or other conditions affecting body's ability to heal.**

Nursing Priority No. 2.

To determine impact of delayed recovery:

- Note length of hospitalization and progress in recovery to date **to compare with expectations for procedure and situation.**

- Determine client's/SO's expectations for recovery and specific stressors related to delay (e.g., return to work or school,

---

Information that appears in brackets has been added by the authors to clarify and enhance the use of nursing diagnoses.

🌐 Cultural   🔄 Collaborative   🏠 Community/Home Care

home responsibilities, child care, financial difficulties, limited support system).

- Determine energy level and current participation in ADLs. Compare with usual level of function.
- Ascertain whether client usually requires assistance in home setting and who provides it, current availability, and capability.
- Obtain psychological assessment of client's emotional status, noting potential problems arising from current situation.

Nursing Priority No. 3.

To promote optimal recovery:

- Inspect incisions or wounds routinely, describing changes (e.g., deepening or healing, wound measurements, presence and type of drainage, development of necrosis).
- Practice and instruct client/caregiver(s) in proper hand hygiene and aseptic technique for incisional care **to reduce incidence of contamination and infection.**
- Collaborate in treatment of complications (e.g., infection, dehiscence).
- Assist with wound care as indicated (e.g., débridement, barrier dressings, wound coverings, skin-protective agents for open or draining wounds).
- Include wound care specialist or stoma therapist as appropriate **to problem-solve healing difficulties.**
- Avoid or limit use of plastics or latex materials. **Client may be sensitive.**
- Provide optimal nutrition and adequate protein intake **to provide a positive nitrogen balance, aiding in healing, and achieving good health.**
- Encourage early ambulation, regular exercise **to promote circulation, improve strength, and reduce risks associated with immobility.**
- Recommend alternating activity with adequate rest periods **to reduce fatigue.**
- Administer medications as indicated (e.g., client may be experiencing stubborn infection requiring intravenous antibiotics or management of chronic pain).
- Instruct client/SO(s) in necessary self-care of incisions and specific symptom management. **With short hospital stays, client/SO(s) usually provide a great deal of postoperative care and monitoring at home.**
- Encourage client to adhere to medical regimen and follow-up care **to monitor healing process and provide for timely intervention as needed.**

Information that appears in brackets has been added by the authors to clarify and enhance the use of nursing diagnoses.

• Refer for outpatient or follow-up care as indicated (e.g., telephone monitoring, home visit, wound care clinic, pain management program).

Nursing Priority No. 4.

To promote wellness (Teaching/Discharge Considerations):

- Demonstrate self-care skills, provide client/SO(s) with health-related information and psychosocial support **to manage symptoms and pain, enhancing well-being.**
- Discuss reality of recovery process in comparison with client's/SO's expectations. **Individuals are often unrealistic regarding energy and time required for healing and own abilities and responsibilities to facilitate process.**
- Involve client/SO(s) in setting incremental goals. **Enhances commitment to plan and reduces likelihood of frustration blocking progress.**
- Refer to physical or occupational therapists, as indicated, **to address exercise program and home-care needs or to identify assistive devices to facilitate independence in ADLs.**
- Identify suppliers for dressings or wound care items and assistive devices as needed.
- Consult dietitian for individual dietary plan **to meet increased nutritional needs that reflect personal situation and resources.**
- Evaluate home situation (e.g., lives alone, bedroom or bathroom on second floor, availability of assistance), where appropriate, **to evaluate for beneficial adjustments, such as moving bedroom to first floor, arranging for commode during recovery, obtaining an in-home emergency call system.**
- Discuss alternative placement (e.g., convalescent or rehabilitation center, as appropriate).
- Identify community resources, as indicated (e.g., visiting nurse, home healthcare agency, Meals on Wheels, respite care). **Facilitates adjustment to home setting.**
- Recommend support group or self-help program for smoking cessation.
- Refer for counseling or support. **May need additional help to overcome feelings of discouragement, deal with changes in life.**

Information that appears in brackets has been added by the authors to clarify and enhance the use of nursing diagnoses.

🌐 Cultural   ⊛ Collaborative   🏠 Community/Home Care

Documentation Focus

Assessment/Reassessment
- Assessment findings, including individual concerns, family involvement, and support factors and availability of resources.
- Cultural expectations.
- Assistive device use or need.

Planning
- Plan of care and who is involved in planning.
- Teaching plan.

Implementation/Evaluation
- Responses of client/SO(s) to plan, interventions, teaching, and actions performed.
- Attainment or progress toward desired outcome(s).
- Modifications to plan of care.

Discharge Planning
- Long-range needs and who is responsible for actions to be taken.
- Specific referrals made.

Sample Nursing Outcomes & Interventions Classifications (NOC/NIC)

NOC—Self-Care: Activities of Daily Living (ADLs)
NIC—Self-Care Assistance

---

impaired Swallowing

Taxonomy II: Nutrition—Class 1 Ingestion (00103)
[Diagnostic Division: Food/Fluid]
Submitted 1986; Nursing Diagnosis Extension and Classification Revision 1998

Definition: Abnormal functioning of the swallowing mechanism associated with deficits in oral, pharyngeal, or esophageal structure or function

Related Factors

Congenital Deficits
Upper airway anomalies; mechanical obstruction (e.g., edema, tracheostomy tube, tumor); history of tube feeding

---

Information that appears in brackets has been added by the authors to clarify and enhance the use of nursing diagnoses.

Neuromuscular impairment (e.g., decreased or absent gag reflex, decreased strength or excursion of muscles involved in mastication, perceptual impairment, facial paralysis); conditions with significant hypotonia

Respiratory disorders; congenital heart disease

Behavioral feeding problems; self-injurious behavior

Failure to thrive; protein energy malnutrition

Neurological Problems

Nasal or nasopharyngeal cavity defects; oropharynx or upper airway anomalies; laryngeal abnormalities; tracheal, laryngeal, or esophageal defects

Gastroesophageal reflux disease; achalasia

Traumas; acquired anatomical defects; cranial nerve involvement; traumatic head injury; developmental delay; cerebral palsy

Prematurity

Defining Characteristics

Subjective

Esophageal Phase Impairment

Reports "something stuck"; odynophagia

Food refusal; volume limiting

Heartburn; epigastric pain

Nighttime coughing or awakening

Objective

Oral Phase Impairment

Weak suck resulting in inefficient nippling

Slow bolus formation; lack of tongue action to form bolus; premature entry of bolus

Incomplete lip closure; food pushed out of or falls from mouth

Lack of chewing

Coughing, choking, or gagging before a swallow

Piecemeal deglutition; abnormality in oral phase of swallow study

Inability to clear oral cavity; pooling in lateral sulci; nasal reflux; sialorrhea; drooling

Long meals with little consumption

Pharyngeal Phase Impairment

Food refusal

Altered head positions; delayed or multiple swallows

Information that appears in brackets has been added by the authors to clarify and enhance the use of nursing diagnoses.

🌐 Cultural 🔵 Collaborative 🏠 Community/Home Care

Inadequate laryngeal elevation; abnormality in pharyngeal phase by swallow study

Choking; coughing; gagging; nasal reflux; gurgly voice quality

Unexplained fevers; recurrent pulmonary infections

Esophageal Phase Impairment

Observed evidence of difficulty in swallowing (e.g., stasis of food in oral cavity, coughing/choking); abnormality in esophageal phase by swallow study

Hyperextension of head (e.g., arching during or after meals)

Repetitive swallowing; bruxism

Unexplained irritability surrounding mealtime

Acidic smelling breath; regurgitation of gastric contents (wet burps); vomitus on pillow; vomiting; hematemesis

Desired Outcomes/Evaluation Criteria— Client Will:

* Pass food and fluid from mouth to stomach safely.
* Maintain adequate hydration as evidenced by good skin turgor, moist mucous membranes, and individually appropriate urine output.
* Achieve and/or maintain desired body weight.

Client/Caregiver Will:

* Verbalize understanding of causative or contributing factors.
* Identify individually appropriate interventions or actions to promote intake and prevent aspiration.
* Demonstrate feeding methods appropriate to the individual situation.
* Demonstrate emergency measures in the event of choking.

Actions/Interventions

Nursing Priority No. 1.

To assess causative/contributing factors and degree of impairment:

∞• Evaluate client's potential for swallowing problems, noting age and medical conditions (e.g., Parkinson's disease, multiple sclerosis, myasthenia gravis, or other neuromuscular conditions). **Swallowing disorders are especially common in the elderly, possibly due to coexistence of variety of neurological, neuromuscular, or other conditions. Infants at risk include those born prematurely or with tracheoesophageal fistula or lip**

Information that appears in brackets has been added by the authors to clarify and enhance the use of nursing diagnoses.

and palate malformation. **Persons with traumatic brain injuries often exhibit swallowing impairments, regardless of gender or age.**

∞• Determine ability to initiate and sustain effective suck. **Weak suck results in inefficient nippling, suggesting ineffective movement of tongue and mouth muscles, impairing ability to swallow.**

• Assess client's cognitive and sensory-perceptual status. **Sensory awareness, orientation, concentration, motor coordination affect desire and ability to swallow safely and effectively.**

• Note symmetry of facial structures and muscle tone.

• Assess strength and excursion of muscles involved in mastication and swallowing.

• Note voice quality and speech. **Abnormal voice (dysphonia) and abnormal speech patterns (dysarthria) are signs of motor dysfunction of structures involved in oral and pharyngeal swallowing.**

• Inspect oropharyngeal cavity for edema, inflammation, altered integrity of oral mucosa, adequacy of oral hygiene.

• Verify proper fit of dentures, if present.

• Ascertain presence and strength of cough and gag reflex. **Although absence of gag reflex is not necessarily predictive of client's eventual ability to swallow safely, it does increase client's potential for aspiration (overt or silent). Coughing, drooling, double swallowing, decreased ability to move food in mouth, and throat clearing with or after swallowing is indicative of swallowing dysfunction and increases risk for aspiration.**

• Review medications **that may affect (1) oropharyngeal function (e.g., benzodiazapines, neuroleptics, anticonvulsants, certain sedatives); (2) esophageal function (e.g., nonsteroidal anti-inflammatory agents, iron preparations, tetracycline, calcium channel blockers); (3) medications that can cause xerostomia (e.g., anticholinergics, opioids, antidepressants, antineoplastics, diuretics), thus impairing swallowing by means of sedation, pharyngeal weakness, inflammation, dry mouth, and so forth.**

• Note hyperextension of head or arching of neck during or after meals or repetitive swallowing, **suggesting inability to complete swallowing process.**

• Auscultate breath sounds **to evaluate the presence of aspiration.**

• Review laboratory test results for underlying problems (e.g., complete blood count **to screen for infectious or inflam-**

Information that appears in brackets has been added by the authors to clarify and enhance the use of nursing diagnoses.

🌐 Cultural ☯ Collaborative 🏠 Community/Home Care

matory conditions or thyroid or other metabolic and nutritional studies **that can affect swallowing.**

⟋• Prepare for or assist with diagnostic testing of swallowing activity (e.g., reflex cough test, swallowing electromyography, transnasal or esophageal endoscopy, videofluorographic swallow studies; fiber-optic endoscopic examination of swallowing) **to identify the pathophysiology of swallowing disorder.**

Nursing Priority No. 2.

To prevent aspiration and maintain airway patency:

• Identify individual factors that can precipitate aspiration or compromise airway.

• Move client to chair for meals, snacks, and drinks when possible; if client must be in bed, raise head of bed as upright as possible with head in anatomical alignment and slightly flexed forward during feeding. Keep client seated upright or head of bed elevated for 30 to 45 minutes after feeding, if possible, **to reduce risk of regurgitation or aspiration.**

• Instruct client to cough and expectorate **when secretion management is of concern.**

• Have suction equipment available during initial feeding attempts and as indicated. Suction oral cavity if client cannot clear secretions **to prevent aspiration.**

• Teach client self-suction when appropriate (e.g., drooling, frequent choking, structural changes in mouth or pharynx. **Promotes airway safety and independence and sense of control with managing secretions.**

Nursing Priority No. 3.

To enhance swallowing ability to meet fluid and caloric body requirements:

⊛• Refer to surgeon, gastroenterologist or neurologist as indicated **for treatment (e.g., reconstructive facial surgery, esophageal dilatation) that may result in improved swallowing.**

⊛• Refer to speech/language pathologist **to identify specific techniques to enhance client efforts and safety measures.**

⚗• Encourage a rest period before meals **to minimize fatigue.**

⚗• Provide analgesics prior to feeding, as indicated, **to enhance comfort, being cautious to avoid decreasing awareness or sensory perception.**

Information that appears in brackets has been added by the authors to clarify and enhance the use of nursing diagnoses.

- Focus client's attention on feeding and swallowing activity. Decrease environmental stimuli and talking, **which may be distracting or promote choking during feeding.**
- Determine food preferences of client **to incorporate as possible, enhancing intake.** Present foods in an appealing, attractive manner.
- Ensure temperature (hot or cold versus tepid) of foods and fluid, **which will stimulate sensory receptors.**
- Provide a consistency of food and fluid that is most easily swallowed. **Risk of choking or aspiration is reduced when food can be formed into a bolus before swallowing, such as gelatin desserts prepared with less water than usual; pudding and custard or liquids are thickened (addition of thickening agent, or yogurt, cream soups prepared with less water); thinned purees (hot cereal with added water); thick drinks, such as nectars; fruit juices that have been frozen into "slush" consistency (thin fluids are most difficult to control); medium-soft boiled or scrambled eggs; canned fruit; soft-cooked vegetables.**
- Avoid milk products and chocolate, **which may thicken oral secretions.**
- Feed one consistency and/or texture of food at a time.
- Place food in unaffected side of client's mouth **(when one side of the mouth is affected by condition, e.g., hemiplegia),** and have client use tongue to assist with moving food bolus to swallowing position.
- Manage size of bites **(e.g., small bites of 1/2 tsp or less are usually easier to swallow).** Use a teaspoon or small spoon **to encourage smaller bites.** Cut all solid foods into small pieces.
- Place food midway in oral cavity; provide medium-sized bites (about 15 mL) **to adequately trigger the swallowing reflex.**
- Provide cognitive cues (e.g., remind client to chew and swallow as indicated) **to enhance concentration and performance of swallowing sequence.** Focus attention on feeding and swallowing activity by decreasing environmental stimuli, **which may be distracting during feeding. Also, if client is talking or laughing while eating, risk of aspiration is increased.**
- Massage the laryngopharyngeal musculature (sides of trachea and neck) gently **to stimulate swallowing.**

Information that appears in brackets has been added by the authors to clarify and enhance the use of nursing diagnoses.

🌐 Cultural 😊 Collaborative 🏠 Community/Home Care

- Observe oral cavity after each bite and have client check around cheeks with tongue for remaining food. Remove food if unable to swallow.
- Incorporate client's eating style and pace when feeding **to avoid fatigue and frustration with process.**
- Allow ample time for eating (feeding).
- Remain with client during meal to reduce anxiety and offer assistance.
- Use a glass with a nose cut-out **to avoid posterior head tilting while drinking.** Refrain from pouring liquid into the mouth or "washing food down" with liquid.
- Monitor intake, output, and body weight to evaluate adequacy of fluid and caloric intake.
- Provide positive feedback for client's efforts.
- Provide oral hygiene following each feeding.
- Consider tube feedings or parenteral solutions, as indicated, **for the client unable to achieve adequate nutritional intake.**
- Consult with dysphagia specialist or rehabilitation team, as indicated.
- Refer to lactation counselor or support group (e.g., La Leche League) **for breastfeeding guidance.**
- Refer to NDs ineffective Breastfeeding; ineffective Infant Feeding Pattern, for additional interventions for infants.

Nursing Priority No. 4.

To promote wellness (Teaching/Discharge Considerations):

- Consult with nutritionist **to establish optimum dietary plan.**
- Place medication in gelatin, jelly, or puddings. Consult with pharmacist **to determine if pills may be crushed or if liquids or capsules are available.**
- Assist client and/or SO(s) in learning specific feeding techniques and swallowing exercises.
- Encourage continuation of facial exercise program **to maintain or improve muscle strength.**
- Instruct client and/or SO(s) in emergency measures in event of choking **to prevent aspiration or more serious complications**.
- Recommend avoiding food intake within 3 hours of bedtime, eliminating alcohol and caffeine intake, reducing weight if

---

Information that appears in brackets has been added by the authors to clarify and enhance the use of nursing diagnoses.

impaired SWALLOWING

needed, using stress-reduction techniques, and elevating head of bed during sleep **to limit potential for gastric reflux and aspiration.**
- Establish routine schedule for monitoring weight.
- Refer to ND risk for imbalanced Nutrition: less than body requirements.

Documentation Focus

Assessment/Reassessment
- Individual findings, including degree and characteristics of impairment, current weight and recent changes.
- Nutritional status.
- Effects on lifestyle and socialization.

Planning
- Plan of care and who is involved in planning.
- Teaching plan.

Implementation/Evaluation
- Response to interventions, teaching, and actions performed.
- Attainment or progress toward desired outcome(s).
- Modifications to plan of care.

Discharge Planning
- Long-term needs and who is responsible for actions to be taken.
- Available resources and specific referrals made.

Sample Nursing Outcomes & Interventions Classifications (NOC/NIC)

NOC—Swallowing Status
NIC—Swallowing Therapy

Information that appears in brackets has been added by the authors to clarify and enhance the use of nursing diagnoses.

⊕ Cultural   ⊕ Collaborative   🏠 Community/Home Care

ineffective family **Therapeutic Regimen Management**

Taxonomy II: Health Promotion—Class 2 Health Management (00080)
[Diagnostic Division: Teaching/Learning]
Submitted 1992

Definition: A pattern of regulating and integrating into family processes a program for the treatment of illness and its sequelae that is unsatisfactory for meeting specific health goals

Related Factors

Complexity of therapeutic regimen or healthcare system
Decisional conflicts
Economic difficulties
Excessive demands; family conflicts

Defining Characteristics

Subjective
Reports difficulty with therapeutic regimen
Reports desire to manage the illness

Objective
Inappropriate family activities for meeting health goals
Acceleration of illness symptoms of a family member
Failure to take action to reduce risk factors; lack of attention to illness

Desired Outcomes/Evaluation Criteria— Family Will:

- Identify individual factors affecting regulation/integration of treatment program.
- Participate in problem-solving of factors.
- Verbalize acceptance of need or desire to change actions to achieve agreed-on outcomes or health goals.
- Demonstrate behaviors and changes in lifestyle necessary to maintain therapeutic regimen.

Information that appears in brackets has been added by the authors to clarify and enhance the use of nursing diagnoses.

Nursing Priority No. 1.

To identify causative/precipitating factors:

- Ascertain family's perception of efforts to date.
- Evaluate family functioning and activities—looking at frequency and effectiveness of family communication, promotion of autonomy, adaptation to meet changing needs, health of home environment and lifestyle, problem-solving abilities, ties to community. **Understanding the family and the context in which it lives allows for more personalized support of the family and choosing coping strategies in partnership with the family to meet individualized goals.**
- Note family health goals and agreement of individual members. **Presence of conflict interferes with problem-solving.**
- Determine understanding of and value of the treatment regimen to the family.
- Identify cultural values or religious beliefs affecting view of situation and willingness to make necessary changes.
- Identify availability and use of resources.

Nursing Priority No. 2.

To assist family to develop strategies to improve management of therapeutic regimen:

- Provide family-centered education addressing management of condition/chronic illness and incorporation of strategies into family's lifestyle. **Helps family make informed decisions, see the connection between illness and treatment; facilitates treatment adherence and improved client outcomes.**
- Assist family members to recognize inappropriate family activities. Help the members identify both togetherness and individual needs and behavior **so that effective interactions can be enhanced and perpetuated.**
- Make a plan jointly with family members to deal with complexity of healthcare regimen or system and other related factors. **Enhances commitment to plan, optimizing outcomes.**
- Identify community resources, as needed, using the three strategies of education, problem-solving, and resource linking **to address specific deficits.**

Information that appears in brackets has been added by the authors to clarify and enhance the use of nursing diagnoses.

⊕ Cultural   ⊛ Collaborative   🏠 Community/Home Care

ineffective family **THERAPEUTIC REGIMEN MANAGEMENT**

Nursing Priority No. 3.

🔒 To promote wellness as related to future health of family members:

- Help family identify criteria to promote ongoing self-evaluation of situation and effectiveness and family progress. **Provides opportunity to be proactive in meeting needs.**
- 🔲 Make referrals to and/or jointly plan with other health, social, and community resources. **Problems are often multifaceted, requiring involvement of numerous providers and agencies.**
- Encourage involvement in disease/condition support groups. **Family resiliency is gained through contact with other families dealing with similar challenges.**
- Provide contact person or case manager for one-to-one assistance, as needed, **to coordinate care, provide support, assist with problem-solving, and so forth.**
- Refer to NDs Caregiver Role Strain; ineffective Self-Health Management, as indicated.

Documentation Focus

Assessment/Reassessment
- Individual findings, including nature of problem and degree of impairment; family values, health goals, and level of participation and commitment of family members.
- Cultural values, religious beliefs.
- Availability and use of resources.

Planning
- Plan of care and who is involved in planning.
- Teaching plan.

Implementation/Evaluation
- Response to interventions, teaching, and actions performed.
- Attainment or progress toward desired outcome(s).
- Modifications of plan of care.

Discharge Planning
- Long-term needs, plan for meeting, and who is responsible for actions.
- Specific referrals made.

Information that appears in brackets has been added by the authors to clarify and enhance the use of nursing diagnoses.

Sample Nursing Outcomes & Interventions Classifications (NOC/NIC)

NOC—Family Health Status
NIC—Family Involvement Promotion

risk for Thermal Injury

Taxonomy II: Safety/Protection—Class 5 Physical Injury (00220)
[Diagnostic Division: Safety]
Submitted 2010

Definition: At risk for damage to skin and mucous membranes due to extreme temperatures

Risk Factors

Exposure to extreme temperatures
Unsafe environment; lack of protective clothing (e.g., flame-retardant sleepwear, gloves, ear covering)
Inattentiveness; smoking; intoxication (alcohol, [other] drug)
Fatigue
Lack of knowledge (patient, caregiver); inadequate supervision
Developmental level (infants, aged); cognitive impairment (e.g., dementia, psychoses)
Neuropathy; neuromuscular impairment (e.g., stroke, amyotrophic lateral sclerosis, multiple sclerosis)
Treatment-related side effects (e.g., pharmaceutical agents)

NOTE: A risk diagnosis is not evidenced by signs and symptoms, as the problem has not occurred; rather, nursing interventions are directed at prevention.

Desired Outcomes/Evaluation Criteria— Client Will:

• Be free of damage to skin or mucous membranes associated with extreme temperatures.
• Demonstrate behaviors, lifestyle changes to reduce risk factors and protect from injury.

Actions/Interventions

This ND is a compilation of a number of situations that can result in injury. Refer to specific NDs, such as Hypothermia;

Information that appears in brackets has been added by the authors to clarify and enhance the use of nursing diagnoses.

🌐 Cultural   ✋ Collaborative   🏠 Community/Home Care

risk for Injury; impaired Skin Integrity; impaired Tissue Integrity; risk for Trauma, as appropriate, for more specific interventions.

Nursing Priority No. 1.

To identify causative/precipitating factors related to risk:

- Identify client at risk (e.g., chronic illness conditions with weakness or prolonged immobility; acute or chronic confusion, mental illness, dementia, head injury; use of multiple medications; use of alcohol or other drugs; cultural, familial, and socioeconomic factors adversely affecting lifestyle and home; exposure to environmental chemicals).
- Note chronological and developmental age of client. **Infants, young children, disabled, debilitated, aged, or impaired individuals are not able to protect themselves and may not recognize and/or react appropriately in dangerous situations.**
- Evaluate client's/SO's level of cognition, competence, decision-making ability and independence.
- Ascertain if client is using alcohol/other drugs or medications **that could impair ability to act in best interest of self or others.**
- Evaluate client's lifestyle practices, noting reports of risk-prone behavior (e.g., smoking in bed, failure to use safety equipment when working with chemicals, allowing child to play with matches, unprotected exposure to sun or cold environment) **that can place client or others at high risk for injury.**
- Ascertain knowledge of safety needs and injury prevention, as well as motivation to prevent injury. **Information may reveal areas of misinformation, lack of knowledge, need for teaching.**

Nursing Priority No. 2.

To assist client/caregiver to reduce or correct individual risk factors:

- Provide client/SO information regarding client's specific situation and consequences of continuing unsafe behaviors **to enhance decision making, clarify expectations and individual needs.**
- Review client's physical and psychological abilities or limitations **to determine adaptations that may be required by current situation.**

Information that appears in brackets has been added by the authors to clarify and enhance the use of nursing diagnoses.

- Provide for client's safety while in facility care (e.g., apply hot and cold treatments judiciously; prevent/monitor smoking; supervise bath temperature in confused individuals, young children, or elderly adults; etc.).
- Be mindful of skin safety issues during surgical procedures:

  Conduct a fire risk assessment at beginning of each surgical procedure and continuously monitor for changes in risk during procedure. **The highest risk procedures involve an ignition source (such as electrocautery device), delivery of supplemental oxygen, and the operation of the ignition source near the oxygen (e.g., head, neck, or upper chest surgery).**

  Provide supplemental oxygen safely, using the lowest concentration possible **to reduce amount of oxygen flowing into surgical field.**

  Verify electrical safety of equipment including intact cords, grounds, and medical engineering verification labels.

  Place dispersive electrode (electrocautery pad) over largest available muscle mass closest to surgical site, ensuring its contact **to prevent electrical burns.**

  Ascertain that alcohol-containing skin prep solutions are not pooled under client or in surgical drapes and had sufficient drying time.

  Protect surrounding skin and tissues appropriately when laser equipment is used in surgical procedures. **Prevents inadvertent skin integrity disruption, hair ignition, and adjacent anatomy injury in area of laser beam use.**

  Apply eye protection before laser activation. **Eye protection for specific laser wavelength must be used to prevent injury.**

- Implement skin care protocol for client receiving radiation therapy:

  Assess skin frequently for side effects of therapy; note breakdown and delayed wound healing. Emphasize importance of reporting open areas to caregiver. **A reddening and/or tanning effect (radiation dermatitis) may develop within the field of radiation.**

  Avoid rubbing the skin or use of soap, lotions, creams, ointments, powders, or deodorants on area; avoid applying heat or attempting to wash off marks/tattoos placed on skin to pinpoint location for radiation therapy. May increase dermal reaction.

- ∞ Avoid application of lotion or oils to skin of infants receiving phototherapy for hyperbilirubinemia **to prevent dermal in-**

Information that appears in brackets has been added by the authors to clarify and enhance the use of nursing diagnoses.

jury and cover male groin with small pad **to protect testes from heat-related injury.**

∞• Provide or instruct in proper care of skin surfaces during exposure to very cold or hot weather. **Although everyone is at risk for frostbite or sunburn, individuals with impaired sensation or cognition and infants/young children require special attention to deal with extremes in weather.**

• Discuss importance of self-monitoring of factors that can contribute to occurrence of injury (e.g., fatigue, anger). **Client/ SO may be able to modify risk through monitoring of actions especially during times when client is likely to be highly stressed.**

🏠• Perform home assessment, if indicated, **to address safety issues.**

🏠• Review specific employment concerns or worksite issues and needs (e.g., properly fitting safety equipment, regular use of safety glasses or goggles, safe storage of hazardous substances).

⊕• Discuss need for and sources of supervision (e.g., before- and after-school programs for children, elder day programs, home-care assistance) **when client or care provider is unable or unwilling to attend to safety concerns.**

Nursing Priority No. 3.

To promote wellness (Teaching/Discharge Criteria):

🏠• Identify individual needs and resources for safety education.

∞• Prevent burn (flame, scalding, chemical, electrical, sunburn) injuries:

Install smoke alarms in kitchen, in every sleeping area, and on every floor of home.

Keep space heaters away from flammable materials and from at-risk persons.

Check all fuel-burning appliances including fireplaces for proper function.

Store combustibles away from all heat-producing appliances.

Prepare and practice an emergency escape plan.

Avoid smoking in bed. Get rid of used cigarettes carefully.

Prevent small children from playing with matches or near open flame or stove.

Turn handles of pots and pans toward side of stove or use back burners.

Set the temperature on water heater to 120°F or use the "low-medium" setting.

Information that appears in brackets has been added by the authors to clarify and enhance the use of nursing diagnoses.

Test water temperature before allowing child/impaired person into tub or shower.

Use cool-water humidifiers instead of hot-steam vaporizers.

Store fireworks, cleaning supplies, and other chemicals out of the reach of children.

Wear gloves, safety glasses, and other protective clothing when handling chemicals.

Avoid storing chemicals in food or drink containers; store in original containers with intact labels.

Check electrical appliances for proper function and follow manufacturer's safety instructions. Discard frayed or damaged electrical cords **to reduce risk of electrical burns**. *Note:* **Most electrical injuries that occur in the home are low-voltage burns and almost exclusively involve either the hands or oral cavity.**

Use child safety plugs in all electrical outlets.

Avoid using electrical appliances while showering or wet.

Avoid lengthy or unnecessary sun exposure/ultraviolet tanning, especially with specific disease conditions or treatments (e.g., systemic lupus, tetracycline or psychotropic drug use, radiation therapy) **to reduce risk of sunburn.**

Advise use of high sun protection factor (SPF) sunblock or sunscreen, particularly on young child and/or client with fair skin (prone to burn).

- Provide telephone numbers and other contact numbers as individually indicated (e.g., fire, police, physician).
- Refer to community resources as indicated (e.g., substance recovery, anger management, and parenting classes) **to address conditions that could exacerbate risk of injury to self or others.**
- Refer to or assist with community education programs **to increase awareness of safety measures and available resources.**
- Identify emergency escape plans and routes for home and community to be **prepared in the event of natural or man-made disaster (e.g., fire, toxic chemical release).**

Documentation Focus

Assessment/Reassessment
- Individual risk factors identified.
- Client's concerns or difficulty making and following through with plan.

Information that appears in brackets has been added by the authors to clarify and enhance the use of nursing diagnoses.

Planning
- Plan of care and who is involved in planning.
- Teaching plan.

Implementation/Evaluation
- Response to interventions, teaching, and actions performed.
- Attainment or progress toward outcomes.

Discharge Planning
- Referrals to other resources.
- Long term need and who is responsible for actions.

Sample Nursing Outcomes & Interventions Classifications (NOC/NIC)

NOC—Tissue Integrity: Skin & Mucous Membrane
NIC—Skin Surveillance

ineffective Thermoregulation

Taxonomy II: Safety/Protection—Class 6 Thermoregulation (00008)
[Diagnostic Division: Safety]
Submitted 1986

Definition: Temperature fluctuation between hypothermia and hyperthermia

Related Factors

Trauma; illness
Extremes of age
Fluctuating environmental temperature
Changes in hypothalamic tissue causing alterations in emission of thermosensitive cells and regulation of heat loss and production
Changes in metabolic rate or activity; changes in level or action of thyroxine and catecholamines
Chemical reactions in contracting muscles

Defining Characteristics

Objective
Fluctuations in body temperature above and below the normal range

---

Information that appears in brackets has been added by the authors to clarify and enhance the use of nursing diagnoses.

Tachycardia; hypertension; increased respiratory rate

Reduction in body temperature below normal range; skin cool to touch; moderate pallor; mild shivering; piloerection; cyanotic nailbeds; slow capillary refill

Increase in body temperature above normal range; skin warm to touch; flushed skin; seizures

Desired Outcomes/Evaluation Criteria— Client/Caregiver Will:

- Verbalize understanding of individual factors and appropriate interventions.
- Demonstrate techniques and behaviors to correct underlying condition or situation.
- Maintain body temperature within normal limits.

Actions/Interventions

Nursing Priority No. 1.

To identify causative/contributing factors:

∞• Note extremes of age (e.g., premature neonate, young child, or aging adult) **as this can directly impact ability to maintain or regulate body temperature.**

- Obtain history concerning present symptoms, correlate with previous episodes or family history, and diagnostic studies. **Thermoregulation is a controlled process that maintains the body's core temperature in the range at which most biochemical processes work best (99°F to 99.6°F [37.2°C to 37.6°C]). Exercise, behavioral impulses, metabolic and hormonal changes influence changes in body temperature, leading to loss or gain of heat.**

- Identify individual factor(s) or underlying condition (e.g., environmental exposure, infectious process, brain injury, effects of drugs or toxins, salt or water depletion, obesity, confined to bed, drug overdose). **Thermoregulation is affected in two ways: (1) endogenous factors (via diseases or conditions of body/organ systems that affect temperature homeostasis) and (2) exogenous factors (via environmental exposures, medications, and nutrition).**

- Monitor laboratory studies (e.g., tests indicative of infection, thyroid or other endocrine tests, organ damage, drug screens).

Information that appears in brackets has been added by the authors to clarify and enhance the use of nursing diagnoses.

Nursing Priority No. 2.

To assist with measures to correct/treat underlying cause:

- Monitor temperature by appropriate route (e.g., tympanic, rectal, oral), using the same site and device over time and noting variation from client's usual or normal temperature.
- Have cooling and warming equipment and supplies readily available during childbirth and following procedures or surgery.
- Maintain ambient temperature in comfortable range **to prevent or compensate for client's heat production or heat loss (e.g., may need to add or remove clothing or blankets, avoid drafts, reduce or increase room temperature and humidity).**
- ∞• Review home management of temperature fluctuations in special population (e.g., newborn infant, person with spinal cord injury, frail elder). **Measures could include use of heating pads, ice bag, radiant heaters or fans; adding or removing clothing or blankets; cool or warm liquids and bath water; occlusive wrap in the delivery room, skin-to-skin contact in newborn; and so forth.**
- Initiate emergent and/or immediate interventions **to restore or maintain body temperature within normal range,** as indicated in NDs Hypothermia; Hyperthermia; risk for imbalanced Body Temperature.
- ⊕• Administer fluids, electrolytes, and medications, as appropriate, **to restore or maintain body and organ function.**
- ⊕• Prepare client for and assist with procedures (e.g., surgical intervention or administering neoplastic agents, antibiotics) **to treat underlying cause of hypothermia or hyperthermia.**

Nursing Priority No. 3.

🏠 To promote wellness (Teaching/Discharge Considerations):

- Review causative or related factors and risk factors, if appropriate, with client/SO(s).
- Provide information concerning disease processes, current therapies, and postdischarge precautions, as appropriate to situation.
- Refer to teaching section in NDs risk for imbalanced Body Temperature; Hypothermia; Hyperthermia, for additional interventions.

Information that appears in brackets has been added by the authors to clarify and enhance the use of nursing diagnoses.

Documentation Focus

Assessment/Reassessment
• Individual findings, including nature of problem, degree of impairment, or fluctuations in temperature.

Planning
• Plan of care and who is involved in planning.
• Teaching plan.

Implementation/Evaluation
• Responses to interventions, teaching, and actions performed.
• Attainment or progress toward desired outcome(s).
• Modifications to plan of care.

Discharge Planning
• Long-term needs and who is responsible for actions to be taken.
• Specific referrals made.

Sample Nursing Outcomes & Interventions Classifications (NOC/NIC)

NOC—Thermoregulation
NIC—Temperature Regulation

---

impaired Tissue Integrity

Taxonomy II: Safety/Protection—Class 2 Physical Injury (00044)
[Diagnostic Division: Safety]
Submitted 1986; Revised 1998 (by small group work 1996)

Definition: Damage to mucous membrane, corneal, integumentary, or subcutaneous tissues

---

Related Factors

Altered circulation
Nutritional factors (e.g., deficit or excess)
Deficient or excess fluid volume
Impaired physical mobility
Chemical irritants [including body excretions, secretions, medications]; radiation

---

Information that appears in brackets has been added by the authors to clarify and enhance the use of nursing diagnoses.

Temperature extremes
Mechanical factors (e.g., pressure, shear, friction); [surgery]
Deficient knowledge
[Infection]

Defining Characteristics

Objective
Damaged tissue (e.g., cornea, mucous membrane, integumentary, subcutaneous)
Destroyed tissue

Desired Outcomes/Evaluation Criteria— Client Will:

- Verbalize understanding of condition and causative factors.
- Identify interventions appropriate for specific condition.
- Demonstrate behaviors and lifestyle changes to promote healing and prevent complications or recurrence.
- Display progressive improvement in wound or lesion healing.

Actions/Interventions

Nursing Priority No. 1.
To identify causative/contributing factors:

- Identify underlying condition or pathology involved in tissue injury (e.g., diabetic neuropathies; peripheral arterial disorders; sensory and perceptual deficits; cognitively impaired, debilitated elderly; emotional or psychological problems; developmental delay; surgery, traumatic injuries; debilitating illness; long-term immobility). **Suggests treatment options, as well as client's desire and ability to protect self, and potential for recurrence of tissue damage.**
- Assess for individual factors **that increase risk of circulatory insufficiency or occlusion and can impede healing, such as (1) trauma that causes internal tissue damage (e.g., burns, high-velocity and penetrating trauma), fractures (especially long-bone fractures) with hemorrhage; (2) external pressures (e.g., from tight dressings, splints or casting, burn eschar); (3) immobility (e.g., long-term bedrest, traction/cast); (4) presence of conditions affecting peripheral circulation and sensation (e.g., atherosclerosis, diabetes, venous insufficiency); (5) lifestyle factors (e.g., smoking, obesity, and sedentary lifestyle); (6) use of**

Information that appears in brackets has been added by the authors to clarify and enhance the use of nursing diagnoses.

medications (e.g., anticoagulants, corticosteroids, immunosuppressives, antineoplastics) that adversely affect healing; (7) malnutrition (deprives the body of protein and calories required for cell growth and repair); and (8) dehydration (impairs transport of oxygen and nutrients).

- Identify specific behaviors, such as occupational hazards or toxic exposures; sport or leisure activity risks; lifestyle choices (e.g., unsafe sex practices); use of restraints or prosthetic devices (e.g., limbs, artificial eye, contact lenses, dentures, artificial airway, indwelling catheter), which can cause pressure on/injure delicate tissues or provide entry point for infectious agents.

- Note race or ethnic background, familial history for genetic, sociocultural, and religious factors that may make individual vulnerable to particular condition or impact treatment.

- Evaluate skin and mucous membranes for hydration status; note presence and degree of edema (1+ to 4+), urine characteristics and output. Determines presence of fluid deficit or overload that can adversely affect cell or tissue strength and organ function. (Refer to ND risk for imbalanced Fluid Volume.)

- Examine eyes for conjunctivitis, hemorrhage, burns, abrasions or lacerations as indicated. Note reports of dry, scratchy eye, vision impairment or pain. May indicate injury to eye tissues requiring more intensive evaluation and interventions. (Refer to ND risk for Dry Eye.)

- Determine nutritional status and impact of malnutrition on situation (e.g., pressure points on emaciated and/or elderly client, obesity, lack of activity, slow healing or failure to heal).

- Note evidence of deep organ or tissue involvement in client with wound (e.g., draining fistula through the integumentary and subcutaneous tissue may signal a bone infection).

- Assess blood supply and sensation (nerve damage) of affected area. Evaluate pulses and calculate ankle-brachial index (ABI) to evaluate actual or potential for impairment of circulation to lower extremities. Result less than 0.9 indicates need for close monitoring and more aggressive intervention (e.g., tighter blood glucose and weight control in diabetic client).

- Note poor hygiene or health practices (e.g., lack of cleanliness, frequent use of enemas, poor dental care) that may be impacting tissue health.

- Assess environmental location of home and work or school, as well as recent travel. Some areas of a country or city may

---

Information that appears in brackets has been added by the authors to clarify and enhance the use of nursing diagnoses.

be more susceptible to certain disease conditions or environmental pollutants.

- Refer to NDs (dependent on individual situation) risk for Peripheral Neurovascular Dysfunction; risk for Perioperative Positioning Injury; impaired physical/bed Mobility; impaired Skin Integrity; [disturbed visual Sensory Perception]; ineffective peripheral Tissue Perfusion; risk for Trauma; risk for Infection for related interventions.

Nursing Priority No. 2.
To assess degree of impairment:

- Obtain a history of condition (e.g., pressure, venous, or diabetic wound; eye or oral lesions), including whether condition is acute or recurrent; original site/characteristics of wound; duration of problem and changes that have occurred over time.
- Assess skin and tissues, bony prominences, pressure areas and wounds for comparative baseline:

Note color, texture, and turgor.

Assess areas of least pigmentation for color changes (e.g., sclera, conjunctiva, nailbeds, buccal mucosa, tongue, palms, and soles of feet).

Note presence, location, and degree of edema (e.g., 4+ pitting).

Record size (depth/width), color, location, temperature, texture of wounds or lesions.

Determine degree and depth of injury or damage to integumentary system (involves epidermis, dermis, and/or underlying tissues), extent of tunneling or undermining, if present. *Note:* Full extent of lesions of mucous membranes or subcutaneous tissue may not be discernible.

Classify burns. Use appropriate measuring tool (e.g., Braden or similar) and staging (I to IV) for ulcers.

Document with drawings and/or photograph wound, lesion(s), burns, as appropriate.

Observe for other distinguishing characteristics of surrounding tissue (e.g., exudate; granulation; cyanosis or pallor; tight, shiny skin).

Describe wound drainage (e.g., amount, color, odor).

- Assist with diagnostic procedures (e.g., x-rays, imaging scans, biopsies, débridement). May be necessary to determine extent of impairment.

Information that appears in brackets has been added by the authors to clarify and enhance the use of nursing diagnoses.

• Obtain specimens of exudate and lesions for Gram's stain, culture and sensitivity, and so forth, when appropriate.
• Determine psychological effects of condition on client/SO(s). **Can be devastating for client's body or self-image and esteem, especially if condition is severe, disfiguring or chronic, as well as costly and burdensome for SO(s)/ caregiver.**

Nursing Priority No. 3.

To assist client to correct/minimize impairment and to promote healing:

• Modify or eliminate factors contributing to condition, if possible. Assist with treatment of underlying condition(s), as appropriate.
• Inspect lesions or wounds daily, or as appropriate, for changes (e.g., signs of infection, complications, or healing). **Promotes timely intervention and revision of plan of care.**
• Provide or encourage optimum nutrition (including adequate protein, lipids, calories, trace minerals, and multivitamins) **to promote tissue health/healing** and adequate hydration **to reduce and replenish cellular water loss and enhance circulation.**
• Encourage adequate periods of rest and sleep **to limit metabolic demands, maximize energy available for healing, and meet comfort needs.**
• Provide or assist with oral care (e.g., teaching oral and dental hygiene, avoiding extremes of hot or cold, changing position of endotrachial and nasogastric tubes, lubricating lips) **to prevent damage to mucous membranes.**
• Promote early mobility. Assist with or encourage position changes, active or passive and assistive exercises **to promote circulation and prevent excessive tissue pressure.**
• Apply appropriate protective and healing devices (e.g., eye pads or goggles, heel protectors, padding or cushions, therapeutic beds and mattresses, as well as appropriate barrier dressings (e.g., semipermeable, occlusive, wet-to-dry, hydrocolloid, hydrogel, polyacrylate moist wound dressing), drainage appliances, and skin-protective agents for open or draining wounds and stomas.
• Practice aseptic technique for cleansing, dressing, or medicating lesions. **Reduces risk of cross-contamination.**
• Use appropriate catheter (e.g., peripheral or central venous) when infusing anticancer or other toxic drugs, and ascertain that intravenous liquid is patent and infusing well **to prevent**

Information that appears in brackets has been added by the authors to clarify and enhance the use of nursing diagnoses.

🌐 Cultural 🔄 Collaborative 🏠 Community/Home Care

infiltration and extravasation with resulting tissue damage.

- Monitor for correct placement of tubes, catheters, and other devices; assess skin tissues around these devices for effects of tape or fasteners or pressure from the devices **to prevent damage to skin and tissues as a result of pressure, friction, or shear forces.**

- Develop regularly timed repositioning schedule for client with mobility and sensation impairments, using turn sheet as needed; encourage and assist with periodic weight shifts for client in chair **to reduce stress on pressure points and encourage circulation to tissues.**

- Use or demonstrate proper turning and transfer techniques **to avoid movements that cause friction or shearing (e.g., pulling client with parallel force, dragging movements).**

- Provide appropriate mattress (e.g., foam, flotation, alternating pressure, or air mattress) and appropriate padding devices (e.g., foam boots, heel protectors, ankle rolls), when indicated.

- Limit use of plastic material (e.g., rubber sheet, plastic-backed linen savers) and remove wet or wrinkled linens promptly. **Moisture potentiates skin and underlying tissues, increasing risk of breakdown and infection.**

- Provide or instruct in proper care of extremities during cold or hot weather. **Individuals with impaired sensation or young children/individuals unable to verbalize discomfort require special attention to deal with extremes in weather (e.g., dressing in layers, wearing gloves, clean, dry socks; properly fitting shoes or boots, face mask in winter; or use of sunscreen and light clothing to protect from dermal injury in summer).**

- Protect client from environmental hazards when vision or hearing or cognitive deficits impact safety.

- Advise smoking cessation and refer for assistance or support, if indicated. **Smoking causes vasoconstriction that interferes with healing.**

- Monitor laboratory studies (e.g., complete blood count, electrolytes, glucose, cultures) **for changes indicative of healing or presence of infection, complications.**

Nursing Priority No. 4.
To promote wellness (Teaching/Discharge Considerations):

- Encourage verbalizations of feelings and expectations regarding condition and potential for recovery of structure and function.

Information that appears in brackets has been added by the authors to clarify and enhance the use of nursing diagnoses.

- Help client and family identify effective successful coping mechanisms and implement them **to reduce pain or discomfort and to improve quality of life.**
- Discuss importance of early detection and reporting of changes in condition or any unusual physical discomforts or changes in pain characteristics. **Promotes early intervention and reduces potential for complications.**
- Emphasize need for adequate nutritional and fluid intake **to optimize healing potential.**
- Instruct in dressing changes (technique and frequency) and proper disposal of soiled dressings **to prevent spread of infectious agent.**
- Review medical regimen (e.g., proper use of topical sprays, creams, ointments, soaks, or irrigations).
- Emphasize importance of follow-up care, as appropriate (e.g., diabetic foot care clinic, wound care specialist or clinic, enterostomal therapist).
- Identify required changes in lifestyle, occupation, or environment **necessitated by limitations imposed by condition or to avoid causative factors.**
- Refer to community or governmental resources, as indicated (e.g., Public Health Department, Occupational Safety and Health Administration, National Association for the Prevention of Blindness).

Documentation Focus

Assessment/Reassessment
- Individual findings, including history of condition, characteristics of wound or lesion, and evidence of other organ or tissue involvement.
- Impact on functioning and lifestyle.
- Availability and use of resources.

Planning
- Plan of care and who is involved in planning.
- Teaching plan.

Implementation/Evaluation
- Responses to interventions, teaching, and actions performed.
- Attainment or progress toward desired outcome(s).
- Modifications to plan of care.

Information that appears in brackets has been added by the authors to clarify and enhance the use of nursing diagnoses.

Discharge Planning

- Long-term needs and who is responsible for actions to be taken.
- Specific referrals made.

Sample Nursing Outcomes & Interventions Classifications (NOC/NIC)

NOC—Tissue Integrity: Skin & Mucous Membranes
NIC—Wound Care

ineffective peripheral Tissue Perfusion

Taxonomy II: Activity/Rest—Class 4 Cardiovascular/
   Pulmonary Responses (00204)
[Diagnostic Division: Circulation]
Submitted 2008; Revised 2010

Definition: Decrease in blood circulation to the periphery that may compromise health

Related Factors:

Deficient knowledge of aggravating factors (e.g., smoking, sedentary lifestyle, trauma, obesity, salt intake, immobility)
Deficient knowledge of disease process (e.g., diabetes, hyperlipidemia; [peripheral artery disease, chronic venous insufficiency])
Hypertension; diabetes mellitus
Sedentary lifestyle
Smoking

Defining Characteristics

Subjective
Extremity pain; claudication
Paresthesia

Objective
Diminished or absent pulses; ankle-brachial index less than 0.90; blood pressure changes in extremities; femoral bruit
Altered skin characteristics (color, elasticity, hair, moisture, nails, sensation, temperature)

Information that appears in brackets has been added by the authors to clarify and enhance the use of nursing diagnoses.

Skin color pale on elevation; capillary refill time of more than
3 seconds; color does not return to leg on lowering it

Shorter total or pain-free distances achieved in the 6-minute
walk test

Edema

Altered motor function

Delayed peripheral wound healing; [ulcerations]

Desired Outcomes/Evaluation Criteria— Client Will: (Include Specific Time Frame)

- Demonstrate increased perfusion as individually appropriate
  (e.g., skin warm and dry, peripheral pulses present and strong,
  absence of edema, free of pain or discomfort).
- Verbalize understanding of condition, therapy regimen, side
  effects of medications, and when to contact healthcare provider.
- Demonstrate behaviors and lifestyle changes to improve circulation (e.g., engage in regular exercise, cessation of smoking, weight reduction, disease management).

Actions/Interventions

Nursing Priority No. 1.

To assess causative/contributing factors:

- Note current situation or presence of conditions (e.g., congestive heart failure, lung disorders, major trauma, septic or
  hypovolemic shock, coagulopathies, sickle cell anemia) **affecting systemic circulation/perfusion.**
- Determine history of conditions associated with thrombus or
  emboli (e.g., problems with coronary or cerebral circulation,
  stroke; high-velocity trauma with fractures, abdominal or orthopedic surgery, long periods of immobility; inflammatory
  diseases; chronic lung disease; diabetes with coexisting peripheral vascular disease; estrogen therapy, cancer and cancer
  therapies, presence of central venous catheters) **to identify
  client at higher risk for venous stasis, vessel wall injury,
  and hypercoagulability.**
- Identify presence of high-risk factors or conditions (e.g.,
  smoking, uncontrolled hypertension, obesity, pregnancy, pelvic tumor, paralysis, hypercholesterolemia, varicose veins, arthritis, sepsis) **that place client at greater risk for developing peripheral vascular disease (including arterial**

Information that appears in brackets has been added by the authors to clarify
and enhance the use of nursing diagnoses.

🌐 Cultural   😊 Collaborative   🏠 Community/Home Care

blockage and chronic venous insufficiency) with associated complications.

- Note location of restrictive clothing, pressure dressings, circular wraps, cast, or traction device **that may restrict circulation to limb.**
- Ascertain impact of condition on functioning and lifestyle. **For example, leg pain may restrict ambulation or person may develop skin ulceration and healing problems that seriously impact quality of life.**

Nursing Priority No. 2.

To evaluate degree of impairment:

- Assess skin color, temperature, moisture, and whether changes are widespread or localized. **Helps in determining location and type of perfusion problem.**
- Compare skin temperature and color with other limb when assessing extremity circulation. **Helps differentiate type of problem (e.g., deep redness in both hands triggered by vibrating machinery is associated with Raynaud's, while edema, redness, swelling in calf of one leg is associated with localized thrombophlebitis).**
- Assess presence, location, and degree of swelling or edema formation. Measure circumference of extremities, noting differences in size. **Useful in identifying or quantifying edema in involved extremity.**
- Measure capillary refill **to determine adequacy of systemic circulation.**
- Note client's nutritional and fluid status. **Protein-energy malnutrition and weight loss make ischemic tissues more prone to breakdown. Dehydration reduces blood volume and compromises peripheral circulation.**
- Inspect lower extremities for skin texture (e.g., atrophic, shiny appearance, lack of hair; or dry/scaly, reddened skin), and skin breaks or ulcerations **that often accompany diminished peripheral circulation.**
- Palpate arterial pulses (bilateral femoral, popliteal, dorsalis pedis, and posterial tibial) using hand-held Doppler if indicated **to determine level of circulatory blockage.**
- Note whether activity alters pulses (**e.g., client with intermittent claudication may have palpable pulses that disappear after ambulation**).
- Determine pulse equality, as well as intensity (e.g., bounding, normal, diminished, or absent), and compare with unaffected

Information that appears in brackets has been added by the authors to clarify and enhance the use of nursing diagnoses.

extremity **to evaluate distribution and quality of blood flow and success or failure of therapy.**

- Evaluate extremity pain reports, noting associated symptoms (e.g., cramping or heaviness, discomfort with walking; progressive temperature or color changes; paresthesias).
- Determine time (day or night) that symptoms are worse, precipitating or aggravating events (e.g., walking), and relieving factors (e.g., rest, sitting down with legs in dependent position, oral analgesics) **to help isolate and differentiate problems such as intermittent chronic claudication versus loss of function and pain due to acute sustained ischemia related to loss of arterial blood flow.**
- Assess motor and sensory function. **Problems with ambulation; hypersensitivity; or loss of sensation, numbness, and tingling are changes that can indicate neurovascular dysfunction or limb ischemia.**
- Check for calf tenderness or pain on dorsiflexion of foot (Homans' sign), swelling and redness. **Indicators of deep vein thrombosis (DVT), although DVT is often present without a positive Homans' sign.**
- Review laboratory studies such as lipid profile, coagulation studies, hemoglobin/hematocrit, renal/cardiac function tests, inflammatory markers (e.g., D dimer, C-reactive protein); and diagnostic studies (e.g., Doppler ultrasound, magnetic resonance angiography, venogram, contrast angiography, resting ankle-brachial index [ABI], leg segmental arterial pressure measurements) **to determine probability, location, and degree of impairment.**

Nursing Priority No. 3.
To maximize tissue perfusion:

- Collaborate in treatment of underlying conditions, such as diabetes, hypertension, cardiopulmonary conditions, blood disorders, traumatic injury, hypovolemia, hypoxemia **to maximize systemic circulation and organ perfusion.**
- Administer medications such as antiplatelet agents, thrombolytics, antibiotics **to improve tissue perfusion or organ function.**
- Administer fluids, electrolytes, nutrients, and oxygen, as indicated, **to promote optimal blood flow, organ perfusion, and function.**
- Assist with or prepare for medical procedures such as endovascular stent placement, surgical revascularization procedures, thrombectomy **to improve peripheral circulation.**

Information that appears in brackets has been added by the authors to clarify and enhance the use of nursing diagnoses.

- Assist with application of elasticized tubular support bandages, adhesive elastic or Velcro wraps (e.g., Circ-Aid), medication-impregnated layered bandage (e.g., Unna boot), multilayer bandage regimens, sequential pneumatic compression devices, and custom-fitted compression stockings, as indicated, **to provide graduated compression of lower extremity in presence of venous stasis ulcer.**
- Refer to wound care specialist if arterial or venous ulcerations are present. **In-depth wound care may include debridement and various specialized dressings that provide optimal moisture for healing, prevention of infection and further injury.**
- Provide interventions **to promote peripheral circulation and limit complications associated with poor perfusion:**

Encourage early ambulation when possible and recommend regular exercise.

Recommend or provide foot and ankle exercises when client unable to ambulate freely **to reduce venous pooling and increase venous return.**

Provide pressure-relieving devices for immobilized client (e.g., air mattress, foam or sheepskin padding, bed or foot cradle).

Assist or instruct client to change position at timed intervals, rather than using presence of pain as signal to change positions.

Elevate legs when sitting; avoid sharp angulation of the hips or knees.

Avoid massaging the leg in presence of thrombosis.

Avoid, or carefully monitor, use of heat or cold, such as hot water bottle, heating pad, or ice pack.

- Refer to NDs risk for Peripheral Neurovascular Dysfunction; risk for impaired Skin Integrity; impaired Tissue Integrity; [disturbed Sensory Perception], for additional interventions as appropriate.

Nursing Priority No. 4.

To promote wellness (Teaching/Discharge Considerations):

- Discuss relevant risk factors (e.g., family history, obesity, age, smoking, hypertension, diabetes, clotting disorders) and potential outcomes of atherosclerosis (e.g., systemic and peripheral vascular disease conditions). **Information necessary for**

Information that appears in brackets has been added by the authors to clarify and enhance the use of nursing diagnoses.

client to make informed choices about remediating risk factors and committing to lifestyle changes.

- Identify necessary changes in lifestyle and assist client to incorporate disease management into activities of daily living. **Promotes independence, enhances self-concept regarding ability to deal with change and manage own needs.**
- Emphasize need for regular exercise program **to enhance circulation and promote general well-being.**
- Refer to dietitian for well-balanced, low-saturated fat, low-cholesterol diet, or other modifications as indicated.
- Discuss care of dependent limbs/foot care, as appropriate. **When circulation is impaired, changes in sensation place client at risk for development of lesions or ulcerations that are often slow to heal.**
- Discourage sitting or standing for extended periods of time, wearing constrictive clothing, or crossing legs when seated, **which restricts circulation and leads to venous stasis and edema.**
- Provide education about relationship between smoking and peripheral vascular circulation, as indicated. **Smoking contributes to development and progression of peripheral vascular disease, and is associated with higher rate of amputation in presence of Buerger's disease.**
- Educate client/SO in reportable symptoms, including any changes in pain level, difficulty walking, nonhealing wounds **to provide opportunity for timely evaluation and intervention.**
- Stress need for regular medical and laboratory follow-up **to evaluate disease progression and response to therapies.**
- Review medication regimen and possible harmful side effects with client/SO. **Client may be on various drugs (e.g., antiplatelet agents, blood viscosity-reducing agents, vasodilators, anticoagulants, or cholesterol-lowering agents) for treatment of the particular vascular disorder. Many of these medications have harmful side effects and require client teaching and ongoing medical monitoring.**
- Emphasize importance of avoiding use of aspirin, some over-the-counter drugs and supplements, or alcohol when taking anticoagulants.
- Refer to community resources such as smoking cessation assistance, weight control program, and exercise group **to provide support for lifestyle changes.**

Information that appears in brackets has been added by the authors to clarify and enhance the use of nursing diagnoses.

🌐 Cultural   ⊕ Collaborative   🏠 Community/Home Care

Documentation Focus

Assessment/Reassessment
- Individual findings, noting nature, extent, and duration of problem, effect on independence and lifestyle.
- Characteristics of pain, precipitators, and what relieves pain.
- Pulse and blood pressure, including above and below suspected lesion as appropriate.

Planning
- Plan of care and who is involved in planning.
- Teaching plan.

Implementation/Evaluation
- Response to interventions, teaching, and actions performed.
- Attainment or progress toward desired outcome(s).
- Modifications to plan of care.

Discharge Planning
- Long-term needs and who is responsible for actions to be taken.
- Available resources, specific referrals made.

Sample Nursing Outcomes & Interventions Classifications (NOC/NIC)

NOC—Tissue Perfusion: Peripheral
NIC—Circulatory Care: Arterial [or] Venous Insufficiency

---

risk for decreased cardiac Tissue Perfusion

Taxonomy II: Activity/Rest—Class 4 Cardiovascular/Pulmonary Responses (00200)
[Diagnostic Division: Circulation]
Submitted 2008

Definition: At risk for decrease in cardiac (coronary) circulation that may compromise health

Risk Factors

Coronary artery spasm; cardiac surgery; cardiac tamponade
Deficient knowledge of modifiable risk factors (e.g., smoking, sedentary lifestyle, obesity); hypertension; hyperlipidemia

---

Information that appears in brackets has been added by the authors to clarify and enhance the use of nursing diagnoses.

Birth control pills
Substance abuse
Diabetes mellitus
Elevated C-reactive protein; hypovolemia, hypoxemia; hypoxia
Family history of coronary artery disease

> **NOTE:** A risk diagnosis is not evidenced by signs and symptoms, as the problem has not occurred; rather, nursing interventions are directed at prevention.

Desired Outcomes/Evaluation Criteria— Client Will:

- Demonstrate adequate coronary perfusion as individually appropriate (e.g., vital signs within client's normal range, free of chest pain or discomfort).
- Identify individual risk factors.
- Verbalize understanding of treatment regimen.
- Demonstrate behaviors and lifestyle changes to maintain or maximize circulation (e.g., cessation of smoking, relaxation techniques, exercise/dietary program).

Actions/Interventions

Nursing Priority No. 1.
To identify individual risk factors:

- Note presence of conditions such as congestive heart failure, major trauma with blood loss, recent cardiac surgery or use of ventricular assist device, chronic anemia, sepsis, **which can affect systemic circulation, tissue oxygenation, and organ function.**
- Note client's age and gender when assessing risk for coronary artery spasm or myocardial infarction. **Risk for heart disorders increases with age. Although men are still considered at higher risk for myocardial infarctions and experience them earlier in life, the rate of mortality among women with coronary artery disease is rising.**
- Identify lifestyle issues such as obesity, smoking, high cholesterol, excessive alcohol intake, use of drugs such as cocaine, and physical inactivity, **which can raise client's risk for coronary artery disease and impaired cardiac tissue perfusion.**
- Determine presence of breathing problems, such as obstructive sleep apnea with oxygen desaturation, **which can pro-**

Information that appears in brackets has been added by the authors to clarify and enhance the use of nursing diagnoses.

duce alveolar hypoventilation, respiratory acidosis and hypoxia, resulting in cardiac dysrhythmias and cardiac dysfunction.

* Determine if client is experiencing usual degree or prolonged stress or may have underlying psychiatric disorder (e.g., anxiety or panic).

* Review client's medications to note current use of vasoactive drugs such as amodirone, dopamine, dobutamine, esmolol, lidocaine, nitroglycerin, vasopressin [not a complete listing] that can exert undesirable side effects, increasing myocardial workload and oxygen consumption.

* Review diagnostic studies (e.g., electrocardiogram, exercise tolerance tests, myocardial perfusion scan; echocardiogram, bubble echocardiogram; angiography, Doppler ultrasound, chest radiography; oxygen saturation, capnometry, or arterial blood gases; electrolytes, lipid profile; blood urea nitrogen/creatinine, cardiac enzymes) to identify conditions requiring treatment and/or response to therapies.

Nursing Priority No. 2.
To determine changes in cardiac status:

* Investigate reports of chest pain, noting changes in characteristics of pain to evaluate for potential myocardial ischemia or inadequate systemic oxygenation or perfusion of organs.

* Monitor vital signs, especially noting blood pressure changes, including hypertension or hypotension, reflecting systemic vascular resistance problems that alter oxygen consumption and cardiac perfusion.

* Assess heart sounds and pulses for dysrhythmias. Can be caused by inadequate myocardial or systemic tissue perfusion, electrolyte or acid-base imbalances.

* Assess for restlessness, fatigue, changes in level of consciousness, increased capillary refill time, diminished peripheral pulses, and pale, cool skin. Signs and symptoms of inadequate systemic perfusion, which reflects cardiac function.

* Inspect for pallor, mottling, cool or clammy skin, and diminished pulses indicative of systemic vasoconstriction resulting from reduced cardiac output.

* Investigate reports of difficulty breathing or respiratory rate outside acceptable parameters, which can be indicative of oxygen exchange problems.

Information that appears in brackets has been added by the authors to clarify and enhance the use of nursing diagnoses.

Nursing Priority No. 3.
To maintain/maximize cardiac perfusion:

- Collaborate in treatment of underlying conditions such as hypovolemia, chronic obstructive pulmonary disease, diabetes, chronic atrial fibrillation **to correct or treat disorders that could influence cardiac perfusion or organ function.**
- Provide supplemental oxygen as indicated **to improve or maintain cardiac and systemic tissue perfusion.**
- Administer fluids and electrolytes as indicated **to maintain systemic circulation and optimal cardiac function.**
- Administer medications (e.g., antihypertensive agents, analgesics, antidysrhythmics, bronchodilators, fibrinolytic agents) **to treat underlying conditions, prevent thromboembolic phenomena, and maintain cardiac tissue perfusion and organ function.**
- Provide periods of undisturbed rest and calming environment **to reduce myocardial workload.**

Nursing Priority No. 4.
To promote wellness (Teaching/Discharge Considerations):

- Discuss cumulative effects of risk factors (e.g., family history, obesity, age, smoking, hypertension, diabetes, clotting disorders) and potential outcomes of atherosclerosis (e.g., systemic and cardiac disease conditions).
- Review modifiable risk factors **to assist client/SO in understanding those areas in which he or she can take action or make healthy-heart choices:**

  Recommend maintenance of normal weight, or weight loss if client is obese. Review specific dietary concerns with client (e.g., reducing animal and dairy fats; increasing plant foods—fruits, vegetables, olive oil, nuts).

  Encourage smoking cessation, when indicated, offering information about smoking-cessation aids and programs.

  Encourage client to engage in regular exercise.

  Discuss cardiac effects of drug use, where indicated (including cocaine, methamphetamines, alcohol).

  Discuss coping and stress tolerance.

  Demonstrate and encourage use of relaxation and stress management techniques.

  Encourage client in high-risk categories (e.g., strong family history, diabetic, prior history of cardiac event) to have regular medical examinations.

Information that appears in brackets has been added by the authors to clarify and enhance the use of nursing diagnoses.

Cultural   Collaborative   Community/Home Care

- Review medications on regular basis **to manage those that affect cardiac function or those given to prevent blood pressure or thromboembolic problems.**
- Refer to educational/community resources, as indicated. **Client/SO may benefit from support to engage in healthier heart activities (e.g., weight loss, smoking cessation, exercise).**
- Instruct in blood pressure monitoring at home, if indicated; advise purchase of home monitoring equipment. **Facilitates management of hypertension, a major risk factor for damage to blood vessels, which contributes to coronary artery disease.**

Documentation Focus

Assessment/Reassessment
- Individual findings, noting specific risk factors.
- Vital signs, cardiac rhythm, presence of dysrhythmias.

Planning
- Plan of care and who is involved in planning.
- Teaching plan.

Implementation/Evaluation
- Response to interventions, teaching, and actions performed.
- Attainment or progress toward desired outcome(s).
- Modifications to plan of care.

Discharge Planning
- Long-term needs and who is responsible for actions to be taken.
- Available resources, specific referrals made.

Sample Nursing Outcomes & Interventions Classifications (NOC/NIC)

NOC—Tissue Perfusion: Cardiac
NIC—Cardiac Precautions

Information that appears in brackets has been added by the authors to clarify and enhance the use of nursing diagnoses.

risk for ineffective cerebral Tissue Perfusion

Taxonomy II: Activity/Rest—Class 4 Cardiovascular/
  Pulmonary Responses (00201)
[Diagnostic Division: Circulation]
Submitted 2008

Definition: At risk for a decrease in cerebral tissue circulation that may compromise health

Risk Factors:

Head trauma; cerebral aneurysm; brain tumor; neoplasm of the
  brain
Carotid stenosis; aortic atherosclerosis; arterial dissection
Atrial fibrillation; sick sinus syndrome; atrial myxoma
Recent myocardial infarction; akinetic left ventricular segment;
  dilated cardiomyopathy; mitral stenosis; mechanical prosthetic valve; infective endocarditis; embolism
Coagulopathy (e.g., sickle cell anemia); disseminated intravascular coagulation; abnormal partial thromboplastin time; abnormal prothrombin time
Hypertension; hypercholesterolemia
Substance abuse
Treatment-related side effects (cardiopulmonary bypass, pharmaceutical agents); thrombolytic therapy

NOTE: A risk diagnosis is not evidenced by signs and symptoms, as the problem has not occurred; rather, nursing interventions are directed at prevention.

Desired Outcomes/Evaluation Criteria— Client Will: (Include Specific Time Frames)

- Display neurological signs within client's normal range.
- Verbalize understanding of condition, therapy regimen, side effects of medications, and when to contact healthcare provider.
- Demonstrate behaviors and lifestyle changes to improve circulation (e.g., cessation of smoking, relaxation techniques, exercise and dietary program).

Information that appears in brackets has been added by the authors to clarify
and enhance the use of nursing diagnoses.

Actions/Interventions

Nursing Priority No. 1.

To assess causative/contributing factors:

* Determine history of conditions associated with thrombus or emboli such as stroke, complicated pregnancy, sickle cell disease, fractures (especially long bones and pelvis) **to identify client at higher risk for decreased cerebral perfusion related to bleeding and/or coagulation problems.**
* Note current situation or presence of conditions (e.g., congestive heart failure, major trauma, sepsis, hypertension) **that can affect multiple body systems and systemic circulation/ perfusion.**
* Ascertain potential for presence of acute neurological conditions, such as traumatic brain injuries, tumors, hemorrhage, anoxic brain injury associated with cardiac arrest, and toxic or viral encephalopathies. **These conditions alter the relationship between intracranial volume and pressure, potentially increasing intracranial pressure and decreasing cerebral perfusion.**
* Investigate client reports of headache, particularly when accompanied by a range of progressive neurological deficits. **May accompany cerebral perfusion deficits associated with conditions such as stroke, transient ischemic attack, brain trauma, or cerebral arteriovenous malformations.**
* Ascertain if client has history of cardiac problems (e.g., recent myocardial infarction, heart failure, heart valve dysfunction or replacement, chronic atrial fibrillation).
* Determine presence of cardiac dysrhythmias. **Can be caused by inadequate myocardial perfusion, electrolyte imbalances, or be associated with brain injury (e.g., bradycardia can accompany traumatic injury; stroke can be precipitated by dysrhythmias).**
* Assess level of consciousness, mental status, speech, and behavior. **Clinical symptoms of decreased cerebral perfusion include fluctuations in consciousness and cognitive function.**
* Evaluate blood pressure. **Chronic or severe acute hypertension can precipitate cerebrovascular spasm and stroke. Low blood pressure or severe hypotension causes inadequate perfusion of brain.**
* Verify proper use of antihypertensive medications. **Individuals may stop medication because of lack of symptoms,**

Information that appears in brackets has been added by the authors to clarify and enhance the use of nursing diagnoses.

presence of undesired side effects, and/or cost of drug, potentiating risk of stroke.

- Review medication regimen noting use of anticoagulants/antiplatelet agents/other drugs **that could cause intracranial bleeding.**
- Review pulse oximetry or arterial blood gases. **Hypoxia is associated with reduced cerebral perfusion.**
- Review laboratory studies **to identify disorders that increase risk of clotting or bleeding or conditions contributing to decreased cerebral perfusion.**
- Review results of diagnostic studies (e.g., ultrasound or other imaging scans such as echocardiography, computed tomography, or magnetic resonance angiography; diffusion and perfusion magnetic resonance imaging) **to determine location and severity of disorder that can cause or exacerbate cerebral perfusion problem.**

Nursing Priority No. 2.

To maximize tissue perfusion:

- Collaborate in treatment of underlying conditions as indicated.
- Restore or maintain fluid balance **to maximize cardiac output and prevent decreased cerebral perfusion associated with hypovolemia.**
- Manage cardiac dysrhythmias via medication administration, pacemaker insertion.
- Restrict fluids, administer diuretics, as indicated, **to prevent decreased cerebral perfusion associated with fluid imbalance, hypertension, and cerebral edema.**
- Maintain head of bed placement (e.g., 0, 15, 30 degrees) as indicated, **to promote optimal cerebral perfusion.**
- Administer vasoactive medications, as indicated, **to increase cardiac output and/or adequate arterial blood pressure to maintain cerebral perfusion.**
- Administer other medications, as indicated (**e.g., steroids may decrease edema, antihypertensives may manage high blood pressure, anticoagulants may prevent cerebral embolus).**
- Prepare client for surgery, as indicated (e.g., carotid endarterectomy, evacuation of hematoma or space-occupying lesion), **to improve cerebral perfusion.**
- Refer to NDs decreased Cardiac Output; decreased Intracranial Adaptive Capacity, for additional interventions.

Information that appears in brackets has been added by the authors to clarify and enhance the use of nursing diagnoses.

Nursing Priority No. 3.

To promote wellness (Teaching/Discharge Considerations):

- Review modifiable risk factors, including hypertension, smoking, diet, physical activity, excessive alcohol intake, illicit drug use, as indicated. **Information can help client make informed choices about remedial risk factors and commit to lifestyle changes, as appropriate.**
- Discuss impact of unmodifiable risk factors such as family history, age, race. **Understanding effects and interrelationship of all risk factors may encourage client to address what can be changed to improve general well-being and reduce individual risk.**
- Assist client to incorporate disease management into activities of daily living. **Promotes independence; enhances self-concept regarding ability to deal with change and manage own needs.**
- Stress necessity of routine follow-up and laboratory monitoring, as indicated, **for effective disease management and possible changes in therapeutic regimen.**
- Refer to educational and community resources, as indicated. **Client/SO may benefit from instruction and support provided by agencies to engage in healthy activities (e.g., weight loss, smoking cessation, exercise).**

Documentation Focus

Assessment/Reassessment

- Individual findings, noting specific risk factors.
- Vital signs, blood pressure, cardiac rhythm.
- Medication regimen.
- Diagnostic studies, laboratory results.

Planning

- Plan of care and who is involved in planning.
- Teaching plan.

Implementation/Evaluation

- Response to interventions, teaching, and actions performed.
- Attainment or progress toward desired outcome(s).
- Modifications to plan of care.

Discharge Planning

- Long-term needs and who is responsible for actions to be taken.
- Available resources, specific referrals made.

Information that appears in brackets has been added by the authors to clarify and enhance the use of nursing diagnoses.

Sample Nursing Outcomes & Interventions Classifications (NOC/NIC)

NOC—Tissue Perfusion: Cerebral
NIC—Cerebral Perfusion Promotion

risk for ineffective peripheral Tissue Perfusion

Taxonomy II: Activity/Rest—Class 4 Cardiovascular/
  Pulmonary Responses
[Diagnostic Division: Circulation]
Submitted 2010

Definition: At risk for a decrease in blood circulation to the periphery that may compromise health

Risk Factors

Age over 60 years; sedentary lifestyle; smoking
Diabetes; hypertension
Endovascular procedures
Deficient knowledge of disease processes (e.g., diabetes, hyperlipidemia)
Deficient knowledge of aggravating factors (e.g., smoking, sedentary lifestyle, trauma, obesity, salt intake, immobility)

NOTE: A risk diagnosis is not evidenced by signs and symptoms, as the problem has not occurred; rather, nursing interventions are directed at prevention.

Desired Outcomes/Evaluation Criteria—Client Will:

• Demonstrate adequate perfusion as individually appropriate (e.g., peripheral pulses present and strong, absence of edema, free of pain or discomfort).
• Verbalize understanding of risk factors and when to contact healthcare provider.
• Demonstrate behaviors or lifestyle changes to improve circulation (e.g., engage in regular exercise, cessation of smoking, weight reduction, disease management).

Information that appears in brackets has been added by the authors to clarify and enhance the use of nursing diagnoses.

🌐 Cultural   🔁 Collaborative   🏠 Community/Home Care

Actions/Interventions

Nursing Priority No. 1.

To identify causative/precipitating factors related to risk:

- Note current situation or presence of conditions that can affect perfusion to all body systems (e.g., client admitted for endovascular procedure such as angiography or placement of stent, history or presence of congestive heart failure, lung disorders, major trauma, septic or hypovolemic shock, coagulopathies, sickle cell anemia) **affecting systemic circulation.**
- Determine history of conditions associated with thrombus or emboli (e.g., problems with coronary or cerebral circulation, stroke; high-velocity trauma with fractures, abdominal or orthopedic surgery, long periods of immobility; inflammatory diseases; chronic lung disease; diabetes with coexisting peripheral vascular disease; estrogen therapy; cancer and cancer therapies; presence of central venous catheters) **to identify client at higher risk for venous stasis, vessel wall injury, and hypercoagulability.**
- Identify presence of high-risk factors or conditions (e.g., smoking, uncontrolled hypertension, obesity, pregnancy, pelvic tumor, paralysis, hypercholesterolemia, varicose veins, arthritis, sepsis). **Places client at greater risk for developing peripheral vascular disease (PVD) with associated complications.**

Nursing Priority No. 2.

To assess for and reduce risk of perfusion complications:

- Evaluate reports of extremity pain promptly, noting any associated symptoms (e.g., cramping or heaviness, discomfort with walking, progressive temperature or color changes, paresthesia) **to help isolate and differentiate problems.**
- Note presence and location of restrictive pressure dressings, circular wraps, cast or traction device **that may impede circulation to limb.**
- Assess skin color and temperature in all extremities **for changes that might indicate circulation problem.**
- Compare skin temperature and color with other limb **if developing problem is suspected.**
- Palpate arterial pulses—bilateral radial, femoral, popliteal, dorsalis pedis, and post-tibial—comparing equality as well

---

Information that appears in brackets has been added by the authors to clarify and enhance the use of nursing diagnoses.

as intensity (i.e., bounding, normal, diminished, or absent). **Helps determine distribution and quality of blood flow.**
- Inspect lower extremities for skin texture (e.g., atrophic; shiny appearance; lack of hair; dry, scaly, reddened skin) and skin breaks or ulcerations **that often accompany diminished peripheral circulation.**
- Note client's nutritional and fluid status. **Malnutrition and weight loss make ischemic tissues more prone to breakdown. Dehydration reduces blood volume and compromises peripheral circulation.**
- Review laboratory studies such as lipid profile, coagulation studies, hemoglobin/hematocrit, renal/cardiac function tests, inflammatory markers (e.g., D dimer, C-reactive protein) **to determine potential for circulatory impairment.**

Nursing Priority No. 3.
To maximize tissue perfusion:
- Collaborate in treatment of underlying conditions, such as diabetes, hypertension, cardiopulmonary conditions, blood disorders, traumatic injury, hypovolemia, hypoxemia **to maximize systemic circulation and organ perfusion.**
- Administer fluids, electrolytes, nutrients, and oxygen, as indicated, **to promote optimal blood flow, organ and peripheral tissue perfusion and function.**
- Provide interventions to promote peripheral circulation and limit complications:

Encourage early ambulation when possible.

Recommend or provide foot and ankle exercises when client unable to ambulate freely.

Provide pressure-relieving/reducing devices for immobilized client (e.g., air mattress, gel or foam padding, bed or foot cradle).

Apply intermittent compression devices or graduated compression stockings to lower extremities **to reduce risk of deep vein thrombosis or tissue ulceration in client who is limited in activity or otherwise at risk.**

Assist with or cue client to change position at timed intervals rather than using presence of pain as signal to change positions **if sensation is/could be impaired.**

Elevate the legs when sitting, but avoid sharp angulation of the hips or knees **to minimize edema formation.**

Discuss/monitor use of heat or cold, such as hot water bottle, heating pad, or ice pack. **Reduces risk of dermal injury.**

Information that appears in brackets has been added by the authors to clarify and enhance the use of nursing diagnoses.

🌐 Cultural   ⚙ Collaborative   🏠 Community/Home Care

- Refer to dietitian or nutritionist to discuss dietary needs (e.g., well-balanced, low-saturated-fat, low-cholesterol diet) or other modifications, as indicated, **to promote weight loss and/or lower cholesterol levels to improve tissue perfusion.**
- Refer to NDs ineffective peripheral Tissue Perfusion; risk for Peripheral Neurovascular Dysfunction; risk for impaired Skin Integrity; impaired Tissue Integrity; [disturbed Sensory Perception], for additional interventions as appropriate.

Nursing Priority No. 4.

To promote wellness (Teaching/Discharge Criteria):

- Discuss relevant risk factors (e.g., family history, obesity, age, smoking, hypertension, diabetes, clotting disorders) and potential outcomes of atherosclerosis (e.g., systemic and peripheral vascular disease conditions). **Information necessary for client to make informed choices about risk factors and commit to lifestyle changes as appropriate.**
- Identify necessary changes in lifestyle and assist client to incorporate disease management into activities of daily living. **Promotes independence, enhances self-concept regarding ability to deal with change and manage own needs.**
- Emphasize need for regular exercise program **to enhance circulation and promote general well-being.**
- Discourage sitting or standing for long periods, wearing constrictive clothing, crossing legs.
- Provide education about relationship between smoking and peripheral vascular circulation, as indicated. **Smoking contributes to development and progression of peripheral vascular disease.**
- Educate client/SO in reportable symptoms, including any changes in pain level, difficulty walking, nonhealing wounds.
- Refer to community resources such as smoking cessation assistance, weight control program, diabetes educator, exercise group **to provide support for lifestyle changes.**

Documentation Focus

Assessment/Reassessment
- Individual risk factors identified.
- Client concerns or difficulty making and following through with plan.

Planning
- Plan of care and who is involved in planning.
- Teaching plan.

Information that appears in brackets has been added by the authors to clarify and enhance the use of nursing diagnoses.

Implementation/Evaluation
• Response to interventions, teaching, and actions performed.
• Attainment or progress toward outcomes.

Discharge Planning
• Referrals to other resources.
• Long-term need and who is responsible for actions.

Sample Nursing Outcomes & Interventions Classifications (NOC/NIC)

NOC—Tissue Perfusion: Peripheral
NIC—Circulatory Care: Arterial Insufficiency

---

impaired Transfer Ability

Taxonomy II: Activity/Rest—Class 2 Activity/Exercise (00090)
[Diagnostic Division: Activity/Rest]
Submitted 1998; Revised 2006

Definition: Limitation of independent movement between two nearby surfaces

---

Related Factors

Insufficient muscle strength; deconditioning; neuromuscular impairment; musculoskeletal impairment (e.g., contractures)
Impaired balance
Pain
Obesity
Impaired vision
Deficient knowledge; cognitive impairment
Environmental constraints (e.g., bed height, inadequate space, wheelchair type, treatment equipment, restraints)

Defining Characteristics

Subjective or Objective
Inability to transfer from bed to chair or chair to bed; from chair to car or car to chair; from chair to floor or floor to chair; on or off a toilet or commode; in or out of bath tub or shower; from bed to standing or standing to bed; from chair to standing or standing to chair; from standing to floor or floor to standing; between uneven levels

---

Information that appears in brackets has been added by the authors to clarify and enhance the use of nursing diagnoses.

🌐 Cultural 🕸 Collaborative 🏠 Community/Home Care

Note: Specify level of independence using a standardized functional scale. (Refer to ND impaired physical Mobility, for suggested functional level classification.)

Desired Outcomes/Evaluation Criteria— Client/Caregiver Will:

- Verbalize understanding of situation and appropriate safety measures.
- Master techniques of transfer successfully.
- Make desired transfers safely.

Actions/Interventions

Nursing Priority No. 1.

To assess causative/contributing factors:

- Determine presence of conditions that contribute to transfer problems. **Neuromuscular and musculoskeletal problems (such as multiple sclerosis, fractures with splints or casts, back injuries, knee/hip replacement surgery, amputation, quadriplegia or paraplegia, contractures or spastic muscles); agedness (diminished faculties, multiple medications, painful conditions, decreased balance, muscle mass, tone, or strength), and effects of dementias, brain injury, and so forth, can seriously impact balance and physical and psychological well-being.**
- Evaluate perceptual and cognitive impairments and ability to follow directions. **Plan of care and choice of interventions is dependent upon nature of condition—acute, chronic, or progressive.**
- Review medication regimen and schedule to determine possible side effects or drug interactions impairing balance and/or muscle tone.

Nursing Priority No. 2.

To assess functional ability:

- Evaluate degree of impairment using functional level classification scale of 0 to 4. **Identifies strengths and deficits (e.g., ability to ambulate with assistive devices or problems with balance, failure to attend to one side, inability to bear weight [client is nonweight-bearing or partial weight-bearing] and may provide information regarding potential for recovery.**

Information that appears in brackets has been added by the authors to clarify and enhance the use of nursing diagnoses.

- Determine presence and degree of perceptual or cognitive impairment and ability to follow directions.
- Note emotional or behavioral responses of client/SO(s) to problems of immobility.

Nursing Priority No. 3.
To promote optimal level of movement:

- Assist with treatment of underlying condition causing dysfunction.
- Consult with physical therapist, occupational therapist, or rehabilitation team **to develop general and specific muscle strengthening and range-of-motion exercises, transfer training and techniques, as well as recommendations and provision of balance, gait, and mobility aids or adjunctive devices.**
- Use appropriate number of people to assist with transfers and correct equipment (e.g., mechanical lift/sling, gait belt, sitting or standing disk pivot) **to safely transfer the client in a particular situation (e.g., chair to bed, chair to car, in or out of shower or tub).**
- Demonstrate and assist with use of side rails, overhead trapeze, transfer boards, transfer or sit-to-stand hoist, specialty slings, safety grab bars, cane, walker, wheelchair, crutches, as indicated, **to protect client and care providers from injury during transfers and movements.**
- Position devices (e.g., call light, bed-positioning switch) within easy reach on the bed or chair. **Facilitates transfer and allows client to obtain assistance for transfer, as needed.**
- Provide instruction or reinforce information for client and caregivers regarding positioning **to improve or maintain balance when transferring.**
- Monitor body alignment, posture, and balance and encourage wide base of support when standing to transfer.
- Use full-length mirror, as needed, **to facilitate client's view of own postural alignment.**
- Demonstrate and reinforce safety measures, as indicated, such as transfer board, gait belt, supportive footwear, good lighting, clearing floor of clutter **to avoid possibility of fall and subsequent injury.**

Nursing Priority No. 4.
To promote wellness (Teaching/Discharge Considerations):

- Assist client/caregivers to learn safety measures as individually indicated. **Actions (e.g., using correct body mechanics**

Information that appears in brackets has been added by the authors to clarify and enhance the use of nursing diagnoses.

🌐 Cultural 🤝 Collaborative 🏠 Community/Home Care

for particular transfer, locking wheelchair before transfer, using properly placed and functioning hoists, ascertaining that floor surface is even and clutter free) are important in facilitating transfers and reducing risk of falls or injury to client and caregiver.

- Refer to appropriate community resources for evaluation and modification of environment (e.g., shower or tub, uneven floor surfaces, steps, use of ramps, standing tables or lifts).
- Refer also to NDs impaired bed/physical/wheelchair Mobility; Unilateral Neglect; risk for Falls; impaired Walking, for additional interventions.

Documentation Focus

Assessment/Reassessment
- Individual findings, including level of function and ability to participate in desired transfers.
- Mobility aids or transfer devices used.

Planning
- Plan of care and who is involved in the planning.
- Teaching plan.

Implementation/Evaluation
- Responses to interventions, teaching, and actions performed.
- Attainment or progress toward desired outcome(s).
- Modifications to plan of care.

Discharge Planning
- Discharge and long-term needs, noting who is responsible for each action to be taken.
- Specific referrals made.
- Sources for and maintenance of assistive devices.

Sample Nursing Outcomes & Interventions Classifications (NOC/NIC)

NOC—Transfer Performance
NIC—Self-Care Assistance: Transfer

Information that appears in brackets has been added by the authors to clarify and enhance the use of nursing diagnoses.

risk for **Trauma**

Taxonomy II: Safety/Protection—Class 2 Physical Injury
(00038)
[Diagnostic Division: Safety]
Submitted 1980

Definition: At risk of accidental tissue injury (e.g.,
wound, burn, fracture)

Risk Factors

Internal

Balancing difficulties; weakness; reduced muscle or hand-eye
coordination

Cognitive or emotional difficulties

Deficient knowledge regarding safe procedures or safety precautions

Economically disadvantaged

History of previous trauma

Poor vision; reduced sensation

External [includes but is not limited to]

Bathing in very hot water (e.g., unsupervised bathing of young
children); pot handles facing toward front of stove

Children playing with dangerous objects; playing with explosives; knives stored uncovered; accessibility of guns

Children riding in the front seat of car; nonuse or misuse of seat
restraints; misuse of necessary headgear (e.g., for bicycles,
motorcycles, skateboarding, skiing)

Contact with rapidly moving machinery; exposure to dangerous
machinery

Contact with intense cold; lack of protection from heat source;
overexposure to radiation

Defective appliances; delayed lighting of gas appliances; potential igniting of gas leaks

Driving a mechanically unsafe vehicle; driving at excessive
speeds; driving without necessary visual aids; driving while
intoxicated

Entering unlighted rooms; obstructed passageways

Experimenting with chemicals; contact with corrosives; inadequately stored corrosives (e.g., lye)

Faulty electrical plugs; frayed wires; overloaded electrical outlets or fuse boxes

---

Information that appears in brackets has been added by the authors to clarify
and enhance the use of nursing diagnoses.

Flammable children's clothing or toys; wearing flowing clothes around open flames

Smoking in bed or near oxygen; inadequately stored combustibles (e.g., matches, oily rags); grease waste collected on stoves

High beds; inappropriate call-for-aid mechanisms for bed-bound client

High-crime neighborhood

Inadequate stair rails; lack of gate at top of stairs; unsafe window protection in homes with young children

Lacks antislip material in bath or shower; slippery floors (e.g., wet or highly waxed); throw rugs; unanchored electric wires

Large icicles hanging from the roof

Physical proximity to vehicle pathways (e.g., driveways, lanes, railroad tracks); unsafe road or walkways

Struggling with restraints

Use of cracked dishware

Use of unsteady ladder or chairs

> **NOTE:** A risk diagnosis is not evidenced by signs and symptoms, as the problem has not occurred; rather, nursing interventions are directed at prevention.

Desired Outcomes/Evaluation Criteria—Client/Caregiver Will:

- Identify and correct potential risk factors in the environment.
- Demonstrate appropriate lifestyle changes to reduce risk of injury.
- Identify resources to assist in promoting a safe environment.
- Recognize need for and seek assistance to prevent accidents or injuries.

Actions/Interventions

This ND is a compilation of a number of situations that can result in injury. Refer to specific NDs—risk for imbalanced Body Temperature; risk for Contamination; impaired Environmental Interpretation Syndrome; risk for Falls; impaired Home Maintenance; Hyperthermia; Hypothermia; risk for Injury; impaired physical Mobility; risk for impaired Parenting; risk for Poisoning; [disturbed Sensory Perception]; impaired Skin Integrity; risk for Suffocation; risk for Thermal Injury;

Information that appears in brackets has been added by the authors to clarify and enhance the use of nursing diagnoses.

impaired Tissue Integrity; risk for self-/other-directed Violence; impaired Walking, as appropriate, for more specific interventions.

Nursing Priority No. 1.

To assess causative/contributing factors:

- Determine factors related to individual situation and extent of risk for trauma. **Influences scope and intensity of interventions to manage threat to safety.**
- ∞• Note client's age, gender and developmental stage, decision-making ability, and level of cognition and competence. **Affects client's ability to protect self and/or others, and influences choice of interventions and teaching.**
- Ascertain knowledge of safety needs and injury prevention, and motivation to prevent injury in home, community, and work setting. **Lack of appreciation of significance of individual hazards increases risk of traumatic injury.**
- Note socioeconomic status and availability and use of resources.
- Assess influence of client's lifestyle and stress **that can impair judgment and greatly increase client's potential for injury.**
- Assess mood, coping abilities, personality styles (i.e., temperament, aggression, impulsive behavior, level of self-esteem). **May result in careless or increased risk-taking without consideration of consequences.**
- Evaluate individual's emotional and behavioral response to violence in surroundings (e.g., neighborhood, television, peer group). **May affect client's view of and regard for own/others' safety.**
- 🏠• Review potential occupational risk factors (e.g., works with dangerous tools and machinery, electricity, explosives; police, fire, EMS officers; working with hazardous chemicals, various inhalants, or radiation).
- Review history of accidents, noting circumstances (e.g., time of day, activities coinciding with accident, who was present, type of injury sustained). **Can provide clues for client's risk for subsequent events and potential for enhanced safety by a change in the people or environment involved (e.g., client may need assistance when getting up at night, or increased playground supervision may be required).**
- Determine potential for abusive behavior by family members/SO(s)/peers.

Information that appears in brackets has been added by the authors to clarify and enhance the use of nursing diagnoses.

- Review diagnostic studies and laboratory tests for impairments or imbalances **that may result in or exacerbate conditions, such as confusion, tetany, and pathological fractures.**

Nursing Priority No. 2.

To enhance safety in healthcare environment:

∞ • Screen client for safety concerns (e.g., risk for falls, cognitive, developmental, vision/other sensory impairments upon admission and during stay in healthcare facility. Assess for and report changes in client's functional status. Perform thorough assessments regarding safety issues when planning for client discharge. **Failure to accurately assess and intervene or refer regarding these issues can place the client at needless risk and creates negligence issues for the healthcare practitioner.**

- Review client's therapeutic regimen on a continual basis when under direct care (e.g., vital signs, medications, treatment modalities, infusions, nutrition, physical environment) **to prevent healthcare-related complications.**

- Provide for routine safety needs:

    Provide adequate supervision and frequent observation.

    Place young children, confused client/person with dementia near nurses' station.

    Orient client to environment.

    Make arrangement for call system for bedridden client in home or hospital setting. Demonstrate use and place device within client's reach.

    Provide for appropriate communication tools (e.g., call light, writing implements and paper; alphabet/picture board).

    Encourage client's use of corrective vision and hearing aids.

    Keep bed in low position or place mattress on floor, as appropriate.

    Use and pad side rails, as indicated.

    Provide seizure precautions.

    Lock wheels on bed and movable furniture. Clear travel paths. Provide adequate area lighting.

    Assist with activities and transfers, as needed.

    Provide well-fitting, nonskid footwear.

    Demonstrate and monitor use of assistive devices, such as transfer devices, cane, walker, crutches, wheelchair, safety bars.

    Provide supervision while client is smoking.

Information that appears in brackets has been added by the authors to clarify and enhance the use of nursing diagnoses.

Provide for appropriate disposal of potentially injurious items (e.g., needles, scalpel blades).

⊗ Follow facility protocol and closely monitor use of restraints, when required (e.g., vest, limb, belt, mitten).

• Emphasize with client importance of obtaining assistance when weak or sedated and when problems of balance, coordination, or postural hypotension are present **to reduce risk of syncope and falls.**

• Demonstrate and encourage use of techniques to reduce or manage stress and vent emotions such as anger, hostility **to reduce risk of violence to self/others.**

⊗• Refer to physical or occupational therapist as appropriate **to identify high-risk tasks, conduct site visits, select, create, or modify equipment; and provide education about body mechanics and musculoskeletal injuries, as well as provide needed therapies.**

⊗• Assist with treatments for underlying medical, surgical, or psychiatric conditions **to improve cognition and thinking processes, musculoskeletal function, awareness of own safety needs, and general well-being.**

Nursing Priority No. 3.
🏠To enhance safety for client in community care setting:

• Provide information to caregivers regarding client's specific disease or condition(s) and associated risks.

• Identify interventions and safety devices to promote safe physical environment and individual safety:

Recommend wearing visual or hearing aids **to maximize sensory input.**

Ensure availability of communication devices (e.g., telephone, computer, alarm system or medical emergency alert device).

Install and maintain electrical and fire safety devices, extinguishers, and alarms.

Review oxygen safety rules.

Identify environmental needs (e.g., decals on glass doors; adequate lighting of stairways, handrails, ramps, bathtub safety tapes) **to reduce risk of falls,** lower temperature on hot water heater **to prevent accidental burns,** etc.

Obtain seat raisers for chairs; ergonomic beds or chairs.

Encourage participation in back safety classes, injury-prevention exercises, mobility or transfer device training.

Install childproof cabinets for medications and toxic household substances, use tamper-proof medication containers.

Information that appears in brackets has been added by the authors to clarify and enhance the use of nursing diagnoses.

Review proper storage and disposal of volatile liquids; installation of proper ventilation for use when mixing or using toxic substances; use of safety glasses or goggles.

Emphasize importance of appropriate use of car restraints, bicycle, motorcycle, skating, or skiing helmets.

Discuss swimming pool fencing and supervision; attending First Aid and cardiopulmonary resuscitation (CPR) classes. Obtain trigger locks or gun safes for firearms.

- Initiate appropriate teaching **when reckless behavior is occurring or likely to occur (e.g., smoking in bed, driving without safety belts, working with chemicals without safety goggles).**
- Refer to counseling or psychotherapy, as needed, especially when individual is "accident prone" or self-destructive behavior is noted. (Refer to NDs risk for other-/self-directed Violence.)

Nursing Priority No. 4.
To promote wellness (Teaching/Discharge Considerations):

- Discuss importance of self-monitoring of conditions or emotions that can contribute to occurrence of injury to self/others (e.g., fatigue, anger, irritability). **Client/SO may be able to modify risk through monitoring of actions or postponement of certain actions, especially during times when client is likely to be highly stressed.**
- Encourage use of warm-up and stretching exercises before engaging in athletic activity **to prevent muscle injuries.**
- Recommend use of seat belts; fitted helmets for cyclists, skate-/snowboarders, skiers; approved infant seat in appropriate position in vehicle; avoidance of hitchhiking; substance abuse programs **to promote transportation and recreation safety.**
- Refer to accident prevention programs (e.g., medication and drug safety, mobility or transfer device training, driving instruction, parenting classes, firearms safety, workplace ergonomics).
- Develop fire safety program (e.g., family fire drills; use of smoke detectors; yearly chimney cleaning; purchase of fire-retardant clothing, especially children's nightwear; safe use of in-home oxygen; fireworks safety).
- Problem-solve with client/parent to provide adequate child supervision after school, during working hours, on school holidays; or day program for frail or confused elder.

Information that appears in brackets has been added by the authors to clarify and enhance the use of nursing diagnoses.

- Explore behaviors related to use of firearms, alcohol, tobacco, and recreational drugs and other substances. **Provides opportunity to review consequences of previously determined risk factors (e.g., potential consequences of illegal activities, effects of smoking on health of family members as well as fire danger; potential for unintentional gunshot injuries, suicide, or homicide; potential for harm related to alcohol and other substances).**
- Identify community resources (e.g., financial, food assistance) **to assist with necessary corrections or improvements and purchases.**
- Recommend involvement in community self-help programs, such as Neighborhood Watch, Helping Hand.
- Promote educational opportunities **geared toward increasing awareness of safety measures (e.g., firearms safety) and resources available to the individual.**
- Seek out and involve businesses in volunteer outreach activities such as building safe playgrounds, community or street cleanup, home repair or improvement for frail elders, and so forth.
- Advocate for and promote solutions for problems of design of buildings, equipment, transportation, and workplace practices **that contribute to accidents.**

Documentation Focus

Assessment/Reassessment
- Individual risk factors, past and recent history of injuries, awareness of safety needs.
- Use of safety equipment or procedures.
- Environmental concerns, safety issues.

Planning
- Plan of care and who is involved in the planning.
- Teaching plan.

Implementation/Evaluation
- Responses to interventions, teaching, and actions performed.
- Attainment or progress toward desired outcome(s).
- Modifications to plan of care.

Discharge Planning
- Long-term needs and who is responsible for actions to be taken.
- Available resources, specific referrals made.

Information that appears in brackets has been added by the authors to clarify and enhance the use of nursing diagnoses.

🌐 Cultural ♨ Collaborative 🏠 Community/Home Care

Sample Nursing Outcomes & Interventions Classifications (NOC/NIC)

NOC—Physical Injury Severity
NIC—Environmental Management: Safety

Unilateral Neglect

Taxonomy II: Perception/Cognition—Class 1 Attention
(00123)
[Diagnostic Division: Neurosensory]
Submitted 1986; Revised 2006

Definition: Impairment in sensory and motor response, mental representation, and spatial attention to body and the corresponding environment, characterized by inattention to one side and overattention to the opposite side. Left-side neglect is more severe and persistent than right-side neglect

Related Factors

Brain injury from: cerebrovascular problems, neurological illness, trauma, tumor
Left hemiplegia from cerebrovascular accident (CVA) of the right hemisphere
Hemianopsia

Defining Characteristics

Subjective
[Reports feeling that part does not belong to own self]

Objective
Marked deviation of the eyes, head, or trunk to the nonneglected side to stimuli and activities on that side
Failure to move eyes, head, limbs, or trunk in the neglected hemisphere despite being aware of a stimulus in that space; failure to notice people approaching from the neglected side
Displacement of sounds to the nonneglected side
Appears unaware of positioning of neglected limb
Lack of safety precautions with regard to the neglected side
Failure to eat food from portion of the plate on the neglected side; failure to dress or groom neglected side

---

Information that appears in brackets has been added by the authors to clarify and enhance the use of nursing diagnoses.

Difficulty remembering details of internally represented familiar scenes that are on the neglected side

Use of only vertical half of page when writing; failure to cancel lines on the half of the page on the neglected side; substitution of letters to form alternative words that are similar to the original in length when reading

Distortion or omission of drawing on the half of the page on the neglected side

Perseveration of visual motor tasks on nonneglected side

Transfer of pain sensation to the nonneglected side

Desired Outcomes/Evaluation Criteria— Client/Caregiver Will:

- Acknowledge presence of sensory-perceptual impairment.
- Identify adaptive and protective measures for individual situation.
- Demonstrate behaviors, lifestyle changes necessary to promote physical safety.

Client Will:

- Verbalize positive realistic perception of self incorporating the current dysfunction.
- Perform self-care within level of ability.

Actions/Interventions

Nursing Priority No. 1.

To assess the extent of altered perception and the related degree of disability:

- Identify underlying reason for alterations in sensory, motor, or behavioral perceptions as noted in Related Factors. **The client with injury to either side of the brain may experience spatial neglect, but it more commonly occurs when brain injury affects the right cortical hemisphere, causing left hemiparesis.**
- Ascertain client's/SO's perception of problem/changes, noting differences in perceptions.
- Assess sensory awareness (e.g., response to stimulus of hot and cold, dull and sharp); note problems with awareness of motion and proprioception.
- Observe client's behavior (as noted in Defining Characteristics) **to determine the extent of impairment.**
- Assess ability to distinguish between right and left.

Information that appears in brackets has been added by the authors to clarify and enhance the use of nursing diagnoses.

🌐 Cultural ♻ Collaborative 🏠 Community/Home Care

- Note physical signs of neglect (e.g., inability to maintain normal posture; disregard for position of affected limb[s], bumping into objects or walls on the left when ambulating, skin irritation/damage on the left side, indicating lack of awareness of injury).
- Explore and encourage verbalization of feelings **to identify meaning of loss and dysfunction to the client and impact it may have on assuming activities of daily living (ADLs).** *Note:* **Expression of loss may be difficult for the client for a variety of reasons. For example, some emotional disturbances and personality changes are caused by the physical effects of brain damage.**
- Assist with/review results of early screening tests. **Tests (often performed at the bedside) may include (and are not limited to) observation to determine if client shows evidence of body neglect such as asymmetric shaving/grooming. Reading test might reveal that client begins reading in the middle of the page, etc.**
- Review results of testing (e.g., computed tomography or magnetic resonance imaging scanning, complete neuropsychological tests) **done to determine cause or type of neglect syndrome (e.g., sensory, motor, representational, personal, spatial, behavioral inattention). Aids in distinguishing neglect from visual field cuts, impaired attention, and planning or visuospatial abilities.**

Nursing Priority No. 2.

To promote optimal comfort and safety for the client in the environment:

- Engage in treatment strategies focused on training of attention to the neglected hemispace:

  Approach client from the unaffected side during acute phase.

  Explain to client that one side is being neglected; repeat as needed.

  Remove excess stimuli from the environment when working with the client **to reduce confusion and reactive stress.**

  Encourage client to turn head and eyes in full rotation and "scan" the environment **to compensate for visual field loss or when neglect therapies include scanning.**

  Position bedside table and objects (e.g., call bell/telephone, tissues) within functional field of vision **to facilitate care.** *Note:* **Therapies may include orienting the client's environment leftward in attempt to help client perceive the neglected space.**

Information that appears in brackets has been added by the authors to clarify and enhance the use of nursing diagnoses.

Position furniture and equipment so travel path is not obstructed. Keep doors wide open or completely closed.

Remove articles in the environment that may create a safety hazard (e.g., footstool, throw rug).

Orient to environment as often as needed and ensure adequate lighting in the environment **to improve client's interpretation of environmental stimuli.**

Monitor affected body part(s) for positioning and anatomical alignment, pressure points, skin irritation or injury, and dependent edema. **Increased risk of injury and ulcer formation necessitates close observation and timely intervention.**

When moving client, describe location of affected areas of body.

Protect affected body part(s) from pressure, injury, and burns, and help client learn to assume this responsibility.

Assist with ambulation or movement, using appropriate mobility and assistive devices **to promote safety of client and caregiver.**

Provide assistance with ADLs (e.g., feeding, bathing, dressing, grooming, toileting), **which helps client tend to affected side or compensate for client's deficits.**

Refer to ND [disturbed Sensory Perception] for additional interventions, as needed.

🍄• Collaborate with rehabilitation team in strategies (e.g., sensory stimulation techniques such as tapping or stroking, patching one half of each eye, auditory stimulation, wedge prism adaptation techniques, virtual reality technology) **to assist client to overcome or compensate for deficits.**

Nursing Priority No. 3.

🏠To promote wellness (Teaching/Discharge Considerations):

• Encourage client to look at and handle affected side **to stimulate awareness.**

• Bring the affected limb across the midline **for client to visualize during care.**

• Provide tactile stimuli to the affected side by touching/ manipulating, stroking, and communicating about the affected side by itself rather than stimulating both sides simultaneously.

• Provide objects of various weight, texture, and size for client to handle **to provide tactile stimulation.**

• Assist client to position the affected extremity carefully and teach to routinely visualize placement of the extremity. Re-

---

Information that appears in brackets has been added by the authors to clarify and enhance the use of nursing diagnoses.

mind with visual cues. If client completely ignores one side of the body, use positioning **to improve perception (e.g., position client facing/looking at the affected side).**

- Encourage client to accept affected limb or side as part of self even when it no longer feels like it belongs.
- Use a mirror to help client adjust position **by visualizing both sides of the body.**
- Use descriptive terms to identify body parts rather than "left" and "right"; for example, "Lift this leg" (point to leg) or "Lift your affected leg."
- Encourage client/SO/family members to discuss situation and impact on life/future. **May help verbalize the reality of changes and provides opportunity to explore solutions to problems and special needs.**
- Acknowledge and accept feelings of despondency, grief, and anger. **When feelings are openly expressed, client can deal with them and move forward.** (Refer to ND Grieving, as appropriate.)
- Reinforce to client the reality of the dysfunction and need to compensate.
- Avoid participating in the client's use of denial.
- Encourage family members and SO(s) to treat client normally and not as an invalid, including client in family activities.
- Place nonessential items (e.g., TV, pictures, hairbrush) on affected side during postacute phase once client begins to cross midline **to encourage continuation of behavior.**
- Refer to and encourage client to use rehabilitative services **to enhance independence in functioning.**
- Identify additional community resources to meet individual needs (e.g., Meals on Wheels, home-care services) **to maximize independence, allow client to return to community setting.**
- Provide informational material and Web sites **to reinforce teaching and promote self-paced learning.**

Documentation Focus

Assessment/Reassessment
- Individual findings, including extent of altered perception, degree of disability, effect on independence and participation in ADLs.
- Results of testing.

Planning
- Plan of care and who is involved in the planning.
- Teaching plan.

Information that appears in brackets has been added by the authors to clarify and enhance the use of nursing diagnoses.

Implementation/Evaluation
* Responses to intervention, teaching, and actions performed.
* Attainment or progress toward desired outcome(s).
* Modifications to plan of care.

Discharge Planning
* Long-term needs and who is responsible for actions to be taken.
* Available resources, specific referrals made.

Sample Nursing Outcomes & Interventions Classifications (NOC/NIC)

NOC—Heedfulness of Affected Side
NIC—Unilateral Neglect Management

impaired **Urinary Elimination**

Taxonomy II: Elimination and Exchange—Class 1 Urinary Function (00016)
[Diagnostic Division: Elimination]
Submitted 1973; Revised 2006

Definition: Dysfunction in urine elimination

Related Factors

Multiple causality; sensory motor impairment; anatomic obstruction; urinary tract infection (UTI); [mechanical trauma; fluid/volume states; psychogenetic factors; surgical diversion]

Defining Characteristics

Subjective
Frequency; urgency
Hesitancy
Dysuria
Nocturia; [enuresis]

Objective
Incontinence
Retention

Information that appears in brackets has been added by the authors to clarify and enhance the use of nursing diagnoses.

🌐 Cultural 🤝 Collaborative 🏠 Community/Home Care

Desired Outcomes/Evaluation Criteria— Client Will:

- Verbalize understanding of condition.
- Identify specific causative factors.
- Achieve normal elimination pattern or participate in measures to correct or compensate for defects.
- Demonstrate behaviors and techniques to prevent urinary infection.
- Manage care of urinary catheter, or stoma, and appliance following urinary diversion.

Actions/Interventions

Nursing Priority No. 1.

To assess causative/contributing factors:

- Identify conditions that may be present, such as urinary tract infection, interstitial cystitis or painful bladder syndrome; dehydration; surgery (including urinary diversion); neurological involvement (e.g., multiple sclerosis [MS], stroke, Parkinson's disease, paraplegia/tetraplegia); mental or emotional dysfunction (e.g., impaired cognition, delirium or confusion, depression, Alzheimer's disease); prostate disorders; recent or multiple pregnancies; pelvic trauma.
- Determine pathology of bladder dysfunction relative to medical diagnosis identified. **Identifies direction for further evaluation and treatment options to discover specifics of individual situation. For example, in such neurological or demyelinating diseases as MS, problem may be related to inability to store urine, empty the bladder, or both.**
- Assist with physical examination (e.g., cough test for incontinence, palpation for bladder retention or masses, prostate size, observation for urethral stricture).
- Note age and gender of client. **Incontinence and urinary tract infections are more prevalent in women and older adults; painful bladder syndrome (PBS) or interstitial cystitis (IC) is more common in women.**
- Investigate pain, noting location, duration, intensity; presence of bladder spasms; or back or flank pain **to assist in differentiating between bladder and kidney as cause of dysfunction.**
- Have client complete Pelvic Pain and Urgency/Frequency (PUF) patient symptom survey, as indicated. **Helps in evaluating the presence and severity of PBS/IC symptoms.**

Information that appears in brackets has been added by the authors to clarify and enhance the use of nursing diagnoses.

- Note reports of exacerbations and spontaneous remissions of symptoms of urgency and frequency, which may or may not be accompanied by pain, pressure, or spasm.
- Determine client's usual daily fluid intake (both amount and beverage choices, use of caffeine). Note condition of skin and mucous membranes, color of urine **to help determine level of hydration.**
- Review medication regimen **for drugs that can alter bladder or kidney function** (e.g., antihypertensive agents such as angiotensin-converting enzyme [ACE] inhibitors, beta-adrenergic blockers; anticholinergics, antihistamines; antiparkinsonian drugs; antidepressants or antipsychotics; sedatives, hypnotics, opioids; caffeine and alcohol).
- Send urine specimen (midstream clean-voided or catheterized) for culture and sensitivities in presence of signs of urinary tract infection—cloudy, foul odor; bloody urine.
- Rule out gonorrhea in men when urethritis with a penile discharge is present and there are no bacteria in the urine.
- Obtain specimen for antibody-coated bacteria assay **to diagnose bacterial infection of the kidney or prostate.**
- Assist with potassium sensitivity test (instillation of potassium solution into bladder), as appropriate. **Eighty percent of patients with PBS/IC will react positively with painful symptoms.**
- Review laboratory tests for hyperglycemia, hyperparathyroidism, or other metabolic conditions; changes in renal function; culture for presence of infection or sexually transmitted disease (STDs); urine cytology for cancer.
- Review results of diagnostic studies (e.g., uroflowmetry; cystometogram; postvoid residual ultrasound (bladder scan); pressure flow and leak point pressure measurement; videourodynamics; electromyography; kidney, ureter, and bladder [KUB] imaging) **to identify presence and type of elimination problem.**

Nursing Priority No. 2.
To assess degree of interference/disability:

- Ascertain client's previous pattern of elimination **for comparison with current situation.** Note reports of problems (e.g., frequency, urgency, painful urination; leaking or incontinence; changes in size and force of urinary stream; problems emptying bladder completely; nocturia or enuresis).
- Ascertain client's/SO's perception of problem and degree of disability (e.g., client is restricting social, employment, or

---

Information that appears in brackets has been added by the authors to clarify and enhance the use of nursing diagnoses.

🌐 Cultural 😊 Collaborative 🏠 Community/Home Care

travel activities; having sexual or relationship difficulties; incurring sleep deprivation; experiencing depression).

- Note influence of culture/ethnicity or gender on client's view of problems of incontinence. **Limited evidence exists to understand and help people cope with the physical and psychosocial consequences of this chronic, socially isolating, and potentially devastating disorder.**
- Have client keep a voiding diary for prescribed number of days to record fluid intake, voiding times, precise urine output, and dietary intake. **Helps determine baseline symptoms, severity of frequency or urgency, and whether diet is a factor (if symptoms worsen).**

Nursing Priority No. 3.

To assist in treating/preventing urinary alteration:

- Refer to specific NDs urinary Incontinence [specify]; Urinary Retention, for additional related interventions.
- Encourage fluid intake up to 3,000 mL/day (within cardiac tolerance), including cranberry juice, **to help maintain renal function, prevent infection and formation of urinary stones, avoid encrustation around catheter, or flush urinary diversion appliance.**
- Discuss possible dietary restrictions (e.g., especially coffee, alcohol, carbonated drinks, citrus, tomatoes, and chocolate) based on individual symptoms.
- Assist with developing toileting routines (e.g., timed voiding, bladder training, prompted voiding, habit retraining), as appropriate. **For adults who are cognitively intact and physically capable of self-toileting, bladder training, timed voiding, and habit retraining may be beneficial.**
- Encourage client to verbalize fears and concerns (e.g., disruption in sexual activity, inability to work). **Open expression allows client to deal with feelings and begin problem-solving.**
- Implement and monitor interventions for specific elimination problem (e.g., pelvic floor exercises or other bladder retraining modalities; medication regimen, including antimicrobials [single-dose is frequently being used for UTI], sulfonamides, antispasmodics); and evaluate client's response **to modify treatment, as needed.**
- Discuss possible surgical procedures and medical regimen, as indicated (e.g., client with benign prostatic hypertrophy bladder or prostatic cancer, PBS/IC). **For example, cystoscopy with bladder hydrodistention may be used for PBS/IC, or**

Information that appears in brackets has been added by the authors to clarify and enhance the use of nursing diagnoses.

an electrical stimulator may be implanted to treat chronic urinary urge incontinence, nonobstructive urinary retention, and symptoms of urgency and frequency.

Nursing Priority No. 4.

To assist in management of long-term urinary alterations:

- Keep bladder deflated by use of an indwelling catheter connected to closed drainage. Investigate alternatives when possible (e.g., intermittent catheterization, surgical interventions, urinary drugs, voiding maneuvers, condom catheter).
- Provide latex-free catheter and care supplies **to reduce risk of latex sensitivity.**
- Check frequently for bladder distention and observe for overflow **to reduce risk of infection and/or autonomic hyperreflexia.**
- Adhere to a regular bladder or diversion appliance emptying schedule **to avoid accidents.**
- Provide for routine diversion appliance care and assist client to recognize and deal with problems, such as alkaline salt encrustation, ill-fitting appliance, malodorous urine, and infection.

Nursing Priority No. 5.

To promote wellness (Teaching/Discharge Considerations):

- Emphasize importance of keeping area clean and dry **to reduce risk of infection and/or skin breakdown.**
- Instruct female clients with UTI to drink large amounts of fluid, void immediately after intercourse, wipe from front to back, promptly treat vaginal infections, and take showers rather than tub baths **to limit risk or avoid reinfection.**
- Recommend smoking cessation program, as appropriate. **Cigarette smoking can be a source of bladder irritation.**
- Encourage SO(s) who participate in routine care to recognize complications (including latex allergy) necessitating medical evaluation or intervention.
- Instruct in proper application and care of appliance for urinary diversion. Encourage liberal fluid intake, avoidance of foods or medications that produce strong odor, use of white vinegar or deodorizer in pouch **to promote odor control.**
- Identify sources for supplies, programs or agencies providing financial assistance. **Lack of access to necessities can be a barrier to management of incontinence, and having help to obtain needed equipment can assist with daily care.**

Information that appears in brackets has been added by the authors to clarify and enhance the use of nursing diagnoses.

- 🝆• Recommend avoidance of gas-forming foods in presence of ureterosigmoidostomy **as flatus can cause urinary incontinence.**
- 🝆• Recommend use of silicone catheter. **Although these catheters are more expensive than rubber catheters, they are more comfortable and generally cause fewer problems with infection when permanent or long-term catheterization is required.**
- 🝆• Demonstrate proper positioning of catheter drainage tubing and bag **to facilitate drainage and prevent reflux.**
- ⊛• Refer client/SO(s) to appropriate community resources, such as ostomy specialist, support group, sex therapist, psychiatric clinical nurse specialist, **to deal with changes in body image and function, when indicated.**

Documentation Focus

Assessment/Reassessment
- Individual findings, including previous and current pattern of voiding, nature of problem, and effect on desired lifestyle.
- Cultural factors or concerns.

Planning
- Plan of care and who is involved in planning.
- Teaching plan.

Implementation/Evaluation
- Response to interventions, teaching, and actions performed.
- Attainment or progress toward desired outcome(s).
- Modifications to plan of care.

Discharge Planning
- Long-term needs and who is responsible for actions to be taken.
- Available resources and specific referrals made.
- Individual equipment needs and sources.

Sample Nursing Outcomes & Interventions Classifications (NOC/NIC)

NOC—Urinary Elimination
NIC—Urinary Elimination Management

Information that appears in brackets has been added by the authors to clarify and enhance the use of nursing diagnoses.

readiness for enhanced Urinary Elimination

Taxonomy II: Elimination and Exchange—Class 1 Urinary Function (00166)
[Diagnostic Division: Elimination]
Submitted 2002

Definition: A pattern of urinary functions that is sufficient for meeting eliminatory needs and can be strengthened

Defining Characteristics

Subjective
Expresses willingness to enhance urinary elimination
Positions self for emptying of bladder

Objective
Urine is straw colored, odorless
Amount of output and specific gravity is within normal limits
Fluid intake is adequate for daily needs

Desired Outcomes/Evaluation Criteria— Client Will:

- Verbalize understanding of condition that has potential for altering elimination.
- Achieve improved elimination pattern emptying bladder, voiding in appropriate amounts.
- Alter lifestyle or environment to accommodate individual needs.

Actions/Interventions

Nursing Priority No. 1.
To assess status and adaptive skills being used by client:

- Identify physical conditions (e.g., surgery, childbirth, recent or multiple pregnancies, pelvic trauma, neurogenic bladder from central nervous system disorders or neuropathies [such as stroke, spinal cord injury, diabetes], prostate disease or surgery, mental or emotional dysfunction) **that can impact client's elimination patterns.**
- Determine client's usual pattern of elimination and compare with current situation **to determine client's readiness for improving elimination patterns and/or how pattern can be**

Information that appears in brackets has been added by the authors to clarify and enhance the use of nursing diagnoses.

🌐 Cultural 🅰 Collaborative 🏠 Community/Home Care

improved. Review voiding diary, if indicated. **Provides baseline for future comparison.**

- Observe voiding patterns, time, color, and amount voided, if indicated (e.g., postsurgical or postpartum client) **to document normalization of elimination.**
- Ascertain methods of self-management (e.g., limiting or increasing liquid intake, acting on urge in timely manner, established voiding schedule, regularly spaced catheterization) **to identify strengths and areas of concern in elimination management.**
- Determine client's usual daily fluid intake. **Amount and timing of fluid intake, as well as beverage choices, are important in managing elimination.**

Nursing Priority No. 2.
To assist client to improve management of urinary elimination:

- Encourage fluid intake, including water and cranberry juice, **to help maintain renal function, prevent infection.**
- Regulate liquid intake at prescheduled times **to promote predictable voiding pattern.**
- Restrict fluid intake 2 to 3 hours before bedtime, if indicated, **to reduce voiding during the night.**
- Assist with modifying current routines, as appropriate. **Client may benefit from additional information in enhancing success, such as responding to cues or urge to void, adjusting schedule of voiding or catheterization (shorter or longer), relaxation and/or distraction techniques, standing or sitting upright during voiding to ensure that bladder is completely empty, and/or practicing pelvic muscle strengthening exercises.**
- Provide assistance or devices, as indicated (e.g., providing means of summoning assistance; placing bedside commode, urinal, or bedpan within client's reach; using elevated toilet seats; mobility devices) **when client is frail or mobility impaired.**
- Modify or recommend diet changes, if indicated, **such as limiting caffeine intake because of its bladder irritant effect or weight loss to reduce overactive bladder symptoms and incontinence by decreasing pressure on the bladder.**
- Modify medication regimens, as appropriate (e.g., administer prescribed diuretics in the morning **to lessen nighttime voiding**). Reduce or eliminate use of hypnotics, if possible, **as client may be too sedated to recognize and respond to urge to void.**

Information that appears in brackets has been added by the authors to clarify and enhance the use of nursing diagnoses.

⊕ • Refer to appropriate resources (e.g., medical supply company, ostomy nurse, rehabilitation team) **for assistance, as desired/ needed to promote self-care.**

Nursing Priority No. 3.
🏠 To promote optimum wellness:

- Encourage continuation of successful toileting program and identify possible alterations to meet individual needs (e.g., use of adult briefs for extended outing or travel with limited access to toilet). **Promotes proactive problem-solving and supports self-esteem and normalization of social interactions and desired lifestyle activities.**
- Instruct client/SO(s)/caregivers in cues that client needs, such as voiding on routine schedule, showing client location of the bathroom, providing adequate room lighting, signs, color coding of door **to assist client in continued continence, especially when in unfamiliar surroundings.**
⊕ • Review with client/SO(s) the signs and symptoms of urinary complications and need for expedient medical follow-up care. **Promotes timely intervention to limit or prevent adverse events.**

Documentation Focus

Assessment/Reassessment
- Individual findings including adaptive skills being used.

Planning
- Plan of care and who is involved in planning.
- Teaching plan.

Implementation/Evaluation
- Responses to treatment plan, interventions, and actions performed.
- Attainment or progress toward desired outcome(s).
- Modifications to plan of care.

Discharge Planning
- Available resources, equipment needs and sources.

Sample Nursing Outcomes & Interventions Classifications (NOC/NIC)

NOC—Urinary Elimination
NIC—Urinary Elimination Management

Information that appears in brackets has been added by the authors to clarify and enhance the use of nursing diagnoses.

[acute/chronic] **Urinary Retention**

Taxonomy II: Elimination and Exchange—Class 1 Urinary Function (00023)
[Diagnostic Division: Elimination]
Submitted 1986

Definition: Incomplete emptying of the bladder

Related Factors

High urethral pressure
Inhibition of reflex arc
Strong sphincter; blockage (e.g., benign prostatic hypertrophy [BPH], perineal swelling, trauma)
[Infections; neurological diseases/trauma]
[Use of pharmaceutical agents with side effect of retention (e.g., opiates, atropine, belladonna, psychotropics, antihistamines)]

Defining Characteristics

Subjective
Sensation of bladder fullness
Dribbling
Dysuria

Objective
Bladder distention
Small or frequent voiding; absence of urine output
Residual urine (150 mL or more)
Overflow incontinence
Reduced stream

Desired Outcomes/Evaluation Criteria— Client Will:

- Verbalize understanding of causative factors and appropriate interventions for individual situation.
- Demonstrate techniques or behaviors to alleviate or prevent retention.
- Void in sufficient amounts with no palpable bladder distention; experience no postvoid residuals greater than 50 mL; have no dribbling or overflow.

Information that appears in brackets has been added by the authors to clarify and enhance the use of nursing diagnoses.

Actions/Interventions

Acute

Nursing Priority No. 1.

To assess causative/contributing factors:

- Note presence of pathological conditions (e.g., urinary tract infection [UTI], neurological disorders or trauma, stone formation, prostate hypertrophy) **that can cause mechanical obstruction, nerve dysfunction, ineffective contraction, or decompensation of detrusor musculature, resulting in ineffective emptying of the bladder and urine retention.**

∞• Note client's gender and age. **Retention is most common among men, where prostate abnormalities or urethral strictures cause outlet obstruction. In either sex, retention may be due to medications (particularly those with anticholinergic effects, including many over-the-counter drugs); severe fecal impaction (which increases pressure on the bladder); or neurogenic bladder in patients with diabetes, multiple sclerosis, Parkinson's disease, or prior pelvic surgery, resulting in bladder denervation.**

- Investigate reports of sudden loss of ability to pass urine or great difficulty passing urine, pain with urination, blood in urine. **May indicate UTI or bladder outlet obstruction.**

- Obtain urine and review results of urinalysis (e.g., presence of red or white blood cells, nitrates, glucose, bacteria) and culture. Blood may be tested for infection, electrolyte imbalance, and (in men) prostate-specific antigen **to determine presence of treatable conditions.**

- Review medications, noting those that can cause or exacerbate retention (e.g., psychotropics, anesthesia, opiates, sedatives, alpha- and beta-adrenergic blockers, anticholinergics, antihistamines, neuroleptics).

- Examine for fecal impaction, surgical site swelling, postpartal edema, vaginal or rectal packing, enlarged prostate, or other factors (e.g., recent removal of indwelling catheter with urethral swelling or spasm) **that may produce a blockage of the urethra.**

- Determine anxiety level (e.g., **client may be too embarrassed to void in presence of others**).

Information that appears in brackets has been added by the authors to clarify and enhance the use of nursing diagnoses.

Nursing Priority No. 2.
To determine degree of interference/disability:

* Ascertain whether client has sensation of bladder fullness and determine level of discomfort. **Sensation and discomfort can vary, depending on underlying cause of retention.**
* Determine if there has been any significant urine output in the last 6 to 8 hours; presence of frequent/small voidings; whether dribbling (overflow) is occurring.
* Palpate height of the bladder. Ascertain whether client has sensation of bladder fullness.
* Note recent amount and type of fluid intake. **Adequate fluid intake is necessary for production of healthy output. If client is not voiding despite adequate fluid intake, fluids may be restricted temporarily to prevent bladder overdistention until adequate urine flow is established.**
* Prepare for and assist with urodynamic testing (e.g., cystometrogram **to measure bladder pressure and volume,** bladder scan **to measure retention volume and/or postvoid residual),** or abdominal leak point pressure test.

Nursing Priority No. 3.
To assist in treating/preventing retention:

* Administer medications as indicated (e.g., antibiotics, stool softeners, pain relievers) **to treat underlying cause.**
* Assist client to sit upright on bedpan or commode or stand **to provide functional position of voiding.**
* Provide privacy **to reduce retention caused by embarrassment or anxiety.**
* Instruct client with mild or moderate obstructive symptoms to "double void" by urinating, resting on toilet for 3 to 5 minutes, and then making a second attempt to urinate. **Promotes more efficient bladder evacuation by allowing the detrusor to contract initially, then rest and contract again.**
* Use ice techniques, spirits of wintergreen, stroking inner thigh, running water in sink or warm water over perineum, if indicated, **to stimulate reflex arc.**
* Remove blockage if possible (e.g., vaginal packing, bowel impaction). Prepare for more aggressive intervention (e.g., surgery, prostatectomy).
* Drain bladder intermittently, using the appropriate catheter (material and size) or catheterize with indwelling catheter **to resolve acute retention.**

Information that appears in brackets has been added by the authors to clarify and enhance the use of nursing diagnoses.

- Reduce recurrences by controlling causative or contributing factors when possible (e.g., ice to perineum **to prevent swelling,** use of stool softeners or laxatives, change of medication or dosage).

Nursing Priority No. 4.
To promote wellness (Teaching/Discharge Considerations):

- Emphasize good voiding habits (e.g., four to six times/day). **Repeated holding of urination for prolonged periods can, over time, overstretch and weaken bladder muscles.**
- Encourage client to report problems immediately **so treatment can be instituted promptly.**
- Emphasize need for adequate fluid intake.

Chronic

Nursing Priority No. 1.
To assess causative/contributing factors:

- Review medical history for diagnoses, such as congenital defects, neurological disorders (e.g., multiple sclerosis, polio), prostatic hypertrophy or surgery, birth canal injury or scarring, spinal cord injury with lower motor neuron injury or bladder stones **that may cause detrusor-sphincter dyssynergia (loss of coordination between bladder contraction and external urinary sphincter relaxation), detrusor muscle atrophy, or chronic overdistention because of outlet obstruction.**
- Determine presence of weak or absent sensory and/or motor impulses (as with stroke, spinal injury, or diabetes) **that predispose client to compromised enervation or interpretation of sensory signals resulting in impaired urination.**
- Evaluate customary fluid intake.
- Assess client's medication regimen (e.g., psychotropic, antihistamines, atropine, belladonna) **to consult with primary care provider regarding client's continued use of drugs that are known to potentiate urinary retention.**

Nursing Priority No. 2.
To determine degree of interference/disability:

- Ascertain effect of condition on functioning and lifestyle. **Chronic urinary retention can limit client's desired life-**

Information that appears in brackets has been added by the authors to clarify and enhance the use of nursing diagnoses.

style (e.g., daily activities, social functioning), and can lead to chronic incontinence and life-threatening complications (e.g., intractable UTIs, kidney failure).

- Measure amount voided and postvoid residuals.
- Determine frequency and timing of voiding and/or dribbling.
- Note size and force of urinary stream.
- Palpate height of bladder.
- Determine presence of bladder spasms.
- Prepare for and assist with urodynamic testing (e.g., uroflow-metry **to assess voiding speed and urine volume,** cystome-trogram **to measure bladder pressure and volume,** bladder scan **to measure retention and/or postvoid residual),** or ab-dominal leak point pressure test.

Nursing Priority No. 3.

To assist in treating/preventing retention:

- Collaborate in treatment of underlying conditions (e.g., BPH, reducing or eliminating medications responsible for retention, repairing perineal scarring or outlet obstruction) **that may correct or reduce severity of retention and associated overflow or total incontinence.**
- Recommend client void or catheterize on frequent, timed schedule **to maintain low bladder pressures.**
- Maintain consistent fluid intake **to wash out bacteria or avoid infections and limit stone formation.**
- Adjust fluid amount and timing, if indicated, **to prevent blad-der distention.**
- Perform and instruct client/SO in Credé's method (client or caregiver applies light pressure or tapping on the bladder) or Valsalva's maneuver (client tries to breathe out without letting air escape through the nose or mouth), if appropriate, **to stim-ulate bladder emptying.** *Note:* **Client with spinal cord in-jury and spastic bladder may be able to "trigger" the blad-der to contract and avoid having to use a catheter.**
- Establish regular voiding or self-catheterization program **to prevent reflux and increased renal pressures.**
- Consult with urologist and prepare for more aggressive inter-vention (e.g., reconstructive surgery, lithotripsy, prostatec-tomy), as indicated, **to remove source of obstruction, re-construct sphincter, or provide for urinary diversion.**
- Refer for consideration of advanced or research-based thera-pies (e.g., implanted sacral, tibial, or pelvic electrical stimu-lating device) **for long-term management of retention.**

Information that appears in brackets has been added by the authors to clarify and enhance the use of nursing diagnoses.

Nursing Priority No. 4.
🏠 To promote wellness (Teaching/Discharge Considerations):

- Establish regular schedule for bladder emptying whether voiding or using catheter.
- Stress need for adequate fluid intake, including use of acidifying fruit juices or ingestion of vitamin C. **Maintains renal function, prevents infection and formation of bladder stones, reduces risk of encrustation around indwelling catheter.**
- Instruct client/SO(s) in clean intermittent self-catheterization techniques **so that more than one individual is able to assist the client in care of elimination needs.**
- Instruct client/SO in care when client has indwelling (urethral or suprapubic catheter) or urinary diversion device (e.g., clean technique, emptying and cleaning of leg bag or drainage bag; irrigation and replacement) **to promote self-care, enhance independence, and prevent complications.**
- Review signs/symptoms of complications requiring medical evaluation/intervention.

Documentation Focus

Assessment/Reassessment
- Individual findings, including nature of problem, degree of impairment, and whether client is incontinent.

Planning
- Plan of care and who is involved in planning.
- Teaching plan.

Implementation/Evaluation
- Response to interventions, teaching, and actions performed.
- Attainment or progress toward desired outcome(s).
- Modifications to plan of care.

Discharge Planning
- Long-term needs and who is responsible for actions to be taken.
- Specific referrals made.

Sample Nursing Outcomes & Interventions Classifications (NOC/NIC)

NOC—Urinary Elimination
NIC—Urinary Retention Care

Information that appears in brackets has been added by the authors to clarify and enhance the use of nursing diagnoses.

risk for **Vascular Trauma**

Taxonomy II: Safety/Protection—Class 2 Physical Injury
[Diagnostic Division: Safety]
Submitted 2008

Definition: At risk for damage to a vein and its surrounding tissues related to the presence of a catheter and/or infused solutions

Risk Factors

Insertion site; impaired ability to visualize the insertion site
Catheter type; catheter width; inadequate catheter fixation
Nature of solution (e.g., concentration, chemical irritant, temperature, pH); infusion rate; length of insertion time

> **NOTE:** A risk diagnosis is not evidenced by signs and symptoms, as the problem has not occurred; rather, nursing interventions are directed at prevention.

Desired Outcomes/Evaluation Criteria— Client Will:

- Identify signs/symptoms to report to healthcare provider.
- Be free of signs/symptoms associated with infusion phlebitis or local infection.
- Develop plan for home therapy and demonstrate appropriate procedures as indicated.

Actions/Interventions

Nursing Priority No. 1.
To assess risk factors:

- Determine presence of medical condition(s) requiring intravenous (IV) therapy (e.g., dehydration, trauma, surgery; long-term antibiotic treatment of severe infections; cancer therapies, pain management when oral drugs not effective or practical).
- ∞• Note client's age, body size, and weight. **Very young or elderly client is at risk because of lack of subcutaneous tissue surrounding veins, and veins may be fragile or ropy, causing difficulties with insertion. Forearm veins may be**

Information that appears in brackets has been added by the authors to clarify and enhance the use of nursing diagnoses.

difficult to see in obese, edematous, or dark-skinned individual.

- Identify particular issues such as client's emotional state, including fear of needles, mental or developmental status that
might interfere with client's ability to cooperate with procedures, IV site choices that interfere with client's mobility, **to
prevent or limit potential for vascular damage.**
- Determine type(s) of solutions being used or planned. **Certain
infusates are associated with greater risk of vein irritation
and pain (e.g., potassium, contrast media); others are associated with significant risk of tissue injury, especially
upon infiltration into surrounding tissues, including certain antibiotics, chemotherapy, or parenteral nutrition.**
- Assess peripheral IV site, when one is already in place, to
determine potential for complications. **Reddened, blanched,
tight, translucent, or cool skin; swelling; pain; numbness;
streak formation; a palpable venous cord or purulent
drainage are indicative of problem with IV requiring immediate intervention.**
- Assess central venous access device (CVAD), if present, to
determine potential for complications. **Inability to aspirate,
slowed or absent solution flow, site pain, engorged veins,
or swelling in upper arm, chest wall, neck, or jaw on side
of catheter insertion may indicate vein- or catheter-related
thrombus, requiring immediate intervention.**

Nursing Priority No. 2.
To reduce potential complications:

- Determine appropriate site choice:

   Inspect and palpate chosen veins to determine size and condition. **Best veins are those that are not scarred, lumpy,
   or fragile, to improve ease of cannulation and effectiveness of infusion.**

   Identify extremities or sites that have impaired circulation or
   injury. **Existing tissue injury, bleeding or edema can inhibit successful IV cannulation and potentiate risk for
   infiltration of infusates.**

   Avoid leg veins in adults **due to potential for thrombophlebitis.**

   Avoid anticubital veins when using peripheral catheter **because placement there limits client's movement and the
   catheter is easily dislodged.**

Information that appears in brackets has been added by the authors to clarify
and enhance the use of nursing diagnoses.

Avoid inserting needle in vein valve site. **Damage to this area can cause blood pooling and increase risk of thrombosis.**

- Use best practice approach to IV insertion:

Determine best type of access when IV therapy is initiated. **Peripheral catheter in forearm is recommended for short-duration, nonirritating solutions of less than 7 days. CVAD is appropriate for infusing many kinds of solutions over long periods of time or when client has suffered multiple peripheral sticks or one extremity is not available (e.g., amputation, dialysis shunt in one arm).**

Use appropriate needle gauge for chosen vein and solution **to deliver solution at appropriate rate, to promote hemo- dilution of fluid(s) at the catheter tip, and to reduce me- chanical and chemical irritation to vein wall.**

Clean site and inject 1% lidocaine per agency protocol **to reduce risk of infection and pain with needle or cannula insertion.**

Stretch and immobilize skin and tissues **to stabilize vein and prevent rolling, requiring multiple sticks.**

Insert needle bevel up during insertion and hold at 3 to 10 degree angle **to prevent "blowing" the vein by piercing the back wall.**

Release tourniquet immediately when insertion is complete **to prevent intravascular pressure from causing bleeding into surrounding tissues.**

Observe for hematoma development and/or reports of pain and discomfort during insertion, **indicating vein damage with bleeding into tissues.**

Secure needle or cannula with tape or other securing device **to prevent dislodging and to extend catheter dwell time.**

Avoid placing tape entirely around arm to anchor catheter; **can impede venous return and cause pooling of fluid, and infiltration or extravasation into surrounding tissues.**

Utilize transparent dressing over insertion site **to protect from external contaminants and to allow easy obser- vation for potential complications.**

- Adhere to recommended infusions, dilutions, and administration rates for medications or irritating substances, such as potassium, **to reduce incidence of tissue irritation and sloughing.**

- Consult with IV/infusion nurse or other medical provider **to problem-solve issues that arise with IVs and/or for inter- ventions for complications.**

Information that appears in brackets has been added by the authors to clarify and enhance the use of nursing diagnoses.

Nursing Priority No. 3.

To promote optimum therapeutic effect:

* Observe IV site on a regular basis and instruct client/caregiver to report any discomfort, bruising, redness, swelling, bleeding or other fluid leaking from site.
* Replace peripheral catheters every 72 to 96 hours (or per agency policy) **to prevent thrombophlebitis and catheter-related infections.**
* Apply pressure to site when IV discontinued for sufficient time **to prevent bleeding, especially in client with coagulopathies or on anticoagulants.**
* Adhere to specific protocols related to infection control. (Refer to ND risk for Infection.)
* Identify community resources and suppliers as indicated **to support home therapy regimen.**

Documentation Focus

Assessment/Reassessment

* Assessment findings pre- and postinsertion, site choice, use of local anesthetic, type and gauge of needle or cannula inserted, number of sticks required, dressing applied.
* Type, amount, and rate of solution administered, presence of additives.
* Client's response to procedure.

Planning

* Plan of care, specific interventions, and who is involved in the planning.
* Teaching plan as appropriate.

Implementation/Evaluation

* Attainment or progress toward desired outcome(s).
* Modifications to plan of care.

Discharge Planning

* Long-term needs, identifying who is responsible for actions to be taken.
* Community resources for equipment and supplies for home therapy.
* Specific referrals made.

Information that appears in brackets has been added by the authors to clarify and enhance the use of nursing diagnoses.

Sample Nursing Outcomes & Interventions classifications (NOC/NIC)

NOC—Risk Control
NIC—Intravenous (IV) Insertion

impaired spontaneous Ventilation

Taxonomy II: Activity/Rest—Class 2 Cardiovascular/
  Pulmonary Response (00033)
[Diagnostic Division: Respiration]
Submitted 1992

Definition: Decreased energy reserves resulting in an inability to maintain independent breathing that is adequate to support life

Related Factors

Metabolic factors; [hypermetabolic state (e.g., infection); nutritional deficits/depletion of energy stores]
Respiratory muscle fatigue
[Airway size or resistance; inadequate secretion management]

Defining Characteristics

Subjective
Dyspnea
Reports apprehension

Objective
Increased metabolic rate
Increased heart rate
Increased restlessness; decreased cooperation
Increased use of accessory muscles
Decreased tidal volume
Decreased PO_2, SaO_2; increased PCO_2

Desired Outcomes/Evaluation Criteria— Client Will:

• Reestablish and maintain effective respiratory pattern via ventilator with absence of retractions or use of accessory muscles,

---

Information that appears in brackets has been added by the authors to clarify and enhance the use of nursing diagnoses.

cyanosis, or other signs of hypoxia; and with arterial blood gases (ABGs)/SaO$_2$ within acceptable range.
• Participate in efforts to wean within individual ability, as appropriate.

Caregiver Will:

• Demonstrate behaviors necessary to maintain respiratory function.

Actions/Interventions

Nursing Priority No. 1.
To determine degree of impairment:
• Identify client with actual or impending respiratory failure (e.g., apnea or slow, shallow breathing; declining mentation or obtunded with need for airway protection).
• Determine presence of conditions that could be associated with hypoventilation. **Causes of (1) central alveolar hypoventilation include congenital defects, drugs, and central nervous system disorders (e.g., stroke, trauma, and neoplasms); (2) obesity hypoventilation syndrome is another well-known cause of hypoventilation; (3) chest wall deformities (e.g., kyphoscoliosis and changes after thoracic surgery) can be associated with alveolar hypoventilation leading to respiratory insufficiency and failure; (4) neuromuscular diseases that can cause alveolar hypoventilation include myasthenia gravis, amyotrophic lateral sclerosis, Guillain-Barré, and muscular dystrophy.**
• Assess spontaneous respiratory pattern, noting rate, depth, rhythm, symmetry of chest movement, use of accessory muscles. **Tachypnea, shallow breathing, demonstrated or reported dyspnea (using a numeric or similar scale); increased heart rate, dysrhythmias; pallor or cyanosis; and intercostal retractions and use of accessory muscles indicate increased work of breathing or impaired gas exchange impairment.**
• Auscultate breath sounds, noting presence or absence and equality of breath sounds, adventitious breath sounds.
• Evaluate ABGs and/or pulse oximetry and capnography **to determine presence and degree of arterial hypoxemia (PaO$_2$ <55) and hypercapnea (CO$_2$ >45), resulting in impaired ventilation requiring ventilatory support.**
• Obtain or review results of pulmonary function studies (e.g., lung volumes, **inspiratory and expiratory pressures, and**

Information that appears in brackets has been added by the authors to clarify and enhance the use of nursing diagnoses.

forced vital capacity), as appropriate, to assess presence and degree of respiratory insufficiency.

- Investigate etiology of current respiratory failure **to determine ventilation needs and most appropriate type of ventilatory support.**
- Review serial chest x-rays and imaging magnetic resonance imaging/computed tomography scan results **to diagnose underlying disorder and monitor response to treatment.**
- Note response to current measures and respiratory therapy (e.g., bronchodilators, supplemental oxygen, nebulizer, intermittent positive-pressure breathing treatments).

Nursing Priority No. 2.

To provide/maintain ventilatory support:

- Collaborate with physician, respiratory care practitioners regarding effective mode of ventilation (e.g., noninvasive oxygenation via continuous positive airway pressure (CPAP) and biphasic positive airway pressure [BiPAP]); or intubation and mechanical ventilation (e.g., continuous mandatory, assist control, intermittent mandatory [IMV], pressure support). **Specific mode is determined by client's respiratory requirements, presence of underlying disease process, and the extent to which client can participate in ventilatory efforts.**
- Ensure that ventilator settings and parameters are correct as ordered by client situation, including respiratory rate, fraction of inspired oxygen (FIO_2 expressed as a percentage; tidal volume); peak inspiratory pressure.
- Observe overall breathing pattern, distinguishing between spontaneous respirations and ventilator breaths. **Client may be completely dependent on the ventilator or able to take breaths but have poor oxygen saturation without the ventilator.**
- Verify that client's respirations are in phase with the ventilator. **Decreases work of breathing; maximizes O_2 delivery.**
- Inflate tracheal or endotracheal (ET) tube cuff properly using minimal leak or occlusive technique. Check cuff inflation periodically per facility protocol and whenever cuff is deflated and reinflated **to prevent risk associated with underinflation or overinflation.**
- Check tubing for obstruction (e.g., kinking or accumulation of water). Drain tubing as indicated; avoid draining toward client or back into the reservoir, **resulting in contamination and providing medium for growth of bacteria.**
- Check ventilator alarms for proper functioning. Do not turn off alarms, even for suctioning. Remove from ventilator and

---

Information that appears in brackets has been added by the authors to clarify and enhance the use of nursing diagnoses.

ventilate manually if source of ventilator alarm cannot be quickly identified and rectified. Verify that alarms can be heard in the nurses' station by care providers.

* Verify that oxygen line is in proper outlet/tank; monitor in-line oxygen analyzer or perform periodic oxygen analysis.
* Verify tidal volume set to volume needed for individual situation and proper functioning of spirometer, bellows, or computer readout of delivered volume. Note alterations from desired volume delivery **to determine alteration in lung compliance or leakage through machine/around tube cuff (if used).**
* Monitor airway pressure **for developing complications or equipment problems.**
* Monitor inspiratory and expiratory ratio.
* Promote maximal ventilation of alveoli; check sigh rate intervals (usually $1\frac{1}{2}$ to 2 times tidal volume). **Reduces risk of atelectasis, helps mobilize secretions.**
* Note inspired humidity and temperature; maintain hydration **to liquify secretions, facilitating removal.**
* Auscultate breath sounds periodically. Investigate frequent crackles or rhonchi that do not clear with coughing or suctioning—**suggestive of developing complications (atelectasis, pneumonia, acute bronchospasm, pulmonary edema).**
* Suction only as needed, using lowest pressure possible **to clear secretions and maintain airway.**
* Note changes in chest symmetry. **May indicate improper placement of ET tube, development of barotrauma.**
* Keep resuscitation bag at bedside **to allow for manual ventilation whenever indicated (e.g., if client is removed from ventilator or troubleshooting equipment problems).**
* Administer sedation as required **to synchronize respirations and reduce work of breathing and energy expenditure, as indicated.**
* Administer and monitor response to medications that promote airway patency and gas exchange.
* Refer to NDs ineffective Airway Clearance; ineffective Breathing Pattern; impaired Gas Exchange, for related interventions.

Nursing Priority No. 3.

To prepare for/assist with weaning process if appropriate:

* Determine physical and psychological readiness to wean, including specific respiratory parameters, absence of infection

---

Information that appears in brackets has been added by the authors to clarify and enhance the use of nursing diagnoses.

 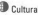

or cardiac failure, client alert and/or able to sustain spontaneous respiration, nutritional status sufficient to maintain work of breathing.

⊕• Determine mode for weaning. **Pressure support mode or multiple daily T-piece trials may be superior to IMV; low-level pressure support may be beneficial for spontaneous breathing trials; and early extubation and institution of noninvasive positive pressure ventilation may have substantial benefits in alert, cooperative client.**

• Explain weaning activities and techniques, individual plan, and expectations. **Reduces fear of unknown.**

• Elevate head of bed or place in orthopedic chair, if possible, or position **to alleviate dyspnea and to facilitate oxygenation.**

• Coach client in "taking control" of breathing (to take slower, deeper breaths, practice abdominal or pursed-lip breathing, assume position of comfort) **to maximize respiratory function and reduce anxiety.**

• Instruct in or assist client to practice effective coughing techniques. **Necessary for secretion management after extubation.**

• Provide quiet environment, calm approach, undivided attention of nurse. **Promotes relaxation, decreasing energy and oxygen requirements.**

• Involve family/SO(s) as appropriate. Provide diversional activity. **Helps client focus on something other than breathing.**

• Instruct client in use of energy-saving techniques during care activities **to limit oxygen consumption and fatigue.**

• Acknowledge and provide ongoing encouragement for client's efforts. Communicate hope for successful weaning response (even partial). **Enhances commitment to continue activity, maximizing outcomes.**

Nursing Priority No. 4.

🏠 To prepare for discharge on ventilator when indicated:

• Ascertain plan for discharge placement (e.g., return home, short-term stay in subacute or rehabilitation center, or permanent placement in long-term care facility).

• Determine specific equipment needs. Identify resources for equipment needs and maintenance and arrange for delivery prior to client discharge.

Information that appears in brackets has been added by the authors to clarify and enhance the use of nursing diagnoses.

- Review layout of home, noting size of rooms, doorways, placement of furniture, number and type of electrical outlets **to identify specific safety needs.**
- Obtain No Smoking signs to be posted in home. Encourage family members to refrain from smoking.
- Have family/SO(s) notify utility companies and fire department about ventilator in home.
- Develop emergency disaster plan to address backup electrical needs and possible evacuation if required.
- Review and provide written or audiovisual materials regarding proper ventilator management, maintenance, and safety **for reference in home setting, enhancing client's/SO's knowledge and level of comfort.**
- Demonstrate airway management techniques and proper equipment cleaning practices.
- Instruct SO(s)/caregivers in other pulmonary physiotherapy measures as indicated (e.g., chest physiotherapy).
- Allow sufficient opportunity for SO(s)/caregivers to practice new skills. Role-play potential crisis situations **to enhance confidence in ability to handle client's needs.**
- Identify signs/symptoms requiring prompt medical evaluation/intervention. **Timely treatment may prevent progression of problem.**
- Provide positive feedback and encouragement for efforts of SO(s)/caregivers. **Promotes continuation of desired behaviors.**
- List names and phone numbers for identified contact persons/resources. **Round-the-clock availability reduces sense of isolation and enhances likelihood of obtaining appropriate information or assistance when needed.**

Nursing Priority No. 5.
To promote wellness (Teaching/Discharge Considerations):

- Discuss impact of specific activities on respiratory status and problem-solve solutions to maximize weaning effort.
- Engage client in specialized exercise program **to enhance respiratory muscle strength and general endurance.**
- Protect client from sources of infection (e.g., monitor health of visitors, roommate, caregivers).
- Recommend involvement in support group; introduce to individuals dealing with similar problems **to provide role models, assistance for problem-solving.**

Information that appears in brackets has been added by the authors to clarify and enhance the use of nursing diagnoses.

- Encourage time out for caregivers **so that they may attend to personal needs, wellness, and growth.**
- Provide opportunities for client/SO(s) to discuss termination of therapy and other end-of-life decisions.
- Refer to individual(s) who are ventilator dependent/have managed home ventilation successfully **to encourage hope for the future.**
- Refer to additional resources (e.g., spiritual advisor, counselor).

Documentation Focus

Assessment/Reassessment
- Baseline findings, subsequent alterations in respiratory function.
- Results of diagnostic testing.
- Individual risk factors and concerns.

Planning
- Plan of care and who is involved in planning.
- Teaching plan.

Implementation/Evaluation
- Client's/SO's responses to interventions, teaching, and actions performed.
- Skill level and assistance needs of SO(s)/family.
- Attainment or progress toward desired outcome(s).
- Modifications to plan of care.

Discharge Planning
- Discharge plan, including appropriate referrals, action taken, and who is responsible for each action.
- Equipment needs and source.
- Resources for support persons or home care providers.

Sample Nursing Outcomes & Interventions Classifications (NOC/NIC)

NOC—Respiratory Status: Ventilation
NIC—Mechanical Ventilation Management: Invasive

Information that appears in brackets has been added by the authors to clarify and enhance the use of nursing diagnoses.

dysfunctional Ventilatory Weaning Response

Taxonomy II: Activity/Rest—Class 4 Cardiovascular/
   Pulmonary Responses (00034)
[Diagnostic Division: Respiration]
Submitted 1992

Definition: Inability to adjust to lowered levels of mechanical ventilator support that interrupts and prolongs the weaning process

Related Factors

Physiological
Ineffective airway clearance
Sleep pattern disturbance
Inadequate nutrition
Uncontrolled pain
[Muscle weakness or fatigue; inability to control respiratory muscles; immobility]

Psychological
Deficient knowledge of the weaning process
Perceived inefficacy about ability to wean
Decreased motivation, self-esteem
Anxiety; fear; insufficient trust in healthcare providers
Hopelessness; powerlessness
[Unprepared for weaning attempt]

Situational
Uncontrolled episodic energy demands
Inappropriate pacing of diminished ventilator support
Inadequate social support
Adverse environment (e.g., noisy, active environment; negative events in the room; low nurse-to-patient ratio; unfamiliar nursing staff)
History of ventilator dependence more than 4 days
History of multiple unsuccessful weaning attempts

Defining Characteristics

Mild

Subjective
Reports feelings of increased need for oxygen; breathing discomfort; fatigue; warmth
Queries about possible machine malfunction

Information that appears in brackets has been added by the authors to clarify and enhance the use of nursing diagnoses.

Objective

Restlessness

Slight increase of respiratory rate from baseline

Increased concentration on breathing

Moderate

Subjective

Reports apprehension

Objective

Slight increase from baseline blood pressure (<20 mmHg) or heart rate (<20 beats/min)

Baseline increase in respiratory rate (<5 breaths/min); minimal respiratory accessory muscle use; decreased air entry on auscultation

Hypervigilance to activities; wide-eyed look

Inability to cooperate or respond to coaching

Diaphoresis

Color changes; pale; slight cyanosis

Severe

Objective

Agitation; decreased level of consciousness

Deterioration in arterial blood gases from current baseline

Increase from baseline blood pressure (≥20 mm Hg), heart rate (≥20 beats/min)

Respiratory rate increases significantly from baseline; full respiratory accessory muscle use; shallow or gasping breaths; paradoxical abdominal breathing

Adventitious breath sounds, audible airway secretions

Asynchronized breathing with the ventilator

Profuse diaphoresis

Cyanosis

Desired Outcomes/Evaluation Criteria—Client Will:

- Actively participate in the weaning process.
- Reestablish independent respiration with arterial blood gases (ABGs) within client's normal range and be free of signs of respiratory failure.
- Demonstrate increased tolerance for activity and participate in self-care within level of ability.

Information that appears in brackets has been added by the authors to clarify and enhance the use of nursing diagnoses.

Nursing Priority No. 1.

To identify contributing factors/degree of dysfunction:

- Determine extent and nature of underlying disorders or factors (e.g., preexisting cardiopulmonary diseases, significant trauma, neuromuscular disorders, multisystem organ failure; ventilator-associated pneumonia; complications from surgical procedures) **that contribute to client's reliance on mechanical support and can affect future weaning efforts.**
- Note length of time client has been receiving ventilator support. Review previous episodes of extubation and reintubation. **Previous unsuccessful weaning attempts (e.g., due to inability to protect airway or clear secretions; oxygen saturation less than 50% on room air) that can influence future weaning interventions.**
- Assess systemic parameters that may affect readiness for weaning using Burns Weaning Assessment Program (BWAP) or similar checklist (e.g., stability of vital signs, factors that increase metabolic rate [e.g., sepsis, fever]; hydration status; need for/recent use of analgesia or sedation; nutritional state; muscle strength; activity level) **to assess systemic parameters that may affect readiness for weaning.** *Note:* **A recent study of the use of BWAP score in five adult critical care units found that a score of 50 or higher was linked to successful weaning outcomes.**
- Ascertain client's awareness and understanding of weaning process, expectations, and concerns. **Client/SO(s) may need specific and repeated instructions during process.**
- Determine psychological readiness, presence and degree of anxiety. **Weaning provokes anxiety regarding ability to breathe on own and likelihood of ventilator dependence. The client must be highly motivated, be able to actively participate in the weaning process, and be physically comfortable enough to work at weaning.**
- Introduce client to individual who has shared similar experiences with successful outcome if desired or indicated **to provide support and encouragement for successful outcome.**
- Review laboratory studies (e.g., complete blood count reflecting number and integrity of red blood cells [**affects oxygen transport**], serum albumin and electrolyte levels indicating nutritional status [**to confirm sufficient energy to meet demands of spontaneous breathing and weaning**]).

Information that appears in brackets has been added by the authors to clarify and enhance the use of nursing diagnoses.

• Review chest x-ray, pulse oximetry or capnography, and/or ABGs. **Before weaning attempts, chest radiograph should show clear lungs or marked improvement in pulmonary congestion. ABGs should document satisfactory oxygenation on an FIO₂ of 40% or less. Capnometry measures end-tidal carbon dioxide values and can be used to confirm correct placement of endotracheal tube and monitor integrity of ventilation equipment.**

Nursing Priority No. 2.
To support weaning process:

• Discuss with client/SO(s) individual plan and expectations. Assure client of nurse's presence and assistance during weaning attempts. **May reduce client's anxiety about process and ultimate outcome and enhance willingness to work at spontaneous breathing.**

• Consult with dietitian, nutritional support team for adjustments in composition of diet **to support respiratory muscle strength and work of breathing and to prevent excessive production of CO₂, which could alter respiratory drive.**

• Implement weaning protocols and mode (e.g., spontaneous breathing trials, automatic tube compensation [ATC], partial client support [SIMV], or pressure support [PSV] during client's spontaneous breathing) **to optimize the work of breathing and to provide support for spontaneous ventilation.**

• Note response to activity/client care during weaning and limit, as indicated. Provide undisturbed rest or sleep periods. Avoid stressful procedures or situations and nonessential activities. **Prevents excessive oxygen consumption or demand with increased possibility of weaning failure.**

• Time medications during weaning efforts **to minimize sedative effects.**

• Provide quiet room, calm approach, undivided attention of nurse. **Enhances relaxation, conserving energy.**

• Involve SO(s)/family, as appropriate (e.g., sitting at bedside, providing encouragement, and helping monitor client status).

• Provide diversional activity (e.g., watching TV, reading aloud) **to focus attention away from breathing when not actively working at breathing exercises.**

• Auscultate breath sounds periodically; suction airway, as indicated.

Information that appears in brackets has been added by the authors to clarify and enhance the use of nursing diagnoses.

- Acknowledge and provide ongoing encouragement for client's efforts.
- Minimize setbacks, focus client attention on gains and progress to date **to reduce frustration that may further impair progress.**

Nursing Priority No. 3

To prepare for discharge on ventilator when indicated:

- Prepare client/SO for alternative actions when client is unable to resume spontaneous ventilation (e.g., tracheostomy with long-term ventilation support in alternate care setting or home, palliative care or end-of-life procedures). **Customized discharge planning for people new to home ventilation is essential. This must include assessment of the environment, assessment of resources, assessment of caregivers, education and training, and a plan of care.**
- Ascertain that all needed equipment is in place, caregivers are trained, and safety concerns have been addressed (e.g., alternative power source, backup equipment, client call or alarm system, established means of client/caregiver communication) **to ease the transfer when client is going home on ventilator.**
- Evaluate caregiver capabilities and burden when client requires long-term ventilator in the home **to determine potential or presence of skill-related problems or emotional issues (e.g., caregiver overload, burnout, or depression).**
- Refer to ND impaired spontaneous Ventilation for additional interventions.

Nursing Priority No. 4.

To promote wellness (Teaching/Discharge Considerations):

- Encourage client/SO(s) to evaluate impact of ventilatory dependence on their lifestyle and what changes they are willing or unwilling to make when client is discharged on ventilator. **Quality-of-life issues must be examined, including issues of privacy and intimacy, and resolved by the ventilator-dependent client and SO(s). All parties need to understand that ventilatory support is a 24-hour job that ultimately affects everyone.**
- Discuss importance of time for self and identify appropriate sources for respite care. (Refer to ND risk for Caregiver Role Strain.)
- Emphasize to client/SO(s) importance of monitoring health of visitors and persons involved in care, avoiding crowds during

---

Information that appears in brackets has been added by the authors to clarify and enhance the use of nursing diagnoses.

flu season, obtaining immunizations, and so forth, **to protect client from sources of infection.**

- Encourage client/SO(s) to discuss advance directives and ascertain that all care providers are aware of the plan of care. **Clarifies parameters for emergency situations, termination of therapy, or other end-of-life decisions, as desired.**
- Recommend involvement in support group (may be online); introduce to other ventilator-dependent individuals who are successfully managing home ventilation, if desired, **to answer questions, provide role model, assist with problem-solving, and offer encouragement and hope for the future.**
- Identify conditions requiring immediate medical intervention **to treat developing complications and prevent respiratory failure.**

Documentation Focus

Assessment/Reassessment
- Baseline findings and subsequent alterations.
- Results of diagnostic testing or procedures.
- Individual risk factors.

Planning
- Plan of care, specific interventions, and who is involved in the planning.
- Teaching plan.

Implementation/Evaluation
- Client response to interventions.
- Attainment or progress toward desired outcome(s).
- Modifications to plan of care.

Discharge Planning
- Status at discharge, long-term needs and referrals, indicating who is to be responsible for each action.
- Equipment needs and supplier.

Sample Nursing Outcomes & Interventions Classifications (NOC/NIC)

NOC—Respiratory Status: Ventilation
NIC—Mechanical Ventilatory Weaning

Information that appears in brackets has been added by the authors to clarify and enhance the use of nursing diagnoses.

NOTE: NANDA has separated the diagnosis of Violence into its two elements: "other-directed" and "self-directed." However, the interventions in general address both situations and have been left in one block following the definitions and supporting data of those two diagnoses.

risk for other-directed Violence

Taxonomy II: Safety/Protection—Class 3 Violence (00138)
[Diagnostic Division: Safety]
Submitted 1980; Revised 1996

Definition: At risk for behaviors in which an individual demonstrates that he or she can be physically, emotionally, and/or sexually harmful to others

Risk Factors

Neurological impairment (e.g., positive EEG, computed tomography, or magnetic resonance imaging scan; neurological findings; head trauma; seizure disorders)

Cognitive impairment (e.g., learning disabilities, attention deficit disorder, decreased intellectual functioning); [organic brain syndrome]

Cruelty to animals; firesetting

Prenatal or perinatal complications

Pathological intoxication; [toxic reaction to pharmaceutical agents]

Psychotic symptomatology (e.g., auditory, visual, command hallucinations; paranoid delusions; loose, rambling, or illogical thought processes); [panic states; rage reactions; manic excitement]

Motor vehicle offenses (e.g., frequent traffic violations, use of a motor vehicle to release anger)

Suicidal behavior; impulsivity; availability of weapon(s)

Body language (e.g., rigid posture, clenching of fists and jaw, hyperactivity, pacing, breathlessness, threatening stances)

History of:

Other-directed violence (e.g., hitting, kicking, scratching, biting someone or spitting at someone; throwing objects at some-

---

Information that appears in brackets has been added by the authors to clarify and enhance the use of nursing diagnoses.

one; attempted rape, rape, sexual molestation; urinating/defecating on a person)

Threats of violence (e.g., verbal threats against property or person, social threats, cursing, threatening notes/letters, threatening gestures, sexual threats)

Violent antisocial behavior (e.g., stealing, insistent borrowing, insistent demands for privileges, insistent interruption of meetings, refusal to eat or take medication, ignoring instructions)

Indirect violence (e.g., tearing off clothes, urinating or defecating on floor, stamping feet, temper tantrum, running in corridors, yelling, writing on walls, ripping objects off walls, throwing objects, breaking a window, slamming doors, sexual advances)

Substance abuse

Childhood abuse or witnessing family violence

risk for self-directed Violence

Taxonomy II: Safety/Protection—Class 3 Violence (00140)
[Diagnostic Division: Safety]
Submitted 1994

Definition: At risk for behaviors in which an individual demonstrates that he or she can be physically, emotionally, and/or sexually harmful to self

Risk Factors

Ages 15 to 19 or 45 and over

Marital status (single, widowed, divorced)

Employment problems (e.g., unemployed, recent job loss/failure); occupation (executive, administrator/owner of business, professional, semiskilled worker)

Conflictual interpersonal relationships

Family background (e.g., chaotic or conflictual, history of suicide)

Sexual orientation (bisexual [active], homosexual [inactive]); engagement in autoerotic sexual acts

Physical health problems (e.g., hypochondriasis, chronic or terminal illness)

Mental health problems (e.g., severe depression, psychosis, severe personality disorder, alcoholism or drug abuse); suicidal ideation or plan; history of multiple suicide attempts

Information that appears in brackets has been added by the authors to clarify and enhance the use of nursing diagnoses.

Emotional problems (e.g., hopelessness, [lifting of depressed mood], despair, increased anxiety, panic, anger, hostility); history of multiple suicide attempts; suicidal ideation; suicidal plan

Lack of personal resources (e.g., poor achievement, poor insight, affect unavailable and poorly controlled)

Lack of social resources (e.g., poor rapport, socially isolated, unresponsive family)

Verbal clues (e.g., talking about death, "better off without me," asking questions about lethal dosages of drugs)

Behavioral clues (e.g., writing forlorn love notes, directing angry messages at an SO who has rejected the person, giving away personal items, taking out a large life insurance policy)

Desired Outcomes/Evaluation Criteria— [Other-Directed or Self-Directed] Client Will:

- Acknowledge realities of the situation.
- Verbalize understanding of why behavior occurs.
- Identify precipitating factors.
- Express realistic self-evaluation and increased sense of self-esteem.
- Participate in care and meet own needs in an assertive manner.
- Demonstrate self-control as evidenced by relaxed posture, nonviolent behavior.
- Use resources and support systems in an effective manner.

Actions/Interventions

Address both "other-directed" and "self-directed"

Nursing Priority No. 1.

To assess causative/contributing factors:

- Determine underlying dynamics as listed in Risk Factors.
- Ascertain client's perception of self and situation. Note use of defense mechanisms (e.g., denial, projection).
- Observe and listen for early cues of distress or increasing anxiety (e.g., irritability, lack of cooperation, demanding behavior, body posture or expression). **May indicate possibility of loss of control, and intervention at this point can prevent a blowup.**
- Identify conditions such as acute or chronic brain syndrome, panic state, hormonal imbalance (e.g., premenstrual syndrome, postpartal psychosis), drug induced, postanesthesia/

Information that appears in brackets has been added by the authors to clarify and enhance the use of nursing diagnoses.

postseizure confusion, traumatic brain injury. **These physical conditions may interfere with ability to control own behavior and will need specific interventions to manage.**

• Review laboratory findings (e.g., blood alcohol, blood glucose, arterial blood gases, electrolytes, renal function tests).

• Observe for signs of suicidal/homicidal intent (e.g., perceived morbid or anxious feeling while with the client; warning from the client: "It doesn't matter," "I'd/They'd be better off dead"; mood swings; "accident-prone" or self-destructive behavior; suicidal attempts; possession of alcohol and/or other drug(s) in known substance abuser). (Refer to ND risk for Suicide.)

• Note family history of suicidal or homicidal behavior. **Children who grow up in homes where violence is accepted tend to grow up to use violence as a means of solving problems.**

• Ask directly if the person is thinking of acting on thoughts or feelings **to determine violent intent.**

• Determine availability of homicidal means.

• Assess client coping behaviors already present. **Client may believe there are no alternatives other than violence, especially if individual has come from a family background of violence.**

• Identify risk factors and assess for indicators of child abuse or neglect: unexplained or frequent injuries, failure to thrive, and so forth.

Nursing Priority No. 2.

To assist client to accept responsibility for impulsive behavior and potential for violence:

• Develop therapeutic nurse-client relationship. Provide consistent caregiver when possible. **Promotes sense of trust, allowing client to discuss feelings openly.**

• Maintain straightforward communication **to avoid reinforcing manipulative behavior.**

• Discuss motivation for change (e.g., failing relationships, job loss, involvement with judicial system). **Crisis situation can provide impetus for change, but requires timely therapeutic intervention to sustain efforts.**

• Help client recognize that client's actions may be in response to own fear **(may be afraid of own behavior or loss of control)**, dependency, and feeling of powerlessness.

• Make time to listen to expressions of feelings. Acknowledge reality of client's feelings and that feelings are okay. (Refer to ND Self-Esteem [specify].)

Information that appears in brackets has been added by the authors to clarify and enhance the use of nursing diagnoses.

- Confront client's tendency to minimize situation or behavior. **In domestic violence situations, individual may be remorseful after incident and will apologize and say that it won't happen again.**
- Review factors (feelings and events) involved in precipitating violent behavior.
- Discuss impact of behavior on others and consequences of actions.
- Acknowledge reality of suicide or homicide as an option. Discuss consequences of actions if they were to follow through on intent. Ask how it will help client to resolve problems. **Provides an opportunity for client to look at reality of choices and potential outcomes.**
- Accept client's anger without reacting on emotional basis. Give permission to express angry feelings in acceptable ways and let client know that staff will be available to assist in maintaining control. **Promotes acceptance and sense of safety.**
- Help client identify more appropriate solutions or behaviors (e.g., motor activities, exercise) **to lessen sense of anxiety and associated physical manifestations.**
- Provide directions for actions client can take, avoiding negatives, such as "Do Nots."

Nursing Priority No. 3.

To assist client in controlling behavior:

- Contract with client regarding safety of self/others.
- Give client as much control as possible within constraints of individual situation. **Enhances self-esteem, promotes confidence in ability to change behavior.**
- Be truthful when giving information and dealing with client. **Builds trust, enhancing therapeutic relationship; prevents manipulative behavior.**
- Identify current and past successes and strengths. Discuss effectiveness of coping techniques used and possible changes. (Refer to ND ineffective Coping.) **Client is often not aware of positive aspects of life, and once recognized, these can be used as a basis for change.**
- Assist client to distinguish between reality and hallucinations or delusions.
- Approach in positive manner, acting as if the client has control and is responsible for own behavior. Be aware, though, that

---

Information that appears in brackets has been added by the authors to clarify and enhance the use of nursing diagnoses.

the client may not have control, especially if under the influence of drugs (including alcohol).

- Maintain distance and do not touch client without permission when situation indicates client does not tolerate such closeness (e.g., post-trauma response).
- Remain calm and state limits on inappropriate behavior (including consequences) in a firm manner.
- Direct client to stay in view of staff/caregiver.
- Administer prescribed medications (e.g., anti-anxiety or antipsychotic), taking care not to oversedate client. **The chemistry of the brain is changed by early violence and has been shown to respond to serotonin, as well as related neurotransmitter systems, which play a role in restraining aggressive impulses.**
- Monitor for possible drug interactions, cumulative effects of drug regimen (e.g., anticonvulsants, antidepressants).
- Give positive reinforcement for client's efforts. **Encourages continuation of desired behaviors.**
- Explore death fantasies when expressed (e.g., "I'll look down and watch them suffer"; "She'll be sorry") or the idea that death is not final (e.g., "I can come back").

Nursing Priority No. 4.

To assist client/SO(s) to correct/deal with existing situation:

- Gear interventions to individual(s) involved, based on age, relationship, and so forth.
- Maintain calm, matter-of fact, nonjudgmental attitude. **Decreases defensive response.**
- Notify potential victims in the presence of serious homicidal threat in accordance with legal and ethical guidelines. **Various Tarasoff statutes exist in many states requiring mental health professionals to report specific threats to both the individual named and law enforcement.**
- Discuss situation with abused or battered person, providing accurate information about choices and effective actions that can be taken.
- Assist individual to understand that angry, vengeful feelings are appropriate in the situation but need to be expressed and not acted on. (Refer to ND Post-Trauma Syndrome, as psychological responses may be very similar.)
- Identify resources available for assistance (e.g., battered women's shelter, social services).

Information that appears in brackets has been added by the authors to clarify and enhance the use of nursing diagnoses.

Nursing Priority No. 5.

To promote safety in event of violent behavior:

- Provide a safe, quiet environment and remove items from the client's environment that could be used to inflict harm to self or others.
- Maintain distance from client who is striking out or hitting and take evasive and controlling actions, as indicated.
- Call for additional staff/security personnel.
- Approach aggressive or attacking client from the front, just out of reach, in a commanding posture with palms down.
- Tell client to *STOP*. **This may be sufficient to help client control own actions.**
- Maintain direct, constant eye contact, when appropriate.
- Speak in a low, commanding voice.
- Provide client with a sense that caregiver is in control of the situation **to provide feeling of safety.**
- Maintain clear route for staff and client and be prepared to move quickly.
- Hold client, using restraints or seclusion, when necessary, until client regains self-control.
- Administer medication, as indicated, **to help client until able to regain self-control.**

Nursing Priority No. 6.

To promote wellness (Teaching/Discharge Considerations):

- Promote client involvement in planning care within limits of situation, allowing for meeting own needs for enjoyment. **Individuals often believe they are not entitled to pleasure and good things in their lives and need to learn how to meet these needs.**
- Assist client to learn assertive rather than manipulative, non-assertive, or aggressive behavior. **Promotes behaviors that help client to engage in positive social activities with others.**
- Discuss reasons for client's behavior with SO(s). Determine desire and commitment of involved parties to sustain current relationships.
- Develop strategies to help parents learn more effective parenting skills (e.g., parenting classes, appropriate ways of dealing with frustrations). **Developing positive relationships has a powerful effect on helping children learn impulse control.**
- Identify support systems (e.g., family/friends, clergy). **In addition to the client, those around him or her need to learn**

Information that appears in brackets has been added by the authors to clarify and enhance the use of nursing diagnoses.

how to be positive role models and display a broader array of skills for resolving problems.

- Refer to formal resources, as indicated (e.g., individual or group psychotherapy, substance abuse treatment program, social services, safe house facility, parenting classes).
- Refer to NDs impaired Parenting; family Coping [specify]; Post-Trauma Syndrome.

Documentation Focus

Assessment/Reassessment
- Individual findings, including nature of concern (e.g., suicidal or homicidal), behavioral risk factors and level of impulse control, plan of action and means to carry out plan.
- Client's perception of situation, motivation for change.
- Family history of violence.
- Availability and use of resources.

Planning
- Plan of care and who is involved in the planning.
- Details of contract regarding violence to self/others.
- Teaching plan.

Implementation/Evaluation
- Actions taken to promote safety, including notification of parties at risk.
- Response to interventions, teaching, and actions performed.
- Attainment or progress toward desired outcome(s).
- Modifications to plan of care.

Discharge Planning
- Long-term needs and who is responsible for actions to be taken.
- Available resources, specific referrals made.

Sample Nursing Outcomes & Interventions Classifications (NOC/NIC)

other-directed Violence
NOC—Aggression Self-Control
NIC—Anger Control Assistance

self-directed Violence
NOC—Impulse Self-Control
NIC—Behavior Management: Self-Harm

Information that appears in brackets has been added by the authors to clarify and enhance the use of nursing diagnoses.

impaired Walking

Taxonomy II: Activity/Rest—Class 2 Activity/Exercise
(00088)
[Diagnostic Division: Activity/Rest]
Submitted 1998; Revised 2006

Definition: Limitation of independent movement within
the environment on foot

Related Factors

Insufficient muscle strength; neuromuscular impairment; mus-
culoskeletal impairment (e.g., contractures)
Limited endurance; deconditioning
Fear of falling; impaired balance, vision
Pain
Obesity
Depressed mood; cognitive impairment
Lack of knowledge
Environmental constraints (e.g., stairs, inclines, uneven sur-
faces, unsafe obstacles, distances, lack of assistive devices or
person, restraints)

Defining Characteristics

Subjective or Objective

Impaired ability to walk required distances, walk on an incline/
decline, walk on uneven surfaces, to navigate curbs, climb
stairs
[Specify level of independence—refer to ND impaired physical
Mobility, for suggested functional level classification]

Desired Outcomes/Evaluation Criteria—
Client Will:

* Be able to move about within environment as needed or desired within limits of ability or with appropriate adjuncts.
* Verbalize understanding of situation or risk factors and safety
measures.

Information that appears in brackets has been added by the authors to clarify
and enhance the use of nursing diagnoses.

Nursing Priority No. 1.

To assess causative/contributing factors:

- Identify conditions or diagnoses (e.g., advanced age, sensory impairments, pain, obesity, chronic fatigue, cognitive dysfunction, acute illness with weakness; *chronic illness* [e.g., cardiopulmonary disorders, cancer], *musculoskeletal injuries or surgery* [e.g., sprains, fractures, tendon or ligament injury; total joint replacement; surgical repair of fractured bone; amputation], *balance problems* [e.g., inner ear infection, brain injury, stroke], *nerve disorders* [e.g., multiple sclerosis, Parkinson's disease, cerebral palsy], *spinal abnormalities* [disease, trauma, degeneration], *impaired circulation or neuropathies* [e.g., peripheral, diabetic, alcoholic], *degenerative bone or muscle disorders* [e.g., osteoporosis, muscular dystrophy, myositis], *foot conditions* [e.g., plantar warts, bunions, ingrown toenails, pressure ulcers]) **that contribute to walking impairment and identify specific needs and appropriate interventions.**
- Note client's particular symptoms related to walking (e.g., unable to bear weight, can't walk usual distance, limping, staggering, stiff leg, leg pain, shuffling, asymmetric or unsteady gait, can walk on certain surfaces, but not on others).
- Determine ability to follow directions and note emotional/behavioral responses **that may be affecting client's ability or desire to engage in activity.**

Nursing Priority No. 2.

To assess functional ability:

- Perform "Get Up and Go" test, as indicated, **to assess client's basic ability to ambulate safely. Factors assessed include sitting balance, ability to transfer from sitting to standing and back to sitting, the pace and stability of ambulation, and the ability to turn without staggering.**
- Determine degree of impairment in relation to suggested functional scale (0 to 4), noting that impairment can be temporary, permanent, or progressive. **Condition may be caused by reversible condition (e.g., weakness associated with acute illness or fractures/surgery with weight-bearing restrictions); or walking impairment can be permanent (e.g., congenital anomalies, amputation, severe rheumatoid arthritis).**

Information that appears in brackets has been added by the authors to clarify and enhance the use of nursing diagnoses.

- Assist with or review results of mobility testing (e.g., gait, timing of walking over fixed distance, distance walked over set period of time [endurance], limb movement analysis, leg strength and speed of walking, ambulatory activity monitoring) **for differential diagnosis and to guide treatment interventions.**
- Note emotional and behavioral responses of client/SO(s) to problems of mobility. **Walking impairments can negatively affect self-concept and self-esteem, autonomy, and independence. Social, occupational, and relationship roles can change, leading to isolation, depression, and economic consequences.**

Nursing Priority No. 3.
To promote safe, optimal level of independence in walking:

- Assist with treatment of underlying condition causing dysfunction, as indicated by individual situation.
- Consult with physical therapist, occupational therapist, or rehabilitation team **for individualized mobility program and identify and develop appropriate devices (e.g., shoe insert, leg brace to maintain proper foot alignment for walking, quad cane, hemiwalker).**
- Demonstrate use of and help client become comfortable with adjunctive devices (e.g., individually prescribed and fitted cane, crutches, walking cast or boot, walker, limb prosthesis, mobility scooter) **to maintain joint stability or immobilization or to maintain alignment or balance during movement.**
- Provide assistance when indicated (e.g., walking on uneven surfaces; client is weak or has to walk a distance; or vision, coordination, or posture are impaired).
- Monitor client's cardiopulmonary tolerance for walking. **Increased pulse rate, chest pain, breathlessness, irregular heartbeat is indicative of need to reduce level of activity.** (Refer to ND Activity Intolerance; decreased Cardiac Output, for related interventions.)
- Encourage adequate rest and gradual increase in walking distance **to reduce fatigue or leg pain associated with walking and improve stamina.** (Refer to NDs Fatigue; risk for Peripheral Neurovascular Dysfunction.)
- Administer medication, as indicated, **to manage pain and maximize level of functioning.** Refer to NDs acute/chronic Pain.

Information that appears in brackets has been added by the authors to clarify and enhance the use of nursing diagnoses.

Cultural Collaborative Community/Home Care

- Implement fall precautions for high-risk clients (e.g., frail or ill elderly, visually or cognitively impaired, person on multiple medications, presence of balance disorders) **to reduce risk of accidental injury.** (Refer to NDs risk for Falls; risk for Disuse Syndrome for related interventions.)
- 🏠• Provide cueing as indicated. **Client may need reminders (e.g., lift foot higher, look where going, walk tall) to concentrate on/perform tasks of walking, especially when balance or cognition is impaired.**
- 🏠• Assist client to obtain needed information, such as handicapped sticker for close-in parking, sources for mobility scooter, or special public transportation options, when indicated.

Nursing Priority No. 4.

🏠To promote wellness (Teaching/Discharge Considerations):

- Involve client/SO(s) in care, assisting them to learn ways of managing deficits **to enhance safety for client and SO(s)/ caregivers.**
- Identify appropriate resources for obtaining and maintaining appliances, equipment, and environmental modifications **to promote mobility.**
- Evaluate client's home (or work) environment for barriers to walking (e.g., uneven surfaces, many steps, no ramps, long distances between places client needs to walk) **to determine needed changes, make recommendations for client safety.**
- Instruct client/SO in safety measures in home, as individually indicated (e.g., maintaining safe travel pathway, proper lighting, wearing glasses, handrails on stairs, grab bars in bathroom, using walker instead of cane when sleepy or walking on uneven surface) **to reduce risk of falls.**
- Discuss need for emergency call/support system (e.g., Lifeline, HealthWatch) **to provide immediate assistance for falls or other home emergencies when client lives alone.**

Documentation Focus

Assessment/Reassessment
- Individual findings, including level of function and ability to participate in specific or desired activities.
- Equipment and assistive device needs.

Planning
- Plan of care and who is involved in the planning.
- Teaching plan.

Information that appears in brackets has been added by the authors to clarify and enhance the use of nursing diagnoses.

Implementation/Evaluation

- Responses to interventions, teaching, and actions performed.
- Attainment or progress toward desired outcome(s).
- Modifications to plan of care.

Discharge Planning

- Discharge and long-term needs, noting who is responsible for each action to be taken.
- Specific referrals made.
- Sources for and maintenance of assistive devices.

Sample Nursing Outcomes & Interventions Classifications (NOC/NIC)

NOC—Ambulation
NIC—Exercise Therapy: Ambulation

Wandering [specify sporadic or continuous]

Taxonomy II: Activity/Rest—Class 3 Energy Balance (00154)
[Diagnostic Division: Safety]
[Submitted 2000]

Definition: Meandering, aimless, or repetitive locomotion that exposes the individual to harm; frequently incongruent with boundaries, limits, or obstacles

---

Related Factors

Cognitive impairment (e.g., memory and recall deficits, disorientation, poor visuoconstructive or visuospatial ability, language defects); sedation

Cortical atrophy

Premorbid behavior (e.g., outgoing, sociable personality; premorbid dementia)

Separation from familiar environment; overstimulating environment

Emotional state (e.g., frustration, anxiety, boredom, depression, agitation)

Physiological state or need (e.g., hunger, thirst, pain, urination, constipation)

Time of day

Information that appears in brackets has been added by the authors to clarify and enhance the use of nursing diagnoses.

Defining Characteristics

Objective

Frequent or continuous movement from place to place

Persistent locomotion in search of something; scanning or searching behaviors

Haphazard locomotion; fretful locomotion; pacing; long periods of locomotion without an apparent destination

Locomotion into unauthorized/private spaces; trespassing

Locomotion resulting in unintended leaving of a premise

Inability to locate significant landmarks in a familiar setting; getting lost

Locomotion that cannot be easily dissuaded; shadowing a caregiver's locomotion

Hyperactivity

Periods of locomotion interspersed with periods of nonlocomotion (e.g., sitting, standing, sleeping)

Desired Outcomes/Evaluation Criteria—Client Will:

- Be free of injury, or unplanned exits.

Caregiver(s) Will:

- Modify environment, as indicated, to enhance safety.
- Provide for maximal independence of client.

Actions/Interventions

Nursing Priority No. 1.

To assess degree of impairment/stage of disease process:

- Ascertain history of client's memory loss and cognitive changes.
- Assist with or review results of specific testing (e.g., Revised Algase Wandering Scale [RAWS], Need-Driven Dementia-Compromised Behavior [NDB], or similar tool), as indicated. **Adjunct tools that quantify wandering in several domains can more easily determine individual risks and safety needs.**
- Evaluate client's mental status during daytime and nighttime, noting when client's confusion is most pronounced and when client sleeps. **Can reveal circumstances under which client is likely to wander.**

Information that appears in brackets has been added by the authors to clarify and enhance the use of nursing diagnoses.

- Identify client's reason for wandering, if possible. **Client may demonstrate searching behavior (e.g., looking for lost item) or be experiencing sensations (e.g., hunger, thirst, discomfort) without ability to express the actual need.**
- Note timing and pattern of wandering behavior. **Client attempting to leave at 5:00 p.m. every day may believe he is going home from work; client may be goal directed (e.g., searching for person or object, escaping from something) or nongoal directed (wandering aimlessly).**
- Monitor client's use or need for assistive devices, such as glasses, hearing aids, cane. **Wandering client is at high risk for falls due to cognitive impairments or forgetting necessary assistive devices or how to properly use them.**
- Determine bowel and bladder elimination pattern, timing of incontinence, presence of constipation **for possible correlation to wandering behavior.**
- Ascertain if client has delusions due to shadows, lights, and noises **to determine necessary changes to environment.**

Nursing Priority No. 2.

🏠 To assist client/caregiver to deal with situations:

- Provide a structured daily routine. **Decreases wandering behavior and minimizes caregiver stress.**
- Encourage participation in family activities and familiar routines, such as folding laundry, listening to music, or shared walking time outdoors. **May reduce anxiety, depression, and restlessness.** *Note:* **Repetitive activity (e.g., folding laundry, or paperwork) may help client with "lapping," wandering to reduce energy expenditure and fatigue.**
- Offer drink of water or snack, bring client to bathroom on a regular schedule. **Wandering may at times be expressing a need.**
- Provide safe place for client to wander, away from safety hazards (e.g., hot water, kitchen stove, open stairway) and other, noisy clients. Arrange furniture, remove scatter rugs, electrical cords, and other high-risk items **to accommodate safe wandering.**
- Make sure that doors or gates have alarms or chimes and that alarms are turned on. Provide door and window locks that are not within line of sight or easily opened **to prevent unsafe exits.**
- Provide 24-hour supervision and reality orientation. **Client can be awake at any time and fail to recognize day/night routines.**

Information that appears in brackets has been added by the authors to clarify and enhance the use of nursing diagnoses.

- Sit with client and visit or reminisce. Provide TV, radio, music **when client is socially gregarious, enjoys conversation, or reminiscence is calming.**
- Avoid overstimulation from activities or new partner/roommate during rest periods when client is in a facility. **Client who is used to wandering in usual living setting may react with increased agitation and emotional outbreaks when admitted to an unfamiliar setting and restricted from wandering.**
- Use pressure-sensitive bed/chair alarms or door mat **to alert caregivers of movement.**
- Avoid using physical or chemical restraints (sedatives) to control wandering behavior. **May increase agitation, sensory deprivation, and falls; may contribute to wandering behavior.**
- Provide consistent staff as much as possible.
- Provide room near monitoring station; check client location on frequent basis.

Nursing Priority No. 3.
To promote wellness (Teaching/Discharge Considerations):

- Identify problems that are remediable and assist client/SO(s) to seek appropriate assistance and access resources. **Encourages problem-solving to improve condition rather than accept the status quo.**
- Provide client ID bracelet or necklace with updated photograph, client name, and emergency contact **to assist with identification efforts, particularly when progressive dementia produces marked changes in client's appearance.**
- Notify neighbors about client's condition and request that they contact client's family or local police if they see client outside alone. **Community awareness can prevent/reduce risk of client being lost or hurt.**
- Register client with community or national resources, such as Alzheimer's Association Safe Return Program, **to assist in identification, location, and safe return of individual with wandering behaviors.**
- Help SO(s) develop plan of care when problem is progressive.
- Refer to community resources, such as day-care programs, support groups, respite care.
- Refer to NDs acute Confusion; chronic Confusion; impaired Environmental Interpretation Syndrome; [disturbed Sensory Perception (specify)]; risk for Injury; risk for Falls.

Information that appears in brackets has been added by the authors to clarify and enhance the use of nursing diagnoses.

Documentation Focus

Assessment/Reassessment

- Assessment findings, including individual concerns, family involvement, and support factors and availability of resources.

Planning

- Plan of care and who is involved in planning.
- Teaching plan.

Implementation/Evaluation

- Responses of client/SO(s) to plan interventions and actions performed.
- Attainment or progress toward desired outcome(s).
- Modifications to plan of care.

Discharge Planning

- Long-term needs and who is responsible for actions to be taken.
- Specific referrals made.

Sample Nursing Outcomes & Interventions Classifications (NOC/NIC)

NOC—Safe Wandering
NIC—Elopement Precautions

Information that appears in brackets has been added by the authors to clarify and enhance the use of nursing diagnoses.

CHAPTER 5

Health Conditions and Client Concerns With Associated Nursing Diagnoses

This chapter presents 460 disorders, health conditions, and life situations reflecting all specialty areas, with associated nursing diagnoses written as client problem/need statements that include the "related to" and "evidenced by" components.

This section will facilitate and help validate the assessment and diagnosis steps of the nursing process. Because the nursing process is perpetual and ongoing, other nursing diagnoses may be appropriate based on changing individual situations. Therefore, the nurse must continually assess, identify, and validate new client needs and evaluate subsequent care. Once the appropriate nursing diagnoses have been selected from this chapter, the reader may refer to Chapter 4, which lists the 217 NANDA diagnoses and review the diagnostic definition, defining characteristics, and related or risk factors for further validation. This step is necessary to determine if the nursing diagnosis is an accurate match, if more data are required, or if another diagnosis needs to be investigated.

To facilitate access to the health conditions or concerns and nursing diagnoses, the client needs have been listed alphabetically and coded to identify nursing specialty areas.

MS: Medical-Surgical
PED: Pediatric
OB: Obstetric
CH: Community/Home
PSY: Psychiatric/Behavioral
GYN: Gynecological

A separate category for geriatrics has not been made because geriatric concerns and conditions are actually subsumed under the other specialty areas, and elderly persons are susceptible to the majority of these problems.

Abdominal hysterectomy   MS
Refer to Hysterectomy

Abdominal perineal resection   MS
Also Refer to Surgery, general
disturbed Body Image may be related to presence of surgical wounds,
    possibly evidenced by verbalizations of feelings or perceptions, fear
    of reaction by others, preoccupation with change.
risk for Constipation: risk factors may include decreased physical ac-
    tivity, slowed gastric motility, abdominal muscle weakness, insuffi-
    cient fluid intake, change in usual foods and/or eating pattern.*
risk for Sexual Dysfunction: risk factors may include altered body struc-
    ture or function (radical resection, treatment procedures), vulnera-
    bility (psychological concern about response of significant other
    [SO](s), and disruption of sexual response pattern (e.g., erection dif-
    ficulty).*

Abortion, elective termination   OB
risk for decisional Conflict: risk factors may include unclear personal
    values/beliefs, lack of experience or interference with decision mak-
    ing, information from divergent sources, deficient support system.*
deficient Knowledge [Learning Need] regarding reproduction, contra-
    ception, self-care, Rh factor may be related to lack of exposure or
    recall, misinterpretation of information, possibly evidenced by re-
    quest for information, statement reflecting misconceptions, inaccu-
    rate follow-through of instructions, development of preventable com-
    plications.
risk for Moral Distress: risk factors may include perception of moral or
    ethical implications of therapeutic procedure, time constraints for
    decision making.*
Anxiety [specify level] may be related to situational or maturational
    crises, unmet needs, unconscious conflict about essential values or
    beliefs, possibly evidenced by increased tension, apprehension, fear
    of unspecific consequences, sympathetic stimulation, focus on self.
acute Pain/impaired Comfort may be related to aftereffects of proce-
    dure, drug effect, possibly evidenced by verbal report, distraction
    behaviors, changes in muscle tone, changes in vital signs.
risk for [maternal] Injury: risk factors may include surgical procedure,
    effects of anesthesia and medications.*

Abortion, spontaneous termination   OB
risk for Bleeding: risk factors may include pregnancy-related compli-
    cations.*
risk for Spiritual Distress: risk factors may include challenged beliefs/
    values, blame for loss directed at self or higher power.*
deficient Knowledge [Learning Need] regarding cause of abortion, self-
    care, contraception, future pregnancy may be related to lack of fa-
    miliarity with new self or healthcare needs, sources for support, pos-
    sibly evidenced by requests for information and statement of concern
    or misconceptions, development of preventable complications.

---

*A risk diagnosis is not evidenced by signs and symptoms, as the problem has
not occurred; rather, nursing interventions are directed at prevention.

Grieving related to perinatal loss, possibly evidenced by crying, expressions of sorrow, or changes in eating habits or sleep patterns.

risk for Sexual Dysfunction: risk factors may include increasing fear of pregnancy and/or repeat loss, impaired relationship with SO(s), self-doubt regarding own femininity.*

Abruptio placentae   OB

risk for Shock: risk factors may include hypotension, hypovolemia.*

Fear related to threat of death (perceived or actual) to fetus and self, possibly evidenced by verbalization of apprehension, increased tension, sympathetic stimulation.

acute Pain may be related to collection of blood between uterine wall and placenta, uterine contractions, possibly evidenced by verbal reports, abdominal guarding, muscle tension, or alterations in vital signs.

risk for disturbed Maternal-Fetal Dyad: risk factors may include complication of pregnancy, compromised oxygen transport.

Abscess, brain (acute)   MS

acute Pain may be related to inflammation, edema of tissues, possibly evidenced by reports of headache, restlessness, irritability, and moaning.

risk for Hyperthermia: risk factors may include illness [inflammatory process], hypermetabolic state, and dehydration.*

acute Confusion may be related to delirium [cerebral edema, altered perfusion, fever], possibly evidenced by fluctuation in cognition or level of consciousness, increased agitation, restlessness, hallucinations.

risk for Suffocation/Trauma: risk factors may include disease process [seizure activity], cognitive difficulties.*

Abscess, skin/tissue   CH/MS

impaired Skin/Tissue Integrity may be related to immunological deficit, infection, possibly evidenced by disruption of skin, destruction of skin layers or tissues, invasion of body structures.

risk for Infection [spread]: risk factors may include broken skin, traumatized tissues, chronic disease, malnutrition, insufficient knowledge.*

Abuse, physical   CH/PSY

Also Refer to Battered child syndrome

risk for Trauma: risk factors may include vulnerable client, recipient of verbal threats, history of physical abuse.*

Powerlessness may be related to interpersonal interactions, lifestyle of helplessness as evidenced by verbal expressions of having no control, reluctance to express true feelings, apathy, passivity.

chronic low Self-Esteem may be related to situational or maturational crisis, overwhelming threat to self, personal vulnerability, inadequate support systems, possibly evidenced by verbalized concern about ability to deal with current situation, chronic worry, anxiety,

---

*A risk diagnosis is not evidenced by signs and symptoms, as the problem has not occurred; rather, nursing interventions are directed at prevention.

depression, poor self-esteem, inability to problem-solve, high illness rate, destructive behavior toward self or others.

Sexual Dysfunction may be related to ineffectual or absent role model, vulnerability, physical abuse possibly evidenced by verbalizations, change in sexual behaviors or activities, inability to achieve desired satisfaction.

Abuse, psychological CH/PSY

ineffective Coping may be related to situational or maturational crisis, overwhelming threat to self, personal vulnerability, inadequate support systems, possibly evidenced by verbalized concern about ability to deal with current situation, chronic worry, anxiety, depression, poor self-esteem, inability to problem-solve, high illness rate, destructive behavior toward self or others.

Powerlessness may be related to abusive relationship, lifestyle of helplessness as evidenced by verbal expressions of having no control, reluctance to express true feelings, apathy, passivity.

Sexual Dysfunction may be related to ineffectual or absent role model, vulnerability, psychological abuse (harmful relationship) possibly evidenced by reported difficulties, inability to achieve desired satisfaction, conflicts involving values, seeking confirmation of desirability.

Achalasia (cardiospasm) MS

impaired Swallowing may be related to neuromuscular impairment, possibly evidenced by observed difficulty in swallowing or regurgitation.

imbalanced Nutrition: less than body requirements may be related to inability and/or reluctance to ingest adequate nutrients to meet metabolic demands and nutritional needs, possibly evidenced by reported or observed inadequate intake, weight loss, and pale conjunctiva and mucous membranes.

acute Pain may be related to spasm of the lower esophageal sphincter, possibly evidenced by reports of substernal pressure, recurrent heartburn, or gastric fullness (gas pains).

Anxiety [specify level]/Fear may be related to recurrent pain, choking sensation, altered health status, possibly evidenced by verbalizations of distress, apprehension, restlessness, or insomnia.

risk for Aspiration: risk factors may include regurgitation or spillover of esophageal contents.*

deficient Knowledge [Learning Need] regarding condition, prognosis, self-care, and treatment needs may be related to lack of familiarity with pathology and treatment of condition, possibly evidenced by requests for information, statement of concern, or development of preventable complications.

Acidosis, metabolic MS

Refer to Diabetic ketoacidosis

---

*A risk diagnosis is not evidenced by signs and symptoms, as the problem has not occurred; rather, nursing interventions are directed at prevention.

Acidosis, respiratory MS

Also Refer to underlying cause or condition

impaired Gas Exchange may be related to ventilation perfusion imbalance (decreased O_2-carrying capacity of blood, altered O_2 supply, alveolar-capillary membrane changes), possibly evidenced by dyspnea with exertion, tachypnea, changes in mentation, irritability, tachycardia, hypoxia, hypercapnia.

Acne CH/PED

impaired Skin Integrity may be related to secretions, infectious process as evidenced by disruptions of skin surface.

disturbed Body Image may be related to change in visual appearance as evidenced by fear of rejection of others, focus on past appearance, negative feelings about body, change in social involvement.

situational low Self-Esteem may be related to adolescence, negative perception of appearance as evidenced by self-negating verbalizations, expressions of helplessness.

Acoustic neuroma MS

Also Refer to Surgery, general

[disturbed auditory Sensory Perception] may be related to altered sensory reception (compression of eighth cranial nerve), possibly evidenced by unilateral sensorineural hearing loss, tinnitus.

risk for Falls: risk factors may include hearing difficulties, dizziness, sense of unsteadiness.*

Acquired immune deficiency syndrome CH

Refer to AIDS

Acromegaly CH

chronic Pain may be related to soft tissue swelling, joint degeneration, peripheral nerve compression possibly evidenced by verbal reports, altered ability to continue previous activities, changes in sleep pattern, fatigue.

disturbed Body Image may be related to biophysical illness or changes, possibly evidenced by verbalization of feelings, concerns, fear of rejection or of reaction of others, negative comments about body, actual change in structure or appearance, change in social involvement.

risk for Sexual Dysfunction: risk factors may include altered body structure, changes in libido.*

Acute respiratory distress syndrome MS

Refer to Respiratory distress syndrome, acute

Adams-Stokes syndrome CH

Refer to Dysrhythmia

ADD PED/PSY

Refer to Attention deficit disorder

---

*A risk diagnosis is not evidenced by signs and symptoms, as the problem has not occurred; rather, nursing interventions are directed at prevention.

Addiction   CH/PSY
Refer to specific substances; Substance dependence/abuse rehabilitation

Addison's disease   MS
deficient [hypotonic] Fluid Volume may be related to vomiting, diarrhea, increased renal losses, possibly evidenced by delayed capillary refill, poor skin turgor, dry mucous membranes, report of thirst.
risk for Electrolyte Imbalance: risk factors may include vomiting, diarrhea, endocrine dysfunction.*
decreased Cardiac Output may be related to hypovolemia and altered electrical conduction (dysrhythmias) and/or diminished cardiac muscle mass, possibly evidenced by alterations in vital signs, changes in mentation, and irregular pulse or pulse deficit.

CH

Fatigue may be related to decreased metabolic energy production, altered body chemistry (fluid, electrolyte, and glucose imbalance), possibly evidenced by unremitting, overwhelming lack of energy, inability to maintain usual routines, decreased performance, impaired ability to concentrate, lethargy, and disinterest in surroundings.
disturbed Body Image may be related to changes in skin pigmentation, mucous membranes, loss of axillary or pubic hair, possibly evidenced by verbalization of negative feelings about body and decreased social involvement.
risk for impaired physical Mobility: risk factors may include neuromuscular impairment (muscle wasting, weakness) and dizziness or syncope.*
imbalanced Nutrition: less than body requirements may be related to glucocorticoid deficiency; abnormal fat, protein, and carbohydrate metabolism; nausea, vomiting, anorexia, possibly evidenced by weight loss, muscle wasting, abdominal cramps, diarrhea, and severe hypoglycemia.
risk for impaired Home Maintenance: risk factors may include effects of disease process, impaired cognitive functioning, and inadequate support systems.*

Adenoidectomy   PED/MS
Refer to Tonsillectomy

Adjustment disorder   PED/PSY
Refer to Anxiety disorders—PED

Adoption/loss of child custody   PSY
risk for complicated Grieving: risk factors may include actual loss of child, expectations for future of child and self, thwarted grieving response to loss.*
risk for Powerlessness: risk factors may include perceived lack of options, no input into decision process, no control over outcome.*

---

*A risk diagnosis is not evidenced by signs and symptoms, as the problem has not occurred; rather, nursing interventions are directed at prevention.

Adrenal crisis, acute

Also Refer to Addison's disease; Shock
deficient [hypotonic] Fluid Volume may be related to failure of regulatory mechanism (damage to or suppression of adrenal gland), inability to concentrate urine, possibly evidenced by decreased venous filling and pulse volume and pressure, hypotension, dry mucous membranes, changes in mentation, decreased serum sodium.
acute Pain may be related to effects of disease process, metabolic imbalances, decreased tissue perfusion, possibly evidenced by reports of severe pain in abdomen, lower back, or legs.
impaired physical Mobility may be related to neuromuscular impairment, decreased muscle strength and control, possibly evidenced by generalized weakness, inability to perform desired activities or movements.
risk for Hyperthermia: risk factors may include presence of illness, infectious process, dehydration.*
risk for ineffective Protection: risk factors may include hormone deficiency, drug therapy, nutritional and metabolic deficiencies.*

Adrenalectomy MS
ineffective Tissue Perfusion (specify) may be related to hypovolemia and vascular pooling (vasodilation), possibly evidenced by diminished pulse, pallor or cyanosis, hypotension, and changes in mentation.
risk for Infection: risk factors may include inadequate primary defenses (incision, traumatized tissues), suppressed inflammatory response, invasive procedures.*
deficient Knowledge [Learning Need] regarding condition, prognosis, self-care and treatment needs may be related to unfamiliarity with long-term therapy requirements, possibly evidenced by request for information and statement of concern or misconceptions.

Adrenal insufficiency CH
Refer to Addison's disease

Affective disorder PSY
Refer to Bipolar disorder; Depressive disorders, major

Affective disorder, seasonal PSY
Also Refer to Depressive disorders, major
[intermittent] ineffective Coping may be related to situational crisis (fall or winter season), disturbance in pattern of tension release, and inadequate resources available, possibly evidenced by verbalizations of inability to cope, changes in sleep pattern (too little or too much), reports of lack of energy, fatigue, lack of resolution of problem, behavioral changes (irritability, discouragement).
risk for imbalanced Nutrition: more/less than body requirements: risk factors may include eating in response to internal cues other than hunger, alteration in usual coping patterns, change in usual activity level, decreased appetite, lack of energy or interest to prepare food.*

---

*A risk diagnosis is not evidenced by signs and symptoms, as the problem has not occurred; rather, nursing interventions are directed at prevention.

Agoraphobia PSY
Also Refer to Phobia

Anxiety [panic] may be related to contact with feared situation (public place, crowds), possibly evidenced by tachycardia, chest pain, dyspnea, gastrointestinal distress, faintness, sense of impending doom.

Agranulocytosis MS

risk for infection: risk factors may include suppressed inflammatory response.*

risk for impaired Oral Mucous Membrane: risk factors may include infection.*

risk for imbalanced Nutrition: less than body requirements: risk factors may include inability to ingest food or fluids (lesions of oral cavity).*

AIDS (acquired immunodeficiency syndrome) MS
Also Refer to HIV positive

risk for Infection [progression to sepsis/onset of new opportunistic infection]: risk factors may include depressed immune system, use of antimicrobial agents, inadequate primary defenses, broken skin, traumatized tissue, malnutrition, environmental exposure, invasive techniques, and chronic disease processes.*

risk for deficient Fluid Volume: risk factors may include excessive losses—copious diarrhea, profuse sweating, vomiting, hypermetabolic state or fever, and restricted intake (nausea, anorexia, lethargy).*

acute/chronic Pain may be related to tissue inflammation or destruction—infections; internal or external cutaneous lesions; rectal excoriation; malignancies; necrosis; peripheral neuropathies, myalgias, and arthralgias, possibly evidenced by verbal reports, self-focusing, or narrowed focus; alteration in muscle tone; paresthesias; paralysis; guarding behaviors; changes in vital signs (acute); restlessness.

risk for ineffective Breathing Pattern/impaired Gas Exchange: risk factors may include muscular impairment—wasting of respiratory musculature, decreased energy, fatigue, respiratory muscle fatigue; retained secretions—tracheobronchial obstruction; pain.*

CH

imbalanced Nutrition: less than body requirements may be related to altered ability to ingest, digest, and/or absorb nutrients (nausea, vomiting, hyperactive gag reflex, gastrointestinal disturbances, fatigue); increased metabolic rate and nutritional needs (fever, infection); possibly evidenced by weight loss, decreased subcutaneous fat and muscle mass, lack of interest in food, aversion to eating, altered taste sensation, abdominal cramping, hyperactive bowel sounds, diarrhea, sore and inflamed buccal cavity, abnormal laboratory results—vitamin, mineral, and protein deficiencies; electrolyte imbalances.

Fatigue may be related to decreased metabolic energy production, increased energy requirements (hypermetabolic state), overwhelming psychological or emotional demands, altered body chemistry (side effects of medication, chemotherapy), sleep deprivation possibly ev-

---

*A risk diagnosis is not evidenced by signs and symptoms, as the problem has not occurred; rather, nursing interventions are directed at prevention.

idenced by unremitting or overwhelming lack of energy, inability to maintain usual routines, decreased performance, impaired ability to concentrate, lethargy, listlessness, and disinterest in surroundings.

<u>ineffective Protection</u> may be related to chronic disease affecting immune and neurological systems, inadequate nutrition, drug therapies, possibly evidenced by deficient immunity, impaired healing, neurosensory alterations, maladaptive stress response, fatigue, anorexia, disorientation.

PSY

<u>Social Isolation</u> may be related to alteration in physical appearance or mental status, altered state of wellness, perceptions of unacceptable social behavior or values, [phobic fear of others (transmission of disease)], possibly evidenced by expressed feelings of aloneness or rejection, absence of supportive SO(s), and withdrawal from usual activities.

<u>chronic Confusion</u> may be related to physiological changes (hypoxemia, central nervous system [CNS] infection by HIV, brain malignancies, and/or disseminated systemic opportunistic infection), altered drug metabolism or excretion, accumulation of toxic elements (renal failure, severe electrolyte imbalance, hepatic insufficiency), possibly evidenced by clinical evidence of organic impairment, altered response to stimuli, memory deficit, and altered personality.

AIDS dementia CH

Also Refer to Dementia, presenile/senile

<u>impaired Environmental Interpretation Syndrome</u> may be related to dementia, depression, possibly evidenced by consistent disorientation, inability to follow simple directions, loss of social functioning from memory decline.

<u>ineffective Protection</u> may be related to immune disorder, inadequate nutrition, drug therapies, possibly evidenced by deficient immunity, impaired healing, neurosensory alterations, maladaptive stress response, fatigue, anorexia, disorientation.

Alcohol abuse/withdrawal CH/MS/PSY

Refer to Drug overdose, acute [depressants]; Delirium tremens; Substance dependency/abuse rehabilitation

Alcohol intoxication, acute MS

Also Refer to Delirium tremens

<u>acute Confusion</u> may be related to substance abuse, hypoxemia, possibly evidenced by hallucinations, exaggerated emotional response, fluctuation in cognition or level of consciousness, increased agitation.

<u>risk for ineffective Breathing Pattern</u>: risk factors may include hypoventilation syndrome, neuromuscular dysfunction, fatigue.*

<u>risk for Aspiration</u>: risk factors may include reduced level of consciousness, depressed cough or gag reflexes, delayed gastric emptying.*

---

*A risk diagnosis is not evidenced by signs and symptoms, as the problem has not occurred; rather, nursing interventions are directed at prevention.

Alcoholism   **CH**
Refer to Substance dependency/abuse rehabilitation

Aldosteronism, primary   **MS**
deficient Fluid Volume may be related to increased urinary losses, possibly evidenced by dry mucous membranes, poor skin turgor, dilute urine, excessive thirst, weight loss.
impaired physical Mobility may be related to neuromuscular impairment, decreased muscle strength, and pain, possibly evidenced by limited range of motion, slowed movement, limited ability to perform gross/fine motor skills.
risk for decreased Cardiac Output: risk factors may include hypovolemia and altered heart rhythm.*

Alkalosis, metabolic   **MS**
Refer to underlying cause or condition, e.g., Renal dialysis

Alkalosis, respiratory   **MS**
Also Refer to underlying cause or condition
impaired Gas Exchange may be related to ventilation-perfusion imbalance (decreased O_2 carrying capacity of blood, altered O_2 supply, alveolar-capillary membrane changes), possibly evidenced by dyspnea, tachypnea, changes in mentation, tachycardia, hypoxia, hypocapnia.

Allergies, seasonal   **CH**
Refer to Hay fever

Alopecia   **CH**
disturbed Body Image may be related to effects of illness or therapy, aging process, change in appearance, possibly evidenced by verbalization of feelings, concerns, fear of rejection or reaction of others, focus on past appearance, preoccupation with change, feelings of helplessness.

ALS   **CH**
Refer to Amyotrophic lateral sclerosis

Alzheimer's disease   **CH**
Also Refer to Dementia, presenile/senile
risk for Injury/Trauma: risk factors may include inability to recognize or identify danger in environment, disorientation, confusion, impaired judgment, weakness, muscular incoordination, balancing difficulties, altered perception, and seizure activity.*
chronic Confusion related to physiological changes (neuronal degeneration), possibly evidenced by inaccurate interpretation of or response to stimuli, progressive or long-standing cognitive impairment, short-term memory deficit, impaired socialization, altered personality, and clinical evidence of organic impairment.
[disturbed Sensory Perception (specify)] may be related to altered sensory reception, transmission, and/or integration (neurological disease-

---

*A risk diagnosis is not evidenced by signs and symptoms, as the problem has not occurred; rather, nursing interventions are directed at prevention.

or deficit), socially restricted environment (homebound, institution-alized), sleep deprivation, possibly evidenced by changes in usual response to stimuli, change in problem-solving abilities, exaggerated emotional responses (anxiety, paranoia, hallucinations), inability to tell position of body parts, diminished or altered sense of taste.

Sleep Deprivation may be related to sensory impairment, changes in activity patterns, psychological stress (neurological impairment), possibly evidenced by wakefulness, disorientation (day/night rever-sal), increased aimless wandering, inability to identify need or time for sleeping, changes in behavior, lethargy; dark circles under eyes and frequent yawning.

ineffective Health Maintenance may be related to deterioration affecting ability in all areas, including coordination and communication, cog-nitive impairment, ineffective individual/family coping, possibly ev-idenced by reported or observed inability to take responsibility for meeting basic health practices, lack of equipment, financial, or other resources, and impairment of personal support system.

PSY

risk for Stress Overload: risk factors may include inadequate resources, chronic illness, physical demands, threats of violence.*

compromised family Coping/Caregiver Role Strain may be related to disruptive behavior of client, family grief about their helplessness watching loved one deteriorate, prolonged disease or disability pro-gression that exhausts the supportive capacity of SO or family, highly ambivalent family relationships,

risk for Relocation Stress Syndrome: risk factors may include little or no preparation for transfer to a new setting, changes in daily routine, sensory impairment, physical deterioration, separation from support systems.*

Amphetamine abuse **PSY**
Refer to Stimulant abuse

Amputation **MS**
risk for ineffective peripheral Tissue Perfusion: risk factors may include reduced arterial or venous blood flow, tissue edema, hematoma for-mation, hypovolemia.*

acute Pain may be related to tissue and nerve trauma, psychological impact of loss of body part, possibly evidenced by reports of inci-sional or phantom pain, observed guarding or protective behavior, narrowed focus or self-focus, and changes in vital signs.

impaired physical Mobility may be related to loss of limb (primarily lower extremity), altered sense of balance, pain, or discomfort, pos-sibly evidenced by reluctance to attempt movement; impaired co-ordination; decreased muscle strength, control, and mass.

situational low Self-Esteem may be related to loss of a body part, change in functional abilities, possibly evidenced by verbalization of feelings of powerlessness, grief, preoccupation with loss, negative feelings about body, focus on past strength, function, or appearance;

---

*A risk diagnosis is not evidenced by signs and symptoms, as the problem has not occurred; rather, nursing interventions are directed at prevention.

change in usual patterns of responsibility or physical capacity to resume role, fear of rejection or reaction by others, and unwillingness to look at or touch residual limb.

Amyotrophic lateral sclerosis (ALS)   MS

impaired physical Mobility may be related to muscle wasting, weakness, possibly evidenced by impaired coordination, limited range of motion, and impaired purposeful movement.

ineffective Breathing Pattern/impaired spontaneous Ventilation may be related to neuromuscular impairment, decreased energy, fatigue, tracheobronchial obstruction, possibly evidenced by shortness of breath, fremitus, respiratory depth changes, and reduced vital capacity.

impaired Swallowing may be related to muscle wasting and fatigue, possibly evidenced by recurrent coughing or choking, and signs of aspiration.

PSY

Powerlessness [specify level] may be related to chronic and debilitating nature of illness, lack of control over outcome, possibly evidenced by expressions of frustration about inability to care for self and depression over physical deterioration.

Grieving may be related to perceived potential loss of self and physiopsychosocial well-being, possibly evidenced by sorrow, choked feelings, expression of distress, changes in eating habits, sleeping patterns, and altered communication patterns or libido.

CH

impaired verbal Communication may be related to physical barrier (neuromuscular impairment), possibly evidenced by impaired articulation, inability to speak in sentences, and use of nonverbal cues (changes in facial expression).

risk for Caregiver Role Strain: risk factors may include illness severity of care receiver, complexity and amount of home-care needs, duration of caregiving required, caregiver is spouse, family/caregiver isolation, lack of respite or recreation for caregiver.*

Anaphylaxis   CH
Also Refer to Shock

ineffective Airway Clearance may be related to airway spasm (bronchial), laryngeal edema, possibly evidenced by diminished breath sounds, presence of adventitious sounds, cough ineffective or absent, difficulty vocalizing, wide-eyed.

decreased Cardiac Output may be related to decreased preload, increased capillary permeability (third spacing) and vasodilation, possibly evidenced by tachycardia, palpitations, changes in blood pressure (BP), anxiety, restlessness.

Anemia   CH
Activity Intolerance may be related to imbalance between O_2 supply (delivery) and demand, possibly evidenced by reports of fatigue and

---

*A risk diagnosis is not evidenced by signs and symptoms, as the problem has not occurred; rather, nursing interventions are directed at prevention.

weakness, abnormal heart rate or BP response, decreased exercise or activity level, and exertional discomfort or dyspnea.

imbalanced Nutrition: less than body requirements may be related to failure to ingest or inability to digest food or absorb nutrients necessary for formation of normal red blood cells (RBCs), possibly evidenced by weight loss or weight below normal for age, height, and body build; decreased triceps skinfold measurement, changes in gums or oral mucous membranes, decreased tolerance for activity, weakness, and loss of muscle tone.

deficient Knowledge [Learning Need] regarding condition, prognosis, self-care and treatment needs may be related to inadequate understanding or misinterpretation of dietary and physiological needs, possibly evidenced by inadequate dietary intake, request for information, and development of preventable complications.

Anemia, iron-deficiency   CH

Also Refer to Anemia

Fatigue may be related to anemia, malnutrition, possibly evidenced by feeling tired, inability to maintain usual routines or level of physical activity.

risk for deficient Fluid Volume: risk factors may include active or chronic blood loss.*

risk for impaired Oral Mucous Membrane: risk factors may include dehydration, malnutrition, vitamin deficiency.*

Anemia, sickle cell   MS

impaired Gas Exchange may be related to decreased O_2-carrying capacity of blood, reduced RBC life span or premature destruction, abnormal RBC structure, increased blood viscosity, pulmonary congestion—impairment of surface phagocytosis; predisposition to bacterial pneumonia/pulmonary infarcts, possibly evidenced by dyspnea, use of accessory muscles, cyanosis or signs of hypoxia, tachycardia, changes in mentation, and restlessness.

ineffective Tissue Perfusion: [specify] may be related to stasis, vaso-occlusive nature of sickling, inflammatory response, atrioventricular shunts in pulmonary and peripheral circulation, myocardial damage (small infarcts, iron deposits, fibrosis), possibly evidenced by signs and symptoms dependent on system involved, such as renal (decreased specific gravity and pale urine in face of dehydration), cerebral (paralysis and visual disturbances), peripheral (distal ischemia, tissue infarctions, ulcerations, bone pain), or cardiac (angina, palpitations).

CH

acute/chronic Pain may be related to intravascular sickling with localized vascular stasis, occlusion, infarction or necrosis and deprivation of O_2 and nutrients, accumulation of noxious metabolites, possibly evidenced by reports of localized, generalized, or migratory joint and/or abdominal or back pain, guarding and distraction behaviors

---

*A risk diagnosis is not evidenced by signs and symptoms, as the problem has not occurred; rather, nursing interventions are directed at prevention.

(moaning, crying, restlessness), facial grimacing, narrowed focus, and changes in vital signs.

deficient Knowledge [Learning Need] regarding disease process, genetic factors, prognosis, self-care and treatment needs may be related to lack of exposure or recall, misinterpretation of information, unfamiliarity with resources, possibly evidenced by questions, statement of concern or misconceptions, exacerbation of condition, inadequate follow-through of therapy instructions, and development of preventable complications.

risk for sedentary Lifestyle: risk factors may include lack of interest or motivation, lack of resources, lack of training or knowledge of specific exercise needs, safety concerns or fear of injury.*

PED

delayed Growth and Development may be related to effects and limitations of physical condition, possibly evidenced by altered physical growth and delay or difficulty performing skills typical of age group.

compromised family Coping may be related to chronic nature of disease and disability, family disorganization, presence of other crises or situations impacting significant person/parent, lifestyle restrictions, possibly evidenced by SO expressing preoccupation with own reaction and displaying protective behavior disproportionate to client's ability or need for autonomy.

Aneurysm, abdominal aortic (AAA)　　MS
Refer to Aortic aneurysm, abdominal

Aneurysm, cerebral　　MS
Refer to Cerebrovascular accident

Aneurysm, ventricular　　MS

decreased Cardiac Output may be related to altered stroke volume, changes in heart rate or rhythm, possibly evidenced by dyspnea, adventitious breath sounds, S_3/S_4 heart sounds, changes in hemodynamic measurements, dysrhythmias.

ineffective Tissue Perfusion [specify] may be related to decreased arterial blood flow, possibly evidenced by BP changes, diminished pulses, edema, dyspnea, dysrhythmias, altered mental status, decreased renal function.

Activity Intolerance may be related to imbalance between oxygen supply and demand, possibly evidenced by weakness, fatigue, abnormal heart rate/BP response to activity, electrocardiogram changes (dysrhythmias, ischemia).

Angina pectoris　　MS

acute Pain may be related to decreased myocardial blood flow, increased cardiac workload/O_2 consumption, possibly evidenced by verbal reports, narrowed focus, distraction behaviors (restlessness, moaning), and autonomic responses (diaphoresis, changes in vital signs).

---

*A risk diagnosis is not evidenced by signs and symptoms, as the problem has not occurred; rather, nursing interventions are directed at prevention.

risk for decreased Cardiac Output: risk factors may include inotropic changes (transient or prolonged myocardial ischemia, effects of medications), alterations in rate, rhythm and electrical conduction, possibly evidenced by changes in hemodynamic readings, dyspnea, restlessness, decreased tolerance for activity, fatigue, diminished peripheral pulses, cool or pale skin, changes in mental status, and continued chest pain.*

Anxiety [specify level] may be related to situational crises, change in health status and/or threat of death, negative self-talk, possibly evidenced by verbalized apprehension, expressed concerns, association of condition with loss of abilities, facial tension, extraneous movements, and focus on self.

CH

Activity Intolerance may be related to imbalance between O_2 supply and demand, possibly evidenced by exertional dyspnea, abnormal pulse or BP response to activity, and electrocardiogram (ECG) changes.

deficient Knowledge [Learning Need] regarding condition, prognosis, self-care and treatment needs may be related to lack of exposure, inaccurate or misinterpretation of information, possibly evidenced by questions, request for information, statement of concern, and inaccurate follow-through of instructions.

risk for sedentary Lifestyle: risk factors may include lack of training or knowledge of specific exercise needs, safety concerns, fear of myocardial injury.*

risk for risk-prone Health Behavior: risk factors may include condition requiring long-term therapy, changes in lifestyle, multiple stressors, assault to self-concept, and altered locus of control.*

Anorexia nervosa   **MS**

imbalanced Nutrition: less than body requirements may be related to psychological restrictions of food intake and/or excessive activity, laxative abuse, possibly evidenced by weight loss, poor skin turgor, decreased muscle tone, denial of hunger, unusual hoarding or handling of food, amenorrhea, electrolyte imbalance, cardiac irregularities, hypotension.

risk for deficient Fluid Volume: risk factors may include inadequate intake of food and liquids, chronic or excessive laxative or diuretic use.*

PSY

disturbed Body Image/chronic low Self-Esteem may be related to perceptual developmental changes, possibly evidenced by verbalized perceptions reflecting altered view of body appearance, refusal to verify actual change.

chronic low Self-Esteem may be related to lack of approval, repeated negative reinforcement, perceived lack of respect from others possibly evidenced by reports feelings of shame or guilt; overly conforming, dependent on others' opinions.

---

*A risk diagnosis is not evidenced by signs and symptoms, as the problem has not occurred; rather, nursing interventions are directed at prevention.

impaired Parenting may be related to issues of control in family, situational or maturational crises, history of inadequate coping methods possibly evidenced by enmeshed family, dissonance among family members, focus on "identified patient," family developmental tasks not being met, family members acting as enablers, ill-defined family rules, functions, or roles.

Antisocial personality disorder   PSY

risk for other-directed Violence: risk factors may include contempt for authority or rights of others, inability to tolerate frustration, need for immediate gratification, easy agitation, vulnerable self-concept, inability to verbalize feelings, use of maladjusted coping mechanisms, history of substance abuse.*

ineffective Coping may be related to very low tolerance for external stress, lack of experience of internal anxiety (e.g., guilt, shame), personal vulnerability, unmet expectations, multiple life changes, possibly evidenced by choice of aggression and manipulation to handle problems or conflicts, inappropriate use of defense mechanisms (e.g., denial, projection), chronic worry, anxiety, destructive behaviors, high rate of accidents.

chronic low Self-Esteem may be related to lack of positive and/or repeated negative feedback, unmet dependency needs, retarded ego development, dysfunctional family system, possibly evidenced by acting-out behaviors (e.g., substance abuse, sexual promiscuity, feelings of inadequacy, nonparticipation in therapy).

compromised/disabled family Coping may be related to family disorganization or role changes, highly ambivalent family relationships, client providing little support in turn for the primary person(s), history of abuse or neglect in the home, possibly evidenced by expressions of concern or complaints, preoccupation of primary person with own reactions to situation, display of protective behaviors disproportionate to client's abilities, or need for autonomy.

impaired Social Interaction may be related to inadequate personal resources (shallow feelings), immature interests, underdeveloped conscience, unaccepted social values, possibly evidenced by difficulty meeting expectations of others, lack of belief that rules pertain to self, sense of emptiness or inadequacy covered by expressions of self-conceit, arrogance, or contempt; behavior unaccepted by dominant cultural group.

Anxiety disorder, generalized   PSY

Anxiety [specify level]/Powerlessness may be related to real or perceived threat to physical integrity or self-concept (may or may not be able to identify the threat), unconscious conflict about essential values or beliefs and goals of life, unmet needs, negative self-talk, possibly evidenced by sympathetic stimulation, extraneous movements (foot shuffling, hand or arm fidgeting, rocking movements, restlessness), persistent feelings of apprehension and uneasiness, a general anxious feeling that client has difficulty alleviating, poor eye

---

*A risk diagnosis is not evidenced by signs and symptoms, as the problem has not occurred; rather, nursing interventions are directed at prevention.

contact, focus on self, impaired functioning, free-floating anxiety, and nonparticipation in decision making.

ineffective Coping may be related to level of anxiety being experienced by the client, personal vulnerability, unmet expectations or unrealistic perceptions, inadequate coping methods and/or support systems, possibly evidenced by verbalization of inability to cope or problem-solve, excessive compulsive behaviors (e.g., smoking, drinking), and emotional or muscle tension, alteration in societal participation, high rate of accidents.

Insomnia may be related to stress, repetitive thoughts, possibly evidenced by reports of difficulty in falling/staying asleep, dissatisfaction with sleep, nonrestorative sleep, lack of energy.

risk for compromised family Coping: risk factors may include inadequate or incorrect information or understanding by a primary person, temporary family disorganization and role changes, prolonged disability that exhausts the supportive capacity of SO(s).*

impaired Social Interaction/Social Isolation may be related to low self-concept, inadequate personal resources, misinterpretation of internal or external stimuli, hypervigilance, possibly evidenced by discomfort in social situations, withdrawal from or reported change in pattern of interactions, dysfunctional interactions, expressed feelings of difference from others, sad, dull affect.

Anxiety disorders   PED/PSY

[severe/panic] Anxiety may be related to situational or maturational crisis, internal transmission and contagion, threat to physical integrity or self-concept, unmet needs, dysfunctional family system, independence conflicts possibly evidenced by somatic complaints, nightmares, excessive psychomotor activity, refusal to attend school, persistent worry or fear of catastrophic doom to family or self.

ineffective Coping may be related to situational or maturational crisis, multiple life changes or losses, personal vulnerability, lack of self-confidence possibly evidenced by inability to problem-solve, persistent or overwhelming fears, inability to meet role expectations, social inhibition, panic attacks.

impaired Social Interaction may be related to excessive self-consciousness, inability to interact with unfamiliar people, altered thought processes possibly evidenced by verbalized or observed discomfort in social situations, inability to receive or communicate a satisfying sense of belonging, caring, or interest; use of unsuccessful social interaction behaviors.

risk for Self-Mutilation/self-directed Violence: risk factors may include panic states, dysfunctional family, history of self-destructive behaviors, emotional disturbance, increasing motor activity.*

compromised/disabled family Coping may be related to situational or developmental crisis (e.g., divorce, addition to the family), unrealistic parental expectations, frequent disruptions in living arrangements, high-risk family situations (neglect or abuse, substance abuse), possibly evidenced by SO reports of frustration with clinging

---

*A risk diagnosis is not evidenced by signs and symptoms, as the problem has not occurred; rather, nursing interventions are directed at prevention.

behaviors, emotional lability, harsh or punitive response to tyrannical behaviors, disproportionate protective behaviors.

Anxiolytic abuse   PSY
Refer to Depressant abuse

Aortic aneurysm, abdominal (AAA)   MS
risk for ineffective Renal Perfusion: risk factors may include hypertension, hypovolemia, hypoxia.*
risk for Infection: risk factors may include turbulent blood flow through arteriosclerotic lesion.*
acute Pain may be related to physical agent [vascular enlargement—dissection or rupture], possibly evidenced by verbal/coded reports, guarding behavior, facial mask, change in vital signs.

Aortic aneurysm repair, abdominal   MS
Also Refer to Surgery, general
Anxiety related to change in health status, threat of death, surgical intervention, possibly evidenced by expressed concerns, apprehension, increased tension, changes in vital signs.
risk for Bleeding: risk factors may include aneurysm, treatment-related side effects—surgery, failure of vascular repair.*
risk for ineffective Renal Perfusion/peripheral Tissue Perfusion: risk factors may include hypertension, treatment-related side effects—surgery, hypovolemia, hypoxia.*

Aortic stenosis   MS
decreased Cardiac Output may be related to altered contractility, altered preload or afterload possibly evidenced by fatigue, dyspnea, changes in vital signs, jugular vein distension, increased central venous pressure (CVP)/PAWP, and syncope.
risk for impaired Gas Exchange: risk factors may include alveolar-capillary membrane changes.*

                                                                         CH
risk for acute Pain: risk factors may include physical agent [episodic ischemia of myocardial tissues and stretching of left atrium].*
Activity Intolerance may be related to imbalance between O_2 supply and demand [decreased or fixed cardiac output], possibly evidenced by exertional dyspnea, reported fatigue or weakness, and abnormal BP or ECG changes or dysrhythmias in response to activity.

Aplastic anemia   CH
Also Refer to Anemia
risk for ineffective Protection: risk factors may include abnormal blood profile (leukopenia, thrombocytopenia), drug therapies (antineoplastics, antibiotics, nonsteroidal anti-inflammatory drugs, anticonvulsants).*
Fatigue may be related to anemia, disease states, malnutrition, possibly evidenced by verbalization of overwhelming lack of energy, inability

---

*A risk diagnosis is not evidenced by signs and symptoms, as the problem has not occurred; rather, nursing interventions are directed at prevention.

to maintain usual routines or level of physical activity, tired, compromised libido, lethargy, increase in physical complaints.

Appendicitis   MS

acute Pain may be related to physical agent [distention of intestinal tissues/inflammation], possibly evidenced by verbal reports, guarding behavior, narrowed focus, and diaphoresis, changes in vital signs.

risk for deficient Fluid Volume: risk factors may include excessive losses through normal routes (vomiting), deviations affecting intake of fluids (nausea, anorexia), and factors influencing fluid needs (hypermetabolic state).*

risk for Infection: risk factors may include tissue destruction [release of pathogenic organisms into peritoneal cavity].*

ARDS   MS

Refer to Respiratory distress syndrome, acute

Arrhythmia, cardiac   MS/CH

Refer to Dysrhythmia, cardiac

Arterial occlusive disease, peripheral   CH

ineffective peripheral Tissue Perfusion may be related to deficient knowledge of disease process, hypertension, smoking, sedentary lifestyle, possibly evidenced by altered skin characteristics, diminished pulses, claudication, delayed peripheral wound healing.

risk for impaired Walking: risk factors may include limited endurance, pain.*

risk for impaired Skin/Tissue Integrity: risk factors may include altered circulation or sensation.*

Arthritis, juvenile rheumatoid   PED/CH

Also Refer to Arthritis, rheumatoid

risk for delayed Development: risk factors may include chronic illness, effects of required therapy.*

risk for Social Isolation: risk factors may include delay in accomplishing developmental task, altered state of wellness, and alterations in physical appearance.*

Arthritis, rheumatoid   CH

acute/chronic Pain may be related to accumulation of fluid, inflammatory process, degeneration of joint, and deformity, possibly evidenced by verbal reports, narrowed focus, guarding or protective behaviors, and physical and social withdrawal.

impaired physical Mobility/Walking may be related to musculoskeletal deformity, pain or discomfort, decreased muscle strength, possibly evidenced by limited range of motion, impaired coordination, reluctance to attempt movement, and decreased muscle strength, control, and mass.

Self-Care Deficit [specify] may be related to musculoskeletal impairment, decreased strength and endurance, limited range of motion,

---

*A risk diagnosis is not evidenced by signs and symptoms, as the problem has not occurred; rather, nursing interventions are directed at prevention.

pain on movement, possibly evidenced by inability to manage activities of daily living (ADLs).

disturbed Body Image/ineffective Role Performance may be related to change in body structure or function, impaired mobility or ability to perform usual tasks, focus on past strength, function, or appearance, possibly evidenced by negative self-talk, feelings of helplessness, change in lifestyle or physical abilities, dependence on others for assistance, decreased social involvement.

Arthritis, septic   CH

acute Pain may be related to joint inflammation, possibly evidenced by verbal or coded reports, guarding behaviors, restlessness, narrowed focus.

impaired physical Mobility may be related to joint stiffness, pain or discomfort, reluctance to initiate movement, possibly evidenced by limited range of motion, slowed movement.

Self-Care Deficit [specify] may be related to musculoskeletal impairment, pain or discomfort, decreased strength, impaired coordination, possibly evidenced by inability to perform desired ADLs.

risk for Infection [spread]: risk factors may include presence of infectious process, chronic disease states, invasive procedures.*

Arthroplasty   MS

risk for Infection: risk factors may include breach of primary defenses (surgical incision), stasis of body fluids at operative site, and altered inflammatory response.*

risk for Bleeding: risk factors may include surgical procedure, trauma to vascular area.*

impaired physical Mobility may be related to decreased strength, pain, musculoskeletal changes, possibly evidenced by impaired coordination and reluctance to attempt movement.

acute Pain may be related to tissue trauma, local edema, possibly evidenced by verbal reports, narrowed focus, guarded movement, and diaphoresis, changes in vital signs.

Arthroscopy, knee   MS

deficient Knowledge [Learning Need] regarding procedure, outcomes, and self-care needs may be related to unfamiliarity with information or resources, misinterpretations, possibly evidenced by questions and requests for information, misconceptions.

risk for impaired Walking: risk factors may include joint stiffness, discomfort, prescribed movement restrictions, use of assistive devices (crutches) for ambulation.*

Asperger's disorder   PED/PSY

impaired Social Interaction may be related to skill deficit about ways to enhance mutuality, communication barriers (poor pragmatic language skills), compulsions, repetitive motor mannerisms, possibly evidenced by observed discomfort in social situations, dysfunctional interactions with others, inability to receive or communicate satisfying sense of belonging.

---

*A risk diagnosis is not evidenced by signs and symptoms, as the problem has not occurred; rather, nursing interventions are directed at prevention.

risk for delayed Development: risk factors may include behavior disorders, lack of eye contact, doesn't pick up on social cues, trouble
with sensory integration.*

impaired Parenting may be related to developmental delay of child,
deficient knowledge of child development, lack of social supports.

risk for Injury: risk factors may include rituals, repetitive motor mannerisms, poor coordination, vulnerability to manipulation of peers.*

Asthma MS
Also Refer to Emphysema

ineffective Airway Clearance may be related to increased production
and retained pulmonary secretions, bronchospasm, decreased energy,
fatigue, possibly evidenced by wheezing, difficulty breathing,
changes in depth and rate of respirations, use of accessory muscles,
and persistent ineffective cough with or without sputum production.

impaired Gas Exchange may be related to altered delivery of inspired
O_2 and air trapping, possibly evidenced by dyspnea, restlessness,
reduced tolerance for activity, cyanosis, and changes in arterial blood
gases (ABGs) and vital signs.

Anxiety [specify level] may be related to perceived threat of death,
possibly evidenced by apprehension, fearful expression, and extraneous movements.

CH

Activity Intolerance may be related to imbalance between O_2 supply
and demand, possibly evidenced by fatigue and exertional dyspnea.

risk for Contamination: risk factors may include presence of atmospheric pollutants, environmental contaminants in the home (e.g.,
smoking or secondhand tobacco smoke).

Athlete's foot CH
impaired Skin Integrity may be related to fungal invasion, humidity,
secretions, possibly evidenced by disruption of skin surface, reports
of painful itching.

risk for Infection [spread]: risk factors may include multiple breaks in
skin, exposure to moist and warm environment.*

Atrial fibrillation CH
Also Refer to Dysrhythmias

Activity Intolerance may be related to imbalance between oxygen supply and demand possibly evidenced by dyspnea, dizziness, presyn-
cope or syncopal episodes.

risk for ineffective cerebral Tissue Perfusion: risk factors may include
arterial fibrillation, embolism, thrombolytic therapy (microemboli).*

Atrial flutter CH
Refer to Dysrhythmias

Atrial tachycardia CH
Refer to Dysrhythmias

---

*A risk diagnosis is not evidenced by signs and symptoms, as the problem has
not occurred; rather, nursing interventions are directed at prevention.

Attention deficit disorder (ADD)   PED/PSY

ineffective Coping may be related to situational or maturational crisis, retarded ego development, low self-concept, possibly evidenced by easy distraction by extraneous stimuli, shifting between uncompleted activities.

chronic low Self-Esteem may be related to retarded ego development, lack of positive or repeated negative feedback, negative role models, possibly evidenced by lack of eye contact, derogatory self-comments, hesitance to try new tasks, inadequate level of confidence.

deficient Knowledge [Learning Need] regarding condition, prognosis, therapy may be related to misinformation or misinterpretations, un-familiarity with resources, possibly evidenced by verbalization of problems or misconceptions, poor school performance, unrealistic expectations of medication regimen.

Autistic disorder   PED/PSY

impaired Social Interaction may be related to abnormal response to sensory input or inadequate sensory stimulation, organic brain dys-function, delayed development of secure attachment or trust, lack of intuitive skills to comprehend and accurately respond to social cues, disturbance in self-concept, possibly evidenced by lack of respon-siveness to others, lack of eye contact or facial responsiveness, treat-ing persons as objects, lack of awareness of feelings in others, in-difference or aversion to comfort, affection, or physical contact, failure to develop cooperative social play and peer friendships in childhood.

impaired verbal Communication may be related to inability to trust others, withdrawal into self, organic brain dysfunction, abnormal in-terpretation or response to and/or inadequate sensory stimulation, possibly evidenced by lack of interactive communication mode, no use of gestures or spoken language, absent or abnormal nonverbal communication, lack of eye contact or facial expression, peculiar patterns of speech (form, content, or speech production), and im-paired ability to initiate or sustain conversation despite adequate speech.

risk for Self-Mutilation: risk factors may include organic brain dys-function, inability to trust others, disturbance in self-concept, inad-equate sensory stimulation or abnormal response to sensory input (sensory overload), history of physical, emotional, or sexual abuse, and response to demands of therapy, realization of severity of con-dition.*

disturbed Personal Identity may be related to organic brain dysfunction, lack of development of trust, maternal deprivation, fixation at pre-symbiotic phase of development, possibly evidenced by lack of awareness of the feelings or existence of others, increased anxiety resulting from physical contact with others, absent or impaired imi-tation of others, repeating what others say, persistent preoccupation with parts of objects, obsessive attachment to objects, marked dis-tress over changes in environment, autoerotic or ritualistic behaviors, self-touching, rocking, swaying.

---

*A risk diagnosis is not evidenced by signs and symptoms, as the problem has not occurred; rather, nursing interventions are directed at prevention.

compromised/disabled family Coping may be related to family members unable to express feelings; excessive guilt, anger, or blaming among family members regarding child's condition; ambivalent or dissonant family relationships; prolonged coping with problem exhausting supportive ability of family members, possibly evidenced by denial of existence or severity of disturbed behaviors, preoccupation with personal emotional reaction to situation, rationalization that problem will be outgrown, attempts to intervene with child are achieving increasingly ineffective results, family withdraws from or becomes overly protective of child.

Barbiturate abuse   CH/PSY
Refer to Depressant abuse

Battered child syndrome   PED/CH
Also Refer to Abuse

risk for Trauma: risk factors may include dependent position in relationship(s), vulnerability (e.g., congenital problems, chronic illness), history of previous abuse or neglect, lack of or nonuse of support systems by caregiver(s).*

interrupted Family Processes/impaired Parenting may be related to poor role model, unrealistic expectations, presence of stressors, and lack of support, possibly evidenced by verbalization of negative feelings, inappropriate caretaking behaviors, and evidence of physical or psychological trauma to child.

                                                      PSY
chronic low Self-Esteem may be related to deprivation and negative feedback of family members, personal vulnerability, feelings of abandonment, possibly evidenced by lack of eye contact, withdrawal from social contacts, discounting own needs, nonassertive or passive, indecisive or overly conforming behaviors.

Post-Trauma Syndrome may be related to sustained or recurrent physical or emotional abuse; possibly evidenced by acting-out behavior, development of phobias, poor impulse control, and emotional numbness.

ineffective Coping may be related to situational or maturational crisis, overwhelming threat to self, personal vulnerability, inadequate support systems, possibly evidenced by verbalized concern about ability to deal with current situation, chronic worry, anxiety, depression, poor self-esteem, inability to problem-solve, high illness rate, destructive behavior toward self or others.

Benign prostatic hyperplasia   CH/MS
[acute/chronic] Urinary Retention/overflow urinary Incontinence may be related to mechanical obstruction (enlarged prostate), decompensation of detrusor musculature, inability of bladder to contract adequately, possibly evidenced by frequency, hesitancy, inability to empty bladder completely, incontinence or dribbling, nocturia, bladder distention, residual urine.

---

*A risk diagnosis is not evidenced by signs and symptoms, as the problem has not occurred; rather, nursing interventions are directed at prevention.

acute Pain may be related to mucosal irritation, bladder distention, colic, urinary infection, and radiation therapy, possibly evidenced by verbal reports (bladder or rectal spasm), narrowed focus, altered muscle tone, grimacing, distraction behaviors, restlessness, and changes in vital signs.

risk for deficient Fluid Volume/Electrolyte Imbalance: risk factors may include postobstructive diuresis, renal or endocrine dysfunction.*

Fear/Anxiety [specify level] may be related to change in health status (possibility of surgical procedure, malignancy); embarrassment or loss of dignity associated with genital exposure before, during, and after treatment, and concern about sexual ability, possibly evidenced by increased tension, apprehension, worry, expressed concerns regarding perceived changes, and fear of unspecific consequences.

Bipolar disorder   PSY

risk for other-directed Violence: risk factors may include irritability, impulsive behavior, delusional thinking, angry response when ideas are refuted or wishes denied, manic excitement, with possible indicators of threatening body language or verbalizations, increased motor activity, overt and aggressive acts, hostility.*

imbalanced Nutrition: less than body requirements may be related to inadequate intake in relation to metabolic expenditures, possibly evidenced by body weight 20% or more below ideal weight, observed inadequate intake, inattention to mealtimes, and distraction from task of eating, laboratory evidence of nutritional deficits or imbalances.

risk for Poisoning [lithium toxicity]: risk factors may include narrow therapeutic range of drug, client's ability (or lack of) to follow through with medication regimen and monitoring, and denial of need for information or therapy.*

Insomnia may be related to psychological stress, lack of recognition of fatigue or need to sleep, hyperactivity, possibly evidenced by denial of need to sleep, interrupted nighttime sleep, one or more nights without sleep, changes in behavior and performance, increasing irritability, restlessness, and dark circles under eyes.

[disturbed Sensory Perception (specify)]/Stress Overload may be related to decrease in sensory threshold, endogenous chemical alteration, psychological stress, sleep deprivation, possibly evidenced by increased distractibility and agitation, anxiety, disorientation, poor concentration, auditory or visual hallucination, bizarre thinking, and motor incoordination.

interrupted Family Processes may be related to situational crises (illness, economics, change in roles), euphoric mood and grandiose ideas or actions of client, manipulative behavior and limit testing, client's refusal to accept responsibility for own actions, possibly evidenced by statements of difficulty coping with situation, lack of adaptation to change, or not dealing constructively with illness, ineffective family decision-making process, failure to send and receive clear messages, and inappropriate boundary maintenance.

---

*A risk diagnosis is not evidenced by signs and symptoms, as the problem has not occurred; rather, nursing interventions are directed at prevention.

Bone cancer   **MS/CH**
Also Refer to Myeloma, multiple; Amputation

acute Pain may be related to bone destruction, pressure on nerves, pos-
    sibly evidenced by verbal or coded report, protective behavior,
    changes in vital signs.

risk for Trauma: risk factors may include increased bone fragility, gen-
    eral weakness, balancing difficulties.*

Bone marrow transplantation   **MS/CH**
Also Refer to Transplantation, recipient

risk for Injury: risk factors may include immune dysfunction or sup-
    pression, abnormal blood profile, action of donor T-cells.*

deficient Diversional Activity may be related to hospitalization or length
    of treatment, restriction of visitors, limitation of activities, possibly
    evidenced by expressions of boredom, restlessness, withdrawal, and
    requests for something to do.

risk for imbalanced Nutrition: less that body requirements: risk factors
    may include increased metabolic needs for healing, altered ability to
    ingest nutrients—nausea, vomiting, anorexia, taste changes, oral le-
    sions.*

Borderline personality disorder   **PSY**
risk for self-/other-directed Violence/Self-Mutilation: risk factors may
    include use of projection as a major defense mechanism, pervasive
    problems with negative transference, feelings of guilt or need to
    "punish" self, distorted sense of self, inability to cope with increased
    psychological or physiological tension in a healthy manner.*

Anxiety [severe to panic] may be related to unconscious conflicts (ex-
    perience of extreme stress), perceived threat to self-concept, unmet
    needs, possibly evidenced by easy frustration and feelings of hurt,
    abuse of alcohol or other drugs, transient psychotic symptoms, and
    performance of self-mutilating acts.

chronic low Self-Esteem/disturbed Personal Identity may be related to
    lack of positive feedback, unmet dependency needs, retarded ego
    development or fixation at an earlier level of development, possibly
    evidenced by difficulty identifying self or defining self-boundaries,
    feelings of depersonalization, extreme mood changes, lack of toler-
    ance of rejection or of being alone, unhappiness with self, striking
    out at others, performance of ritualistic self-damaging acts, and belief
    that punishing self is necessary.

Social Isolation may be related to immature interests, unaccepted social
    behavior, inadequate personal resources, and inability to engage in
    satisfying personal relationships, possibly evidenced by alternating
    clinging and distancing behaviors, difficulty meeting expectations of
    others, experiencing feelings of difference from others, expressing
    interests inappropriate to developmental age, and exhibiting behavior
    unaccepted by dominant cultural group.

Botulism (food-borne)   **MS**
deficient Fluid Volume may be related to active losses—vomiting, di-
    arrhea, decreased intake—nausea, dysphagia, possibly evidenced by

---

*A risk diagnosis is not evidenced by signs and symptoms, as the problem has
not occurred; rather, nursing interventions are directed at prevention.

reports of thirst, dry skin and mucous membranes, decreased BP and urine output, change in mental state, increased hematocrit (Hct).

impaired physical Mobility may be related to neuromuscular impairment, possibly evidenced by limited ability to perform gross or fine motor skills.

Anxiety [specify level]/Fear may be related to threat of death, interpersonal transmission, possibly evidenced by expressed concerns, apprehension, awareness of physiological symptoms, focus on self.

risk for impaired spontaneous Ventilation: risk factors may include neuromuscular impairment, presence of infectious process.*

CH

Contamination may be related to lack of proper precautions in food storage or preparation as evidenced by gastrointestinal and neurological effects of exposure to biological agent.

Bowel obstruction   MS
Refer to Ileus

Brain tumor   MS

acute Pain may be related to pressure on brain tissues, possibly evidenced by reports of headache, facial mask of pain, narrowed focus, and changes in vital signs.

impaired Memory may be related to altered circulation to and/or destruction of brain tissue, possibly evidenced by memory loss, personality changes, impaired ability to make decisions or conceptualize, and inaccurate interpretation of environment.

[disturbed Sensory Perception (specify)] may be related to altered sensory reception/integration, possibly evidenced by changes in sensory acuity, change in behavior pattern, poor concentration/problem-solving abilities, disorientation.

risk for deficient Fluid Volume: risk factors may include recurrent vomiting from irritation of vagal center in medulla and decreased intake.*

Self-Care Deficit [specify] may be related to sensory or neuromuscular impairment interfering with ability to perform tasks, possibly evidenced by unkempt and disheveled appearance, body odor, and verbalization or observation of inability to perform ADLs.

Breast cancer   MS/CH
Also Refer to Cancer

Anxiety [specify level] may be related to change in health status, threat of death, stress, interpersonal transmission, possibly evidenced by expressed concerns, apprehension, uncertainty, focus on self, diminished productivity.

deficient Knowledge [Learning Need] regarding diagnosis, prognosis, and treatment options may be related to lack of exposure or unfamiliarity with information resources, information misinterpretation, cognitive limitation, anxiety, possibly evidenced by verbalizations, statements of misconceptions, inappropriate behaviors.

---

*A risk diagnosis is not evidenced by signs and symptoms, as the problem has not occurred; rather, nursing interventions are directed at prevention.

risk for disturbed Body Image: risk factors may include significance of body part with regard to sexual perceptions.*

risk for Sexual Dysfunction: risk factors may include health-related changes, medical treatments, concern about relationship with SO.*

Bronchitis   CH

ineffective Airway Clearance may be related to excessive, thickened mucus secretions, possibly evidenced by presence of rhonchi, tachypnea, and ineffective cough.

Activity Intolerance [specify level] may be related to imbalance between O_2 supply and demand, general weakness, exhaustion—interruption in usual sleep pattern due to cough, discomfort, dyspnea, possibly evidenced by reports of fatigue, dyspnea, and abnormal vital sign response to activity.

acute Pain may be related to inflammation of lung parenchyma, persistent cough, cellular reactions to circulating toxins, aching associated with fever, possibly evidenced by reports of pleuritic chest pain, guarding affected area, distraction behaviors, and restlessness.

Bronchopneumonia   MS/CH

Also Refer to Bronchitis

ineffective Airway Clearance may be related to tracheal bronchial inflammation, edema formation, increased sputum production, pleuritic pain, decreased energy, fatigue, possibly evidenced by changes in rate and depth of respirations, abnormal breath sounds, use of accessory muscles, dyspnea, cyanosis, effective or ineffective cough—with or without sputum production.

impaired Gas Exchange may be related to alveolar-capillary membrane changes—inflammatory effects, ventilation-perfusion mismatch—collection of secretions affecting O_2 exchange across alveolar membrane, and hypoventilation, altered release of oxygen at cellular level—fever, shifting oxyhemogloblin curve, possibly evidenced by restlessness, changes in mentation, dyspnea, tachycardia, pallor, cyanosis, and ABGs or oximetry evidence of hypoxia.

risk for Infection [spread]: risk factors may include decreased ciliary action, stasis of secretions, presence of existing infection, immunosuppression, chronic disease, malnutrition.*

Bulimia nervosa   PSY/MS

Also Refer to Anorexia nervosa

impaired Dentition may be related to dietary habits, poor oral hygiene, chronic vomiting, possibly evidenced by erosion of tooth enamel, multiple caries, abraded teeth.

impaired Oral Mucous Membrane may be related to malnutrition or vitamin deficiency, poor oral hygiene, chronic vomiting, possibly evidenced by sore, inflamed buccal mucosa, swollen salivary glands, ulcerations of mucosa, reports of constant sore mouth or throat.

risk for deficient Fluid Volume/Bleeding: risk factors may include consistent self-induced vomiting, chronic or excessive laxative or diuretic use, esophageal erosion or tear (Mallory-Weiss syndrome).*

---

*A risk diagnosis is not evidenced by signs and symptoms, as the problem has not occurred; rather, nursing interventions are directed at prevention.

deficient Knowledge [Learning Need] regarding condition, prognosis, complication, treatment may be related to lack of exposure or recall, unfamiliarity with information about condition, learned maladaptive coping skills, possibly evidenced by verbalization of misconception of relationship of current situation and bingeing and purging behaviors, distortion of body image, verbalized need for information, desire to change behaviors.

Burns (dependent on type, degree, and severity of the injury) MS/CH

risk for deficient Fluid Volume/Bleeding: risk factors may include loss of fluids through wounds, capillary damage and evaporation, hypermetabolic state, insufficient intake, hemorrhagic losses.*

risk for ineffective Airway Clearance: risk factors may include tracheobronchial obstruction—mucosal edema and loss of ciliary action with smoke inhalation; circumferential full-thickness burns of the neck, thorax, and chest, with compression of the airway or limited chest excursion, trauma—direct upper airway injury by flame, steam, chemicals, or gases; fluid shifts, pulmonary edema, decreased lung compliance.*

risk for Infection: risk factors may include loss of protective dermal barrier, traumatized tissue, necrosis, decreased hemoglobin (Hb), suppressed inflammatory response, environmental exposure, invasive procedures.*

acute/chronic Pain may be related to destruction of skin, tissues, and nerves; edema formation, and manipulation of injured tissues, possibly evidenced by verbal reports, narrowed focus, distraction and guarding behaviors, facial mask of pain, and changes in vital signs.

risk for imbalanced Nutrition: less than body requirements: risk factors may include hypermetabolic state as much as 50% to 60% higher than normal proportional to the severity of injury, protein catabolism, anorexia, restricted oral intake.*

Post-Trauma Syndrome may be related to life-threatening event, possibly evidenced by reexperiencing the event, repetitive dreams or nightmares, psychic or emotional numbness, and sleep disturbance.

ineffective Protection may be related to extremes of age, inadequate nutrition, anemia, impaired immune system, possibly evidenced by impaired healing, deficient immunity, fatigue, anorexia.

PED

deficient Diversional Activity may be related to long-term hospitalization, frequent lengthy treatments, and physical limitations, possibly evidenced by expressions of boredom, restlessness, withdrawal, and requests for something to do.

risk for delayed Development: risk factors may include effects of physical disability, separation from SO(s), and environmental deficiencies.*

---

*A risk diagnosis is not evidenced by signs and symptoms, as the problem has not occurred; rather, nursing interventions are directed at prevention.

Bursitis   CH

acute/chronic Pain may be related to inflammation of affected joint, possibly evidenced by verbal reports, guarding behavior, and narrowed focus.

impaired physical Mobility may be related to inflammation and swelling of joint and pain, possibly evidenced by diminished range of motion, reluctance to attempt movement, and imposed restriction of movement by medical treatment.

Calculi, urinary   CH/MS

acute Pain may be related to increased frequency or force of ureteral contractions, tissue trauma, edema formation, cellular ischemia, possibly evidenced by reports of sudden, severe, colicky pain, guarding and distraction behaviors, self-focus, and changes in vital signs.

impaired Urinary Elimination may be related to stimulation of the bladder by calculi, renal or ureteral irritation, mechanical obstruction of urinary flow, inflammation, possibly evidenced by urgency and frequency, oliguria, hematuria.

risk for deficient Fluid Volume: risk factors may include stimulation of renal-intestinal reflexes—nausea, vomiting, and diarrhea, changes in urinary output, postobstructive diuresis.*

risk for Infection: risk factors may include stasis of urine.*

deficient Knowledge [Learning Need] regarding condition, prognosis, self-care, and treatment needs may be related to lack of exposure or recall and information misinterpretation, possibly evidenced by requests for information, statements of concern, and recurrence or development of preventable complications.

Cancer   MS

Also Refer to Chemotherapy

Fear/Death Anxiety may be related to situational crises, threat to or change in health or socioeconomic status, role functioning, interaction patterns, threat of death, separation from family, interpersonal transmission of feelings, possibly evidenced by expressed concerns, feelings of inadequacy or helplessness, insomnia, increased tension, restlessness, focus on self, sympathetic stimulation

Grieving may be related to potential loss of physiological well-being (body part or function), change in lifestyle, perceived potential death, possibly evidenced by anger, sadness, withdrawal, choked feelings, changes in eating or sleep patterns, activity level, libido, and communication patterns.

acute/chronic Pain may be related to the disease process (compression of nerve tissue, infiltration of nerves or their vascular supply, obstruction of a nerve pathway, inflammation), or side effects of therapeutic agents, possibly evidenced by verbal reports, self-focusing or narrowed focus, alteration in muscle tone, facial mask of pain, distraction or guarding behaviors, autonomic responses, and restlessness.

Fatigue may be related to decreased metabolic energy production, increased energy requirements (hypermetabolic state), overwhelming

---

*A risk diagnosis is not evidenced by signs and symptoms, as the problem has not occurred; rather, nursing interventions are directed at prevention.

---

psychological or emotional demands, and altered body chemistry—side effects of medications, chemotherapy, radiation therapy, biotherapy, possibly evidenced by unremitting or overwhelming lack of energy, inability to maintain usual routines, decreased performance, impaired ability to concentrate, lethargy, listlessness, and disinterest in surroundings.

impaired Home Maintenance may be related to debilitation, lack of resources, and/or inadequate support systems, possibly evidenced by verbalization of problem, request for assistance, and lack of necessary equipment or aids.

PSY/PED

risk for interrupted Family Processes: risk factors may include situational or transitional crises—long-term illness, change in roles or economic status; developmental—anticipated loss of a family member.*

readiness for enhanced family Coping possibly evidenced by verbalizations of impact of crisis on own values, priorities, goals, or relationships.

Candidiasis   CH
Also Refer to Thrush

impaired Skin/Tissue Integrity may be related to infectious lesions, possibly evidenced by disruption of skin surfaces and mucous membranes.

acute Pain/impaired Comfort may be related to exposure of irritated skin and mucous membranes to excretions (urine, feces), possibly evidenced by verbal or coded reports, restlessness, guarding behaviors.

risk for Sexual Dysfunction: risk factors include presence of infectious process and vaginal discomfort.*

Cannabis abuse   CH
Refer to Stimulant abuse

Cardiac catheterization   MS
Anxiety [specify level] may be related to threat to or change in health status, stress, family heredity possibly evidenced by expressed concerns, apprehension, uncertainty, focus on self.

risk for decreased Cardiac Output: risk factors may include altered heart rate and rhythm (vasovagal response, ventricular dysrhythmias), decreased myocardial contractility (ischemia).*

risk for decreased cardiac Tissue Perfusion: risk factors may include coronary artery spasm, hypovolemia, hypoxia, [thrombosis, emboli].*

risk for Adverse Reaction to Iodinated Contrast Media: risk factors may include underlying disease—heart disease, concurrent use of medications (e.g., beta-blockers, metformin), history of allergies.*

Cardiac surgery   MS/PED
risk for decreased Cardiac Output: risk factors may include altered myocardial contractility secondary to temporary factors—ventricular

---

*A risk diagnosis is not evidenced by signs and symptoms, as the problem has not occurred; rather, nursing interventions are directed at prevention.

wall surgery, recent myocardial infarction, response to certain medications or drug interactions; altered preload—hypovolemia, and afterload—systemic vascular resistance; altered heart rate or rhythm—dysrhythmias.*

risk for Bleeding/deficient Fluid Volume: risk factors may include intraoperative bleeding with inadequate blood replacement; bleeding related to insufficient heparin reversal, fibrinolysis, or platelet destruction; or volume depletion effects of intraoperative or postoperative diuretic therapy.*

risk for impaired Gas Exchange: risk factors may include alveolar-capillary membrane changes (atelectasis), intestinal edema, inadequate function or premature discontinuation of chest tubes, and diminished O_2-carrying capacity of the blood.*

acute Pain/impaired Comfort may be related to tissue inflammation or trauma, edema formation, intraoperative nerve trauma, and myocardial ischemia, possibly evidenced by reports of incisional discomfort, pain in chest and donor site; paresthesia or pain in hand, arm, shoulder; anxiety, restlessness, irritability; distraction behaviors; and changes in heart rate and BP.

impaired Skin/Tissue Integrity related to mechanical trauma (surgical incisions, puncture wounds) and edema evidenced by disruption of skin surface and tissues.

Cardiogenic shock   MS
Refer to Shock, cardiogenic

Cardiomyopathy   CH/MS
decreased Cardiac Output may be related to altered contractility, possibly evidenced by dyspnea, fatigue, chest pain, dizziness, syncope.

Activity Intolerance may be related to imbalance between O_2 supply and demand, possibly evidenced by weakness, fatigue, dyspnea, abnormal heart rate and BP response to activity, ECG changes.

ineffective Role Performance may be related to changes in physical health, stress, demands of job/life, possibly evidenced by change in usual patterns of responsibility, role strain, change in capacity to resume role.

Carotid endarterectomy   MS
Also Refer to Surgery, general

risk for ineffective cerebral Tissue Perfusion: risk factors may include carotid stenosis, embolism, thrombolytic therapy.*

Carpal tunnel syndrome   CH/MS
acute/chronic Pain may be related to pressure on median nerve, possibly evidenced by verbal reports, reluctance to use affected extremity, guarding behaviors, expressed fear of re-injury, altered ability to continue previous activities.

impaired physical Mobility may be related to neuromuscular impairment and pain, possibly evidenced by decreased hand strength, weakness, limited range of motion, and reluctance to attempt movement.

---

*A risk diagnosis is not evidenced by signs and symptoms, as the problem has not occurred; rather, nursing interventions are directed at prevention.

risk for Peripheral Neurovascular Dysfunction: risk factors may include mechanical compression (e.g., brace, repetitive tasks or motions), immobilization.*

deficient Knowledge [Learning Need] regarding condition, prognosis, treatment, and safety needs may be related to lack of exposure or recall, information misinterpretation, possibly evidenced by questions, statements of concern, request for information, inaccurate follow-through of instructions, development of preventable complications.

Casts CH/MS

Also Refer to Fractures

risk for Peripheral Neurovascular Dysfunction: risk factors may include presence of fracture(s), mechanical compression (cast), tissue trauma, immobilization, vascular obstruction.*

risk for impaired Skin Integrity: risk factors may include pressure of cast, moisture or debris under cast, objects inserted under cast to relieve itching, and altered sensation or circulation.*

Self-Care Deficit [specify] may be related to impaired ability to perform self-care tasks, possibly evidenced by statements of need for assistance and observed difficulty in performing ADLs.

Cataract CH

[disturbed visual Sensory Perception] may be related to altered sensory reception or status of sense organs, and therapeutically restricted environment (surgical procedure, patching), possibly evidenced by diminished acuity, visual distortions, and change in usual response to stimuli.

risk for Trauma: risk factors may include poor vision, reduced hand-eye coordination.*

Anxiety [specify level]/Fear may be related to alteration in visual acuity, threat of permanent loss of vision/independence, possibly evidenced by expressed concerns, apprehension, and feelings of uncertainty.

deficient Knowledge [Learning Need] regarding ways of coping with altered abilities, therapy choices, lifestyle changes may be related to lack of exposure or recall, misinterpretation, or cognitive limitations, possibly evidenced by requests for information, statement of concern, inaccurate follow-through of instructions, development of preventable complications.

Cat scratch disease CH

acute Pain may be related to effects of circulating toxins (fever, headache, and lymphadenitis), possibly evidenced by verbal reports, guarding behavior, and changes in vital signs.

Hyperthermia may be related to inflammatory process, possibly evidenced by increased body temperature, flushed warm skin, tachypnea, and tachycardia.

Celiac disease CH

imbalanced Nutrition: less than body requirements may be related to inability to absorb nutrients (mucosal damage, loss of villi, prolif-

---

*A risk diagnosis is not evidenced by signs and symptoms, as the problem has not occurred; rather, nursing interventions are directed at prevention.

eration of crypt cells, shortened transit time through gastrointestinal tract), possibly evidenced by weight loss, abdominal distention, steatorrhea, evidence of anemia, vitamin deficiencies.

Diarrhea may be related to irritation, malabsorption, possibly evidenced by abdominal pain, hyperactive bowel sounds, at least three loose stools per day.

risk for deficient Fluid Volume: risk factors may include mild to massive steatorrhea, diarrhea.*

Cellulitis   CH/MS

risk for Infection [abscess, bacteremia]: risk factors may include broken skin, chronic disease, presence of pathogens, insufficient knowledge to avoid exposure to pathogens.*

acute Pain/impaired Comfort may be related to inflammatory process, circulating toxins possibly evidenced by reports of localized pain or headache, guarding behaviors, restlessness, changes in vital signs.

impaired Tissue Integrity may be related to trauma, inflammation and/or invasion of tissues by infectious bacterial agent, or altered circulation; possibly evidenced by redness, warmth, edema, tenderness or pain under the surface of skin, or deep in tissues.

Cerebrovascular accident (CVA)   MS

ineffective cerebral Tissue Perfusion may be related to interruption of blood flow (occlusive disorder, hemorrhage, cerebral vasospasm or edema), possibly evidenced by altered level of consciousness, changes in vital signs, changes in motor or sensory responses, restlessness, memory loss, as well as sensory, language, intellectual, and emotional deficits.

impaired physical Mobility may be related to neuromuscular involvement (weakness, paresthesia, flaccid or hypotonic paralysis, spastic paralysis), perceptual or cognitive impairment, possibly evidenced by inability to purposefully move involved body parts, limited range of motion, impaired coordination, and/or decreased muscle strength or control.

impaired verbal [and/or written] Communication may be related to impaired cerebral circulation, neuromuscular impairment, loss of facial/oral muscle tone and control, generalized weakness, fatigue, possibly evidenced by impaired articulation, does not or cannot speak (dysarthria), inability to modulate speech, find and/or name words, identify objects and/or inability to comprehend written or spoken language, inability to produce written communication.

Self-Care Deficit [specify] may be related to neuromuscular impairment, decreased strength or endurance, loss of muscle control or coordination, perceptual or cognitive impairment, pain, discomfort, and depression, possibly evidenced by stated or observed inability to perform ADLs, requests for assistance, disheveled appearance, and incontinence.

---

*A risk diagnosis is not evidenced by signs and symptoms, as the problem has not occurred; rather, nursing interventions are directed at prevention.

risk for impaired Swallowing: risk factors may include muscle paralysis and perceptual impairment.*

risk for Unilateral Neglect: risk factors may include sensory loss of part of visual field with perceptual loss of corresponding body segment.*

impaired Home Maintenance may be related to condition of individual family member, insufficient finances, family organization or planning; unfamiliarity with resources, and inadequate support systems, possibly evidenced by members expressing difficulty in managing home in a comfortable manner, requesting assistance with home maintenance, disorderly surroundings, and overtaxed family members.

situational low Self-Esteem/disturbed Body Image may be related to functional impairment, loss, focus on past function/strength, and cognitive or perceptual changes, possibly evidenced by actual change in function, self-negating verbalizations, reports perceptions reflecting altered view of body function.

Grieving: may be related to loss of processes of body [neuromuscular impairments], loss of job/role function, status/independence, possibly evidenced by psychological distress, despair, anger, disorganization.

Cervix, dysfunctional   OB
Refer to Dilation of cervix, premature

Cesarean birth   OB
Also Refer to Cesarean birth, unplanned; Cesarean birth, postpartal

deficient Knowledge [Learning Need] regarding surgical procedure and expectation, postoperative routines and therapy, and self-care needs may be related to lack of information/misinterpretation, possibly evidenced by statements of concern, questions, and misconceptions.

risk for deficient Fluid Volume/Bleeding: risk factors may include restrictions of oral intake, blood loss; pregnancy-related complications.*

risk for impaired Attachment: risk factors may include separation, existing health conditions of mother or infant, lack of privacy.*

Cesarean birth, postpartal   OB
Also Refer to Postpartal period

risk for impaired Attachment: risk factors may include developmental transition or gain of a family member, situational crisis (e.g., surgical intervention, physical complications interfering with initial acquaintance and interaction, negative self-appraisal).*

acute Pain/impaired Comfort may be related to surgical trauma, effects of anesthesia, hormonal effects, bladder or abdominal distention, possibly evidenced by verbal reports (e.g., incisional pain, cramping, afterpains, spinal headache), guarding or distraction behaviors, irritability, facial mask of pain.

---

*A risk diagnosis is not evidenced by signs and symptoms, as the problem has not occurred; rather, nursing interventions are directed at prevention.

risk for situational low Self-Esteem: risk factors may include perceived "failure" at life event, maturational transition, perceived loss of control in unplanned delivery.*

risk for Injury: risk factors may include biochemical or regulatory functions (e.g., orthostatic hypotension, development of pregnancy-induced hypertension or eclampsia), effects of anesthesia, thromboembolism, abnormal blood profile (anemia or excessive blood loss, rubella sensitivity, Rh incompatibility), tissue trauma.*

risk for Infection: risk factors may include tissue trauma, broken skin, decreased Hb, invasive procedures and/or increased environmental exposure, prolonged rupture of amniotic membranes, malnutrition.*

Self-Care Deficit [specify] may be related to effects of anesthesia, decreased strength and endurance, physical discomfort, possibly evidenced by verbalization of inability to perform desired ADL(s).

Cesarean birth, unplanned OB

Also Refer to Cesarean birth, postpartal

deficient Knowledge [Learning Need] regarding underlying procedure, pathophysiology, and self-care needs may be related to incomplete or inadequate information, possibly evidenced by request for information, verbalization of concerns or misconceptions, and inappropriate or exaggerated behavior.

Anxiety [specify level] may be related to actual or perceived threat to mother/fetus, emotional threat to self-esteem, unmet needs or expectations, interpersonal transmission, possibly evidenced by increased tension, apprehension, feelings of inadequacy, sympathetic stimulation, and narrowed focus, restlessness.

Powerlessness may be related to interpersonal interaction, perception of illness-related regimen, lifestyle of helplessness, possibly evidenced by verbalization of lack of control, lack of participation in care or decision making, passivity.

risk for disturbed Maternal-Fetal Dyad: risk factors may include compromised oxygen transport, complication of pregnancy.*

risk for acute Pain: risk factors may include increased or prolonged contractions, psychological reaction.*

risk for Infection: risk factors may include invasive procedures, rupture of amniotic membranes, break in skin, decreased Hb, exposure to pathogens.*

Chemotherapy MS/CH

Also Refer to Cancer

risk for deficient Fluid Volume: risk factors may include gastrointestinal losses (vomiting, diarrhea); interference with adequate intake (stomatitis, anorexia), losses through abnormal routes (indwelling tubes, wounds, fistulas), hypermetabolic state.*

imbalanced Nutrition: less than body requirements may be related to inability to ingest adequate nutrients—nausea, stomatitis, gastric irritation, taste distortions, and fatigue; hypermetabolic state, poorly controlled pain, possibly evidenced by weight loss (wasting),

---

*A risk diagnosis is not evidenced by signs and symptoms, as the problem has not occurred; rather, nursing interventions are directed at prevention.

aversion to eating, reported altered taste sensation, sore and inflamed buccal cavity, diarrhea and/or constipation.

impaired Oral Mucous Membrane may be related to side effects of therapeutic agents or radiation, dehydration, and malnutrition, possibly evidenced by ulcerations, leukoplakia, decreased salivation, and reports of pain.

disturbed Body Image may be related to anatomical or structural changes, loss of hair and weight, possibly evidenced by negative feelings about body, preoccupation with change, feelings of helplessness or hopelessness, and change in social environment.

ineffective Protection may be related to inadequate nutrition, drug or radiation therapy, abnormal blood profile, disease state (cancer), possibly evidenced by impaired healing, deficient immunity, anorexia, fatigue.

readiness for enhanced Hope possibly evidenced by expressed desire to enhance belief in possibilities and sense of meaning to life.

Cholecystectomy   MS

acute Pain may be related to interruption in skin and tissue layers with mechanical closure (sutures or staples) and invasive procedures (including T-tube, nasogastric [NG] tube), possibly evidenced by verbal reports, guarding or distraction behaviors, and changes in vital signs.

ineffective Breathing Pattern may be related to pain, muscular impairment, decreased energy, fatigue, possibly evidenced by fremitus, tachypnea, and decreased respiratory depth and vital capacity, holding breath, reluctance to cough.

risk for deficient Fluid Volume/Bleeding: risk factors may include losses from vomiting or NG aspiration, medically restricted intake, altered coagulation.*

Cholelithiasis   CH

acute Pain may be related to obstruction or ductal spasm, inflammatory process, tissue ischemia, necrosis, possibly evidenced by verbal reports, guarding or distraction behaviors, self- or narrowed focus, and changes in vital signs.

risk for imbalanced Nutrition: less than body requirements: risk factors may include self-imposed or prescribed dietary restrictions, nausea and vomiting, dyspepsia, pain; loss of nutrients; impaired fat digestion—obstruction of bile flow.*

deficient Knowledge [Learning Need] regarding pathophysiology, therapy choices, and self-care needs may be related to lack of information or recall, misinterpretation, possibly evidenced by verbalization of concerns, questions, and recurrence of condition.

Chronic obstructive lung disease   CH/MS

ineffective Airway Clearance may be related to bronchospasm, increased production of tenacious secretions, retained secretions, and decreased energy, fatigue, possibly evidenced by presence of wheezes, crackles, tachypnea, dyspnea, changes in depth of respi-

---

*A risk diagnosis is not evidenced by signs and symptoms, as the problem has not occurred; rather, nursing interventions are directed at prevention.

rations, use of accessory muscles, persistent cough, and chest x-ray findings.

impaired Gas Exchange may be related to altered O_2 delivery (obstruction of airways by secretions or bronchospasm, air trapping) and alveoli destruction, possibly evidenced by dyspnea, restlessness, confusion, abnormal ABG values—hypoxia, hypercapnia, changes in vital signs, and reduced tolerance for activity.

Activity Intolerance may be related to imbalance between O_2 supply and demand and generalized weakness, possibly evidenced by verbal reports of fatigue, exertional dyspnea, and abnormal vital sign response.

imbalanced Nutrition: less than body requirements may be related to inability to ingest adequate nutrients (dyspnea, fatigue, medication side effects, sputum production, anorexia), possibly evidenced by weight loss, reported altered taste sensation, decreased muscle mass or subcutaneous fat, poor muscle tone, and aversion to eating/lack of interest in food.

risk for Infection: risk factors may include decreased ciliary action, stasis of secretions, and debilitated state or malnutrition.*

Circumcision   PED

deficient Knowledge [Learning Need] regarding surgical procedure, prognosis, and treatment may be related to lack of exposure, misinterpretation, unfamiliarity with information resources, possibly evidenced by request for information, verbalization of concern/misconceptions, inaccurate follow-through of instructions.

acute Pain may be related to trauma to/edema of tender tissues, possibly evidenced by crying, changes in sleep pattern, refusal to eat.

impaired Urinary Elimination may be related to tissue injury or inflammation or development of urethral fistula, possibly evidenced by edema, difficulty voiding.

risk for Bleeding: risk factors may include decreased clotting factors immediately after birth, previously undiagnosed problems with bleeding or clotting.*

risk for Infection: risk factors may include immature immune system, invasive procedure, tissue trauma, environmental exposure.*

Cirrhosis   MS/CH

Also Refer to Substance dependence/abuse rehabilitation; Hepatitis, acute viral

risk for impaired Liver Function: risk factors may include viral infection, alcohol abuse.*

imbalanced Nutrition: less than body requirements may be related to inability to ingest or absorb nutrients (anorexia, nausea, indigestion, early satiety), abnormal bowel function, impaired storage of vitamins, possibly evidenced by aversion to eating, observed lack of intake, poor muscle tone, muscle wasting, weight loss, and imbalances in nutritional studies.

excess Fluid Volume may be related to compromised regulatory mechanism (e.g., syndrome of inappropriate antidiuretic hormone,

---

*A risk diagnosis is not evidenced by signs and symptoms, as the problem has not occurred; rather, nursing interventions are directed at prevention.

decreased plasma proteins, malnutrition) and excess sodium and/or fluid intake, possibly evidenced by generalized or abdominal edema, weight gain, dyspnea, BP changes, positive hepatojugular reflex, change in mentation, altered electrolytes, changes in urine specific gravity, and pleural effusion.

risk for impaired Skin Integrity: risk factors may include altered circulation and metabolic state, poor skin turgor, skeletal prominence, presence of edema or ascites, and accumulation of bile salts in skin.*

risk for Bleeding: risk factors may include abnormal blood profile, altered clotting factors—decreased production of prothrombin, fibrinogen, and factors VIII, IX, and X; impaired vitamin K absorption; release of thromboplastin, portal hypertension, development of esophageal varices.*

risk for acute Confusion: risk factors may include alcohol abuse, increased serum ammonia level, and inability of liver to detoxify certain enzymes or drugs.*

Self-Esteem [specify]/disturbed Body Image may be related to biophysical changes, altered physical appearance, uncertainty of prognosis, changes in role function, personal vulnerability, self-destructive behavior (alcohol-induced disease), possibly evidenced by verbalization of changes in lifestyle, fear of rejection/reaction of others, negative feelings about body or abilities, and feelings of helplessness, hopelessness, powerlessness.

risk for ineffective Protection: risk factors may include abnormal blood profile (altered clotting factors), portal hypertension, development of esophageal varices.*

Cocaine hydrochloride poisoning, acute   MS
Also Refer to Stimulant abuse; Substance dependence/abuse rehabilitation

ineffective Breathing Pattern may be related to pharmacological effects on respiratory center of the brain, possibly evidenced by tachypnea, altered depth of respiration, shortness of breath, and abnormal ABGs.

risk for decreased Cardiac Output: risk factors may include drug effect on myocardium (degree dependent on drug purity and quality used), alterations in electrical rate, rhythm, or conduction, preexisting myocardiopathy.*

CH

risk for impaired Liver Function: risk factors may include cocaine abuse.*

imbalanced Nutrition: less than body requirements may be related to anorexia, insufficient or inappropriate use of financial resources, possibly evidenced by reported inadequate intake, weight loss or less than normal weight gain, lack of interest in food, poor muscle tone, signs or laboratory evidence of vitamin deficiencies.

risk for Infection: risk factors may include injection techniques, impurities of drugs, localized trauma/nasal septum damage, malnutrition, altered immune state.*

---

*A risk diagnosis is not evidenced by signs and symptoms, as the problem has not occurred; rather, nursing interventions are directed at prevention.

ineffective Coping may be related to personal vulnerability, negative role modeling, inadequate support systems, ineffective or inadequate coping skills with substitution of drug, possibly evidenced by use of harmful substance despite evidence of undesirable consequences.

[disturbed Sensory Perception (specify)] may be related to exogenous chemical, altered sensory reception, transmission, or integration (hallucination), altered status of sense organs, possibly evidenced by responding to internal stimuli from hallucinatory experiences, bizarre thinking, anxiety, panic, changes in sensory acuity (sense of smell or taste).

Coccidioidomycosis (San Joaquin/Valley Fever)

acute Pain may be related to inflammation, possibly evidenced by verbal reports, distraction behaviors, and narrowed focus.

Fatigue may be related to decreased energy production, states of discomfort, possibly evidenced by reports of overwhelming lack of energy, inability to maintain usual routine, emotional lability or irritability, impaired ability to concentrate, and decreased endurance or libido.

deficient Knowledge [Learning Need] regarding nature and course of disease, therapy and self-care needs may be related to lack of information, possibly evidenced by statements of concern and questions.

Colitis, ulcerative

Diarrhea may be related to inflammation or malabsorption of the bowel, presence of toxins, segmental narrowing of the lumen, possibly evidenced by increased bowel sounds and peristalsis, frequent watery stools (acute phase), changes in stool color, abdominal pain, urgency, cramping.

acute/chronic Pain may be related to inflammation of the intestines, hyperperistalsis, prolonged diarrhea, and anal/rectal irritation, fissures, fistulas, possibly evidenced by verbal reports, guarding or distraction behaviors—restlessness, self-focusing.

risk for deficient Fluid Volume: risk factors may include excessive losses through normal routes—severe frequent diarrhea, vomiting; capillary plasma loss; hypermetabolic state—inflammation, fever; restricted intake—nausea, anorexia.*

imbalanced Nutrition: less than body requirements may be related to altered intake or absorption of nutrients—medically restricted intake, fear that eating may cause diarrhea; and hypermetabolic state, possibly evidenced by weight loss, decreased subcutaneous fat and muscle mass, poor muscle tone, hyperactive bowel sounds, steatorrhea, pale conjunctiva and mucous membranes, and aversion to eating.

ineffective Coping may be related to chronic nature and indefinite outcome of disease, multiple stressors repeated over time, situational

---

*A risk diagnosis is not evidenced by signs and symptoms, as the problem has not occurred; rather, nursing interventions are directed at prevention.

---

crisis, personal vulnerability, severe pain, inadequate sleep, lack of or ineffective support systems, possibly evidenced by verbalization of inability to cope, discouragement, anxiety, preoccupation with physical self, chronic worry, emotional tension, depression, and recurrent exacerbation of symptoms.

risk for Powerlessness: risk factors may include unresolved dependency conflicts, feelings of insecurity or resentment, repression of anger and aggressive feelings, lacking a sense of control in stressful situations, sacrificing own wishes for others, and retreat from aggression or frustration.*

Colostomy   MS

risk for impaired Skin Integrity: risk factors may include absence of sphincter at stoma, character and flow of effluent and flatus from stoma, reaction to product or removal of adhesive, and improperly fitting or care of appliance.*

risk for Diarrhea/Constipation: risk factors may include interruption or alteration of normal bowel function/placement of ostomy, changes in dietary or fluid intake, and effects of medication.*

CH

deficient Knowledge [Learning Need] regarding changes in physiological function, and self-care and treatment needs may be related to lack of exposure or recall, information misinterpretation, possibly evidenced by questions, statement of concern, and inaccurate follow-through of instruction or performance of ostomy care, development of preventable complications.

disturbed Body Image may be related to biophysical changes (presence of stoma, loss of control of bowel elimination) and psychosocial factors (altered body structure, disease process—cancer, colitis, and associated treatment regimen, possibly evidenced by verbalization of change in perception of self, negative feelings about body, fear of rejection/reaction of others, not touching or looking at stoma, and refusal to participate in care.

impaired Social Interaction may be related to fear of embarrassing situation secondary to altered bowel control with loss of contents, odor, possibly evidenced by reduced participation and verbalized or observed discomfort in social situations.

risk for Sexual Dysfunction: risk factors may include altered body structure and function, radical resection and treatment procedures, vulnerability, psychological concern about response of SO(s), and disruption of sexual response pattern—erection difficulty.*

Coma   MS

risk for Suffocation: risk factors may include cognitive impairment/loss of protective reflexes and purposeful movement.*

risk for deficient Fluid Volume/imbalanced Nutrition: less than body requirements: risk factors may include inability to ingest food or fluids, increased needs—hypermetabolic state.*

---

*A risk diagnosis is not evidenced by signs and symptoms, as the problem has not occurred; rather, nursing interventions are directed at prevention.

[total] Self-Care Deficit may be related to cognitive impairment and absence of purposeful activity, evidenced by inability to perform ADLs.

risk for ineffective cerebral Tissue Perfusion: risk factors may include head trauma, substance abuse, embolism, cerebral aneurysm, brain tumor/neoplasm.*

risk for Infection: risk factors may include stasis of body fluids (oral, pulmonary, urinary), invasive procedures, and nutritional deficits.*

Coma, diabetic   MS
Refer to Diabetic ketoacidosis; Coma

Complex regional pain syndrome   MS
acute/chronic Pain may be related to continued nerve stimulation, possibly evidenced by verbal reports, distraction or guarding behaviors, narrowed focus, changes in sleep patterns, and altered ability to continue previous activities.

ineffective peripheral Tissue Perfusion may be related to reduction of arterial blood flow (arteriole vasoconstriction), possibly evidenced by extremity pain, altered skin characteristics, diminished pulses, and edema.

[disturbed tactile Sensory Perception] may be related to altered sensory reception (neurological deficit, pain), possibly evidenced by change in usual response to stimuli, abnormal sensitivity of touch, physiological anxiety, and irritability.

risk for ineffective Role Performance: risk factors may include situational crisis, chronic disability, debilitating pain.*

risk for compromised family Coping: risk factors may include temporary family disorganization and role changes and prolonged disability that exhausts the supportive capacity of SO(s).*

Concussion, brain   CH
acute Pain may be related to trauma to or edema of cerebral tissue, possibly evidenced by reports of headache, guarding or distraction behaviors, and narrowed focus.

risk for deficient Fluid Volume: risk factors may include vomiting, decreased intake, and hypermetabolic state (fever).*

risk for impaired Memory: risk factors may include neurological disturbances.*

deficient Knowledge [Learning Need] regarding condition, treatment/safety needs, and potential complications may be related to lack of recall, misinterpretation, cognitive limitation, possibly evidenced by questions or statement of concerns, development of preventable complications.

Conduct disorder (childhood, adolescence)   PSY/PED
risk for self-/other-directed Violence: risk factors may include retarded ego development, antisocial character, poor impulse control, dysfunctional family system, loss of significant relationships, history of suicidal or acting-out behaviors.*

---

*A risk diagnosis is not evidenced by signs and symptoms, as the problem has not occurred; rather, nursing interventions are directed at prevention.

defensive Coping may be related to inadequate coping strategies, maturational crisis, multiple life changes or losses, lack of control of impulsive actions, and personal vulnerability, possibly evidenced by inappropriate use of defense mechanisms, inability to meet role expectations, poor self-esteem, failure to assume responsibility for own actions, hypersensitivity to slight or criticism, and excessive smoking, drinking, or drug use.

ineffective Impulse Control may be related to chronic low self-esteem, anger, disorder of development, mood, personality possibly evidenced by acting without thinking, irritability, temper outbursts.

chronic low Self-Esteem may be related to life choices perpetuating failure, personal vulnerability, possibly evidenced by self-negating verbalizations, anger, rejection of positive feedback, frequent lack of success in life events.

CH

compromised/disabled family Coping may be related to excessive guilt, anger, or blaming among family members regarding child's behavior; parental inconsistencies; disagreements regarding discipline, limit setting, and approaches; and exhaustion of parental resources (prolonged coping with disruptive child), possibly evidenced by unrealistic parental expectations, rejection or overprotection of child; and exaggerated expressions of anger, disappointment, or despair regarding child's behavior or ability to improve or change.

impaired Social Interaction may be related to retarded ego development, developmental state (adolescence), lack of social skills, low self-concept, dysfunctional family system, and neurological impairment, possibly evidenced by dysfunctional interaction with others (difficulty waiting turn in games or group situations, not seeming to listen to what is being said), difficulty playing quietly and maintaining attention to task or play activity, often shifting from one activity to another and interrupting or intruding on others.

Congestive heart failure   MS
Refer to Heart failure, chronic

Conn's syndrome   MS/CH
Refer to Aldosteronism, primary

Constipation   CH
Constipation may be related to weak abdominal musculature, gastrointestinal obstructive lesions, pain on defecation, diagnostic procedures, pregnancy, possibly evidenced by change in character and frequency of stools, feeling of abdominal or rectal fullness or pressure, changes in bowel sounds, abdominal distention.

impaired Comfort may be related to abdominal fullness or pressure, straining to defecate, and trauma to delicate tissues, possibly evidenced by verbal reports, reluctance to defecate, and distraction behaviors.

deficient Knowledge [Learning Need] regarding dietary needs, bowel function, and medication effect may be related to lack of information, misconceptions, possibly evidenced by development of problem and verbalization of concerns or questions.

risk for decreased Cardiac Output: risk factors may include decreased myocardial contractility, diminished circulating volume (preload), alterations in electrical conduction, and increased systemic vascular resistance (SVR) (afterload).*

acute Pain may be related to direct chest tissue and bone trauma, invasive tubes and lines, donor site incision, tissue inflammation and edema formation, intraoperative nerve trauma, possibly evidenced by verbal reports, changes in vital signs, and distraction behaviors (restlessness), irritability.

[disturbed Sensory Perception (specify)] may be related to restricted environment (postoperative or acute), sleep deprivation, effects of medications, continuous environmental sounds and activities, and psychological stress of procedure, possibly evidenced by disorientation, alterations in behavior, exaggerated emotional responses, and visual or auditory distortions.

CH

ineffective Role Performance may be related to situational crises (dependent role), recuperative process, uncertainty about future, possibly evidenced by delay or alteration in physical capacity to resume role, change in usual role or responsibility, change in self or others' perception of role.

Crohn's disease MS/CH

Also Refer to Colitis, ulcerative

imbalanced Nutrition: less than body requirements may be related to intestinal pain after eating, decreased transit time through bowel, fear that eating may cause diarrhea possibly evidenced by weight loss, decreased subcutaneous fat and muscle mass, poor muscle tone, aversion to eating, and observed lack of intake.

Diarrhea may be related to inflammation, irritation—particular dietary intake, malabsorption of the bowel, presence of toxins, segmental narrowing of the lumen, possibly evidenced by hyperactive bowel sounds, increased peristalsis, cramping, and frequent loose liquid stools.

deficient Knowledge [Learning Need] regarding condition, nutritional needs, and prevention of recurrence may be related to misinterpretation of information, lack of recall, unfamiliarity with resources, possibly evidenced by statements of concern, questions, inaccurate follow-through of instructions, and development of preventable complications or exacerbation of condition.

Croup PED/CH

ineffective Airway Clearance may be related to presence of thick, tenacious mucus and swelling or spasms of the epiglottis, possibly evidenced by harsh, brassy cough; tachypnea, use of accessory breathing muscles, and presence of wheezes.

deficient Fluid Volume may be related to decreased ability or aversion to swallowing, presence of fever, and increased respiratory losses,

---

*A risk diagnosis is not evidenced by signs and symptoms, as the problem has not occurred; rather, nursing interventions are directed at prevention.

possibly evidenced by dry mucous membranes, poor skin turgor, and scanty, concentrated urine.

Croup, membranous   PED/CH
Also Refer to Croup

risk for Suffocation: risk factors may include inflammation of larynx with formation of false membrane.*

Anxiety [specify level]/Fear may be related to change in environment, perceived threat to self (difficulty breathing), and transmission of anxiety of adults, possibly evidenced by restlessness, facial tension, glancing about, and sympathetic stimulation.

C-Section   OB
Refer to Cesarean birth; Cesarean birth, unplanned

Cushing's syndrome   CH/MS
risk for excess Fluid Volume: risk factors may include compromised regulatory mechanism (fluid and sodium retention).*

risk for Infection: risk factors may include immunosuppressed inflammatory response, skin and capillary fragility, and negative nitrogen balance.*

imbalanced Nutrition: less than body requirements may be related to inability to utilize nutrients (disturbance of carbohydrate metabolism), possibly evidenced by decreased muscle mass and increased resistance to insulin.

Self-Care Deficit [specify] may be related to muscle wasting, generalized weakness, fatigue, and demineralization of bones, possibly evidenced by statements of or observed inability to complete or perform ADLs.

disturbed Body Image may be related to change in structure or appearance (effects of disease process, drug therapy), possibly evidenced by negative feelings about body, feelings of helplessness, and changes in social involvement.

Sexual Dysfunction may be related to loss of libido, impotence, and cessation of menses, possibly evidenced by verbalization of concerns and/or dissatisfaction with and alteration in relationship with SO.

risk for Trauma [fractures]: risk factors may include increased protein breakdown, negative protein balance, demineralization of bones.*

CVA   MS/CH
Refer to Cerebrovascular accident

Cystic fibrosis   CH/PED
ineffective Airway Clearance may be related to excessive production of thick mucus and decreased ciliary action, possibly evidenced by abnormal breath sounds, ineffective cough, cyanosis, and altered respiratory rate and depth.

risk for Infection: risk factors may include stasis of respiratory secretions and development of atelectasis.*

---

*A risk diagnosis is not evidenced by signs and symptoms, as the problem has not occurred; rather, nursing interventions are directed at prevention.

imbalanced Nutrition: less than body requirements may be related to impaired digestive process and absorption of nutrients, possibly evidenced by failure to gain weight, muscle wasting, and retarded physical growth.

deficient Knowledge [Learning Need] regarding pathophysiology of condition, medical management, and available community resources may be related to insufficient information, misconceptions, possibly evidenced by statements of concern and questions, inaccurate follow-through of instructions, development of preventable complications.

compromised family Coping may be related to chronic nature of disease and disability, inadequate or incorrect information or understanding by a primary person, possibly evidenced by significant person attempting assistive or supportive behaviors with less than satisfactory results, protective behavior disproportionate to client's abilities, or need for autonomy.

Cystitis CH

acute Pain may be related to inflammation and bladder spasms, possibly evidenced by verbal reports, distraction behaviors, and narrowed focus.

impaired Urinary Elimination may be related to inflammation or irritation of bladder, possibly evidenced by frequency, nocturia, and dysuria.

deficient Knowledge [Learning Need] regarding condition, treatment, and prevention of recurrence may be related to inadequate information, misconceptions, possibly evidenced by statements of concern and questions, recurrent infections.

Cytomegalic inclusion disease CH
Refer to Cytomegalovirus infection

Cytomegalovirus (CMV) infection CH
[risk for disturbed visual Sensory Perception]: risk factors may include inflammation of the retina.*

risk for fetal Infection: risk factors may include transplacental exposure, contact with blood or body fluids.*

Deep Vein Thrombosis (DVT) CH/MS
Refer to Thrombophlebitis

Degenerative joint disease CH
Refer to Arthritis, rheumatoid

Dehiscence (abdominal) MS
impaired Skin Integrity may be related to altered circulation, altered nutritional state (obesity, malnutrition), and physical stress on incision, possibly evidenced by poor or delayed wound healing and disruption of skin surface or wound closure.

risk for Infection: risk factors may include inadequate primary defenses (separation of incision, traumatized intestines, environmental exposure).*

---

*A risk diagnosis is not evidenced by signs and symptoms, as the problem has not occurred; rather, nursing interventions are directed at prevention.

risk for impaired Tissue Integrity: risk factors may include exposure of abdominal contents to external environment.*

Fear/[severe] Anxiety may be related to crises, perceived threat of death, possibly evidenced by fearfulness, restless behaviors, and sympathetic stimulation.

deficient Knowledge [Learning Need] regarding condition, prognosis, and treatment needs may be related to lack of information or recall, misinterpretation of information, possibly evidenced by development of preventable complication, requests for information, and statement of concern.

Dehydration   PED/CH

deficient Fluid Volume [specify] may be related to etiology as defined by specific situation, possibly evidenced by dry mucous membranes, poor skin turgor, decreased pulse volume and pressure, and thirst.

risk for impaired Oral Mucous Membrane: risk factors may include dehydration and decreased salivation.*

deficient Knowledge [Learning Need] regarding fluid needs may be related to lack of information, misinterpretation, possibly evidenced by questions, statement of concern, and inadequate follow-through of instructions, development of preventable complications.

Delirium tremens (acute alcohol withdrawal) MS/PSY

[severe to panic] Anxiety/Fear may be related to cessation of alcohol intake, physiological withdrawal, threat to self-concept, perceived threat of death, possibly evidenced by increased tension, apprehension, feelings of inadequacy, shame, self-disgust, or remorse; fear of unspecified consequences, identifies object of fear.

[disturbed Sensory Perception (specify)] may be related to exogenous factors—alcohol consumption and sudden cessation; endogenous—electrolyte imbalance, elevated ammonia and blood urea nitrogen (BUN); sleep deprivation, and psychological stress, possibly evidenced by disorientation, restlessness, irritability, exaggerated emotional responses, bizarre thinking, and visual or auditory distortions or hallucinations.

risk for decreased Cardiac Output: risk factors may include direct effect of alcohol on heart muscle, altered SVR, presence of dysrhythmias.*

risk for Trauma: risk factors may include alterations in balance, reduced muscle coordination, cognitive impairment, and involuntary clonic/tonic muscle activity.*

imbalanced Nutrition: less than body requirements may be related to poor dietary intake, effects of alcohol on organs involved in digestion, interference with absorption or metabolism of nutrients and amino acids, possibly evidenced by reports of inadequate food intake, altered taste sensation, lack of interest in food, debilitated state, decreased subcutaneous fat and muscle mass, signs or laboratory findings of mineral and electrolyte deficiency.

---

*A risk diagnosis is not evidenced by signs and symptoms, as the problem has not occurred; rather, nursing interventions are directed at prevention.

Delivery, precipitous/out of hospital   OB

Also Refer to Labor, precipitous; Labor stages I–II

risk for deficient Fluid Volume: risk factors may include presence of nausea, vomiting, lack of intake, excessive vascular loss.*

risk for Infection: risk factors may include broken or traumatized tissue, increased environmental exposure, rupture of amniotic membranes.*

risk for fetal Injury: risk factors may include rapid descent and pressure changes, compromised circulation, environmental exposure.*

Delusional disorder   PSY

risk for self-/other-directed Violence: risk factors may include perceived threats of danger, increased feelings of anxiety, acting out in an irrational manner.*

[severe] Anxiety may be related to inability to trust, possibly evidenced by rigid delusional system, frightened of other people and own hostility.

Powerlessness may be related to lifestyle of helplessness, feelings of inadequacy, interpersonal interaction, possibly evidenced by verbal expressions of no control or influence over situation(s), use of paranoid delusions, aggressive behavior to compensate for lack of control.

impaired Social Interaction may be related to mistrust of others, delusional thinking, lack of knowledge or skills to enhance mutuality, possibly evidenced by discomfort in social situations, difficulty in establishing relationships with others, expression of feelings of rejection, no sense of belonging.

Dementia, presenile/senile   CH/PSY

Also Refer to Alzheimer's disease

impaired Memory may be related to neurological disturbances, possibly evidenced by observed experiences of forgetting, inability to determine if a behavior was performed, inability to perform previously learned skills, inability to recall factual information or recent or past events.

Fear may be related to decreases in functional abilities, public disclosure of disabilities, further mental or physical deterioration, possibly evidenced by social isolation, apprehension, irritability, defensiveness, suspiciousness, aggressive behavior.

Self-Care Deficit [specify] may be related to cognitive decline, physical limitations, frustration over loss of independence, depression, possibly evidenced by impaired ability to perform ADLs.

risk for Trauma: risk factors may include changes in muscle coordination or balance, impaired judgment, seizure activity.*

risk for sedentary Lifestyle: risk factors may include lack of interest or motivation, lack of resources, lack of training or knowledge of specific exercise needs, safety concerns or fear of injury.*

---

*A risk diagnosis is not evidenced by signs and symptoms, as the problem has not occurred; rather, nursing interventions are directed at prevention.

risk for Caregiver Role Strain: risk factors may include illness severity of care receiver, duration of caregiving required, complexity or amount of caregiving tasks, care receiver exhibiting deviant or bizarre behavior; family/caregiver isolation, lack of respite or recreation, spouse is caregiver.*

Grieving may be related to awareness of something "being wrong," predisposition for anxiety and feelings of inadequacy, family perception of potential loss of loved one, possibly evidenced by expressions of distress, anger at potential loss, choked feelings, crying, alteration in activity level, communication patterns, eating habits, and sleep patterns.

Depressant abuse   CH/PSY
Also Refer to Drug overdose, acute (depressants)

ineffective Denial may be related to weak, underdeveloped ego, unmet self-needs, possibly evidenced by inability to admit impact of condition on life, minimizes symptoms or problem, refuses healthcare attention.

ineffective Coping may be related to weak ego, possibly evidenced by abuse of chemical agents, lack of goal-directed behavior, inadequate problem-solving, destructive behavior toward self.

imbalanced Nutrition: less than body requirements may be related to use of substance in place of nutritional food, possibly evidenced by loss of weight, pale conjunctiva and mucous membranes, electrolyte imbalances, anemias.

risk for Injury: risk factors may include changes in sleep, decreased concentration, loss of inhibitions.*

Depression, postpartum   OB/PSY
Also Refer to Depressive disorders

risk for impaired Attachment: risk factors may include anxiety associated with the parent role, inability to meet personal needs, perceived guilt regarding relationship with infant.*

Fatigue may be related to stress, sleep deprivation, depression as evidenced by reports overwhelming lack of energy, inability to maintain usual routines, increase in physical complaints.

situational low Self-Esteem may be related to developmental changes, disturbed body image, possibly evidenced by evaluation of self as unable to deal with situation, self-negating verbalizations, reports helplessness.

Depressive disorders, major depression, dysthymia   PSY
risk for self-directed Violence: risk factors may include depressed mood and feeling of worthlessness and hopelessness.*

[moderate to severe] Anxiety may be related to stress, unconscious conflict about essential values or goals of life, unmet needs, threat

---

*A risk diagnosis is not evidenced by signs and symptoms, as the problem has not occurred; rather, nursing interventions are directed at prevention.

to self-concept, interpersonal transmission or contagion, possibly evidenced by feelings of inadequacy, sleep disturbances, fatigue, difficulty concentrating, diminished productivity/ability to problem-solve, rumination.

Insomnia may be related to biochemical alterations (decreased serotonin), unresolved fears and anxieties, and inactivity, possibly evidenced by difficulty in falling or remaining asleep, early morning awakening or awakening later than desired, reports of not feeling rested, physical signs (e.g., dark circles under eyes, excessive yawning).

Social Isolation/impaired Social Interaction may be related to alterations in mental status or thought processes (depressed mood), inadequate personal resources, decreased energy, inertia, difficulty engaging in satisfying personal relationships, feelings of worthlessness, low self-concept, inadequacy or absence of significant purpose in life, and knowledge or skill deficit about social interactions, possibly evidenced by decreased involvement with others, expressed feelings of difference from others, remaining in home/room/bed, refusing invitations or suggestions for social involvement, and dysfunctional interaction with peers, family, and/or others.

interrupted Family Processes may be related to situational crises of illness of family member with change in roles or responsibilities, developmental crises (e.g., loss of family member or relationship), possibly evidenced by statements of difficulty coping with situation, family system not meeting needs of its members, difficulty accepting or receiving help appropriately, ineffective family decision-making process, and failure to send and to receive clear messages.

risk for impaired Religiosity: risk factors may include ineffective support or coping, lack of social interaction, depression.*

risk for Injury [effects of electroconvulsive therapy]: risk factors may include effects of therapy on the cardiovascular, respiratory, musculoskeletal, and nervous systems; and pharmacological effects of anesthesia.*

Dormatitis, seborrheic   CH

impaired Skin Integrity may be related to chronic inflammatory condition of the skin, possibly evidenced by disruption of skin surface with dry or moist scales, yellowish crusts, erythema, and fissures.

Diabetes, gestational   OB

Also Refer to Diabetes mellitus

risk for unstable Blood Glucose Level: risk factors may include pregnancy, dietary intake, lack of diabetes management, inadequate blood glucose monitoring.*

risk for disturbed Maternal-Fetal Dyad: risk factors may include impaired glucose metabolism, compromised oxygen transport—changes in circulation; treatment-related side effects.*

---

*A risk diagnosis is not evidenced by signs and symptoms, as the problem has not occurred; rather, nursing interventions are directed at prevention.

deficient Knowledge [Learning Need] regarding diabetic condition, prognosis, and treatment needs may be related to lack of resources or exposure to information, misinformation, possibly evidenced by questions, statements of misconceptions, inaccurate follow-through of instructions, development of preventable complications.

Diabetes mellitus CH/PED

deficient Knowledge [Learning Need] regarding disease process, treatment, and individual care needs may be related to unfamiliarity with information, lack of recall, misinterpretation, possibly evidenced by requests for information, statements of concern, misconceptions, inadequate follow-through of instructions, or development of preventable complications.

risk for unstable Blood Glucose Level: risk factors may include lack of adherence to diabetes management, medication management, inadequate blood glucose monitoring, physical activity level, health status, stress, rapid growth periods.*

risk-prone Health Behavior may be related to inadequate comprehension, multiple stressors, as evidenced by minimizes health status change, failure to achieve optimal sense of control.

risk for Infection: risk factors may include decreased leukocyte function, circulatory changes, and delayed healing.*

[risk for disturbed Sensory Perception (specify)]: risk factors may include endogenous chemical alteration (glucose, insulin, and/or electrolyte imbalance).*

compromised family Coping may be related to inadequate or incorrect information or understanding by primary person(s), other situational or developmental crises or situations the significant person(s) may be facing, lifelong condition requiring behavioral changes impacting family, possibly evidenced by family expressions of confusion about what to do, verbalizations that they are having difficulty coping with situation, family does not meet physical or emotional needs of its members; SO(s) preoccupied with personal reaction (e.g., guilt, fear), display protective behavior disproportionate (too little or too much) to client's abilities or need for autonomy.

Diabetic ketoacidosis CH/MS

deficient Fluid Volume [specify] may be related to hyperosmolar urinary losses, gastric losses and inadequate intake, possibly evidenced by increased urinary output, dilute urine; reports of weakness, thirst, sudden weight loss, hypotension, tachycardia, delayed capillary refill, dry mucous membranes, poor skin turgor.

unstable Blood Glucose Level may be related to medication management, lack of diabetes management, inadequate blood glucose monitoring, presence of infection, possibly evidenced by elevated serum glucose level, presence of ketones in urine, nausea, weight loss, blurred vision, irritability.

---

*A risk diagnosis is not evidenced by signs and symptoms, as the problem has not occurred; rather, nursing interventions are directed at prevention.

Fatigue may be related to decreased metabolic energy production, altered body chemistry (insufficient insulin), increased energy demands (hypermetabolic state—infection), possibly evidenced by overwhelming lack of energy, inability to maintain usual routines, decreased performance, impaired ability to concentrate, listlessness.

risk for Infection: risk factors may include high glucose levels, decreased leukocyte function, stasis of body fluids, invasive procedures, alterations in circulation.*

Dialysis, general CH
Also Refer to Dialysis, peritoneal; Hemodialysis

imbalanced Nutrition: less than body requirements may be related to inadequate ingestion of nutrients—dietary restrictions, anorexia, nausea, vomiting, stomatitis, sensation of feeling full with continuous ambulatory peritoneal dialysis; loss of peptides and amino acids (building blocks for proteins) during dialysis, possibly evidenced by reported inadequate intake, aversion to eating, altered taste sensation, poor muscle tone, weakness, sore and inflamed buccal cavity, pale conjunctiva and mucous membranes.

Grieving may be related to actual or perceived loss, chronic and/or fatal illness, and thwarted grieving response to a loss, possibly evidenced by verbal expression of distress or unresolved issues, denial of loss, altered eating habits, sleep and dream patterns, activity levels, libido, crying, labile affect; feelings of sorrow, guilt, and anger.

disturbed Body Image/situational low Self-Esteem may be related to situational crisis and chronic illness with changes in usual roles and body image, possibly evidenced by verbalization of changes in lifestyle, focus on past function, negative feelings about body, feelings of helplessness and powerlessness, extension of body boundary to incorporate environmental objects (e.g., dialysis setup), change in social involvement, overdependence on others for care, not taking responsibility for self-care, lack of follow-through, and self-destructive behavior.

Self-Care Deficit [specify] may be related to perceptual or cognitive impairment (accumulated toxins), intolerance to activity, decreased strength and endurance, pain, discomfort, possibly evidenced by reported inability to perform ADLs, disheveled or unkempt appearance, strong body odor.

Powerlessness may be related to illness-related regimen and healthcare environment, possibly evidenced by verbal expression of having no control, depression over physical deterioration, nonparticipation in care, anger, and passivity.

compromised/disabled family Coping may be related to inadequate or incorrect information or understanding by a primary person, temporary family disorganization and role changes, client providing little support in turn for the primary person, and prolonged disease and disability progression that exhausts the supportive capacity of significant persons, possibly evidenced by expressions of concern or reports about response of SO(s)/family to client's health problem,

---

*A risk diagnosis is not evidenced by signs and symptoms, as the problem has not occurred; rather, nursing interventions are directed at prevention.

preoccupation of SO(s) with own personal reactions, display of intolerance or rejection, and protective behavior disproportionate (too little or too much) to client's abilities or need for autonomy.

Dialysis, peritoneal   MS/CH
Also Refer to Dialysis, general

risk for excess Fluid Volume: risk factors may include inadequate osmotic gradient of dialysate, fluid retention—malpositioned, kinked, or clotted catheter; bowel distention, peritonitis, scarring of peritoneum; excessive oral or intravenous (IV) intake.*

risk for Trauma: risk factors may include improper placement during insertion or manipulation of catheter.*

acute Pain/impaired Comfort may be related to catheter irritation, improper catheter placement, presence of edema, abdominal distention, inflammation or infection, rapid infusion or infusion of cold or acidic dialysate, possibly evidenced by verbal reports, guarding or distraction behaviors, and self-focus.

risk for Infection [peritoneal]: risk factors may include contamination of catheter or infusion system, skin contaminants, sterile peritonitis (response to composition of dialysate).*

risk for ineffective Breathing Pattern: risk factors may include increased abdominal pressure restricting diaphragmatic excursion, rapid infusion of dialysate, pain or discomfort, inflammatory process—atelectasis/pneumonia.*

Diaper rash   PED
Refer to Candidiasis

Diarrhea   PED/CH
deficient Knowledge [Learning Need] regarding causative and contributing factors, and therapeutic needs may be related to lack of information, misconceptions, possibly evidenced by statements of concern, questions, and development of preventable complications.

risk for deficient Fluid Volume: risk factors may include excessive losses through gastrointestinal tract, altered intake.*

acute Pain may be related to abdominal cramping and irritation or excoriation of skin, possibly evidenced by verbal reports, facial grimacing, and changes in vital signs.

impaired Skin Integrity may be related to effects of excretions on delicate tissues, possibly evidenced by reports of discomfort and disruption of skin surface or destruction of skin layers.

Digitalis toxicity   MS/CH
decreased Cardiac Output may be related to altered myocardial contractility or electrical conduction, properties of digitalis (long half-life and narrow therapeutic range), concurrent medications, age and general health status, and electrolyte and acid-base balance, possibly evidenced by changes in rate, rhythm, or conduction (development or worsening of dysrhythmias); changes in mentation, worsening of heart failure, elevated serum drug levels.

---

*A risk diagnosis is not evidenced by signs and symptoms, as the problem has not occurred; rather, nursing interventions are directed at prevention.

risk for imbalanced Fluid Volume: risk factors may include excessive losses from vomiting or diarrhea, decreased intake, nausea, decreased plasma proteins, malnutrition, continued use of diuretics; excess sodium and fluid retention.*

deficient Knowledge [Learning Need] regarding condition/therapy and self-care needs may be related to information misinterpretation and lack of recall, possibly evidenced by inaccurate follow-through of instructions and development of preventable complications.

Dilation and curettage (D and C)   OB/GYN
Also Refer to Abortion, elective or spontaneous termination

deficient Knowledge [Learning Need] regarding surgical procedure, possible postprocedural complications, and therapeutic needs may be related to lack of exposure or unfamiliarity with information, possibly evidenced by requests for information and statements of concern, misconceptions.

Dilation of cervix, premature   OB
Also Refer to Labor, preterm

Anxiety [specify level] may be related to situational crisis, threat of death or fetal loss, possibly evidenced by increased tension, apprehension, feelings of inadequacy, sympathetic stimulation, and repetitive questioning.

risk for disturbed Maternal-Fetal Dyad: risk factors may include surgical intervention, use of tocolytic drugs.*

risk for fetal Injury: risk factors may include premature delivery, surgical procedure.*

Grieving may be related to perceived potential fetal loss, possibly evidenced by expression of distress, guilt, anger, choked feelings.

Dislocation/subluxation of joint   CH
acute Pain may be related to lack of continuity of bone/joint, muscle spasms, edema, possibly evidenced by verbal or coded reports, guarded or protective behaviors, narrowed focus, changes in vital signs.

risk for Injury: risk factors may include nerve impingement, improper fitting of splint device.*

impaired physical Mobility may be related to immobilization device, activity restrictions, pain, edema, decreased muscle strength, possibly evidenced by limited range of motion, limited ability to perform motor skills, gait changes.

Disseminated intravascular coagulation (DIC)   MS
risk for deficient Fluid Volume: risk factors may include failure of regulatory mechanism (coagulation process) and active loss—hemorrhage.*

ineffective Tissue Perfusion [specify] may be related to alteration of arterial or venous flow (microemboli throughout circulatory system, and hypovolemia), possibly evidenced by changes in respiratory rate and depth, changes in mentation, decreased urinary output, and development of acral cyanosis or focal gangrene.

---

*A risk diagnosis is not evidenced by signs and symptoms, as the problem has not occurred; rather, nursing interventions are directed at prevention.

Anxiety [specify level]/Fear may be related to sudden change in health status/threat of death, interpersonal transmission or contagion, possibly evidenced by sympathetic stimulation, restlessness, focus on self, and apprehension.

risk for impaired Gas Exchange: risk factors may include reduced O_2-carrying capacity, development of acidosis, fibrin deposition in microcirculation, and ischemic damage of lung parenchyma.*

acute Pain may be related to bleeding into joints/muscles, with hematoma formation, and ischemic tissues with areas of acral cyanosis or focal gangrene, possibly evidenced by verbal reports, narrowed focus, alteration in muscle tone, guarding or distraction behaviors, restlessness, changes in vital signs.

Dissociative disorders   PSY

[severe/panic] Anxiety/Fear may be related to a maladaptation or ineffective coping continuing from early life, unconscious conflict(s), threat to self-concept, unmet needs, or phobic stimulus, possibly evidenced by maladaptive response to stress (e.g., dissociating self or fragmentation of the personality), increased tension, feelings of inadequacy, and focus on self, projection of personal perceptions onto the environment.

risk for self-/other-directed Violence: risk factors may include dissociative state/conflicting personalities, depressed mood, panic states, and suicidal or homicidal behaviors.*

disturbed Personal Identity may be related to psychological conflicts (dissociative state), childhood trauma or abuse, threat to physical integrity or self-concept, and underdeveloped ego, possibly evidenced by alteration in perception or experience of the self, loss of one's own sense of reality or the external world, poorly differentiated ego boundaries, confusion about sense of self, confusion regarding purpose or direction in life, memory loss, presence of more than one personality within the individual.

compromised family Coping may be related to multiple stressors repeated over time, prolonged progression of disorder that exhausts the supportive capacity of significant person(s), family disorganization and role changes, high-risk family situation, possibly evidenced by family/SO(s) describing inadequate understanding or knowledge that interferes with assistive or supportive behaviors, relationship and marital conflict.

Diverticulitis   CH

acute Pain may be related to inflammation of intestinal mucosa, abdominal cramping, and presence of fever or chills, possibly evidenced by verbal reports, guarding or distraction behaviors, changes in vital signs, and narrowed focus.

Diarrhea/Constipation may be related to altered structure or function and presence of inflammation, possibly evidenced by signs and symptoms dependent on specific problem (e.g., increase or decrease in frequency of stools and change in consistency).

---

*A risk diagnosis is not evidenced by signs and symptoms, as the problem has not occurred; rather, nursing interventions are directed at prevention.

deficient Knowledge [Learning Need] regarding disease process, potential complications, therapeutic and self-care needs may be related to lack of information/misconceptions, possibly evidenced by statements of concern, request for information, and development of preventable complications.

risk for Powerlessness: risk factors may include chronic nature of disease process and recurrent episodes despite cooperation with medical regimen.*

Down syndrome
PED/CH

Also Refer to Mental retardation

delayed Growth and Development may be related to effects of physical or mental disability, possibly evidenced by altered physical growth, delay or inability in performing skills and self-care or self-control activities appropriate for age.

risk for Trauma: risk factors may include cognitive difficulties and poor muscle tone or coordination, weakness.*

imbalanced Nutrition: less than body requirements may be related to poor muscle tone and protruding tongue, possibly evidenced by weak and ineffective sucking or swallowing and observed lack of adequate intake with weight loss or failure to gain.

interrupted Family Processes may be related to situational or maturational crises requiring incorporation of new skills into family dynamics, possibly evidenced by confusion about what to do, verbalized difficulty coping with situation, unexamined family myths.

risk for complicated Grieving: risk factors may include loss of "the perfect child," chronic condition requiring long-term care, and unresolved feelings.*

risk for impaired Attachment: risk factors may include ill infant/child who is unable to effectively initiate parental contact due to altered behavioral organization, inability of parents to meet personal needs.*

risk for Social Isolation: risk factors may include withdrawal from usual social interactions and activities, assumption of total child care, and becoming overindulgent or overprotective.*

Drug overdose, acute (depressants)
MS/PSY

Also Refer to Substance dependence/abuse rehabilitation

ineffective Breathing Pattern/impaired Gas Exchange may be related to neuromuscular impairment or CNS depression, decreased lung expansion, possibly evidenced by changes in respirations, cyanosis, and abnormal ABGs.

risk for Trauma/Suffocation/Poisoning: risk factors may include CNS depression or agitation, hypersensitivity to the drug(s), psychological stress.*

risk for self-/other-directed Violence: risk factors may include suicidal behaviors, toxic reactions to drug(s).*

risk for Infection: risk factors may include drug injection techniques, impurities in injected drugs, localized trauma; malnutrition, altered immune state.*

---

*A risk diagnosis is not evidenced by signs and symptoms, as the problem has not occurred; rather, nursing interventions are directed at prevention.

Drug withdrawal   CH/MS
[disturbed Sensory Perception (specify)] may be related to biochemical
    imbalance, altered sensory integration possibly evidenced by sensory
    distortions, poor concentration, irritability, hallucinations.
risk for Injury: risk factors may include CNS agitation (depressants).*
risk for Suicide: risk factors may include alcohol or other substance
    abuse, legal or disciplinary problems, depressed mood (stimulants).*
acute Pain/impaired Comfort may be related to biochemical changes
    associated with cessation of drug use possibly evidenced by reports
    of muscle aches, fever, diaphoresis, rhinorrhea, lacrimation, malaise.
[Self-Care Deficit (specify)] may be related to perceptual or cognitive
    impairment, therapeutic management (restraints) possibly evidenced
    by inability to meet own physical needs.
Insomnia may be related to cessation of substance use, fatigue possibly
    evidenced by reports of insomnia/hypersomnia, decreased ability to
    function, increased irritability.
Fatigue may be related to altered body chemistry (drug withdrawal),
    sleep deprivation, malnutrition, poor physical condition possibly ev-
    idenced by verbal reports of overwhelming lack of energy, inability
    to maintain usual level of physical activity, inability to restore energy
    after sleep, compromised concentration.

Duchenne's muscular dystrophy   PED/CH
Refer to Muscular dystrophy [Duchenne's]

DVT   CH/MS
Refer to Thrombophlebitis

Dysmenorrhea   GYN
acute Pain may be related to exaggerated uterine contractility, pos-
    sibly evidenced by verbal reports, guarding or distraction behaviors,
    narrowed focus, and changes in vital signs.
risk for Activity Intolerance: risk factors may include severity of pain
    and presence of secondary symptoms (nausea, vomiting, syncope,
    chills), depression.*
ineffective Coping may be related to chronic, recurrent nature of prob-
    lem, anticipatory anxiety, and inadequate coping methods, possibly
    evidenced by muscular tension, headaches, general irritability,
    chronic depression, and verbalization of inability to cope, report of
    poor self-concept.

Dysrhythmia, cardiac   MS
risk for decreased Cardiac Output: risk factors may include altered elec-
    trical conduction and reduced myocardial contractility.*
deficient Knowledge [Learning Need] regarding medical condition and
    therapy needs may be related to lack of information or recall, mis-
    interpretation, and unfamiliarity with information resources, possibly
    evidenced by questions, statement of misconception, failure to im-
    prove on previous regimen, and development of preventable com-
    plications.

---

*A risk diagnosis is not evidenced by signs and symptoms, as the problem has
not occurred; rather, nursing interventions are directed at prevention.

risk for Poisoning, [digitalis toxicity]: risk factors may include limited range of therapeutic effectiveness, lack of education or proper precautions, reduced vision, cognitive limitations.*

Eating disorders   CH/PSY
Refer to Anorexia nervosa; Bulimia nervosa; Obesity

Eclampsia   OB
Also Refer to Pregnancy-induced hypertension
Anxiety [specify]/Fear may be related to situational crisis, threat of change in health status or death (self/fetus), separation from support system, interpersonal contagion possibly evidenced by expressed concerns, apprehension, increased tension, decreased self-assurance, difficulty concentrating.
risk for maternal Injury: risk factors may include tissue edema, hypoxia, tonic/clonic convulsions, abnormal blood profile and/or clotting factors.*
impaired physical Mobility may be related to prescribed bedrest, discomfort, anxiety possibly evidenced by difficulty turning, postural instability.
risk for Self-Care Deficit [specify]: risk factors may include weakness, discomfort, physical restrictions.*

Ectopic pregnancy (tubal)   OB
Also Refer to Abortion, spontaneous termination
acute Pain may be related to distention or rupture of fallopian tube, possibly evidenced by verbal reports, guarding or distraction behaviors, facial mask of pain, and diaphoresis, changes in vital signs.
risk for Bleeding/deficient Fluid Volume: risk factors may include pregnancy-related complications, hemorrhagic losses and decreased or restricted intake.*
Anxiety [specify level]/Fear may be related to threat of death and possible loss of ability to conceive, possibly evidenced by increased tension, apprehension, sympathetic stimulation, restlessness, and focus on self.

Eczema (dermatitis)   CH
acute Pain/impaired Comfort may be related to cutaneous inflammation and irritation, possibly evidenced by verbal reports, irritability, and scratching.
risk for Infection: risk factors may include broken skin and tissue trauma.*
Social Isolation may be related to alterations in physical appearance, possibly evidenced by expressed feelings of rejection and decreased interaction with peers.

Edema, pulmonary   MS
excess Fluid Volume may be related to decreased cardiac functioning, excessive fluid/sodium intake, possibly evidenced by dyspnea, presence of crackles (rales), pulmonary congestion on x-ray, restlessness, anxiety, and increased CVP and pulmonary pressures.

---

*A risk diagnosis is not evidenced by signs and symptoms, as the problem has not occurred; rather, nursing interventions are directed at prevention.

impaired Gas Exchange may be related to altered blood flow and decreased alveolar/capillary exchange (fluid collection or shifts into interstitial space or alveoli), possibly evidenced by hypoxia, restlessness, and confusion.

Anxiety [specify level]/Fear may be related to perceived threat of death (inability to breathe), possibly evidenced by responses ranging from apprehension to panic state, restlessness, and focus on self.

Electroconvulsive therapy   PSY

Decisional Conflict may be related to lack of relevant or multiple and divergent sources of information, mistrust of regimen or healthcare personnel, sense of powerlessness, support system deficit.

risk for Injury: risk factors may include effects of therapeutic procedure, and pharmacological effects of anesthesia.*

acute Confusion may be related to CNS effects of electric shock, medications, and anesthesia, possibly evidenced by fluctuation in cognition, agitation.

impaired Memory may be related to neurological disturbance, possibly evidenced by reported or observed experiences of forgetting, difficulty recalling recent events or factual information.

Emphysema   CH/MS

impaired Gas Exchange may be related to alveolar-capillary membrane changes and destruction, possibly evidenced by dyspnea, restlessness, changes in mentation, abnormal ABG values.

ineffective Airway Clearance may be related to increased production or retained tenacious secretions, decreased energy level, and muscle wasting, possibly evidenced by abnormal breath sounds (rhonchi), ineffective cough, changes in rate and depth of respirations, and dyspnea.

Activity Intolerance may be related to imbalance between O_2 supply and demand, possibly evidenced by reports of fatigue, weakness, exertional dyspnea, and abnormal vital sign response to activity.

imbalanced Nutrition: less than body requirements may be related to inability to ingest food (shortness of breath, anorexia, generalized weakness, medication side effects), possibly evidenced by lack of interest in food, reported altered taste, loss of muscle mass and tone, fatigue, and weight loss.

risk for Infection: risk factors may include inadequate primary defenses (stasis of body fluids, decreased ciliary action), chronic disease process, and malnutrition.*

Powerlessness may be related to illness-related regimen and healthcare environment, possibly evidenced by verbal expression of having no control, depression over physical deterioration, nonparticipation in therapeutic regimen, anger, and passivity.

Encephalitis   MS

risk for ineffective cerebral Tissue Perfusion: risk factors may include cerebral edema altering or interrupting cerebral arterial or venous

---

*A risk diagnosis is not evidenced by signs and symptoms, as the problem has not occurred; rather, nursing interventions are directed at prevention.

E

blood flow, hypovolemia, exchange problems at cellular level (acidosis).*

Hyperthermia may be related to increased metabolic rate, illness, and dehydration, possibly evidenced by increased body temperature, flushed, warm skin; and increased pulse and respiratory rates.

acute Pain may be related to inflammation or irritation of the brain and cerebral edema, possibly evidenced by verbal reports of headache, photophobia, distraction behaviors, restlessness, and changes in vital signs.

risk for Trauma/Suffocation: risk factors may include restlessness, clonic/tonic activity, altered sensorium, cognitive impairment, generalized weakness, ataxia, vertigo.*

Endocarditis   MS

risk for decreased Cardiac Output: risk factors may include inflammation of lining of heart and structural change in valve leaflets.*

Anxiety [specify level] may be related to change in health status and threat of death, possibly evidenced by apprehension, expressed concerns, and focus on self.

acute Pain may be related to generalized inflammatory process and effects of embolic phenomena, possibly evidenced by verbal reports, narrowed focus, distraction behaviors, and changes in vital signs.

risk for Activity Intolerance: risk factors may include imbalance between O_2 supply and demand, debilitating condition.*

risk for ineffective Tissue Perfusion [specify]: risk factors may include embolic interruption of arterial flow (embolization of thrombi or valvular vegetations).*

Endometriosis   GYN

acute/chronic Pain may be related to pressure of concealed bleeding, formation of adhesions, possibly evidenced by verbal reports (pain between or with menstruation), guarding or distraction behaviors, and narrowed focus.

Sexual Dysfunction may be related to pain secondary to presence of adhesions, possibly evidenced by verbalization of problem, and altered relationship with partner.

deficient Knowledge [Learning Need] regarding pathophysiology of condition and therapy needs may be related to lack of information/misinterpretations, possibly evidenced by statements of concern and misconceptions.

Enteral feeding   MS/CH

imbalanced Nutrition: less than body requirements may be related to conditions that interfere with nutrient intake or increase nutrient need or metabolic demand—cancer and associated treatments, anorexia, surgical procedures, dysphagia, or decreased level of consciousness, possibly evidenced by body weight 10% or more under ideal, decreased subcutaneous fat or muscle mass, poor muscle tone, changes in gastric motility and stool characteristics.

---

*A risk diagnosis is not evidenced by signs and symptoms, as the problem has not occurred; rather, nursing interventions are directed at prevention.

---

risk for Infection: risk factors may include invasive procedure with surgical placement of feeding tube, malnutrition, chronic disease, improper preparation, handling or contamination of the feeding solution.*

risk for Aspiration: risk factors may include presence of feeding tube, bolus tube feedings, increased intragastric pressure, delayed gastric emptying, medication administration.*

risk for imbalanced Fluid Volume: risk factors may include active loss or failure of regulatory mechanisms specific to underlying disease process or trauma, inability to obtain or ingest fluids.*

Fatigue may be related to decreased metabolic energy production, increased energy requirements—hypermetabolic state, healing process; altered body chemistry—medications, chemotherapy, possibly evidenced by overwhelming lack of energy, inability to maintain usual routines/accomplish routine tasks, lethargy, impaired ability to concentrate.

Enteritis   MS/CH
Refer to Colitis, ulcerative; Crohn's disease

Epididymitis   MS
acute Pain may be related to inflammation, edema formation, and tension on the spermatic cord, possibly evidenced by verbal reports, guarding or distraction behaviors (restlessness), and changes in vital signs.

risk for Infection, [spread]: risk factors may include presence of inflammation, infectious process, insufficient knowledge to avoid spread of infection.*

deficient Knowledge [Learning Need] regarding pathophysiology, outcome, and self-care needs may be related to lack of information, misinterpretations, possibly evidenced by statements of concern, misconceptions, and questions.

Epilepsy   CH
Refer to Seizure disorder

Erectile dysfunction   CH
Sexual Dysfunction may be related to altered body function possibly evidenced by reports of disruption of sexual response pattern, inability to achieve desired satisfaction.

situational low Self-Esteem may be related to functional impairment; rejection of other(s).

Failure to thrive, infant/child   PED
imbalanced Nutrition: less than body requirements may be related to inability to ingest, digest, or absorb nutrients (defects in organ function or metabolism, genetic factors), physical deprivation, psychosocial factors, possibly evidenced by lack of appropriate weight gain or weight loss, poor muscle tone, pale conjunctiva, and laboratory tests reflecting nutritional deficiency.

---

*A risk diagnosis is not evidenced by signs and symptoms, as the problem has not occurred; rather, nursing interventions are directed at prevention.

delayed Growth and Development may be related to inadequate care-taking (physical or emotional neglect or abuse), indifference, inconsistent responsiveness, multiple caretakers, environmental and stimulation deficiencies, possibly evidenced by altered physical growth, flat affect, listlessness, decreased response, delay or difficulty in performing skills or self-control activities appropriate for age group.

risk for impaired Parenting: risk factors may include lack of knowledge, inadequate bonding, unrealistic expectations for self or infant, and lack of appropriate response of child to relationship.*

deficient Knowledge [Learning Need] regarding pathophysiology of condition, nutritional needs, growth and development expectations, and parenting skills may be related to lack of information, misinformation or misinterpretation, possibly evidenced by verbalization of concerns, questions, and misconceptions, or development of preventable complications.

Fatigue syndrome, chronic CH

Fatigue may be related to disease state, inadequate sleep, possibly evidenced by verbalization of unremitting and overwhelming lack of energy, inability to maintain usual routines, listless, compromised concentration.

chronic Pain may be related to chronic physical disability, possibly evidenced by verbal reports of headache, sore throat, arthralgias, abdominal pain, muscle aches, altered ability to continue previous activities, changes in sleep pattern.

Self-Care Deficit [specify] may be related to tiredness, pain/discomfort, possibly evidenced by reports of inability to perform desired ADLs.

risk for ineffective Role Performance: risk factors may include health alterations, stress.*

Femoral popliteal bypass MS

Also Refer to Surgery, general

risk for ineffective peripheral Tissue Perfusion: risk factors may include interruption of arterial blood flow, hypovolemia.*

risk for Peripheral Neurovascular Dysfunction: risk factors may include vascular obstruction, immobilization, mechanical compression, dressings.*

impaired Walking may be related to surgical incisions, dressings, possibly evidenced by inability to walk desired distance, climb stairs, negotiate inclines.

Fetal alcohol syndrome PED

risk for Injury [CNS damage]: risk factors may include external chemical factors (alcohol intake by mother), placental insufficiency, fetal drug withdrawal in utero or postpartum, and prematurity.*

disorganized infant Behavior may be related to prematurity, environmental overstimulation, lack of containment or boundaries, possibly evidenced by change from baseline physiological measures, tremors, startles, twitches, hyperextension of arms and legs, deficient self-regulatory behaviors, deficient response to visual or auditory stimuli.

*A risk diagnosis is not evidenced by signs and symptoms, as the problem has not occurred; rather, nursing interventions are directed at prevention.

risk for impaired Parenting: risk factors may include mental and/or physical illness, inability of mother to assume the overwhelming task of unselfish giving and nurturing, presence of stressors (financial or legal problems), lack of available or ineffective role model, interruption of bonding process, lack of appropriate response of child to relationship.*

PSY

ineffective [maternal] Coping may be related to personal vulnerability, low self-esteem, inadequate coping skills, and multiple stressors (repeated over period of time), possibly evidenced by inability to meet basic needs, fulfill role expectations, or problem-solve, and excessive use of drug(s).

dysfunctional Family Processes may be related to lack of or insufficient support from others, mother's drug problem and treatment status, together with poor coping skills, lack of family stability, overinvolvement of parents with children and multigenerational addictive behaviors, possibly evidenced by abandonment, rejection, neglectful relationships with family members, and decisions and actions by family that are detrimental.

Fetal demise · OB

Grieving may be related to death of fetus/infant (wanted or unwanted), possibly evidenced by verbal expressions of distress, anger, loss, crying, alteration in eating habits or sleep pattern.

situational low Self-Esteem may be related to perceived "failure" at a life event, possibly evidenced by negative self-appraisal in response to life event in a person with a previous positive self-evaluation, verbalization of negative feelings about the self (helplessness, uselessness), difficulty making decisions.

risk for Spiritual Distress: risk factors may include loss of loved one, low self-esteem, poor relationships, challenged belief and value system (birth is supposed to be the beginning of life, not of death) and intense suffering.*

Fibromyalgia syndrome, primary · CH

acute/chronic Pain may be related to idiopathic diffuse condition possibly evidenced by reports of achy pain in fibrous tissues (muscles, tendons, ligaments), muscle stiffness or spasm, disturbed sleep, guarding behaviors, fear of re-injury or exacerbation, restlessness, irritability, self-focusing, reduced interaction with others.

Fatigue may be related to disease state, stress, anxiety, depression, sleep deprivation possibly evidenced by verbalization of overwhelming lack of energy, inability to maintain usual routines or desired level of physical activity, tired, feelings of guilt for not keeping up with responsibilities, increase in physical complaints, listless.

risk for Hopelessness: risk factors may include chronic debilitating physical condition, prolonged activity restriction (possibly self-induced) creating isolation, lack of specific therapeutic cure, prolonged stress.*

---

*A risk diagnosis is not evidenced by signs and symptoms, as the problem has not occurred; rather, nursing interventions are directed at prevention.

Also Refer to Casts; Traction

risk for Trauma [additional injury]: risk factors may include loss of
skeletal integrity, movement of skeletal fragments, use of traction
apparatus, and so on.*

acute Pain may be related to muscle spasms, movement of bone fragments, soft tissue trauma, edema, traction or immobility device,
stress, and anxiety, possibly evidenced by verbal reports, distraction
behaviors, self-focusing or narrowed focus, facial mask of pain,
guarding or protective behavior, alteration in muscle tone, and
changes in vital signs.

risk for Peripheral Neurovascular Dysfunction: risk factors may include
reduction or interruption of blood flow (direct vascular injury, tissue
trauma, excessive edema, thrombus formation, hypovolemia).*

impaired physical Mobility may be related to musculoskeletal impairment, pain, discomfort, restrictive therapies–extremity immobilization, bedrest; and psychological immobility, possibly evidenced by
inability to purposefully move within the physical environment, imposed restrictions, reluctance to attempt movement, limited range of
motion, and decreased muscle strength or control.

risk for impaired Gas Exchange: risk factors may include altered blood
flow, blood or fat emboli, alveolar-capillary membrane changes (interstitial pulmonary edema, congestion).*

deficient Knowledge [Learning Need] regarding healing process, therapy requirements, potential complications, and self-care needs may
be related to lack of exposure or recall, misinterpretation of information, possibly evidenced by statements of concern, questions, and
misconceptions.

Frostbite   **MS/CH**

impaired Tissue Integrity may be related to altered circulation and thermal injury, possibly evidenced by damaged or destroyed tissue.

acute Pain may be related to diminished circulation with tissue ischemia
or necrosis, and edema formation, possibly evidenced by verbal reports, guarding or distraction behaviors, narrowed focus, and
changes in vital signs.

risk for Infection: risk factors may include traumatized tissue or tissue
destruction, altered circulation, and compromised immune response
in affected area.*

Gallstones   **CH**

Refer to Cholelithiasis

Gangrene, dry   **MS**

ineffective peripheral Tissue Perfusion may be related to interruption
in arterial flow, possibly evidenced by cool skin temperature, change
in color (black), atrophy of affected part, and presence of pain.

acute Pain may be related to tissue hypoxia and necrotic process, possibly evidenced by verbal reports, guarding or distraction behaviors,
narrowed focus, and changes in vital signs.

---

*A risk diagnosis is not evidenced by signs and symptoms, as the problem has
not occurred; rather, nursing interventions are directed at prevention.

Gas, lung irritant   MS/CH

ineffective Airway Clearance may be related to irritation and inflammation of airway, possibly evidenced by marked cough, abnormal
breath sounds (wheezes), dyspnea, and tachypnea.

risk for impaired Gas Exchange: risk factors may include irritation and
inflammation of alveolar membrane (dependent on type of agent and
length of exposure).*

Anxiety [specify level] may be related to change in health status and
threat of death, possibly evidenced by verbalizations, increased tension, apprehension, and sympathetic stimulation.

Gastritis, acute   MS

acute Pain may be related to irritation or inflammation of gastric mucosa, possibly evidenced by verbal reports, guarding or distraction
behaviors, and changes in vital signs.

risk for deficient Fluid Volume/Bleeding: risk factors may include excessive losses through vomiting and diarrhea, reluctance to ingest or
restrictions of oral intake; gastrointestinal disorder, continued bleeding.*

Gastritis, chronic   CH

risk for imbalanced Nutrition: less than body requirements: risk factors
may include inability to ingest adequate nutrients (prolonged nausea,
vomiting, anorexia, epigastric pain).*

deficient Knowledge [Learning Need] regarding pathophysiology, psychological factors, therapy needs, and potential complications may
be related to lack of information or recall, unfamiliarity with information resources, information misinterpretation, possibly evidenced
by verbalization of concerns, questions, and continuation of problem
or development of preventable complications.

Gastroenteritis   MS

Diarrhea may be related to toxins, contaminants, travel, infectious process, parasites possibly evidenced by at least three loose, liquid
stools/day, hyperactive bowel sounds, abdominal pain.

risk for deficient Fluid Volume: risk factors may include excessive
losses (diarrhea, vomiting), hypermetabolic state (infection), decreased intake (nausea, anorexia), extremes of age or weight.*

risk for Infection [transmission]: risk factors may include insufficient
knowledge to prevent contamination (inappropriate hand hygiene
and food handling).*

Gastroesophageal reflux disease (GERD)   CH

acute/chronic Pain may be related to acidic irritation of mucosa, muscle
spasm, recurrent vomiting possibly evidenced by reports of heartburn, distraction behaviors.

impaired Swallowing may be related to GERD, esophageal defects,
achalasia possibly evidenced by reports of heartburn or epigastric
pain, "something stuck" when swallowing, food refusal or volume
limiting, nighttime coughing or awakening.

---

*A risk diagnosis is not evidenced by signs and symptoms, as the problem has
not occurred; rather, nursing interventions are directed at prevention.

risk for imbalanced Nutrition: less than body requirements: risk factors may include limiting intake, recurrent vomiting.*

risk for Insomnia: risk factors may include nighttime heartburn, regurgitation of stomach contents.*

risk for Aspiration: risk factors may include incompetent lower esophageal sphincter, regurgitation of gastric acid.*

Gender identity disorder   PSY

(For individuals experiencing persistent and marked distress regarding uncertainty about issues relating to personal identity, e.g., sexual orientation and behavior.)

Anxiety [specify level] may be related to unconscious or conscious conflicts about essential values and beliefs (ego-dystonic gender identification), threat to self-concept, unmet needs, possibly evidenced by increased tension, helplessness, hopelessness, feelings of inadequacy, uncertainty, insomnia and focus on self, and impaired daily functioning.

ineffective Role Performance/disturbed Personal Identity may be related to crisis in development in which person has difficulty knowing or accepting to which sex he or she belongs or is attracted, sense of discomfort and inappropriateness about anatomical sex characteristics, possibly evidenced by confusion about sense of self, purpose or direction in life, sexual identification or preference, verbalization of desire to be or insistence that person is the opposite sex, change in self-perception of role, and conflict in roles.

ineffective Sexuality Pattern may be related to ineffective or absent role models and conflict with sexual orientation and/or preferences, lack of or impaired relationship with an SO, possibly evidenced by verbalizations of discomfort with sexual orientation or role, and lack of information about human sexuality.

risk for compromised/disabled family Coping: risk factors may include inadequate or incorrect information or understanding, SO unable to perceive or to act effectively in regard to client's needs, temporary family disorganization and role changes, and client providing little support in turn for primary person.*

readiness for enhanced family Coping possibly evidenced by family member's attempts to describe growth or impact of crisis on own values, priorities, goals, or relationships, family member is moving in direction of health-promoting and enriching lifestyle that supports client's search for self and choosing experiences that optimize wellness.

Genetic disorder   CH/OB

Anxiety may be related to presence of specific risk factors (e.g., exposure to teratogens), situational crisis, threat to self-concept, conscious or unconscious conflict about essential values and life goals, possibly evidenced by increased tension, apprehension, uncertainty, feelings of inadequacy, expressed concerns.

deficient Knowledge [Learning Need] regarding purpose and process of genetic counseling may be related to lack of awareness of

---

*A risk diagnosis is not evidenced by signs and symptoms, as the problem has not occurred; rather, nursing interventions are directed at prevention.

ramifications of diagnosis, process necessary for analyzing available options, and information misinterpretation, possibly evidenced by verbalization of concerns, statement of misconceptions, request for information.

risk for interrupted Family Processes: risk factors may include situational crisis, individual/family vulnerability, difficulty reaching agreement regarding options.*

Spiritual Distress may be related to intense inner conflict about the outcome, normal grieving for the loss of the "perfect" child, anger that is often directed at God or greater power, religious beliefs and moral convictions, possibly evidenced by verbalization of inner conflict about beliefs, questioning of the moral and ethical implications of therapeutic choices, viewing situation as punishment, anger, hostility, and crying.

risk for complicated Grieving: risk factors may include preloss psychological symptoms, predisposition for anxiety and feelings of inadequacy, frequency of major life events.*

Gigantism CH
Refer to Acromegaly

Glaucoma CH
[disturbed visual Sensory Perception] may be related to altered sensory reception—increased intraocular pressure, atrophy of optic nerve head, possibly evidenced by progressive loss of visual field.

Anxiety [specify level] may be related to change in health status, presence of pain, possibility or reality of loss of vision, unmet needs, and negative self-talk, possibly evidenced by apprehension, uncertainty, and expressed concern regarding changes in life event.

Glomerulonephritis PED
excess Fluid Volume may be related to failure of regulatory mechanism (inflammation of glomerular membrane inhibiting filtration), possibly evidenced by weight gain, edema or anasarca, intake greater than output, and BP changes.

acute Pain may be related to effects of circulating toxins and edema or distention of renal capsule, possibly evidenced by verbal reports, guarding or distraction behaviors, and changes in vital signs.

imbalanced Nutrition: less than body requirements may be related to anorexia and dietary restrictions, possibly evidenced by aversion to eating, reported altered taste, weight loss, and decreased intake.

deficient Diversional Activity may be related to treatment modality or restrictions, fatigue, and malaise, possibly evidenced by statements of boredom, restlessness, and irritability.

risk for disproportionate Growth: risk factors may include infection, malnutrition, chronic illness.*

Goiter CH
disturbed Body Image may be related to visible swelling in neck, possibly evidenced by verbalization of feelings, fear of reaction of others, actual change in structure, change in social involvement.

---

*A risk diagnosis is not evidenced by signs and symptoms, as the problem has not occurred; rather, nursing interventions are directed at prevention.

Anxiety may be related to change in health status and progressive growth of mass, perceived threat of death.

risk for imbalanced Nutrition: less than body requirements: risk factors may include decreased ability to ingest or difficulty swallowing.*

risk for ineffective Airway Clearance: risk factors may include tracheal compression or obstruction.*

Gonorrhea   CH
Also Refer to Sexually transmitted infection (STI)

risk for Infection [dissemination, bacteremia]: risk factors may include presence of infectious process in highly vascular area and lack of recognition of disease process.*

acute Pain may be related to irritation or inflammation of mucosa and effects of circulating toxins, possibly evidenced by verbal reports of genital or pharyngeal irritation, perineal or pelvic pain, guarding or distraction behaviors.

deficient Knowledge [Learning Need] regarding disease cause, transmission, therapy, and self-care needs may be related to lack of information, misinterpretation, denial of exposure, possibly evidenced by statements of concern, questions, misconceptions, and inaccurate follow-through of instructions, development of preventable complications.

Gout   CH
acute Pain may be related to inflammation of joint(s), possibly evidenced by verbal reports, guarding or distraction behaviors, and changes in vital signs.

impaired physical Mobility may be related to joint pain and inflammation, possibly evidenced by reluctance to attempt movement, limited range of motion, and therapeutic restriction of movement.

deficient Knowledge [Learning Need] regarding cause, treatment, and prevention of condition may be related to lack of information or misinterpretation, possibly evidenced by statements of concern, questions, misconceptions, and inaccurate follow-through of instructions.

Guillain-Barré syndrome (acute polyneuritis)   MS
risk for ineffective Breathing Pattern/Airway Clearance: risk factors may include weakness or paralysis of respiratory muscles, impaired gag or swallow reflexes, decreased energy, fatigue.*

[disturbed Sensory Perceptual (specify)] may be related to altered sensory reception, transmission, or integration (altered status of sense organs, sleep deprivation), therapeutically restricted environment, endogenous chemical alterations (electrolyte imbalance, hypoxia), and psychological stress, possibly evidenced by reported or observed change in usual response to stimuli, altered communication patterns, and measured change in sensory acuity and motor coordination.

impaired physical Mobility may be related to neuromuscular impairment, pain or discomfort, possibly evidenced by impaired

---

*A risk diagnosis is not evidenced by signs and symptoms, as the problem has not occurred; rather, nursing interventions are directed at prevention.

coordination, partial or complete paralysis, decreased muscle strength and control.

Anxiety [specify level]/Fear may be related to situational crisis, change in health status or threat of death, possibly evidenced by increased tension, restlessness, helplessness, apprehension, uncertainty, fearfulness, focus on self, and sympathetic stimulation.

risk for Disuse Syndrome: risk factors include paralysis and pain.*

Hallucinogen abuse   CH/PSY

Also Refer to Substance dependence/abuse rehabilitation

Anxiety/Fear may be related to situational crisis, threat to or change in health status, perceived threat of death, inexperience or unfamiliarity with effects of drug possibly evidenced by assumptions of "losing my mind or control," apprehension, preoccupation with feelings of impending doom, sympathetic stimulation.

Self-Neglect may be related to substance use, executive processing ability, possibly evidenced by inadequate personal/environmental hygiene, nonadherence to health activities.

[Self-Care Deficit (specify)] may be related to perceptual or cognitive impairment, therapeutic management (restraints) possibly evidenced by inability to meet own physical needs.

Hay fever   CH

impaired Comfort may be related to irritation or inflammation of upper airway mucous membranes and conjunctiva, possibly evidenced by verbal reports, irritability, and restlessness.

deficient Knowledge [Learning Need] regarding underlying cause, appropriate therapy, and required lifestyle changes may be related to lack of information, possibly evidenced by statements of concern, questions, and misconceptions.

Heart failure, chronic   MS

decreased Cardiac Output may be related to altered myocardial contractility, inotropic changes; alterations in rate, rhythm, and electrical conduction; and structural changes (valvular defects, ventricular aneurysm), possibly evidenced by tachycardia, dysrhythmias, changes in BP, extra heart sounds, decreased urine output, diminished peripheral pulses, cool, ashen skin; orthopnea, crackles; dependent or generalized edema and chest pain.

excess Fluid Volume may be related to reduced glomerular filtration rate (GFR), increased antidiuretic hormone production, and sodium and water retention, possibly evidenced by orthopnea and abnormal breath sounds, S_3 heart sound, jugular vein distention, positive hepatojugular reflex, weight gain, hypertension, oliguria, generalized edema.

risk for impaired Gas Exchange: risk factors may include alveolar-capillary membrane changes (fluid collection or shifts into interstitial space or alveoli).*

                                                                     CH

Activity Intolerance may be related to imbalance between O_2 supply and demand, generalized weakness, and prolonged bedrest, seden-

---

*A risk diagnosis is not evidenced by signs and symptoms, as the problem has not occurred; rather, nursing interventions are directed at prevention.

tary lifestyle, possibly evidenced by reported or observed weakness, fatigue, changes in vital signs, presence of dysrhythmias, dyspnea, pallor, and diaphoresis.

risk for impaired Skin Integrity: risk factors may include prolonged chair or bedrest, edema, vascular pooling, decreased tissue perfusion.*

deficient Knowledge [Learning Need] regarding cardiac function/disease process, therapy and self-care needs may be related to lack of information or misinterpretation, possibly evidenced by questions, statements of concern, misconceptions; development of preventable complications or exacerbations of condition.

Heatstroke   MS

Hyperthermia may be related to prolonged exposure to hot environment, vigorous activity with failure of regulating mechanism of the body, possibly evidenced by high body temperature (>105°F [40.6°C]), flushed, hot skin; tachycardia, and seizure activity.

decreased Cardiac Output may be related to functional stress of hypermetabolic state, altered circulating volume and venous return, and direct myocardial damage secondary to hyperthermia, possibly evidenced by decreased peripheral pulses, dysrhythmias, tachycardia, and changes in mentation.

Hemodialysis   MS/CH

Also Refer to Dialysis, general

risk for Injury [loss of vascular access]: risk factors may include clotting or thrombosis, infection, disconnection and hemorrhage.*

risk for deficient Fluid Volume/Bleeding: risk factors may include excessive fluid losses or shifts via ultrafiltration, fluid restrictions, altered coagulation, disconnection of shunt.*

risk for excess Fluid Volume: risk factors may include rapid or excessive fluid intake—IV, blood, plasma expanders, saline given to support BP during procedure.*

ineffective Protection may be related to chronic disease state, drug therapy, abnormal blood profile, inadequate nutrition, possibly evidenced by altered clotting, impaired healing, deficient immunity, fatigue, anorexia.

Hemophilia   PED

risk for deficient [isotonic] Fluid Volume: risk factors may include impaired coagulation/hemorrhagic losses.*

risk for acute/chronic Pain: risk factors may include nerve compression from hematomas, nerve damage, or hemorrhage into joint space.*

risk for impaired physical Mobility: risk factors may include joint hemorrhage, swelling, degenerative changes, and muscle atrophy.*

ineffective Protection may be related to abnormal blood profile, possibly evidenced by altered clotting.

compromised family Coping may be related to prolonged nature of condition that exhausts the supportive capacity of significant

---

*A risk diagnosis is not evidenced by signs and symptoms, as the problem has not occurred; rather, nursing interventions are directed at prevention.

person(s), possibly evidenced by protective behaviors disproportionate to client's abilities or need for autonomy.

Hemorrhoidectomy — MS/CH

acute Pain may be related to edema or swelling, and tissue trauma, possibly evidenced by verbal reports, guarding or distraction behaviors, focus on self, and changes in vital signs.

risk for Urinary Retention: risk factors may include perineal trauma, edema or swelling, and pain.*

deficient Knowledge [Learning Need] regarding therapeutic treatment and potential complications may be related to lack of information or misconceptions, possibly evidenced by statements of concern and questions.

Hemorrhoids — CH/OB

acute Pain may be related to inflammation and edema of prolapsed varices, possibly evidenced by verbal reports, and guarding or distraction behaviors.

Constipation may be related to pain on defecation and reluctance to defecate, possibly evidenced by frequency less than usual pattern, and hard, formed stools.

Hemothorax — MS

Also Refer to Pneumothorax

risk for Trauma/Suffocation: risk factors may include concurrent disease or injury process, dependence on external device (chest drainage system), and lack of safety education or precautions.*

Anxiety [specify level] may be related to change in health status and threat of death, possibly evidenced by increased tension, restlessness, expressed concern, sympathetic stimulation, and focus on self.

Hepatitis, acute viral — MS/CH

impaired Liver Function related to viral infection as evidenced by jaundice, hepatic enlargement, abdominal pain, marked elevations in serum liver function tests.

Fatigue may be related to decreased metabolic energy production, discomfort, altered body chemistry—changes in liver function, effect on target organs, possibly evidenced by reports of lack of energy, inability to maintain usual routines, decreased performance, and increased physical complaints.

imbalanced Nutrition: less than body requirements may be related to inability to ingest adequate nutrients—nausea, vomiting, anorexia, hypermetabolic state, altered absorption and metabolism, possibly evidenced by aversion to eating or lack of interest in food, altered taste sensation, observed lack of intake, and weight loss.

acute Pain/impaired Comfort may be related to inflammation and swelling of the liver, arthralgias, urticarial eruptions, and pruritus, possibly evidenced by verbal reports, guarding or distraction behaviors, focus on self, and changes in vital signs.

---

*A risk diagnosis is not evidenced by signs and symptoms, as the problem has not occurred; rather, nursing interventions are directed at prevention.

risk for Infection: risk factors may include inadequate secondary defenses and immunosuppression, malnutrition, insufficient knowledge to avoid exposure to pathogens.*

risk for impaired Tissue Integrity: risk factors may include bile salt accumulation in the tissues.*

risk for impaired Home Management: risk factors may include debilitating effects of disease process and inadequate support systems (family, financial, role model).*

deficient Knowledge [Learning Need] regarding disease process and transmission, treatment needs, and future expectations may be related to lack of information or recall, misinterpretation, unfamiliarity with resources, possibly evidenced by questions, statement of concerns, misconceptions, inaccurate follow-through of instructions, or development of preventable complications.

Hernia, hiatal CH

chronic Pain may be related to regurgitation of acidic gastric contents, possibly evidenced by verbal reports, facial grimacing, and focus on self.

deficient Knowledge [Learning Need] regarding pathophysiology, prevention of complications and self-care needs may be related to lack of information, misconceptions, possibly evidenced by statements of concern, questions, and recurrence of condition.

Herniated nucleus pulposus (ruptured intervertebral disk) CH/MS

acute/chronic Pain may be related to nerve compression or irritation and muscle spasms, possibly evidenced by verbal reports, guarding or distraction behaviors, preoccupation with pain, self-focus or narrowed focus, changes in vital signs when pain is acute, altered muscle tone or function, changes in eating or sleeping patterns and libido, physical or social withdrawal.

impaired physical Mobility may be related to pain (muscle spasms), discomfort, therapeutic restrictions—bedrest, traction, or braces; muscular impairment, and depressive mood state, possibly evidenced by reports of pain on movement, reluctance to attempt or difficulty with purposeful movement, decreased muscle strength, impaired coordination, and limited range of motion.

deficient Diversional Activity may be related to length of recuperation period and therapy restrictions, physical limitations, pain, and depression, possibly evidenced by statements of boredom, disinterest, "nothing to do," restlessness, irritability, withdrawal.

Heroin withdrawal CH/MS

acute Pain/impaired Comfort may be related to cessation of drug, muscle tremors/twitching, possibly evidenced by reports of muscle aches, hot or cold flashes, diaphoresis, lacrimation, rhinorrhea, drug cravings.

[severe] Anxiety may be related to CNS hyperactivity possibly evidenced by apprehension, pervasive anxious feelings, jittery, restlessness, weakness, insomnia, anorexia.

---

*A risk diagnosis is not evidenced by signs and symptoms, as the problem has not occurred; rather, nursing interventions are directed at prevention.

risk for ineffective Self-Health Management: risk factors may include protracted withdrawal, economic difficulties, family or social support deficits, perceived barriers or benefits.*

Herpes, herpes simplex CH

acute Pain may be related to presence of localized inflammation and open lesions, possibly evidenced by verbal reports, distraction behaviors, and restlessness.

risk for [secondary] Infection: risk factors may include broken or traumatized tissue, altered immune response, and untreated infection or treatment failure.*

risk for Sexual Dysfunction: risk factors may include lack of knowledge, values conflict, and/or fear of transmitting the disease.*

Herpes zoster (shingles) CH

acute Pain may be related to inflammation and local lesions along sensory nerve(s), possibly evidenced by verbal reports, guarding or distraction behaviors, narrowed focus, restlessness, and changes in vital signs.

deficient Knowledge [Learning Need] regarding pathophysiology, therapeutic needs, and potential complications may be related to lack of information, misinterpretation, possibly evidenced by statements of concern, questions, and misconceptions.

High-altitude pulmonary edema (HAPE) MS

Also Refer to Mountain sickness, acute

impaired Gas Exchange may be related to ventilation perfusion imbalance, alveolar-capillary membrane changes, altered O_2 supply, possibly evidenced by dyspnea, confusion, cyanosis, tachycardia, abnormal ABGs.

excess Fluid Volume may be related to compromised regulatory mechanism, possibly evidenced by shortness of breath, anxiety, edema, abnormal breath sounds, pulmonary congestion.

High-altitude sickness MS

Refer to Mountain sickness, acute; High-altitude pulmonary edema

HIV infection CH

Also Refer to AIDS

risk-prone Health Behavior may be related to life-threatening, stigmatizing condition or disease, assault to self-esteem, altered locus of control, inadequate support systems, possibly evidenced by verbalization of nonacceptance or denial of diagnosis, failure to take action that prevents health problems.

deficient Knowledge [Learning Need] regarding disease, prognosis, and treatment needs may be related to lack of exposure or recall, information misinterpretation, unfamiliarity with information resources, or cognitive limitation, possibly evidenced by statement of misconception, request for information, inappropriate or exaggerated behaviors (hostile, agitated, hysterical, apathetic), inaccurate follow-

---

*A risk diagnosis is not evidenced by signs and symptoms, as the problem has not occurred; rather, nursing interventions are directed at prevention.

through of instructions, or development of preventable complications.

risk for ineffective Self-Health Management: risk factors may include complexity of healthcare system and access to care, economic difficulties; complexity of therapeutic regimen—confusing or difficult dosing schedule, duration of regimen; mistrust of regimen and/or healthcare personnel, client and provider interactions; health beliefs or cultural influences, perceived seriousness, susceptibility, or benefits of therapy; decisional conflicts, powerlessness.*

risk for complicated Grieving: risk factors may include preloss psychological symptoms, predisposition for anxiety and feelings of inadequacy, frequency of major life events.*

Hodgkin's disease   CH/MS
Also Refer to Cancer; Chemotherapy

Anxiety [specify level]/Fear may be related to threat of self-concept and threat of death, possibly evidenced by apprehension, insomnia, focus on self, and increased tension.

deficient Knowledge [Learning Need] regarding diagnosis, pathophysiology, treatment, and prognosis may be related to lack of information/misinterpretation, possibly evidenced by statements of concern, questions, and misconceptions.

acute Pain/impaired Comfort may be related to manifestations of inflammatory response (fever, chills, night sweats) and pruritus, possibly evidenced by verbal reports, distraction behaviors, and focus on self.

risk for ineffective Breathing Pattern/Airway Clearance: risk factors may include tracheobronchial obstruction (enlarged mediastinal nodes and/or airway edema).*

Hospice/End-of-life care   CH
acute/chronic Pain may be related to biological, physical, psychological agent; chronic physical disability, possibly evidenced by verbal or coded report, preoccupation with pain, changes in appetite/eating, sleep pattern, altered ability to continue desired activities, guarded or protective behaviors, restlessness, irritability, narrowed focus—altered time perception, impaired thought processes.

Activity Intolerance/Fatigue may be related to generalized weakness, bedrest or immobility, pain, progressive disease state or debilitating condition, depressive state, imbalance between O_2 supply and demand, possibly evidenced by inability to maintain usual routine, verbalized lack of desire or interest in activity, decreased performance, lethargy.

Grieving/Death Anxiety may be related to anticipated loss of physiological well-being, change in body function, perceived threat of death or dying process, possibly evidenced by changes in communication pattern, denial of potential loss; choked feelings, anger, fear of loss of physical or mental abilities; negative death images or unpleasant thoughts about any event related to death or dying; anticipated pain related to dying; powerlessness over issues related to dying, worrying

*A risk diagnosis is not evidenced by signs and symptoms, as the problem has not occurred; rather, nursing interventions are directed at prevention.

about impact of one's own death on SO(s), being the cause of other's grief and suffering, concerns of overworking the caregiver as terminal illness incapacitates.

compromised/disabled family Coping/Caregiver Role Strain may be related to prolonged disease/disability progression, temporary family disorganization and role changes, unrealistic expectations, inadequate or incorrect information or understanding by primary person, possibly evidenced by client expressing despair about family reactions or lack of involvement, history of poor relationship between caregiver and care receiver; altered caregiver health status; SO attempting assistive or supportive behaviors with less than satisfactory results, apprehension about future regarding caregiver's ability to provide care; SO describing preoccupation about personal reactions; displaying intolerance, abandonment, rejection; family behaviors that are detrimental to well-being.

risk for Spiritual Distress: risk factors may include physical or psychological stress, energy-consuming anxiety; situational losses; blocks to self-love, low self-esteem, inability to forgive.*

risk for Moral Distress: risk factors may include conflict among decision makers, cultural conflicts, end-of-life decisions, loss of autonomy, physical distance of decision makers.*

Hydrocephalus   PED/MS

ineffective cerebral Tissue Perfusion may be related to decreased arterial or venous blood flow (compression of brain tissue), possibly evidenced by changes in mentation, restlessness, irritability, reports of headache, pupillary changes, and changes in vital signs.

[disturbed visual Sensory Perception] may be related to pressure on sensory or motor nerves, possibly evidenced by reports of double vision, development of strabismus, nystagmus, pupillary changes, and optic atrophy.

risk for impaired physical Mobility: risk factors may include neuromuscular impairment, decreased muscle strength, and impaired coordination.*

risk for decreased Intracranial Adaptive Capacity: risk factors may include brain injury, changes in perfusion pressure or intracranial pressure.*

CH

risk for Infection: risk factors may include invasive procedure, presence of shunt.*

deficient Knowledge [Learning Need] regarding condition, prognosis, and long-term therapy needs and medical follow-up may be related to lack of information, misperceptions, possibly evidenced by questions, statement of concern, request for information, and inaccurate follow-through of instruction, or development of preventable complications.

Hyperactivity disorder   PED/PSY

ineffective Impulse Control may be related to compunction, possibly evidenced by acting without thinking, temper outbursts.

---

*A risk diagnosis is not evidenced by signs and symptoms, as the problem has not occurred; rather, nursing interventions are directed at prevention.

defensive Coping may be related to mild neurological deficits, dysfunctional family system, abuse or neglect, possibly evidenced by denial of obvious problems, projection of blame or responsibility, grandiosity, difficulty in reality testing perceptions.

impaired Social Interaction may be related to retarded ego development, negative role models, neurological impairment, possibly evidenced by discomfort in social situations; interrupts or intrudes on others, difficulty waiting turn in games or group activities, difficulty maintaining attention to task.

disabled family Coping may be related to excessive guilt, anger, or blaming among family members, parental inconsistencies, disagreements regarding discipline, limit-setting approaches; exhaustion of parental expectations, possibly evidenced by unrealistic parental expectations, rejection or overprotection of child, exaggerated expression of feelings, despair regarding child's behavior.

Hyperbilirubinemia   PED

neonatal Jaundice may be related to, difficulty transitioning to extrauterine life, feeding pattern not well established, abnormal weight loss, possibly evidenced by abnormal blood profile—elevated BUN, yellow-orange skin/sclera.

risk for Injury [effects of treatment]: risk factors may include physical properties of phototherapy and effects on body regulatory mechanisms, invasive procedure (exchange transfusion), abnormal blood profile, chemical imbalances.*

deficient Knowledge [Learning Need] regarding condition prognosis, treatment and safety needs may be related to lack of exposure or recall and information misinterpretation, possibly evidenced by questions, statement of concern, and inaccurate follow-through of instructions, or development of preventable complications.

Hyperemesis gravidarum   OB

deficient Fluid Volume may be related to excessive gastric losses and reduced intake, possibly evidenced by dry mucous membranes, decreased, concentrated urine; decreased pulse volume and pressure, thirst, and hemoconcentration.

risk for Electrolyte Imbalance: risk factors may include vomiting, dehydration.*

imbalanced Nutrition: less than body requirements may be related to inability to ingest, digest, or absorb nutrients (prolonged vomiting), possibly evidenced by reported inadequate food intake, lack of interest in food or aversion to eating, and weight loss.

risk for ineffective Coping: risk factors may include situational or maturational crisis (pregnancy, change in health status, projected role changes, concern about outcome).*

Hypertension   CH

deficient Knowledge [Learning Need] regarding condition, therapeutic regimen, and potential complications may be related to lack of information or recall, misinterpretation, cognitive limitations, and/or

---

*A risk diagnosis is not evidenced by signs and symptoms, as the problem has not occurred; rather, nursing interventions are directed at prevention.

denial of diagnosis, possibly evidenced by statements of concern, questions, and misconceptions, inaccurate follow-through of instructions, and lack of BP control.

risk-prone Health Behavior may be related to condition requiring change in lifestyle, altered locus of control, and absence of feelings, denial of illness, possibly evidenced by verbalization of nonacceptance of health status change and lack of movement toward independence.

risk for Activity Intolerance: risk factors may include generalized weakness, imbalance between oxygen supply and demand.*

risk for Sexual Dysfunction: risk factors may include side effects of medication.*

MS

risk for decreased Cardiac Output: risk factors may include increased afterload (vasoconstriction), fluid shifts, hypovolemia, myocardial ischemia, ventricular hypertrophy or rigidity.*

acute Pain may be related to increased cerebrovascular pressure, possibly evidenced by verbal reports (throbbing pain located in suboccipital region, present on awakening and disappearing spontaneously after being up and about), reluctance to move head, avoidance of bright lights and noise, increased muscle tension.

Hypertension, pulmonary   CH/MS
Refer to Pulmonary hypertension

Hyperthyroidism   CH
Also Refer to Thyrotoxicosis

Fatigue may be related to hypermetabolic imbalance with increased energy requirements, irritability of CNS, and altered body chemistry, possibly evidenced by verbalization of overwhelming lack of energy to maintain usual routine, decreased performance, emotional lability or irritability, and impaired ability to concentrate.

Anxiety [specify level] may be related to increased stimulation of the CNS (hypermetabolic state, pseudocatecholamine effect of thyroid hormones), possibly evidenced by increased feelings of apprehension, overexcitement or distress, irritability or emotional lability, shakiness, restless movements, tremors.

risk for imbalanced Nutrition: less than body requirements: risk factors may include inability to ingest adequate nutrients for hypermetabolic rate and constant activity level, impaired absorption of nutrients—vomiting, diarrhea, hyperglycemia, relative insulin insufficiency.*

risk for Dry Eye: risk factors may include periorbital edema, altered protective mechanisms of eye—reduced ability to blink; eye dryness.*

Hypoglycemia   CH
acute Confusion may be related to inadequate glucose for cellular brain function and effects of endogenous hormone activity, possibly evidenced by increased restlessness, misperceptions, fluctuation in cognition/level of consciousness.

---

*A risk diagnosis is not evidenced by signs and symptoms, as the problem has not occurred; rather, nursing interventions are directed at prevention.

risk for unstable Blood Glucose Level: risk factors may include dietary intake, lack of adherence to diabetes management, inadequate blood glucose monitoring, medication management.*

deficient Knowledge [Learning Need] regarding pathophysiology of condition, therapy, and self-care needs may be related to lack of information or recall, misinterpretations, possibly evidenced by development of hypoglycemia and statements of questions, misconceptions.

Hypoparathyroidism (acute) MS

risk for Injury: risk factors may include neuromuscular excitability or tetany and formation of renal stones.*

acute Pain may be related to recurrent muscle spasms and alteration in reflexes, possibly evidenced by verbal reports, distraction behaviors, and narrowed focus.

risk for ineffective Airway Clearance: risk factors may include spasm of the laryngeal muscles.*

Anxiety [specify level] may be related to threat to, or change in, health status, physiological responses.

H

Hypothermia (systemic) CH

Also Refer to Frostbite

Hypothermia may be related to exposure to cold environment, inadequate clothing, age extremes (very young or elderly), damage to hypothalamus, consumption of alcohol or medications causing vasodilation, possibly evidenced by reduction in body temperature below normal range, shivering, cool skin, pallor.

deficient Knowledge [Learning Need] regarding risk factors, treatment needs, and prognosis may be related to lack of information or recall, misinterpretation, possibly evidenced by statement of concerns, misconceptions, occurrence of problem, and development of complications.

Hypothyroidism CH

Also Refer to Myxedema

impaired physical Mobility may be related to weakness, fatigue, muscle aches, altered reflexes, and mucin deposits in joints and interstitial spaces, possibly evidenced by decreased muscle strength or control, and impaired coordination.

Fatigue may be related to decreased metabolic energy production, possibly evidenced by verbalization of unremitting or overwhelming lack of energy, inability to maintain usual routines, impaired ability to concentrate, decreased libido, irritability, listlessness, decreased performance, increase in physical complaints.

[disturbed Sensory Perception (specify)] may be related to mucin deposits and nerve compression, possibly evidenced by paresthesias of hands and feet or decreased hearing.

Constipation may be related to decreased physical activity, slowed peristalsis, possibly evidenced by frequency less than usual pattern,

---

*A risk diagnosis is not evidenced by signs and symptoms, as the problem has not occurred; rather, nursing interventions are directed at prevention.

decreased bowel sounds, hard dry stools, and development of fecal impaction.

Hysterectomy

GYN/MS
Also Refer to Surgery, general

acute Pain may be related to tissue trauma and abdominal incision, edema or hematoma formation, possibly evidenced by verbal reports, guarding or distraction behaviors, and changes in vital signs.

risk for impaired Urinary Elimination/[acute] Urinary Retention: risk factors may include mechanical trauma, surgical manipulation, presence of localized edema or hematoma, or nerve trauma with temporary bladder atony.*

risk for Sexual Dysfunction: risk factors may include concerns regarding altered body function or structure, perceived changes in femininity, changes in hormone levels, loss of libido, and changes in sexual response pattern.*

risk for complicated Grieving: risk factors may include preloss psychological symptoms, predisposition for anxiety and feelings of inadequacy, frequency of major life events. *

Ileocolitis

MS/CH
Refer to Crohn's disease

Ileostomy

MS/CH
Refer to Colostomy

Ileus

MS

acute Pain may be related to distention or edema, and ischemia of intestinal tissue, possibly evidenced by verbal reports, guarding or distraction behaviors, narrowed focus, and changes in vital signs.

Diarrhea/Constipation may be related to presence of obstruction or changes in peristalsis, possibly evidenced by changes in frequency and consistency or absence of stool, alterations in bowel sounds, presence of pain, and cramping.

risk for deficient Fluid Volume: risk factors may include increased intestinal losses (vomiting and diarrhea), and decreased intake.*

Impetigo

PED/CH

impaired Skin Integrity may be related to presence of infectious process and pruritus, possibly evidenced by open or crusted lesions.

acute Pain may be related to inflammation and pruritus, possibly evidenced by verbal reports, distraction behaviors, and self-focusing.

risk for [secondary] Infection: risk factors may include broken skin, traumatized tissue, altered immune response, and virulence and contagious nature of causative organism.*

risk for Infection [transmission]: risk factors may include virulent nature of causative organism, insufficient knowledge to prevent infection of others.*

---

*A risk diagnosis is not evidenced by signs and symptoms, as the problem has not occurred; rather, nursing interventions are directed at prevention.

Infection, prenatal

Also Refer to AIDS

risk for maternal/fetal Infection: risk factors may include inadequate
primary defenses (e.g., broken skin, stasis of body fluids), inadequate
secondary defenses (e.g., decreased Hb, immunosuppression), inadequate acquired immunity, environmental exposure, malnutrition,
rupture of amniotic membranes.*

deficient Knowledge regarding treatment/prevention, prognosis of condition may be related to lack of exposure to information and/or unfamiliarity with resources, misinterpretation possibly evidenced by
verbalization of problem, inaccurate follow-through of instructions,
development of preventable complications or continuation of infec
tious process.

impaired Comfort may be related to body response to infective agent,
properties of infection (e.g., skin or tissue irritation, development of
lesions), possibly evidenced by verbal reports, restlessness, withdrawal from social contacts.

Infection, wound

risk for Infection [sepsis]: risk factors may include presence of infection, broken skin, traumatized tissues, chronic disease (e.g., diabetes,
anemia), stasis of body fluids, invasive procedures, altered immune
response.*

impaired Skin/Tissue Integrity may be related to altered circulation,
presence of infection, wound drainage, nutritional deficit, possibly
evidenced by delayed healing, damaged tissues, invasion of body
structures.

risk for delayed Surgical Recovery: risk factors may include presence
of infection, activity restrictions or limitations, nutritional deficiencies.*

Inflammatory bowel disease

Refer to Colitis, ulcerative; Crohn's disease

Infertility

situational low Self-Esteem may be related to functional impairment
(inability to conceive), unrealistic self-expectations, sense of failure
possibly evidenced by self-negating verbalizations, expressions of
helplessness, perceived inability to deal with situation.

chronic Sorrow may be related to perceived physical disability (inability
to conceive) possibly evidenced by expressions of anger, disappointment, emptiness, self-blame, helplessness, sadness, feelings interfering with client's ability to achieve maximum well-being.

risk for Spiritual Distress: risk factors may include energy-consuming
anxiety, low self-esteem, deteriorating relationship with SO, viewing
situation as deserved or punishment for past behaviors.*

Influenza

acute Pain/impaired Comfort may be related to inflammation and effects
of circulating toxins, possibly evidenced by verbal reports, distraction behaviors, and narrowed focus.

---

*A risk diagnosis is not evidenced by signs and symptoms, as the problem has
not occurred; rather, nursing interventions are directed at prevention.

risk for deficient Fluid Volume: risk factors may include excessive gastric losses, hypermetabolic state, and altered intake.*

Hyperthermia may be related to effects of circulating toxins and dehydration, possibly evidenced by increased body temperature, warm, flushed skin; and tachycardia.

risk for ineffective Breathing: risk factors may include response to infectious process, decreased energy, fatigue.*

Insulin shock   MS/CH
Refer to Hypoglycemia

Intestinal obstruction   MS
Refer to Ileus

Irritable bowel syndrome   CH
acute Pain may be related to abnormally strong intestinal contractions, increased sensitivity of intestine to distention, hypersensitivity to hormones gastrin and cholecystokinin, skin or tissue irritation, perirectal excoriation, possibly evidenced by verbal reports, guarding behavior, expressive behavior (restlessness, moaning, irritability).

Constipation may be related to motor abnormalities of longitudinal muscles and changes in frequency and amplitude of contractions, dietary restrictions, stress, possibly evidenced by change in bowel pattern, decreased frequency, sensation of incomplete evacuation, abdominal pain, distention.

Diarrhea may be related to motor abnormalities of longitudinal muscles and changes in frequency and amplitude of contractions, possibly evidenced by precipitous passing of liquid stool on rising or immediately after eating, rectal urgency, incontinence, bloating.

Kawasaki disease   PED
Hyperthermia may be related to increased metabolic rate and dehydration, possibly evidenced by increased body temperature greater than normal range, flushed skin, increased respiratory rate, and tachycardia.

acute Pain may be related to inflammation and edema or swelling of tissues, possibly evidenced by verbal reports, restlessness, guarding behaviors, and narrowed focus.

impaired Skin Integrity may be related to inflammatory process, altered circulation, and edema formation, possibly evidenced by disruption of skin surface, including macular rash and desquamation.

impaired Oral Mucous Membrane may be related to inflammatory process, dehydration, and mouth breathing, possibly evidenced by pain, hyperemia, and fissures of lips.

risk for decreased Cardiac Output: risk factors may include structural changes, inflammation of coronary arteries and alterations in rate, rhythm, or conduction.*

Kidney stone(s)   CH
Refer to Calculi, urinary

---

*A risk diagnosis is not evidenced by signs and symptoms, as the problem has not occurred; rather, nursing interventions are directed at prevention.

Labor, induced/augmented

deficient Knowledge [Learning Need] regarding procedure, treatment
needs, and possible outcomes may be related to lack of exposure/
recall, information misinterpretation, and unfamiliarity with information resources, possibly evidenced by questions, statements of
concern/misconception, and exaggerated behaviors.

risk for maternal Injury: risk factors may include adverse effects or
response to therapeutic interventions.*

risk for impaired fetal Gas Exchange: risk factors may include altered
placental perfusion or cord prolapse.*

acute Pain may be related to altered characteristics of chemically stimulated contractions, psychological concerns, possibly evidenced by
verbal reports, increased muscle tone, distraction or guarding behaviors, and narrowed focus.

Labor, precipitous

Anxiety [specify level] may be related to situational crisis, threat to self
or fetus, interpersonal transmission, possibly evidenced by increased
tension; scared, fearful, restless, jittery; sympathetic stimulation.

risk for impaired Skin/Tissue Integrity: risk factors may include rapid
progress of labor, lack of necessary equipment.*

acute Pain may be related to occurrence of rapid, strong muscle contractions; psychological issues, possibly evidenced by verbalizations
of inability to use learned pain-management techniques, sympathetic
stimulation, distraction behaviors (e.g., moaning, restlessness).

Labor, preterm

Activity Intolerance may be related to muscle or cellular hypersensitivity, possibly evidenced by continued uterine contractions or irritability.

risk for Poisoning: risk factors may include dose-related toxic or side
effects of tocolytics.*

risk for fetal Injury: risk factors may include delivery of premature or
immature infant.*

Anxiety [specify level] may be related to situational crisis, perceived
or actual threats to self or fetus, and inadequate time to prepare for
labor, possibly evidenced by increased tension, restlessness, expressions of concern, and changes in vital signs.

deficient Knowledge [Learning Need] regarding preterm labor treatment needs and prognosis may be related to lack of information and
misinterpretation, possibly evidenced by questions, statements of
concern, misconceptions, inaccurate follow-through of instruction,
and development of preventable complications.

Labor, stage I (active phase)

acute Pain/impaired Comfort may be related to contraction-related hypoxia, dilation of tissues, and pressure on adjacent structures combined with stimulation of both parasympathetic and sympathetic
nerve endings, possibly evidenced by verbal reports, guarding or

L

---

*A risk diagnosis is not evidenced by signs and symptoms, as the problem has
not occurred; rather, nursing interventions are directed at prevention.

distraction behaviors (restlessness), muscle tension, and narrowed focus.

impaired Urinary Elimination may be related to altered intake, dehydration, fluid shifts, hormonal changes, hemorrhage, severe intrapartal hypertension, mechanical compression of bladder, and effects of regional anesthesia, possibly evidenced by changes in amount or frequency of voiding, urinary retention, slowed progression of labor, and reduced sensation.

risk for ineffective [individual/couple] Coping: risk factors may include situational crises, personal vulnerability, use of ineffective coping mechanisms, inadequate support systems, and pain.*

Labor, stage II (expulsion) OB

acute Pain may be related to strong uterine contractions, tissue stretching/dilation and compression of nerves by presenting part of the fetus, and bladder distention, possibly evidenced by verbalizations, facial grimacing, guarding or distraction behaviors (restlessness), narrowed focus, and diaphoresis.

Cardiac Output [fluctuation] may be related to changes in SVR, fluctuations in venous return (repeated or prolonged Valsalva's maneuvers, effects of anesthesia or medications, dorsal recumbent position occluding the inferior vena cava and partially obstructing the aorta), possibly evidenced by decreased venous return, changes in vital signs (BP, pulse), urinary output, fetal bradycardia.

risk for impaired fetal Gas Exchange: risk factors may include mechanical compression of head or cord, maternal position or prolonged labor affecting placental perfusion, and effects of maternal anesthesia, hyperventilation.*

risk for impaired Skin/Tissue Integrity: risk factors may include untoward stretching or lacerations of delicate tissues (precipitous labor, hypertonic contractile pattern, adolescence, large fetus) and application of forceps.*

risk for Fatigue: risk factors may include pregnancy, stress, anxiety, sleep deprivation, increased physical exertion, anemia, environmental humidity or temperature, lights.*

Laminectomy, cervical MS

Also Refer to Laminectomy, lumbar

risk for Perioperative-Positioning Injury: risk factors may include immobilization, muscle weakness, obesity, advanced age.*

risk for ineffective Airway Clearance: risk factors may include retained secretions, pain, muscle weakness.*

risk for impaired Swallowing: risk factors may include operative edema, pain, neuromuscular impairment.*

Laminectomy, lumbar MS

Also Refer to Surgery, general

ineffective Tissue Perfusion [specify] may be related to diminished or interrupted blood flow—edema of operative site, hematoma forma-

---

*A risk diagnosis is not evidenced by signs and symptoms, as the problem has not occurred; rather, nursing interventions are directed at prevention.

tion; hypovolemia, possibly evidenced by paresthesia, numbness, decreased range of motion or muscle strength.

risk for [spinal] Trauma: risk factors may include temporary weakness of spinal column, balancing difficulties, changes in muscle tone or coordination.*

acute Pain may be related to traumatized tissues—surgical manipulation, harvesting bone graft, localized inflammation, and edema, possibly evidenced by altered muscle tone, verbal reports, and distraction or guarding behaviors, changes in vital signs, diaphoresis, pallor.

impaired physical Mobility may be related to imposed therapeutic restrictions, neuromuscular impairment, and pain, possibly evidenced by limited range of motion, decreased muscle strength or control, impaired coordination, and reluctance to attempt movement.

risk for [acute] Urinary Retention: risk factors may include pain and swelling in operative area and reduced mobility/restrictions of position.*

Laryngectomy   MS
Also Refer to Cancer; Chemotherapy

ineffective Airway Clearance may be related to partial or total removal of the glottis, temporary or permanent change to neck breathing, edema formation, and copious and thick secretions, possibly evidenced by dyspnea or difficulty breathing, changes in rate and depth of respiration, use of accessory respiratory muscles, weak or ineffective cough, abnormal breath sounds, and cyanosis.

impaired Skin/Tissue Integrity may be related to surgical removal of tissues and grafting, effects of radiation or chemotherapeutic agents, altered circulation or reduced blood supply, compromised nutritional status, edema formation, and pooling or continuous drainage of secretions, possibly evidenced by disruption of skin and tissue surface and destruction of skin and tissue layers.

impaired Oral Mucous Membrane may be related to dehydration or absence of oral intake, decreased saliva production, poor or inadequate oral hygiene, pathological condition (oral cancer), mechanical trauma (oral surgery), difficulty swallowing and pooling or drooling of secretions, and nutritional deficits, possibly evidenced by xerostomia (dry mouth), oral discomfort, thick, mucoid saliva; decreased saliva production, dry and crusted or coated tongue, inflamed lips, absent teeth and gums, poor dental health and halitosis.

CH

impaired verbal Communication may be related to anatomical deficit (removal of vocal cords), physical barrier (tracheostomy tube), and required voice rest, possibly evidenced by inability to speak, change in vocal characteristics, and impaired articulation.

risk for Aspiration: risk factors may include impaired swallowing, facial and neck surgery, presence of tracheostomy, tube feedings.*

Laryngitis   CH/PED
Refer to Croup

---

*A risk diagnosis is not evidenced by signs and symptoms, as the problem has not occurred; rather, nursing interventions are directed at prevention.

Latex allergy

Latex Allergy Response may be related hypersensitivity to natural latex rubber protein, possibly evidenced by contact dermatitis—erythema, blisters; delayed hypersensitivity—eczema, irritation; hypersensitivity—generalized edema, wheezing, bronchospasm, hypotension, cardiac arrest.

Anxiety [specify level]/Fear may be related to threat of death, possibly evidenced by expressed concerns, hypervigilance, restlessness, focus on self.

risk for risk-prone Health Behavior: risk factors may include health status requiring change in occupation.*

Lead poisoning, acute

Also Refer to Lead poisoning, chronic

Contamination may be related to flaking or peeling paint (young children), improperly lead-glazed ceramic pottery, unprotected contact with lead (e.g., battery manufacture or recycling, bronzing, soldering or welding), imported herbal products or medicinals, possibly evidenced by abdominal cramping, headache, irritability, decreased attentiveness, constipation, tremors.

risk for Trauma: risk factors may include loss of coordination, altered level of consciousness, clonic or tonic muscle activity, neurological damage.*

risk for deficient Fluid Volume: risk factors may include excessive vomiting, diarrhea, or decreased intake.*

deficient Knowledge [Learning Need] regarding sources of lead and prevention of poisoning may be related to lack of information/misinterpretation, possibly evidenced by statements of concern, questions, and misconceptions.

Lead poisoning, chronic

Also Refer to Lead poisoning, acute

Contamination may be related to flaking or peeling paint (young children), improperly lead-glazed ceramic pottery, unprotected contact with lead (e.g., battery manufacture or recycling, bronzing, soldering or welding), imported herbal products or medicinals, possibly evidenced by chronic abdominal pain, headache, personality changes, cognitive deficits, seizures, neuropathy.

imbalanced Nutrition: less than body requirements may be related to decreased intake (chemically induced changes in the gastrointestinal tract), possibly evidenced by anorexia, abdominal discomfort, reported metallic taste, and weight loss.

chronic Pain may be related to deposition of lead in soft tissues and bone, possibly evidenced by verbal reports, distraction behaviors, and focus on self.

risk for delayed Development/disproportionate Growth: risk factors may include lead poisoning.*

---

*A risk diagnosis is not evidenced by signs and symptoms, as the problem has not occurred; rather, nursing interventions are directed at prevention.

Also Refer to Chemotherapy

risk for Infection: risk factors may include inadequate secondary defenses (alterations in mature white blood cells [WBCs], increased number of immature lymphocytes, immunosuppression, and bone marrow suppression), invasive procedures, and malnutrition.*

Anxiety [specify level]/Fear may be related to change in health status, threat of death, and situational crisis, possibly evidenced by sympathetic stimulation, apprehension, feelings of helplessness, focus on self, and insomnia.

Activity Intolerance [specify level] may be related to reduced energy stores, increased metabolic rate, imbalance between O_2 supply and demand—anemia, hypoxia; therapeutic restrictions—isolation, bedrest; effect of drug therapy, possibly evidenced by generalized weakness, reports of fatigue and exertional dyspnea, abnormal heart rate or BP response.

acute Pain may be related to physical agents (infiltration of tissues/organs/CNS, expanding bone marrow) and chemical agents (antileukemic treatments), psychological manifestations—anxiety, fear possibly evidenced by verbal reports (abdominal discomfort, arthralgia, bone pain, headache), distraction behaviors, narrowed focus, and changes in vital signs.

risk for deficient Fluid Volume/Bleeding: risk factors may include excessive losses (vomiting, diarrhea, coagulopathy), decreased intake (nausea, anorexia), increased fluid need (hypermetabolic state/fever), predisposition for kidney stone formation, tumor lysis syndrome.*

risk for Infection: risk factors may include inadequate secondary defenses (alterations in mature WBCs, increased number of immature lymphocytes, immunosuppression, and bone marrow suppression), invasive procedures, and malnutrition.*

ineffective Protection may be related to abnormal blood profiles, drug therapy—cytotoxic agents, steroids; radiation treatments possibly evidenced by deficient immunity, impaired healing, altered clotting, weakness

Fatigue may be related to disease state, anemia possibly evidenced by verbalizations, inability to maintain usual routines, listlessness.

imbalanced Nutrition: less than body requirements may be related to inability to ingest nutrients possibly evidenced by lack of interest in food, anorexia, weight loss, abdominal fullness, pain.

Also Refer to condition(s) requiring or contributing to need for facility placement

Anxiety [specify level]/Fear may be related to change in health status, role functioning, interaction patterns, socioeconomic status, environment; unmet needs, recent life changes, and loss of friends/SO(s), possibly evidenced by apprehension, restlessness, insomnia,

---

*A risk diagnosis is not evidenced by signs and symptoms, as the problem has not occurred; rather, nursing interventions are directed at prevention.

repetitive questioning, pacing, purposeless activity, expressed concern regarding changes in life events, and focus on self.

Grieving may be related to perceived, actual, or potential loss of physiopsychosocial well-being, personal possessions, and SO(s), as well as cultural beliefs about aging and debilitation, possibly evidenced by denial of feelings, depression, sorrow, guilt, alterations in activity level, sleep patterns, eating habits, and libido.

risk for Poisoning [drug toxicity]: risk factors may include effects of aging (reduced metabolism, impaired circulation, precarious physiological balance, presence of multiple diseases and organ involvement), and use of multiple prescribed and over-the-counter drugs.*

impaired Memory may be related to neurological disturbances, hypoxia, fluid imbalance possibly evidenced by inability to recall events/factual information, reports experience of forgetting.

Insomnia may be related to internal factors (illness, psychological stress, inactivity) and external factors (environmental changes, facility routines), possibly evidenced by reports of difficulty in falling asleep/not feeling rested, interrupted sleep, awakening earlier than desired, change in behavior or performance, increasing irritability, and listlessness.

risk for Sexual Dysfunction: risk factors may include biopsychosocial alteration of sexuality, interference in psychological/physical well-being, self-image, and lack of privacy/SO(s).*

risk for Relocation Stress Syndrome: risk factors may include temporary or permanent move that may be voluntary or involuntary, lack of predeparture counseling, multiple losses, feeling of powerlessness, lack of or inappropriate use of support system, changes in psychosocial or physical health status.*

risk for impaired Religiosity: risk factors may include life transition, ineffective support or coping, lack of social interaction, depression.*

Lupus erythematosus, systemic (SLE)   CH

Fatigue may be related to inadequate energy production or increased energy requirements (chronic inflammation), overwhelming psychological or emotional demands, states of discomfort, and altered body chemistry (including effects of drug therapy), possibly evidenced by reports of unremitting and overwhelming lack of energy, inability to maintain usual routines, decreased performance, lethargy, and decreased libido.

acute Pain may be related to widespread inflammatory process affecting connective tissues, blood vessels, serosal surfaces and mucous membranes, possibly evidenced by verbal reports, guarding or distraction behaviors, self-focusing, and changes in vital signs.

impaired Skin/Tissue Integrity may be related to chronic inflammation, edema formation, and altered circulation, possibly evidenced by presence of skin rash or lesions, ulcerations of mucous membranes, and photosensitivity.

disturbed Body Image may be related to presence of chronic condition with rash, lesions, ulcers, purpura, mottled erythema of hands, alo-

*A risk diagnosis is not evidenced by signs and symptoms, as the problem has not occurred; rather, nursing interventions are directed at prevention.

pecia, loss of strength, and altered body function, possibly evidenced by hiding body parts, negative feelings about body, feelings of helplessness, and change in social involvement.

Lyme disease   CH/MS

acute/chronic Pain may be related to systemic effects of toxins, presence of rash, urticaria, and joint swelling or inflammation, possibly evidenced by verbal reports, guarding behaviors, autonomic responses, and narrowed focus.

Fatigue may be related to increased energy requirements, altered body chemistry, and states of discomfort evidenced by reports of overwhelming lack of energy, inability to maintain usual routines, decreased performance, lethargy, and malaise.

risk for decreased Cardiac Output: risk factors may include alteration in cardiac rate, rhythm, or conduction.*

Macular degeneration   CH

[disturbed visual Sensory Perception] may be related to altered sensory reception, possibly evidenced by reported or measured change in sensory acuity, change in usual response to stimuli.

Anxiety [specify level]/Fear may be related to situational crisis, threat to or change in health status and role function, possibly evidenced by expressed concerns, apprehension, feelings of inadequacy, diminished productivity, impaired attention.

risk for impaired Home Maintenance: risk factors may include impaired cognitive functioning, inadequate support systems.*

risk for impaired Social Interaction: risk factors may include limited physical mobility, environmental barriers.*

Mallory-Weiss syndrome   MS

Also Refer to Achalasia

risk for deficient Fluid Volume: risk factors may include excessive vascular losses, presence of vomiting, and reduced intake.*

deficient Knowledge [Learning Need] regarding causes, treatment, and prevention of condition may be related to lack of information or misinterpretation, possibly evidenced by statements of concern, questions, and recurrence of problem.

Mastectomy   MS

impaired Skin/Tissue Integrity may be related to surgical removal of skin and tissue, altered circulation, presence of edema, drainage, changes in skin elasticity and sensation, and tissue destruction (radiation), possibly evidenced by disruption of skin surface and destruction of skin layers and subcutaneous tissues.

impaired physical Mobility may be related to neuromuscular impairment, pain, and edema formation, possibly evidenced by reluctance to attempt movement, limited range of motion, and decreased muscle mass and strength.

bathing/dressing Self-Care Deficit may be related to temporary decreased range of motion of one or both arms, possibly evidenced by statements of inability to perform or complete self-care tasks.

M

*A risk diagnosis is not evidenced by signs and symptoms, as the problem has not occurred; rather, nursing interventions are directed at prevention.

disturbed Body Image/situational low Self-Esteem may be related to loss of body part denoting femininity, fear of rejection or reaction of others, behaviors inconsistent with self-value system possibly evidenced by not looking at or touching area, self-negating verbalizations, preoccupation with loss, and change in social involvement or relationship.

risk for complicated Grieving: risk factors may include preloss psychological symptoms, predisposition for anxiety and feelings of inadequacy, frequency of major life events.*

Mastitis   OB/GYN

acute Pain may be related to erythema and edema of breast tissues, possibly evidenced by verbal reports, guarding or distraction behaviors, self-focusing, changes in vital signs.

risk for Infection [spread/abscess formation]: risk factors may include traumatized tissues, stasis of fluids, and insufficient knowledge to prevent complications.*

deficient Knowledge [Learning Need] regarding pathophysiology, treatment, and prevention may be related to lack of information or misinterpretation, possibly evidenced by statements of concern, questions, and misconceptions.

risk for ineffective Breastfeeding: risk factors may include inability to feed on affected side or interruption in breastfeeding.*

Mastoidectomy   PED/MS

risk for Infection [spread]: risk factors may include preexisting infection, surgical trauma, and stasis of body fluids in close proximity to brain.*

acute Pain may be related to inflammation, tissue trauma, and edema formation, possibly evidenced by verbal reports, distraction behaviors, restlessness, self-focusing, and changes in vital signs.

[disturbed auditory Sensory Perception] may be related to presence of surgical packing, edema, and surgical disturbance of middle ear structures, possibly evidenced by reported/tested hearing loss in affected ear.

Measles   CH/PED

acute Pain may be related to inflammation of mucous membranes, conjunctiva, and presence of extensive skin rash with pruritus, possibly evidenced by verbal reports, distraction behaviors, self-focusing, and changes in vital signs.

Hyperthermia may be related to presence of viral toxins and inflammatory response, possibly evidenced by increased body temperature, flushed, warm skin; and tachycardia.

risk for [secondary] Infection: risk factors may include altered immune response and traumatized dermal tissues.*

deficient Knowledge [Learning Need] regarding condition, transmission, and possible complications may be related to lack of information, misinterpretation, possibly evidenced by statements of concern,

---

*A risk diagnosis is not evidenced by signs and symptoms, as the problem has not occurred; rather, nursing interventions are directed at prevention.

questions, misconceptions, and development of preventable complications.

Melanoma, malignant   MS/CH
Refer to Cancer; Chemotherapy

Meningitis, acute meningococcal   MS
risk for Infection [spread]: risk factors may include hematogenous dissemination of pathogen, stasis of body fluids, suppressed inflammatory response (medication-induced), and exposure of others to pathogens.*

risk for ineffective cerebral Tissue Perfusion: risk factors may include cerebral edema altering or interrupting cerebral arterial or venous blood flow, hypovolemia, exchange problems at cellular level (acidosis).*

Hyperthermia may be related to infectious process (increased metabolic rate) and dehydration, possibly evidenced by increased body temperature, warm, flushed skin; and tachycardia.

acute Pain may be related to inflammation or irritation of the meninges with spasm of extensor muscles (neck, shoulders, and back), possibly evidenced by verbal reports, guarding or distraction behaviors, narrowed focus, photophobia, and changes in vital signs.

risk for Trauma/Suffocation: risk factors may include alterations in level of consciousness, possible development of clonic/tonic muscle activity (seizures), and generalized weakness, prostration, ataxia, vertigo.*

Meniscectomy   MS/CH
impaired Walking may be related to pain, joint instability, and imposed medical restrictions of movement, possibly evidenced by impaired ability to move about environment as needed or desired.

deficient Knowledge [Learning Need] regarding postoperative expectations, prevention of complications, and self-care needs may be related to lack of information, possibly evidenced by statements of concern, questions, and misconceptions.

Menopause   GYN
ineffective Thermoregulation may be related to fluctuation of hormonal levels, possibly evidenced by skin flushed/warm to touch, diaphoresis, night sweats, cold hands or feet.

Fatigue may be related to change in body chemistry, lack of sleep, depression, possibly evidenced by reports of lack of energy, tired, inability to maintain usual routines, decreased performance.

risk for Sexual Dysfunction: risk factors may include perceived altered body function, changes in physical response, myths or inaccurate information, impaired relationship with SO.*

risk for stress urinary Incontinence: risk factors may include degenerative changes in pelvic muscles and structural support.*

readiness for enhanced Self-Health Management possibly evidenced by expressed desire for management of life cycle changes, increased control of health practice.

M

---

*A risk diagnosis is not evidenced by signs and symptoms, as the problem has not occurred; rather, nursing interventions are directed at prevention.

Also Refer to Down syndrome

impaired verbal Communication may be related to developmental delay, impairment of cognitive and motor abilities, possibly evidenced by impaired articulation, difficulty with phonation, and inability to modulate speech or find appropriate words (dependent on degree of retardation).

risk for Self-Care Deficit [specify]: risk factors may include impaired cognitive ability and motor skills.*

risk for imbalanced Nutrition: more than body requirements: risk factors may include decreased metabolic rate coupled with impaired cognitive development, dysfunctional eating patterns, and sedentary activity level.*

risk for sedentary Lifestyle: risk factors may include lack of interest or motivation, lack of resources, lack of training or knowledge of specific exercise needs, safety concerns, fear of injury.*

impaired Social Interaction may be related to impaired thought processes, communication barriers, and knowledge or skill deficit about ways to enhance mutuality, possibly evidenced by dysfunctional interactions with peers, family, and/or SO(s), and verbalized or observed discomfort in social situation.

compromised family Coping may be related to chronic nature of condition and degree of disability that exhausts supportive capacity of SO(s), other situational or developmental crises or situations SO(s) may be facing, unrealistic expectations of SO(s), possibly evidenced by preoccupation of SO with personal reaction, SO(s) withdraw(s) or enter(s) into limited interaction with individual, protective behavior disproportionate (too much or too little) to client's abilities or need for autonomy.

impaired Home Maintenance may be related to impaired cognitive functioning, insufficient finances/family organization or planning, lack of knowledge, and inadequate support systems, possibly evidenced by requests for assistance, expression of difficulty in maintaining home, disorderly surroundings, and overtaxed family members.

risk for Sexual Dysfunction: risk factors may include biopsychosocial alteration of sexuality, ineffectual or absent role models, misinformation or lack of knowledge, lack of SO(s), and lack of appropriate behavior control.*

Metabolic syndrome   **CH/MS**

risk for unstable Blood Glucose Level: risk factors may include dietary intake, weight gain, physical activity level.*

sedentary Lifestyle may be related to deficient knowledge of health benefits of physical exercise, lack of interest/motivation or resources; possibly evidenced by verbalized preference for activities low in physical activity, choice of a daily routine lacking physical exercise.

compromised family Coping may be related to chronic nature of condition and degree of disability that exhausts supportive capacity of SO(s), other situational or developmental crises or situations SO(s)

---

*A risk diagnosis is not evidenced by signs and symptoms, as the problem has not occurred; rather, nursing interventions are directed at prevention.

may be facing, unrealistic expectations of SO(s), possibly evidenced by preoccupation of SO with personal reaction, SO(s) withdraw(s) or enter(s) into limited interaction with individual, protective behavior disproportionate (too much or too little) to client's abilities or need for autonomy.

impaired Home Maintenance may be related to impaired cognitive functioning, insufficient finances and family organization or planning, lack of knowledge, and inadequate support systems, possibly evidenced by requests for assistance, expression of difficulty in maintaining home, disorderly surroundings, and overtaxed family members.

risk for ineffective Tissue Perfusion [specify]: risk factors may include arterial plaque formation (elevated triglycerides, low levels of HDL), prothrombotic state, proinflammatory state.*

Miscarriage   OB
Refer to Abortion, spontaneous termination

Mitral stenosis   MS/CH
Activity Intolerance may be related to imbalance between O_2 supply and demand, possibly evidenced by reports of fatigue, weakness, exertional dyspnea, and tachycardia.

impaired Gas Exchange may be related to altered blood flow, possibly evidenced by restlessness, hypoxia, and cyanosis (orthopnea/paroxysmal nocturnal dyspnea).

decreased Cardiac Output may be related to impeded blood flow as evidenced by jugular vein distention, peripheral or dependent edema, orthopnea, paroxysmal nocturnal dyspnea.

deficient Knowledge [Learning Need] regarding pathophysiology, therapeutic needs, and potential complications may be related to lack of information or recall, misinterpretation, possibly evidenced by statements of concern, questions, inaccurate follow-through of instructions, and development of preventable complications.

Mononucleosis, infectious   CH
Fatigue may be related to decreased energy production, states of discomfort, and increased energy requirements (inflammatory process), possibly evidenced by reports of overwhelming lack of energy, inability to maintain usual routines, lethargy, and malaise.

acute Pain/impaired Comfort may be related to inflammation of lymphoid and organ tissues, irritation of oropharyngeal mucous membranes, and effects of circulating toxins, possibly evidenced by verbal reports, distraction behaviors, and self-focusing.

Hyperthermia may be related to inflammatory process, possibly evidenced by increased body temperature, warm, flushed skin; and tachycardia.

deficient Knowledge [Learning Need] regarding disease transmission, self-care needs, medical therapy, and potential complications may be related to lack of information, misinterpretation, possibly

---

*A risk diagnosis is not evidenced by signs and symptoms, as the problem has not occurred; rather, nursing interventions are directed at prevention.

evidenced by statements of concern, misconceptions, and inaccurate follow-through of instructions.

Mood disorders PSY
Refer to Depressive disorders

Mountain sickness, acute (AMS) CH/MS
acute Pain may be related to reduced O_2 tension, possibly evidenced by reports of headache.

Fatigue may be related to stress, increased physical exertion, sleep deprivation, possibly evidenced by overwhelming lack of energy, inability to restore energy even after sleep, compromised concentration, decreased performance.

risk for deficient Fluid Volume: risk factors may include increased water loss (e.g., overbreathing dry air), exertion, altered fluid intake (nausea).*

Multiple personality PSY
Refer to Dissociative disorders

Multiple sclerosis CH
Fatigue may be related to decreased energy production or increased energy requirements to perform activities, psychological or emotional demands, pain or discomfort, medication side effects, possibly evidenced by verbalization of overwhelming lack of energy, inability to maintain usual routine, decreased performance, impaired ability to concentrate, increase in physical complaints.

[disturbed visual, kinesthetic, tactile Sensory Perception] may be related to delayed or interrupted neuronal transmission, possibly evidenced by impaired vision, diplopia, disturbance of vibratory or position sense, paresthesias, numbness, and blunting of sensation.

impaired physical Mobility may be related to neuromuscular impairment; discomfort or pain; sensoriperceptual impairments; decreased muscle strength, control and/or mass; deconditioning, as evidenced by limited ability to perform motor skills; limited range of motion; gait changes, postural instability.

Powerlessness/Hopelessness may be related to illness-related regimen, unpredictability of disease, and lifestyle of helplessness, possibly evidenced by verbal expressions of having no control or influence over the situation, depression over physical deterioration that occurs despite client compliance with regimen, nonparticipation in care or decision making when opportunities are provided, passivity, decreased verbalization and affect, isolating behaviors.

impaired Home Maintenance may be related to effects of debilitating disease, impaired cognitive and/or emotional functioning, insufficient finances, and inadequate support systems, possibly evidenced by reported difficulty, observed disorderly surroundings, and poor hygienic conditions.

compromised/disabled family Coping may be related to situational crises/temporary family disorganization and role changes, client pro-

---

*A risk diagnosis is not evidenced by signs and symptoms, as the problem has not occurred; rather, nursing interventions are directed at prevention.

viding little support in turn for SO(s), prolonged disease or disability progression that exhausts the supportive capacity of SO(s), feelings of guilt, anxiety, hostility, despair, and highly ambivalent family relationships, possibly evidenced by client expressing or confirming concern or report about SO's response to client's illness, SO(s) preoccupied with own personal reactions, intolerance, abandonment, neglectful care of the client, and distortion of reality regarding client's illness.

Mumps   PED/CH

acute Pain may be related to presence of inflammation, circulating toxins, and enlargement of salivary glands, possibly evidenced by verbal reports, guarding or distraction behaviors, self-focusing, and changes in vital signs.

Hyperthermia may be related to inflammatory process (increased metabolic rate) and dehydration, possibly evidenced by increased body temperature, warm, flushed skin; and tachycardia.

risk for deficient Fluid Volume: risk factors may include hypermetabolic state and painful swallowing, with decreased intake.*

Muscular dystrophy (Duchenne's)   PED/CH

impaired physical Mobility may be related to musculoskeletal impairment or weakness, possibly evidenced by decreased muscle strength, control, and mass, limited range of motion, and impaired coordination.

delayed Growth and Development may be related to effects of physical disability, possibly evidenced by altered physical growth and altered ability to perform self-care or self-control activities appropriate to age.

risk for imbalanced Nutrition: more than body requirements: risk factors may include sedentary lifestyle and dysfunctional eating patterns.*

compromised family Coping may be related to situational crisis, emotional conflicts around issues about hereditary nature of condition and prolonged disease or disability that exhausts supportive capacity of family members, possibly evidenced by preoccupation with personal reactions regarding disability and displaying protective behavior disproportionate (too little or too much) to client's abilities or need for autonomy.

Myasthenia gravis   MS

ineffective Breathing Pattern/Airway Clearance may be related to neuromuscular weakness and decreased energy, fatigue, possibly evidenced by dyspnea, changes in rate and depth of respiration, ineffective cough, and adventitious breath sounds.

impaired verbal Communication may be related to neuromuscular weakness, fatigue, and physical barrier (intubation), possibly evidenced by facial weakness, impaired articulation, hoarseness, and inability to speak.

impaired Swallowing may be related to neuromuscular impairment of laryngeal or pharyngeal muscles, and muscular fatigue, possibly

---

*A risk diagnosis is not evidenced by signs and symptoms, as the problem has not occurred; rather, nursing interventions are directed at prevention.

evidenced by reported or observed difficulty swallowing, coughing, choking, and evidence of aspiration.

Anxiety [specify level]/Fear may be related to situational crisis, threat to self-concept, change in health or socioeconomic status or role function; separation from support systems, lack of knowledge, and inability to communicate, possibly evidenced by expressed concerns, increased tension, restlessness, apprehension, sympathetic stimulation, crying, focus on self, uncooperative behavior, withdrawal, anger, and noncommunication.

CH

deficient Knowledge [Learning Need] regarding drug therapy, potential for crisis (myasthenic or cholinergic), and self-care management may be related to inadequate information, misinterpretation, possibly evidenced by statements of concern, questions, and misconceptions; development of preventable complications.

impaired physical Mobility may be related to neuromuscular impairment, possibly evidenced by reports of progressive fatigability with repetitive or prolonged muscle use, impaired coordination, and decreased muscle strength/control.

[disturbed visual Sensory Perception] may be related to neuromuscular impairment, possibly evidenced by visual distortions (diplopia) and motor incoordination.

Myeloma, multiple   MS/CH
Also Refer to Cancer

acute/chronic Pain may be related to destruction of tissues or bone, side effects of therapy, possibly evidenced by verbal or coded reports, guarding or protective behaviors, changes in appetite or weight, sleep; reduced interaction with others.

impaired physical Mobility may be related to loss of integrity of bone structure, pain, deconditioning, depressed mood, possibly evidenced by verbalizations, limited range of motion, slowed movement, gait changes.

risk for ineffective Protection: risk factors may include presence of cancer, drug therapies, radiation treatments, inadequate nutrition.*

Myocardial infarction   MS
Also Refer to Myocarditis

acute Pain may be related to ischemia of myocardial tissue, possibly evidenced by verbal reports, guarding or distraction behaviors (restlessness), facial mask of pain, self-focusing, and diaphoresis, changes in vital signs.

Anxiety [specify level]/Fear may be related to threat of death, threat of change of health status, role functioning and lifestyle; interpersonal transmission or contagion, possibly evidenced by increased tension, fearful attitude, apprehension, expressed concerns or uncertainty, restlessness, sympathetic stimulation, and somatic complaints.

risk for decreased Cardiac Output: risk factors may include changes in rate and electrical conduction, reduced preload/increased SVR and

---

*A risk diagnosis is not evidenced by signs and symptoms, as the problem has not occurred; rather, nursing interventions are directed at prevention.

altered muscle contractility/depressant effects of some medications, infarcted or dyskinetic muscle, structural defects.*

CH

risk for sedentary Lifestyle: risk factors may include lack of resources, lack of training or knowledge of specific exercise needs, safety concerns, fear of injury.*

Myocarditis MS
Also Refer to Myocardial infarction

Activity Intolerance may be related to imbalance in O_2 supply and demand (myocardial inflammation or damage), cardiac depressant effects of certain drugs, and enforced bedrest, possibly evidenced by reports of fatigue, exertional dyspnea, tachycardia and palpitations in response to activity, ECG changes—dysrhythmias, and generalized weakness.

risk for decreased Cardiac Output: risk factors may include degeneration of cardiac muscle.*

deficient Knowledge [Learning Need] regarding pathophysiology of condition, outcomes, treatment, and self-care needs and lifestyle changes may be related to lack of information, misinterpretation, possibly evidenced by statements of concern, misconceptions, inaccurate follow-through of instructions, and development of preventable complications.

Myringotomy PED/MS
Refer to Mastoidectomy

Myxedema CH
Also Refer to Hypothyroidism

disturbed Body Image may be related to change in structure or function (loss of hair, thickening of skin, masklike facial expression, enlarged tongue, menstrual and reproductive disturbances), possibly evidenced by negative feelings about body, feelings of helplessness, and change in social involvement.

imbalanced Nutrition: more than body requirements may be related to decreased metabolic rate and activity level, possibly evidenced by weight gain greater than ideal for height and frame.

risk for decreased Cardiac Output: risk factors may include altered electrical conduction and myocardial contractility.*

Narcolepsy CH
Insomnia may be related to medical condition, possibly evidenced by hypersomnia, reports of unsatisfying nighttime sleep, vivid visual or auditory illusions or hallucinations at onset of sleep, sleep interrupted by vivid or frightening dreams.

risk for Trauma: risk factors may include sudden loss of muscle tone, momentary paralysis (cataplexy), sudden inappropriate sleep episodes.*

risk for chronic low Self-Esteem: risk factors may include negative evaluation of self, personal vulnerability, chronic physical condition,

---

*A risk diagnosis is not evidenced by signs and symptoms, as the problem has not occurred; rather, nursing interventions are directed at prevention.

impaired work or social performance, problems with social relationships, reduced quality of life.*

Necrotizing cellulitis, fasciitis MS
Also Refer to Cellulitis, Sepsis

Hyperthermia may be related to inflammatory process, response to circulatory toxins, possibly evidenced by body temperature above normal range; flushed, warm skin: tachycardia, altered mental status.

impaired Tissue Integrity may be related to inflammation, edema, ischemia, possibly evidenced by damaged or destroyed tissue, dermal gangrene.

Neglect/Abuse CH/PSY
Refer to Abuse; Battered child syndrome

Neonatal, normal newborn PED
risk for impaired Gas Exchange: risk factors may include prenatal or intrapartal stressors, excess production of mucus, or cold stress.*

risk for Hypothermia: risk factors may include large body surface in relation to mass, limited amounts of insulating subcutaneous fat, non-renewable sources of brown fat and few white fat stores, thin epidermis with close proximity of blood vessels to the skin, inability to shiver, and movement from a warm uterine environment to a much cooler environment.*

risk for impaired Attachment: risk factors may include developmental transition (gain of a family member), anxiety associated with the parent role, lack of privacy (healthcare interventions, intrusive family/visitors).*

risk for imbalanced Nutrition: less than body requirements: risk factors may include rapid metabolic rate, high caloric requirement, increased insensible water losses through pulmonary and cutaneous routes, fatigue, and a potential for inadequate or depleted glucose stores.*

risk for Infection: risk factors may include inadequate secondary defenses (inadequate acquired immunity, e.g., deficiency of neutrophils and specific immunoglobulins), and inadequate primary defenses (e.g., environmental exposure, broken skin, traumatized tissues, decreased ciliary action).*

Neonatal, premature newborn PED
impaired Gas Exchange may be related to alveolar-capillary membrane changes (inadequate surfactant levels), altered blood flow (immaturity of pulmonary arteriole musculature), altered O_2 supply (immaturity of CNS and neuromuscular system, tracheobronchial obstruction), altered O_2-carrying capacity of blood (anemia), and cold stress, possibly evidenced by respiratory difficulties, inadequate oxygenation of tissues, and acidemia.

ineffective Breathing Pattern may be related to immaturity of the respiratory center, poor positioning, drug-related depression and metabolic imbalances, decreased energy, fatigue, possibly evidenced by dyspnea, tachypnea, periods of apnea, nasal flaring and use of accessory muscles, cyanosis, abnormal ABGs, and tachycardia.

---

*A risk diagnosis is not evidenced by signs and symptoms, as the problem has not occurred; rather, nursing interventions are directed at prevention.

risk for ineffective Thermoregulation: risk factors may include immature CNS development (temperature regulation center), decreased
ratio of body mass to surface area, decreased subcutaneous fat, limited brown fat stores, inability to shiver or sweat, poor metabolic
reserves, muted response to hypothermia, and frequent medical or
nursing manipulations and interventions.*

risk for deficit Fluid Volume: risk factors may include extremes of age
and weight, excessive fluid losses (thin skin, lack of insulating fat,
increased environmental temperature, immature kidney, and failure
to concentrate urine).*

risk for disorganized infant Behavior: risk factors may include prematurity (immaturity of CNS system, hypoxia), lack of containment or
boundaries, pain, overstimulation, separation from parents.*

Nephrectomy   MS

acute Pain may be related to surgical tissue trauma with mechanical
closure (suture), possibly evidenced by verbal reports, guarding or
distraction behaviors, self-focusing, and changes in vital signs.

risk for deficient Fluid Volume: risk factors may include excessive vascular losses and restricted intake.*

ineffective Breathing Pattern may be related to incisional pain with
decreased lung expansion, possibly evidenced by tachypnea, fremitus, changes in respiratory depth and chest expansion, and changes
in ABGs.

Constipation may be related to reduced dietary intake, decreased mobility, gastrointestinal obstruction (paralytic ileus), and incisional
pain with defecation, possibly evidenced by decreased bowel sounds,
reduced frequency/amount of stool, and hard, formed stool.

Nephrolithiasis   MS/CH
Refer to Calculi, urinary

Nephrotic syndrome   MS/CH

excess Fluid Volume may be related to compromised regulatory mechanism with changes in hydrostatic or oncotic vascular pressure and
increased activation of the renin-angiotensin-aldosterone system,
possibly evidenced by edema, anasarca, effusions, ascites, weight
gain, intake greater than output, and BP changes.

imbalanced Nutrition: less than body requirements may be related to
excessive protein losses and inability to ingest adequate nutrients
(anorexia), possibly evidenced by weight loss and muscle wasting
(may be difficult to assess due to edema), lack of interest in food,
and observed inadequate intake.

risk for Infection: risk factors may include chronic disease and steroidal
suppression of inflammatory responses.*

risk for impaired Skin Integrity: risk factors may include presence of
edema and activity restrictions.*

*A risk diagnosis is not evidenced by signs and symptoms, as the problem has
not occurred; rather, nursing interventions are directed at prevention.

Neuralgia, trigeminal CH

acute Pain may be related to neuromuscular impairment with sudden violent muscle spasm, possibly evidenced by verbal reports, guarding or distraction behaviors, self-focusing, and changes in vital signs.

deficient Knowledge [Learning Need] regarding control of recurrent episodes, medical therapies, and self-care needs may be related to lack of information or recall and misinterpretation, possibly evidenced by statements of concern, questions, and exacerbation of condition.

Neuritis CH

acute/chronic Pain may be related to nerve damage usually associated with a degenerative process, possibly evidenced by verbal reports, guarding or distraction behaviors, self-focusing, and changes in vital signs.

deficient Knowledge [Learning Need] regarding underlying causative factors, treatment, and prevention may be related to lack of information, misinterpretation, possibly evidenced by statements of concern, questions, and misconceptions.

Nicotine withdrawal CH

readiness for enhanced Self-Health Management possibly evidenced by expressed concerns, desire to seek higher level of wellness.

risk for imbalanced Nutrition: more than body needs: risk factors may include return of appetite, normalization of basal metabolic rate, eating in response to internal cues.*

risk for ineffective Self-Health Management: risk factors may include economic difficulties, lack of support systems, continued environmental exposure.*

Nonketotic hyperglycemic-hyperosmolar coma MS

deficient Fluid Volume may be related to excessive renal losses, inadequate oral intake, extremes of age, presence of infection possibly evidenced by sudden weight loss, dry skin and mucous membranes, poor skin turgor, hypotension, increased pulse, fever, change in mental status (confusion to coma).

imbalanced Nutrition: less than body requirements may be related to decreased preload (hypovolemia), altered heart rhythm (hyper- or hypokalemia) possibly evidenced by decreased hemodynamic pressures (e.g., CVP), ECG changes, dysrhythmias.

decreased Cardiac Output may be related to inadequate utilization of nutrients (insulin deficiency), decreased oral intake, hypermetabolic state, possibly evidenced by recent weight loss, imbalance between glucose and insulin levels.

risk for Trauma: risk factors may include weakness, cognitive limitations or altered consciousness, loss of large- or small-muscle coordination (risk for seizure activity).*

---

*A risk diagnosis is not evidenced by signs and symptoms, as the problem has not occurred; rather, nursing interventions are directed at prevention.

imbalanced Nutrition: more than body requirements may be related to food intake that exceeds body needs, psychosocial factors, socioeconomic status, possibly evidenced by weight of 20% or more over optimum body weight, excess body fat by skinfold or other measurements, reported or observed dysfunctional eating patterns, intake more than body requirements.

sedentary Lifestyle may be related to lack of interest or motivation, lack of resources, lack of training or knowledge of specific exercise needs, safety concerns, fear of injury, possibly evidenced by demonstration of physical deconditioning, choice of a daily routine lacking physical exercise.

Activity Intolerance may be related to imbalance between O_2 supply and demand, and sedentary lifestyle, possibly evidenced by fatigue or weakness, exertional discomfort, and abnormal heart rate or BP response.

risk for Sleep Deprivation: risk factors may include inadequate daytime activity, discomfort, sleep apnea.*

disturbed Body Image/chronic low Self-Esteem may be related to view of self in contrast to societal values; family or subcultural encouragement of overeating; control, sex, and love issues; perceived failure at ability to control weight, possibly evidenced by negative feelings about body; fear of rejection or reaction of others; feeling of hopelessness, powerlessness; and lack of follow-through with treatment plan.

impaired Social Interaction may be related to self-concept disturbance, absence of or ineffective supportive SO(s), limited mobility, possibly evidenced by reluctance to participate in social gatherings, verbalized or observed discomfort in social situations, dysfunctional interactions with others, feelings of rejection.

Obsessive-compulsive disorder   PSY

[severe] Anxiety may be related to earlier life conflicts possibly evidenced by repetitive actions, recurring thoughts, decreased social and role functioning.

risk for impaired Skin/Tissue Integrity: risk factors may include repetitive behaviors related to cleansing (e.g., hand washing, brushing teeth, showering).*

risk for ineffective Role Performance: risk factors may include psychological stress, health-illness problems.*

Opioid abuse   CH/PSY
Refer to Depressant abuse

Organic brain syndrome   CH
Refer to Alzheimer's disease

---

*A risk diagnosis is not evidenced by signs and symptoms, as the problem has not occurred; rather, nursing interventions are directed at prevention.

Osteoarthritis (degenerative joint disease) CH
Refer to Arthritis, rheumatoid
(Although this is a degenerative process versus the inflammatory process of rheumatoid arthritis, nursing concerns are the same.)

Osteomyelitis MS/CH
acute Pain may be related to inflammation and tissue necrosis, possibly evidenced by verbal reports, guarding or distraction behaviors, self-focus, and changes in vital signs.

Hyperthermia may be related to increased metabolic rate and infectious process, possibly evidenced by increased body temperature and warm, flushed skin.

ineffective [bone] Tissue Perfusion may be related to inflammatory reaction with thrombosis of vessels, destruction of tissue, edema, and abscess formation, possibly evidenced by bone necrosis, continuation of infectious process, and delayed healing.

risk for impaired Walking: risk factors may include inflammation and tissue necrosis, pain, joint instability.*

deficient Knowledge [Learning Need] regarding pathophysiology of condition, long-term therapy needs, activity restriction, and prevention of complications may be related to lack of information, misinterpretation, possibly evidenced by statements of concern, questions, and misconceptions, and inaccurate follow-through of instructions.

Osteoporosis CH
risk for Trauma: risk factors may include loss of bone density and integrity increasing risk of fracture with minimal or no stress.*

acute/chronic Pain may be related to vertebral compression on spinal nerve, muscles, and ligaments; spontaneous fractures, possibly evidenced by verbal reports, guarding or distraction behaviors, self-focus, and changes in sleep pattern.

impaired physical Mobility may be related to pain and musculoskeletal impairment, possibly evidenced by limited range of motion, reluctance to attempt movement, expressed fear of re-injury, and imposed restrictions or limitations.

Palsy, cerebral (spastic hemiplegia) PED/CH
impaired physical Mobility may be related to muscular weakness or hypertonicity, increased deep tendon reflexes, tendency to contractures, and underdevelopment of affected limbs, possibly evidenced by decreased muscle strength, control, mass; limited range of motion; and impaired coordination.

compromised family Coping may be related to permanent nature of condition, situational crisis, emotional conflicts, temporary family disorganization, and incomplete information or understanding of client's needs, possibly evidenced by verbalized anxiety or guilt regarding client's disability, inadequate understanding and knowledge base, and displaying protective behaviors disproportionate (too little or too much) to client's abilities or need for autonomy.

---

*A risk diagnosis is not evidenced by signs and symptoms, as the problem has not occurred; rather, nursing interventions are directed at prevention.

delayed Growth and Development may be related to effects of physical disability, possibly evidenced by altered physical growth, delay or difficulty in performing skills (motor, social, expressive), and altered ability to perform self-care or self-control activities appropriate to age.

Pancreatitis — MS
acute Pain may be related to obstruction of pancreatic or biliary ducts, chemical contamination of peritoneal surfaces by pancreatic exudate, autodigestion of pancreas, extension of inflammation to the retroperitoneal nerve plexus, possibly evidenced by verbal reports, guarding or distraction behaviors, self-focusing, grimacing, changes in vital signs, and alteration in muscle tone.

risk for deficient Fluid Volume/Bleeding: risk factors may include excessive gastric losses (vomiting, nasogastric [NG] suctioning), increase in size of vascular bed (vasodilation, effects of kinins), thirdspace fluid transudation, ascites formation, alteration of clotting process.*

risk for unstable Blood Glucose Level: risk factors may include decreased insulin production, increased glucagon release, physical health status, stress.*

imbalanced Nutrition: less than body requirements may be related to vomiting, decreased oral intake, prescribed dietary restrictions, altered ability to digest nutrients (loss of digestive enzymes), possibly evidenced by reported inadequate food intake, aversion to eating, reported altered taste sensation, weight loss, and reduced muscle mass.

risk for Infection: risk factors may include inadequate primary defenses (stasis of body fluids, altered peristalsis, change in pH secretions), immunosuppression, nutritional deficiencies, tissue destruction, and chronic disease.*

Panic disorder — PSY
Fear may be related to unfounded morbid dread of a seemingly harmless object/situation, possibly evidenced by physiological symptoms, mental/cognitive behaviors indicative of panic, withdrawal from/ total avoidance of situations placing client in contact with feared object.

[severe to panic] Anxiety may be related to unidentified stressors, limitations placed on ritualistic behavior, possibly evidenced by episodes of immobilizing apprehension, behaviors indicative of panic, expressed feelings of terror or inability to cope.

Paranoid personality disorder — PSY
risk for self-/other-directed Violence: risk factors may include perceived threats of danger, paranoid delusions, and increased feelings of anxiety.*

[severe] Anxiety may be related to inability to trust (has not mastered task of trust versus mistrust), possibly evidenced by rigid delusional

*A risk diagnosis is not evidenced by signs and symptoms, as the problem has not occurred; rather, nursing interventions are directed at prevention.

system (serves to provide relief from stress that justifies the delusion), frightened of other people and own hostility.

Powerlessness may be related to feelings of inadequacy, lifestyle of helplessness, maladaptive interpersonal interactions (e.g., misuse of power, force, abusive relationships), sense of severely impaired self-concept, and belief that individual has no control over situation(s), possibly evidenced by paranoid delusions, use of aggressive behavior to compensate, and expressions of recognition of damage paranoia has caused self and others.

[disturbed Sensory Perception (specify)] may be related to psychological stress, possibly evidenced by change in behavior pattern/usual response to stimuli.

compromised family Coping may be related to temporary or sustained family disorganization or role changes, prolonged progression of condition that exhausts the supportive capacity of SO(s), possibly evidenced by family system not meeting physical, emotional, or spiritual needs of its members; inability to express or to accept wide range of feelings, inappropriate boundary maintenance, SO(s) describe(s) preoccupation with personal reactions.

Paraplegia   MS/CH
Also Refer to Quadriplegia

impaired Transfer Ability may be related to loss of muscle function and control, injury to upper extremity joints (overuse).

[disturbed kinesthetic/tactile Sensory Perception] may be related to neurological deficit with loss of sensory reception and transmission, psychological stress, possibly evidenced by reported or measured change in sensory acuity, change in usual response to stimuli, anxiety, disorientation, bizarre thinking; exaggerated emotional responses.

reflex urinary Incontinence/impaired Urinary Elimination may be related to disruption of bladder innervation, bladder atony, fecal impaction possibly evidenced by bladder distention, retention, incontinence or overflow, urinary tract infections, kidney stone formation, renal dysfunction.

situational low Self-Esteem may be related to situational crisis, loss of body functions, change in physical abilities, perceived loss of self/identity, possibly evidenced by negative feelings about body or self, feelings of helplessness, powerlessness, delay in taking responsibility for self-care or participation in therapy, and change in social involvement.

Sexual Dysfunction may be related to loss of sensation, altered function, and vulnerability, possibly evidenced by seeking of confirmation of desirability, verbalization of concern, alteration in relationship with SO, and change in interest in self or others.

Parathyroidectomy   MS
acute Pain may be related to presence of surgical incision and effects of calcium imbalance (bone pain, tetany), possibly evidenced by verbal reports, guarding or distraction behaviors, self-focus, and changes in vital signs.

risk for excess Fluid Volume: risk factors may include preoperative renal involvement, stress-induced release of antidiuretic hormone, and changing calcium and electrolyte levels.*

risk for ineffective Airway Clearance: risk factors may include edema formation and laryngeal nerve damage.*

deficient Knowledge [Learning Need] regarding postoperative care, complications, and long-term needs may be related to lack of information or recall, misinterpretation, possibly evidenced by statements of concern, questions, and misconceptions.

Parenteral feeding   MS/CH

imbalanced Nutrition: less than body requirements may be related to conditions that interfere with nutrient intake or increase nutrient need or metabolic demand—cancer and associated treatments, anorexia, surgical procedures, dysphagia, or decreased level of consciousness, possibly evidenced by body weight 10% or more under ideal, decreased subcutaneous fat or muscle mass, poor muscle tone.

risk for Infection: risk factors may include insertion of venous catheter, malnutrition, chronic disease, improper preparation or handling of feeding solution.*

risk for Injury [multifactor]: risk factors may include catheter-related complications (air emboli, septic thrombophlebitis).*

risk for imbalanced Fluid Volume: risk factors may include active loss or failure of regulatory mechanisms specific to underlying disease process or trauma, complications of therapy—high glucose solutions/hyperglycemia—hyperosmolar nonketotic coma and severe dehydration; inability to obtain or ingest fluids.*

Fatigue may be related to decreased metabolic energy production, increased energy requirements—hypermetabolic state, healing process; altered body chemistry—medications, chemotherapy; possibly evidenced by overwhelming lack of energy, inability to maintain usual routines/accomplish routine tasks, lethargy, impaired ability to concentrate.

Parkinson's disease   CH

impaired Walking may be related to neuromuscular impairment (muscle weakness, tremors, bradykinesia) and musculoskeletal impairment (joint rigidity), possibly evidenced by inability to move about the environment as desired, increased occurrence of falls.

impaired Swallowing may be related to neuromuscular impairment, muscle weakness, possibly evidenced by reported or observed difficulty in swallowing, drooling, evidence of aspiration (choking, coughing).

impaired verbal Communication may be related to muscle weakness and incoordination, possibly evidenced by impaired articulation, difficulty with phonation, and changes in rhythm and intonation.

risk for Stress Overload: risk factors may include inadequate resources, chronic illness, physical demands.*

Caregiver Role Strain may be related to illness, severity of care receiver, psychological or cognitive problems in care receiver, caregiver is

*A risk diagnosis is not evidenced by signs and symptoms, as the problem has not occurred; rather, nursing interventions are directed at prevention.

spouse, duration of caregiving required, lack of respite or recreation for caregiver, possibly evidenced by feeling stressed, depressed, worried; lack of resources or support, family conflict.

Pelvic inflammatory disease OB/GYN/CH

risk for Infection [spread]: risk factors may include presence of infectious process in highly vascular pelvic structures, delay in seeking treatment.*

acute Pain may be related to inflammation, edema, and congestion of reproductive and pelvic tissues, possibly evidenced by verbal reports, guarding or distraction behaviors, self-focus, and changes in vital signs.

Hyperthermia may be related to inflammatory process and hypermetabolic state, possibly evidenced by increased body temperature; warm, flushed skin; and tachycardia.

risk for situational low Self-Esteem: risk factors may include perceived stigma of physical condition (infection of reproductive system).*

deficient Knowledge [Learning Need] regarding cause, complications of condition, therapy needs, and transmission of disease to others may be related to lack of information, misinterpretation, possibly evidenced by statements of concern, questions, misconceptions, and development of preventable complications.

Periarteritis nodosa MS/CH

Refer to Polyarteritis [nodosa]

Pericarditis MS

acute Pain may be related to tissue inflammation and presence of effusion, possibly evidenced by verbal reports of pain affected by movement or position, guarding or distraction behaviors, self-focus, and changes in vital signs.

Activity Intolerance may be related to imbalance between O_2 supply and demand (restriction of cardiac filling and ventricular contraction, reduced cardiac output), possibly evidenced by reports of weakness, fatigue, exertional dyspnea, abnormal heart rate or BP response, and signs of heart failure.

risk for decreased Cardiac Output: risk factors may include accumulation of fluid (effusion), restricted cardiac filling and contractility.*

Anxiety [specify level] may be related to change in health status and perceived threat of death, possibly evidenced by increased tension, apprehension, restlessness, and expressed concerns.

Perinatal loss/death of child OB/CH

Grieving may be related to death of fetus or infant, possibly evidenced by verbal expressions of distress, anger, loss, guilt; crying; change in eating habits or sleep.

situational low Self-Esteem may be related to perceived failure at a life event, inability to meet personal expectations, possibly evidenced by negative self-appraisal in response to situation or personal actions,

P

---

*A risk diagnosis is not evidenced by signs and symptoms, as the problem has not occurred; rather, nursing interventions are directed at prevention.

expressions of helplessness, hopelessness, evaluation of self as unable to deal with situation.

risk for ineffective Role Performance: risk factors may include stress, family conflict, inadequate support system.*

risk for interrupted Family Processes: risk factors may include situational crisis, developmental transition [loss of child], family roles shift.*

risk for Spiritual Distress: risk factors may include blame for loss directed at self or higher power, intense suffering, alienation from SO or support systems. *

Peripheral arterial occlusive disease   CH
Refer to Arterial occlusive disease

Peripheral vascular disease (atherosclerosis)   CH
ineffective peripheral Tissue Perfusion may be related to reduction or interruption of arterial or venous blood flow, possibly evidenced by changes in skin temperature and color, lack of hair growth, BP and pulse changes in extremity, presence of bruits, and reports of claudication.

Activity Intolerance may be related to imbalance between O_2 supply and demand, possibly evidenced by reports of muscle fatigue, weakness and exertional discomfort (claudication).

risk for impaired Skin/Tissue Integrity: risk factors may include altered circulation with decreased sensation and impaired healing.*

Peritonitis   MS
risk for Infection [spread/septicemia]: risk factors may include inadequate primary defenses (broken skin, traumatized tissue, altered peristalsis), inadequate secondary defenses (immunosuppression), and invasive procedures.*

deficient Fluid Volume [mixed] may be related to fluid shifts from extracellular, intravascular, and interstitial compartments into intestines and/or peritoneal space, excessive gastric losses (vomiting, diarrhea, NG suction), fever, hypermetabolic state, and restricted intake, possibly evidenced by dry mucous membranes; poor skin turgor; delayed capillary refill; weak peripheral pulses; diminished urinary output; dark, concentrated urine; hypotension; and tachycardia.

acute Pain may be related to chemical irritation of parietal peritoneum, trauma to tissues, abdominal distention—accumulation of fluid in abdominal or peritoneal cavity, possibly evidenced by verbal reports, muscle guarding, rebound tenderness, distraction behaviors, facial mask of pain, self-focus, changes in vital signs.

risk for imbalanced Nutrition: less than body requirements: risk factors may include nausea, vomiting, intestinal dysfunction, metabolic abnormalities, increased metabolic needs.*

Pheochromocytoma   MS
Anxiety [specify level] may be related to excessive physiological (hormonal) stimulation of the sympathetic nervous system, situational

P

---

*A risk diagnosis is not evidenced by signs and symptoms, as the problem has not occurred; rather, nursing interventions are directed at prevention.

crises, threat to or change in health status, possibly evidenced by apprehension, shakiness, restlessness, focus on self, fearfulness, diaphoresis, and sense of impending doom.

deficient Fluid Volume [mixed] may be related to excessive gastric losses (vomiting, diarrhea), hypermetabolic state, diaphoresis, and hyperosmolar diuresis, possibly evidenced by hemoconcentration, dry mucous membranes, poor skin turgor, thirst, and weight loss.

decreased Cardiac Output/ineffective Tissue Perfusion [specify] may be related to altered preload—decreased blood volume, altered SVR, and increased sympathetic activity (excessive secretion of catecholamines), possibly evidenced by cool, clammy skin; change in BP (hypertension, postural hypotension), visual disturbances, severe headache, and angina.

deficient Knowledge [Learning Need] regarding pathophysiology of condition, outcome, preoperative and postoperative care needs may be related to lack of information or recall, possibly evidenced by statements of concern, questions, and misconceptions.

Phlebitis CH
Refer to Thrombophlebitis

Phobia PSY
Also Refer to Anxiety disorder, generalized

Fear may be related to learned irrational response to natural or innate origins (phobic stimulus), unfounded morbid dread of a seemingly harmless object or situation, possibly evidenced by sympathetic stimulation and reactions ranging from apprehension to panic, withdrawal from or total avoidance of situations that place individual in contact with feared object.

impaired Social Interaction may be related to intense fear of encountering feared object, activity or situation; and anticipated loss of control, possibly evidenced by reported change of style or pattern of interaction, discomfort in social situations, and avoidance of phobic stimulus.

Placenta previa OB
risk for deficient Fluid Volume: risk factors may include excessive vascular losses (vessel damage and inadequate vasoconstriction).*

impaired fetal Gas Exchange: may be related to altered blood flow, altered O_2-carrying capacity of blood (maternal anemia), and decreased surface area of gas exchange at site of placental attachment, possibly evidenced by changes in fetal heart rate or activity and release of meconium.

Fear may be related to threat of death (perceived or actual) to self or fetus, possibly evidenced by verbalization of specific concerns, increased tension, sympathetic stimulation.

risk for deficient Diversional Activity: risk factors may include imposed activity restrictions, bedrest.*

---

*A risk diagnosis is not evidenced by signs and symptoms, as the problem has not occurred; rather, nursing interventions are directed at prevention.

Pleurisy   CH

acute Pain may be related to inflammation or irritation of the parietal
   pleura, possibly evidenced by verbal reports, guarding or distraction
   behaviors, self-focus, and changes in vital signs.

ineffective Breathing Pattern may be related to pain on inspiration, possibly evidenced by decreased respiratory depth, tachypnea, and dyspnea.

risk for Infection [pneumonia]: risk factors may include stasis of pulmonary secretions, decreased lung expansion, and ineffective
   cough.*

Pneumonia   CH/MS

Refer to Bronchitis; Bronchopneumonia

Pneumothorax   MS

Also Refer to Hemothorax

ineffective Breathing Pattern may be related to decreased lung expansion (fluid and air accumulation), musculoskeletal impairment, pain,
   inflammatory process, possibly evidenced by dyspnea, tachypnea,
   altered chest excursion, respiratory depth changes, use of accessory
   muscles and nasal flaring, cough, cyanosis, and abnormal ABGs.

risk for decreased Cardiac Output: risk factors may include compression
   or displacement of cardiac structures.*

acute Pain may be related to irritation of nerve endings within pleural
   space by foreign object (chest tube), possibly evidenced by verbal
   reports, guarding or distraction behaviors, self-focus, and changes in
   vital signs.

Polyarteritis (nodosa)   MS/CH

ineffective Tissue Perfusion [specify] may be related to reduction or
   interruption of blood flow, possibly evidenced by organ tissue infarctions, changes in organ function, and development of organic
   psychosis.

Hyperthermia may be related to widespread inflammatory process, possibly evidenced by increased body temperature and warm, flushed
   skin.

acute Pain may be related to inflammation, tissue ischemia, and necrosis
   of affected area, possibly evidenced by verbal reports, guarding or
   distraction behaviors, self-focus, and changes in vital signs.

Grieving may be related to perceived loss of self, possibly evidenced
   by expressions of sorrow and anger, altered sleep and/or eating patterns, changes in activity level, and libido.

Polycythemia vera   CH

Activity Intolerance may be related to imbalance between O_2 supply
   and demand, possibly evidenced by reports of fatigue, weakness.

ineffective Tissue Perfusion [specify] may be related to reduction or
   interruption of arterial or venous blood flow (insufficiency, thrombosis, or hemorrhage), possibly evidenced by pain in affected area,

---

*A risk diagnosis is not evidenced by signs and symptoms, as the problem has
not occurred; rather, nursing interventions are directed at prevention.

impaired mental ability, visual disturbances, and color changes of skin or mucous membranes.

Polyradiculitis   MS
Refer to Guillain-Barré syndrome

Postoperative recovery period   MS
ineffective Breathing Pattern may be related to neuromuscular and perceptual or cognitive impairment, decreased lung expansion and energy, and tracheobronchial obstruction, possibly evidenced by changes in respiratory rate and depth, reduced vital capacity, apnea, cyanosis, and noisy respirations.

risk for imbalanced Body Temperature: risk factors may include exposure to cool environment, effect of medications/anesthetic agents, extremes of age or weight, and dehydration.*

risk for acute Confusion: risk factors may include pharmaceutical agents—anesthesia, pain.

risk for deficient Fluid Volume: risk factors may include restriction of oral intake, loss of fluid through abnormal routes (indwelling tubes, drains) and normal routes (vomiting, loss of vascular integrity, changes in clotting ability), extremes of age and weight.*

acute Pain may be related to disruption of skin, tissue, and muscle integrity; musculoskeletal/bone trauma; and presence of tubes and drains, possibly evidenced by verbal reports, alteration in muscle tone, facial mask of pain, distraction or guarding behaviors, narrowed focus, and changes in vital signs.

impaired Skin/Tissue Integrity may be related to mechanical interruption of skin and tissues, altered circulation, effects of medication, accumulation of drainage, and altered metabolic state, possibly evidenced by disruption of skin surface, skin layers, and tissues.

risk for Infection: risk factors may include broken skin, traumatized tissues, stasis of body fluids, presence of pathogens or contaminants, environmental exposure, and invasive procedures.*

Postpartal period   OB/CH
readiness for enhanced Family Processes possibly evidenced by expressing willingness to enhance family dynamics.

risk for deficient Fluid Volume/Bleeding: risk factors may include excessive blood loss during delivery, reduced intake, inadequate replacement, nausea, vomiting, increased urine output, and insensible losses.*

acute Pain/impaired Comfort may be related to tissue trauma and edema, muscle contractions, bladder fullness, and physical or psychological exhaustion, possibly evidenced by reports of cramping (afterpains), self-focusing, alteration in muscle tone, distraction behaviors, and changes in vital signs.

impaired Urinary Elimination may be related to hormonal effects (fluid shifts, continued elevation in renal plasma flow), mechanical trauma, tissue edema, and effects of medication and anesthesia, possibly evidenced by frequency, dysuria, urgency, incontinence, or retention.

---

*A risk diagnosis is not evidenced by signs and symptoms, as the problem has not occurred; rather, nursing interventions are directed at prevention.

Constipation may be related to decreased muscle tone associated with diastasis recti, prenatal effects of progesterone, dehydration, excess analgesia or anesthesia, pain (hemorrhoids, episiotomy, or perineal tenderness), prelabor diarrhea and lack of intake, possibly evidenced by frequency less than usual pattern, hard-formed stool, straining at stool, decreased bowel sounds, and abdominal distention.

Insomnia may be related to pain or discomfort, intense exhilaration and excitement, anxiety, exhausting process of labor and delivery, and needs/demands of family members, possibly evidenced by verbal reports of difficulty in falling or staying asleep, dissatisfaction with sleep, lack of energy, nonrestorative sleep.

risk for impaired Attachment/Parenting: risk factors may include lack of support between or from SO(s), ineffective or no role model, anxiety associated with the parental role, unrealistic expectations, presence of stressors (e.g., financial, housing, employment).*

Postpartum psychosis   OB/PSY
Also Refer to Depression, postpartum

ineffective Coping may be related to situational/maturational crisis, inadequate level of confidence in ability to cope, inadequate level of perception of control, possibly evidenced by inability to meet basic needs, inability to problem-solve, sleep pattern disturbance, poor concentration.

risk for other-directed Violence: risk factors may include mood swings, increased anxiety, despondency, hopelessness, psychotic symptomatology.*

Post-traumatic stress disorder   PSY
Post-Trauma Syndrome related to having experienced a traumatic life event, possibly evidenced by reexperiencing the event, somatic reactions, psychic or emotional numbness, altered lifestyle, impaired sleep, self-destructive behaviors, difficulty with interpersonal relationships, development of phobia, poor impulse control/irritability, and explosiveness.

risk for other-directed Violence: risk factors may include startle reaction, an intrusive memory causing a sudden acting out of a feeling as if the event were occurring, use of alcohol or other drugs to ward off painful effects and produce psychic numbing, breaking through the rage that has been walled off, response to intense anxiety or panic state, and loss of control.*

ineffective Coping may be related to personal vulnerability, inadequate support systems, unrealistic perceptions, unmet expectations, overwhelming threat to self, and multiple stressors repeated over a period of time, possibly evidenced by verbalization of inability to cope or difficulty asking for help, muscular tension, headaches, chronic worry, and emotional tension.

complicated Grieving may be related to actual or perceived object loss (loss of self as seen before the traumatic incident occurred, as well as other losses incurred in/after the incident), loss of physiopsychosocial well-being, thwarted grieving response to a loss, and lack of

*A risk diagnosis is not evidenced by signs and symptoms, as the problem has not occurred; rather, nursing interventions are directed at prevention.

resolution of previous grieving responses, possibly evidenced by verbal expression of distress at loss, anger, sadness, labile affect; alterations in eating habits, sleep/dream patterns, libido; reliving of past experiences, expression of guilt, and alterations in concentration.

interrupted Family Processes may be related to situational crisis, failure to master developmental transitions, possibly evidenced by expressions of confusion about what to do and that family is having difficulty coping; family system not meeting physical, emotional, or spiritual needs of its members; not adapting to change or dealing with traumatic experience constructively; and ineffective family decision-making process.

Pregnancy (prenatal period) 1st trimester   OB/CH

risk for imbalanced Nutrition: less than body requirements: risk factors may include changes in appetite, insufficient intake (nausea, vomiting, inadequate financial resources and nutritional knowledge), meeting increased metabolic demands (increased thyroid activity associated with the growth of fetal and maternal tissues).*

impaired Comfort may be related to hormonal influences, physical changes, possibly evidenced by verbal reports (nausea, breast changes, leg cramps, hemorrhoids, nasal stuffiness), alteration in muscle tone, inability to relax.

risk for disturbed Maternal-Fetal Dyad: risk factors may include environmental and hereditary factors and problems of maternal well-being that directly affect the developing fetus (e.g., malnutrition, substance use).*

[maximally compensated] Cardiac Output may be related to increased fluid volume and maximal cardiac effort, hormonal effects of progesterone and relaxin (places the client at risk for hypertension and/or circulatory failure), and changes in peripheral resistance (afterload), possibly evidenced by variations in BP and pulse, syncopal episodes, presence of pathological edema.

readiness for enhanced family Coping possibly evidenced by movement toward health-promoting and enriching lifestyle, choosing experiences that optimize pregnancy experience and wellness.

risk for Constipation: risk factors may include changes in dietary and fluid intake, smooth muscle relaxation, decreased peristalsis, and effects of medications (e.g., iron).*

Fatigue/Insomnia may be related to increased carbohydrate metabolism, altered body chemistry, increased energy requirements to perform ADLs, discomfort, anxiety, inactivity, possibly evidenced by reports of overwhelming lack of energy, inability to maintain usual routines, difficulty falling asleep, dissatisfaction with sleep, decreased quality of life.

risk for ineffective Role Performance: risk factors may include maturational crisis, developmental level, history of maladaptive coping, absence of support systems.*

deficient Knowledge [Learning Need] regarding normal physiological/psychological changes and self-care needs may be related to lack of

---

*A risk diagnosis is not evidenced by signs and symptoms, as the problem has not occurred; rather, nursing interventions are directed at prevention.

information or recall, and misinterpretation of normal physiological and psychological changes and their impact on the client/family, possibly evidenced by questions, statements of concern, misconceptions, and inaccurate follow-through of instructions, development of preventable complications.

Pregnancy (prenatal period) 2nd trimester   OB/CH

Also Refer to Pregnancy 1st trimester

risk for disturbed Body Image: risk factors may include perception of biophysical changes, response of others.*

ineffective Breathing Pattern may be related to impingement of the diaphragm by enlarging uterus, possibly evidenced by reports of shortness of breath, dyspnea, and changes in respiratory depth.

risk for [decompensated] Cardiac Output: risk factors may include increased circulatory demand, changes in preload (decreased venous return) and afterload (increased peripheral vascular resistance), and ventricular hypertrophy.*

risk for excess Fluid Volume: risk factors may include changes in regulatory mechanisms, sodium and water retention.*

Sexual Dysfunction may be related to conflict regarding changes in sexual desire and expectations, fear of physical injury to woman or fetus, possibly evidenced by reported difficulties, limitations, or changes in sexual behaviors or activities.

Pregnancy (prenatal period) 3rd trimester   OB/CH

Also Refer to Pregnancy 1st and 2nd trimesters

deficient Knowledge [Learning Need] regarding preparation for labor and delivery, infant care may be related to lack of exposure or experience, misinterpretations of information, possibly evidenced by request for information, statement of concerns, misconceptions.

impaired Urinary Elimination may be related to uterine enlargement, increased abdominal pressure, fluctuation of renal blood flow, and GFR, possibly evidenced by urinary frequency, urgency, dependent edema.

risk for ineffective Coping/compromised family Coping: risk factors may include situational or maturational crisis, personal vulnerability, unrealistic perceptions, absent or insufficient support systems.*

risk for disturbed Maternal-Fetal Dyad: risk factors may include presence of hypertension, infection, substance use or abuse, altered immune system, abnormal blood profile, tissue hypoxia, premature rupture of membranes.*

Pregnancy, adolescent   OB/CH

Also Refer to Pregnancy 1st, 2nd, and 3rd trimesters

interrupted Family Processes may be related to situational or developmental transition (economic, change in roles, gain of a family member), possibly evidenced by family expressing confusion about what to do, unable to meet physical, emotional, or spiritual needs of the members; family inability to adapt to change or to deal with traumatic experience constructively, does not demonstrate respect for

---

*A risk diagnosis is not evidenced by signs and symptoms, as the problem has not occurred; rather, nursing interventions are directed at prevention.

individuality and autonomy of its members, ineffective family decision-making process, and inappropriate boundary maintenance.

Social Isolation may be related to alterations in physical appearance, perceived unacceptable social behavior, restricted social sphere, stage of adolescence, and interference with accomplishing developmental tasks, possibly evidenced by expressions of feelings of aloneness, rejection, or difference from others; uncommunicative, withdrawn, no eye contact, seeking to be alone, unacceptable behavior, and absence of supportive SO(s).

situational/chronic low Self-Esteem may be related to situational or maturational crisis, biophysical changes, and fear of failure at life events, absence of support systems, possibly evidenced by self-negating verbalizations, expressions of shame, guilt, fear of rejection or reaction of other, hypersensitivity to criticism, and lack of follow-through or nonparticipation in prenatal care.

deficient Knowledge [Learning Need] regarding pregnancy, developmental or individual needs, future expectations may be related to lack of exposure, information misinterpretation, unfamiliarity with information resources, lack of interest in learning, possibly evidenced by questions, statement of concern, misconception, sense of vulnerability, denial of reality, inaccurate follow-through of instruction, and development of preventable complications.

risk for impaired Parenting may be related to chronological age and developmental stage; unmet social, emotional, or maturational needs of parenting figures; unrealistic expectation of self/infant/partner; ineffective role model or social support; lack of role identity; and presence of stressors (e.g., financial, social).*

Pregnancy, high-risk   OB/CH
Also Refer to Pregnancy 1st, 2nd, and 3rd trimesters

Anxiety [specify level] may be related to situational crisis, threat of maternal or fetal death (perceived or actual), interpersonal transmission and contagion, possibly evidenced by increased tension, apprehension, feelings of inadequacy, somatic complaints, difficulty sleeping.

deficient Knowledge [Learning Need] regarding high-risk situation/ preterm labor may be related to lack of exposure to or misinterpretation of information, unfamiliarity with individual risks and own role in risk prevention and management, possibly evidenced by request for information, statement of concerns, misconceptions, inaccurate follow-through of instructions.

risk of maternal Injury: risk factors may include preexisting medical conditions, complications of pregnancy.*

risk for Activity Intolerance: risk factors may include presence of circulatory or respiratory problems, uterine irritability.*

risk for ineffective Self-Health Management: risk factors may include client value system, health beliefs and cultural influences, issues of control, presence of anxiety, complexity of therapeutic regimen, economic difficulties, perceived susceptibility.*

---

*A risk diagnosis is not evidenced by signs and symptoms, as the problem has not occurred; rather, nursing interventions are directed at prevention.

Pregnancy-induced hypertension (preeclampsia)   OB/CH

Also Refer to Eclampsia

deficient Fluid Volume may be related to a plasma protein loss, decreasing plasma colloid osmotic pressure allowing fluid shifts out of vascular compartment, possibly evidenced by edema formation, sudden weight gain, hemoconcentration, nausea, vomiting, epigastric pain, headaches, visual changes, decreased urine output.

decreased Cardiac Output may be related to hypovolemia/decreased venous return, increased SVR, possibly evidenced by variations in BP and hemodynamic readings, edema, shortness of breath, change in mental status.

risk for disturbed Maternal-Fetal Dyad: risk factors may include vasospasm of spiral arteries and relative hypovolemia.*

deficient Knowledge [Learning Need] regarding pathophysiology of condition, therapy, self-care and nutritional needs, and potential complications may be related to lack of information or recall, misinterpretation, possibly evidenced by statements of concern, questions, misconceptions, inaccurate follow-through of instructions, or development of preventable complications.

Premenstrual dysphoric disorder   GYN/PSY

chronic/acute Pain may be related to cyclic changes in female hormones affecting other systems (e.g., vascular congestion or spasms), vitamin deficiency, fluid retention, possibly evidenced by increased tension, apprehension, jitteriness, verbal reports, distraction behaviors, somatic complaints, self-focusing, physical and social withdrawal.

excess Fluid Volume may be related to abnormal alterations of hormonal levels, possibly evidenced by edema formation, weight gain, and periodic changes in emotional status, irritability.

[moderate to panic] Anxiety may be related to cyclic changes in female hormones affecting other systems, possibly evidenced by feelings of inability to cope or loss of control, depersonalization, increased tension, apprehension, jitteriness, somatic complaints, and impaired functioning.

ineffective Coping may be related to personal vulnerability, threat to self-concept, multiple stressors, possibly evidenced by reports inability to cope, inadequate problem-solving, sleep pattern disturbance.

deficient Knowledge [Learning Need] regarding pathophysiology of condition and self-care/treatment needs may be related to lack of information, misinterpretation, possibly evidenced by statements of concern, questions, misconceptions, and continuation of condition, exacerbating symptoms.

Premenstrual tension syndrome (PMS)   GYN/CH

Refer to Premenstrual dysphoric disorder

---

*A risk diagnosis is not evidenced by signs and symptoms, as the problem has not occurred; rather, nursing interventions are directed at prevention.

Pressure ulcer or sore CH

Also Refer to Ulcer, decubitus

ineffective peripheral Tissue Perfusion may be related to reduced or interrupted blood flow, possibly evidenced by presence of inflamed, necrotic lesion.

deficient Knowledge [Learning Need] regarding cause/prevention of condition and potential complications may be related to lack of information, misinterpretation, possibly evidenced by statements of concern, questions, misconceptions, and inaccurate follow-through of instructions.

Preterm labor OB/CH

Refer to Labor, preterm

Prostatectomy MS

impaired Urinary Elimination may be related to mechanical obstruction (blood clots, edema, trauma, surgical procedure, pressure or irritation of catheter and balloon) and loss of bladder tone, possibly evidenced by dysuria, frequency, dribbling, incontinence, retention, bladder fullness, suprapubic discomfort.

risk for Bleeding/deficient Fluid Volume: risk factors may include trauma to highly vascular area with excessive vascular losses, restricted intake, postobstructive diuresis.*

acute Pain may be related to irritation of bladder mucosa and tissue trauma or edema, possibly evidenced by verbal reports (bladder spasms), distraction behaviors, self-focus, and changes in vital signs.

disturbed Body Image may be related to perceived threat of altered body or sexual function, possibly evidenced by preoccupation with change or loss, negative feelings about body, and statements of concern regarding functioning.

CH

risk for Sexual Dysfunction: risk factors may include situational crisis (incontinence, leakage of urine after catheter removal, involvement of genital area) and threat to self-concept or change in health status.*

Pruritus CH

impaired Comfort/acute Pain may be related to cutaneous hyperesthesia and inflammation, possibly evidenced by verbal reports, distraction behaviors, and self-focus.

risk for impaired Skin Integrity: risk factors may include mechanical trauma (scratching) and development of vesicles or bullae that may rupture.*

Psoriasis CH

impaired Skin Integrity may be related to increased epidermal cell proliferation and absence of normal protective skin layers, possibly evidenced by scaling papules and plaques.

disturbed Body Image may be related to cosmetically unsightly skin lesions, possibly evidenced by hiding affected body part, negative

---

*A risk diagnosis is not evidenced by signs and symptoms, as the problem has not occurred; rather, nursing interventions are directed at prevention.

feelings about body, feelings of helplessness, and change in social involvement.

Pulmonary edema   MS
impaired Gas Exchange may be related to alveolar-capillary membrane changes (fluid collection or shifts into interstitial space or alveoli) possibly evidenced by dyspnea, restlessness, irritability, abnormal rate/depth of respirations, lethargy, confusion.

[moderate to severe] Anxiety may be related to change in health status, threat of death, interpersonal transmission possibly evidenced by expressed concerns, distress, apprehension, extraneous movement.

risk for impaired spontaneous Ventilation: risk factors may include respiratory muscle fatigue, problems with secretion management.*

Pulmonary edema, high-altitude   MS
Refer to High-altitude pulmonary edema

Pulmonary embolus   MS
ineffective Breathing Pattern may be related to tracheobronchial obstruction (inflammation, copious secretions, or active bleeding), decreased lung expansion, inflammatory process, possibly evidenced by changes in depth and/or rate of respiration, dyspnea, use of accessory muscles, altered chest excursion, abnormal breath sounds (crackles, wheezes), and cough (with or without sputum production).

impaired Gas Exchange may be related to ventilation-perfusion imbalance, alveolar-capillary membrane changes (atelectasis, airway or alveolar collapse, pulmonary edema or effusion, excessive secretions or active bleeding), possibly evidenced by profound dyspnea, restlessness, apprehension, somnolence, cyanosis, and changes in ABGs or pulse oximetry (hypoxemia and hypercapnia).

Fear/Anxiety [specify level] may be related to severe dyspnea and inability to breathe normally, perceived threat of death, threat to or change in health status, physiological response to hypoxemia and acidosis, and concern regarding unknown outcome of situation, possibly evidenced by restlessness, irritability, withdrawal or attack behavior, sympathetic stimulation (cardiovascular excitation, pupil dilation, sweating, vomiting, diarrhea), crying, voice quivering, and impending sense of doom.

Pulmonary hypertension   CH/MS
impaired Gas Exchange may be related to changes in alveolar membrane, increased pulmonary vascular resistance, possibly evidenced by dyspnea, irritability, decreased mental acuity, somnolence, abnormal ABGs.

decreased Cardiac Output may be related to increased pulmonary vascular resistance, decreased blood return to left side of heart, possibly evidenced by increased heart rate, dyspnea, fatigue.

Activity Intolerance may be related to imbalance between O_2 supply and demand, possibly evidenced by reports of weakness, fatigue, abnormal vital signs with activity.

---

*A risk diagnosis is not evidenced by signs and symptoms, as the problem has not occurred; rather, nursing interventions are directed at prevention.

Anxiety may be related to change in health status, stress, threat to self-concept, possibly evidenced by expressed concerns, uncertainty, awareness of physiological symptoms, diminished productivity or ability to problem-solve.

Purpura, idiopathic thrombocytopenic   CH

ineffective Protection may be related to abnormal blood profile, drug therapy (corticosteroids or immunosuppressive agents), possibly evidenced by altered clotting, fatigue, deficient immunity.

Activity Intolerance may be related to decreased O_2-carrying capacity/imbalance between O_2 supply and demand, possibly evidenced by reports of fatigue, weakness.

deficient Knowledge [Learning Need] regarding therapy choices, outcomes, and self-care needs may be related to lack of information/misinterpretation, possibly evidenced by statements of concern, questions, and misconceptions.

Pyelonephritis   MS

acute Pain may be related to acute inflammation of renal tissues, possibly evidenced by verbal reports, guarding/distraction behaviors, self-focus, and changes in vital signs.

Hyperthermia may be related to inflammatory process and increased metabolic rate, possibly evidenced by increase in body temperature; warm, flushed skin; tachycardia; and chills.

impaired Urinary Elimination may be related to inflammation or irritation of bladder mucosa, possibly evidenced by dysuria, urgency, and frequency.

deficient Knowledge [Learning Need] regarding therapy needs and prevention may be related to lack of information, misinterpretation, possibly evidenced by statements of concern, questions, misconceptions, and recurrence of condition.

Quadriplegia   MS/CH
Also Refer to Paraplegia

ineffective Breathing Pattern may be related to neuromuscular impairment of innervation of diaphragm—lesions at or above C5, complete or mixed loss of intercostal muscle function, reflex abdominal spasms, gastric distention, possibly evidenced by decreased respiratory depth, dyspnea, cyanosis, and abnormal ABGs.

risk for Trauma [additional spinal injury]: risk factors may include temporary weakness or instability of spinal column.*

Grieving may be related to perceived loss of self, anticipated alterations in lifestyle and expectations, and limitation of future options or choices, possibly evidenced by expressions of distress, anger, sorrow, choked feelings, and changes in eating habits, sleep, communication patterns.

[total] Self-Care Deficit related to neuromuscular impairment, evidenced by inability to perform self-care tasks.

bowel Incontinence/Constipation may be related to disruption of nerve innervation, perceptual impairment, changes in dietary and fluid in-

---

*A risk diagnosis is not evidenced by signs and symptoms, as the problem has not occurred; rather, nursing interventions are directed at prevention.

take, change in activity level, side effects of medication possibly evidenced by inability to evacuate bowel voluntarily; increased abdominal pressure or distention; dry, hard-formed stool; change in bowel sounds.

impaired bed/wheelchair Mobility may be related to loss of muscle function and control possibly evidenced by inability to reposition self, impaired ability to operate wheelchair.

risk for Autonomic Dysreflexia: risk factors may include altered nerve function (spinal cord injury at T6 or above), bladder, bowel, or skin stimulation (tactile, pain, thermal).*

impaired Home Maintenance may be related to permanent effects of injury, inadequate or absent support systems and finances, and lack of familiarity with resources, possibly evidenced by expressions of difficulties, requests for information and assistance, outstanding debts or financial crisis, and lack of necessary aids and equipment.

Rape   CH

deficient Knowledge [Learning Need] regarding required medical and legal procedures, prophylactic treatment for individual concerns (STDs, pregnancy), community resources and supports may be related to lack of information, possibly evidenced by statements of concern, questions, misconceptions, and exacerbation of symptoms.

Rape-Trauma Syndrome related to actual or attempted sexual penetration without consent, possibly evidenced by wide range of emotional reactions, including anxiety, fear, anger, embarrassment, and multisystem physical complaints.

risk for impaired Tissue Integrity: risk factors may include forceful sexual penetration and trauma to fragile tissues.*

PSY

ineffective Coping may be related to personal vulnerability, unmet expectations, unrealistic perceptions, inadequate support systems or coping methods, multiple stressors repeated over time, overwhelming threat to self, possibly evidenced by verbalizations of inability to cope or difficulty asking for help, muscular tension, headaches, emotional tension, chronic worry.

Sexual Dysfunction may be related to biopsychosocial alteration of sexuality (stress of post-trauma response), vulnerability, loss of sexual desire, impaired relationship with SO, possibly evidenced by alteration in achieving sexual satisfaction, change in interest in self or others, preoccupation with self.

Raynaud's phenomenon   CH

acute/chronic Pain may be related to vasospasm or altered perfusion of affected tissues, ischemia or destruction of tissues, possibly evidenced by verbal reports, guarding of affected parts, self-focusing, and restlessness.

ineffective peripheral Tissue Perfusion may be related to periodic reduction of arterial blood flow to affected areas, possibly evidenced

---

*A risk diagnosis is not evidenced by signs and symptoms, as the problem has not occurred; rather, nursing interventions are directed at prevention.

by pallor, cyanosis, coolness, numbness, paresthesia, slow healing of lesions.

deficient Knowledge [Learning Need] regarding pathophysiology of condition, potential for complications, therapy and self-care needs may be related to lack of information, misinterpretation, possibly evidenced by statements of concern, questions, and misconceptions; development of preventable complications.

Reflex sympathetic dystrophy (RSD)   CH
Refer to Complex regional pain syndrome

Regional enteritis   CH
Refer to Crohn's disease

Renal failure, acute   MS
excess Fluid Volume may be related to compromised regulatory mechanisms–decreased kidney function, possibly evidenced by weight gain, edema or anasarca, intake greater than output, venous congestion, changes in BP and CVP, and altered electrolyte levels, decreased Hb and Hct; pulmonary congestion on x-ray.

risk for imbalanced Nutrition: less than body requirements: risk factors may include inability to ingest or digest adequate nutrients—anorexia, nausea, vomiting, ulcerations of oral mucosa, and increased metabolic needs; protein catabolism, therapeutic dietary restrictions.*

risk for Infection: risk factors may include depression of immunological defenses, invasive procedures and devices, and changes in dietary intake, malnutrition.*

risk for acute Confusion: risk factors may include accumulation of toxic waste products and altered cerebral perfusion.*

Renal failure, chronic   CH/MS
Also Refer to Dialysis, general

risk for decreased Cardiac Output: risk factors may include fluid imbalances affecting circulating volume, myocardial workload, SVR; alterations in rate, rhythm, cardiac conduction—electrolyte imbalances, hypoxia; accumulation of toxins—urea; soft tissue calcification—deposits of calcium phosphate.*

risk for Bleeding: risk factors may include abnormal blood profile—suppressed erythropoietin production or secretion, decreased RBC production and survival, altered clotting factors; increased capillary fragility.*

risk for acute Confusion: risk factors may include electrolyte imbalance, increased BUN/creatinine, azotemia.

risk for impaired Skin Integrity: risk factors may include altered metabolic state and circulation (anemia with tissue ischemia), altered sensation (peripheral neuropathy), decreased skin turgor, reduced activity or immobility, accumulation of toxins in the skin.*

risk for impaired Oral Mucous Membrane: risk factors may include decreased or lack of salivation, fluid restrictions, chemical irritation, conversion of urea in saliva to ammonia.*

---

*A risk diagnosis is not evidenced by signs and symptoms, as the problem has not occurred; rather, nursing interventions are directed at prevention.

Renal transplantation   MS

risk for excess Fluid Volume: risk factors may include compromised regulatory mechanism (implantation of new kidney requiring adjustment period for optimal functioning).*

disturbed Body Image may be related to failure and subsequent replacement of body part and medication-induced changes in appearance, possibly evidenced by preoccupation with loss or change, negative feelings about body, and focus on past strength or function.

Fear may be related to potential for transplant rejection or failure and threat of death, possibly evidenced by increased tension, apprehension, concentration on source, and verbalizations of concern.

risk for Infection: risk factors may include broken skin, traumatized tissue, stasis of body fluids, immunosuppression, invasive procedures, nutritional deficits, and chronic disease.*

    CH

risk for ineffective Coping/compromised family Coping: risk factors may include situational crises, family disorganization and role changes, prolonged disease exhausting supportive capacity of SO(s)/family, therapeutic restrictions, long-term therapy needs.*

Respiratory distress syndrome, acute   MS

ineffective Airway Clearance may be related to loss of ciliary action, increased amount and viscosity of secretions, and increased airway resistance, possibly evidenced by presence of dyspnea, changes in depth and rate of respiration, use of accessory muscles for breathing, wheezes and crackles, cough with or without sputum production.

impaired Gas Exchange may be related to changes in pulmonary capillary permeability with edema formation, alveolar hypoventilation and collapse, with intrapulmonary shunting, possibly evidenced by tachypnea, use of accessory muscles, cyanosis, hypoxia per ABGs or oximetry, anxiety, and changes in mentation.

risk for deficient Fluid Volume: risk factors may include active loss from diuretic use and restricted intake.*

risk for decreased Cardiac Output: risk factors may include alteration in preload (hypovolemia, vascular pooling, diuretic therapy, and increased intrathoracic pressure, use of ventilator and positive end-expiratory pressure [PEEP]).*

Anxiety [specify level]/Fear may be related to physiological factors (effects of hypoxemia), situational crisis, change in health status and threat of death possibly evidenced by increased tension, apprehension, restlessness, focus on self, and sympathetic stimulation.

risk for [barotrauma] Injury: risk factors may include increased airway pressure associated with mechanical ventilation (PEEP).*

Respiratory distress syndrome (premature infant)   PED

Also Refer to Neonatal, premature newborn

impaired Gas Exchange may be related to alveolar-capillary membrane changes (inadequate surfactant levels), altered O_2 supply

---

*A risk diagnosis is not evidenced by signs and symptoms, as the problem has not occurred; rather, nursing interventions are directed at prevention.

(tracheobronchial obstruction, atelectasis), altered blood flow (immaturity of pulmonary arteriole musculature), altered O_2-carrying capacity of blood (anemia), and cold stress, possibly evidenced by tachypnea, use of accessory muscles—retractions, expiratory grunting, pallor, or cyanosis, abnormal ABGs, and tachycardia.

impaired spontaneous Ventilation may be related to respiratory muscle fatigue and metabolic factors, possibly evidenced by dyspnea, increased metabolic rate, restlessness, use of accessory muscles, and abnormal ABGs.

risk for Infection: risk factors may include inadequate primary defenses (decreased ciliary action, stasis of body fluids, traumatized tissues), inadequate secondary defenses (deficiency of neutrophils and specific immunoglobulins), invasive procedures, and malnutrition (absence of nutrient stores, increased metabolic demands).*

risk for ineffective Gastrointestinal Perfusion: risk factors may include persistent fetal circulation and exchange problems.*

risk for impaired Attachment: risk factors may include premature or ill infant who is unable to effectively initiate parental contact (altered behavioral organization), separation, physical barriers, anxiety associated with the parental role and demands of infant.*

Respiratory syncytial virus (RSV)   PED

impaired Gas Exchange may be related to inflammation of airways, ventilation perfusion imbalance, apnea, possibly evidenced by dyspnea, abnormal arterial blood gases/hypoxia.

ineffective Airway Clearance may be related to infection, retained secretions, exudate in the alveoli, possibly evidenced by dyspnea, adventitious breath sounds, ineffective cough.

risk for deficient Fluid Volume: risk factors may include increased insensible losses (fever, diaphoresis), decreased oral intake.*

Retinal detachment   CH

[disturbed visual Sensory Perception] related to decreased sensory reception, possibly evidenced by visual distortions, decreased visual field, and changes in visual acuity.

deficient Knowledge [Learning Need] regarding therapy, prognosis, and self-care needs may be related to lack of information or misconceptions, possibly evidenced by statements of concern and questions.

risk for impaired Home Maintenance: risk factors may include visual limitations, activity restrictions.*

Reye's syndrome   PED

deficient Fluid Volume may be related to failure of regulatory mechanism (diabetes insipidus), excessive gastric losses (pernicious vomiting), and altered intake, possibly evidenced by increased/dilute urine output, sudden weight loss, decreased venous filling, dry mucous membranes, decreased skin turgor, hypotension, and tachycardia.

ineffective cerebral Tissue Perfusion may be related to diminished arterial or venous blood flow and hypovolemia, possibly evidenced by memory loss, altered consciousness, and restlessness or agitation.

---

*A risk diagnosis is not evidenced by signs and symptoms, as the problem has not occurred; rather, nursing interventions are directed at prevention.

risk for Trauma: risk factors may include generalized weakness, reduced coordination, and cognitive deficits.*

ineffective Breathing Pattern may be related to decreased energy and fatigue, cognitive impairment, tracheobronchial obstruction, and inflammatory process (aspiration pneumonia), possibly evidenced by tachypnea, abnormal ABGs, cough, and use of accessory muscles.

Rheumatic fever   PED

acute Pain may be related to migratory inflammation of joints, possibly evidenced by verbal reports, guarding or distraction behaviors, self-focus, and changes in vital signs.

Hyperthermia may be related to inflammatory process, hypermetabolic state, possibly evidenced by increased body temperature; warm, flushed skin; and tachycardia.

Activity Intolerance may be related to generalized weakness, joint pain, medical restrictions, and bedrest, possibly evidenced by reports of fatigue, exertional discomfort, and abnormal heart rate in response to activity.

risk for decreased Cardiac Output: risk factors may include cardiac inflammation or enlargement and altered contractility.*

Rickets (osteomalacia)   PED

delayed Growth and Development may be related to dietary deficiencies or indiscretions, malabsorption syndrome, and lack of exposure to sunlight, possibly evidenced by altered physical growth and delay or difficulty in performing motor skills typical for age.

deficient Knowledge [Learning Need] regarding cause, pathophysiology, therapy needs, and prevention may be related to lack of information, possibly evidenced by statements of concern, questions, misconceptions, and inaccurate follow-through of instructions.

Ringworm, tinea   CH
Also Refer to Athlete's Foot

impaired Skin Integrity may be related to fungal infection of the dermis, possibly evidenced by disruption of skin surfaces—presence of lesions.

deficient Knowledge [Learning Need] regarding infectious nature, therapy, and self-care needs may be related to lack of information, misinformation, possibly evidenced by statements of concern, questions, and recurrence or spread.

Rubella   PED/CH

acute Pain/impaired Comfort may be related to inflammatory effects of viral infection and presence of desquamating rash, possibly evidenced by verbal reports, distraction behaviors, restlessness.

deficient Knowledge [Learning Need] regarding contagious nature, possible complications, and self-care needs may be related to lack of information, misinterpretations, possibly evidenced by statements of concern, questions, and inaccurate follow-through of instructions.

R

---

*A risk diagnosis is not evidenced by signs and symptoms, as the problem has not occurred; rather, nursing interventions are directed at prevention.

Scabies

impaired Skin Integrity may be related to presence of invasive parasite and development of pruritus, possibly evidenced by disruption of skin surface and inflammation.

deficient Knowledge [Learning Need] regarding communicable nature, possible complications, therapy, and self-care needs may be related to lack of information, misinterpretation, possibly evidenced by questions and statements of concern about spread to others.

Scarlet fever

Hyperthermia may be related to effects of circulating toxins, possibly evidenced by increased body temperature; warm, flushed skin; and tachycardia.

acute Pain/impaired Comfort may be related to inflammation of mucous membranes and effects of circulating toxins (malaise, fever), possibly evidenced by verbal reports, distraction behaviors, guarding (decreased swallowing), and self-focus.

risk for deficient Fluid Volume: risk factors may include hypermetabolic state (hyperthermia) and reduced intake.*

Schizophrenia (schizophrenic disorders)

[disturbed Sensory Perception (specify)] may be related to biochemical/electrolyte imbalance, psychological stress, possibly evidenced by disorientation to space/time, hallucinations, change in behavior pattern.

impaired verbal Communication may be related to altered perceptions, alteration in self-concept, psychological barriers, e.g., psychosis possibly evidenced by inappropriate verbalizations, difficulty in comprehending usual communication pattern, difficulty in use of facial expressions.

Social Isolation may be related to alterations in mental status, mistrust of others, delusional thinking, unacceptable social behaviors, inadequate personal resources, and inability to engage in satisfying personal relationships, possibly evidenced by difficulty in establishing relationships with others, dull affect, uncommunicative or withdrawn behavior, seeking to be alone, inadequate or absent significant purpose in life, and expression of feelings of rejection.

ineffective Health Maintenance/impaired Home Maintenance may be related to impaired cognitive or emotional functioning, altered ability to make deliberate and thoughtful judgments, altered communication, and lack or inappropriate use of material resources, possibly evidenced by inability to take responsibility for meeting basic health practices in any or all functional areas and demonstrated lack of adaptive behaviors to internal or external environmental changes, disorderly surroundings, accumulation of dirt and unwashed clothes, repeated hygienic disorders.

risk for self-/other-directed Violence: risk factors may include disturbances of thinking or feeling (depression, paranoia, suicidal ideation), lack of development of trust and appropriate interpersonal re-

---

*A risk diagnosis is not evidenced by signs and symptoms, as the problem has not occurred; rather, nursing interventions are directed at prevention.

lationships, catatonic or manic excitement, toxic reactions to drugs (alcohol).*

ineffective Coping may be related to personal vulnerability, inadequate support system(s), unrealistic perceptions, inadequate coping methods, and disintegration of thought processes, possibly evidenced by impaired judgment, cognition, and perception; diminished problem-solving or decision-making capacities; poor self-concept; chronic anxiety; depression; inability to perform role expectations; and alteration in social participation.

interrupted Family Processes/disabled family Coping may be related to ambivalent family system or relationships, change of roles, and difficulty of family member in coping effectively with client's maladaptive behaviors, possibly evidenced by deterioration in family functioning, ineffective family decision-making process, difficulty relating to each other, client's expressions of despair at family's lack of reaction or involvement, neglectful relationships with client, extreme distortion regarding client's health problem including denial about its existence or severity, or prolonged overconcern.

Self-Care Deficit [specify] may be related to perceptual and cognitive impairment, immobility (withdrawal, isolation, and decreased psychomotor activity), and side effects of psychotropic medications, possibly evidenced by inability or difficulty in areas of feeding self, keeping body clean, dressing appropriately, toileting self, and/or changes in bowel or bladder elimination.

Sciatica   CH

acute/chronic Pain may be related to peripheral nerve root compression, possibly evidenced by verbal reports, guarding or distraction behaviors, and self-focus.

impaired physical Mobility may be related to neurological pain and muscular involvement, possibly evidenced by reluctance to attempt movement and decreased muscle strength and mass.

Scleroderma   CH

Also Refer to Lupus erythematosus, systemic (SLE)

impaired physical Mobility may be related to musculoskeletal impairment and associated pain, possibly evidenced by decreased strength, decreased range of motion, and reluctance to attempt movement.

ineffective Tissue Perfusion [specify)] may be related to reduced arterial blood flow (arteriolar vasoconstriction), possibly evidenced by changes in skin temperature and color, ulcer formation, and changes in organ function (cardiopulmonary, gastrointestinal, renal).

imbalanced Nutrition: less than body requirements may be related to inability to ingest, digest, or absorb adequate nutrients (sclerosis of the tissues rendering mouth immobile, decreased peristalsis of esophagus or small intestine, atrophy of smooth muscle of colon), possibly evidenced by weight loss, decreased intake, and reported or observed difficulty swallowing.

S

---

*A risk diagnosis is not evidenced by signs and symptoms, as the problem has not occurred; rather, nursing interventions are directed at prevention.

risk-prone Health Behavior may be related to disability requiring change in lifestyle, inadequate support systems, assault to self-concept, and altered locus of control, possibly evidenced by verbalization of nonacceptance of health status change and lack of movement toward independence or future-oriented thinking.

disturbed Body Image may be related to skin changes with induration, atrophy, and fibrosis, loss of hair, and skin and muscle contractures, possibly evidenced by verbalization of negative feelings about body, focus on past strength or function or appearance, fear of rejection or reaction by others, hiding body part, and change in social involvement.

Scoliosis   PED

disturbed Body Image may be related to altered body structure, use of therapeutic device(s), and activity restrictions, possibly evidenced by negative feelings about body, change in social involvement, and preoccupation with situation or refusal to acknowledge problem.

deficient Knowledge [Learning Need] regarding pathophysiology of condition, therapy needs, and possible outcomes may be related to lack of information, misinterpretation, possibly evidenced by statements of concern, questions, misconceptions, and inaccurate follow-through of instructions.

risk-prone Health Behavior may be related to lack of comprehension of long-term consequences of behavior, possibly evidenced by failure to take action, minimizes health status change, and evidence of failure to improve.

Seizure disorder   CH

deficient Knowledge [Learning Need] regarding condition and medication control may be related to lack of information, misinterpretations, scarce financial resources, possibly evidenced by questions, statements of concern, misconceptions, incorrect use of anticonvulsant medication, recurrent episodes or uncontrolled seizures.

chronic low Self-Esteem/disturbed Personal Identity may be related to stigma associated with condition, perception of being out of control or helpless, possibly evidenced by verbalization about changed lifestyle, fear of rejection, negative feelings about "brain" or self, change in usual pattern of responsibility, denial of problem resulting in lack of follow-through or nonparticipation in therapy.

impaired Social Interaction may be related to unpredictable nature of condition and self-concept disturbance, possibly evidenced by decreased self-assurance, verbalization of concern, discomfort in social situations, inability to receive or communicate a satisfying sense of belonging or caring, and withdrawal from social contacts and activities.

risk for Trauma/Suffocation: risk factors may include weakness, balancing difficulties, cognitive limitations, altered consciousness, loss of large or small muscle coordination (during seizure).*

---

*A risk diagnosis is not evidenced by signs and symptoms, as the problem has not occurred; rather, nursing interventions are directed at prevention.

Sepsis MS

Also Refer to Sepsis, puerperal

risk for deficient Fluid Volume: risk factors may include marked increase in vascular compartment, massive vasodilation, capillary permeability, vascular shifts to interstitial space, and reduced intake.*

risk for decreased Cardiac Output: risk factors may include decreased preload—venous return and circulating volume; altered afterload—increased SVR; negative inotropic effects of hypoxia, complement activation, and lysosomal hydrolase.*

risk for impaired Gas Exchange: risk factors may include effects of endotoxins on the respiratory center in the medulla—hyperventilation and respiratory alkalosis; hypoventilation; changes in vascular resistance, alveolar-capillary membrane changes—increased capillary permeability leading to pulmonary congestion; interference with oxygen delivery and utilization in the tissues—endotoxin-induced damage to the cells and capillaries.*

risk for Shock: risk factors may include infection/sepsis, hypovolemia—fluid shifts/third spacing; hypotension, hypoxemia.*

Sepsis, puerperal OB

Also Refer to Sepsis

risk for Infection [spread/septic shock]: risk factors may include presence of infection, broken skin, and/or traumatized tissues, rupture of amniotic membranes, high vascularity of involved area, stasis of body fluids, invasive procedures, and/or increased environmental exposure, chronic disease (e.g., diabetes, anemia, malnutrition), altered immune response, and untoward effect of medications (e.g., opportunistic or secondary infection).*

Hyperthermia may be related to inflammatory process, hypermetabolic state, dehydration, effect of circulating endotoxins on the hypothalamus, possibly evidenced by increase in body temperature; warm, flushed skin; increased respiratory rate; and tachycardia.

risk for impaired Attachment: risk factors may include interruption in bonding process, physical illness, perceived threat to own survival.*

risk for ineffective peripheral Tissue Perfusion: risk factors may include interruption or reduction of blood flow (presence of infectious thrombi).*

S

Serum sickness CH

acute Pain may be related to inflammation of the joints and skin eruptions, possibly evidenced by verbal reports, guarding or distraction behaviors, and self-focus.

deficient Knowledge [Learning Need] regarding nature of condition, treatment needs, potential complications, and prevention of recurrence may be related to lack of information, misinterpretation, possibly evidenced by statements of concern, questions, misconceptions, and inaccurate follow-through of instructions.

---

*A risk diagnosis is not evidenced by signs and symptoms, as the problem has not occurred; rather, nursing interventions are directed at prevention.

Sexually transmitted infection (STI)   GYN/CH

risk for Infection [transmission]: risk factors may include contagious nature of infecting agent and insufficient knowledge to avoid exposure to or transmission of pathogens.*

impaired Skin/Tissue Integrity may be related to invasion of or irritation by pathogenic organism(s), possibly evidenced by disruptions of skin or tissues and inflammation of mucous membranes.

deficient Knowledge [Learning Need] regarding condition, prognosis/ complications, therapy needs, and transmission may be related to lack of information, misinterpretation, lack of interest in learning, possibly evidenced by statements of concern, questions, misconceptions; inaccurate follow-through of instructions; and development of preventable complications.

Shock   MS

Also Refer to Shock, cardiogenic; Shock, hypovolemic/hemorrhagic

ineffective Tissue Perfusion [specify] may be related to changes in circulating volume and/or vascular tone, possibly evidenced by changes in skin color and temperature and pulse pressure, reduced BP, changes in mentation, and decreased urinary output.

Anxiety [specify level] may be related to change in health status and threat of death, possibly evidenced by increased tension, apprehension, sympathetic stimulation, restlessness, and expressions of concern.

Shock, cardiogenic   MS

Also Refer to Shock

decreased Cardiac Output may be related to structural damage, decreased myocardial contractility, and presence of dysrhythmias, possibly evidenced by ECG changes, variations in hemodynamic readings, jugular vein distention, cold or clammy skin, diminished peripheral pulses, and decreased urinary output.

risk for impaired Gas Exchange: risk factors may include ventilation perfusion imbalance, alveolar-capillary membrane changes.*

Shock, hypovolemic/hemorrhagic   MS

Also Refer to Shock

deficient Fluid Volume may be related to excessive vascular loss, inadequate intake or replacement, possibly evidenced by hypotension, tachycardia, decreased pulse volume and pressure, change in mentation, and decreased, concentrated urine.

Shock, septic   MS

Refer to Sepsis

Sick sinus syndrome   MS

Also Refer to Dysrhythmia, cardiac

decreased Cardiac Output may be related to alterations in rate, rhythm, and electrical conduction, possibly evidenced by ECG evidence of dysrhythmias, reports of palpitations or weakness, changes in mentation or consciousness, and syncope.

---

*A risk diagnosis is not evidenced by signs and symptoms, as the problem has not occurred; rather, nursing interventions are directed at prevention.

risk for Trauma: risk factors may include changes in cerebral perfusion with altered consciousness, loss of balance.*

SLE

CH

Refer to Lupus erythematosus, systemic

Smallpox

MS

risk of Infection [spread]: risk factors may include contagious nature of organism, inadequate acquired immunity, presence of chronic disease, immunosuppression.*

deficient Fluid Volume may be related to hypermetabolic state, decreased intake (pharyngeal lesions, nausea), increased losses (vomiting), fluid shifts from vascular bed, possibly evidenced by reports of thirst, decreased BP, venous filling and urinary output; dry mucous membranes, decreased skin turgor, change in mental state, elevated Hct.

impaired Tissue Integrity may be related to immunological deficit, possibly evidenced by disruption of skin surface, cornea, mucous membranes.

Anxiety [specify level]/Fear may be related to threat of death, interpersonal transmission and contagion, separation from support system, possibly evidenced by expressed concerns, apprehension, restlessness, focus on self.

CH

interrupted Family Processes may be related to temporary family disorganization, situational crisis, change in health status of family member, possibly evidenced by changes in satisfaction with family, stress-reduction behaviors, mutual support; expression of isolation from community resources.

ineffective community Coping may be related to man-made disaster (bioterrorism), inadequate resources for problem-solving, possibly evidenced by deficits of community participation, high illness rate, excessive community conflicts, expressed vulnerability or powerlessness.

Snow blindness

CH

[disturbed visual Sensory Perception] may be related to altered status of sense organ (irritation of the conjunctiva, hyperemia), possibly evidenced by intolerance to light (photophobia) and decreased or loss of visual acuity.

acute Pain may be related to irritation and vascular congestion of the conjunctiva, possibly evidenced by verbal reports, guarding or distraction behaviors, and self-focus.

Anxiety [specify level] may be related to situational crisis and threat to or change in health status, possibly evidenced by increased tension, apprehension, uncertainty, worry, restlessness, and focus on self.

Somatoform disorders

PSY

ineffective Coping may be related to severe level of anxiety that is repressed, personal vulnerability, unmet dependency needs, fixation

---

*A risk diagnosis is not evidenced by signs and symptoms, as the problem has not occurred; rather, nursing interventions are directed at prevention.

in earlier level of development, retarded ego development, and inadequate coping skills, possibly evidenced by verbalized inability to cope or problem-solve, high illness rate, multiple somatic complaints of several years' duration, decreased functioning in social and occupational settings, narcissistic tendencies with total focus on self and physical symptoms, demanding behaviors, history of "doctor shopping," and refusal to attend therapeutic activities.

chronic Pain may be related to severe level of repressed anxiety, low self-concept, unmet dependency needs, history of self or loved one having experienced a serious illness, possibly evidenced by verbal reports of severe or prolonged pain, guarded movement or protective behaviors, facial mask of pain, fear of re-injury, altered ability to continue previous activities, social withdrawal, demands for therapy or medication.

[disturbed Sensory Perception (specify)] may be related to psychological stress (narrowed perceptual fields, expression of stress as physical problems), poor quality of sleep, presence of chronic pain, possibly evidenced by reported change in voluntary motor or sensory function (paralysis, anosmia, aphonia, deafness, blindness, loss of touch or pain sensation), *la belle indifférence* (lack of concern over functional loss).

impaired Social Interaction may be related to inability to engage in satisfying personal relationships, preoccupation with self and physical symptoms, altered state of wellness, chronic pain, and rejection by others, possibly evidenced by preoccupation with own thoughts, sad or dull affect, absence of supportive SO(s), uncommunicative or withdrawn behavior, lack of eye contact, and seeking to be alone.

Spinal cord injury (SCI)   MS/CH
Refer to Paraplegia; Quadriplegia

Sprain of ankle or foot   CH
acute Pain may be related to trauma to and swelling in joint, possibly evidenced by verbal reports, guarding or distraction behaviors, self-focusing, and changes in vital signs.

impaired Walking may be related to musculoskeletal injury, pain, and therapeutic restrictions, possibly evidenced by reluctance to attempt movement, inability to move about environment easily.

Stapedectomy   MS
risk for Trauma: risk factors may include increased middle ear pressure with displacement of prosthesis and balancing difficulties, dizziness.*

risk for Infection: risk factors may include surgically traumatized tissue, invasive procedures, and environmental exposure to upper respiratory infections.*

acute Pain may be related to surgical trauma, edema formation, and presence of packing, possibly evidenced by verbal reports, guarding or distraction behaviors, and self-focus.

---

*A risk diagnosis is not evidenced by signs and symptoms, as the problem has not occurred; rather, nursing interventions are directed at prevention.

STI   **CH**
Refer to Sexually transmitted infection

Stimulant abuse   **CH**
Also Refer to Cocaine hydrochloride poisoning, acute; Substance
  dependence/abuse rehabilitation
imbalanced Nutrition: less than body requirements may be related to
    anorexia, insufficient or inappropriate use of financial resources, pos-
    sibly evidenced by reported inadequate intake, weight loss or less
    than normal weight gain; lack of interest in food, poor muscle tone,
    signs or laboratory evidence of vitamin deficiencies.
risk for Infection: risk factors may include injection techniques, impu-
    rities of drugs; localized trauma or nasal septum damage, malnutri-
    tion, altered immune state.*
Insomnia may be related to CNS sensory alterations, psychological
    stress possibly evidenced by constant alertness, racing thoughts pre-
    venting rest, denial of need to sleep, reported inability to stay awake,
    initial insomnia then hypersomnia.

                                            PSY
Fear/Anxiety [specify] may be related to paranoid delusions associated
    with stimulant use possibly evidenced by feelings or beliefs that oth-
    ers are conspiring against or are about to attack or kill client.
ineffective Coping may be related to personal vulnerability, negative
    role modeling, inadequate support systems; ineffective or inadequate
    coping skills with substitution of drug, possibly evidenced by use of
    harmful substance despite evidence of undesirable consequences.
[disturbed Sensory Perception (specify)] may be related to exogenous
    chemical, altered sensory reception, transmission, or integration (hal-
    lucination), altered status of sense organs, possibly evidenced by
    responding to internal stimuli from hallucinatory experiences, bizarre
    thinking, anxiety or panic changes in sensory acuity (sense of smell/
    taste).

Substance dependence/abuse rehabilitation   **PSY/CH**
(following acute detoxification)
ineffective Denial may be related to threat of unpleasant reality, lack
    of emotional support from others, overwhelming stress, possibly ev-
    idenced by lack of acceptance that drug use is causing the present
    situation, delay in seeking or refusal of healthcare attention to the
    detriment of health, use of manipulation to avoid responsibility for
    self, projection of blame or responsibility for problems.
ineffective Coping may be related to personal vulnerability, negative
    role modeling, inadequate support systems, previous ineffective or
    inadequate coping skills with substitution of drug(s), possibly evi-
    denced by impaired adaptive behavior and problem-solving skills,
    decreased ability to handle stress of illness or hospitalization, finan-
    cial affairs in disarray, employment or school difficulties—losing
    time on job or not maintaining steady employment, poor work or

S

---

*A risk diagnosis is not evidenced by signs and symptoms, as the problem has
not occurred; rather, nursing interventions are directed at prevention.

school performances, on-the-job injuries; verbalization of inability to cope or ask for help.

Powerlessness may be related to substance addiction with or without periods of abstinence, episodic compulsive indulgence, attempts at recovery, and lifestyle of helplessness, possibly evidenced by ineffective recovery attempts, statements of inability to stop behavior, requests for help, constantly thinking about drug and/or obtaining drug, alteration in personal, occupational, and social life.

imbalanced Nutrition: less than body requirements may be related to insufficient dietary intake to meet metabolic needs for psychological, physiological, or economic reasons, possibly evidenced by weight less than normal for height and body build; decreased subcutaneous fat or muscle mass; reported altered taste sensation; lack of interest in food; poor muscle tone; sore, inflamed buccal cavity; laboratory evidence of protein or vitamin deficiencies.

Sexual Dysfunction may be related to altered body function (neurological damage and debilitating effects of drug use), possibly evidenced by progressive interference with sexual functioning, a significant degree of testicular atrophy, gynecomastia, impotence or decreased sperm counts in men; and loss of body hair; thin, soft skin; spider angiomas; amenorrhea; and increase in miscarriages in women.

dysfunctional Family Processes may be related to abuse and history of alcoholism or drug use, inadequate coping skills, lack of problem-solving skills, genetic predisposition or biochemical influences, possibly evidenced by feelings of anger, frustration, or responsibility for alcoholic's behavior; suppressed rage, shame, embarrassment, repressed emotions, guilt, vulnerability, disturbed family dynamics or deterioration in family relationships, family denial or rationalization, closed communication systems, triangulating family relationships, manipulation, blaming, enabling to maintain substance use, inability to accept or receive help.

OB

risk for fetal Injury: risk factors may include drug or alcohol use, exposure to teratogens.*

deficient Knowledge [Learning Need] regarding condition, effects on pregnancy, prognosis, treatment needs may be related to lack or misinterpretation of information, lack of recall, cognitive limitations, interference with learning, possibly evidenced by statements of concern, questions, misconceptions, inaccurate follow-through of instructions, development of preventable complications, continued use despite complications.

compromised/disabled Family Coping may be related to codependency issues, situational crisis of pregnancy and drug abuse, family disorganization, exhausted supportive capacity of family members possibly evidenced by denial or belief that all problems are due to substance use, financial difficulties, severely dysfunctional family, codependent behaviors.

---

*A risk diagnosis is not evidenced by signs and symptoms, as the problem has not occurred; rather, nursing interventions are directed at prevention.

Also Refer to Postoperative recovery period

deficient Knowledge [Learning Need] regarding surgical procedure, expectations, postoperative routines, therapy, and self-care needs may be related to lack of information or recall, misinterpretation, possibly evidenced by statements of concern, questions, and misconceptions.

Anxiety [specify level]/Fear may be related to situational crisis, unfamiliarity with environment, change in health status, threat of death and separation from usual support systems, possibly evidenced by increased tension, apprehension, decreased self-assurance, fear of unspecific consequences, focus on self, sympathetic stimulation, and restlessness.

risk for Perioperative-Positioning Injury: risk factors may include disorientation, sensory and perceptual disturbances due to anesthesia, immobilization, musculoskeletal impairments, obesity, emaciation, edema.*

risk for Injury: risk factors may include wrong client, procedure, site, implants, equipment or materials; interactive conditions between individual and environment; external environment—physical design, structure of environment, exposure to equipment, instrumentation, positioning, use of pharmaceutical agents; internal environment—tissue hypoxia, abnormal blood profile or altered clotting factors, broken skin.*

risk for Infection: risk factors may include broken skin, traumatized tissues, stasis of body fluids; presence of pathogens or contaminants, environmental exposure, invasive procedures.*

risk for imbalanced Body Temperature: risk factors may include exposure to cool environment, use of medications, anesthetic agents; extremes of age, weight; dehydration.*

ineffective Breathing Pattern may be related to chemically induced muscular relaxation, perception or cognitive impairment, decreased lung expansion, energy; tracheobronchial obstruction.

risk for deficient Fluid Volume: risk factors may include preoperative fluid deprivation, nausea, blood loss, and excessive gastrointestinal losses (vomiting or gastric suction), extremes of age and weight.*

Synovitis (knee)   CH

acute Pain may be related to inflammation of synovial membrane of the joint with effusion, possibly evidenced by verbal reports, guarding or distraction behaviors, self-focus, and changes in vital signs.

impaired Walking may be related to pain and decreased strength of joint, possibly evidenced by reluctance to attempt movement, inability to move about environment as desired.

Syphilis, congenital   PED

Also Refer to Sexually transmitted infection (STI)

acute Pain may be related to inflammatory process, edema formation, and development of skin lesions, possibly evidenced by irritability or crying that may be increased with movement of extremities and changes in vital signs.

---

*A risk diagnosis is not evidenced by signs and symptoms, as the problem has not occurred; rather, nursing interventions are directed at prevention.

impaired Skin/Tissue Integrity may be related to exposure to pathogens during vaginal delivery, possibly evidenced by disruption of skin surfaces and rhinitis.

delayed Growth and Development may be related to effect of infectious process, possibly evidenced by altered physical growth and delay or difficulty performing skills typical of age group.

deficient Knowledge [Learning Need] regarding pathophysiology of condition, transmissibility, therapy needs, expected outcomes, and potential complications may be related to caretaker/parental lack of information, misinterpretation, possibly evidenced by statements of concern, questions, and misconceptions.

Syringomyelia   MS

[disturbed Sensory Perception (specify)] may be related to altered sensory perception (neurological lesion), possibly evidenced by change in usual response to stimuli and motor incoordination.

Anxiety [specify level]/Fear may be related to change in health status, threat of change in role functioning and socioeconomic status, and threat to self-concept, possibly evidenced by increased tension, apprehension, uncertainty, focus on self, and expressed concerns.

impaired physical Mobility may be related to neuromuscular and sensory impairment, possibly evidenced by decreased muscle strength, control, and mass; and impaired coordination.

Self-Care Deficit [specify] may be related to neuromuscular and sensory impairments, possibly evidenced by statement of inability to perform care tasks.

Tay-Sachs disease   PED

delayed Growth and Development may be related to effects of physical condition, possibly evidenced by altered physical growth, loss of or failure to acquire skills typical of age, flat affect, and decreased responses.

[disturbed visual Sensory Perception] may be related to neurological deterioration of optic nerve, possibly evidenced by loss of visual acuity.

CH

[family] Grieving may be related to expected eventual loss of infant/ child, possibly evidenced by expressions of distress, denial, guilt, anger, and sorrow; choked feelings; changes in sleep and eating habits; and altered libido.

[family] Powerlessness may be related to absence of therapeutic interventions for progressive and fatal disease, possibly evidenced by verbal expressions of having no control over situation or outcome and depression over physical and mental deterioration.

risk for Spiritual Distress: risk factors may include challenged belief and value system by presence of fatal condition with racial or religious connotations and intense suffering.*

compromised family Coping may be related to situational crisis, temporary preoccupation with managing emotional conflicts and personal

---

*A risk diagnosis is not evidenced by signs and symptoms, as the problem has not occurred; rather, nursing interventions are directed at prevention.

suffering, family disorganization, and prolonged and progressive nature of disease, possibly evidenced by preoccupations with personal reactions, expressed concern about reactions of other family members, inadequate support of one another, and altered communication patterns.

Thrombophlebitis CH/MS/OB
ineffective peripheral Tissue Perfusion may be related to interruption of venous blood flow, venous stasis, possibly evidenced by changes in skin color and temperature over affected area, development of edema, pain, diminished peripheral pulses, slow capillary refill.

acute Pain/impaired Comfort may be related to vascular inflammation and irritation, edema formation, accumulation of lactic acid, possibly evidenced by verbal reports, guarding or distraction behaviors, restlessness, and self-focus.

risk for impaired physical Mobility: risk factors may include pain and discomfort and restrictive therapies or safety precautions.*

deficient Knowledge [Learning Need] regarding pathophysiology of condition, therapy/self-care needs, and risk of embolization may be related to lack of information, misinterpretation, possibly evidenced by statements of concern, questions, inaccurate follow-through of instructions, and development of preventable complications.

Thrombosis, venous MS
Refer to Thrombophlebitis

Thrush CH
impaired Oral Mucous Membrane may be related to presence of infection as evidenced by white patches or plaques, oral discomfort, mucosal irritation, bleeding.

Thyroidectomy MS
Also Refer to Hyperthyroidism; Hypoparathyroidism; Hypothyroidism
risk for ineffective Airway Clearance: risk factors may include tracheal obstruction—edema, hematoma formation, laryngeal spasms.*

impaired verbal Communication may be related to tissue edema, pain or discomfort, and vocal cord injury or laryngeal nerve damage, possibly evidenced by impaired articulation, does not or cannot speak, and use of nonverbal cues and gestures.

risk for Injury [tetany]: risk factors may include chemical imbalance—hypocalcemia, increased release of thyroid hormones; excessive CNS stimulation.*

risk for [head/neck] Trauma: risk factors may include loss of muscle control and support, and position of suture line.*

acute Pain may be related to presence of surgical incision and manipulation of tissues and muscles, postoperative edema, possibly evidenced by verbal reports, guarding or distraction behaviors, narrowed focus, and changes in vital signs.

T

*A risk diagnosis is not evidenced by signs and symptoms, as the problem has not occurred; rather, nursing interventions are directed at prevention.

Thyrotoxicosis

Also Refer to Hyperthyroidism

risk for decreased Cardiac Output: risk factors may include uncontrolled hypermetabolic state increasing cardiac workload, changes in venous return and SVR, and alterations in rate, rhythm, and electrical conduction.*

Anxiety [specify level] may be related to physiological factors or CNS stimulation—hypermetabolic state and pseudocatecholamine effect of thyroid hormones; possibly evidenced by increased feelings of apprehension, shakiness, loss of control, panic, changes in cognition, distortion of environmental stimuli, extraneous movements, restlessness, and tremors.

deficient Knowledge [Learning Needs] regarding condition, treatment needs, and potential for complications or crisis situation may be related to lack of information or recall, misinterpretation, possibly evidenced by statements of concern, questions, and misconceptions, and inaccurate follow-through of instructions.

TIA

Refer to Transient ischemic attack

Tic douloureux

Refer to Neuralgia, trigeminal

Tonsillectomy

Anxiety [specify level]/Fear may be related to separation from supportive others, unfamiliar surroundings, and perceived threat of injury or abandonment, possibly evidenced by crying, apprehension, trembling, and sympathetic stimulation (pupil dilation, increased heart rate).

risk for ineffective Airway Clearance: risk factors may include sedation, collection of secretions and blood in oropharynx, and vomiting.*

risk for deficient Fluid Volume: risk factors may include operative trauma to highly vascular site, hemorrhage.*

acute Pain may be related to physical trauma to oronasopharynx, presence of packing, possibly evidenced by restlessness, crying, and facial mask of pain.

Tonsillitis

acute Pain may be related to inflammation of tonsils and effects of circulating toxins, possibly evidenced by verbal reports, guarding or distraction behaviors, reluctance or refusal to swallow, self-focus, and changes in vital signs.

Hyperthermia may be related to presence of inflammatory process, hypermetabolic state and dehydration, possibly evidenced by increased body temperature; warm, flushed skin; and tachycardia.

deficient Knowledge [Learning Need] regarding cause, transmission, treatment needs, and potential complications may be related to lack of information, misinterpretation, possibly evidenced by statements

---

*A risk diagnosis is not evidenced by signs and symptoms, as the problem has not occurred; rather, nursing interventions are directed at prevention.

of concern, questions, inaccurate follow-through of instructions, and recurrence of condition.

Total joint replacement
MS

Also Refer to Surgery, general

risk for Infection: risk factors may include inadequate primary defenses (broken skin, exposure of joint), inadequate secondary defenses or immunosuppression (long-term corticosteroid use), invasive procedures, surgical manipulation, implantation of foreign body, and decreased mobility.*

impaired physical Mobility may be related to pain and discomfort, musculoskeletal impairment, and surgery and restrictive therapies, possibly evidenced by reluctance to attempt movement, difficulty purposefully moving within the physical environment, reports of pain or discomfort on movement, limited range of motion, and decreased muscle strength and control.

risk for ineffective peripheral Tissue Perfusion: risk factors may include reduced arterial or venous blood flow, direct trauma to blood vessels, tissue edema, improper location or dislocation of prosthesis, and hypovolemia.*

acute Pain may be related to physical agents (traumatized tissues, surgical intervention, degeneration of joints, muscle spasms) and psychological factors (anxiety, advanced age), possibly evidenced by verbal reports, guarding or distraction behaviors, self-focus, and changes in vital signs.

risk for Constipation: risk factors may include insufficient physical activity, decreased mobility, weakness, insufficient fiber or fluid intake, dehydration, poor eating habits, decreased gastrointestinal motility, effects of medications—anesthesia, opiate analgesics; environmental changes, inadequate toileting.*

Toxemia of pregnancy
OB

Refer to Pregnancy-induced hypertension

Toxic shock syndrome
MS

Also Refer to Septicemia

Hyperthermia may be related to inflammatory process, hypermetabolic state and dehydration, possibly evidenced by increased body temperature; warm, flushed skin; and tachycardia.

deficient Fluid Volume may be related to increased gastric losses (diarrhea, vomiting), fever and hypermetabolic state, and decreased intake, possibly evidenced by dry mucous membranes; increased pulse; hypotension; delayed venous filling; decreased, concentrated urine; and hemoconcentration.

acute Pain may be related to inflammatory process, effects of circulating toxins, and skin disruptions, possibly evidenced by verbal reports, guarding or distraction behaviors, self-focus, and changes in vital signs.

impaired Skin/Tissue Integrity may be related to effects of circulating toxins and dehydration, possibly evidenced by development of

T

---

*A risk diagnosis is not evidenced by signs and symptoms, as the problem has not occurred; rather, nursing interventions are directed at prevention.

desquamating rash, hyperemia, and inflammation of mucous membranes.

Traction   MS
Also Refer to Casts; Fractures

acute Pain may be related to direct trauma to tissue/bone, muscle spasms, movement of bone fragments, edema, injury to soft tissue, traction or immobility device, anxiety, possibly evidenced by verbal reports, guarding or distraction behaviors, self-focus, alteration in muscle tone, and changes in vital signs.

impaired physical Mobility may be related to neuromuscular and skeletal impairment, pain, psychological immobility, and therapeutic restrictions of movement, possibly evidenced by limited range of motion, inability to move purposefully in environment, reluctance to attempt movement, and decreased muscle strength and control.

risk for Infection: risk factors may include invasive procedures—including insertion of foreign body through skin and bone; presence of traumatized tissue, and reduced activity with stasis of body fluids.*

deficient Diversional Activity may be related to length of hospitalization or therapeutic intervention and environmental lack of usual activity, possibly evidenced by statements of boredom, restlessness, and irritability.

Transfusion reaction, blood   MS
Also Refer to Anaphylaxis

risk for imbalanced Body Temperature: risk factors may include infusion of cold blood products, systemic response to toxins.*

Anxiety [specify level] may be related to change in health status and threat of death, exposure to toxins, possibly evidenced by increased tension, apprehension, sympathetic stimulation, restlessness, and expressions of concern.

risk for impaired Skin Integrity: risk factors may include immunological response.*

Transient ischemic attack (TIA)   CH

ineffective cerebral Tissue Perfusion may be related to interruption of blood flow (e.g., vasospasm), possibly evidenced by altered mental status, behavioral changes, language deficit, change in motor or sensory response.

Anxiety/Fear may be related to change in health status, threat to self-concept, situational crisis, interpersonal contagion, possibly evidenced by expressed concerns, apprehension, restlessness, irritability.

risk for ineffective Denial risk factors may include change in health status requiring change in lifestyle, fear of consequences, lack of motivation.*

Transplantation, recipient   MS

Anxiety/Fear may be related to unconscious conflict about essential values/beliefs, situational crisis, threat of death (organ rejection), un-

---

*A risk diagnosis is not evidenced by signs and symptoms, as the problem has not occurred; rather, nursing interventions are directed at prevention.

familiarity with environmental experience, possibly evidenced by reports apprehension/increased tension, uncertainty, worried, insomnia, increased vital signs.

risk for Infection: risk factors may include medically chronic disease, induced immunosuppression, suppressed inflammatory response, invasive procedures, broken skin/traumatized tissues.

(Refer to specific conditions relative to compromise of failure of individual transplanted organs, e.g., Renal failure, acute; Heart Failure, chronic; Pancreatitis.)

CH

ineffective Coping/compromised family Coping may be related to situational crisis, high degree of threat, uncertainty, family disorganization or role changes, prolonged disease exhausting supportive capacity of family/SO, possibly evidenced by reports of inability to cope, sleep pattern disturbance, fatigue, poor concentration, protective behaviors disproportionate to client's needs, SO describes preoccupation with personal reaction.

risk for ineffective Protection: risk factors may include drug therapies, compromised immune system, effects of debilitating disease.*

readiness for enhanced Self-Health Management possibly evidenced by expressed desire to manage treatment/prevent sequelae, no unexpected acceleration of illness symptoms.

risk for ineffective Self-Health Management: risk factors may include complexity of therapeutic regimen and healthcare system, economic difficulties, family patterns of healthcare.

Traumatic brain injury (TBI)   CH

ineffective cerebral Tissue Perfusion may be related to interruption of blood flow — hemorrhage, hematoma, cerebral edema (localized or generalized response to injury, metabolic alterations, drug or alcohol overdose), decreased systemic BP—hypovolemia, cardiac dysrhythmias; hypoxia, possibly evidenced by altered level of consciousness, memory loss, changes in motor or sensory responses, restlessness, changes in vital signs.

risk for decreased Intracranial Adaptive Capacity: risk factors may include brain injuries, systemic hypotension with intracranial hypertension.*

risk for ineffective Breathing Pattern: risk factors may include neuromuscular dysfunction—injury to respiratory center of brain; perception or cognitive impairment, tracheobronchial obstruction.*

[disturbed Sensory Perception (specify)] may be related to altered sensory reception, transmission and/or integration—neurological trauma or deficit, possibly evidenced by disorientation to time, place, person; change in usual response to stimuli, motor incoordination, altered communication patterns, visual or auditory distortions, altered thought processes or bizarre thinking, exaggerated emotional responses, change in behavior pattern.

risk for Infection: risk factors may include traumatized tissues, broken skin, invasive procedures, decreased ciliary action, stasis of body

---

*A risk diagnosis is not evidenced by signs and symptoms, as the problem has not occurred; rather, nursing interventions are directed at prevention.

fluids, nutritional deficits, suppressed inflammatory response—steroid use; altered integrity of closed system—cerebrospinal fluid leak.*

risk for imbalanced Nutrition: less than body requirements: risk factors may include altered ability to ingest nutrients—decreased level of consciousness; weakness of muscles for chewing or swallowing, hypermetabolic state.*

CH

impaired physical Mobility may be related to perceptual or cognitive impairment, decreased strength and endurance, restrictive therapies or safety precautions possibly evidenced by inability to purposefully move within physical environment—bed mobility, transfer, ambulation; impaired coordination, limited range of motion, decreased muscle strength or control.

risk for impaired Memory/chronic Confusion: risk factors may include head injury, neurological disturbances.

interrupted Family Processes may be related to situational transition and crisis, uncertainty about ultimate outcome, expectations possibly evidenced by difficulty adapting to change or dealing with traumatic experience constructively, family not meeting needs of all members, difficulty accepting or receiving help appropriately, inability to express or to accept feelings of members.

Self-Care Deficit [specify] may be related to neuromuscular or musculoskeletal impairment, weakness, pain, perceptual or cognitive impairment possibly evidenced by inability to perform desired or appropriate ADLs.

Trichinosis   CH

acute Pain may be related to parasitic invasion of muscle tissues, edema of upper eyelids, small localized hemorrhages, and development of urticaria, possibly evidenced by verbal reports, guarding or distraction behaviors (restlessness), and changes in vital signs.

deficient Fluid Volume may be related to hypermetabolic state (fever, diaphoresis), excessive gastric losses (vomiting, diarrhea), and decreased intake (difficulty swallowing), possibly evidenced by dry mucous membranes; decreased skin turgor; hypotension; decreased venous filling; decreased, concentrated urine; and hemoconcentration.

ineffective Breathing Pattern may be related to myositis of the diaphragm and intercostal muscles, possibly evidenced by resulting changes in respiratory depth, tachypnea, dyspnea, and abnormal ABGs.

deficient Knowledge [Learning Need] regarding cause and prevention of condition, therapy needs, and possible complications may be related to lack of information, misinterpretation, possibly evidenced by statements of concern, questions, and misconceptions.

Tuberculosis (pulmonary)   CH

risk for Infection [spread/reactivation]: risk factors may include inadequate primary defenses (decreased ciliary action and stasis of

---

*A risk diagnosis is not evidenced by signs and symptoms, as the problem has not occurred; rather, nursing interventions are directed at prevention.

secretions, tissue destruction with extension of infection), lowered resistance, suppressed inflammatory response, malnutrition, environmental exposure, insufficient knowledge to avoid exposure to pathogens, or inadequate therapeutic intervention.*

ineffective Airway Clearance may be related to thick, viscous, or bloody secretions; fatigue with poor cough effort, and tracheal or pharyngeal edema, possibly evidenced by abnormal respiratory rate, rhythm, and depth; adventitious breath sounds (rhonchi, wheezes), stridor, and dyspnea.

risk for impaired Gas Exchange: risk factors may include decrease in effective lung surface, atelectasis, destruction of alveolar-capillary membrane, bronchial edema, thick, viscous secretions.*

Activity Intolerance may be related to imbalance between O_2 supply and demand, possibly evidenced by reports of fatigue, weakness, and exertional dyspnea.

imbalanced Nutrition: less than body requirements may be related to inability to ingest adequate nutrients (anorexia, effects of drug therapy, fatigue, insufficient financial resources), possibly evidenced by weight loss, reported lack of interest in food/altered taste sensation, and poor muscle tone.

risk for ineffective Self-Health Management: risk factors may include complexity of therapeutic regimen, economic difficulties, family patterns of healthcare, perceived seriousness or benefits (especially during remission), side effects of therapy.*

Tympanoplasty   MS
Refer to Stapedectomy

Typhus (tick-borne/Rocky Mountain spotted fever)   CH/MS
Hyperthermia may be related to generalized inflammatory process (vasculitis), possibly evidenced by increased body temperature; warm, flushed skin; and tachycardia.

acute Pain may be related to generalized vasculitis and edema formation, possibly evidenced by verbal reports, guarding or distraction behaviors, self-focus, and changes in vital signs.

[ineffective Tissue Perfusion (specify)] may be related to reduction or interruption of blood flow (generalized vasculitis, thrombi formation), possibly evidenced by reports of headache or abdominal pain, changes in mentation, and areas of peripheral ulceration or necrosis.

Ulcer, decubitus   CH/MS
impaired Skin/Tissue Integrity may be related to altered circulation, nutritional deficit, fluid imbalance, impaired physical mobility, irritation of body excretions or secretions, and sensory impairments, evidenced by tissue damage or destruction.

acute Pain may be related to destruction of protective skin layers and exposure of nerves, possibly evidenced by verbal reports, distraction behaviors, and self-focus.

U

---

*A risk diagnosis is not evidenced by signs and symptoms, as the problem has not occurred; rather, nursing interventions are directed at prevention.

risk for Infection: risk factors may include broken or traumatized tissue, increased environmental exposure, and nutritional deficits.*

Ulcer, peptic (acute)   MS/CH
risk for Shock: risk factors may include hypovolemia, hypotension.*

Fear/Anxiety [specify level] may be related to change in health status and threat of death, possibly evidenced by increased tension, restlessness, irritability, fearfulness, trembling, tachycardia, diaphoresis, lack of eye contact, focus on self, verbalization of concerns, withdrawal, and panic or attack behavior.

acute Pain may be related to caustic irritation and destruction of gastric tissues, reflex muscle spasms in stomach wall possibly evidenced by verbal reports, distraction behaviors, self-focus, and changes in vital signs.

deficient Knowledge [Learning Need] regarding condition, therapy and self-care needs, and potential complications may be related to lack of information, recall, misinterpretation, possibly evidenced by statements of concern, questions, misconceptions; inaccurate followthrough of instructions; and development of preventable complications or recurrence of condition.

Ulcer, venous stasis   CH
impaired Skin/Tissue Integrity may be related to altered venous circulation, edema formation, inflammation, decreased sensation possibly evidenced by destruction of skin layers, invasion of body structures.

ineffective peripheral Tissue Perfusion may be related to interruption of venous flow—small vessel vasoconstrictive reflex, possibly evidenced by skin discoloration, edema formation, altered sensation, delayed healing.

Unconsciousness   MS
Refer to Coma

Urinary diversion   MS/CH
risk for impaired Skin Integrity: risk factors may include absence of sphincter at stoma, character and flow of urine from stoma, reaction to product or chemicals, and improperly fitting appliance or removal of adhesive.*

disturbed Body Image related factors may include biophysical factors (presence of stoma, loss of control of urine flow), and psychosocial factors (altered body structure, disease process and associated treatment regimen, such as cancer), possibly evidenced by verbalization of change in body image, fear of rejection or reaction of others, negative feelings about body, not touching or looking at stoma, refusal to participate in care.

acute Pain may be related to physical factors (disruption of skin or tissues, presence of incisions and drains), biological factors (activity of disease process, such as cancer, trauma), and psychological factors (fear, anxiety), possibly evidenced by verbal reports, self-focusing,

---

*A risk diagnosis is not evidenced by signs and symptoms, as the problem has not occurred; rather, nursing interventions are directed at prevention.

guarding or distraction behaviors, restlessness, and changes in vital signs.

impaired Urinary Elimination may be related to surgical diversion, tissue trauma, and postoperative edema, possibly evidenced by loss of continence, changes in amount and character of urine, and urinary retention.

Urolithiasis   MS/CH
Refer to Calculi, urinary

Uterine bleeding, dysfunctional   GYN/MS
Anxiety [specify level] may be related to perceived change in health status and unknown etiology, possibly evidenced by apprehension, uncertainty, fear of unspecified consequences, expressed concerns, and focus on self.

Activity Intolerance may be related to imbalance between O_2 supply and demand/decreased O_2-carrying capacity of blood (anemia), possibly evidenced by reports of fatigue or weakness.

Uterus, rupture of, in pregnancy   OB
deficient Fluid Volume may be related to excessive vascular losses, possibly evidenced by hypotension, increased pulse rate, decreased venous filling, and decreased urine output.

decreased Cardiac Output may be related to decreased preload (hypovolemia), possibly evidenced by cold, clammy skin; decreased peripheral pulses; variations in hemodynamic readings; tachycardia; and cyanosis.

acute Pain may be related to tissue trauma and irritation of accumulating blood, possibly evidenced by verbal reports, guarding or distraction behaviors, self-focus, and changes in vital signs.

Anxiety [specify level] may be related to threat of death of self or fetus, interpersonal contagion, physiological response (release of catecholamines), possibly evidenced by fearful, scared affect; sympathetic stimulation, stated fear of unspecified consequences, and expressed concerns.

Vaginismus   GYN/CH
acute Pain may be related to muscle spasm and hyperesthesia of the nerve supply to vaginal mucous membrane, possibly evidenced by verbal reports, distraction behaviors, and self-focus.

Sexual Dysfunction may be related to physical and/or psychological alteration in function (severe spasms of vaginal muscles), possibly evidenced by verbalization of problem, inability to achieve desired satisfaction, and alteration in relationship with SO.

Vaginitis   GYN/CH
impaired Tissue Integrity may be related to irritation and inflammation and mechanical trauma (scratching) of sensitive tissues, possibly evidenced by damaged or destroyed tissue, presence of lesions.

acute Pain may be related to localized inflammation and tissue trauma, possibly evidenced by verbal reports, distraction behaviors, and self-focus.

deficient Knowledge [Learning Need] regarding hygienic and therapy needs and sexual behaviors and transmission of infection may be related to lack of information, misinterpretation, possibly evidenced by statements of concern, questions, and misconceptions.

VAP (ventilator-aquired pneumonia) MS

Refer to Bronchopneumonia

Varices, esophageal MS

Also Refer to Ulcer, peptic (acute)

risk for Bleeding/deficient Fluid Volume: risk factors may include presence of varices, reduced intake, and gastric losses (vomiting), vascular loss.*

Anxiety [specify level]/Fear may be related to change in health status and threat of death, possibly evidenced by increased tension, apprehension, sympathetic stimulation, restlessness, focus on self, and expressed concerns.

Varicose veins CH

chronic Pain may be related to venous insufficiency and stasis, possibly evidenced by verbal reports.

disturbed Body Image may be related to change in structure (presence of enlarged, discolored tortuous superficial leg veins), possibly evidenced by hiding affected parts and negative feelings about body.

risk for impaired Skin/Tissue Integrity: risk factors may include altered circulation, venous stasis, and edema formation.*

Venereal disease CH

Refer to Sexually transmitted infection (STI)

Ventricular fibrillation MS

Also Refer to Dysrhythmias

decreased Cardiac Output may be related to altered electrical conduction and reduced myocardial contractility possibly evidenced by absence of measurable cardiac output, loss of consciousness, no palpable pulses.

Ventricular tachycardia MS

Also Refer to Dysrhythmias

risk for decreased Cardiac Output: risk factors may include altered electrical conduction and reduced myocardial contractility.*

West Nile fever CH/MS

Hyperthermia may be related to infectious process, possibly evidenced by elevated body temperature, skin flushed and warm to touch, tachycardia, increased respiratory rate.

acute Pain may be related to infectious process and circulating toxins, possibly evidenced by reports of headache, myalgia, eye pain, abdominal discomfort.

risk for deficient Fluid Volume: risk factors may include hypermetabolic state, decreased intake, anorexia, nausea, losses from normal routes (vomiting, diarrhea).*

risk for impaired Skin Integrity: risk factors may include hyperthermia, decreased fluid intake, alterations in skin turgor, bedrest, circulating toxins.*

W

---

*A risk diagnosis is not evidenced by signs and symptoms, as the problem has not occurred; rather, nursing interventions are directed at prevention.

Wilms' tumor

Also Refer to Cancer; Chemotherapy

Anxiety [specify level]/Fear may be related to change in environment and interaction patterns with family members and threat of death with family transmission and contagion of concerns, possibly evidenced by fearful or scared affect, distress, crying, insomnia, and sympathetic stimulation.

risk for Injury: risk factors may include nature of tumor (vascular, mushy with very thin covering) with increased danger of metastasis when manipulated.*

interrupted Family Processes may be related to situational crisis of life-threatening illness, possibly evidenced by a family system that has difficulty meeting physical, emotional, and spiritual needs of its members, and inability to deal with traumatic experience effectively.

deficient Diversional Activity may be related to environmental lack of age-appropriate activity (including activity restrictions) and length of hospitalization and treatment, possibly evidenced by restlessness, crying, lethargy, and acting-out behavior.

Wound, gunshot

(Depends on site and speed/character of bullet.)

risk for deficient Fluid Volume: risk factors may include excessive vascular losses, altered intake or restrictions.*

acute Pain may be related to destruction of tissue (including organ and musculoskeletal), surgical repair, and therapeutic interventions, possibly evidenced by verbal reports, guarding or distraction behaviors, self-focus, and changes in vital signs.

impaired Tissue Integrity may be related to mechanical factors (yaw of projectile and muzzle blast), possibly evidenced by damaged or destroyed tissue.

risk for Infection: risk factors may include tissue destruction and increased environmental exposure, invasive procedures, and decreased Hb.*

risk for Post-Trauma Syndrome: risk factors may include nature of incident (catastrophic accident, assault, suicide attempt) and possibly injury or death of other(s) involved.*

---

*A risk diagnosis is not evidenced by signs and symptoms, as the problem has not occurred; rather, nursing interventions are directed at prevention.

NANDA-I's Taxonomy II

The 13 domains and their classes are:

DOMAIN 1 HEALTH PROMOTION. The awareness of well-being or normality of function and the strategies used to maintain control of and enhance that well-being or normality of function

Class 1 Health Awareness: Recognition of normal function and well-being

Class 2 Health Management: Identifying, controlling, performing, and integrating activities to maintain health and well-being

DOMAIN 2 NUTRITION. The activities of taking in, assimilating, and using nutrients for the purposes of tissue maintenance, tissue repair, and the production of energy

Class 1 Ingestion: Taking food or nutrients into the body

Class 2 Digestion: The physical and chemical activities that convert foodstuffs into substances suitable for absorption and assimilation

Class 3 Absorption: The act of taking up nutrients through body tissues

Class 4 Metabolism: The chemical and physical processes occurring in living organisms and cells for the development and use of protoplasm, production of waste and energy, with the release of energy for all vital processes

Class 5 Hydration: The taking in and absorption of fluids and electrolytes

DOMAIN 3 ELIMINATION AND EXCHANGE. Secretion and excretion of waste products from the body

Class 1 Urinary Function: The process of secretion, reabsorption, and excretion of urine

Class 2 Gastrointestinal Function: The process of absorption and excretion of the end products of digestion

Class 3 Integumentary Function: The process of secretion and excretion through the skin

Class 4 Respiratory Function: The process of exchange of gases and removal of the end products of metabolism

DOMAIN 4 ACTIVITY/REST. The production, conservation, expenditure, or balance of energy resources

Class 1 Sleep/Rest: Slumber, repose, ease, relaxation, or inactivity

Class 2 Activity/Exercise: Moving parts of the body (mobility), doing work, or performing actions often (but not always) against resistance

Class 3 Energy Balance: A dynamic state of harmony between intake and expenditure of resources

Class 4 Cardiovascular/Pulmonary Responses: Cardiopulmonary mechanisms that support activity/rest

Class 5 Self-Care: Ability to perform activities to care for one's body and bodily functions

DOMAIN 5 PERCEPTION/COGNITION. The human information processing system including attention, orientation, sensation, perception, cognition, and communication

Class 1 Attention: Mental readiness to notice or observe

Class 2 Orientation: Awareness of time, place, and person

Class 3 Sensation/Perception: Receiving information through the senses of touch, taste, smell, vision, hearing, and kinesthesia and the comprehension of sense data resulting in naming, associating, and/or pattern recognition

Class 4 Cognition: Use of memory, learning, thinking, problem-solving, abstraction, judgment, insight, intellectual capacity, calculation, and language

Class 5 Communication: Sending and receiving verbal and nonverbal information

DOMAIN 6 SELF-PERCEPTION. Awareness about the self

Class 1 Self-Concept: The perception(s) about the total self

Class 2 Self-Esteem: Assessment of one's own worth, capability, significance, and success

Class 3 Body Image: A mental image of one's own body

DOMAIN 7 ROLE RELATIONSHIPS. The positive and negative connections or associations between people or groups of people and the means by which those connections are demonstrated

Class 1 Caregiving Roles: Socially expected behavior patterns by people providing care who are not healthcare professionals

Class 2 Family Relationships: Associations of people who are biologically related or related by choice

Class 3 Role Performance: Quality of functioning in socially expected behavior patterns

DOMAIN 8 SEXUALITY. Sexual identity, sexual function, and reproduction

Class 1 Sexual Identity: The state of being a specific person in regard to sexuality and/or gender

Class 2 Sexual Function: The capacity or ability to participate in sexual activities

Class 3 Reproduction: Any process by which human beings are produced

DOMAIN 9 COPING/STRESS TOLERANCE. Contending with
life events/life processes

Class 1 Post-Trauma Responses: Reactions occurring after
physical or psychological trauma

Class 2 Coping Responses: The process of managing environmental stress

Class 3 Neurobehavioral Stress: Behavioral responses reflecting nerve and brain function

DOMAIN 10 LIFE PRINCIPLES. Principles underlying
conduct, thought, and behavior about acts, customs,
or institutions viewed as being true or having intrinsic
worth

Class 1 Values: The identification and ranking of preferred
mode of conduct or end states

Class 2 Beliefs: Opinions, expectations, or judgments
about acts, customs, or institutions viewed as being true
or having intrinsic worth

Class 3 Value/Belief/Action Congruence: The correspon-
dence or balance achieved among values, beliefs, and
actions

DOMAIN 11 SAFETY/PROTECTION. Freedom from danger,
physical injury, or immune system damage; preservation
from loss; and protection of safety and security

Class 1 Infection: Host responses following pathogenic invasion

Class 2 Physical Injury: Bodily harm or hurt

Class 3 Violence: The exertion of excessive force or power
so as to cause injury or abuse

Class 4 Environmental Hazards: Sources of danger in the
surroundings

Class 5 Defensive Processes: The processes by which the
self protects itself from the non-self

Class 6 Thermoregulation: The physiological process of
regulating heat and energy within the body for purposes
of protecting the organism

DOMAIN 12 COMFORT. Sense of mental, physical, or social
well-being or ease

Class 1 Physical Comfort: Sense of well-being or ease and/
or freedom from pain

Class 2 Environmental Comfort: Sense of well-being or
ease in/with one's environment

Class 3 Social Comfort: Sense of well-being or ease with
one's social situations

DOMAIN 13 GROWTH/DEVELOPMENT. Age-appropriate increases in physical dimensions, maturation of organ systems, and/or progression through the developmental milestones

Class 1 Growth: Increases in physical dimensions or maturity of organ systems

Class 2 Development: Progression or regression through a sequence of recognized milestones in life

Definitions of Taxonomy II Axes

AXIS 1 DIAGNOSTIC CONCEPT: Defined as the principal element or the fundamental and essential part, the root, of the diagnostic statement describing the *human response* that is the core of the diagnosis.

AXIS 2 SUBJECT OF THE DIAGNOSIS: The person(s) for whom a nursing diagnosis is determined. Values are:

Individual: A single human being distinct from others; a person.

Family: Two or more people having continuous or sustained relationships, perceiving reciprocal obligations, sensing common meaning, and sharing certain obligations toward others; related by blood and/or choice.

Group: A number of people with shared characteristics.

Community: A group of people living in the same locale under the same governance, such as neighborhoods, cities, or census tracts. When the unit of care is not explicitly stated, it becomes the individual by default.

AXIS 3 JUDGMENT: A descriptor or modifier that limits or specifies the meaning of the diagnostic concept. Values are:

Complicated: Intricately involved, complex

Compromised: Damaged, made vulnerable

Decreased: Lessened (in size, amount, or degree)

Defensive: Used or intended to defend or protect

Deficient: Insufficient, inadequate

Delayed: Late, slow, or postponed

Disabled: Limited, handicapped

Disorganized: Not properly arranged or controlled

Disproportionate: Too large or too small in comparison with norm

Disturbed: Agitated, interrupted, interfered with

Dysfunctional: Not operating normally

Effective: Producing the intended or desired effect

Enhanced: Improved in quality, value, or extent

Excessive: Greater than necessary or desirable

Failure: Cessation of proper functioning or performance

Imbalanced: Out of proportion or balance

Impaired: Damaged, weakened

Ineffective: Not producing the intended or desired effect

Insufficient: Quantity or quality that is not able to fulfill a need or requirement

Interrupted: Having its continuity broken

Low: Below the norm

Organized: Properly arranged or controlled

Perceived: Observed through the senses

Readiness for: In a suitable state for an activity or situation

Risk for: Increased danger, probability, or vulnerability

Situational: Related to a particular circumstance

AXIS 4 LOCATION: Consists of parts/regions of the body and/or their related functions—all tissues, organs, anatomical sites or structures. Values are:

Auditory	*Neurovascular*
Bladder	*Olfactory*
Body	*Oral*
Bowel	*Peripheral*
Cardiac	*Peripheral vascular*
Cardiopulmonary	*Renal*
Cerebral	*Skin*
Dentition	*Tactile*
Gastrointestinal	*Tissue*
Gustatory	*Urinary*
Intracranial	*Vascular*
Kinesthetic	*Verbal*
Liver	*Visual*
Mucous membranes	

AXIS 5 AGE: The age of the person who is the subject of the diagnosis. Values are:

Fetus	*School-Age child*
Neonate	*Adolescent*
Infant	*Adult*
Toddler	*Older adult*
Preschool child	

AXIS 6 TIME: The duration of the diagnostic concept. Values are:

Acute: Lasting less than 6 months

Chronic: Lasting more than 6 months

Intermittent: Stopping or starting again at intervals, periodic, cyclic

Continuous: Uninterrupted, going on without stop

AXIS 7 STATUS OF THE DIAGNOSIS: The actuality or potentiality of the problem/syndrome or the categorization of the diagnosis as a health promotion diagnosis. Values are:

Actual: Existing in fact or reality, existing at the present time

---

Health Promotion: Behavior motivated by the desire to increase well-being and actualize human health potential (Pender, Murdaugh, & Parsons, 2006)

Risk: Vulnerability, especially as a result of exposure to factors that increase the chance of injury or loss

---

Permission from NANDA International. (2012). *NANDA-I Nursing Diagnoses: Definitions & Classification 2012–2014*. Oxford: Wiley-Blackwell.

Bibliography

Books

Aacovou, I: The Role of the Nurse in the Rehabilitation of Patients with Radical Changes in Body Image Due to Burn Injuries. Psychiatric Department, Makarios Hospital, Nicosia, Cyprus, 2004.

Aboujoude, E, and Koran, LM: Impulse Control Disorders. Cambridge University Press, New York, 2010.

Ackley, BJ, and Ladwig, GB: Nursing Diagnosis Handbook: An Evidence-Based Guide to Planning Care, ed. 9. Mosby Elsevier, St Louis, MO, 2011.

Adams, S: Shock, systemic inflammatory response and multiple organ dysfunction. In Brooker, C, and Nicol, M (eds): Nursing Adults: The Practice of Caring. Mosby, Edinburgh, Scotland, 2003.

American Nurses Association: Nursing's Social Policy Statement. Washington, DC, 1995.

American Nurses Association: Nursing's Social Policy Statement, ed. 2. Washington, DC, 2003, p 6.

American Nurses Association: Social Policy Statement. Kansas City, MO, 1980.

American Nurses Association: Standards of Clinical Nursing Practice. Kansas City, MO, 1991.

American Psychological Association: When Children Experience Trauma: A Guide for Parents and Families. American Psychological Association, Washington, DC, (No date).

Andrade, C, and Clifford, P: Outcome Based Massage, ed. 2. Lippincott, Philadelphia, 2001.

Andrews, C, Creamer, M, Crino, R, et al: The Treatment of Anxiety Disorders: Clinician Guides and Patient Manuals. Cambridge University Press, Cambridge, UK, 2002.

Androwich, I, Burkhart, L, and Gettrust, KV: Community and Home Health Nursing. Delmar, Albany, NY, 1996.

Association of Perioperative Registered Nurses (AORN): AORN Standards and Recommended Practices for Perioperative Nursing. Association of Perioperative Registered Nurses (AORN), Denver, CO, 2001.

Banasik, JL, and Copstead, LEC (eds): Pathophysiology, ed. 3. Elsevier Saunders, St Louis, MO, 2005.

Bastable, SB: Essentials of Patient Education. Jones and Bartlett, Sudbury, MA, 2005.

Becker, RE, and Yudofsky, SC: Sexual and gender identity disorders. In Essentials of Clinical Psychiatry. American Psychiatric Press, Washington, DC, 1999.

Beers, MH, and Berkow, R: The Merck Manual of Diagnosis and Therapy, ed. 17. Merck Research Laboratories, Whitehouse Station, NJ, 1999.

Bellis, TJ: When the Brain Can't Hear: Unraveling the Mystery of Auditory Processing Disorder. Atria Books, New York, 2003.

Blach, DA, and Ignatavicius, DD: Interventions for clients with vascular problems. In Ignatavicius, DD, and Workman, ML (eds): Medical-Surgical Nursing: Critical Thinking for Collaborative Care, ed. 5. Elsevier Saunders, St Louis, MO, 2006.

Boston Women's Health Book Collective: Our Bodies, Ourselves for the New Century, ed. 7. Peter Smith Publisher, Gloucester, MA, 1998.

Branden, N: The Six Pillars of Self-Esteem. Bantam Books, New York, 1995.

Carey, CF, Lee, HH, and Woeltje, KF (eds): The Washington Manual of Medical Therapeutics, ed. 29. Lippincott-Raven, Philadelphia, 1998.

Cassileth, BR: The Alternative Medicine Handbook: The Complete Reference Guide to Alternative and Complementary Therapies. WW Norton, New York, 1998.

Cavanaugh, BM: Nurse's Manual of Laboratory and Diagnostic Tests, ed. 4. FA Davis, Philadelphia, 2003.

Clinebell, HJ: Growth resources in transactional analysis. In Contemporary Growth Therapies. Abingdon Press, Nashville, TN, 1981.

Condon, RE, and Nyhus, LM (eds): Manual of Surgical Therapeutics, ed. 9. Little, Brown, Boston, 1996.

Cox, H, Sridaromont, K, King, M, et al: Clinical Applications of Nursing Diagnosis: Adult, Child, Women's Psychiatric, Gerontic, and Home Health Considerations, ed. 4. FA Davis, Philadelphia, 2002.

Creasy, R, Resnk, R, and Iams, JD (auth/eds): Maternal-Fetal Medicine: Principles and Practice, ed. 6. WB Saunders, Philadelphia, 2008.

Cummings, B: Managing stress: Coping with life's challenges. In Health: The Basics, ed. 5. Pearson Education, Upper Saddle River, NJ, 2003.

D'Apolito, K, McGrath, J, and O'Brien, A: Infant and Family Centered Developmental Care Guidelines, ed. 3. National Association of Neonatal Nurses, Des Plaines, IL, 2000.

de Chesnay, M: Vulnerable populations: Vulnerable people. In de Chesnay, M and Anderson, BA (eds): Caring for the Vulnerable: Perspectives in Nursing Theory, Practice, and Research, ed. 3. Jones & Bartlett Learning, Burlington, MA, 2012.

Deglin, JH, Vallerand, AH, and Sanoski, CA: Davis's Drug Guide for Nurses, ed. 12. FA Davis, Philadelphia, 2011.

Doenges, M, and Moorhouse, M: Maternal/Newborn Plans of Care, ed. 3. FA Davis, Philadelphia, 1999.

Doenges, M, Moorhouse, M, and Murr, A: Nursing Care Plans Across the Life Span, ed. 8. FA Davis, Philadelphia, 2010.

Doenges, M, Moorhouse, M, and Murr, A: Nursing Diagnosis Manual: Planning, Individualizing, and Documenting Client Care, ed. 2. FA Davis, Philadelphia, 2008.

Doenges, ME, Townsend, MC, and Moorhouse, MF: Psychiatric Care Plans: Guidelines for Planning and Documenting Client Care, ed. 3. FA Davis, Philadelphia, 1998.

Editorial Staff: Complications and high-risk conditions of the prenatal period. In Straight A's in Maternal-Neonatal Nursing, ed. 2. Wolters Kluwer, Lippincott Williams & Wilkins, Philadelphia, 2008.

Editorial Staff: Cultural Childbearing Practices. Monograph in Lippincott Manual of Nursing Practice Pocket Guides: Maternal-Neonatal Nursing. Lippincott Williams & Wilkins, Philadelphia, 2007.

Editorial Staff: RDAs for Pregnant Women. Monograph in Lippincott Manual of Nursing Practice Pocket Guides: Maternal-Neonatal Nursing. Lippincott Williams & Wilkins, Philadelphia, 2007.

Editorial Staff: Renal system. In Pathophysiology Made Incredibly Easy! ed. 3. Lippincott Williams & Wilkins, Philadelphia, 2006.

Engel, J: Pocket Guide to Pediatric Assessment, ed. 4. Mosby, St Louis, MO, 2002.

Felver, L, and Kirkhorn, MJ: Fluid, electrolyte, and acid-base homeostasis. In Copstead, LEC, and Banasik, JL, (eds): Pathophysiology, ed. 3. Elsevier Saunders, St Louis, MO, 2005.

Finchman, FD, and Bradbury, TN (eds): The Psychology of Marriage: Basic Issues & Applications. Guilford Press, New York, 1990.

Fink, JB, Hess, DR, et al: Respiratory Care: Principles and Practices. W. B. Saunders, Philadelphia, 2002.

Ghosh, TB, Victor, BS, Hales, RR, et al: Suicide. The American Psychiatric Press Textbook of Psychiatry, ed. 2. American Psychiatric Press, Washington, DC, 1994.

Goleman, D: Emotional Intelligence: Why It Can Matter More than IQ. Bantam Books, New York, 1995.

Goleman, D: Emotional Intelligence: Why It Matters More than IQ, 10th Anniversary ed, Bantam, New York, 2006.

Gorman, L, Sultan, D, and Raines, M: Davis's Manual of Psychosocial Nursing for General Patient Care. FA Davis, Philadelphia, 1996.

Gorski, LA: Intravenous therapy. In Ackley, BJ, et al (eds): Evidence-Based Nursing Care Guidelines: Medical-Surgical Interventions. Mosby Elsevier, St Louis, MO, 2008.

Guyton, AC, and Hall, JE: Textbook of Medical Physiology, ed. 12. W. B. Saunders, Philadelphia, 2010.

Hallenbeck, J: Treatment of Nausea and Vomiting in Palliative Care Perspectives. Oxford University Press, New York, 2003.

Hareven, TK (ed): Aging and Generational Relations over the Life Course: A Historical and Cross-Cultural Perspective. Walter De Gruyter, Inc., New York, 1995.

Harkulich, JT, et al: Teacher's Guide: A Manual for Caregivers of Alzheimer's Disease in Long-Term Care. Embassy Printing, Cleveland Heights, OH, Copyright pending.

Harvard Medical School: Sexuality in Midlife and Beyond: A Special Health Report from Harvard Medical School. Harvard Health Publications, Cambridge, MA, 2003.

Hess, C: Clinical Guide to Wound Care, ed. 4. Lippincott Williams & Wilkins, Philadelphia, 2002.

Hogstel, MO, and Curry, LC: Health Assessment Through the Life Span, ed. 4. FA Davis, Philadelphia, 2005.

Holloway, B, Moredich, C, and Aduddell, K: OB Peds Women's Health Notes: Nurse's Clinical Pocket Guide. FA Davis, Philadelphia, 2006.

Hyde, K, and DeLamater, K: Understanding Human Sexuality, ed. 7. McGraw-Hill, New York, 2002.

Ignatavicius, DD, and Workman, ML (eds): Medical-Surgical Nursing: Critical Thinking for Collaborative Care. Elsevier Saunders, St Louis, MO, 2006.

Jaffe, MS, and McVan, BF: Laboratory and Diagnostic Test Handbook. FA Davis, Philadelphia, 1997.

Johnson, M, and Maas, M: Nursing Outcomes Classification (NOC), ed. 2. Mosby, St Louis, MO, 2000.

Kastenbaum, R: Death-related anxiety. In Michelson, L, and Ascher, I, (eds): Anxiety and Stress Disorders. Guilford Press, New York, 1987.

King, L: Toward a Theory for Nursing: General Concepts of Human Behavior. Wiley, New York, 1971.

Kolcaba, K: Comfort Theory and Practice. Springer, New York, 2003.

Kuhn, MA: Pharmacotherapeutics: A Nursing Process Approach, ed. 4. FA Davis, Philadelphia, 1998.

Kumagi, KAS, Chin, PA, Finocchiaro, D, et al: Physical Management of the Neurologically Involved Client: Techniques for Bed Mobility and Transfers. Rehabilitation Nursing Practice, McGraw-Hill, New York, 1998.

Kunert, PK, and Porth, CM: Stress and adaptation. In Porth, CM, and Martin, G (eds): Pathophysiology: Concepts of Altered Health States. Lippincott, Philadelphia, 2002.

Ladewig, P, London, M, and Davidson, M: Contemporary Maternal-Newborn Nursing Care, ed. 5. Prentice Hall, Upper Saddle River, NJ, 2002.

Lampe, S: Focus Charting, ed. 7. Creative Healthcare Management, Minneapolis, MN, 1997.

Lauderdale, J: Transcultural perspectives in childbearing. In Andrews, MM, and Boyle, JS (eds): Transcultural Concepts in Nursing Care, ed. 5. Wolters Kluwer Health, Lippincott Williams & Wilkins, Philadelphia, 2007.

Lawrence, RA, and Lawrence, R: Breastfeeding: A Guide for the Medical Profession, ed. 6. Mosby, St Louis, 2005.

Lee, D, Barrett, C, and Ignatavicius, D: Fluids and Electrolytes: A Practical Approach, ed. 4. FA Davis, Philadelphia, 1996.

Leeuwen, AM, Kranpitz, TR, and Smith, L: Davis's Comprehensive Handbook of Diagnostic Tests with Nursing Implications, ed. 2. FA Davis, Philadelphia, 2006.

Leiniger, MM: Transcultural Nursing: Theories, Research, and Practices, ed. 3. McGraw-Hill, Hilliard, OH, 1996.

Lipson, JG, Dibble, S, and Minarik, P (eds): Culture & Nursing Care: A Pocket Guide. UCSF Nursing Press, San Francisco, 1999.

Littlejohns, L, and Bader, M: Monitoring Technologies in Critically Ill Neuroscience Patients. Jones and Bartlett, Boston, 2009.

London, ML, Ladewig, PW, Ball, JW, et al: Maternal and Child Nursing, ed. 3. Prentice Hall, Upper Saddle River, NJ, 2003.

Lowdermilk, D, Cashion, M, and Perry, S: Maternity & Women's Health Care, ed. 10. Elsevier-Mosby, St Louis, MO, 2012.

Lutz, CA, and Pryztulski, KR: Nutrition and Diet Therapy, ed. 3. FA Davis, Philadelphia, 2001.

Manning, JE: Fluid and blood resuscitation. In Tintinalli, JE (ed): Emergency Medicine: A Comprehensive Study Guide. McGraw-Hill, New York, 2004.

McCaffrey, M, and Passero, C: Pain: Clinical Manual, ed. 2. Mosby, St Louis, MO, 1999.

McCance, KL, and Huether, SE: Pathophysiology: The Biologic Basis for Disease in Adults and Children, ed. 3. Mosby, St Louis, MO, 1997.

McCloskey, JC, and Bulechek, GM (eds): Nursing Interventions Classification, ed. 3. Mosby, St Louis, MO, 2000.

McCormack B, and Yorkey, M: Ten great things that exercise can do for you. Chapter 24 in Fit Over 40 for Dummies. Wiley, Hoboken, NJ, 2000.

McLeod, ME: Interventions for clients with diabetes mellitus. In Ignativicius, DD, and Workman, ML (eds): Medical-Surgical Nursing: Critical Thinking for Collaborative Care, ed. 5. Elsevier Saunders, Philadelphia, 2006.

Meek, J (ed): The American Academy of Pediatrics New Mother's Guide to Breastfeeding. Bantam Books, New York, 2002.

Mentes, JC: Evidence-Based Practice Guideline Hydration Management. University of Iowa Gerontological Nursing Interventions Research Center, Research Dissemination Core, Iowa City, IA, 2004.

Mentgen, J, and Bulbrook, MJT: Healing Touch, Level I Notebook. Healing Touch, Lakewood, CO, 1994.

Metheny, N: Fluid and Electrolyte Balance: Nursing Considerations, ed. 5. Jones & Barthlett, Sudbury, MA, 2010.

Moir, A, and Jessel, D: Brain Sex: The Real Difference Between Men & Women. Dell, New York, 1991.

Moller, MD, and Murphy, MF: Recovering from Psychosis: A Wellness Approach. Psychiatric Rehabilitation Nurses Inc., Nine Mile Falls, WA, 1998.

Morbacher, R, and Kendall-Tackett, K: Breastfeeding Made Simple: Seven Natural Laws for Nursing Mothers, ed. 2. New Harbinger Publications, Oakland, CA, 2010.

Mountstephen, M: How to Detect Developmental Delay and What to Do Next: Practical Applications for Home and School. Jessica Kinsley Publishers, Philadelphia, 2011.

Murray-Swank, A, Lucksted, A, Medoff, AR, et al: Religiosity, Psychosocial Adjustment, and Subjective Burden of Persons Who Care for Those with Mental Illness. Psychiatric Services, American Psychiatric Association, Arlington, VA, 2006.

NANDA International: Nursing Diagnoses: Definitions and Classification 2012–2014. Wiley-Blackwell, Oxford, 2012.

Neeld, EH: Finding Daylight After Loss Shatters Your Life. Seven Choices. Grand Central Publishing, New York, 2003.

Neifert, M: Great Expectations: The Essential Guide to Breastfeeding. Sterling, New York, 2009.

Newfield, SA, Hinz, MD, Tilley DS, et al: Cox's Clinical Applications of Nursing Diagnosis: Adult, Child, Women's Psychiatric, Gerontic, and Home Health Considerations, ed. 5. FA Davis, Philadelphia, 2007.

[No authors listed] Early Identification of Alzheimer's Disease and Related Dementias: Clinical Practice Guideline, US Department of Health and Human Services, Public Health Service Agency for Health Care Policy and Research, Rockville, MD, November 1996.

O'Neill, JA, Grasfeld, J, Fonkalsrud, E, et al (eds): Necrotizing enterocolitis (NEC). In Principles of Pediatric Surgery, ed. 2. Mosby, St Louis, MO, 2003.

Ossman, N, and Campbell, M: Adult Positions, Transitions, and Transfers: Reproducible Instruction Cards for Caregivers. Communication Skill Builders/Therapy Skill Builders, Elsevier, St. Louis, 1995.

Pearce, JC: The Biology of Transcendence: A Blueprint of the Human Spirit. Park Street Press, Rochester, VT, 2004.

Pender, NJ, Murdaugh, CC, and Parsons, MA: Health Promotion in Nursing Practice, ed. 5. Prentice Hall, Upper Saddle River, NJ, 2006.

Peplau, HE: Interpersonal Relations in Nursing: A Conceptual Frame of Reference for Psychodynamic Nursing. Putnam, New York, 1952.

Phillips, CR: Family-Centered Maternity Care. Jones & Bartlett, Sudbury, MA, 2003.

Porth, CM, and Kunert, PK: Pathophysiology: Concepts of Altered Health States. JB Lippincott, Philadelphia, 2002.

Purnell, LD and Paulanka, BJ: Transcultural Health Care: A Culturally Competent Approach. FA Davis, Philadelphia, 1998.

Purnell, LD, and Paulanka, BJ: Transcultural Health Care: A Culturally Competent Approach, ed. 3. FA Davis, Philadelphia, 2008.

Ricci, SS, and Kyle, T: Maternity and Pediatric Nursing. Lippincott Williams & Wilkins, Philadelphia, 2008.

Rimmer, JH: Aging, Mental Retardation, and Physical Fitness. Center on Health Promotion Research for Persons with Disabilities, University of Illinois at Chicago, 1996.

Riodan, J, Auerbach, K: Breastfeeding and Human Lactation, ed. 4. Jones & Bartlett, Boston, 2010.

Seligman, M, Reivich, K, Jaycox, LH, et al: The Optimistic Child. Houghton Mifflin, Boston, 1996.

Shore, LS: Nursing Diagnosis: What It Is and How to Do It: A Programmed Text. Medical College of Virginia Hospitals, Richmond, 1988.

Singer Kaplan, H: Sexual Desire Disorders: Dysfunctional Regulation of Sexual Motivation. Routledge, London, 1995.

Sommers, MS, Johnson, SA, and Beery, TA: Diseases and Disorders: A Nursing Therapeutics Manual, ed. 3. FA Davis, Philadelphia, 2007.

Sparks, SM, and Taylor, CM: Nursing Diagnoses Reference Manual, ed. 5. Springhouse, Springhouse, PA, 2001.

Springhouse (ed): Phototherapy. In Lippincott's Nursing Procedures, ed. 5. Lippincott Williams & Wilkins, Philadelphia, 2008.

Stanley, M, Blair, KA, and Beare, PG: Gerontological Nursing: Promoting Successful Aging with Older Adults, ed. 3. FA Davis, Philadelphia, 2005.

Stark, J: The renal system. In Alspach, JG (ed): Core Corriculum for Critical Care Nursing. Saunders, St Louis, MO, 2006.

Stuart, GW, and Laraia, MT: Principles and Practice of Psychiatric Nursing, ed. 7. Mosby, St Louis, MO, 2001.

Tabloski, PA (ed): Gerontological Nursing. Pearson Prentice-Hall, Upper Saddle River, NJ, 2006.

Townsend, MC: Essentials of Psychiatric Mental Health Nursing Concepts of Care in Evidence-Based Practice, ed. 5. FA Davis, Philadelphia, 2010.

Townsend, M: Nursing Diagnoses in Psychiatric Nursing: Care Plans and Psychotropic Medications, ed. 6. FA Davis, Philadelphia, 2004.

Townsend, MC: Psychiatric Mental Health Nursing Concepts of Care, ed. 4. FA Davis, Philadelphia, 2003.

Townsend, MC: Psychiatric Mental Health Nursing Concepts of Care, ed. 5. FA Davis, Philadelphia, 2005.

US Dept of Health and Human Services: Continuing Education Program on SIDS Risk Reduction. National Institutes of Health, Washington, DC, 2005.

Valdivia, R: The Implications of Culture on Developmental Delay. ERIC Clearinghouse on Disabilities and Gifted Education, Reston, VA, 1999.

Venes, D (ed): Taber's Cyclopedic Medical Dictionary, ed. 21. FA Davis, Philadelphia, 2009.

Wilkinson, R, and Marmot, M: Social Determinants of Health: The Solid Facts, ed. 3. World Health Organization (WHO), Copenhagen, 2003.

Workman, ML: Interventions for clients with electrolyte imbalances. In Ignatavicius, DD, and Workman, ML (eds): Medical-Surgical Nursing: Critical Thinking for Collaborative Care, ed. 5. Elsevier Saunders, St Louis, MO, 2006.

Wright, N, Morton, J, and Kim, J: Best Medicine: Human Milk in the NICU, ed. 5. Hale, Amarillo, TX, 2002.

Yura, H, and Walsh, MB: The Nursing Process: Assessing, Planning, Implementing, Evaluating, ed. 5. Appleton & Lange, Norwalk, CT, 1988.

Articles

Abrams, RC, Lachs, M, McAvay, G, et al: Predictors of self-neglect in community-dwelling elders. Am J Psychiatry 159:1724–30, 2002.

Ackerman, MH, and Mick, DJ: Instillation of normal saline before suctioning patients with pulmonary infections: A prospective randomized controlled trial. Am J Crit Care 7(4):261, 1998.

Agency for Healthcare Research and Quality (AHRQ): Acute pain management: Operative or medical procedures and trauma: Clinical practice guidelines. Clin Pharm 11:5, 1992.

Akton, GB, Kumpfer, KL, Turner, CW, et al: Effectiveness of a family skills training program for substance abuse prevention with inner city African-American families. Subst Use Misuse 31(2):157–75, 1996.

Aldabal, L, and Bahammam, AS: Metabolic, endocrine, and immune consequences of sleep deprivation. Open Respir Med 2011; 31–41, 2011.

Alexander, JW, Solomkin, JS, and Edwards, MJ: Updated recommendations for control of surgical site infections. Ann Surg 253(6):1082–93, 2011.

Algase, DL, Beel-Bates, C, and Beattie, E: Wandering in long term care. Ann Long Term Care 11(1):33–9, 2003.

Altman, KW, Yu, G-P, and Schaefer, SD: Consequence of dysphagia in the hospitalized patient. Arch Otolaryngeal Head Neck Surg 136(8):784–9, 2010.

American Academy of Pediatrics on Infectious Diseases: Prevention of human papillomavirus infection: Provisional recommendations for girls and women with quadrivalent human papillomavirus vaccine. Pediatrics 120(3):666–8, 2007.

American Academy of Pediatrics, Task Force on Sleep Position and SIDS: Changing concepts of sudden infant death syndrome: Implications for infant sleeping environment and sleep position. Pediatrics 105:650, 2000.

American Academy of Pediatrics. Clinical practice guideline: Diagnosis and management of childhood obstructive sleep apnea syndrome. Pediatrics 109:704–12, 2002.

American Academy of Pediatrics: The changing concept of sudden infant death syndrome: Diagnostic coding shifts, controversies regarding the sleeping environment, and new variations to consider in reducing risk. Pediatrics 116(5):1245–55, 2005.

American Diabetes Association: Preventative foot care in people with diabetes. Diabetes Care 26(Suppl 1):578–9, 2003.

American Diabetes Association: Standards of medical care in diabetes—2011: Foot care recommendations. Diabetes Care 34(Suppl 1):S11–61, 2011.

American Dietetic Association: Nutrition across the spectrum of aging. J Am Diet Assoc 105(2):616–33, 2005.

American Heart Association, the Council on Clinical Cardiology, the Councils on Cardiovascular Nursing, et al: Core components of cardiac rehabilitation secondary prevention programs: 2007 update. Circulation 115:2675–82, 2007.

Anderson, NR: The role of the home healthcare nurse in smoking cessation: Guidelines for successful intervention. Home Healthcare Nurse 24(7):424–31, 2006.

Aslibekyan, S, Levitan, EB, and Mittleman, MA: Prevalent cocaine use and myocardial infarction. Am J Cardiology 102(8):966–9, 2008.

Association of Perioperative Registered Nurses (AORN) Standards, Recommended Practices and Guidelines: Latex. AORN J 79(3):653–72, 2004.

Astle, SM: Restoring electrolyte balance. RN 68(5):31–4, 2005.

Austin, S: Seven legal tips for safe nursing practice. Nursing 38(3):34–9, 2008.

Ayers, DM, and Montgomery, M: Putting a stop to dysfunctional uterine bleeding, Nursing 39(1):44–50, 2009.

Azlin, B, Hatta, S, Norzila, Z, et al: Health locus of control among noncompliant hypertensive patients undergoing pharmacotherapy. Malaysian J Psychiatry 16(1):20–9, 2007.

Baer, HR, and Wolf, SL: Modified Emory Functional Ambulation Profile: An outcome measure for the rehabilitation of poststroke gait dysfunction. Stroke 32:973–9, 2001.

Bagai, A, Thavendiranathan, P, and Detsky, AS: Does this patient have hearing impairment? JAMA 295(4):416–28, 2006.

Baldacchino, D, and Draper, P: Spiritual coping strategies: A review of the nursing research literature. J Adv Nurs 34(5):833–41, 2001.

Baldwin, K: Stroke: It's a knock-out punch. Nursing Made Incredibly Easy! 4(2):10–23, 2006.

Bale, E, and Berrecloth, R: The obese patient. Anaesthetic issues: Airway and positioning, J Periop Pract 8:294–9, 2010.

Bakker, M, De Lange, FP, Helmich, RC, et al: Cerebral correlates of motor imagery of normal and precision gait. Neuroimage 41:998–1010, 2006.

Barry, J, McQuade, C, and Livingstone, T: Using nurse case management to promote self-efficiency in individuals with rheumatoid arthritis. Rehabil Nurs 23(6):300, 1998.

Barthlen, GM: Sleep disorders: Obstructive sleep apnea, restless leg syndrome, and insomnia in geriatric patients. Geriatrics 57(11):34–9, 2002.

Bartley, MK: Keep venous thromboembolism at bay. Nursing 36(10):36–41, 2006.

Bartol, T: Putting a patient with diabetes in the driver's seat. Nursing 32(2):53–5, 2002.

Barton-Burke, M: Cancer-related fatigue and sleep disturbances: Further research on the prevalence of these two symptoms in long-term cancer survivors can inform education, policy, and clinical practice. Am J Nurs 106(3 Suppl):72–77, 2006.

Bates, B, Choi, JY, Duncan PW, et al: Veterans Affairs/Department of Defense Clinical Practice Guidelines for the Management of Adult Stroke Rehabilitation Care: An executive summary. Stroke 36(9):2049–56, 2005.

Bauer, J, and Steinhauer, R: A readied response: The emergency plan. RN 65(6):40, 2002.

Bauldoff, GS, and Diaz, PT: Improving outcomes for COPD patients. Nurse Practitioner: Am J Primary Care 31(8):26–43, 2006.

Bausewein, C, Farquhar, M, Booth, S, et al: Measurement of breathlessness in advanced disease: A systematic review. Respir Med 101(3):399–410, 2007.

Beattie, S: Bedside emergency: Hemorrhage. RN 70(8): 30–4, 2007.

Beattie, S: In from the cold. RN 69(11):22–7, 2006.

Beatty, GE: Shedding light on Alzheimer's. The Nurse Practitioner: The American J of Primary Health Care 31(9):32–43, 2006.

Beauchamp-Johnson, BM: Scale down bariatric surgery risks. Nurse Management 37(9):27–32, 2006.

Beck, AC, and Beck, AT: Cognitive therapy for depression. Clin Psychol 48(3):3–5, 1995.

Beck, AT, Brown, G, and Berchick, RJ: Relationship between hopelessness and ultimate suicide: A replication with psychiatric outpatients. Am J Psychiatry 147:190–5, 1990.

Becker, B: To stand or not to stand. Rehab Management 18(2):28–34, 2005.

Beckett, N: Clinical nurses characterizations of patient coping problems. Int J Nurs Knowledge 2(2):72–8, 1991.

Bennett, JA: Dehydration: Hazards and benefits. Geriatr Nurs 21(2):84–8. 2000.

Berge, JM, and Holm, KE: Boundary ambiguity in parents with chronically ill children: Integrating theory and research. Fam Relations 56(2):123–34, 2007.

Bergman, J: The importance of skin-to-skin contact for every newborn. Breastfeeding Today 6(4):4–6, 2011.

Bin-Nun, A, Bromiker, R, and Wilschanski, M: Oral probiotics prevent necrotizing enterocolitis in very low birth weight neonates. J Pediatr 147(2):192–6, 2005.

Bissinger, RL, Annibale, DJ: Thermoregulation in very low-birthweight infants during the golden hour results and implications. Adv Neonatal Care 10(5):230–8, 2010.

Black, J, Baharestani, MM, and Cudigan, J: From the NPUAP: National Pressure Ulcer Advisory Panel's updated pressure ulcer staging system. Dermatol Nurs 19(4):343–9, 2007.

Blank-Reid, C: Abdominal trauma: Dealing with the damage. Nursing 37(4 Suppl: ED Insider):4–11, 2007.

Blann, LE: Early intervention for children and families with special needs. MCN, Am J Maternal/Child Nurs 30(4):263–7, 2005.

Bliss DZ, Jung, HJ, Savik, K, et al: Supplementation with dietary fiber improves fecal incontinence. Nurs Res 50(4):203–13, 2001.

Bockhold, KM: Who's afraid of hepatitis C? Am J Nurs 100(5):26–32, 2000.

Bodden, J: Treatment options in the hemodynamically unstable patient with a pelvic fracture. Orthop Nurs 28(3):109–14, 2009.

Boesch, C, Myers, J, Habersaat, A, et al: Maintenance of exercise capacity and physical activity patterns after cardiac rehabilitation. J Cardiopulm Rehab 25(1):14–21, 2005.

Bohrer, GJ: Anxiety, emotional and physical discomfort. NurseWeek 3(1):21–2, 2002.

Boissoneault, G: MCI and dementia: Diagnosis and treatment. JAAPA 23(1):18–22, 2010.

Bokinskie, JC, and Evanson, TA: The stranger among us: Ministering health to migrants. J Christian Nurs 26(4):202–9, 2009.

Bonanno, G, Galea, S, Buchiarelli, A, et al: What predicts psychological resilience after disaster? The role of demographics, resources, and life stress. J Consult Clin Psychol 75(5):671–82, 2007.

Bond, AE, Nelson, K, Germany, CL, et al: The left ventricular assist device. Am J Nurs 103(1):33–40, 2003.

Borbasi, S, Jones, J, Lockwood, C, et al: Health professionals' perspective of providing care to people with dementia in the acute setting: Toward better practice. Geriatric Nurs 27(5):300–8, 2006.

Bortz, W: Disuse and aging, 2009. J Gerontol A Bio Sci Med Sci 65(4):382–5, 2010.

Bostwick, JM: The many faces of confusion: Timing and collateral history often holds the key to diagnosis. Postgrad Med 108(6):60–72, 2000.

Bowman, A, Breiner, JE, Doerschug, KC, et al: Implementation of an evidence-based feeding protocol and aspiration risk reduction algorithm. Crit Care Nurs Q 28(4):324–33, 2005.

Braden, BJ: The Braden Scale for predicting pressure sore risk: Reflections after 25 years. Adv Skin Wound Care 25(2):61, 2003.

Brain Trauma Foundation Team: Indications for intracranial monitoring: Guidelines for the Management of Severe Traumatic Brain Injury. J Neurotrauma 24(Suppl 1):S37–S44, 2007.

Bramson, L, Lee, JW, Montgomery, S, et al: Effect of early skin-to-skin mother-infant contact during the first three hours following birth on exclusive breast-feeding during the maternity hospital stay. J Hum Lact 26(2):130–7, 2010.

Brantley, PJ, Mehan, DJ, and Ames, SC: Minor stressors and generalized anxiety disorder among low-income patients attending primary care clinics. J Nerv Ment Dis 87:435–40, 1999.

Bray, B, Van Sell, SL, and Miller-Anderson, M: Stress incontinence: It's no laughing matter. RN 70(4):25–9, 2007.

Breaslau, N: The epidemiology of trauma, PTSD, and other posttrauma disorders. Trauma Violence Abuse 10(3):198–210, 2009.

Breitenbach, JE: Putting an end to perfusion confusion. Nursing Made Incredibly Easy! 5(3):50–60, 2007.

Bridges, E, and Thomas, K: Noninvasive measurement of body temperature in critically ill patients. Crit Care Nurse 29(3):94–7, 2009.

Bright, L: Strategies to improve the patient safety outcome indicator: Preventing or reducing falls. Home Healthcare Nurse 23(1):29–36, 2005.

Brooks, RL, and Goldstein, S: Risk, resilience and futurists: Changing the lives of our children. Education Horizons 9(3):14–5, 2006.

Broscious, SK, and Castagnola, J: Chronic kidney disease: Acute man-ifestations and role of critical care nurses. Crit Care Nurse 26(4):17–27, 2009.

Bryson, GL, and Wynand, A: Evidence-based clinical update: General anesthesia and the risk of delirium and postoperative cognitive dys-function. Can J Anaesth 53(7):669–77, 2006.

Buchman, AS, Boyle, PA, Leurgans, SE, et al: Cognitive function is associated with the development of mobility impairments in community-dwelling elders. Am J Geriatr Psychiatry 19(6):571–80, 2011.

Buckle, J: Alternative/complementary therapies. Crit Care Nurse 18(5):54, 1998.

Burgio, KL, Locher, JL, and Goode, PS: Combined behavioral and drug therapy for urge incontinence in older women. Obstet Gynecol Sur-vey 55(8):485–6, 2000.

Burkhart, L: A click away: Documenting spiritual care. J Cardiovasc Nurs 22(1):6–12, 2005.

Burkhart, I, and Solari-Twadell, PA. Spirituality and religiousness: Dif-ferentiating the diagnosis through a review of the nursing literature. Nurs Diag Int J Nurs Lang Class 12:45–54, 2001.

Burnett, J, Regev, T, Pratti, LL, et al: Social network: A profile of the elder who self-neglects. J Elder Abuse Negl 18(4):35–49, 2006.

Burns, A, Byrne, J, and Ballard, C: Sensory stimulation in dementia: An effective option for managing behavioral problems. Br Med J 325:1312–3, 2002.

Burns, SM: Mechanical ventilation of patients with acute respiratory distress syndrome and patents requiring weaning: The evidence guid-ing practice. Crit Care Nurse 25(4):14–24, 2005.

Burns, SM, Fisher, C, and Tribble, SSE: Multifactor clinical score and outcome of mechanical ventilation weaning trials: Burns Wean As-sessment Program. Am J Crit Care 19.431–9, 2010.

Butcher, HK, and McGonigal-Kenney, M: Depression & dispiritedness in later life. Am J Nurs 105(12):52–61, 2005.

Butler, AC, and Beck, AT: Cognitive therapy for depression. Clin Psy-chol. 48(3):3–5, 1995.

Butts, JB: Outcomes of comfort touch in institutionalized elderly female residents. Geriatr Nurs 22(4):180–4, 2001.

Calamaro, C, and Waite, R: Cultural proficiency, research, and evidence-based practice: Implications for the nurse practitioner. J Pediatric Health Care 23(1):69–72, 2008.

Calianno, C, and Holton, SJ: Fighting the triple threat of lower extrem-ity ulcers. Nursing 37(3):57–63, 2007.

Calianno, C: Patient hygiene, part 2—Skin care: Keeping the outside healthy. Nursing 32(6):1–13, 2002.

Callen, J, and Pinelli, J: A review of the literature examining the benefits and challenges, incidence and duration, and barriers to breastfeeding in preterm infants. Adv Neonatal Care 5(2):72–88, 2005.

Campbell, H, Tadros, G, Hanna, G, et al: Diogenes syndrome: Frontal lobe dysfunction or multi-factorial disorder. Geriatr Med 35(3):77–9, 2005.

Capão, FJA, Rocha-Sousa, A, Falcão-Reis, et al: Modern sports eye injuries. Br J Ophthalmol 87(11):1336–9, 2003.

Capazuti, E, Boltz, M, Renz, S, et al: Nursing home involuntary relocation: Clinical outcomes and perceptions of residents and families. J Am Med Dir Assoc 7(8):486–92, 2006.

Caprio, S, Daniels, SR, Drewnowski, A, et al: Influence of race, ethnicity, and culture on childhood obesity: Implications for prevention and treatment: A consensus statement of Shaping America's Health and the Obesity Society. Diabetes Care 31(11):2211–21, 2008.

Carl, W, and Havens, J: The cancer patient with severe mucositis. Cur Rev Pain 4(3):197–202, 2000.

Carls, C: The prevalence of stress urinary incontinence in high school and college-age female athletes in the Midwest: Implications for education and prevention. Urol Nurs 27(1):21–4, 2007.

Carnevale, FA, Alexander, E, and Renneck, J: Daily living with distress and enrichment: The moral experience of families with ventilator-assisted children at home. Pediatr 117(1):e48–e60. 2006.

Carrington, AL, Abott, CA, Grifiths, J, et al: Peripheral vascular and nerve function associated with lower limb amputation in people with and without diabetes. Clin Sci 101(3):261–6, 2001.

Casa, DJ, McDermott, BP, Lee, EC, et al: Cold water immersion: The gold standard for exertional heatstroke treatment. Exerc Sport Sci Rev 35(3):141–9, 2007.

Catania, K, Huang, C, James, P, and Ohr, M: PUPPI: The pressure ulcer prevention protocol interventions. Am J Nurs 107(4):44–51, 2007.

Cayley, WE: Diagnosing the cause of chest pain. Am Fam Physician (72):2012–21, 2005.

Centers for Disease Control and Prevention: Recommended immunization schedules for persons aged 0–18 years—United States. MMWR, 55(51–52):Q1–Q4, 2006.

Chang, M, and Kelley, A: Patient education: Addressing cultural diversity and health literacy issues. Urol Nurs 27(5):411–7, 2007.

Chatters, IM, Taylor, RJ, and Lincoln, KD: Advances in the measurement of religiosity among older African Americans: Implications for health and mental health researchers. J Ment Health Aging 8(1):181–200, 2001.

Cheatham, ML: Abdominal compartment syndrome: Pathophysiology and definitions. Scand J Trauma, Resusc Emer Med 17:10, 2009.

Cheever, KH: An overview of pulmonary arterial hypertension: Risks, pathogenesis, clinical manifestations, and management. J Cardiovasc Nurs 20(2):108–16, 2005.

Chengappa, KN: Clozapine reduces severe self-mutilation and aggression in psychotic patients with borderline personality disorder. J Clin Psychiatry 60(7):477–84, 1999.

Cherif, M and Younis, EI: Liver transplantation. Clin Fam Prac 2(1):117, 2000.

Chey, WD, and Wong, BCY: American College of Gastroenterology guideline on the management of Helicobacter Pylori infection. Am J Gastroenterol 102:1808–25, 2007.

Chiaro, C: Preventing relocation stress, easing children's transition. Special report. Colorado Springs Business Journal, 2003.

Chibulka, NT, White, DM, Woehrle, J, et al: Hip pain and mobility deficits-hip osteoarthritis: Clinical practice guidelines linked to the International Classification of Functioning Disabilityand Health from the Orthopaedic Section of the American Physical Therapy Association. J Orthop Sports Phys Ther 39(4):A1–25, 2009.

Chilton, BA: Recognizing spirituality. Image: J Nurs Scholarship 30(4):400, 1998.

Clarke, L, and Whittaker, M: Self-mutilation: Culture, contexts, and nursing responses. J Clin Nurs 7(2):129–37, 1998.

Cleary-Goldman, J, et al: Impact of maternal age on obstetric outcome. Obstet & Gynecol 105(5):983–90, 2005.

Cmiel, CA: Noise control: A nursing team's approach to sleep promotion. Am J Nurs 104(2):40–8, 2004.

Coaten, R: Movement matters. Natl Healthcare J 5:53, 2002.

Cochran, H: Diagnose and treat primary insomnia. Nurse Pract: Am J Primary Health Care 28(9):13–27, 2003.

Cohen, D: Optional but necessary. Rehab Manage 18(10):26–9, 2005.

Cohen, D: Providing an assist. Rehabil Manage 21(8):16–9, 2008.

Cole, C, and Richards, K: Sleep disruption in older adults. Am J Nurs, 107 (5):40–9, 2007.

Cole, MG, and Dependukuri, N: Risk factors for depression among the elderly community subjects: A systematic review and meta-analysis. Am J Psychiatr 160(6):1147–56, 2003.

Collins, M, and Claros, E: Recognizing the face of dehydration. Nursing 41(8):26–31, 2011.

Cook, LS: Choosing the right intravenous catheter. Home Healthcare Nurse 25(8):523–31, 2007.

Coppieters, MW, van de Velde, M, and Sappaerts, KH: Positioning in anaesthesiology: Toward a better understanding of stretch-induced perioperative neuropathies. Anesthesiology 97:75–81, 2002.

Cormier, M: The role of hepatitis C support groups. Gastroenterol Nurs 28(3 Suppl): S4–S9, 2005.

Cowan, LG, and Stechmiller, J: Prevalence of wet-to-dry dressings in wound care. Adv Skin Wound Care 22(12):567–73, 2009.

Crawford, A, and Harris, H: I.V. fluids: What nurses need to know. Nursing 41(5):30–8, 2011.

Creswell, C, and Chalder, T: Defensive coping styles in chronic fatigue syndrome. J Psychosom Res 51(4): 607–10, 2001.

Crowe, AV, Howse, M, and Bell, GM: Substance abuse and the kidney. QJM 93(3):147–152, 2000.

Curzio, J, and McCowan, M: Getting research into practice: Developing oral hygiene standards. Br J Nurs 9(7):434–8, 2000.

Czernuszenko, A: Risk factors for falls in post-stroke patients treated in a neurorehabilitation ward. Neurol Neurochir Pol 41(1):28–35, 2007.

Dallam, SJ: The identification and management of self-mutilating patients in primary care. Nurse Pract 22(5):151–65, 1997.

Daly, SEJ, and Hartmann, PD: Infant demand and milk supply. Part 1: Infant demand and milk production in lactating women. J Hum Lact 11(1):21–6, 1995.

D'Arcy, Y: Conquering PAIN: Have you tried these new techniques? Nursing 35(3):36–41, 2005.

D'Arcy, Y: Eye on capnography. Men in Nursing 2(2):25–9, 2007.

D'Arcy, Y: Managing pain in a patient who's drug-dependent. Nursing 37(3):36–40, 2007.

Davison, SN, and Simpson, C: Hope and advance care planning in patients with end stage renal disease: Qualitative interview study. BMJ 333:886–9, 2006.

Day, MR, and Leahy-Warren, P: Self-neglect 1: Recognizing features and risk factors. Nursing Times 104(25):28–9, 2008.

Day, MR, and Leahy-Warren, P: Self-neglect 2: Nursing assessment and management. Nursing Times 104(24):26–7, 2008.

Deckelbaum, RJ, and Williams, CL: Childhood obesity: The health issue. Obes Res 9(4 Suppl):S239–S43, 2001.

DeJong, MJ: Emergency! Hyponatremia. Am J Nurs 98(12):36, 1998.

Dellinger, RP, Levy, MM, Carlet, JM, et al: Surviving sepsis campaign: Guidelines for management for severe sepsis and septic shock: 2008. Crit Care Med 36(1):296–327, 2008.

Denison, B: Touch the pain away: New research on therapeutic touch and persons with fibromyalgia syndrome. Holist Nurs Pract 18(3):142–51, 2004.

Diel-Oplinger, L, and Kaminski, MF: Choosing the right fluid to counter hypovolemic shock. Nursing 34(3):52–54, 2004.

diMaria-Ghalili, RA, and Amelia, E: Nutrition in older adults: Interventions and assessment can help curb the growing threat of malnutrition. Am J Nurs 105(3):4050, 2005.

Dougherty, AL, Mohrie, CR, Galarneau, MR, et al: Battlefield extremity injuries in Operation Iraqi Freedom. Injury 40(7):772–7, 2009.

Doughty, D, and Kisanga, J: Regulatory guidelines for bladder management in long-term care: Are you in compliance with F-Tag 315? J Wound, Ostomy Cont Nurs 37(4):399–411, 2010.

Douglas, SL, and Daly BJ: Caregivers of long-term ventilator patients: Physical and psychological outcomes. Chest 123:1073–81, 2003.

Drew N: Combating the social isolation of chronic mental illness, J Psychosoc Nurs 29(6):14–17, 1991.

Ducharme, S: Autonomic dysreflexia (sexuality and SCI). Paraplegia News, Nov 1, 2006.

Duncan, LG, Coatsworth, JD, and Greenberg, MT: Pilot study to gauge acceptability of a mindfulness based, family-focused preventive intervention. J Prim Prev 30(5):605–18, 2009.

Dunn, D: Age-smart care: Preventing perioperative complications in older adults. Nursing 4(3):30–9, 2006.

Dunn, D: Preventing perioperative complications in special populations. Nursing 35(11):36–43, 2005.

Durston, S: What you need to know about viral hepatitis. Nursing 35(8):36–41, 2005.

Dutton, RP: Current concepts in hemorrhagic shock. Anesthesiol Clin North Am 25(1):23–34, 2007.

Dworak, PA, and Levy, A: Strolling along. Rehab Manage 18(9):26–31, 2005.

Editorial Staff: Patho Puzzler: Don't let your head explode over increased ICP. Nursing Made Incredibly Easy! 5(2):21–5, 2007.

Eisenhauer, C: Media review: The new glucose revolution: The authoritative guide to the glycemic index—The dietary solution for lifelong health. Fam Community Health 30(1):86, 2007.

Elbright, PR, Patterson, ES, and Render, ML: The "New Look" approach to patient safety: A guide for clinical specialist leadership. Clin Nurs Spec 16(5):247–53, 2002.

Eldar-Avidan, D, Haj-Yahia, M, and Greenbaum, C: Divorce is a part of my life . . . resilience, survival, and vulnerability: Young adults' perception of the implications of parental divorce. J Marital Fam Ther 35(1):30–46, 2009.

Elgart, HN, Johnson, KL, and Munro, N: Assessment of fluids and electrolytes. AACN Clin Issues 15(4):607–21, 2004.

Ellis, A: Showing people they are not worthless individuals. Voices: The Art and Science of Psychotherapy 1(2):74–7, 1965.

Elpern, EH, Covert, B, and Kleinpell, R: Moral distress of staff nurses in a medical intensive care unit. Am J Crit Care 14:523–39, 2005.

El-Zayadi, AR: Heavy smoking and liver. World J Gastroenterol 12(38):6089–101, 2006.

Enslein, J, Tripp-Reimer, R, Kelley, LS, et al: Evidence-based protocol. Interpreter facilitation for persons with limited English proficiency. J Gerontol Nurs 28(7):5–13, 2002.

Epstein, CD, and Peerless, JR: Weaning readiness and fluid balance in older critically ill surgical patients. Am J Crit Care 15(1):54–64, 2006.

Epstein, SK: Weaning from mechanical ventilation. Respir Care 47(4):454–66, 2002.

Estes, K, and Thomure, J: Aspirin for the primary prevention of adverse cardiovascular events. Crit Care Nurs Q 31(4):324–39, 2008.

Evans, LK, and Cotter, VT: Avoiding restraints in patients with dementia: Understanding, prevention, and management are the keys. Am J Nurs 108(3):40–9, 2007.

Evans, S, Tsao, JC, Sternlieb, S, et al: Using the biopsychosocial model to understand the health benefits of yoga. J Complement Integr Med 6(1):1–22, 2009.

Fagring, AJ, Gaston-Johansson, F, and Danielson, E: Description of unexplained chest pain and its influence on daily life in men and women. Eur J Cardiovasc Nurs (4):337–44, 2005.

Fallot, RD: Assessment of spirituality and implications for service planning. New Dir Ment Health Serv 80:13–23, 1998.

Fegin, R, Barnetz, Z, and Davidson-Arad, B: Quality of life in family members coping with chronic illness in a relative: An exploratory study. Fam Syst Health 26(3):267–81, 2008.

Feifel, H, and Branscomb, BA: Who's afraid of death? J Abnorm Psychol 81(3):282–8, 1973.

Feigenbaum, K: Update on gastroparesis. Gastroenterol Nurs 29(3):239–44, 2006.

Feldman, R, Eidelman, AI, Sirota, L, and Weller, A: Comparison of skin-to-skin (kangaroo) and traditional care: Parenting outcomes and preterm infant development. Pediatr 110(1):16–26, 2002.

Ferry, M: Strategies for ensuring good hydration in the elderly. Nutrition Reviews 63(Suppl):22–9, 2005.

Finfer, S, Bellomo, R, Boyce, N, et al: A comparison of albumin and saline for fluid resuscitation in the intensive care unit. N Engl J Med 350(22):2247–56, 2004.

Fish, KB: Suicide awareness at the elementary school level. J Psychosoc Nurs Ment Health Serv 38(7):20–3, 2000.

Fishbain, DA, Cole, RB, Cutler, RB, et al: A structured evidenced-based review on the meaning of non-organic physical signs: Waddell's Signs. Pain Med 4(2):141–81, 2003.

Fitzgerald, MA: LAB LOGIC: Hyponatremia associated with SSRI use in a 65-year-old woman. The Nurse Pract 33(2):2–11, 2008.

Flannery, J: Using the levels of cognitive functioning assessment scale with traumatic brain injury in an acute care setting. Rehabil Nurs 23(2):88, 1998.

Fleck, CA: Why wet to dry? J Am Coll Cert Wound Spec 1(4):109–13, 2009.

Flegal, KM, Ogden, CL, Wei, R, et al: Prevalence of overweight in US children: Comparison of US growth charts from the Centers for Disease Control and Prevention with other reference values for body mass index. Am J Clin Nutr 73(6):1086–93.

Fort, CW: How to combat 3 deadly trauma complications. Nursing 33(5):58–63, 2003.

Foss, CM, et al: Exercise testing for evaluation of hypoxemia and/or desaturation: Revision & update. Resp Care 46(5):514–22, 2001.

Franke, J: Stress, burnout, and addiction. Tex Med 95(3):43–52, 1999.

Friedman, MM: Improving infection control in home care: From ritual to science-based practice. Home Healthcare Nurse 18(2):99–106, 2002.

Fronk, C, Huntington, R, and Chadwick, BA: Expectations for traditional family roles: Palestinian adolescents in the West Bank and Gaza. Sex Roles: A Journal of Research 41(9):705–35, 1999.

Frost, KL, and Topp, R: A physical activity RX for the hypertensive patient. Nurse Pract: Am J Primary Health Care 31(4):29–37, 2006.

Fulmer, T: Elder abuse and neglect assessment. Gerontal Nurs 29(1):8–9, 2003.

Gabany, E, and Shellenbarger, T: Caring for families with deployment stress. Am J Nurs 110(11):36–41, 2010.

Galea, S, Nandi, A, and Vlahov, D: The epidemiology of post-traumatic stress disorders after disasters. Epidemiol Rev 27(1):78–91, 2005.

Gallaher, S, Langlois, C, Spect, DW, et al: Preplanning with protocols for skin and wound care in obese patients. Adv Skin Wound Care 17(8):442–3, 2004.

Galligan, M: Proposed guidelines for skin-to-skin treatment of neonatal hypothermia. Amer J Matern Child Nurs 31(5):298–304, 2006.

Gance-Cleveland, B: Motivational interviewing as a strategy to increase families' adherence to treatment regimens. J Specialists Pediatr Nurs 10(3):151–5, 2005.

Garcia, J, and Wills, L: Sleep disorders in children and teens: Helping patients and their families get some sleep. Postgrad Med 107(3):161–88, 2002.

Garcia, JM, and Chambers, E: Managing dysphagia through diet modifications. Am J Nurs 110(11):26–33, 2010.

Garon, BR, Sierzant, T, and Ormiston, C: Silent aspiration: Results of 2,000 video fluoroscopic evaluations. J Neurosci Nurs 41(4):178–85, 2009.

Garzon, DL, Thrasher, C, and Tiernan, K: Providing optimal care for children with developmental disorders. Nurse Pract 35(10):30–9, 2010.

Gemma, M, Tommasino, C, Cerri, M, et al: Intracranial effects of endotracheal suctioning in the acute phase of head injury. J Neurosurgical Anesth 14(1):50–4, 2002.

Giasson, M, and Bouchard, L: Effect of therapeutic touch on the well-being of persons with terminal cancer. J Holistic Nurs 16(3):383–98, 1998.

Girot, M: Smoking and stroke. Presse Med 38(7–8):1120–5, 2009.

Given, B, Sherwood, P, and Given, C: What knowledge and skills do caregivers need? Am J Nurs 108(9 Suppl):S28–S34, 2008.

Gjerdongen, D: Expectant parents' anticipated changes in workload after the birth of their first child. J Fam Pract 49(11):993–7, 2000.

Glare, PA, Dunwoodie, D, Clark, K, et al: Treatment of nausea and vomiting in terminally ill cancer patients. Drugs 68(18):2575–90, 2008.

Goertz, S: Eye of diagnostics: Gauging fluid balance with osmolality. Nursing 36(10):70–71, 2006.

Goldberg, SM: Identifying intestinal obstruction: Better safe than sorry. Nurs Crit Care 3(5):18–23, 2008.

Goldman, LR: Linking research and policy to ensure children's environmental health. Environ Health Perspect 106(13):957–61, 1998.

Goldrich, G: Understanding the 12-lead ECG, part I. Nursing 36(11):36–41, 2006.

Goldrick, BA, and Goetz, AM: 'Tis the season for influenza. Nurse Pract Am J Primary Health Care 31(12):24–33, 2006.

Good, KK, Verble, JA, Secrest, J, et al: Postoperative hypthermia—The chilling consequences. AORN 83(5):1055–66, 2006.

Gordon, BN: Child temperament and adult behavior: An exploration of "goodness of fit." Child Psychiatry Hum Dev 11(3):167–78, 1981.

Gorman, D, Calhoun, K, Carassco, M, et al: Take a rapid treatment approach to cardiogenic shock. Nurs Crit Care 3(4):18–27, 2008.

Gorman-Smith, D, Henry, DB, and Tolan, PH: Exposure to community violence and violence perpetration: The protective effects of family functioning. J Clin Child Psychol 33(3):439–49, 2004.

Gosdon, MJ: Using technology to reduce medication errors. Nursing 39(6):57–8, 2009.

Graf, C: Functional decline in hospitalized older adults. Am J Nurs 106(1):58–67, 2006.

Graf, C: The Lawton Instrumental Activities of Daily Living Scale. Am J Nurs 108(4):52–46, 2008.

Grant, JE, Levine, L, Kim, D, et al: Impulse control disorders in adult psychiatric inpatients. AM J Psychiatry 162: 2184–8, 2005.

Gray, M: Assessment and management of urinary incontinence. Nurse Pract: Am J Primary Health Care 30(7):32–43, 2005.

Gray, M: Context for WOC practice: Synthesizing the evidence to guide facility wide policies for wound, ostomy and continence care. J Wound, Ostomy Continence Nurs 36(2):123–5, 2005.

Gray, M: Overactive bladder: An overview. J Wound, Ostomy Continence Nurs 32(Suppl 3):1–5, 2005.

Gray, M: Urinary retention: Management in the acute care setting (part 2). Am J Nurs 100(8):36–44, 2000.

Gray, M, Bliss, DZ, Doughty, DB, et al: Incontinence-associated dermatitis: A consensus. J Wound, Ostomy Continence Nurs 34(1):45–54, 2007.

Gray, R, Wykes, T, Gournay, K, et al: From compliance to concordance: A review of literature on interventions to enhance compliance with antipsychotic medications. J Psychiatr Ment Health Nurs 9(3):277–84, 2002.

Gregory, CM: Caring for caregivers: Proactive planning eases burdens on caregivers. Lifelines 1(2):51, 1997.

Greiter, H: The spiritual side of nursing. RN 65(5):43–4, 2002.

Grundstein, A, Dowd, J, and Mentemeyer, V: Quantifying the heat related hazard for children in motor vehicles. American Meteorological Society (AMS) 91(9):1183, 2001.

Grzankowski, JA: Altered thought processes related to traumatic brain injury and their nursing implications. Rehabil Nurs 22(1):24–31, 1997.

Guerrant, RL, Van Gilder, T, Steiner, TS, et al: Practice guidelines for the management of infectious diarrhea. Clin Infect Dis 32(3):331–51, 2001.

Guigoz, Y: The Mini Nutritional Assessment (MNA) review of the literature—What does it tell us? J Nutr Health Aging 10(6):466–85, 2006.

Gura, T: "I'll do it tomorrow." Scientific American Mind 19:32–9, 2009.

Gussy, MG, Waters, EG, Walsh, O, et al: Early childhood caries: Current evidence for aetiology and prevention. J Paediatr Child Health 42:37–43, 2006.

Hadaway, LC: Reopen the pipeline for IV therapy. Nursing 35(8):54–61, 2005.

Hadaway, LC: Targeting therapy with central venous access devices. Nursing 38(6):34–40, 2008.

Hahn, J: Cueing in to client language. Reflections 25(1):8–11, 1999.

Haigler, DH, Bauer, LJ, and Travis, SS: "Caring for you, caring for me": A ten-year caregiver educational initiative of the Rosalynn Carter Institute for Human Development. Health Soc Work 31(2):149–52, 2006.

Halpin-Landry, JE, and Goldsmith, S: Feet first: Diabetes care. Am J Nurs 99(2):26, 1999.

Hankins, J: The role of albumin in fluid and electrolyte balance. J Infusion Nurs 29(5):260–5, 2006.

Hanley, C: Delirium in the acute care setting: MEDSURG Nurs 13(4):217–25, 2004.

Hanna, DR: The lived experience of moral distress: Nurses who assisted with elective abortions. Research and Theory for Nursing Practice 19(1):95–124, 2005.

Hanneman, SK, and Gusick, M: Frequency of oral care and positioning of patients in critical care: A replication study. Am J Crit Care 14(5):378–86, 2005.

Harris, SM, Adams, MS, Zubatsky, M, et al: A caregiver perspective of how Alzheimer's disease and related disorders affect couple intimacy. Aging Mental Health 15(8):950–60, 2011.

Harvey, S: Assessment of the clinical effectiveness of the pulmonary catheters in the management of patients in intensive care (PAC-Man): A randomised controlled trial. Lancet 366(9484):472–7, 2005.

Hatzmann, J, Heymans, HS, Ferrer-i-Carbonell, A, et al: Hidden consequences of success in pediatrics: Parental health-related quality of life. Pediatr 122(5):1030–8, 2008.

Hauk, FR, Thompson, JM, Tanabe, KO, et al: Breastfeeding and reduced risk of Sudden Infant Death Syndrome: A meta-analysis. Pediatr 128(1):1–8, 2011.

Haye, BD, Klein-Schwartz, W, and Gonzales, LF: Causes of therapeutic errors in older adults: Evaluation of National Poison Center data. J Am Geriatr Soc 57(4):653–8, 2009.

Hedges, ST, et al: Evidence-based treatment recommendations for uremic bleeding. Nat Clin Pract Nephrol 3(3):138–53, 2007.

Held-Warmkessel, J, and Schiech, L: Responding to 4 gastrointestinal complications in cancer patients. Nursing 38(7):3238, 2008.

Henneman, EA: Liberating patients from mechanical ventilation: A team approach. Crit Care Nurs 21(3):25–33, 2001.

Hensley, LG: Treatment for survivors of rape: Issues and interventions. J of Mental Health Counseling 24(4):330–47, 2002.

Herr, K, Coyne, PJ, Key, T, et al: Pain assessment in the nonverbal patient: Position statement with clinical practice recommendations. Pain Management Nursing 7(2):44–52, 2006.

Herson, L, Hart, K, Gordon, M, et al: Identifying and overcoming barriers to providing sexuality information in the clinical setting. Rehabil Nurs 24(4):148, 1999.

Herter, R, and Kazer, MW: Best practices in urinary catheter care. Home Healthcare Nurs 28(6):342–9, 2010.

Hertz, JE, Koren, ME, Rossett, J, et al: Early identification of relocation risk in older adults with critical illness. Crit Care Quarterly 31(1):59–64, 2008.

Hill, PD, Aldag, JC, Zinaman, M, et al: Predictors of preterm infant feeding methods and perceived insufficient milk supply at week 12 postpartum. J Hum Lact 23(1):32–8, 2007.

Hiner, BC: Valsalva Maneuver. Clin Med Res 3(2):55, 2005.

Ho, J, and Birnham, C: Acculturation gaps in Vietnamese immigrant families: Impact on family relationships. Int J Intercult Relat 34(1):22–3, 2010.

Hodgson, N, Freedman, VA, Granger, DA, et al: Biobehavioral correlates of relocation in the frail elderly: Salivary cortisol, affect, and cognitive function. J Am Geriatr Soc 52(11):1856–62, 2004.

Holcomb, S: Topics in Progressive Care: Third-spacing: When body fluid shifts. Nursing Crit Care 4(2):9–12, 2009.

Holcomb, SS: Acute abdomen: What a pain! Nursing 38(9):34–40, 2008.

Holcomb, SS: Caring for the patient with chronic hepatitis C. Nursing 38(12):32–7, 2008.

Holley, JL: Hypovolemia and dehydration in the oncology patient—A viewpoint of salt and water imbalance. J Support Oncol 4:455–6, 2006.

Holm, K, and Foreman, M: Analysis of measures of functional and cognitive ability for aging adults with cardiac and vascular disease. J Cardiovasc Nurs 21(5 Suppl 1):S40–S5, 2006.

Honkus, VL: Sleep deprivation in critical care units. Crit Care Nurs Q, 26(3), 179–91, 2003.

Horowitz, C, Davis, MH, Palermo, AG, et al: Approaches to eliminating sociocultural disparities in health. Health Care Financing Review 21(4):57–74, 2000.

Horsley, T, Clifford, T, Barrowman, N, et al: Benefits and harms associated with the practice of bed sharing. Arch Pediatr Adolesc Med 161(3):237–45, 2007.

Houghton, D: HAI prevention: The power is in your hands. Nurs Manage 37(Suppl 5):1–7, 2006.

Hoyt, DP, and Magoon, TM: A validation study of the Taylor Manifest Anxiety Scale. J of Clinical Psychology 10(4):357–61, 1954.

Hughes, L: Physical and psychological variables that influence pain in patients with fibromyalgia. Orthop Nurs 25(2):112–9, 2006.

Hunt, R: Community-based nursing. Am J Nurs 98(10):44, 1998.

Hunter, A, Denman-Vitale, S, and Garzon, L: Global infections: Recognition, management, and prevention. Nurse Pract: Am J Primary Health Care 32(2):34–41, 2007.

Hunter, JD, and Damani, Z: Intra-abdominal hypertension and the abdominal compartment syndrome. Anaesthesia 59(9):899–907, 2004.

Huston, CJ: Emergency! Dental luxation and avulsion. Am J Nurs 97(9):48, 1997.

Hutchison, CP: Healing touch: An energetic approach. Am J Nurs 99(4):43, 1999.

Infusion Nurses Society: Infusion nursing standards of practice. J Infusion Nurs 29(1 Suppl):S1–S92, 2006.

Inouye, SK, Studenski, S, and Tinetti, ME: Geriatric syndromes: Clinical, research and policy implications of a core geriatric concept. J Am Geriatr Society 55(5):780–91, 2007.

Institute for Clinical Systems Improvement (ICSI): Perioperative protocol. Health care protocol. Institute for Clinical Systems Improvement (ICSI) Oct:105, 2005.

Iregui, M, Malen, J, Tuteur, P, et al: Determinants of outcome for patients admitted to a long-term ventilator unit. South Med J 95(3):310–7, 2002.

Irwin, RS: Introduction to the diagnosis and management of cough: ACCP evidence-based clinical practice guidelines. Chest 29(1 Suppl):255–75, 2006.

Isaacs, A: Depression and your patient. Am J Nurs 98(7):26, 1998.

Iscoe, KE, Campbell, JE, Jamnik, V, et al: Efficacy of continuous real-time blood glucose monitoring during and after prolonged high-intensity cycling exercise: Spinning with a continuous glucose monitoring system. Diabetes Technol Ther 8(6):627–35, 2006.

Iyasu, S, Randall, L, Welty, K, et al: Risk factors for sudden infant death syndrome among Northern Plains Indians. JAMA 288(21):2717, 2002.

Jacelon, CS, and Henneman, EA: Profiles in dignity: Nursing perspectives on nursing and critically ill older patients. Crit Care Nurse 24(4):30–5, 2004.

Jacobs, DG, Jacobs, DO, and Kudsk, KA: Practice management guidelines for nutritional support of the trauma patient. J Trauma 57(3):660–78, 2004.

Jenko, M, and Moffitt, S: Transcultural nursing principles. J Hospice & Palliative Nursing 8(3):172–80, 2006.

Jennings-Ingle, S: The sobering facts about alcohol withdrawal syndrome. Nursing Made Incredibly Easy! 5(1):50–60, 2007.

Johnson, CV, and Hayes, JA: Troubled spirits: Prevalence and predictors of religious and spiritual concerns among university students and counseling center clients. J Counseling Psychol 50:409–19, 2003.

Johnson, J, Pearson, V, and McDivitt, L: Stroke rehabilitation: Assessing stroke survivors' long-term learning needs. Rehabil Nurs 22(5):243, 1997.

Johnson, JG, Cohen, P, Chen, H, et al: Parenting behaviors associated with risk for personality disorder during adulthood. Arch Gen Psychiatry 63(5):579–87, 2006.

Jones, TS: A bolt out of the blue: Dealing with the aftermath of spinal cord injury. Nursing Made Incredibly Easy! 3(6):14–28, 2005.

Jurich, AP: The nature of suicide. Clinical update (insert in Family Therapy Magazine) 3(6):1–8, 2003.

Kalvemark, S, Hoglund, AT, Hansson, MG, et al: Living with conflicts—Ethical dilemmas and moral distress in the health care system. Soc Sci Med, 58(6):1075–84, 2004.

Kamel, HK, Phlavan, M, Malekquodarzi, B, et al: Utilizing pain assessment scales increases the frequency of diagnosing pain among elderly nursing home residents. J Pain Symptom Manage 21(6):450–5, 2001.

Kania, DS, and Scott, CM: Postexposure prophylaxis considerations for occupational and nonoccupational exposures. Adv Emerg Nurs J 29(1):20–32, 2007.

Kaplow, R: AACN synergy model for patient care: A framework to optimize outcomes. Crit Care Nurse (Suppl):27–30, February 2003.

Kare, J, and Shneiderman, A: Hyperthermia and hypothermia in the older population. Top Emerg Med 23(3):39–52, 2011.

Katerndahl, D: Panic and plaques: Panic disorder and coronary artery disease in patients with chest pain. J Am Board Fam Pract 17(2):114–26, 2004.

Kearney, PM, and Griffin, T: Between joy and sorrow: Being a parent of a child with a developmental disability. J Adv N 34:582–92, 2001.

Keegan, L: Getting comfortable with alternative and complementary therapies. Nursing 28(4):50, 1998.

Keeney, CE, and Head, BA: Palliative nursing care of the patient with cancer-related fatigue. J Hospice Palliative Nurs 13(5):270–8, 2011.

Kehl-Pruett, W: Deep vein thrombosis in hospitalized patients: A review of evidence-based guidelinesfor prevention. Dimens Crit Care Nurs 25(2):53–9, 2006.

Keller, DM: Iodinated contrast media raises risk for thyroid dysfunction. Ann Intern Med 172:153 9, 2012.

Keller, LO, Schaffer, MA, and Lia-Hoagberg, MA: Assessment, program planning, and evaluation in population-based public health practice. J Public Health Manage Pract 8(5):30–43, 2002.

Kelso, LA: Cirrhosis: Caring for patients with end-stage liver failure. Nurs Pract: Am J Primary Health Care, 33(7):24–30, 2008.

Kersting, K: A new approach to complicated grief. Monitor on Psych 35(10):51, 2004.

Kilgore, WD, Kilgore, DB, Day, LM, et al: The effects of 53 hours of sleep deprivation on moral judgment. Sleep 30(3):345–52, 2006.

Kimerling, R, Ouimette, P, Prins, A, et al: Brief report: Utility of a short screening scale for DSM-IV PTSD in primary care. J Gen Intern Med 21(1):65–7, 2006.

Kirton, C: The HIV/AIDS epidemic: A case of good news/bad news. Nursing Made Incredibly Easy! 3(2):28–40, 2005.

Kiser, LJ, Donahue, A, Hodgkinson, S, et al: Strengthening family coping resources: The feasibility of a multifamily group intervention for families exposed to trauma. J Trauma Stress 23(6):802–6, 2010.

Kline, A: Pinpointing the cause of pediatric respiratory distress. Nursing 33(9):58–63, 2003.

Klonowski, EI, and Masodi, JE: The patient with Crohn's disease. RN 62(3):32, 1999.

Knight, DJW, and Mahajan, RP: Patient positioning in anaesthesia. Contin Educ Anaesth Crit Care Pain 4(5):160–3, 2004.

Knobel, R, and Holditch-Davis, D: Thermoregulation and heat loss prevention after birth and during neonatal intensive care unit stabilization of extremely low birth weight infants. J Obstet Gynecol Neonatal Nurs 36(3):280–7, 2007.

Kohtz, C, and Thompson, M: Preventing contrast medium-induced nephropathy. Am J Nurs 107(9):40–9, 2007.

Kolcaba, K, and DiMarco, MA: Comfort theory and its application to pediatric nursing. Pediatr Nurse 31(3):187–94, 2005.

Kolcaba, KY, and Fisher EM: A holistic perspective on comfort care as an advance directive. Crit Care Nurs Q 18(4):66–67, 1996.

Kopala, B, and Burkhart, L: Ethical dilemma and moral distress: Proposed new NANDA diagnoses. Int J Nurs Terminologies Classifications 16(1): 3–13, 2005.

Korinko, A, and Yurick, A: Maintaining skin integrity during radiation therapy. Am J Nurs 97(2):40, 1997.

Kouch, M: Managing symptoms for a "good death." Nursing 36(11):58–63, 2006.

Kourouche, S, Curtis, K, Watson, WL, et al: Identifying risk and raising awareness in older person trauma: A trauma center initiative. J Trauma Nurs 18(3):163–70, 2011.

Krassioukov, AF, Furlan, JC, and Fehlings, MG: Autonomic dysreflexia in acute spinal cord injury: An under-recognized clinical entity. J Neruotrauma 20(8):707–16, 2003.

Krishnan, P, and Hawranik, P: Diagnosis and management of geriatric insomnia: A guide for nurse practitioners. J Am Acad Nurse Pract 20(12):590–9, 2008.

Kubo, K, Akima, H, Ushiyama, J, et al: Effects of resistance training during bed rest on the viscoelastic properties of tendon structures of tendon structures in the lower limb. Scand J Med Sci Sports 14(5):296–302, 2004.

Kwon, P: Hope, defense mechanisms, and adjustment: Implications for false hope and defensive hopelessness. J Personality 70(2):207–31, 2002.

Lambing, A: Bleeding disorders: Patient history key to diagnosis. Nurse Pract: Am J Primary Health Care 32(12):16–24, 2007.

Lamblass, M: Treating pediatric overweight through reductions in sedentary behavior: A review of the literature. J Pediatr Health Care, 23(1):29–36, 2008.

Langemo, D, Hanson, D, Hunter, S, et al: Incontinence and incontinence-associated dermatitis. J Prev Healing 24(3):126–40, 2011.

Lapointe, LA: Coagulopathies in trauma patients. AACN Adv Pract in Acute Crit Care 13(2):192–203, 2002.

Larden, CN, Palmer, ML, and Janssen, P: Efficacy of therapeutic touch in treating pregnant inpatients who have a chemical dependency. J Holist Nurs 22(4):320–32, 2004.

Laroche, HH, Hofer, TP, and Davis, MM: Adult fat intake associated with the presence of children in households: Findings from NHANES III. J Am Board Fam Med 20(1):9–15, 2007.

Larsen, LS: Effectiveness of a counseling intervention to assist family caregivers of chronically ill relatives. J Psychosoc Nurs Ment Health Serv 36(8):26, 1998.

Larson, CE: Evidence-based practice: Safety and efficacy of oral re-hydration therapy for the treatment of diarrhea and gastroenteritis in pediatrics. Pediatr Nurs 26(2):177–9, 2000.

Laskowski-Jones, L: Responding to trauma: Your priorities in the first hour. Nursing 36(9):52–8, 2006.

Lauder, W, Anderson, I, and Barclay, A: A framework for good practice in interagency interventions with cases of self-neglect. J Psychiatr Ment Health Nurs 12(2):192–8, 2005.

Lauder, W, Anderson, I, and Barclay, A: Housing and self-neglect: The responses of health, social care and environmental health agencies. J Interprof Care 19(4):317–25, 2005.

Laudet, AB, Morgen, K, and White, WL: The role of social supports, spirituality, religiousness, life meaning and affiliation with 12-Step fellowships in quality of life satisfaction among individuals in re-covery from alcohol and drug problems. Alcohol Treat Q 24(1–2):33–73, 2006.

Lauer, T: Rape trauma syndrome in intimate relationships. Family Therapy Magazine 5(1):36–41, 2006.

LeBlanc, K, and Baranoski, S: Prevention and management of skin tears. Adv Skin Wound Care 22(7):325–32, 2009.

Leiter, JC, and Bohm, I: Mechanisms of pathogenesis in the Sudden Infant Death Syndrome. Resp Physiol Neurobiol 159(2):127–38, 2007.

Lenehan, GP: Latex allergy: Separating fact from fiction. Nursing 32(3):58–64, 2002.

Lichtenstein, B, Laska, MK, and Clair, JM: Chronic sorrow in the HIV-positive patient: Issues of race, gender, and social support. AIDS Patient Care STDs 16(1):27–38, 2002.

Liken, MA: Caregivers in crisis: Moving a relative with Alzheimer's to assisted living. Clin Nurs Res 10(1):53–69, 2001.

Liken, MA: Experiences of family caregivers of a relative with Alzheimer's disease. J Psychosoc Nurs 39(12):32–7, 2001.

Livneh, H, and Antonak, RF: Psychosocial adaptation to chronic illness and disability: A primer for counselors . J Counseling Dev 83(1):12–20, 2005.

Lloyd-Jones, D, Adams, R, Carnethon, M, et al: Heart disease and stroke statistics--2009 update: A report from the American Heart Association Statistics Committee and Stroke Statistics Subcommit-tee. Circulation 119(3):480–6, 2009.

Locher, J, Burgio, KL, Goode, PS, et al: Effects of age and casual attribution to aging on health-related behaviors associated with uri-nary incontinence in older women. Gerontologist 42(4):515–21, 2002.

Lohve, V, Miaskowski, C, and Rusteen, T: The relationship between hope and caregiver strain in family caregivers of parents with ad-vanced cancer. Cancer Nurs 35(2):99–105, 2011.

Lopez, NJ, Smith, PC, and Guiterrez, J: Periodontal therapy may reduce the risk of preterm low birth weight in women with periodontal dis-ease: A randomized controlled trial. J Periodontol 73(8):911–24, 2002.

Lorente L, Lecuona M, Jimenez A, et al: Ventilator-associated pneu-monia using a heated humidifier or a heat and moisture exchanger: A randomized controlled trial. Crit Care 10:4, 2006.

Lorio, AK: Transfer dependent. Rehab Management 18(7):22–6, 2005.

Lowes, L, and Lynn, P: Chronic sorrow in parents of children with newly diagnosed diabetes: A review of the literature and discussion of the implications for nursing practice. J Adv Nurs 32(1):41–8, 2000.

Lund, CH, Osborn, JW, and Kuller, J: Neonatal skin care: Clinical outcomes of the AWHONN/NANN evidence-based clinical practice guideline. J Neonatal Nurs 30(1):30–40, 2001.

Luo, L: Aging and memory: A cognitive approach. Can J Psychiatry 53(6):346–53, 2008.

Lyman, B: Metabolic complications associated with parenteral nutrition. J Infusium Nurs 25(1):36–44, 2002.

MacIntyre, NR: Evidence-based guidelines for weaning and discontinuation of ventilatory support. S Chest 120(6 Suppl):S385–484. 2001.

Major, DA: Utilizing role theory to help employed parents cope with children's chronic illness. Health Res Educ 18(1):45–57, 2001.

Malinowski, A, and Stamler, LL: Comfort: Exploration of the concept in nursing. JAN 39(6):599–606, 2002.

Mallick, MJ, and Whipple, TW: Validity of the nursing diagnosis of relocation stress syndrome. Nurs Res 49(2):97–100, 2000.

Manaviat, MR, Rashidi, M, Afkhami-Ardekani, M, et al: Prevalance of dry eyes syndrome and diabetic retinopathy in type 2 diabetic patients. BMC Ophthamol June 2(8):10, 2008.

Mann, AR: Manage the power of pain. Men in Nurs 1(4):20–8, 2006.

Manno, MS: Preventing adverse drug events. Nursing 36(3):56–61, 2006.

Manoguerra, AS, and Cobaugh, DJ: Guideline on the use of ipecac syrup in the out-of-hospital management of ingested poisons. Clin Toxicol 43(1):1–10, 2005.

Massarratt, S: Smoking and the gut. Arch Iranian Med 11(3):205–305, 2008.

Masters, KJ, Bellonci, C, Bernet, W, et al: Summary of the practice parameter for the prevention and management of aggressive behavior in child and adolescent psychiatric institutions with special reference to seclusion and restraint. J Am Acad Child Adolesc Psychiatry 40(11):1356–8, 2001.

Matthews, TJ, and MacDorman, MF: SIDS deaths by race/ethnic origin of the mother: Infant mortality statistics from the 2004 period linked birth/infant death data set. National Vital Statistics 55(12), 2007.

Matzo, M, Sherman, DW, Mazanec, P, et al: Teaching cultural consideration at the end of life. End of Life Nursing Education Consortium program recommendations. J Contin Educ Nurs 33(6):270–8, 2002.

Mauk, KL: Medications for management of overactive bladder. ARN Network, June/July:3–7, 2005.

McAllister, M: Promoting physiologic-physical adaptation in chronic obstructive pulmonary disease: Pharmacotherapeutic evidence-based research and guidelines. Home Healthcare Nurse 23(8):523–31, 2005.

McCaffrey, R: Make POVN prevention a priority. OR Nurse 2012 1(2):39–45, 2007.

McCaffrey, R, and Rozzano, L: The effect of music on pain and acute confusion in older adults undergoing hip and knee surgery. Holistic Nurs Pract 20(5):218–24, 2006.

McCain, D, and Sutherland, S: Nursing essentials: Skin grafts for patients with burns. Am J Nurs 98(7):34, 1998.

McClave, SA, Lukan, JK, Lowen, JA, et al: Poor validity of residual volumes as a marker for risk of aspiration in critically ill patients. Crit Care Med 33(2):324–30, 2005.

McCool, FD, and Rosen, MJ: Nonpharmacologic airway clearance therapies. Chest 129(Suppl):S250–9, 2006.

McCoy ML: Care of the congestive heart failure patient: The care, cure, and core model. J Pract Nurs 56(1):5–6, 30, 2006.

McCullagh, MC: Home modification. Am J Nurs 106(10):54–63, 2006.

McCullough, K, Estes, J, McCullough, G, et al: RN compliance with SPL dysphagia recommendations in acute care. Top Geriatr Rehabil 23(4):330–40, 2008.

McEnany, G: Sexual dysfunction in the pharmacologic treatment of depression: When "don't ask, don't tell" is an unsuitable approach to care. J Am Psych Nurs Assoc 4(1):24–9, 1998.

McGuire, J: Transitional off-loading: An evidence-based approach to pressure redistribution in the diabetic foot. Adv Skin Wound Care 23(4):175–88, 2010.

McIntyre, LL: Parent training for young children with developmental disabilities: Randomized control trial. Am J Ment Retard 113(5):356–68, 2008.

McLean, SE, Jensen, LA, Schroeder, DG, et al: Improving adherence to a mechanical ventilation weaning protocol for critically ill adults: Outcomes after an implementation program. Am J Crit Care 15(3):299–309, 2006.

McLeod, DL, and Wright, LM: Conversations of spirituality: Spirituality in family systems nursing Making the case with four clinical vignettes. J Fam Nurs 7(4):391–415, 2001.

McNett, MM, and Gianakis, A: Nursing interventions for critically ill traumatic brain injury patients. J Neurosci Nurs 42(2):71–7, 2010.

McWilliams, JR: An evidenced based pediatric fall assessment tool for home health. Home Healthcare Nurse 20(29):98–105, 2011.

Meleski, DD: Families with chronically ill children. Am J Nurs 102(5):47–54, 2002.

Melnyk, BM: Intervention studies involving parents of hospitalized young children: An analysis of the past and future recommendations. J Pediatr Nurs 15(1):4–13, 2000.

Mentes, J, and Claros, E: Oral hydration in older adults. Am J Nurs 106(6):40–9, 2006.

Mentes, JC, Wakefield, B, and Culp, K: Use of a urine color chart to monitor hydration status in nursing home residents. Biol Res Nurs 7(3):197–203, 2006.

Merkelj, I: Urinary incontinence in the elderly. South Med J 94(10):952–7, 2001.

Metheny, NA, Boltz, M, Greenberg, SA: Preventing aspiration in older adults with dysphagia. Am J Nurs 108(2):45–6, 2008.

Michael, KM, Allen, JK, and Macko, RE: Fatigue after stroke: Relationship to mobility, fitness, ambulatory activity, social support, and falls efficacy. Rehabil Nurs 31(5):210–7, 2006.

Miller, CK, Ulbrecht, JS, Lyons, J, et al: A reduced-carbohydrate diet improves outcomes in patients with metabolic syndrome: A transitional study. Top Clin Nutr 22(1):82–91, 2007.

Miller, D: Is advanced maternal age an independent risk factor for uteroplacental insufficiency? Am J Obstet Gynecol 192(6):1974–82, 2005.

Miller, J: Keeping your patient hemodynamically stable. Nursing 27(5):36–41, 2007.

Miller, SK, and Alpert, PT: Assessment and differential diagnosis of abdominal pain. Nurse Pract: Am J Primary Health Care 31(7):39–47, 2006.

Milne, JL, and Krissovich, M: Behavioral therapies at the primary care level: The current state of knowledge. J Wound, Ostomy Continence Nurs 31(6):367–76, 2004.

Mintz, TG: Relocation stress syndrome in older adults. Social Work Today 5(6):38, 2005.

Mizuno, K, Tsugi, T, Takebayashi, T, et al: Prism adaptation therapy enhances rehabilitation of stroke patients with unilateral spatial neglect: A randomized controlled trial. Neurorehabil Neural Repair 25(8):711–20, 2011.

Moe, SM: Disorders involving calcium, phosphorus, and magnesium. Primary Care 35(2):215–37, 2008.

Mohr, WK: Cross-ethnic variations in the care of psychiatric patients: A review of contributing factors and practice considerations. J Psychosoc Nurs Ment Health Serv 36(5):16, 1998.

Moore, K: Hypothermia in trauma. J Trauma Nurs 15(2):62–4, 2008.

Morgan, A, Ward, E, and Murdoch, B: Clinical characteristics of acute dysphagia in pediatric patients following traumatic brain injury. J Head Trauma Rehabil 19(3):226–40, 2004.

Morin, CM, Vallieres, A, Guay, B, et al: Cognitive behavioral therapy, singly and combined with medication, for persistent insomnia. JAMA 301(19):2005–15, 2009.

Moshang, J: The growing problem of type 2 diabetes. LPN2005 1(3):26–34, 2005.

Mosocco, D: Clipboard: Childhood vaccines. Home Healthcare Nurse 25(1):7–8, 2007.

Moss, SE, Klein, R, and Klein BE: Long-term incidence of dry eye in an older population. Optom Vis Sci 85(8):668–74, 2008.

Mullen-Fortino, M, and O'Brien, M: Caring for the patient after coronary artery bypass graft. Nursing 38(3):46–52, 2008.

Muller, AC, and Bell, AE: Diagnostic update: Electrolyte update: Potassium, chloride and magnesium. Nurs Crit Care 3(1):5–7, 2008.

Munro, C, and Grap, MJ: Oral health and care in the intensive care unit: State of science. Am J Crit Care 13(1):25–33, 2004.

Murabito, JM, Evans, JC, Larson, MG, et al: The ankle-brachial index in the elderly and risk of stroke, coronary disease and death. Arch Intern Med 163(16):1939–42, 2003.

Muraoka, M, Mine, K, and Matsumoto, K: Psychogenic vomiting: The relation between patterns of vomiting and psychiatric diagnoses. Gut 31(5):526–8, 1990.

Murphy, K: Anxiety: When is it too much? Nursing Made Incredibly Easy! 3(5):22–31, 2005.

Murray, TW, Chalmers, JM, and Spenser, JA: A longitudinal study of medication exposure and xerostomia among older people. Gerontol 23(4):205–13, 2006.

Mussi, C, Ungar, A, Salvioli, G, et al: Orthostatic hypotension as a cause of syncope in patients older than 65 years admitted to emergency departments for transient loss of consciousness. J Gerontol A Biol Sci Med Sci 64(7):801–6, 2009.

Nadolski, M: Getting a good night's sleep: Diagnosing and treating insomnia. Plast Surg Nurs 25(4):167–73, 2005.

Narayan, MC: Culture's effects on pain assessment and management. Am J Nurs 110(4):38–48, 2010.

Naylor, MD, Stephens, C, Bowles, KH, et al: Cognitively impaired older adults. Am J Nurs 105(2):52–61, 2005.

Neal-Boylan, L: Health assessment of the very old person at home. Home Healthcare Nurse 25(6):388–98, 2007.

Nelson, A: Safe patient handling & movement. Am J Nurs 103(3):32–43, 2003.

Nelson, DP, LeMaster, TH, Plost, GN, et al: Recognizing sepsis in the adult patient. Am J Nurs 109(3):40–50, 2009.

Newman, DK: Assessment of the patient with an overactive bladder. J Wound, Ostomy Continence Nurs 32(3 Suppl):5–10, 2005.

Newman, DK, and Palmer, MH: The state of the science on urinary incontinence. Am J Nurs 103(2 Suppl):2–53, 2003.

Newman, R: The road to resilience. Monitor on Psychology 33(9):62. 2002.

Ng, LF, Lim, JB, and Wong, HB: Effects of head posture on cerebral hemodynamics: Its influences on intracranial pressure, cerebral perfusion pressure, and cerebral oxygenation. Neurosurg 54(3):593–9, 2004.

Ngo-Metzer, Q, Massagli, MP, Clarridge, BR, et al: Linguistic and cultural barriers to care: Perspectives of Chinese and Vietnamese immigrants. J Gen Int Med (JGIM) 18(1):44–52, 2003.

Nichols, S: Mindreading and the core architecture of moral psychology. Cognition, 84:221–36, 2002.

Nieves, J, and Capone-Swearer, D: The clot that changes lives. Nursing Critical Care 1(3):18–28, 2006.

Ninan, PT: Dissolving the burden of generalized anxiety disorder. J Clin Psych 62(Suppl 9):5–10, 2001.

No author listed: Changing concepts of sudden infant death syndrome: Implications for infant sleeping environment and sleep position. Task Force on Infant Sleep Position and Sudden Infant Death Syndrome. Pediatr 105(3):650–56, 2000.

No author listed: Taking Control of Stress. Harvard Health Publications: Big Sandy, TX, Special Supplement, 2007.

No author listed: Understanding transcultural nursing. Nursing 35(1):14–23. Supplement Career Directory, 2005.

Nsier, S, Makris, C, Mathieu, D, et al: Intensive care unit-acquired infection as a side effect of sedation. Crit Care 14(2):R30, 2010.

Nusbaum, N: Safety versus autonomy: Dilemmas and strategies in protection of vulnerable community-dwelling elderly. Annals Long-Term Care 12(5):50–53, 2004.

Nye, CL, Zucker, RA, and Fitzgerald, HE: Early family-based intervention in the path to alcohol problems, rationale and relationship between treatment process characteristics and child and parenting outcomes. J Stud Alcohol (13 Suppl):S10–S21, 1999.

Oddy, WH, Li, J, Landsborough, L, et al: The association of maternal overweight and obesity with breastfeeding duration. J Pediatr 149(2):185–91, 2006.

Odom-Forren, J: Preventing surgical site infections. Nursing 36(6):59–63, 2006.

Odom-Forren, J: Surgical-site infection: Still a reality. Nurs Manage 36(11 Suppl: OR Insider):16–20, 2005.

O'Grady, NP, Barie, PS, Bartlett, JG, et al: Guidelines for evaluation of new fever in critically ill adult patients: 2008 update from the American College of Critical Care Medicine and the Infectious Disease Society of America. Crit Care Med 36(4):1330–49, 2008.

Okan, K, Woo, K, Ayello, EA, et al: The role of moisture balance in wound healing. Advances for skin & wound care. J Prev Healing 20(1):39–53, 2007.

Olson, DM, Borel, CO, Lasowitz, DT, et al: Quiet time: A nursing intervention to promote sleep in neurocritical care units. Am J Crit Care 10(2):74–8, 2001.

O'Lynn, C, and Krautscheid, L: How should I touch you? A qualitative study of attitudes on intimate touch in nursing care. Am J Nurs 111(3):24–31, 2011.

O'Malley, P: The undertreatment of pain: Ethical and legal implications for the clinical nurse specialist. Clin Nurs Spec 19(5):236–7, 2005.

O'Shea, RS, Dasarthy, S, and McCullough, RS: Alcoholic liver disease. Am J Gastroenterol 105(1):14–32, 2010.

Pacorbo-Hidalgo, PL, Garcia-Fernandez, FP, and Lopez-Medina, IM: Risk assessment scales for pressure ulcers prevention: A systematic review. J Adv Nurs 54(1):94–110, 2006.

Paice, J: Managing psychological conditions in palliative care. Am J Nurs 102(11):36–43, 2002.

Palmer, CA, Burnett, DJ, and Dean, B: It's more than just candy: Important relationships between nutrition and oral health. Nutr Today 4:154–64, 2010.

Palmer, JB, Drennen, JC, and Baba, M: Evaluation and treatment of swallowing impairments. Am Fam Physician 61(8):2453–62, 2000.

Palmer, JL, and Metheny, NA: How to try this: Preventing aspiration in older adults with dysphagia. Am J Nurs 108:1–40, 2008.

Panzera, AK: Interstitial cystitis/painful bladder syndrome. Urol Nurs 27(1):13–19, 2007.

Parkins, JM, and Gfroer, SD: Chronic pain: The impact on academic, social, and emotional functioning. Natl Assoc Sch Psychol: Communique 38(1):24–5, 2009.

Parkman, CA, and Calfee, BE: Advance directives, honoring your patient's end-of-life wishes. Nursing 27(4):48, 1997.

Parsons, KS, Galinsky, TL, and Waters, T: Suggestions for preventing musculoskeletal disorders in home healthcare workers, Part 1: Lift and transfer assistance for partially weight-bearing home care patients. Home Healthcare Nurse 24(3):158–64, 2006.

Parsons, KS, Galinsky, TL, and Waters, T: Suggestions for preventing musculoskeletal disorders in home healthcare workers. Part 2: Lift and transfer assistance for non-weight-bearing home care patients. Home Healthcare Nurse 24(4):227–33, 2006.

Parzella, MA: Renal vulnerability to drug toxicity: Drug table. CJASN 4(7):1275–83, 2009.

Pasero, C, and McCaffrey, M: No self-report means no pain-intensity rating. Am J Nurs 105(10):50–3, 2005.

Patel, M, Chipman, J, Carlin, BW, et al: Sleep in the intensive care setting. Crit Care Nurs Q 31(4):309–18, 2008.

Patterson, M, Mechan, P, Hughes, N, et al: Safe vertical transfer of patient with extremity cast or splint. Orthop Nurs 28(2 Suppl):S18–S23, 2006.

Pearsen, OR, Busse, ME, van Deursen, RWM, et al: Quantification of walking mobility in neruological disorders. QJM: Int J Med 97:463–75, 2004.

Peden, AR, Hall, LA, Rayens, MK, et al: Reducing negative thinking and depressive symptoms in college women. J Nurs Scholar 32(2):145–51, 2000.

Perry, A: Quality of life. Rehabil Manage 18(7):18–21, 2005.

Peters, M, Fitzpatrick, R, Doll, H, et al: The impact of perceived lack of support provided by health and social care services to caregivers of people with motor neuro disease. Amyotroph Lateral Scler 13(2):223–8, 2012.

Pharoah, PO, and Platt, MJ: Sudden Infant Death Syndrome in twins and singletons. Twin Res Hum Gen 10(4):644–8, 2007.

Phillips, CD, and McLeroy, KR: Health in rural America: Remembering the importance of place. Am J Public Health 94(10):1661–3, 2004.

Phillips, NA: Female sexual dysfunction: Evaluation and treatment. Am Fam Phys 62(1):127–36;141–2, 2000.

Pieper, B, Sieggreen, M, Freeland, B, et al: Discharge information needs of patients after surgery. J Wound, Ostomy Continence Nurs 33(3):281–90, 2006.

Pierce, LL: Barriers to access: Frustrations of people who use a wheelchair for full-time mobility. Rehabil Nurs 23(3):120, 1998.

Pignone, MP, Ammerman, A, Fernandez, L, et al: Counseling to promote a healthy diet in adults: A summary of the evidence for the US Preventive Services Task Force. Am J Prev Med 24(1):75, 2003.

Pirie, S: Patient care in the preoperative environment. J Perioper Pract 20(7):245–8, 2010.

Pisacane, A, Continisio, GI, Aldinucci, M, et al: A controlled trial of the father's role in breastfeeding promotion. Pediatr 116(4):e494–8, 2005.

Plummer, P, Morris, ME, and Dunai, J: Assessment of unilateral neglect. Phys Ther 83(8):732–40, 2003.

Poe, SS, Cvach, MM, Gartrell, DG, et al: An evidence-based approach to fall risk assessment, prevention, and management: Lessons learned. J Nurs Care Quality 20(2):107–16, 2005.

Power, N, and Franck, L: Parent participation in care of hospitalized children: A systematic review. J Adv Nurs 62(6):622–41, 2008.

Powers, SR, and Scully, C: Oral malodour (halitosis). BMJ 333(7569):632–5, 2006.

Prahlow, JA, Prahlow, TJ, and Rakow, RJ: Case study: Asphyxia caused by inspissated oral and nasopharyngeal secretions. Am J Nurs 109(6):38–43, 2009.

Pringle-Specht, JK: Nine myths of incontinence in older adults. Am J Nurs, 105(6):58–68, 2005.

Pruitt, B: Weaning patients from mechanical ventilation. Nursing 36(9):36–41, 2006.

Pryor, J, and Jannings, W: Preparing patients to self-manage faecal continence following spinal cord injury. J Aust Rehabil Nurs Assoc 7:2, 2004.

Purgason, K: Broken hearts: Differentiating stress-induced cardiomyopathy from acute myocardial infarction in the patient presenting with acute coronary syndrome. Dimensions Crit Care Nurs 25(6):247–53, 2006.

Quigley, PA, Bulat, T, and Hart-Hughes, S: Strategies to reduce risk of fall-related injuries in rehabilitation nursing. Rehabil Nurs 32(3):120–5, 2007.

Rabe, KF, Hurd, S, Anzueto, A, et al: Global strategy for the diagnosis, management, and prevention of chronic obstructive pulmonary disease. Am J Respir Crit Care Med 176:532–5, 2007.

Ragsdale, JA: Hereditary hemorrhagic telangiectasia from epistaxis to life-threatening GI bleeding. Gastroenterol Nurs 30(4):293–9, 2007.

Raina, P, O'Donnell, M, Rosenbaum, P, et al: The health and well-being of caregivers of children with cerebral palsy. Pediatr 115(6):e626–36, 2005.

Rangel-Castillo, L, and Robertson, CS: Management of intracranial hypertension. Crit Care Clin 22(4):713–32, 2006.

Ranney, R: Classification of peridontal diseases. Peridontology 2:13–25, 2000.

Rasin, J, and Barrick, AL: Bathing persons with dementia. Am J Nurs 104(3):30–4, 2004.

Reddy, L: Heads up on cerebral bleeds. Nursing 3(5 Suppl: E D):4–9, 2006.

Reddy, M, Gill, SS, and Rochan, PA: Preventing pressure ulcers: A systematic review. JAMA 296(8):974–84, 2006.

Rehman, HU: Involuntary weight loss in the elderly. Clin Geriatr Med 13(37):45, 2008.

Reitz, A, Stohrer, M, Kramer, G, et al: European experience of 200 cases treated with Botulinum-A toxin injections into the detrusor muscle for urinary incontinence due to neurogenic detrusor overactivity. European Urol 45(4):510–5, 2004.

Reznikoff, PTM. Perceived peer and family relationships, hopelessness and locus of control as factors in adolescent suicide attempts. Suicide and life-threatening behavior 12(3):141–50,1982.

Ricci, R, Calhoun, J, and Chatterjee, A: Orientation bias in unilateral neglect: Representational contributions. Cortex 36(5):671–7, 2000.

Rice, J, Hicks, PB, and Wiche, V: Life care planning: A role for social workers. Soc Work Health Care 31(1):85–94, 2000.

Riely, M: Facilitating children's grief. J Sch Nurs 19(4):212–8, 2003.

Riesch, SK, Anderson, LS, Pridham, KA, et al: Furthering the understanding of parent-child relationships: A nursing scholarship review series, Part 5: Parent-adolescent and teen parent-child relationships. J Spec Pediatr Nurs 15(3):182–201, 2010.

Riggs, JM: Manage heart failure. Nursing Crit Care 1(4):18–28, 2006.

Ristolainen, L, Heiononen, A, Waller, B, et al: Gender differences in sport injury risk and types of injuries: A retrospective twelve-month study on cross-country skiers, long distance runners and soccer players. J Sports Sci Med 8:443–51, 2009.

Roberts, I, Yates, D, Sandercock, P, et al: Effect of intravenous corticosteroids on death within 14 days in 10,008 adults with a clinically significant head injury (MRC CRASH trial): Randomized placebo-controlled trial. Lancet 364:1321–8, 2004.

Robertson, RG, and Montagnini, M: Geriatric failure to thrive. Am Fam Phys 70(2):343–50, 2004.

Robinson, AW: Getting to the heart of denial. Am J Nurs 99(5):38, 1999.

Roger, VL, Go, AS, and Lloyd-Jones, DM. Heart disease and stroke statistics—2011 update: A report from the American Heart Association. Circulation 123; e18–209, 2011.

Rogers, S, Ryan, M, and Slepoy, L: Successful ventilator weaning: A collaborative effort. Rehabil Nurs 23(5):265, 1998.

Romero, DV, Treston, J, and O'Sullivan, AL: Hand-to-hand combat: Preventing MRSA infection: Advances in skin & wound care: J Prev Healing 19(6):328–33, 2006.

Rosen, L: Sit on it. Rehabil Manage 18(2):36–41, 2005.

Rosenberger, PH, Jokl, P, Cameron, A, et al: Shared decision making, preoperative expectations, and postoperative reality: Differences in physician and patient predictions and ratings of knee surgery outcomes. Arthroscopy 21(5):562–9, 2005.

Rosenthal, K: Guarding against vascular site infection. Nurs Manage 37(4):54–66, 2006.

Rosenthal, K: Tailor your IV insertion-techniques for special populations. Nursing 35(5):36–41, 2005.

Ross, LA: Spiritual aspects of nursing. J Adv Nurs 19(3):439–47, 1994.

Rousseau, P: Hope in the terminally ill. West J Med 173(2):117–8. 2000.

Rovner, ES, and Wein, AJ: Treatment options for stress urinary incontinence. Rev Urol 6(Suppl 3):S29–S47, 2004.

Rowe, MA: People with dementia who become lost. Am J Nurs 103(7):32, 2003.

Rueter, MA, and Koerner, AF: The effect of family communication patterns on adopted adolescent adjustment. J Marriage Fam 70(3):715–27, 2008.

Ryan, RM, and Deci, EL: Self-determination theory and the facilitation of intrinsic motivation, social development, and well being. Am Psychol 55(1):68–76, 2000.

Saatciolgllu, O, Rahsan, E, and Dkuran, C: Role of family in alcohol and substance abuse. Psychiatry and Clinical Neurosciences 60(2):125–32, 2006

Sachdeva, A, Dalton, M, and Amaragiri, SV: Elastic compression stockings for prevention of deep vein thrombosis. Cochrane Database Syst Rev. 7(7):CD001484, 2010.

Sacks, FM, and Katan, M: Randomized clinical trials on the effects of dietary fat and carbohydrate on plasma proteins and cardiovascular disease. Am J Med 113(Suppl 9B):13–24, 2002.

Sahel, JA, Bandello, F, Ausutin, A, et al: Health-related quality of life and utility in patients with age-related mascular degeneration. Arch Ophthalmol 124(7):945–51, 2007.

Sahuquillo, J, Vilatra, A: Cooling the injured brain: How does moderate hypothermia influence the pathophysiology of traumatic brain injury? Curr Pharm Des 13:2310–22, 2007.

Sakowitz, O, and Unterberg, A: Detecting and treating microvascular ischemia after subarachnoid hemorrhage. Curr Opin Crit Car 12(2):103–11, 2006.

Salmon, DA, Moulton, LH, Omer, SB, et al: Factors associated with refusal of childhood vaccines among parents of school-aged children: A case-control. Arch Pediatr Adolesc Med 159(5):470–6, 2005.

Saltz, LB: Progress in cancer care—The hype, the hope, and the gap between perception and reality. J Clin Oncol 26(31):520–1, 2008.

Samarel N, Fawcett J, Davis MM, and Ryan FM: Effects of dialogue and therapeutic touch on preoperative and postoperative experiences of breast cancer surgery: An exploratory study. Oncol Nurs Forum 25(8):1369–76, 1998.

Sampselle, CM: Behavioral interventions in young and middle-age women: Simple interventions to combat a complex problem. Am J Nurs 103(3Suppl):S9–S19, 2003.

Sampselle, CM, Wyman, JF, Thomas KK, et al: Continence for women: Evaluation of AWHONN's third research utilization project. JOGNN 29:9–17, 2000.

Sauerbeck, LR: Primary stroke prevention. Am J Nurs 106(11):40–9, 2006.

Scanlon, C: Defining standards for end-of-life care. Am J Nurs 97(11):58, 1997.

Scharer, K, and Brooks, G: Mothers of chronically ill neonates and primary nurses in the NICU: Transfer of care. Neonatal Network 13(5):37–46, 1994.

Scheck, A: Therapists on the team: Diabetic wound prevention is everybody's business. Rehabil Nurs 16(7):18, 1999.

Schenck, CH, and Mahowald, MW: Parasomnias: Managing bizarre sleep-related behavior disorders. Postgrad Med 107(3):145–60, 2002.

Schiffman, RF: Drug and subtance use in adolescents MCN, Am J Maternal/Child Nurs 29(1):21–7, 2004.

Schillinger, D, Matchinger, EL, and Wang, F: Language, literacy, and communication regarding medication in an anticoagulation clinic: A comparison of verbal vs. visual assessment. J Health Commun 11(7):651–4, 2006.

Schlessinger, DA, and Ulitsch, E: The eyes have it. OR Nurse 3(4):26-32, 2009.

Schmelling, S: Home, adapted home. Rehabil Manage 18(6):12–9, 2005.

Schraeder, C, Lamb, G, Shelton, P, et al: Community nursing organizations: A new frontier. Am J Nurs 97(1):63, 1997.

Schulman, C, and Schiech, C: End points of resuscitation: Choosing the right parameters to monitor. Dimens Crit Care Nurs 21(1):2–10, 2002.

Schulz, R, and Sherwood, PR: Physical and mental health effects of family caregiving. Am J Nurs 108(9 Suppl):S23–S27, 2008.

Schumacher, K, Beck, CA, and Marren, JM: Family caregivers: Caring for older adults, working with their families. Am J Nurs 106(8):40–9, 2006.

Schutte-Rodin, Broch, L, Buysse, D, et al: Clinical guideline for the evaluation and management of chronic insomnia in adults. J Clin Sleep Med 15(4):487–504, 2008.

Schuyler, D: Cognitive therapy for depression. Primary Psychiatry 10(5):33–6, 2003.

Schwebel, DC, and Barton, BK: Contributions of multiple risk factors to child injury. J Pediatr Psychol 30(7):553–61, 2005.

Selekman, MD: Adolescent self-harm: A growing epidemic. Family Therapy Magazine 1(2):34–40. 2004.

Sendecka, M, Baryluk, A, Poltz-Dacewicz, M: Prevalence and risk factors of dry eye syndrome. Prezql Epidemiol 58(1):227–33, 2004.

Sendelbach, S, and Guthrie, PF: Acute confusion/delirium. J Gerontol Nurs 35(11):11–18. 2009.

Shahar, E, Whitney, CW, Redline, S, et al: Sleep-disordered breathing and cardiovascular disease: Cross sectional results of the sleep heart health study 163:19–23, 2001.

Sharts-Hopko, NC: Issues in pediatric immunization. MCN 34(2):80–8, 2009.

Sherratt, K, Thornton, and A, Hatton, C: Emotional and behavioral responses to music in people with dementia: An observational study. Aging Ment Health 8(3):223–41, 2004.

Ship, KM: Gait disturbances in older age: The reasons arc many and varied, but researchers agree that identifying the source and preserving mobility are primary concerns. Duke Med Health News 16(8):3–4, 2010.

Shovein, JT, Camozo, RJ, and Hyams, I: Hepatitis A: How benign is it? Am J Nurs 100(3):43–7, 2000.

Sieggreen, M: A contemporary approach to peripheral arterial disease. Health Pract: Am J of Primary Health Care 31(7):14–25, 2006.

Sieggreen, M: Understanding critical limb ischemia. Nursing 38(10):50–5, 2008.

Sieggreen, MY: Getting a leg up on managing venous ulcers. Nursing Made Incredibly Easy! 4(6):52–60, 2006.

Sinacore, DR: Managing the diabetic foot. Rehabil Manag 11(4):60, 1998.

Singh, H, Houy, TL, Singh, N, et al: Gastrointestinal prophylaxis in critically ill patients. Crit Care Nurs Q 31(4):291–301, 2008.

Singleton, JK: Nurses' perspectives of encouraging client's care of self in a short-term rehabilitation unit within a long-term care facility. Rehabil Nurs 21(1):23–30, 35, 2000.

Sittner, BJ, Hudson, DB, and DeFrain, J: Using the concept of family strengths to enhance nursing care. MCN 32(6):353–7, 2007.

Sloan, PD, Ivey, J, Helton, M, et al: Nutritional issues in long term care. JAMDA 9(7):476–85, 2001.

Smatlak, P, and Knebel, AR: Clinical evaluation of noninvasive monitoring of oxygen saturation in critically ill patients. Am J Crit Care 7(5):370, 1998.

Smeltzer, MD. Making a point about open fractures. Nursing 40(2):124 30, 2010.

Smith, AM, and Schwirian, PM: The relationship between caregiver burden and TBI survivors' cognition and functional ability after discharge. Rehabil Nurs 23(5):252, 1998.

Smith, DW, Arnstein, P, Rosa, KC, et al: Effects of integrating therapeutic touch into a cognitive behavioral pain treatment program. Report of a pilot clinical trial. J Holist Nurs 20(4):367–87, 2002.

Smith, JM: Indwelling catheter management: From habit-based to evidence-based practice. Ostomy Wound Manage 49(12):34–45, 2003.

Smith, JS: The psychology of burns. J Trauma Nurs 13(3):105–6, 2006.

Smith, R, Curci, M, and Silverman, A: Pain management: The global connection. Nurs Manage 33(6):26–9, 2002.

Smith, SM, Mathews-Oliver, SA, Zwart, SR, et al: Nutritional status is altered in the self-neglecting elderly. J Nutr 136(10):2534–41, 2006.

Smith Hammond, CA, and Goldstein, LB: Cough and aspiration of food and liquids due to oral-pharyngeal dysphagia: AACP evidence-based clinical practice guidelines, EBP compendium. Chest 129(1 Suppl):154S–168S, 2006.

Smochek, MR, Oblaczynsk, C, Lauck, DL, et al: Interventions for risk for suicide and risk for violence. Nurs Diagn. Int J Nurs Lang Class 11(2):60, April–June 2000.

Sommer, KD, and Sommer, NW: When your patient is hearing impaired. RN 65(12):28–32, 2002.

Sommers, J, and Vodanovich, SJ: Boredom proneness: Its relationship to psychological-and physical-health symptoms. J Clin Psych 56(1):149–55, 2000.

Song, A-J, and Algase, D: Premorbid characteristics and wandering behavior in persons with dementia. Arch Psychiatr Nurs 22(6):318–27, 2008.

Spahn, DR, Cerny, V, Coats, TJ, et al: Management of bleeding following major trauma: A European guideline. Crit Care 11(1):17, 2006.

Spaniol, JR, Knight, AR, Zebley, JL, et al: Fluid resuscitation therapy for hemorrhagic shock. J Trauma Nurs 14(3):152–60, 2007.

Spielman, AJ, Caruso, LS, and Glovinsky, PB: A behavioral perspective on insomnia treatment. Psychiatr Clin North Am 10(4):541–3, 1987.

Spurlock, WR: Spiritual well-being and caregiver burden in Alzheimer's caregivers. Geriatr Nurs 26(3):154–61, 2005.

Stabin, MG, and Breitz, H: Breast milk secretion of radiopharmaceuticals; Mechanisms, findings, and radiation dosimetry. J Nuclear Med 41(5):863–73, 2000.

Stawicki, SP: Mechanical ventilation: Weaning and extubation. OPUS 12 Scientist 1(2):13–16, 2007.

Stegeman, CA: Oral manifestations of diabetes. Home Healthcare Nurse 23(4):233–40, 2005.

Stein, PS, and Henry, RG: Poor oral hygiene in long-term care. Am J Nurs 109(6):44–50, 2009.

Steiner, ME, and Despotis, GJ: Transfusion algorithims and how they apply to blood conservation: The high-risk cardiac surgical patient. Oncol Clin North Am 21(1):177, 2007.

Stiefel, KA, Damron, S, Sowers, NJ, et al: Improving oral hygiene for the seriously ill patient: Implementing research-based practice. Medsurg Nurs 9(1):40–3, 2000.

Stockman, J: In too deep: Understanding deep vein thrombosis. Nursing Made Incredibly Easy! 6(2):29–38, 2008.

Stuban, SL: Home mechanical ventilation. Am J Nurs 110(5):63–7, 2010.

Sullivan, CS, Logan, J, and Kolasa, KM: Medical nutrition therapy for the bariatric patient. Nutrition Today 41(5):207–12, 2006.

Summer, CH: Recognizing and responding to spiritual distress. Am J Nurs 98(1):26, 1998.

Sund-Lavander, M, Grodzinsky, E, Lloyd, D, et al: Errors in body temperature measurement in febrile intensive care patients. In J Nurs Pract 10(5):216–23, 2004.

Sur, DK, and Bukont, EL: Evaluating fever of unidentifiable source in young children. Am Fam Physician 75(12):1805–11, 2007.

Swan, L. Unilateral spatial neglect. Phys Ther 81(9):1572–80, 2001.

Swann, J: Managing dressing problems in older adults in long-term care. Nurs Resident Care 10(11):564–7, 2008.

Szymanski, L, and King, B: Practice parameters for the assessment and treatment of children, adolescents, and adults with mental retardation and comorbid mental disorders. J Am Acad Child Adolesc Psychiatry 38(12 Suppl):5S–31S, 1999.

Tan, G, Waldman, K, and Bostick, R: Psychosocial issues, sexuality, and cancer. Sexuality Disabil 20(4):297–318, 2002.

Talerico, KA: Relocation to a long-term care facility: Working with patients and families before, during, and after. J Psychosoc Nurs 42(3):10–16, 2004.

Teasdale, G, and Jennett, B: Assessment of coma and impaired consciousness: A practical scale. Lancet 2(7872):81–4. 1974.

ter Wolbeek, M, van Doornem, LJP, Kavelaars, A, et al: Severe fatigue in adolescents: A common phenomenon? Pediatrics 117(6):e1078–86, 2006.

Thomas, SP: Identifying and intervening with girls at risk for violence. J Sch Nurs 19(3):130–9, 2003.

Townsend-Roccichelli, J, Sandford, JT, and VandeWaa, E: Managing sleep disorders in the elderly. Am J Primary Health 35(5):30–7, 2010.

Traustadottir, T, Bosch, PR, Matt, K, et al: The HPA axis response to stress in women: Effects of aging and fitness. Psychoneuroendocrinology 30(4):392–402, 2005.

Travis, S: "Caring for you, caring for me": A ten-year caregiver educational initiative of the Rosalynn Carter Institute for Human Development. Health and Social Work, May 1, 2006.

Trendall, J: Concept analysis: Chronic fatigue. J AdvNurs 32(5):1126–31, 2005.

Trenouth, MJ, and Campbell, AN. Questionnaire evaluation of feeding methods for cleft lip and palate neonates. Int J Pediatr Dent 6(4):241–4, 1996.

Trieger, N: Oral care in the intensive care unit. Am J Crit Care 13(1):24, 2004.

Tsirlin, I, Dupierrix, E, Chokron, S, et al: Uses of virtual reality for diagnosis, rehabilitation and study of unilateral spacial neglect: Review and analysis. Cyber Psychol Behav 12(2):175–81, 2009.

Turkowski, BB: Managing insomnia. Orthop Nurs 25(5):339–45, 2006.

Turnbough, L, and Wilson, L. Take your medicine: Nonadherence issues in patients with ulcerative colitis. Gastroenterol Nurs 30(3):212–7, 2007.

Unoki, T, Serita, A, and Grap, MJ: Automatic tube compensation during weaning from mechanical ventilation: Evidence and clinical implications. Crit Care Nurs 28(4):34–42, 2008.

Urbenjaphol, P, Jitpanya, C, and Khaorophthum, S: Effects of the Sensory Stimulation Program on recovery in unconscious patients with traumatic brain injury. J Neurosci Nurs 41(3):E10–16. 2009.

Urkin, J, and Merrick, J: The choking game or suffocation roulette in adolescence. Int J Adolesc Med Health 18(2):207–8, 2006.

Vacca, VM, and Vilolett, S: Teamwork integral to treating cerebral arteriovenous malformation. Nurs Crit Care 3(3):20–7, 2008.

Vayda, EP, Patterson, MB, and Whitehouse, PJ: The future of dementia: A case of hardening of the categories. Am J Geriatr Psychiatry 18(9):755–8, 2010.

Verbunt, JA, Seelen, HA, Vlaeyen, JW, et al: Disuse and deconditioning in chronic low back pain: Concepts and hypotheses on contributing mechanisms. Eur J Pain 7(9):9–21, 2003.

Vocat, R, Staub, F, Stroppini, T, et al: Anosognosia for hemiplegia: A clinical-anatomical prospective study. Brain, 133:3578–97, 2010.

Wadland, DL: Maintaining skin integrity in the OR. OR Nurse 2011 4(2):26–32, 2010.

Walker, CA, Curry, LC, and Hogstel, MO: Relocation stress syndrome in older adults transitioning from home to long term care facility: Myth or reality? J Psychosoc Nurs Ment Health Serv 45(1):38–45, 2007.

Wallhagen, MI, Pettengill, E, and Whiteside, M: Sensory impairment in older adults. Part 1: Hearing loss. Am J Nurs 106(10):40–9, 2006.

Wallston, BS, and Wallston, KA: Locus of control and health: A review of the literature. Health Education Monographs, University of South Florida, Spring 1978, 107–17 (rev Jan 11, 1999).

Warms, CA, Marshal, JM, Hoffman, AJ, et al: There are a few things you did not ask about my pain: Writing in the margins of a survey questionnaire. Rehabil Nurs 30(6):248–56, 2006.

Watkins, E: Combining cognitive therapy with medication in bipolar disorder. Advances in Psychiatric Treatment 9:106–10, 2003.

Watson, L: Childhood constipation. Community Pract 83(7):40–2, 2010.

Watson, R, Modeste, N, Catolico, O, et al: The relationship between caregiver burden and self-care deficits in former rehabilitation patients. Rehabil Nurs 23(5):258, 1998.

Waugh, KG: Measuring the right angle. Rehabil Manage 18(1):40–7, 2005.

Wehling-Weepie, AK, and McCarthy, A: A healthy lifestyle program: Promoting child health in schools. J School Nurs 18(6):322, 2002.

Weinhouse, GL, and Schwab, RJ: Sleep in the critically ill patient. Sleep, 29:707–15, 2006.

Welch, MB, Brummett, CM, Welch, TD, et al: Preoperative peripheral nerve injuries: A retrospective study of 380,680 cases during a 10–year period at a single institution. Anesthesiology 111(3):490–7, 2009.

Wheeler, MS: Pain assessment and management in the patient with mild to moderate cogntive impairment. Home Healthcare Nurse 24(6):354–9, 2006.

Wheeler, SL, and Houston, K: The role of diversional activities in the general medical hospital setting. Holistic Nurs Practice 19(2):67–9, 2005.

Whetstone, L, and Morrissey, S: Children at risk: The association between perceived weight status and suicidal thoughts and attempts in middle school youth. J School Health 77(2): 59–66, 2007.

White, R: Nurse assessment of oral health: A review of practice and education. Br J Nurs 9(5):260–6, 2000.

Whiteman, K, and McCormick, C: When your patient is in liver failure. Nursing 35(4):58–63, 2005.

Whiteside, MM, Wallhagen, MI, and Pettengill, E: Sensory impairment in older adults. Part 2: Vision loss. Am J Nurs 106(11):52–61, 2006.

Whitfield, W: Research in religion and mental health. Naming of parts—Some reflections. Int J Psychiatr Nurs Res 8(1), 891–6, 2002.

Widerstrom-Noga, E, Cruz-Almeida, Y, and Krassioukov, A: Is there a relationship between chronic pain and autonomic dysreflexia in persons with cervical spinal cord injury? J Neurotrauma 21(2):195–204, 2004.

Williams, AM, and Deaton, SB: Phantom limb pain: Elusive, yet real. Rehabil Nurs 22(2):73, 1997.

Wilson, L, and Kolcaba, K: Practical application of comfort theory in the perianesthesia setting. J Perianesthesia Nurs 19(3):164–74, 2004.

Wing, R, and Phalen, S: Long-term weight loss maintenance. Am J Clin Nutr 82(1 Suppl):222–5, 2005.

Winkelman, C, and Chlan, L: Bed rest in health and critical illness: A body systems approach. AACN Advanced Critical Care 20(3):254–66, 2009.

Wipke-Tevis, DD, and Sae-Sia, W: Caring for vascular leg ulcers. Home Healthcare Nurse 22(4):237–47, 2004.

Wittchen, HU, and Hover, J: Generalized anxiety disorder: Nature and course. J Clin Psychiatry 62(Suppl 11):15–19, 2001.

Woods, A: X marks the spot: Understanding metabolic syndrome. Nursing Made Incredibly Easy! 1(1):19–26, 2001.

Woods, DL, Ruth, F, Craven, RF, et al: The effect of therapeutic touch and cortisol in persons with Alzheimer's disease. Altern Ther Health Med 11(1):104–14, 2005.

Woods, DL, and Dimond, M: The effect of therapeutic touch on agitated behavior and cortisol in persons with Alzheimer's disease. Biol Res Nurs 4(2):104–14, 2002.

Wotton, K, Crannitch, K, and Munt, R: Prevalence, risk factors and strategies to prevent dehydration in older adults. Contemp Nurs 31(1):44–56, 2008.

Wright, MNJ, Martin, M, Goff, T, et al: Cocaine and thrombosis: A narrative systematic review of clinical and in vivo studies. Subst Abuse Treat Prevent Policy 2:27, 2007. doi: 10.1186/1747-597X-2-27

Wung, S, and Kozik, T: Electrocardiographic evaluation of cardiovascular status. J Cardiovasc Nurs 23(2):169–74, 2008.

Wyman, JF: Behavioral interventions for the patient with overactive bladder. J Wound, Ostomy Continence Nurs 32(3 Suppl):11–15, 2005.

Wyman, JF: Treatment of urinary incontinence in men and older women: The evidence shows the efficacy of a variety of techniques. Am J Nurs 103(3 Suppl):26–35, 2003.

Wyman, JF, Fantl, JA, McClish, DK, et al: Comparative efficacy of behavioral interventions in the management of female urinary incontinence. Am J Obstet Gynecol 179(4):999, 1998.

Yawn, B, Wollan, PC, Jacobsen, SJ, et al: Identification of women's coronary heart disease risk factors prior to first myocardial infarction. J Women's Health 13(10):1087–96, 2004.

Yedidia, M, and Tiedmann, A: How do family caregivers describe their needs for professional help? Am J Nurs 108(9 Suppl):S15–S37, 2008.

Zarit, S, and Femia, E: Behavioral and psychosocial interventions for family caregivers. Am J Nurs 108(9):47–53, 2008.

Ziere, G, Dieleman, JP, Hofman, A, et al: Polypharmacy and falls in the middle age and elderly population. Br J Clin Pharmacol 61(2):218–23, 2006.

Zikmund-Fisher, BJ: Deficits and variations in patients' experience with making 9 common medical decisions: The DECISIONS Survey. Med Decis Making 30(5 Suppl):S85–S95, 2010.

Zimmerman, JH, and Maddrey, WJ: Acetaminophen (paracetamol) hepatotoxicity with regular intake of alcohol: Analyses of instances of therapeutic misadventure. Hepatology 22(3):767–73, 1995.

Zink, EK, and McQuillan, K: Managing traumatic brain injury. Nursing 35(9):36–43, 2005.

Zurakowski, T: The practicalities and pitfalls of polypharmacy. The Nurse Pract 34(4):36–41, 2009.

Zwakhalen, SMG, Hamers, JPH, Abu-Saad, HH, et al: Pain in elderly people with severe dementia: A systematic review of behavioural pain assessment tools. BMC Geriatrics 6(3):1–37, 2006.

Electronic Resources

Adams, L. (No date). Taking personal responsibility. Retrieved April 2012, from http://www.gordontraining.com/free-workplace-articles/taking-personal-responsibility/

Adams, L. (2003). Being a leader doesn't make you one. Retrieved April 2012, from http://www.gordontraining.com/free-workplace-articles/being-a-leader-doesnt-make-you-one/

Adams, L. (2006). Climate—The emotional one that is. Retrieved March 2012, from http://www.gordontraining.com/free-workplace-articles/climate-the-emotional-one-that-is/

Adams, L. (2008). How to deal with adversity. Retrieved April 2012, from http://www.gordontraining.com/free-workplace-articles/how-do-you-deal-with-adversity/

Adams, L. (2011). The language of love. Retrieved March 2012, from http://www.gordontraining.com/free-parenting-articles/the-language-of-love/

Advance for Nurses Patient Handouts. Retrieved March 2012, from http://nursing.advanceweb.com/article/keeping-your-children-safe-from-accidental-poisoning-html-2.aspx

Agency for Healthcare Research and Quality (AHRQ). (2003). Pharmacologic management of heart failure and left ventricular systolic dysfunction: Effect in female, black, and diabetic patients, and cost-effectiveness. Summary, Evidence Report/Technology Assessment. Rockville, MD. Retrieved March 2012, from http://archive.ahrq.gov/clinic/tp/hrtfailtp.htm

Agency for Healthcare Research and Quality (AHRQ). (2010). Exercise-induced bronchoconstriction and asthma: EPC Evidence Reports. Retrieved September 2010, from http://www.ahrq.gov/clinic/tp/eibeiatp.htm#Report

Agency for Healthcare Research and Quality (AHRQ). (2010). Screening for family and intimate partner violence. The Guide to Clinical Preventive Services 2010–2011. Retrieved February 2012, from http://www.ahrq.gov/clinic/pocketgd1011/pocketgd1011.pdf

Agency for Healthcare Research and Quality (AHRQ). (2001). Treatment of pulmonary disease following cervical spinal cord injury: Evidence report/technology assessment number 27. Retrieved September 2012 from http://archive.ahrq.gov/clinic/epcsums/spinalsum.htm

Alaoui, S. (2011). Women's status in Islam: The line between culture and religion. Retrieved May 2012, from http://prospectjournal.ucsd.edu/index.php/2011/02/womens-status-in-islam-the-line-between-culture-and-religion/

Alexopoulos, GS, Jeste, DV, Chung, H, et al. (2005). Treatment of dementia and agitation: A guide for families and caregivers. A Post-graduate Medicine Special Report. Retrieved February 2012, from http://www.psychguides.com/sites/psychguides.com/files/docs/Dementia%20Handout.pdf

Alzheimer's Disease and Related Disorders Association (ADRDA). (2003, update 2011). About Alzheimer's disease. Retrieved September 2011, from http://www.alz.org/professionals_and_researchers_resources_for_your_patients.asp

Alzheimer's Disease and Related Disorders Association (ADRDA). (2009). Disease tests for Alzheimer's disease and dementia. Retrieved July 2011, from http://www.alz.org/alzheimers_disease_steps_to_diagnosis.asp

Alzheimer's Disease and Related Disorders Association (ADRDA). (No date). Treatments for Alzheimer's disease. Retrieved July 2011, from http://www.alz.org/alzheimers_disease_treatments_for_behavior.asp

Alzheimer's Foundation of America: About Alzheimer's: Physicians and care professionals educational materials. (update 2011). Retrieved January 2012, from http://www.alzfdn.org/AboutAlzheimers/definition.html

Ambalayanan, N. (2008). Fluid, electrolyte, and nutrition management of the newborn. Retrieved August 2011, from http://emedicine.medscape.com/article/976386-overview

Ameres, MJ, and Yeh, B. (2005). Pain after surgery. Retrieved March 2012, from http://www.emedicinehealth.com/pain_after_surgery/page2_em.htm

American Academy of Family Physicians (2011). Breastfeeding (position paper). Retrieved May 2011, from www.aafp.org/online/en/home/policy/policies/b/breastfeedingpositionpaper.html

American Academy of Pediatrics (1999). Ten steps to support parents' choice to breastfeed their baby. Retrieved May 2011, from www.aap.org/breastfeeding/tenSteps.pdf

American College of Cardiology Foundation and American Heart Association. (2009). 2009 Focused Update: ACCF/AHA Guidelines for the diagnosis and management of heart failure in adults. Retrieved June 2011, from http://circ.ahajournals.org/cgi/reprint/CIRCULATIONAHA.109.192064

American Heart Association. (No date). AHA scientific position: Risk factors and coronary heart disease. Retrieved March 2012, from http://www.ehow.com/facts_5615891_aha-factors-coronary-heart-disease.html

American Heart Association. (2009). What is peripheral vascular disease? Retrieved March 2012, from http://www.heart.org/idc/groups/heart-public/@wcm/@hcm/documents/downloadable/ucm_300323.pdf

American Liver Foundation: Wellness Education Toolkit. (2011). Your liver: Your life: What everybody needs to know about liver wellness. Retrieved July 2011, from http://www.yourliver.org/Liver-Wellness-Presentation.pdf

American Liver Foundation (2006).You are at risk for liver damage or disease if . . . . NIH Fact Sheet. Retrieved January 2012, from http://www.yourliver.org/risk.html

American Lung Association. (2010). State of lung disease in diverse communities 2010. Retrieved June 2011, from http://www.lungusa.org/assets/documents/publications/lung-disease-data/solddc_2010

American Medical Directors Association (AMDA). (2009). Dehydration and fluid maintenance in the long-term care setting. Retrieved September 2011, from http://www.guideline.gov/content.aspx?id=15590

American Medical Directors Association (AMDA). (2008). Delirium and acute problematic behavior in the long-term care setting. Retrieved July 2011, from http://www.guideline.gov/content.aspx?id=12379

American Medical Directors Association (AMDA). (2009). Pain management in the long-term care setting. Retrieved March 2012, from http://www.guideline.gov/content.aspx?id=15593

American Nurses Association (ANA). Position Statement: Latex Allergy. Retrieved January 2011, from http://www.nursingworld.org/MainMenuCategories/HealthcareandPolicyIssues/ANAPositionStatements/Archives.aspx

American Public Health Association. (2012). Environmental Health Competency Project: Draft recommendations for non-technical competencies at the local level. Retrieved May 2012, from http://www.apha.org/programs/standards/healthcompproject/corenontechnicalcompetencies.htmtx

American Public Health Association. (2008). Public health in America. Retrieved May 2012, from http://www.health.gov/phfunctions/public.htm

American Society of Health-System Pharmacists Fact Sheet. (No date). Preventing accidental poisoning. Retrieved March 2012, from http://www.safemedication.com/safemed/MedicationTipsTools/WhatYouShouldKnow/PreventingAccidentalPoisoning.aspx

American Speech-Language-Hearing Association (ASHA). (No date). Noise. Information sheet. Retrieved July 2011, from http://www.asha.org/public/hearing/Noise/

American Speech-Language-Hearing Association (ASHA). (No date). Voice Disorders. Retrieved July 2011, from http://www.asha.org/public/speech/disorders/voice.htm

American Speech-Language-Hearing Association (ASHA). (No date). Speech for clients with tracheostomies or ventilators. Information sheet. Retrieved July 2011, from http://www.asha.org/public/speech/disorders/tracheostomies.htm

American Speech-Language-Hearing Association (ASHA). (2000). Tip sheet: "I can hear, but I can't understand what's being said." Retrieved July 2011, from http://www.asha.org/about/news/tipsheets/Hearing_loss_and_aging.htm

American Speech-Language-Hearing Association (ASHA). (No date). What is language? What is speech? Information sheet. Retrieved July 2011, from http://www.asha.org/public/speech/development/language_speech.htm

Amitai, A, and Sinert, D. (2011). Ventilator management. Retrieved April 2012, from http://emedicine.medscape.com/article/810126-overview

Anderson, HS. (2011). Mild cognitive impairment. Retrieved January 2012, from http://emedicine.medscape.com/article/1136393-overview

Angel Eyes (The Colorado SIDS Program). (2008). Epidemiology/risk reduction. Retrieved August 2011, from www.angeleyes.org/index-2.html

Anubhuti, R. (No date). The question about death and death anxiety. Retrieved May 2012, from http://www .hypnos .co .uk /hypnomag / rattan.htm

Arnold, JL. (2006, update 2011). Personal protective equipment. Article for patient education, eMedicineHealth Web site. Retrieved July 2011, from http://www .emedicinehealth .com /personal _protective _equipment/article_em.htm

Association for Psychological Science (APS). Patients' health motivates workers to wash their hands. Retrieved April 2012, from http://www .psychologicalscience .org/index .php /news/releases/patients-health-motivates-workers-to-wash-their-hands.html

Aziz, F, and Comeroto, AJ. (2012). Abdominal angina. Retrieved February 2012, from http://emedicine .medscape .com /article /188618-overview

Ballen, K. (No date). Therapeutic Touch healing hospice clients and their families. Retrieved February 2012, from http://www .infinityinSt com/ articles/ttouch_hospice.html

Barclay, L. (2009). Hospital-supervised exercise may prevent need for surgery in patients with claudication. Retrieved March 2012, from http://www.medscape.org/viewarticle/587997?src=rss

Barrett, AM, and John, ST. (2007, update 2010). Retrieved July 2011, from http://emedicine.medscape.com/article/1136474-overview

Bartol, T. (2004). How can I get them to do what they are "supposed" to do? Or—Moving our mindset from "leave the driving to us" to "putting you in the driver's seat." Retrieved February 2012, from http://www.medscape.com/viewarticle/493600_4

Basson, MD. (2010). Constipation in adults. Retrieved July 2011, from http://www .emedicinehealth .com /constipation _in _adults/article _em .htm

Bates, B. (2009). Hepatitis C will be "the big virus" over next 20 years. Article for Internal Medicine News Digital Network. Retrieved July 2011, from http://www .internalmedicinenews .com /search /search-single-view /hepatitis-c-will-be-the-big-virus-over-next-20-years / f8b9e54e16.html

Bates, B. (2007). Simple questions can help uncover urinary incontinence. Family Practice News. Retrieved April 2012, from http:// www.familypracticenews.com/news/across-specialties/single-article /simple-questions-can-help-uncover-urinary-incontinence / 033e1d0bc0.html

Bazemore, PH, Wilson, WH, and Bigelow, DA. (2011). Retrieved April 2012, from http://emedicine.medscape.com/article/293530-overview

Beattie, L. (No date). Optimism and the power of positive thinking: Change your thoughts, change your life! Retrieved May 2012, from http://www .sparkpeople.com/resource/wellness_articles.asp?id=835

Beaumont, LR. (2009). Developing the essential social skills to recognize, interpret and respond constructively to yourself and others. Retrieved March 2012, from http://emotionalcompetency.com/

Beckett, C. (2000). Family theory as a framework for assessment. Retrieved April 2012, from http://jan .ucc .nau .edu/~nur350-c /class/2 _family/theory/lesson2-1-3.html

Behrman, AJ, and Howarth, M. (2011). Latex allergy. Retrieved February 2012, from http://emedicine .medscape .com /article /756632-overview

Beland, N. (2005). How to be happy. Women's Health. Retrieved April May 2012, from http://www.womenshealthmag.com/health/how-to-be-happier

Belknap, KA. (2004). Fact Sheet on wheelchairs for children. Retrieved February 2012, from http://www.abledata.com/abledata_docs/children_wheelchair.htm

Bhimji, S, and Hale, KM (No date listed). Peripheral vascular disease. Retrieved March 2012, from http://www .emedicinehealth .com / peripheral_vascular_disease/article_em.htm

Bienenfeld, D. (2010). Malingering. Retrieved March 2012, from http://emedicine.medscape.com/article/293206-overview

Blackwell, A. (2009). Five powerful ways to regain control of your life. Retrieved March 2012, from http://www.thebridgemaker.com/five-powerful-ways-to-regain-control-of-your-life-now/

Blagen, M, and Yang, J. (2008). Courage and hope as factors for client change: Important cultural implications and spiritual considerations. Retrieved February 2012, from http://counselingoutfitters.com/vistas /vistas08/Blagen.htm

Blanicka, P. (2002). Reframing: The essence of mediation. Retrieved April 2012, from http://www.mediate.com/articles/blanciak.cfm

Bolstad, R, and Blamlett, M. (No date). The transforming conflict. Retrieved February 2012, from http://www .nlpca .com /DCweb / Transforming_Conflict.html

Bolstad, R, and Blamlett, M. (No date). Win-win. Retrieved March 2012, from http://www.nlpca.com/DCweb/win_win_.html?itemid=171

Bonham, PA, and Flemister, BG. (2008). Guideline for management of wounds in patients with lower-extremity arterial disease. Retrieved March 2012, from http://www.guideline.gov/content.aspx?id=12613

Boyles, S. (2005). Spouse caregivers most likely to be abusive. Retrieved February2012, from http://www.webmd.com/balance/news/ 20050211/spouse-caregivers-most-likely-to-be-abusive

Brain Trauma Foundation, Inc. (2007). American Association of Neurological Surgeons. Guidelines for the management of severe traumatic brain injury: Blood pressure and oxygenation. Retrieved March 2012, from http://www.guideline.gov/content.aspx?id=10989

Branden, N. (2010). FAQs about self-esteem. Retrieved April 2012, from http://www.self-esteem-nase.org/faq.php

Brandler, ES, and Sinert, R. (2010). Cardiogenic shock in emergency medicine. Retrieved March 2012, from http://emedicine .medscape .com/article/759992-overview

Brandt, AL. Transition issues for the elderly and their families. Retrieved February 2012, from http://www .ec-online .net /knowledge / articles/brandttransitions.html

Brannon, S, Vij, S, and Gentili, A. (2011). Geriatric sleep disorder. Retrieved January 2012, from http://emedicine .medscape .com / article/292498-overview#a0101

Braye, S, Orr, D, and Peron-Shoot, M. (2011). Self-neglect and adult safeguarding: Findings from research. Retrieved February 2012, from http://www.scie.org.uk/publications/reports/report46.pdf

Breazeale, T. (2007). Attachment parenting: A practical approach for the reduction of attachment disorders and the promotion of emotionally secure children. A master's thesis submitted to the Faculty of Bethel College. Retrieved May 2012, from http://www.visi.com/~jlb/thesis/ch1.html

Brhel, R. (2008). The age of gentle discipline. Retrieved March 2012, from http://theattachedfamily.com/membersonly/?p=177

Bronte-Tinkew, K, Burkhauser, M, and Metz, A. (2008). Elements of promising practice in teen fatherhood programs: Evidence-based and evidence-informed research findings on what works. Retrieved March 2012, from http://www.childtrends.org/Files//Child_Trends-2008_05_08_SP_PromisingPracTeenFH.pdf

Bryg, RG. (2009). Heart failure: Recognizing caregiver burnout. Retrieved May 2012, from http://www.webmd.com/heart-disease/heart-failure/heart-failure-recognizing-burnout-caregiver

Brynes, G. (2006). Dealing with dementia: Help for relatives, friends, and caregivers. Retrieved February 2012, from http://www.ncpamd.com/dementia.htm

Burgess, AW, and Holstrom, LL. (2003). Dancing in the darkness. Retrieved April 2012, from http://www.dancinginthedarkness.com/articles.php?show=11&arc=83

Burns, SL. (1997–2008). The medical basis of stress, depression, anxiety, sleep problems and drug use. Retrieved April 2012, from http://www.teachhealth.com/

Calver, P, Braungardt, T, Kupchik, N, et al. (2005). The big chill: Improving the odds after cardiac arrest. CE Home Study Program for RNweb. Retrieved November 2011, from http://www.modernmedicine.com/modernmedicine/article/articleDetail.jsp?id=158219

Campagnolo, DI. (2009). Autonomic dysreflexia in spinal cord injury. Retrieved January 2011, from http://emedicine.medscape.com/article/322709/

Cascio, J. (2005). Bias in writings on gender identity disorders. Retrieved February 2012, from http://www.trans health.com/2002/bias-gender-identity-disorder/

Cavazos, JE, and Spitz, M. (2011). Epilepsy and seizures. Retrieved April 2012, from http://emedicine.medscape.com/article/1184846-overview

Centers for Disease Control and Prevention (CDC). (2010). CDC vision for the 21st century: "Health protection . . . health equality." Retrieved May 2012, from http://www.cdc.gov/about/organization/mission.htm

Centers for Disease Control and Prevention (CDC). (2004). 2004 Surgeon General's report: Highlights: Smoking among adults in the United States: Coronary heart disease and stroke. Retrieved March 2012, from http://www.cdc.gov/tobacco/data_statistics/sgr/2004/highlights/heart_disease/index.htm

Centers for Disease Control and Prevention (CDC). (2007). Adult and child immunization schedules. Fact sheet for National Immunization Program. Retrieved November 2011, from http://www.cdc.gov/vaccines/recs/schedules/default.htm#child

Centers for Disease Control and Prevention (CDC). (2010). CDC and Healthcare Infection Control Practices: Ventilator-associated pneumonia (VAP) event. Retrieved January 2012, from http://www.cdc.gov/nhsn/PDFs/pscManual/6pscVAPcurrent.pdf

Centers for Disease Control and Prevention (CDC). (2009). Healthy homes: Health issues related to community design (Fact sheets). Retrieved September 2011, from http://www.cdc/gov/healthyplaces/newhealthyhomes.htm

Centers for Disease Control and Prevention (CDC)/SAFEUSA. (2012). Preventing choking among infants and young children. Retrieved April 2012, from https://www.rke.vaems.org/wvems/Libraryfiles/Misc/A_12.pdf

Centers for Disease Control and Prevention (CDC). (2011). Sudden Unexpected Infant Deaths and Sudden Infant Death Syndrome: Various pages. Retrieved August 2011, from http://www.cdc.gov/SIDS/index.htm

Centers for Disease Control and Prevention (CDC). (2010 update). Vaccines and immunizations. Retrieved February 2012, from http://www.cdc.gov/vaccines/default.htm

Centers for Disease Control and Prevention (CDC). (2010 update). Various pages regarding the National Children's Study, the National Biomonitoring Program, the National Report on Human Exposure to Environmental Chemicals. Retrieved August 2011, from http://www.cdc.gov/biomonitoring/environmental_chemicals.html

Centers for Disease Control and Prevention (CDC). (2011). What would happen if we stopped vaccinations? Fact sheet for National Immunization Program. Retrieved November 2011, from http://www.cdc.gov/vaccines/vac-gen/whatifstop.htm

Centers for Disease Control and Prevention (CDC). (2006, update 2009). When should a mother avoid breastfeeding? Retrieved July 2011, from http://www.cdc.gov/breastfeeding/disease/contraindicators.htm

Centers for Disease Control and Prevention (CDC), Injury Center. (No date). Youth violence: Risk and protective factors. Retrieved January 2012, from http://www.cdc.gov/violenceprevention/youthviolence/riskprotectivefactors.html

Centers for Disease Control and Prevention (CDC). (2000–2007). Latex allergy prevention. Article for National Institute for Occupational Safety and Health (NIOSH) Web site. Retrieved January 2011, from http://www.cdc.gov/niosh/docs/98-113/

Centers for Disease Control and Prevention (CDC). (No date). Oral health: Preventing cavities, gum disease, tooth loss, and oral cancers: At a glance 2011. Retrieved August 2011, from http://www.cdc.gov/chronicdisease/resources/publications/AAG/doh.htm#links

Centers for Disease Control and Prevention (CDC): National Center for Injury Prevention and Control. (2011). Intimate partner violence. Retrieved January 2012, from http://www.cdc.gov/violenceprevention/intimatepartnerviolence

Centers for Disease Control and Prevention (CDC): National Center for Injury Prevention and Control. (2011). Sexual violence. Retrieved January 2012, from http://www.cdc.gov/ViolencePrevention/pdf/SV_Factsheet-a.pdf

Centers for Disease Control and Prevention (CDC). (2000). Unintentional Poisoning – Keep Yourself and Others Safe. Retrieved March 2012, from http://www.cdc.gov/Features/poisonprevention/

Centre for Addiction and Mental Health. (2010). Factors that influence a couples relationship. Retrieved April 2012, from http://www.camh.net/Care_Treatment/Resources_clients_families_friends/Couple_Therapy/couple_therapy_factors.html

Bach, M. (2012). Therapeutic Touch. Retrieved February 2012, from http://takingcharge.csh.umn.edu/explore-healing-practices/therapeutic-touch

---

Bush, GW. Champion aspirations for human dignity. (2002). Retrieved February 2012, from http://georgewbush-whitehouse.archives.gov/ nsc/nss/2002/nss2.html

Chang, L. (2009). Overflow incontinence. Retrieved April 2012, from http:/ /www.webmd.com/urinary-incontinence-oab/overflow-incontinence

Chang, L. (2012). Urge incontinence. Retrieved April 2012, from ttp://www .webmd.com/urinary-incontinence-oab/america-asks-11/urge?page=1

Chawla, B. (2009). Psychosocial difficulties of parents with young children with severe disabilities. Retrieved February 2012, from http://www .parenting-journals .com /84 /prominent-psychosocial-difficulties-that-parents-of-young-children-with-severe-disabilities-may-cope-with-during-their-child%e2%80%99s-early-years/

Cheshire, Jr, WP. (2007). Grey matters when eloquence is inarticulate. An article for Ethics & Medicine: An International Journal of Bioethics 22(3). Retrieved February 2012, from www .cbhd .org / resources/neuroethics/cheshire_2007-01-26.htm

Child Information Gateway. (2008). Long term consequences of child abuse and neglect. Retrieved March 2012, from http://www .childwelfare.gov/pubs/factsheets/long_term_consequences.cfm

Cincinnati Children's Hospital Medical Center. (2006). Evidence-based clinical guideline for acute gastroenteritis (AGE) in children in children aged 2 months through 5 years. Retrieved September 2011, from http://www .guideline .gov /content .aspx?id=9529 www .guideline.gov

Clark, CM. (No date). Relations between social support and physical health. Retrieved February 2012, from http://www .personalityresearch .org / papers/clark.html

Cluett, J. (2010). Types of pain medicine. Retrieved March 2012, from http://orthopedics .about .com /od /medicati3 /p /medications .htm

Cohn, M. (2008). Importance of an effective community relations program. Retrieved February 2012, from http://cohnpr.com/Articles/ CommunityRelations.html

Comerota, AJ. (2012). Abdominal angina. Retrieved February 2012, from http://emedicine.medscape.com/article/188618-overview

Consumer Product Safety Commission (CPSC). (No date). Safety for older consumers' home safety checklist. Retrieved January 2012, from http://www.cpsc.gov/cpscpub/pubs/701.pdf

Cortese, MM, and Parashar, UD. (2009). Prevention of Rotavirus Gastroenteritis Among Infants and Children Recommendations of the Advisory Committee on Immunization Practices (ACIP). Retrieved February 2012, from http://www .cdc .gov /mmwr /preview / mmwrhtml/rr5802a1.htm?s_cid=rr5802a1_e

Craig, KJ, Brown, KJ, and Baum, A. (2000). Environmental factors in the etiology of anxiety. In Neuropsychopharmcology: The Fifth Generation of Progress. Retrieved September 2011, from http://www .acnp.org/publications/psycho4generation.aspx

Croft, H, (reviewer). (2008). Admitting powerlessness. Retrieved March 2012, from http://www .healthyplace .com /relationships / serendipity/admitting-powerlessness/menu-id-1529/

Cunha, BA. (2009). Chronic fatigue syndrome. Retrieved September 2011, from http://emedicine .medscape .com /article /235980-overview

Cunha, JP. (No date). Fever. Retrieved April 2012, from http://www
.medicinenet.com/aches_pain_fever/article.htm

Cunha, JP. (2011). Heat exhaustion and heatstroke. Retrieved November 2011, from http://www .emedicinehealth .com /heat _exhaustion _and_heat_stroke/article_em.htm

Cunha, JP. (2011). Vomiting and nausea. Retrieved February 2012, from http://www.emedicinehealth.com/vomiting_and_nausea/article _em.htm

Cunha, JP, and Shiel, WC. (2011). Medical shock. Retrieved March 2012, from http://www.medicinenet.com/shock/article.htm

Curtis, R. (2002). Outdoor action guide to hypothermia and cold weather injuries. Retrieved November 2011, from http://nasdonline .org/static_content/documents/1420/d001215.pdf

Curtis, R. (1997). Outdoor action guide to heat related illnesses & fluid balance. Retrieved November 2011, from www.princeton.edu/~oa/ safety/hypocold.html

Dagi, TF, and Schecter, W (2008). Preparation of the operating room. Retrieved January 2012, from http://www .acssurgery .com /acs / chapters/ch0108.htm

Dahl, AA. (2012). Dry eye syndrome (Dry Eyes, Keratoconjunctivitis Sicca). Retrieved May 2012, from http://www.medicinenet.com/dry _eyes/article.htm

Davidson, J, and Wood, C, (2004). A conflict resolution model. Retrieved May 2012, from http://findarticles.com/p/articles/ mi_m0NQM/is_1_43/ai_114784808/

Davidson, T, and Frey, R (2006). Self-mutilation. Gale Encyclopedia of Children's Health: Infancy through Adolescence. Retrieved May 2012, from http://www.encyclopedia.com/topic/Self-Mutilation.aspx

Davies, EJ, et al. (2010). Exercise-based rehabilitation for heart failure. Cochrane Database of Systematic Reviews 2010. Retrieved January 2011 from http://onlinelibrary .wiley .com /o /cochrane /clsysrev / articles/CD003331/frame.html

Davis, JL. (2009). Coping with anxiety. Retrieved April 2012, from http://www.webmd.com/anxiety-panic/guide/coping-with-anxiety

Davis, N. (2007). [Short online summaries from]: Multi-Sensory Trauma Processing, A Manual for Understanding and Treating PTSD and Job-Related Trauma. Retrieved March 2012, from http:// drnancydavis.com/about/incidents-that-traumatize-rescue-workers

Dawodu, ST. (2006). Swallowing disorders. Retrieved April 2012, from http://emedicine.medscape.com/article/317667-overview

Dawadu, ST, Scott M, Chase, M, et al. (2011). Nutritional management in the rehabilitation setting. Retrieved September 2011, from http:// emedicine.medscape.com/article/318180-overview

Dawn, W. (2000). Long-term support for family and friends with chronic illness. Retrieved January 2012, from http://voices .yahoo .com/longterm-support-family-friends-chronic-383411.html

Dennis, BP, and Small, EB. (2003). Incorporating cultural diversity in nursing care: An action plan. ABNF Journal. Retrieved February 2012, from http://findarticles.com/p/articles/mi_m0MJT/is_1_14/ai _98250419/

DeNoon, D. (2006). C. Diff: New threat from old bug: Epidemic gut infection causing rapid rise in life-threatening disease. Retrieved August 2011, from http://www .webmd .com /digestive-disorders / news/20061012/c-diff-new-threat-from-old-bug

Developers: World Health Organization (WHO); National Heart, Lung and Blood Institute (NHLBI); Global Initiative for Chronic Obstructive Lung Disease (GOLD). (2001, update 2010). Global strategy for the diagnosis, management, and prevention of chronic obstructive pulmonary disease. Retrieved 2011 from http://www.goldcopd.org/Guidelineitem.asp?l1=2&l2=1&intId=2003

Dion, R. (2005). Overcoming relocation stress. Military OneSource, PTSD Support Services. Retrieved March 2012, from http://www.ptsdsupport.net/relocation_stress.html

Diskin, A. (2006, update 2009). Gastroenteritis in emergency medicine. Retrieved August 2011, from http://emedicine.medscape.com/article/775277-overview

Dombeck, M, and Wells-Moran, J. (update 2006). Coping strategies and defense mechanisms: Basic and intermediate defenses. Retrieved January 2012, from http://www .mentalhelp .net /poc /view _doc .php?type=doc&id=9791&cn=353

Dombeck, M, and Wells-Moran, J. (update 2006). Setting boundaries appropriately: Assertiveness training. Retrieved April 2012, from http://www.mentalhelp.net/poc/view_doc.php?type=doc&id=9778

Dorsey, CJ. (2003). The theory of self care management in vulnerable populations. Retrieved February 2012, from http://www.allbusiness.com/professional-scientific/scientific-research/728539-1.html

Dowshen, S. (2010). Your child's growth. Retrieved January 2012, from http://kidshealth .org /parent /growth /growing /childs _growth .html#

Dugdale, DD. (2010). Bowel incontinence. Retrieved April 2011, from http://www.nlm.nih.gov/medlineplus/ency/article/003135.htm

Dumitru, I. (2011). Heart Failure. Retrieved June 2011, from http://emedicine.medscape.com/article/163062-overview#showall

Duncan, LG, Duncan, J, Coatsworth, D, et al: Pilot study to gauge acceptability of a mindfulness based, family-focused preventive intervention. J Prim Prev 30(5): 605–18, 2009. http://www.ncbi.nlm.nih.gov/pmc/articles/PMC2730448/. doi: 10.1007/s10935-009-0185-9

Dunn, S. (update 2004). Researching your options: Pros and cons of researching your cancer. Retrieved February 2012 from http://www.cancerguide.org/pros_cons.html

Eby, N, and Car, M. (2004). Violence and brain injuries. Quality Matters. Retrieved April 2012, from http://www .vahealth .org /Injury / projectradarva/documents/older/pdf/QMSpr04.pdf

Edelstein, JA, Li, J, Silverberg, MA, et al. (2005). Hypothermia. Retrieved July 2011, from http://emedicine .medscape .com /article / 770542-overview

Elinopoulos, C. (2010). Deconditioning and sarcopenia. Retrieved February 2012, from http://www .ltlmagazine .com /article /deconditioning-and-sarcopenia

Emergency Nurses Association. (No date). Water safety. Retrieved January 2012, from www.ena.org

Erickson, B. (No date). What is anticipatory grief? Retrieved March 2012, from http://www .strengthforcaring .com /manual /grief-death-and-dying-end-of-life-care/what-is-anticipatory-grief/

Family Caregiver Alliance: National Center on Caregiving: Fact Sheets. (No date). Caring for adults with cognitive and memory impairments.

Retrieved January 2012, from http://www.caregiver.org/caregiver/jsp/content_node.jsp?nodeid=392

Farkas, H. (2011). Chronic pain. Retrieved March 2012, from http://www.emedicinehealth.com/chronic_pain/article_em.htm

Fayyaz, J, and Lessnau, K-D. (2012). Hypoventilation syndromes. Retrieved April 2012, from http://emedicine.medscape.com/article/304381-overview

Ferry, R. (2010). Fever in children. Retrieved November 2011, from http://www.emedicinehealth.com/fever_in_children/article_em.htm

Ferry, RJ. (2011). Constipation in children. Retrieved July 2011, from http://www.emedicinehealth.com/constipation_in_children/article_em.htm

Forrette, TL. (2006). Transitioning from mechanical ventilation. Retrieved April 2012, from http://www.medscape.org/viewarticle/528367

Foster, CS, Yuksel, E, Anzaar, F, et al. (2012). Dry eye syndrome. Retrieved May 2012, from http://emedicine.medscape.com/article/1210417-overview

Fowler, B. (2000). Inability to cope in Asperger's Syndrome. Retrieved January 2012, from http://www.suite101.com/article.cfm/aspergers_syndrome/47938

Frazier, L. (No date). The Bill of Rights vs the Patient's Bill of Rights. Retrieved February 2012, from http://www.ehow.com/about_5325243_bill-vs-patients-bill-rights.html

Frey, RJ. (2002). Generalized anxiety disorder. Retrieved March 2012, from http://www.minddisorders.com/Flu-Inv/Generalized-anxiety-disorder.html#b

Fulop, T, Agraharkar, M, Rondon-Berrios, H, et al. (2009). Hypomagnesemia. Retrieved August 2011, from http://emedicine.medscape.com/article/246366-overview

Futrell, M, and Melillo, KD. (2008). Wandering: Evidence-based protocol. Retrieved April 2012, from http://guideline.gov/content.aspx?id=12992

Galletta, GM, and Khandwalla, HM. (2006). Obesity and weight control. Retrieved February 2012, from http://www.emedicinehealth.com/weight_loss_and_control/article_em.htm

Garbee, DD, and Gentry, J. (2001). Coping with the stress of surgery (patient strategies). AORN Journal. Retrieved February 2012, from http://findarticles.com/p/articles/mi_m0FSL/is_5_73/ai_74571582/

Gary, JP. (2011). Exercise-induced asthma. Retrieved June 2011, from http://emedicine.medscape.com/article/1938228-overview#showall

Gavin, ML. (2010). Household safety: Preventing suffocation. Retrieved April 2012, from http://kidshealth.org/parent/firstaid_safe/home/safety_suffocation.html

Geriatric Nursing Resources for Care of Older Adults. (2008). Nursing Standard of Practice Protocol: Assessment and management of mealtime difficulties. Retrieved February 2012, from http://consultgerirn.org/topics/mealtime_difficulties/want_to_know_more

Gerlach, P. (2011). Perspective on family role and rule problems. Retrieved February 2012, from http://sfhelp.org/fam/roles_rules.htm

Gerstein, PS. (2011). Delirium, dementia, and amnesia in emergency medicine. Retrieved July 2011, from http://emedicine.medscape.com/article/793247-overview

Gettinger-Dinner, L. (2007). Suicide risk assessment: What providers need to know. Retrieved May 2012, from http://news.nurse.com/apps/pbcs.dll/article?AID=200770420001

Gill, C. (1995). A brief history: Attitudes and treatment of persons with disabilities. Retrieved January 2012, from http://www.jik.com/ilarts .html

Glass, JS, and Mann, MA. (2004). Harmonious families: Using family counseling and adventure based learning opportunities to enhance growth. Retrieved April 2012, from http://www.shsu.edu/~piic/ spring%202006/Glass.html

Goleman, D. (1995, October 3). Early violence leaves its mark on the brain. New York Times. Retrieved April 2012, from http://www.cirp .org/library/psych/goleman/

Goodwin, RS. (2009). Prevention of aspiration pneumonia: A research-based protocol. Retrieved February 2011, from http://www .pspinformation.com/disease/aspiration/pneu.shtml

Gordon, T. (No date). Getting what you need every time – Method III. Retrieved December 2011, from http://www.gordontraining.com/ free-parenting-articles/get-what-you-need-every-time-method-iii/

Gordon, T. (No date). Description, definition, synonyms, organizer terms, types of training. Retrieved February 2012, from ttp://wik.ed .uiuc.edu/index.php/Thomas_Gordon

Gordon, T. (No date). Families need rules. Retrieved March 2012, from http://www .gordontraining .com /free-parenting-articles /families-need-rules/

Gordon, T. (No date). How children really react to control. Retrieved January 2012, from http://www .naturalchild .org /guest /thomas _gordon.html

Gordon, T. (No date). Origins of the Gordon model. Retrieved March 2012, from http://www.gordontraining.com/thomas-gordon/origins-of-the-gordon-model/

Gordon, T. (No date). What every parent should know. Retrieved January 2012, from http://www.gordontraining.com/artman2/uploads/1 /What_Every_Parent_Should_Know_1.pdf

Gore, TA, and Lucas, JZ. (2011). Posttraumatic stress disorder. Retrieved March 2012, from http://emedicine.medscape.com/article/ 288154-treatment

Greenstein, DB. (2011). Caring for children with special needs—Developmental delays. Retrieved August 2011, from www.ces.ncsu .edu/depts/fcs/pdfs/NC12.pdf

Grenz, K, Bynum, G, Pine, D, et al. (2005, update 2011). Preventive services for children and adolescents. Institute for Clinical Systems Improvement (ICSI). Retrieved August 2011, from http://www.icsi .org /preventive _services _for _children _ _guideline _ /preventive _services_for_children_and_adolescents_2531.htm

Griffin, M. (2009). Decision making: Complexities and variables. Electronic Shriver Sarcoma Update Newsletter. Retrieved September 2012 from http://sarcomahelp.org/learning_center/articles/decisions .html

Grinstead, SF. (2009). Chronic pain management must address resistance and denial. Retrieved February 2012, from http://www .recoveryview .com /2009 /06 /resistance-and-denial-management-needed-for-effective-chronic-pain-management/

Gum, RM, (update 2011). CBRNE - Chemical warfare mass casualty management. Retrieved July 2011, from http://emedicine.medscape .com/article/831375-overview

---

Guandalini, S. (2010). Diarrhea. Retrieved August 2011, from http://emedicine.medscape.com/article/928598-overview

Guvakov, D, Weiss, S, and Cheung, A. (2011). Hypothermia: Laboratory and other studies for hypothermia table. Retrieved November 2011, from http://pier.acponline.org/physicians/public/d598/diagnosis/d598-s3.html

Hahn, JF, Olsen, CL, Tomaselli, N, et al. (No date). Wounds: Nursing care and product selection—Part 1 (CE offering). Retrieved March 2012, from http://ce.nurse.com/ce80-60/wounds-part-1-nursing-care-and-product-selection/coursepage/

Hamdy, O, Cirkowitz, E, Uwaifo, GI, et al. (2012). Obesity. Retrieved February 2012, from http://emedicine.medscape.com/article/123702-overview

Harbaugh, BL. (2005). Correlates of family-nurse boundary ambiguity in parents of hospitalized children. Retrieved February 2012, from http://stti.confex.com/stti/bcscience38/techprogram/paper_19687.htm

Harder, AF. (2002). Stages of the family life cycle. Retrieved February 2012, from http://www.childhoodaffirmations.com/general/family/stages.html

Hastings, K. (2007). What's in your coping toolbox. Retrieved December 2011, from http://karenhastings.articlealley.com/whats-in-your-coping-toolbox--by-karen-hastings-122024.htm

HealthPartners Dental Group and Clinics. (2009). Guidelines for the diagnosis and treatment of peridontal diseasaes. Retrieved March 2012, from http://www.guideline.gov/content.aspx?id=14335

Health Sciences Centre. (2012). Suffocation/Choking. Fact sheet for Manitoba Health Schools. Retrieved April 2012, from http://www.gov.mb.ca/healthyschools/topics/safety.html

Healthwise Staff. (2009). Tooth Decay: Prevention. Retrieved August 2011, from http://www.webmd.com/oral-health/tc/tooth-decay-prevention

Helman, RS, and Habal, R. (2010). Heatstroke. Retrieved April 2011, from http://emedicine.medscape.com/article/166320-overview

Henderson, D, and Henderson, K. (No date). A very simplistic explanation of free radicals and antioxidants. Retrieved February 2012, from http://www.menieres-disease.ca/health_reports/free_radicals_anti_oxidants.htm

Henkin, RI. (2012). Taste and Smell Clinic research and clinical overview. Retrieved March 2012, from http://www.tasteandsmell.com/clinical.htm

Hertz, G, and Cataletto, ME. (2011). Sleep dysfunction in women. Retrieved January 2012, from http://emedicine.medscape.com/article/1189087-overview

Hingley, AT. (2000). Preventing childhood poisoning. Retrieved March 2012, from http://www.kidsource.com/kidsource/content3/fda.poisoning.all.safety.html

Hollander, T. (2008). 13 signs of anger and how to manage them in sobriety. Retrieved February 2012, from http://www.selfhelpmagazine.com/article/alcohol-anger

Holson, D, and Gathers, S. (2010). Constipation in Emergency Medicine. Retrieved July 2011, from http://emedicine.medscape.com/article/774726-overview

Hopkins, L. (2005). Assertive communication: 6 tips for effective use. Retrieved April 2012, from http://ezinearticles .com /?Assertive-Communication---6-Tips-For-Effective-Use&id=10259

Hopper, J. (2012). Mindfulness and kindness: Inner sources of freedom and happiness. Retrieved April 2012, from http://www .jimhopper .com/mindfulness/

Hospital and Palliative Nurses Association. (2005). Spiritual distress. Patient/Family Teaching Sheets. Retrieved May 2012, from http://www.hpna.org/pdf/PatientShcct_SpiritualDistress.pdf

Huang, LH, Anchalla, KP, Ellsbury, DL, et al. Dehydration. (2009). Retrieved September 2011, from http://emedicine .medscape .com / article/906999-overview

Hunt, J. (No date). What is attachment parenting? Retrieved February 2012, from http://www.naturalchild.org/jan_hunt/attachment_parenting.html

Hunter, TS (2011). Diabetic peripheral neuropathy. Retrieved March 2012, from http://drugtopics .modernmedicine .com /drugtopics / author/authorInfo.jsp?id=6455

Hyman, SE. (1999). Thinking about violence in our schools, Discussion at the White House. National Institute of Mental Health. Retrieved May 2012, from http://www .namigc .org /content /fact _sheets / childrenadolescents/MentalIllnesses/vioweb.htm

Institute of Public Care. (2008). What works in promoting good outcomes for children in need through enhanced parenting skills? Retrieved March 2012, from http://www.ssiacymru.org.uk/media/pdf/ g/d/5_-_parenting_skills_formattcd_.pdf

Jacobson, JA. (2008). Radiation and Imaging. Monograph from the online Merck Manual for Health Care Professionals. Retrieved May 2012, from http://www .merckmanuals .com /professional /special _subjects /principles _of _radiologic _imaging /radiation _and _imaging .html#v1124912

Jagminas, L. (2006, update 2011). CBRNE—Chemical decontamination. Retrieved July 2011, from http://emedicine .medscape .com / article/831175-overview

Jochman, C. (2009). Fear of change—How to see change as a positive impact in life. Retrieved February 2012, from http://www.suite101 .com/content/fear-of-change-a178729

Johns Hopkins Vasculitis Center. (2011). Buerger's disease. Retrieved March 2012, from http://www.hopkinsvasculitis.org/types-vasculitis /buergers-disease/

Jordon, D. (2009). "We were powerless over our addiction": Why the first step is so controversial. Retrieved March 2012, from http://www .sunshinecoasthealthcentre .ca /drugrehab /exploring-addiction / powerlessness-addiction/18082009

Institute for Clinical Systems Improvement (ICSI). (2008). Guideline: Prevention of falls (acute care protocol). Retrieved September 2011, from http://www .guideline .gov /content .aspx-?id=16005

Institute for Clinical Systems Improvement (ICSI). (2009). Assessment and management of chronic pain. Retrieved July 2011, from http://www.guideline.gov/content.aspx?id=15525

Kam, K. (2010). Sleep and the night shift: Could you have work sleep disorder? Retrieved January 2012, from http://www .webmd .com / sleep-disorders/excessive-sleepiness-10/night-shift-sleep

Kanaparthi, LK, Lessnau, KD, and Peralta, R. (2012). Distributive shock. Retrieved March 2012, from http://emedicine.medscape.com /article/168689-overview

Kaplan, M, and Krueger, R. (2010). Diagnosis, assessment, and treatment of hypersexuality. Retrieved May 2012, from http:// www .thefreelibrary .com /Diagnosis%2c+Assessment%2c+and +treatment+of+hypersexuality.-a0226161876

Kates, LW, and Schraga, ED. (2011). Cooling techniques for hyper- thermia. Retrieved July 2011, from http://emedicine.medscape.com /article/149546-overview

Kearney, P. (updated 2010). Chronic grief (or is it periodic grief?) Grief in a family context. Retrieved April 2012, from http://www.indiana .edu/~famlygrf/units/chronic.html

Kedlaya, D, and Kuang, T. (2011). Assistive devices to improve inde- pendence. Retrieved April 2012, from http://emedicine .medscape .com/article/325247-overview#showall

Kemle, K. (2011). Falls in older adults: Averting disaster. Retrieved July 2011, from http://www .clinicaladvisor .com /falls-in-older- adults-averting-a-disaster/article/195485/

Kidd, M. (2007). What do patients fear most? Retrieved September 2011, from http://www.medscape.com/view/article/561455

Kirshner, D, and Jacobs, DH. (2005). Aphasia. Retrieved July 2011, from http://emedicine.medscape.com/article/1135944-overview

Kirshner, HS, and Jacobs, DH. (2010). Confusional states and acute memory disorders. Retrieved February 2012, from http://emedicine .medscape.com/article/1135767-overview.

Kizer, KW, and Blum, LN. (2005). Safe practices for better health care. Abstract for a portion of the Consensus Report. Retrieved January 2012, from http://www.ahrq.gov/qual/nqfpract.htm

Klimes, R. (1994–2012). Managing stress: Living without stress over- load. CE offering for LearnWell.org Web site. Retrieved April 2012, from http://www.learnwell.org/stress.htm

Kochan, JP, and Kanamalla, US. (2011). Cerebral revascularization im- aging. Retrieved March 2012, from http://emedicine.medscape.com /article/420186-overview

Koh, HK, et al. (2007). Inhaled corticosteroids compared to placebo for prevention of exercise-induced bronchoconstriction. Cochrane Da- tabase of Systematic Reviews. Retrieved September 2010, from http://www2.cochrane.org/reviews/en/ab002739.

Kolcaba, K. (2006). FAQs (frequently asked questions). On the comfort line. Web site devoted to the concept of comfort in nurs- ing. Retrieved July 2011, from http://www.thecomfortline.com/ home/faq.html

Kolecki, P, and Meckhoff, CR. (2010). Hypovolemic shock. Retrieved September 2012, from http://emedicine .medscape .com /article / 760145-overview

Kotelnikov, V. (No date). Personal beliefs, values and basic assump- tions and attitudes—Understanding what drives you and others. Re- trieved February 2012, from ttp://www.1000ventures.com/business _guide/crosscuttings/character_beliefs-values.html

Kresevic, DM. (2008). Nursing Standard of Practice Protocol: Assess- ment of function in acute care. Retrieved March 2012, from http:// consultgerirn.org/topics/function/want_to_know_more

Krull, E. (2010). Family conflict power struggles. Psych Central. Retrieved 2012, from http://blogs.psychcentral.com/family/2010/01/family-conflict-power-struggles/

Laberge, M. (No date). Thermoregulation. Retrieved April 2012, from http://www.enotes.com/thermoregulation-reference/thermoregulation

LaGrand, L. (2008). Five best ways to develop your coping skills. Retrieved December 2011, from http://www.articlesbase.com/self-help-articles/five-best-ways-to-develop-your-coping-skills-609070.html

Lansang, RS. (2008). Bowel Management. Retrieved July 2011, from http://emedicine.medscape.com/article/321172-overview

Larson, N. (2011). After rape, getting a medical exam is essential. Retrieved April 2012, from http://womenshealth.about.com/lw/Health-Medicine/Womens-Health/After-Rape-Getting-a-Medical-nbsp-Exam-is-Essential.htm

Lashley, FR. (2006). Emerging infectious diseases at the beginning of the 21st century. Online Journal of Issues in Nursing 11(1). Retrieved January 2011, from http://www.medscape.com/viewarticle/528306

Lathrop, D. (2000). Ramp the planet! Retrieved February 2012, from http://www.spinlife.com/

Lawhorne, LS. (2009). Altered nutritional status: Guideline. Retrieved February 2012, from http://www.guideline.gov/content.aspx?id=15590

Lawrence, S. (No date). Exploring Porges' theory of social engagement using a music stimulation program for an 8 year old boy with autism. Retrieved May 2012, from http://www.thelisteningprogram.com/PDF/News/ABT_Porges.pdf

Lawrence, S. (2005). When health fears are overblown. Retrieved September 2011, from http://www.webmd.com/balance/features/when-health-fears-are-overblown

Lawson, J. (2011). Accepting powerlessness. Retrieved March 2012, from http://www.livestrong.com/article/14716-accepting-powerlessness/

Lawson, J. (2011). Enabling personality. Retrieved March 2012, from http://www.livestrong.com/article/14675-enabling-personality/

Lawson, J. (2011). Improving assertive behavior. Retrieved April 2012, from http://www.livestrong.com/article/14699-improving-assertive-behavior/Improviong

Lederer, E, Ouseph, R, Nayak, V, et al. (2011). Hyperkalemia. Retrieved August 2011, from http://emedicine.medscape.com/article/240903-overview

Lederer, E, Ouseph, R, and Yazel, L. (2009). Hypokalemia. Retrieved August 2011, from http://emedicine.medscape.com/article/242008-overview

Lee, D, and Marks, JW. (update 2010). Acetaminophen (Tylenol) liver damage. Retrieved January 2010, from http://www.medicinenet.com/tylenol_liver_damage/article.htm

Lenneman, A. (2011). Shock, cardiogenic. Retrieved June 2011, from http://emedicine.medscape.com/article/152191-overview

Leopold, D, Holbrook, EH, Noell, CA. (2009). Disorders of taste and smell. Retrieved March 2012, from http://emedicine.medscape.com/article/861242-overview

Lien, CA. (No date). Thermoregulation in the elderly. Syllabus on Geriatric Anesthesiology. American Society of Anesthesologists Web site. Retrieved April 2011, from http://asatest .asahq .org /clinical / geriatrics/thermo.htm

Lindamer, LA, Lebowitz, B, Hough, RL, et al. (2009). Establishing an implementation network: Lessons learned from community-based participatory research. Retrieved February 2012, from http://www .implementationscience.com/content/4/1/17

Linwood, AS. (2006). Parent-Child Relations. Retrieved January 2012, from http://www.healthline.com/galecontent/parent-child-relationships

London, S. (2011). Resistant infections are increasing in hospitals. Retrieved July 2011, from http://www.familypracticenews.com/news/ more-top-news /single-view /resistant-infections-are-increasing-in-hospitals/3dae4b6c94.html

Lopez-Rowe, V. (2011). Peripheral arterial occlusive disease. Retrieved March 2012, from http://emedicine .medscape .com /article /460178-overview

Lubit, R. 2011). Acute treatment of disaster survivors. Retrieved March 2012, from http://emedicine.medscape.com/article/295003-overview

Lukitsch, I, and Pham, TQ. (2010). Hypernatremia. Retrieved August 2010, from http://emedicine.medscape.com/article/241094-overview

Luis, PD. (2007) Urinary incontinence (various pages). The Merck Manual for Health Care Professionals. Retrieved April 2012, from http://www .merckmanuals .com /professional /genitourinary _disorders /voiding _disorders/urinary_incontinence.html

Malignant Hyperthermia Association of the United States (MHAUS). Guideline statement for malignant hyperthermia in the perioperative environment. Retrieved November 2011 from http://www.aSt org/ pdf/Standards_of_Practice/Guideline_Malignant_Hyperthermia.pdf

Mandlie, K. (2011). How parenting styles affect our children's development. Retrieved March 2012, from http://yourkidsed.com.au/info /how-parenting-styles-influence-our-childrens-development

Marano, HE. (2003, update 2009). Ending procrastination. Retrieved April 2012, from http://www.psychologytoday.com/articles/200310 /ending-procrastination

Marks, JW. (2011). Constipation. Retrieved July 2011, from http://www .medicinenet.com/constipation/article.htm

Marks, JW. (2010). Dysphagia (Difficulty Swallowing). Retrieved April 2012, from http://www.medicinenet.com/swallowing/article.htm

Martinuzzi, B. (2007). The breaking point. Retrieved April 2012, from http://www.mindtools.com/pages/article/newTCS_93.htm

Maryland Department of Human Services. (2009). In-home family preservation services. Retrieved February 2012, from http://dhr.maryland .gov/ssa/family/

Mayo Clinic—Rochester. (2006). Mild cognitive impairment prevalent in elderly population: Risk increases as age goes up and education goes down. Retrieved February 2012, from http://www .eurekalert .org/pub_releases/2006-04/mc-mci033006.php

Mayo Clinic Staff. (1998–2012). Dry eye. Various pages. Retrieved May 2012, from https://www.mayoclinic.com/health/dry-eyes/DS00463

Mayo Clinic Staff. (1998–2012). Alzheimer's: Understand and control wandering. RetrievedApril 2012, from http://www.mayoclinic.com/ health/alzheimers/HQ00218

Mayo Clinic Staff. (2007, update 2011). Dehydration. Retrieved September 2011, from http://www.mayoclinic.com/health/dehydration/ DS00561#

Mayo Clinic Staff. (2011). Denial: When it helps, when it hurts. Retrieved February 2012, from http://www.mayoclinic.com/health/denial/SR00043

Mayo Clinic Staff. (No date.) Antibiotic-associated diarrhea. Retrieved August 2011, from http://www .mayoclinic .com /health /antibiotic-associated-diarrhea/DS00454

Mayo Clinic Staff. (2011). Urinary incontinence surgery: When other treatments aren't enough. Retrieved April 2012, from http://www .mayoclinic.com/health/urinary-incontinence-surgery/WO00126

Mayo Clinic Staff (2011). Self-Esteem: 4 Steps to Feeling Better About Yourself. Retrieved May 2012, from http://health.msn.com/healthy-living/manage-stress/articlepage.aspx?cp-documentid=100167125

McDaniel, ND. (2007). Beyond Viagra: The hidden roots and risks of erectile dysfunction. Retrieved April 2012, from www.lifescript.com /channels /healthy _living /Mens _Health /beyond _viagra _the _hidden _roots_and_risks_of_erectile_dysfunction.asp

McDonald, M, and Evans, N. (2008). Infection Control Guidelines for Healthcare Professionals. Retrieved November 2011, from http://www.nursingceu.com/courses/257/index_nceu.htm

McGee, J. (No date). Self-injury. Retrieved May 2012, from http://www .smilelifework.org/node/3/adolescent

McGovern, C. (2003). Skin, hair and nail assessment. Unit 2 (lecture materials). Villanova University College of Nursing. Retrieved March 2012, from http://www10.homepage.villanova.edu/marycarol .mcgovern/2104/SkinHairNail2.htm

McKay, SL, Fravel, J, and Scanlon, C. (2009). Management of constipation. Retrieved July 2011, from http://guidelines .gov /content .aspx?id=15434

Meadows, M. (2008). Nutrition: Healthy eating. Retrieved February 2012, from http://www .medicinenet .com /script /main /art .asp ?articlekey=61982

Menna, A. (2004). Rape trauma syndrome: The journey to healing belongs to everyone. Retrieved April 2012, from www.giftfromwithin .org/html/journey.html

Messina, J. (2007). Eliminating manipulation: Tools for handling control issues. Retrieved February 2012, from http://coping .us / toolsforhandlingcontrol/eliminatemanipulation.html

Miller-Huey, R. (No date). Hydration in elders: More than just a glass of water. Retrieved September 2011, from www .caregiver .com / articles/general/hydration_in_elders.htm

Mills, J. (1999). The ontology of religiosity: The oceanic feeling and the value of the lived experience. Retrieved April 2012, from http:/ /evans-experientialism.freewebspace.com/mills_jon.htm

Moore, A. (2004). Hedonism. The Stanford Encyclopedia of Philosophy Retrieved May 2012, from http://plato .stanford .edu /entries / hedonism/

Moran, G. (No date). Dignity, uniqueness and rights. Retrieved February 2012, from http://www.nyu.edu/classes/gmoran/EXC-RIGH.pdf

Morris-Kukowski, CL, and Egland, AG. (2009). Toxicity, deadly in a single dose. Retrieved March 2012, from http://emedicine.medscape .com/article/1011108-overview

Moses, S. (2011). Peripheral arterial occlusive disease. Retrieved March 2012, from http://www.fpnotebook.com/surgery/cv/prphrlartrloclsvds.htm

Moses, S. (2012). Unna's boot. Family Practice Notebook. Retrieved March 2012, from http://www.fpnotebook.com/surgery/pharm/unsbt.htm

Muche, JA, and McCarty, S. (2011). Geriatric rehabilitation. Retrieved March 2012, from http://emedicine.medscape.com/article/318521-overview

Mukherjee, S, Mihas, AA, Heuman, DM, et al. (2011). Alcoholic hepatitis. Article for Internal Medicine News Digital Network. Retrieved July 2011, from http://emedicine.medscape.com/article/170539-overview

Murphy, E. (No date). Coping with disability. Retrieved January 2012, from http://www.mainlinehealth.org/oth/Page.asp?PageID=OTH000413

Murray, D. (2012). Increasing your milk supply naturally. Retrieved September 2012, from http://breastfeeding.about.com/od/milksupplyproblems/a/Increasing-Your-Milk-Supply-Naturally.htm

Nagin, MJ. (2009). Relactation—How to increase your milk supply. Retrieved September 2012, from http://breastfeeding.about.com/od/lactation/a/relactation.htm

National Ag Safety Database (NASD). (2002). Sleep deprivation: Cause and consequences. Fact sheet for Nebraska Rural Health and Safety Coalition. Retrieved April 2012, from http://nasdonline.org/document/871/d000705/sleep-deprivation-causes-and-consequences.html

National Aphasia Association (NAA). (No date). More aphasia facts. Retrieved July 2011, from http://www.aphasia.org/Aphasia%20Facts/aphasia_facts.html

National Aphasia Association (NAA). (2001). Understanding primary progressive aphasia. Retrieved July 2011, from http://www.aphasia.org/Aphasia%20Facts/understanding_primary_progressive_aphasia.html

National Association for Continence (NAFC). (2010). What is incontinence? (Various pages). Retrieved April 2012, from http://www.nafc.org/bladder-bowel-health/what-is-incontinence/

National Cancer Institute. (2011). Chronic nausea and vomiting in advanced cancer. Retrieved February 2012, from http://www.cancer.gov/cancertopics/pdq/supportivecare/nausea/Patient/page5

National Cancer Institute. (2012). Oral complications of chemotherapy and head/neck radiation: Various sections. Retrieved March 2012, from http://www.cancer.gov/cancertopics/pdq/supportivecare/oralcomplications/HealthProfessional/page1/AllPages

National Cancer Institute. (update 2011). Risk factors for complicated grief and other negative bereavement outcomes. Retrieved March 2012, from http://www.cancer.gov/cancertopics/pdq/supportivecare/bereavement/HealthProfessional/page4

National Center on Elder Abuse. (2002). Preventing elder abuse by family caregivers. Retrieved May 2012, from http://www.ncea.aoa.gov/main_site/pdf/family/caregiver.pdf

National Center for Injury Prevention and Control. (No date). Drowning prevention. Retrieved January 2012, from http://www.cdc.gov/Features/dsDrowningRisks/

National Collaborating Centre for Mental Health, Social Care Institute for Excellence, National Institute for Health and Clinical Excellence. (2006). Dementia: Supporting people with dementia and their careers in health and social care; National Clinical Guideline. Retrieved July 2011, from http://www.guideline.gov/content.aspx?id=10178

National Digestive Diseases Information Clearinghouse (NDDIC). (update 2007). Constipation. Retrieved July 2011, from http://digestive .niddk.nih.gov/ddiseases/pubs/constipation/

National Digestive Diseases Information Clearinghouse (NDDIC). (update 2008). Viral hepatitis: A through E and beyond. Retrieved January 2012, from digestive.niddk.nih.gov/ddiseases/pubs/viralhepatitis/

National Digestive Diseases Information Clearinghouse (NDDIC). (No date). Diarrhea. Retrieved August 2011, from http://digestive.niddk .nih.gov/ddiseases/pubs/diarrhea/

National Institute of Drug Abuse. (2009). InfoFacts: Treatment approaches for drug addiction. Retrieved January 2012, from http:// www.drugabuse.gov/publications/drugfacts/treatment-approaches- drug-addiction

National Institute of Mental Health. (2009). Anxiety disorders. Retrieved January 2012, from http://www.nimh.nih.gov/health/ publications/anxiety-disorders/introduction.shtml

National Institute of Mental Health. (2012). Generalized Anxiety disorders. Retrieved May 2012, from http://www.minddisorders.com/ Flu-Inv/Generalized-anxiety-disorder.html

National Institute of Neurological Disorders and Stroke (NINDS). (2007). Brain basics. Understanding sleep. Retrieved January 2012, from www.ninds.nih.gov/disorders/brain_basics/understanding _sleep.htm

National Institute of Neurological Disorders and Stroke (NINDS). (2011). Post-Polio Syndrome Fact Sheet. Retrieved September 2011, from http://www.ninds.nih.gov/disorders/post_polio/detail_post _polio.htm

National Institute of Neurological Disorders and Stroke (NINDS). (2012). Swallowing disorders information page. Retrieved April 2012, from http://www.ninds.nih.gov/disorders/swallowing_disorders/swallowing _disorders.htm

National Institute on Aging. (2010). Hyperthermia: Too hot for your health. Retrieved November 2011, from http://www.nih.gov/news/ health/jul2010/nia-22.htm

National Kidney and Urologic Diseases Information Clearinghouse (NKUDIC). (2011). Urodynamic testing. Retrieved April 2012, from http://kidney.niddk.nih.gov/kudiseases/pubs/urodynamic/index.htm

National Multiple Sclerosis Society. (No date). Understanding the unique role of fatigue in multiple sclerosis. Retrieved September 2011, from http://www.nationalmssociety.org/about-multiple- sclerosis/what-we-know-about-ms/symptoms/index.aspx

National Sleep Foundations. (No date). Various Fact Sheets regarding women, adolescents, the elderly and sleep needs. Retrieved April 2012, from http://www.sleepfoundation.org/

National Stroke Association (NSA). (2009 update). Various public information monographs regarding controllable risk factors. Retrieved March 2012, from http://www.stroke.org/site/PageServer?pagename=cont

Nauert, R. (2007). Amphetamine, cocaine usage increase risk of stroke among young adults. Article reporting result of study at UT Southwestern. Retrieved March 2012, from http://www.utsouthwestern .edu/newsroom/news-releases/year-2007/amphetamine-cocaine- usage-increase-risk-of-stroke-among-young-adults.html

Newman, DK. (2009). Using the BladderScan for bladder volume assessment. Retrieved April 2012, from http://www.seekwellness.com/incontinence/using_the_bladderscan.htm

No author listed. (No date). Assertiveness: What is assertiveness? Retrieved March 2012, from http://students .georgiasouthern .edu / counseling/selfhelp/assert.htm

No author listed. (No date). Breastfeeding guidelines following radiopharmaceutical administration. Retrieved August 2011, from http://nuclearpharmacy.uams.edu/resources/breastfeeding.asp

No author listed. (No date). Developmental delays: A pediatrician's guide to your children's health and safety. Retrieved August 2011, from www.keepkidshealthy.com/welcome/conditions/developmentaldelays.html

No author listed. (No date). Impulse Control Disorders. PsychoSolve Website. Retrieved May 2012, from http://www.newharbinger.com/PsychSolve/ImpulseControlDisorders/tabid/132/Default.aspx

No author listed. (No date). Sometimes grief becomes complicated, unresolved or stuck. Retrieved March 2012, from http://www.4therapy.com /life-topics /grief-loss /sometimes-grief-becomes-complicated-unresolved-or-stuck-2249

No author listed. (No date). Symptom: Walking symptoms. Retrieved April 2012, from http://wrongdiagnosis.com/sym/walking_symptoms.htm

No author listed. (1995). Individual differences in cognitive processes of planning: A personality variable? The Psychological Record. Retrieved April 2012, from http://www .thefreelibrary .com / Individual+differences+in+cognitive+processes+of+planning%3A +a...-a017150075

No author listed. (2005). The Therapeutic Touch process. Retrieved February 2012, from http://www .therapeutic-touch .org/newsarticle .php?newsID=19

No author listed. (update 2005). Evidence-based clinical practice guideline of community-acquired pneumonia in children 60 days to 17 years of age. Retrieved June 2011, from http://www.guideline.gov/content.aspx?id=9690

No author listed. (update 2009). Autonomic dysreflexia. Fact sheet for Northeast Rehabilitation Health Network. Retrieved February 2012, from http://www.sci-info-pages.com/ad.html

No author listed. (2011). Grief, bereavement, and coping with loss: Treatment. Retrieved March 2012, from http://www .cancer .gov / cancertopics /pdq /supportivecare /bereavement /HealthProfessional / page5

No author listed. (2011). Psychiatric disorders/psychotic disorders: Thought disorders. WikiBooks. Retrieved April 2012, from http://en .wikibooks.org/wiki/Psychiatric_Disorders/Psychotic_Disorders

No author listed. (update 2011). Factors that affect complicated grief. Retrieved March 2012, from http://www .cancer.gov /cancertopics / pdq/supportivecare/bereavement/Patient/page4

No author listed. (update 2011). Types of grief reactions. Retrieved March 2012, from http://www .cancer .gov /cancertopics /pdq / supportivecare/bereavement/HealthProfessional/page3

Novello, NP, and Blumstein, HA. (2010). Hypermagnesemia in emergency medicine. Retrieved August 2011, from http://emedicine .medscape.com/article/766604-overview

Nuespiel, DR, and Stubbs, EH (2011). Nightmares. Retrieved March 2012, from http://emedicine.medscape.com/article/914428-overview

O'Brien, T. (2008). Parent empowerment program (PEP). Retrieved March 2012, from http://www.tim-obrien.com/empowerment.php?doc=details

O'Connell-Gifford, E. (2011). The use of photo documentation. Retrieved April 2012, from Medline Healthy Skin Magazine http://issuu.com/medlineindustries/docs/healthyskinv8i2

Olade, R. (2010). Cardiac catheterization (left heart). Retrieved June 2011, from http://emedicine.medscape.com/article/1819224-overview

Oliver, RI. (2009). Resuscitation and early management burns. Retrieved September 2011, from http://emedicine.medscape.com/article/1277360-overview

Osborne, H. (2004). In other words—helping patients make difficult decisions. Retrieved February 2012, from http://www.healthliteracy.com/article.asp?PageID=3808

Oswalt, A. (2008). Urie Bronfenbrenner and child development. Retrieved March 2012, from http://www.mentalhelp.net/poc/view_doc.php?type=doc&id=7930&cn=28

Paik, N-J. (2012). Dysphagia. Retrieved August 2012, from http://emedicine.medscape.com/article/324096-overview

Palmer, RM. (2004). Management of common clinical disorders in geriatric patients: Delirium. Retrieved April 2012, from http://www.acpmedicine.com/acp/chapters/ch0809.htm

Parker, LC. (2012). Top 10 care essentials for ventilator patients. Retrieved April 2012, from http://www.medscape.com/viewarticle/761358-2

Patel, K, Basson, MD, Borsa, JJ, et al. (2011). Deep vein thrombosis. Retrieved March 2012, from http://emedicine.medscape.com/article/1911303-overview

Paul, M. (No date). Relationships: The art of listening. Retrieved February 2012, from http://ezinearticles.com/?Relationships---The-Art-of-Listening&id=2459633

Paula, R. (2006, update 2011). Abdominal compartment syndrome. Retrieved February 2012, from http://emedicine.medscape.com/article/829008-overview

Paula, R. (2008). Compartment syndrome, extremity. Retrieved March 2012, from http://kristinandjerry.name/cmru/rescue_info/Medical%20Issues/Compartment%20Syndrome%20-%20Extremity%20-%20Paula.htm

Patterson, B. (2009). A Buddhist approach to grief counseling. Retrieved February 2012, from http://bethspatterson.wordpress.com/2009/09/06/a-buddhist-approach-to-grief-counseling/

Perone, LM, Webb, LK, and Jackson, ZV. (2007). Retrieved April 2012, from http://findarticles.com/p/articles/mi_m0JAX/is_3_55/ai_n18791408/

Peterson, R, and Green, S. (2009). Families first—Keys to successful family functioning: Problem solving. Retrieved February 2012, from http://www.pubs.ext.vt.edu/350/350-091/350-091.html

Pickhardt, C. (2002). Role conflict of the single parent. Retrieved May 2012, from http://www.carlpickhardt.com/page48.html

Pilgrim, G. (2011). Therapeutic communication techniques. Retrieved February 2012, from http://www.buzzle.com/articles/therapeutic-communication-techniques.html

Pinksy, MR, Faresi, FA, Brenner, BE, et al. (2011). Septic shock. Retrieved March 2012, from http://emedicine.medscape.com/article/168402-overview

Planned Parenthood. (2006). Sexual health—Sexuality. Retrieved May 2007, from http://plannedparenthood .org /sexual-health /sexual-health-relationship/sexuality.htm

Plunkett, S. (No date). Family developmental theory. Retrieved February 2012, from http://hhd .csun .edu /hillwilliams /542 /Family %20Developmental%20Theory.htm

Policastro, MA, Sinert, R, and Guerrero, P. (2011). Urinary obstruction. Retrieved April 2012, from http://emedicine.medscape.com/article/ 778456-overview#showall

Pozza, AM, and Kemp, S. (2011). Pediatric type 2 Diabetes Mellitus. Retrieved February 2012, from http://emedicine .medscape .com / article/925700-overview

Pychyl, TA (2009). Retrieved February 2012, from http://www .psychologytoday .com /blog /dont-delay /200903 /proactive-coping-strategy-self-regulation-and-enhanced-well-being

Rader, J, Jones, D, and Miller, L. (No date). Wheelchair seating: For older adults. Part 1: A guide for caregivers. Retrieved February 2012, from http://www .kfmc .org /providers /nh /tools /restraints /peer / wheelchairpositioning.pdf

Rajen, M. (2006). Toxins everywhere. Article for New Straits Times. Retrieved July 2011, from http://neurotalk .psychcentral .com / thread10246.html

Ranganath, S, and Strohbehn, K. (2009). Fecal Incontinence. Retrieved April 2011, from http://emedicine .medscape .com /article /268674-overview

Rangel-Castilla, L, Gasco, J, Hanbali, F, et al. (2011). Closed head trauma. Retrieved January 2012, from http://emedicine .medscape .com/article/251834-overview

Rape, Abuse, & Incest National Network (RAINN). (2009). Ways to reduce your risk of sexual assault (various pages). Retrieved April 2012, from http://www .rainn .org /get-information /sexual-assault-prevention

Rape Crisis Staff. (No date). Phases of recovery. Retrieved April 2012, from http://rapecrisis .org .za /information-for-survivors /phases-of-recovery/

Rape Victim Advocates. (2008). Rape trauma syndrome. Retrieved April 2012, from http://www.rapevictimadvocates.org/trauma.asp

Rape Victim Advocates. (2008). When the survivor is male. Retrieved April 2012, from http://www.rapevictimadvocates.org/male.asp

Reasoner, R. (2000). The true meaning of self-esteem. Retrieved May 2012, from http://www.jamestown.k12.nd.us/school/gussner/teacher /rasmussen/counselorconnectiontopics/selfesteem.pdf

Richards, JR, Derlet, RW, Albertson, TE. (2011). Methamphetamine toxicity. Retrieved March 2012, from http://emedicine .medscape .com/article/820918-overview

Ries, AL, Bauldoff, GS, Carlin, BW, et al. (2007). Pulmonary rehabilitation: Joint ACCP/AACVPR evidence-based clinical practice guidelines. National Guideline Clearinghouse. Retrieved June 2011, from http://www.guideline.gov/content.aspx?id=10856

Ringrose, H. (2001). Dysfunctional families. Retrieved February 2012, from http://www .suite101 .com /article .cfm /gifted _talented _teens / 56964

Rosland, AM, Heisler, M, Piette, JD (2011). The impact of family behaviors and communication patterns on chronic illness outcomes: A

systematic review. Retrieved February 2012, from http://www
.bioportfolio .com /resources /pmarticle /198478 /The-Impact-Of-
Family-Behaviors-And-Communication-Patterns-On-Chronic-
Illness-Outcomes.html

Russo, MB, and Shaikh, S. (2005). Sleep: Understanding the basics.
Retrieved April 2012, from http://sleepdisorders.about.com

Saisan, J, Smith, M, and Segal, J. (update 2012). Relationship help:
Tips for building romantic relationships that last. Retrieved April
2012, from http://www.helpguide.org/mental/improve_relationships
.htm

Salem, R. (2003). Empathic listening. Retrieved February 2012, from
http://www.beyondintractability.org/essay/empathic_listening/

Saulino, MF, and Vacarro, AR. (2011). Rehabilitation of persons with
spinal cord injuries. Retrieved January 2011, from http://emedicine
.medscape.com/article/1265209/

Savrock, J. (2006): Counseling distressed students may be improved by
religious/spiritual discussion. Retrieved May 2012, from http://www
.ed.psu.edu/news/spiritual.asp

Scheinfeld, NS, Mokashi, A, Lin, A. (2010). Protein-energy malnutrition. Retrieved February 2012, from http://emedicine.medscape.com
/article/1104623-overview

Schmidt, RJ, and Somam, SS. (2009). Renovascular hypertension. Retrieved March 2012, from http://emedicine .medscape .com /article /
245140-overview

Schoenborn, C. (2004). Marital status and health: United States, 1999–
2002. Advance Data from Vital and Health Statistics, no. 351. Retrieved February 2012, from http://www .cdc .gov /nchs /data /ad /
ad351.pdf

Schulman, A. (2008). Bioethics and the question of human dignity.
Bioethics and Human Dignity. Retrieved February 2012, from http:/
/bioethics .georgetown .edu /pcbe /reports /human _dignity /chapter1
.html

Schwartz, SM. (2012). Obesity in children. Retrieved February 2012,
from http://emedicine.medscape.com/article/985333-overview

Scott, E. (update 2008). Coping skills for parents and kids. Retrieved
February 2012, from http://stress .about .com /od /parentingskills /a /
coping_skills.htm

Search and Rescue Research Staff. (2011). Alzheimer's disease and
related disorders SAR research: Wandering characteristics. Retrieved
April 2012, from http://www .dbs-sar .com /SAR _Research /
Wandering_Characteristics.htm

Searle, J. (No date). Eating and swallowing. Fact sheet regarding Huntington's disease. Retrieved April 2012, from http://huntingtondisease
.tripod.com/swallowing/id22.html

Seepersad, S. (No date). Critical analysis paper. Understanding loneliness using attachment and systems theories and developing an applied intervention. Retrieved May 2012, from http://www
.webofloneliness .com /uploads /7 /3 /2 /3 /7323413 /critical _analysis
_paper_loneliness.pdf

Seligman, M. (No date). Positive health. Retrieved February 2012, from
.http://www .authentichappiness .sas .upenn .edu /newsletter .aspx-
?id=1559

Selvarajah, A. (2000). Self-esteem: The problem behind all problems.
Retrieved May 2012, from http://www .selfgrowth .com /articles /
selvarajah13.html

Semchyshyn, N, and Sengelmann, RD. (2012). Surgical complications. Retrieved April 2012, from http://emedicine.medscape.com/article/1128404-overview#all

Sexuality Information and Education Council of the United States (SIECUS). (No date). Sexuality education Q & A. Retrieved April 2012, from http://www .siecus .org /index .cfm?fuseaction=page .viewpage &pageid=521&grandparentid=477&parentid=514

Sharma, VP. (1996). Normal mourning and "complicated grief." Retrieved March 2012, from http://www.Mindpub.com/art045.htm

Sharma, YRS. (No date). Research studies on spiritual philosophy/science. Retrieved February 2012, from http://www.selfgrowth.com /articles/research_studies_on_spiritual_philosophyscience

Sherman, C. (2002). Antisuicidal effect of psychotropics remains uncertain. Clin Psychiatry News 30(8). Retrieved May 2012, from http:/ /www .baumhedlundlaw .com /media /ssri /paxil /FDAHearing / ANTISUICIDAL%20EFFECT%20REMAINS%20UNCERTAIN .pdf

Sheslow, DV. (2008). Developing your child's self-esteem. Retrieved January 2012, from http://kidshealth.org/parent/emotions/feelings/ self_esteem.html#cat145

Siddiqi, NH. (2011). Contrast Medium Reactions. Retrieved May 2012, from 1. http://emedicine.medscape.com/article/422855-overview#a1

Simon, EE, and Hamrahian, SM. (2009). Hyponatremia. Retrieved August 2011, from http://emedicine .medscape .com /article /242166-overview

Sims, DD. (No date). Mending the family circle: Coping with the death of a loved one. Retrieved January 2012, from http://www .touchstonesongrief .com /touchstones /articles /SURVIVING%20THE %20DEATH%20OF%20A%20LOVED%20ONE.pdf

Sinclair, C. (2001). Brain organization as seen in unilateral spatial neglect. Retrieved February 2012, from http://serendip.brynmawr.edu /bb/neuro/neuro01/web2/Sinclair.html

Singh, MK, Patel, J, and Gallagher, RM. (2012). Chronic pain syndrome. Retrieved March 2012, from http://emedicine.medscape.com /article/310834-overview

Smith, CE, and Soreide, E. (2005). Hypothermia in trauma victims. Retrieved November 2011, from http://www.asahq.org/Knowledge-Base /Diseases-and-Conditions /ASA /Hypothermia-in-Trauma-Victims.aspx

Smith, CM, and Cotter, V. (2008). Age-related changes in health. In Evidence-based geriatric nursing protocols for best practice. Retrieved April 2012, from http://www.guideline.gov/

Smith, K. (2002). Public heath nursing. Retrieved December 2011, from http://www.encyclopedia.com/doc/1G2-3404000702.html

Solomon, A. (2000). Relocation stress: The warning signs. Psych Bytes. Retrieved March 2012, from http://www .therapyinla .com /psych / psych0100.html

Sophy, C. (No date). Four tips to help you set and enforce family boundaries. Retrieved February 2012, from http://ezinearticles.com/?Four-Tips-To-Help-You-Set-And-Enforce-Family-Boundaries&id=76369

South Carolina Department of Health and Environmental Control. (2006). Hydration management. Retrieved March 2012, from http://ddsn.sc.gov

/providers /manualsandguidelines /Documents /HealthCareGuidelines / HydrationManagement.pdf

Spratt, EG, Ibeziako, PI, and DeMaso, D. (2012). Somatoform disorder. Retrieved September 2012 from http://emedicine.medscape.com/ article/918628-overview

Spinowitz, BS, and Rodriguez, J. (2011). Renal artery stenosis. Retrieved March 2012, from http://emedicine.medscape.com/article/ 245023-overview

State of Alaska Cold Injuries and Cold Water Near Drowning Guidelines. (2006). Retrieved November 2011, from ttp://www.hypothermia.org/ protocol.htm

Stephens, E. (2010). Peripheral vascular disease. Retrieved March 2012, from http://emedicine.medscape.com/article/761556-overview

Stoppler, MC. (2011). Heatstroke. Retrieved November 2011, from http://www.medicinenet.com/script/main/art.asp?articlekey=10110

Stoppler, MC. (2011). Incontinence. Retrieved April 2012, from http:/ /www.emedicinehealth.com/incontinence/article_em.htm

Stoppler, MC. (2009). Poison proofing your home. Retrieved March 2011, from http://www.emedicinehealth.com/poison_proofing_your _home/article_em.htm

Styles, S, and Vega, CP. (2007). AHA Updates: Recommendations for antibiotic prophylaxis for dental procedures. Retrieved August 2011, from www.medscape.com/viewarticle/555596

Sullivan, S. (2006). Faith and poverty: Personal religiosity and organized religion in the lives of low-income urban mothers. Retrieved April 2012, from http://www.bc.edu/centers/boisi/publicevents/ browse_events_by_date/s06/sullivan.html

Suneja, M, and Muster, HA. (2010). Hypocalcemia. Retrieved August 2011, from http://emedicine.medscape.com/article/241893-overview

Swaminathan, A, and Naderi, S. (2010). Pneumonia, aspiration. Retrieved February 2011, from http://cmedicine.medscape.com/article /807600-overview

Tan, WA, Powell, S, and Nanjundappa, A. (2011). Abdominal aortic aneurysm rupture imaging. Retrieved March 2012, from http:// emedicine.medscape.com/article/416397-overview

Task Force on Pulmonary Embolism, European Society of Cardiology. (2000). Guidelines on diagnosis and management of acute pulmonary embolism. Retrieved March 2012, from http://eurheartj .oxfordjournals.org/content/21/16/1301.full.pdf

Teasell, R, and Marshall, S, et al. (2008). The National Center for Evidence-Based Practice in Communication Disorders. Evidence-based review of moderate to severe acquired brain injury. Retrieved February 2012, from http://www.ncepmaps.org/Review-332.php

Texas Medical Association. (2009). Effective and ineffective coping: The process of stress. Retrieved May 2012, from http://www.texmed .org/template.aspx?id=4479

The Advocates for Human Rights. Sexual assault response teams. Retrieved April 2012, from http://www.stopvaw.org/sexual_assault _response_teams.html

The College of Physicians of Philadelphia. (2011). Cultural perspectives on vaccination. Retrieved November 2011, from http://www .historyofvaccines.org/content/articles/cultural-perspectives-vaccination

Thompson-Tormaschy, T. (2007). What's the big deal about "I"-Messages? Retrieved March 2012, from http://psychcentral.com/lib/2007/whats-the-big-deal-about-i-messages/

Tilton, SR. (2008). Review of the State-Trait Inventory (STAI). NewsTones 48(2). Retrieved February 2012, from http://www.theaaceonline.com/stai.pdf

Tolan, RW, and Stewart, JM. (2011). Pediatric chronic fatigue syndrome. Retrieved September 2011, from http://emedicine.medscape.com/article/1844636-overview

Turek, P. (2011). Male sexual health issues and treatment. Retrieved May 2012, from http://www.theturekclinic.com/male-sexual-health.html

Turnbull, GB. (2008). The importance of coordinating ostomy care and teaching across settings. Retrieved February 2012, from http://www.o-wm.com/article/454

Tversky, A, and Kahneman, D. (1981). The framing of decisions and the psychology of choice. Retrieved February 2012, from http://rangevoting.org/TverskyK81.html

US Department of Health and Human Services, Department of Agriculture. (2010). The Dietary Guidelines for Americans, 2010. Various parts. Retrieved February 2012, from http://www.health.gov/paguidelines/pdf/paguide.pdf

US Department of Health and Human Services. (2010). 2008 Physical Guidelines Physical Guidelines for Americans. Retrieved September 2010, from http://www.cnpp.usda.gov/DietaryGuidelines.htm

Vanderhyder, D. (2008). Stress management for caregivers of Alzheimer's using guided imagery. Retrieved January 2012 from http://caregiverhelp.blogspot.com/2008/06/stress-management-for-caregivers-of.html

Vasavada, SP, Carmel, ME, and Rackley, R. (2012). Urinary incontinence. Retrieved April 2012, from http://emedicine.medscape.com/article/452289-overview

Vasconcellos, J. et al. (No date). In defense of self-esteem. Retrieved April 2012, from http://www .self-esteem-nase .org /amember / newsarticles/InDefenseofSelf-Esteem.pdf

Veterans Health Administration, Department of Defense. (2001). Clinical practice guidelines for the management of medically unexplained symptoms: Chronic pain and fatigue. Retrieved September 2011, from http://www.healthquality.va.gov/mus/mus_fulltext.pdf

VHA National Center for Patient Safety (NCPS) Fall Prevention and Management. (2009). Retrieved September 2011, from http://www.patientsafety.gov/CogAids/FallPrevention/index.html#page=page-1

Viele, CS, Quin, AM, and Daly, CF. (2006). Dehydration and electrolyte requirements in oncology care. Cancer Care Quarterly. Retrieved September 2011, from http://www .mediabistro .com /portfolios / samples_files/162412_5KaA4NawhyfT53_1903z44at_.pdf

Vivo, M. (2009). Using parent effectiveness training to help families in crisis. Retrieved February 2012, from http://www .adolescent-substance-abuse .com /substance-abuse /using-parent-effectiveness-training-to-help-families-in-crisis.htm

Von Wager, K. (No date). Identity crisis—Theory and research. Retrieved March 2007, from http://psychology .about .com /od / theoriesofpersonality/a/identitycrisis.htm

Walant, K. (2000). A little self-care goes a long way. Retrieved May 2012, from http://www.naturalchild.org/guest/karen_walant2.html

Watson, S. (No date). Understanding inappropriate behavior. Retrieved March 2012, from http://specialed.about.com/od/behavioremotional/a/behavsupport.htm

WebHealthCentre. (2012). Suffocation and artificial respiration. Retrieved April 2012, from http://www .webhealthcentre .com / HealthyLiving/first_aid_suffoc.aspx

Williams, ME. (2009). The basic geriatric respiratory examination. Retrieved June 2011, from http://www .medscape .org /viewarticle / 703696_2,

Wilmont, WW, and Bergstrom, MJ. (2003). Relationship theories— Self-other relationship. Retrieved April 2012, from http://www .encyclopedia.com/doc/1G2-3406900352.html

Wilner, AN. (2008). Patients' cultural and spiritual beliefs influence their diagnosis, treatment and management. Retrieved February 2012, from http://www.medscape.com/viewarticle/574203

Woolston, C. (2006). Aging and stress. Article for Caremark Health Resources. Retrieved April 2012, from http://consumer .healthday .com/encyclopedia/article.asp?AID=645997

World Gastroenterological Organization (WGO). (2008). Acute diarrhea. Retrieved August 2011, from http://www .guideline .gov / popups/printView.aspx?id=12679

World Health Organization (WHO). (2007). WHO global report on falls prevention in older age. Section 2.5. p 10. Retrieved January 2012, from http://www.stopfalls.org/files/WHO_Report.pdf

World Health Organization (WHO). (No date). Hospital hygiene and infection control. Retrieved November 2011, from www .who .int/ water_sanitation_health/medicalwaste/148to158.pdf

World Health Organization (WHO). (2004). Palliative care & symptom management: Nausea & vomiting. Retrieved February 2012, from http://www.who.int/hiv/pub/imai/genericpalliativecare082004.pdf

Yeats, WR, Bernstein, BE, Bessman, E, et al. (update 2012). Anxiety Disorders. Retrieved January 2012, from http://emedicine.medscape .com/article/286227-overview

Zeidler, MR, Becker, K, Ouellette, DR, et al. (2011). Insomnia. Retrieved July 2011, from http://emedicine .medscape .com /article / 1187829-overview

Zuger, A. (2001). Adherence by any measure still matters. Journal Watch. Retrieved May 2012, from http://aids-clinical-care .jwatch .org/cgi/content/full/2001/701/1

Index

Contrast media, iodinated, adverse reaction to, risk for, 82–85
Coping
   community
      ineffective, 288–290
      readiness for enhanced, 294–296
   defensive, 275–279
   family
      compromised, 272–275
      disabled, 279–282
      readiness for enhanced, 296–299
   ineffective, 283–287
   readiness for enhanced, 290–294
Coronary artery bypass surgery, 1083
Crohn's disease, 1083
Croup, 1083–1084
   membranous, 1084
Cushing's syndrome, 1084
CVA (cerebrovascular accident), 1073–1074
Cystic fibrosis, 1084–1085
Cystitis, 1085
Cytomegalic inclusion disease. *See* Cytomegalovirus (CMV) infection
Cytomegalovirus (CMV) infection, 1085

D

Death anxiety, 299–303
Death of child, 1144–1145
Decision-making, readiness for enhanced, 303–305
Decision-making, in nursing process, 5
Decisional conflict, 306–309
Decreased cardiac output, 172–179
Decreased cardiac tissue perfusion, risk for, 963–967
Decreased intracranial adaptive capacity, 555–559
Decubitus ulcer, 1179–1180
Deep vein thrombosis (DVT). *See* Thrombophlebitis
Defensive coping, 275–279
Deficient community health, 466–469
Deficient diversional activity, 334–337
Deficient fluid volume, risk for, 413–417
Deficient hyper/hypotonic fluid volume, 399–404
Deficient isotonic fluid volume, 404–409
Deficient knowledge, 569–573
Degenerative joint disease. *See* Arthritis, rheumatoid
Dehiscence (abdominal), 1085–1086
Dehydration, 1086
Delayed development, risk for, 317–321
Delayed growth and development, 459–466
Delayed surgical recovery, 926–931
Delirium tremens, 1086
Delivery, precipitous/out of hospital, 1087
Delusional disorder, 1087
Dementia
   AIDS, 1049
   presenile/senile, 1087–1088

Joint
   degenerative disease of. *See* Arthritis, rheumatoid
   dislocation/subluxation of, 1093
   replacement of, total, 1175
Juvenile rheumatoid arthritis, 1059

K

Kawasaki disease, 1120
Kidney stones, 1069
Knee synovitis, 1171
Knowledge
   deficient, 569–573
   readiness for enhanced, 573–576

L

Labor
   induced/augmented, 1121
   precipitous, 1121
   preterm, 1121
   stage I (active phase), 1121–1122
   stage II (expulsion), 1122
Laminectomy
   cervical, 1122
   lumbar, 1122–1123
Laryngectomy, 1123
Laryngitis, 1083–1084
Latex allergy, 1124
Latex allergy response, 576–580
   risk for, 581–583
Lead poisoning, acute, 1124
Lead poisoning, chronic, 1124
Leukemia, acute, 1125
Leukemia, chronic, 1125
Lifestyle, sedentary, 584–588
Liver function, impaired, risk for, 588–593
Loneliness, risk for, 593–596
Long-term care, 1125–1126
Lumbar laminectomy, 1122–1123
Lupus erythematosus, systemic (SLE), 1126–1127
Lyme disease, 1127

M

Macular degeneration, 1127
Mallory-Weiss syndrome, 1127
Mastectomy, 1127–1128
Mastitis, 1128
Mastoidectomy, 1128
Maternal-fetal dyad, disturbed, risk for, 596–603
Measles, 1128–1129
Medical/surgical assessment tool, adult, 22–33

Pregnancy
  adolescent, 1151–1152
  high-risk, 1152
  1st trimester, 1150–1151
  2nd trimester, 1151
  3rd trimester, 1151
Pregnancy-induced hypertension (preeclampsia), 1153
Premenstrual dysphoric disorder, 1153
Premenstrual tension syndrome (PMS). *See* Premenstrual dysphoric
  disorder
Prenatal assessment tool, 36–37
Prenatal infection, 1119
Prenatal period. *See* Pregnancy
Pressure ulcer or sore, 1154
Preterm labor, 1121
Problem-sensing, 14
Prostatectomy, 1154
Prostatic hyperplasia, benign, 1063–1064
Protection, ineffective, 723–725
Pruritus, 1154
Psoriasis, 1154–1155
Psychiatric nursing assessment tool, 34–35
Psychological abuse, 1044
Psychosis, postpartum, 1149
Puerperal sepsis, 1165
Pulmonary edema, 1097–1098, 1155
  high-altitude, 1112
Pulmonary embolus, 1155
Pulmonary hypertension, 1155–1156
Purpura, idiopathic thrombocytopenic, 1156
Pyelonephritis, 1156

Q
Quadriplegia, 1156–1157

R
Rape, 1157
Rape-trauma syndrome, 726–731
Raynaud's phenomenon, 1157–1158
Readiness for enhanced breastfeeding, 162–166
Readiness for enhanced childbearing process, 200–209
Readiness for enhanced comfort, 216–221
Readiness for enhanced communication, 228–232
Readiness for enhanced community coping, 294–296
Readiness for enhanced coping, 290–294
Readiness for enhanced decision-making, 303–305
Readiness for enhanced family coping, 296–299
Readiness for enhanced family processes, 376–380
Readiness for enhanced fluid balance, 395–399
Readiness for enhanced hope, 482–485
Readiness for enhanced immunization status, 503–507

Risk for violence
    other-directed, 1024–1025
    self-directed, 1025–1031
Risk-prone health behavior, 470–473
Rocky Mountain spotted fever, 1179
Role conflict, parental, 777–780
Role performance, ineffective, 780–784
Rubella, 1161